# What experts are saying about The PDR Family Guide to Prescription Drugs

"The premier professional drug reference now gives consumers their best guide to medical problems and the medications prescribed for them.... Clear, readable, comprehensive."

**Barrie R. Cassileth, PhD**
**Adjunct Professor**
**University of North Carolina and**
**Duke University Medical Center**

"A must for every household where there are concerns about the safe use of medications. It is an ideal way to clarify and supplement the information provided by your health care provider."

**Jack M. Rosenberg, PharmD, PhD**
**Professor of Clinical Pharmacy and**
**Pharmacology**
**Director Division of Pharmacy Practice**
**Arnold & Marie Schwartz College of Pharmacy**
**and Health Sciences**
**Long Island University**

"An easy-to-read guide to medications, side effects, and efficacy.... Now one can get understandable medical information which can help keep health costs down, yet give patients a fine comfort level with the medicines they take."

**Leon G. Smith, MD, FACP**
**Director of Medicine**
**Saint Michael's Medical Center**

"As individuals increasingly empower themselves in a variety of areas in our society, so too are they requiring more information and input into their own medical care decisions. This book is a great resource for the patient in his or her dialogue with the physician."

**Joseph R. Cruse, MD**
**Founding Medical Director**
**The Betty Ford Center**

"A valuable and timely adjunct in this age of consumer education, patient rights, and quality health care for all....*The PDR Family Guide*, written in clear, understandable terms with easily accessible cross references, is an ideal way for consumers to learn more about their prescribed medications."

**Roberta S. Abruzzese, EdD, RN, FAAN**
**Editor, *Decubitus: The Journal of Skin Ulcers***

"An excellent supplement to the education that should occur during every health care visit. The *Guide* allows people to find answers when and where they need them — any time of the day or night in their own home."

**Barbara P. Yawn, MD,MS**
**Associate Professor of Clinical Family Medicine**
**and Community Health**
**University of Minnesota**

# Other Books and Services from Medical Economics

### The PDR® Family Guide to Nutrition and Health™

This new home handbook from *Physicians' Desk Reference*® offers you a realistic, medically proven way of upgrading your family's diet without needless denial. Covers weight loss, heart health, cancer prevention, stress, energy, fitness, and more—with easy, practical steps you can take at every stage of life, from infancy through retirement. Includes a complete guide to nutritional supplements and drugs, a comprehensive fat and calorie counter, a full-color drug identification guide, and more. Fully illustrated, with 800 fact-filled pages. To order, call toll-free 1-800-331-0072.

### The PDR® Family Guide to Women's Health and Prescription Drugs™

For a frank, in-depth look at all of a woman's unique health concerns, add this essential *PDR® Family Guide* to your home health library. From menstrual problems to menopause, you'll find the latest information on a full range of gynecological infections and disorders, plus up-to-the-minute facts on AIDS-prevention, recovery from rape, contraceptive technology, osteoporosis, heart disease, diet, cancer, and more. A total of 900 pages of vital medical information. To order, call toll-free 1-800-331-0072.

### Professional References

Physicians' Desk Reference®
PDR For Nonprescription Drugs®
PDR For Ophthalmology®
PDR Guide to Drug Interactions, Side Effects, Indications™
PDR® Generics™
PDR® Medical Dictionary
PDR® Nurse's Handbook™
PDR® Nurse's Dictionary™
Pocket PDR® (Handheld Electronic Database)
PDR® Electronic Library™ (CD-ROM)
PDR® Drug REAX™

Medical Device Register®
Directory of Healthcare Group Purchasing Organizations™
Directory of Hospital Personnel™
HMO/PPO Directory™
Product Development Directory™

Red Book® (Pharmaceutical Prices)
The Red Book® Database

# THE PDR®
## FAMILY GUIDE
### TO PRESCRIPTION DRUGS®

**FOURTH EDITION**

Crown Trade Paperbacks
New York

# Publisher's Note

The drug information contained in this book is based on product labeling published in the 1996 edition of *Physicians' Desk Reference®*, supplemented with facts from other sources the publisher believes reliable. While diligent efforts have been made to assure the accuracy of this information, the book does not list every possible action, adverse reaction, interaction, and precaution; and all information is presented without guarantees by the authors, consultants, and publisher, who disclaim all liability in connection with its use.

This book is intended only as a reference for use in an ongoing partnership between doctor and patient in the vigilant management of the patient's health. It is not a substitute for a doctor's professional judgment, and serves only as a reminder of concerns that may need discussion. All readers are urged to consult with a physician before beginning or discontinuing use of any prescription drug or undertaking any form of self-treatment.

Brand names listed in this book are intended to represent only the more commonly used products. Inclusion of a brand name does not signify endorsement of the product; absence of a name does not imply a criticism or rejection of the product. The publisher is not advocating the use of any product described in this book, does not warrant or guarantee any of these products, and has not performed any independent analysis in connection with the product information contained herein.

Published by Crown Trade Paperbacks, 201 East 50th Street, New York, New York,10022. Member of the Crown Publishing Group.

Random House, Inc. New York, Toronto, London, Sydney, Auckland
http://www.randomhouse.com/
CROWN TRADE PAPERBACKS and colophon are trademarks of Crown Publishers, Inc.

Three previous editions of this title were published by Medical Economics Company, Inc in 1993, 1994, and 1995.
Printed in the United States of America

Library of Congress Cataloging-in-Publication Data is available upon request.

ISBN 0-609-80068-X

10 9 8 7 6 5 4 3 2 1

Fourth Edition

PHYSICIANS' DESK REFERENCE®, PDR®, PDR For Ophthalmology®, PDR For Nonprescription Drugs®, The PDR® Family Guide to Prescription Drugs®, and Pocket PDR® are registered trademarks used herein under license. PDR® Generics™, PDR® Family Guides™, The PDR® Family Guide to Women's Health and Prescription Drugs™, The PDR® Family Guide to Nutrition and Health™, PDR Guide to Interactions, Side Effects, Indications™, PDR® Nurse's Handbook™, PDR® Electronic Library™, PDR® Drug Interactions/Side Effects/Indications Diskettes™, and PDR® Drug REAX™ are trademarks used herein under license.

**Officers of Medical Economics:** *President and Chief Executive Officer:* William A. Schlegel; *President and Chief Operating Officer of Corporate Business Groups:* Curtis B. Allen; *Vice President, Corporate Human Resources:* Pamela M. Bilash; *Senior Vice President, Chief Financial Officer:* Paul Hilger; *Senior Vice President, Corporate Operations:* John R. Ware; *Senior Vice President, Corporate Business Development:* Raymond M. Zoeller; *Vice President, Information Services and Chief Information Officer:* Edward J. Zecchini.

Bulk copy inquiries are invited. Contact the Commercial Sales Department at 1-800-442-6657.

# Contents

# The PDR® Family Guide to Prescription Drugs®

## FOURTH EDITION

**Editor-in-Chief:** David W. Sifton
**Product Manager:** Karen B. Sperber
**Director of Professional Services:** Mukesh Mehta, R Ph
**Art Director:** Robert Hartman

---

**Assistant Editors:** Ann Ben Larbi; Gwynned L. Kelly; Thelma Perin

**Writers:** Lynn H. Buechler; Gregory A. Freeman

**Managing Pharmaceutical Editor:** Marion Gray, R Ph

**Pharmaceutical Consultant:** Kathryn M. Martin, PharmD

**Illustrations:** Christopher Wikoff, MAMS

**Editorial Production:** Vice President of Production: David Pitler; Contracts and Support Services Director: Marjorie A. Duffy; Director of Production, Annuals: Carrie Williams; Manager of Production, Annuals: Kimberly Hiller-Vivas; Electronic Publishing Coordinator: Joanne M. Pearson; Electronic Publishing Designer: Kevin J. Leckner; Senior Digital Imaging Coordinator: Shawn W. Cahill; Digital Imaging Coordinator: Frank J. M<sup>c</sup>Elroy, III

## Medical Economics Company

**Executive Vice President, Directory Services:** Paul A. Konowitch

**Vice President of Product Management:** Stephen B. Greenberg

Trade Sales Manager: Robin B. Bartlett; Trade Sales Account Executive: Bill Gaffney; Marketing Communications Manager: Maryann Malorgio; Manager, Database Administration: Lynne Handler; Manager, Electronic Publishing: David Levy; Administrative Assistants: Sandra Loeffler, Helene Wattman, Linda Levine

# Foreword

Like its predecessors, this new edition of *The PDR Family Guide to Prescription Drugs* strives to make the many benefits of modern pharmaceuticals—as well as their undeniable risks—as clear and simple as can be. Unlike other books in the field, *The PDR Family Guide* discloses all important side effects specifically attributed to the drug by the manufacturer, no matter how rare. As a safeguard against error, it also provides you with full information on standard dosage recommendations. It tells exactly what to do when you miss a dose of your medication, while alerting you to the warning signs of an overdose. And to help you find all these facts as quickly as possible, it lists each medication under its familiar brand name—with a cross-reference in case the drug is dispensed generically.

Still, despite the depth and detail of the information you'll find here, *The PDR Family Guide* is not a replacement for your doctor's advice. Instead, it serves as a reminder of the basic instructions and caveats that all too often are forgotten by the time a patient leaves the doctor's office, as well as providing you with a checklist of the problems and conditions that you must be certain the doctor knows about—facts that might call for a change in your prescription.

In this way, the book is designed to serve as an aid in an ongoing dialogue between you and your doctor—a collaboration that's necessary for any treatment to work. Just as the doctor must tell you how and why to use a particular drug, you must tell the doctor how it affects you, reporting any reactions or drug interactions you suspect you may have. And while it's up to the doctor to devise your treatment strategy, it's up to you to make sure that the right doses are administered at the right times, and that the prescribed course of therapy is completed as planned.

*Physicians' Desk Reference* has been providing doctors with the information needed for safe, effective drug therapy for fully 50 years. Designed especially for healthcare professionals, it presents the facts in a detailed, technical format approved by the Food and Drug Administration. Now, to make the key facts buried in this wealth of data accessible to everyone, *The PDR Family Guide* has stripped away the medical shorthand and technical terminology, and presented the core of this information in a simple, standard format designed for maximum convenience and ease of use by the consumer.

Almost all the information you'll find in *The Family Guide's* consumer drug profiles has been extracted from PDR itself. When necessary, however, selected facts have been added from other sources—in particular, the databases maintained by PDR's sister company, MICROMEDEX, INC. Generally, this extra information describes uses for a drug that are still awaiting formal FDA approval, or supplies instructions meant specifically for the patient, such as how to make up a missed dose.

Finally, to give you added perspective, the book includes a series of chapters that provide a general overview of many common ailments and the ways they can be treated today. As with the drug profiles, these chapters are designed to supplement the information you receive from your doctor, and to aid you in discussing your treatment.

Modern drug therapy is a vast and complicated field—so complicated that, for many questions about medicines, the answer varies with each patient. *The PDR Family Guide to Prescription Drugs* gives you general guidelines for safe drug use; but only your doctor, evaluating the unique details of your case, can give you the exact instructions best suited for you. The goal of this book is simply to alert you to the most pertinent questions to ask, and to help clarify your doctor's answers—in short, to give you the tools you need to supervise your own medical care as effectively as possible. We wish you good health.

Robert W. Hogan, MD
Chair, Board of Medical Consultants

# How to Use This Book

Modern medicines spare us all an incredible amount of suffering. If you doubt it, imagine a world without antibiotics to cure infections, analgesics to alleviate pain, or any of the many drugs we use to ease stiff joints and help weakened hearts.

But today's potent medicines are not without their risks. For certain people, at certain times, some drugs can cause problems. And for all people, misusing a medication is an invitation to trouble. The purpose of this book is to alert you to those times and those conditions which should make you wary, and to help you use all of your medications safely and effectively.

This book is not a substitute for a visit to the doctor. Only a doctor can weigh all the diverse aspects of your condition and choose the treatment most likely to meet your needs. What we hope this book can do, however, is help you sort out the facts and questions that deserve further discussion. Your doctor, after all, can respond only to the problems and concerns you mention. And a seemingly unimportant question could turn out to be a crucial aspect of your particular case.

The book is divided into two major parts. In the first section, you'll find profiles of the more frequently prescribed medications. The second section gives you an overview of common diseases and disorders, and the types of treatments to expect.

## The Drug Profiles

The profiles in this section are designed to give you detailed information on the nation's most frequently prescribed prescription drugs, plus a few widely used over-the-counter medications. Though the section covers more than 1,000 products, it is not all-inclusive. If you do not find a profile for a particular prescription you've received, you shouldn't be concerned. There are a number of specialized, yet valuable drugs in current use that have been omitted here due to lack of space.

Most prescription products have two names — a generic chemical name and a manufacturer's brand name. Both are listed alphabetically in this book, with a profile of the drug appearing under the more familiar of the two. In most instances, that means the brand name. In a few cases — such as insulin, for example — the generic name heads the profile. In either case, the drug's other name gives you a cross-reference to the profile.

If there is more than one brand of a drug, you'll usually find the profile under the name that's most frequently prescribed. For example, information on amoxicillin can be found in the profile of Amoxil, the nation's leading brand. Other brands of amoxicillin, such as Wymox and Polymox, are cross-referenced to the Amoxil entry.

The drug profiles begin with correct pronunciation of the name, followed by the other brand and generic names for the drug. The information that follows these names is divided into 10 sections. Here's what you'll find in each.

## Why is this drug prescribed?

This section provides an overview of the major diseases and disorders for which the drug is generally given. It names each basic problem, but does not go into technical details. For instance, the information here will confirm that a particular antibiotic is used to fight, say, upper respiratory tract infections. The section does not, however, attempt to list all the specific germs that the antibiotic is capable of eliminating.

## Most important fact about this drug

Highlighted here is one key point — out of the dozens found in a typical profile — that is especially worthwhile to remember. We've placed it here for the sake of emphasis. Never regard this section as a definitive summary of the drug.

## How should you take this medication?

Some drugs should never be taken with meals. Others must be. This section details such special instructions including how and when to take the medication, and any dietary restrictions that may apply. Also found here is advice on what to do when you forget a dose, and any special storage requirements that apply.

## What side effects may occur?

Shown here are the potential side effects that the manufacturer has listed in the drug's FDA-approved product labeling. Virtually any drug will occasionally cause an unwanted reaction. However, even the most common of these reactions is generally seen in only a small minority of patients. For that reason, presence of a long list of possible side effects does not mean that the drug is unusually dangerous or trouble-prone. In fact, your odds of experiencing even one of these effects are typically very low. Not listed are the side effects that can be detected only by a physician or analysis in a laboratory.

## Why should this drug not be prescribed?

A few drugs are known to be harmful under certain specific conditions, which are detailed here — the most common being hypersensitivity to the drug itself. If you think one of these restrictions applies to you, you should alert your doctor immediately. If you're correct, he or she may decide to use an alternative treatment.

## Special warnings about this medication

This cautionary information is presented as a double check. If it includes any problems or conditions that your doctor may be unaware of, be sure to bring them to his or her attention. Chances are that no change in treatment will be called for; but it's worth making sure. In any event, do not take this information as a signal to change your dosage or discontinue the drug without consulting your doctor. Such a change might well do more harm than good.

## Possible food and drug interactions when taking this medication

In this section you'll find a list of specific drugs — and types of drugs — that have been known to interact with the medicine being profiled. Generally, the list includes a few examples of each type. However, it is far from inclusive. If you're not certain whether a medication you're taking falls into one of these categories, be sure to check with your doctor or pharmacist.

Remember, too, that the chances of an interaction — and its intensity if one occurs— vary from person to person. In many cases, the benefits of the two medicines may outweigh the results of an interaction. Don't stop taking either drug without first consulting your doctor.

## Special information if you are pregnant or breastfeeding

Very few medicines have been definitively proved safe for use during pregnancy. On the other hand, only a handful are known to be inevitably harmful. Most drugs fall in-between, in a gray area where no harm has been reported, but neither has safety been conclusively proved. With many of these drugs, the small theoretical risk they pose may be overshadowed by your need for treatment. This section will tell you whether a drug has been confirmed safe, is known to be dangerous, or is part of that large group about which scientists are not really sure.

## Recommended dosage

Shown here are excerpts of the dosage guidelines your doctor uses. They generally present a range of doses recommended for typical cases, and sometimes include a recommended maximum. The information is presented as a convenient double check in case you suspect a misunderstanding or a typographical error on your prescription label. It is not useful for determining an exact dosage yourself. The dose that's best for you depends on numerous factors — such as your age, weight, physical condition, and response to the drug — that can be properly evaluated only by your doctor.

### Overdosage

As another safety measure, this section lists, when available, the signs of an overdose. If the symptoms listed in this section lead you to suspect an overdose, your best response is to seek emergency medical attention immediately.

## The Disease Overviews

Though each drug profile gives you a thorough run-down on a particular medication, none of the profiles addresses the larger question of alternative therapies. To accomplish that, this second major section presents a series of brief, highly condensed surveys of major health problems and the treatments currently used to combat them. Only generally accepted treatments are included, and none is described in detail. The aim is merely to give you insight into the problem itself, and to brief you on the range of treatments your doctor has at his or her disposal.

When reviewing this material, it's important to remember that every drug and every treatment has specific benefits and drawbacks, and that your doctor must weigh these against the unique details of your personal physical condition when prescribing a medication. It's more than likely that your prescription is the best — and in some cases, the only — remedy that's right for you. But if you have reason to suspect that it's not working as intended, you shouldn't hesitate to ask your doctor about it. If one of the alternatives mentioned here is appropriate for you, he or she may decide it's time to try it.

## Other Features

The book includes several other sections that you'll find useful when faced with certain specific problems. For instance, there are two indices near the end of the book.

**The Disease and Disorder Index** enables you to quickly identify drugs available for a particular medical condition. Arranged alphabetically by ailment, it lists all the medications profiled in the book.

**The General Index,** found at the very end of the book, includes all key topics covered in the Disease Overviews, as well as the names of all medications described in the Drug Profiles.

Also available are the following special sections.

### Product Identification Guide

It's wise to keep all your prescription medications in their original bottles or vials. However, if they do somehow get mixed up, you may find this section helpful for sorting them out. It includes actual-size photographs of the leading products discussed in the book, arranged alphabetically by brand name. Manufacturers occasionally change the color and shape of a product, so if a prescription does not match the photo shown here, check with your pharmacist before assuming there's been a mistake.

### The Appendices

This section provides you with two important safeguards that every home should always have handy. One is a brief guide to safe medication use. The other—for ready reference in an emergency— is a directory of regional poison control centers.

## The Doctor-Patient Partnership

Although doctors today can often work miracles with advanced technology and sophisticated medicines, they still need the help of the patient to make most treatments work. No matter how potent the medication, it can still prove worthless if you fail to take it properly. Likewise, if you react badly to a drug, or have a condition that makes it dangerous, there is nothing any doctor can do about it unless you report the problem.

This book is offered as an aid in this cooperative effort with your doctor. We hope it suggests the right questions to ask, while allaying any unwarranted concerns you might have. Most of all, we hope it helps in some small way to make all of your treatments as effective as they can possibly be. □

# Drug Identification Guide

## ACCUPRIL

**QUINAPRIL HCL**
PARKE-DAVIS

5 MG       10 MG

20 MG       40 MG

## ACCUTANE

**ISOTRETINOIN**
ROCHE

10 MG       20 MG

40 MG

## ACHROMYCIN V

**TETRACYCLINE HCL**
LEDERLE

250 MG

500 MG

## ACTIGALL

**URSODIOL**
CIBAGENEVA

300 MG

## ADALAT

**NIFEDIPINE**
BAYER

10 MG

20 MG

## ADIPEX-P

**PHENTERMINE HCL**
GATE

37.5 MG

## ALDACTAZIDE

**SPIRONOLACTONE/
HYDROCHLOROTHIAZIDE**
G. D. SEARLE

25 MG / 25 MG

50 MG / 50 MG

## ALDACTONE

**SPIRONOLACTONE**
G. D. SEARLE

25 MG       50 MG

100 MG

## ALDOMET

**METHYLDOPA**
MERCK

125 MG       250 MG

500 MG

## ALTACE

**RAMIPRIL**
HOECHST MARION ROUSSEL

1.25 MG

2.5 MG

5 MG

10 MG

## ALUPENT

**METAPROTERENOL SULFATE**
BOEHRINGER INGELHEIM

10 MG

## AMARYL

**GLIMEPIRIDE**
HOECHT MARION ROUSSEL

1 MG

2 MG

4 MG

## AMBIEN

**ZOLPIDEM TARTRATE**
G. D. SEARLE

5 MG

10 MG

## AMOXIL

**AMOXICILLIN**
SMITHKLINE BEECHAM

250 MG

500 MG

125 MG

250 MG
CHEWABLE

## ANAFRANIL

**CLOMIPRAMINE HCL**
CIBAGENEVA

25 MG

50 MG

75 MG

## ANAPROX

**NAPROXEN SODIUM**
ROCHE

275 MG

## ANAPROX DS

**NAPROXEN SODIUM**
ROCHE

550 MG

## ANEXSIA

**HYDROCODONE BITARTRATE/
ACETAMINOPHEN**
MONARCH

5 MG / 500 MG

7.5 MG / 650 MG

## ANSAID

**FLURBIPROFEN**
UPJOHN

50 MG

100 MG

## ANTIVERT

**MECLIZINE HCL**
ROERIG

12.5 MG

25 MG

50 MG

## ANSAID

**FLURBIPROFEN**
UPJOHN

50 MG       100 MG

## APRESAZIDE

**HYDRALAZINE HCL/
HYDROCHLOROTHIAZIDE**
CIBAGENEVA

25 MG / 25 MG

50 MG / 50 MG

100 MG / 50 MG

## ARMOUR THYROID

**THYROID**
FOREST

30 MG       60 MG

## ARTANE

**TRIHEXYPHENIDYL HCL**
LEDERLE LABORATORIES

2 MG       5 MG

## ASACOL

**MESALAMINE**
PROCTER & GAMBLE

400 MG
DELAYED-RELEASE TABLETS

## ATARAX

**HYDROXYZINE HCL**
ROERIG

10 MG   25 MG

50 MG

## ATIVAN

**LORAZEPAM**
WYETH-AYERST

0.5 MG   1 MG

2 MG

## AUGMENTIN

**AMOXICILLIN/
CLAVULANATE POTASSIUM**
SMITHKLINE BEECHAM

250 MG / 125 MG

500 MG / 125 MG

125 MG/31.25 MG
CHEWABLE

250 MG/62.5 MG
CHEWABLE

## AXID

**NIZATIDINE**
ELI LILLY

150 MG

300 MG

## AZULFIDINE EN-TABS

**SULFASALAZINE**
PHARMACIA

500 MG

## BACTRIM

**SULFAMETHOXAZOLE/
TRIMETHOPRIM**
ROCHE

400 MG / 80 MG

## BACTRIM DS

**SULFAMETHOXAZOLE/
TRIMETHOPRIM**
ROCHE

800 MG / 160 MG

## BEEPEN-VK

**PENICILLIN V POTASSIUM**
SMITHKLINE BEECHAM

250 MG

500 MG

## BELLATAL

**BELLADONNA ALKALOIDS
W/ PHENOBARBITAL**
RICHWOOD

## BENADRYL

**DIPHENHYDRAMINE HCL**
PARKE - DAVIS

50 MG

## BENTYL

**DICYCLOMINE HCL**
HOECHST MARION ROUSSEL

10 MG

20 MG

## BIAXIN

**CLARITHROMYCIN**
ABBOTT

250 MG

500 MG

## BLOCADREN

**TIMOLOL MALEATE**
MERCK

5 MG   10 MG

20 MG

## BREVICON

**NORETHINDRONE /
ETHINYL ESTRADIOL**
G.D. SEARLE

0.5 MG/0.035 MG

## BRICANYL

**TERBUTALINE SULFATE**
HOECHST MARION ROUSSEL

2.5 MG   5 MG

## BRONTEX

**CODEINE PHOSPHATE /
GUAIFENESIN**
P&G PHARMACEUTICALS

10 MG / 300 MG

## BUMEX

**BUMETANIDE**
ROCHE

0.5 MG   1 MG

2 MG

## BUSPAR

**BUSPIRONE HCL**
BRISTOL-MYERS SQUIBB

5 MG   10 MG

## CALAN

**VERAPAMIL HCL**
G. D. SEARLE

40 MG   80 MG

120 MG

## CALAN SR

**VERAPAMIL HCL**
G. D. SEARLE

120 MG

180 MG

240 MG

## CAPOTEN

**CAPTOPRIL**
BRISTOL-MYERS SQUIBB

12.5 MG   25 MG

50 MG

100 MG

## CAPOZIDE

**CAPTOPRIL/
HYDROCHLOROTHIAZIDE**
BRISTOL-MYERS SQUIBB

25 MG/
15 MG   25 MG/
25 MG

50 MG/
15 MG

50 MG/
25 MG

## CARAFATE

**SUCRALFATE**
HOECHST MARION ROUSSEL

1 GM

## CARDENE

**NICARDIPINE HCL**
ROCHE

20 MG

30 MG

## CARDENE SR

**NICARDIPINE HCL**
ROCHE

30 MG

45 MG

60 MG

## CARDIZEM

**DILTIAZEM HCL**
HOECHST MARION ROUSSEL

30 MG   60 MG

90 MG

120 MG

## CARDIZEM CD

**DILTIAZEM HCL**
HOECHST MARION ROUSSEL

120 MG

180 MG

240 MG

300 MG

### CARDIZEM SR
**DILTIAZEM HCL**
HOECHST MARION ROUSSEL

60 MG

90 MG

120 MG

### CARDURA
**DOXAZOSIN MESYLATE**
ROERIG

1 MG     2 MG

4 MG     8 MG

### CATAFLAM
**DICLOFENAC POTASSIUM**
CIBAGENEVA

50 MG

### CATAPRES
**CLONIDINE HCL**
BOEHRINGER INGELHEIM

0.1 MG     0.2 MG

0.3 MG

### CECLOR
**CEFACLOR**
ELI LILLY

250 MG

500 MG

### CEFTIN
**CEFUROXIME AXETIL**
GLAXO WELLCOME

125 MG

250 MG

500 MG

### CEFZIL
**CEFPROZIL**
BRISTOL-MYERS SQUIBB

250 MG

500 MG

### CIPRO
**CIPROFLOXACIN HCL**
BAYER

250 MG

500 MG

750 MG

### CLARITIN
**LORATADINE**
SCHERING

10 MG

### CLARITIN D
**LORATADINE/
PSEUDOEPHEDRINE SULFATE**
SCHERING

5 MG/120 MG

### CLINORIL
**SULINDAC**
MERCK

150 MG     200 MG

### CLOMID
**CLOMIPHENE CITRATE**
HOECHST MARION ROUSSEL

50 MG

### CLOZARIL
**CLOZAPINE**
SANDOZ

25 MG     100 MG

### CO-GESIC
**HYDROCODONE
BITARTRATE/
ACETAMINOPHEN**
CENTRAL

5 MG / 500 MG

### COGENTIN
**BENZTROPINE MESYLATE**
MERCK

0.5 MG     1 MG

2 MG

### COGNEX
**TACRINE HCL**
PARKE-DAVIS

10 MG

20 MG

30 MG

40 MG

### COLESTID
**COLESTIPOL HCL**
UPJOHN

### COMPAZINE
**PROCHLORPERAZINE**
SMITHKLINE BEECHAM

5 MG     10 MG

25 MG

10 MG
SUSTAINED RELEASE

15 MG
SUSTAINED RELEASE

### CORGARD
**NADOLOL**
BRISTOL-MYERS SQUIBB

20 MG     40 MG

80 MG

120 MG

160 MG

### CORZIDE
**NADOLOL/
BENDROFLUMETHIAZIDE**
BRISTOL MYERS SQUIBB

40 MG / 5 MG

### COUMADIN
**WARFARIN SODIUM**
DUPONT PHARMA

1 MG     2 MG

2.5 MG     4 MG

5 MG     7.5 MG

10 MG

### COZAAR
**LOSARTAN POTASSIUM**
MERCK

25 MG     50 MG

### CYCRIN
**MEDROXYPROGESTERONE
ACETATE**
ESI LEDERLE

10 MG

### CYLERT
**PEMOLINE**
ABBOTT

18.75 MG     37.5 MG

75 MG

37.5 MG
CHEWABLE

### CYTOTEC
**MISOPROSTOL**
G. D. SEARLE

100 MCG     200 MCG

### CYTOXAN
**CYCLOPHOSPHAMIDE**
BRISTOL-MYERS SQUIBB
ONCOLOGY

25 MG | 50 MG

### DALMANE
**FLURAZEPAM HCL**
ROCHE

15 MG

30 MG

### DARVOCET-N 100
**ACETAMINOPHEN/
PROPOXYPHENE NAPSYLATE**
ELI LILLY

650 MG/100 MG

### DARVON
**PROPOXYPHENE HCL**
ELI LILLY

65 MG

### DARVON COMPOUND-65
**PROPOXYPHENE HCL/
ASPIRIN/CAFFEINE**
ELI LILLY

65 MG/389 MG/32.4 MG

### DARVON-N
**PROPOXYPHENE
NAPSYLATE**
ELI LILLY

100 MG

### DAYPRO
**OXAPROZIN**
G. D. SEARLE

600 MG

### DECADRON
**DEXAMETHASONE**
MERCK

0.5 MG | 0.75 MG

4 MG

### DECONAMINE
**CHLORPHENIRAMINE
MALEATE/
PSEUDOEPHEDRINE HCL**
BERLEX

4 MG / 60 MG

### DELTASONE
**PREDNISONE**
UPJOHN

5 MG

10 MG

20 MG

### DEMEROL
**MEPERIDINE HCL**
SANOFI WINTHROP

50 MG | 100 MG

### DEMULEN 1/35
**ETHYNODIOL DIACETATE/
ETHINYL ESTRADIOL**
G. D. SEARLE

1 MG/35 MCG

### DEMULEN 1/50
**ETHYNODIOL DIACETATE/
ETHINYL ESTRADIOL**
G. D. SEARLE

1 MG/50 MCG

### DEPAKENE
**VALPROIC ACID**
ABBOTT

250 MG

### DEPAKOTE
**DIVALPROEX SODIUM**
ABBOTT

125 MG

125 MG

250 MG

500 MG

### DESOGEN
**DESOGESTREL / ETHINYL
ESTRADIOL**
ORGANON

0.15 MG/0.03 MG

### DESYREL
**TRAZODONE HCL**
APOTHECON

50 MG | 100 MG

150 MG
DIVIDOSE

300 MG
DIVIDOSE

### DEXEDRINE
**DEXTROAMPHETAMINE
SULFATE**
SMITHKLINE BEECHAM

5 MG

5 MG
EXTENDED RELEASE

15 MG
EXTENDED RELEASE

### DIABETA
**GLYBURIDE**
HOECHST MARION ROUSSEL

1.25 MG | 2.5 MG

5 MG

### DIABINESE
**CHLORPROPAMIDE**
PFIZER

100 MG | 250 MG

### DIAMOX
**ACETAZOLAMIDE**
LEDERLE

125 MG

250 MG

500 MG

### DIDRONEL
**ETIDRONATE DISODIUM**
PROCTER & GAMBLE

200 MG

400 MG

### DIFLUCAN
**FLUCONAZOLE**
ROERIG

50 MG | 100 MG

150 MG | 200 MG

### DILANTIN
**PHENYTOIN**
PARKE-DAVIS

30 MG

100 MG

50 MG
CHEWABLE

### DILAUDID
**HYDROMORPHONE HCL**
KNOLL

2 MG | 4 MG

8 MG

### DIPENTUM
**OLSALAZINE SODIUM**
PHARMACIA

250 MG

### DISALCID
**SALSALATE**
RIKER

500 MG

500 MG

750 MG

### DITROPAN
**OXYBUTYNIN CHLORIDE**
HOECHST MARION ROUSSEL

5 MG

## DIURIL

**CHLOROTHIAZIDE**
MERCK

250MG    500MG

## DOLOBID

**DIFLUNISAL**
MERCK

250 MG

500 MG

## DONNATAL

**BELLADONNA ALKALOIDS/
PHENOBARBITAL**
A. H. ROBINS

EXTENDED RELEASE

## DORAL

**QUAZEPAM**
WALLACE

7.5 MG    15 MG

## DORYX

**DOXYCYCLINE HYCLATE**
PARKE-DAVIS

100 MG

## DURICEF

**CEFADROXIL
MONOHYDRATE**
BRISTOL-MYERS SQUIBB

500 MG

1GM

## DYAZIDE

**HYDROCHLOROTHIAZIDE /
TRIAMTERENE**
SMITHKLINE BEECHAM

25 MG / 37.5 MG

## DYCILL

**DICLOXACILLIN SODIUM**
SMITHKLINE BEECHAM

250 MG

500 MG

## DYNACIRC

**ISRADIPINE**
SANDOZ

2.5 MG

5 MG

## E.E.S. 400 FILMTAB

**ERYTHROMYCIN
ETHYLSUCCINATE**
ABBOTT

400 MG

## E-MYCIN

**ERYTHROMYCIN**
KNOLL

250 MG    333 MG

## EFFEXOR

**VENLAFAXINE HCL**
WYETH-AYERST

25 MG    37.5 MG

50 MG    75 MG

100 MG

## ELAVIL

**AMITRIPTYLINE HCL**
ZENECA

10 MG    25 MG

50 MG    75 MG

100 MG

150 MG

## ELDEPRYL

**SELEGILINE HCL**
SOMERSET

5 MG

## EMPIRIN W/ CODEINE NO.3

**ASPIRIN/CODEINE
PHOSPHATE**
ALLEN & HANBURYS

325 MG / 30 MG

## ENDEP

**AMITRIPTYLINE HCL**
ROCHE

10 MG    50 MG

100 MG

## ENTEX LA

**PHENYLPROPANOLAMINE
HCL/GUAIFENESIN**
PROCTER & GAMBLE

75 MG / 400 MG

## EPITOL

**CARBAMAZEPINE**
LEMMON

200 MG

## EQUANIL

**MEPROBAMATE**
WYETH-AYERST

200 MG    400 MG

## ERYPED CHEWABLE

**ERYTHROMYCIN
ETHYLSUCCINATE**
ABBOTT

200 MG

## ERY-TAB

**ERYTHROMYCIN**
ABBOTT

250 MG

333 MG

500 MG

## ERYC

**ERYTHROMYCIN**
PARKE-DAVIS

250 MG
DELAYED-RELEASE CAPSULE

## ERYTHROMYCIN FILMTAB

**ERYTHROMYCIN**
ABBOTT

250 MG

500 MG

## ESGIC

**BUTALBITAL /
ACETAMINOPHEN/ CAFFEINE**
FOREST

50 MG /325 MG / 40 MG

## ESGIC PLUS

**BUTALBITAL /
ACETAMINOPHEN/ CAFFEINE**
FOREST

50 MG /500 MG / 40 MG

## ESIDRIX

**HYDROCHLOROTHIAZIDE**
CIBAGENEVA

25 MG    50 MG

## ESKALITH

**LITHIUM CARBONATE**
SMITHKLINE BEECHAM

300 MG

## ESKALITH CR

**LITHIUM CARBONATE**
SMITHKLINE BEECHAM

450 MG

## ESTRACE

**ESTRADIOL**
BRISTOL-MYERS SQUIBB

0.5 MG    1 MG    2 MG

## EULEXIN

**FLUTAMIDE**
SCHERING

125 MG

## EXGEST LA
**PHENYLPROPANOLAMINE HCL / GUAIFENESIN**
CARNRICK

75 MG/400 MG

## FAMVIR
**FAMCICLOVIR**
SMITHKLINE BEECHAM

500 MG

## FASTIN
**PHENTERMINE HCL**
SMITHKLINE BEECHAM

30 MG

## FELBATOL
**FELBAMATE**
WALLACE

400 MG

600 MG

## FELDENE
**PIROXICAM**
PRATT

10 MG

20 MG

## FIORINAL
**BUTALBITAL/ASPIRIN/ CAFFEINE**
SANDOZ

50 MG / 325 MG / 40 MG

50 MG / 325 MG / 40 MG

## FIORINAL W/CODEINE
**BUTALBITAL/ASPIRIN/ CAFFEINE/CODEINE**
SANDOZ

50 MG / 325 MG /
40 MG / 30 MG

## FIORICET
**ACETAMINOPHEN/ BUTALBITAL/CAFFEINE**
SANDOZ

325 MG / 50 MG / 40 MG

## FIORICET W/CODEINE
**ACETAMINOPHEN/ BUTALBITAL/CAFFEINE/ CODEINE**
SANDOZ

325 MG / 50 MG /
40 MG / 30 MG

## FLAGYL
**METRONIDAZOLE**
G.D. SEARLE.

250 MG

375 MG

500 MG

## FLEXERIL
**CYCLOBENZAPRINE HCL**
MERCK

10 MG

## FLOXIN
**OFLOXACIN**
MCNEIL

200 MG

300 MG

400 MG

## FOSAMAX
**ALENDRONATE SODIUM**
MERCK

10 MG    40 MG

## FULVICIN-P/G
**GRISEOFULVIN**
SCHERING

250 MG

330 MG

## GANTRISIN
**SULFISOXAZOLE**
ROCHE

500 MG

## GENORA 1/35
**ETHINYL ESTRADIOL/ NORETHINDRONE**
RUGBY

0.035 MG/1 MG

## GENORA 1/50
**NORETHINDRONE/ MESTRANOL**
RUGBY

1MG/0.05 MG

## GLUCOTROL
**GLIPIZIDE**
PRATT

5 MG    10 MG

## GLYNASE PRESTAB
**GLYBURIDE , MICRONIZED**
UPJOHN

1.5 MG    3 MG

6 MG

## GRISACTIN
**GRISEOFULVIN**
WYETH-AYERST

250 MG

500 MG

## GRISACTIN ULTRA
**GRISEOFULVIN**
ESI LEDERLE

250 MG

330 MG

## HALCION
**TRIAZOLAM**
UPJOHN

0.125 MG    0.25 MG

## HALDOL
**HALOPERIDOL**
MCNEIL

0.5 MG    1 MG

2 MG    5 MG

10 MG    20 MG

## HISMANAL
**ASTEMIZOLE**
JANSSEN

10 MG

## HYDERGINE
**ERGOLOID MESYLATES**
SANDOZ

1 MG

1 MG

## HYDROCET
**HYDROCODONE BITARTRATE/ ACETAMINOPHEN**
CARNRICK

5 MG / 500 MG

## HYDRODIURIL
**HYDROCHLOROTHIAZIDE**
MERCK

25 MG    50 MG

100 MG

## HYGROTON

**CHLORTHALIDONE**
RHONE-POULENC RORER

25 MG     50 MG

100 MG

## HYTRIN

**TERAZOSIN HCL**
ABBOTT

1 MG     2 MG

5 MG     10 MG

## ILOSONE

**ERYTHROMYCIN ESTOLATE**
DISTA

250 MG

## IMDUR

**ISOSORBIDE MONONITRATE**
KEY

60 MG

120 MG

## IMITREX

**SUMATRIPTAN SUCCINATE**
CERENEX

25 MG     50 MG

## INDERAL

**PROPRANOLOL HCL**
WYETH-AYERST

10 MG     20 MG

40 MG     60 MG

80 MG

## INDERAL LA

**PROPRANOLOL HCL**
WYETH-AYERST

60 MG

80 MG

120 MG

160 MG

## INDERIDE

**PROPRANOL HCL/
HYDROCHLOROTHIAZIDE**
WYETH-AYERST

40 MG / 25 MG     80 MG / 25 MG

## INDERIDE LA

**PROPRANOL HCL/
HYDROCHLOROTHIAZIDE**
WYETH-AYERST

80 MG / 50 MG

120 MG / 50 MG

160 MG / 50 MG

## INDOCIN

**INDOMETHACIN**
MERCK

25 MG

50 MG

75 MG
SUSTAINED RELEASE

## IONAMIN

**PHENTERMINE RESIN**
FISONS

15 MG

30 MG

## ISMO

**ISOSORBIDE MONONITRATE**
WYETH-AYERST

20 MG

## ISOLLYL

**ASPIRIN/BUTALBITAL/
CAFFEINE**
RUGBY

325 MG / 50 MG / 40 MG

## ISOPTIN

**VERAPAMIL HCL**
KNOLL

40 MG     80 MG

120 MG

## ISOPTIN SR

**VERAPAMIL HCL**
KNOLL

120 MG

180 MG

240 MG

## ISORDIL

**ISOSORBIDE DINITRATE**
WYETH-AYERST

2.5 MG     5 MG
SUBLINGUAL

10 MG
SUBLINGUAL

40 MG
EXTENDED RELEASE

40 MG
EXTENDED RELEASE

5 MG     10 MG

20 MG     30 MG

40 MG

## K-DUR

**POTASSIUM CHLORIDE**
KEY

10 MEQ

20 MEQ

## KAON-CL 10

**POTASSIUM CHLORIDE**
SAVAGE

750 MG

## KEFLEX

**CEPHALEXIN**
DISTA

250 MG

500 MG

## KEFTAB

**CEPHALEXIN HCL**
DISTA

500 MG

## KLONOPIN

**CLONAZEPAM**
ROCHE

0.5 MG     1 MG

2 MG

## KLOR-CON

**POTASSIUM CHLORIDE**
UPSHER-SMITH

8 MEQ     10 MEQ

## LAMICTAL

**LAMOTRIGINE**
GLAXO WELLCOME

25 MG     100 MG

150 MG     200 MG

## LANOXIN

**DIGOXIN**
BURROUGHS WELLCOME

0.125 MG     0.25 MG

## LASIX

**FUROSEMIDE**

HOECHST MARION ROUSSEL

20 MG          40 MG

80 MG

## LEDERCILLIN VK

**PENICILLIN V POTASSIUM**

LEDERLE

250 MG          500 MG

## LESCOL

**FLUVASTATIN SODIUM**

SANDOZ

20 MG

40 MG

## LEVOTHROID

**LEVOTHYROXINE SODIUM**

FOREST

50 MCG          100 MCG

150 MCG

## LEVLEN

**LEVONORGESTREL/
ETHINYL ESTRADIOL**

BERLEX

0.15 MG/0.03 MG

## LEVOXYL

**LEVOTHYROXINE SODIUM**

DANIELS

50 MCG          100 MCG

150 MCG

## LEVSIN

**HYOSCYAMINE SULFATE**

SCHWARZ

0.125 MG

## LEVSIN / SL

**HYOSCYAMINE SULFATE**

SCHWARZ

0.125 MG

## LEVSINEX

**HYOSCYAMINE SULFATE**

SCHWARZ

0.375 MG

## LIBRIUM

**CHLORDIAZEPOXIDE HCL**

ROCHE

5 MG

10 MG

25 MG

## LIBRAX

**CHLORDIAZEPOXIDE HCL/
CLIDINIUM BR**

ROCHE

5 MG/2.5 MG

## LIBRITABS

**CHLORDIAZEPOXIDE**

ROCHE

25 MG

## LITHONATE

**LITHIUM CARBONATE**

SOLVAY

300 MG

## LITHOTABS

**LITHIUM CARBONATE**

SOLVAY

300 MG

## LODINE

**ETODOLAC**

WYETH-AYERST

200 MG

300 MG

400 MG

## LOESTRIN 1/20

**NORETHINDRONE ACETATE/
ETHINYL ESTRADIOL**

PARKE-DAVIS

1 MG / 20 MCG

## LOESTRIN 1.5/30

**NORETHINDRONE ACETATE/
ETHINYL ESTRADIOL**

PARKE-DAVIS

1.5 MG / 30 MCG

## LOMOTIL

**DIPHENOXYLATE HCL/
ATROPINE SULFATE**

G. D. SEARLE

2.5 MG / 0.025 MG

## LO/OVRAL

**NORGESTREL /
ETHINYL ESTRADIOL**

WYETH-AYERST

0.3 MG/0.03 MG

## LOPID

**GEMFIBROZIL**

PARKE-DAVIS

600 MG

## LOPRESSOR

**METOPROLOL TARTRATE**

CIBAGENEVA

50 MG

100 MG

## LOPURIN

**ALLOPURINOL**

KNOLL

100 MG          300 MG

## LORABID

**LORACARBEF**

ELI LILLY

200 MG

400 MG

## LORCET PLUS

**HYDROCODONE
BITARTRATE/
ACETAMINOPHEN**

FOREST

7.5 MG / 650 MG

## LORTAB

**HYDROCODONE BITARTRATE /
ACETAMINOPHEN**

UCB

2.5 MG / 500 MG

5 MG / 500 MG

7.5 MG / 500 MG

## LOTENSIN

**BENAZEPRIL HCL**

CIBAGENEVA

5 MG          10 MG

20 MG          40 MG

## LOTENSIN HCT

**BENAZEPRIL HCL/
HYDROCHLOROTHIAZIDE USP**

CIBAGENEVA

5 MG/6.25 MG

10 MG/12.5 MG

20 MG/12.5 MG

20 MG/25 MG

## LOZOL

**INDAPAMIDE**

RHONE-POULENC RORER

1.25 MG          2.5 MG

## LURIDE SF LOZI-TABS

**SODIUM FLUORIDE**

COLGATE-HOYT

1 MG

## LUVOX

**FLUVOXAMINE MALEATE**

SOLVAY

50 MG

100 MG

## MACRODANTIN

**NITROFURANTOIN**
PROCTER & GAMBLE

25 MG

50 MG

100 MG

## MACROBID

**NITROFURANTOIN
MONOHYDRATE
MACROCRYSTALS**
PROCTER & GAMBLE

75 MG / 25 MG

## MATERNA

**VITAMINS & MINERALS**
LEDERLE

## MAXAQUIN

**LOMEFLOXACIN HCL**
G. D. SEARLE

400 MG

## MAXZIDE

**TRIAMTERENE/
HYDROCHLOROTHIAZIDE**
LEDERLE

37.5 MG/     75 MG/
25 MG        50 MG

## MEDROL

**METHYLPREDNISOLONE**
UPJOHN

2 MG     4 MG

8 MG     16 MG

---

## MELLARIL

**THIORIDAZINE HCL**
SANDOZ

25 MG     50 MG

100 MG     150 MG

200 MG

## METHERGINE

**METHYLERGONOVINE
MALEATE**
SANDOZ

0.2 MG

## METHOTREXATE SODIUM

**METHOTREXATE SODIUM**
LEDERLE

2.5 MG

## MEVACOR

**LOVASTATIN**
MERCK

10 MG     20 MG

40 MG

## MEXITIL

**MEXILETINE HCL**
BOEHRINGER INGELHEIM

150 MG

200 MG

250 MG

---

## MICRO-K EXTENCAPS

**POTASSIUM CHLORIDE**
A. H. ROBINS

8 MEQ

10 MEQ

## MICRONASE

**GLYBURIDE**
UPJOHN

1.25 MG     2.5 MG

5 MG

## MIDRIN

**ISOMETHEPTENE
MUCATE/
DICHLORALPHENAZONE/
ACETAMINOPHEN**
CARNRICK

65 MG / 100 MG / 325 MG

## MILTOWN

**MEPROBAMATE**
WALLACE

200 MG     400 MG

600 MG

## MINIPRESS

**PRAZOSIN HCL**
PFIZER

1 MG

2 MG

5 MG

---

## MINOCIN

**MINOCYCLINE HCL**
LEDERLE

50 MG

100 MG

## MODICON

**NORETHINDRONE/ ETHINYL
ESTRADIOL**
ORTHO

0.5 MG / 0.035 MG

## MODURETIC

**AMILORIDE HCL/
HYDROCHLOROTHIAZIDE**
MERCK

5 MG / 50 MG

## MONOKET

**ISOSORBIDE MONONITRATE**
SCHWARZ

10 MG     20 MG

## MONOPRIL

**FOSINOPRIL SODIUM**
BRISTOL-MYERS SQUIBB

10 MG     20 MG

## MOTRIN

**IBUPROFEN**
UPJOHN

400 MG

600 MG

800 MG

---

## MS CONTIN

**MORPHINE SULFATE**
PURDUE FREDERICK

15 MG     30 MG

60 MG     100 MG

200 MG

## MYSOLINE

**PRIMIDONE**
WYETH-AYERST

50 MG     250 MG

## NAPROSYN

**NAPROXEN**
ROCHE

250 MG

375 MG

500 MG

## NARDIL

**PHENELZINE SULFATE**
PARKE-DAVIS

15 MG

## NATALINS RX

**VITAMINS, PRENATAL**
BRISTOL-MYERS SQUIBB

## NAVANE

**THIOTHIXENE**
ROERIG

5 MG

10 MG

## NEORAL

### CYCLOSPORINE
SANDOZ

25 MG

100 MG

## NEPTAZANE

### METHAZOLAMIDE
LEDERLE

25 MG     50 MG

## NEURONTIN

### GABAPENTIN
PARKE-DAVIS

100 MG     300 MG

400 MG

## NIZORAL

### KETOCONAZOLE
JANSSEN

200 MG

## NOLVADEX

### TAMOXIFEN CITRATE
ZENECA

10 MG

## NORDETTE

### LEVONORGESTREL / ETHINYL ESTRADIOL
WYETH-AYERST

0.15 MG / 0.03 MG

---

## NORGESIC

### ORPHENADRINE CITRATE/ ASPIRIN/CAFFEINE
3M PHARMACEUTICALS

25 MG / 385 MG / 30 MG

## NORGESIC FORTE

### ORPHENADRINE CITRATE/ ASPIRIN/ CAFFEINE
3M PHARMACEUTICALS

50 MG / 770 MG / 60 MG

## NORINYL/1+35

### ETHINYL ESTRADIOL/ NORETHINDRONE
G.D. SEARLE

0.035 MG / 1 MG

## NORINYL/1+50

### MESTRANOL/ NORETHINDRONE
G.D. SEARLE

0.05 MG/1 MG

## NOROXIN

### NORFLOXACIN
MERCK

400 MG

## NORMODYNE

### LABETALOL HCL
SCHERING

100 MG     200 MG

300 MG

---

## NORPACE

### DISOPYRAMIDE PHOSPHATE
G. D. SEARLE

100 MG

150 MG

## NORPACE CR

### DISOPYRAMIDE PHOSPHATE
G. D. SEARLE

100 MG

150 MG

## NORPRAMIN

### DESIPRAMINE HCL
HOECHST MARION ROUSSEL

10 MG     25 MG

50 MG     75 MG

100 MG     150 MG

## NORVASC

### AMLODIPINE BESYLATE
PFIZER

2.5 MG     5 MG

10 MG

## OBY-CAP

### PHENTERMINE HCL
RICHWOOD

30 MG

---

## OGEN

### ESTROPIPATE
UPJOHN

0.625 MG

1.25 MG

2.5 MG

## OMNIPEN

### AMPICILLIN
WYETH-AYERST

250 MG

500 MG

## ORASONE

### PREDNISONE
SOLVAY

1 MG

## ORETIC

### HYDROCHLOROTHIAZIDE
ABBOTT

50 MG

## ORINASE

### TOLBUTAMIDE
UPJOHN

## ORTHO-CEPT

### DESOGESTREL / ETHINYL ESTRADIOL
ORTHO

0.15 MG / 0.03 MG

## ORTHO-CYCLEN

### NORGESTIMATE / ETHINYL ESTRADIOL
ORTHO

0.25 MG / 0.035 MG

---

## ORTHO TRI-CYCLEN

### NORGESTIMATE / ETHINYL ESTRADIOL
ORTHO

0.18 MG / 0.035 MG

0.25 MG / 0.035 MG

0.215 MG / 0.035 MG

## ORTHO-NOVUM 1/35

### NORETHINDRONE / ETHINYL ESTRADIOL
ORTHO

1 MG / 0.035 MG

## ORTHO-NOVUM 1/50

### NORETHINDRONE / MESTRANOL
ORTHO

1 MG / 0.05 MG

## ORTHO-NOVUM 10/11

### NORETHINDRONE / MESTRANOL
ORTHO

0.5 MG / 0.035 MG

1 MG / 0.035 MG

## ORTHO-NOVUM 7/7/7

### NORETHINDRONE / MESTRANOL
ORTHO

0.5 MG / 0.035 MG

0.75 MG / 0.035 MG

1 MG / 0.035 MG

## ORUDIS

**KETOPROFEN**
WYETH-AYERST

25 MG

50 MG

75 MG

## ORUVAIL

**KETOPROFEN**
WYETH-AYERST

100 MG

150 MG

200 MG
EXTENDED RELEASE CAPSULES

## OVCON 35

**NORETHINDRONE / ETHINYL
ESTRADIOL**
BRISTOL-MYERS SQUIBB

0.4 MG / 0.035 MG

## OVCON 50

**NORETHINDRONE/ ETHINYL
ESTRADIOL**
BRISTOL-MYERS SQUIBB

1 MG / 0.05 MG

## OVRAL

**NORGESTREL /
ETHINYL ESTRADIOL**
WYETH-AYERST

0.5 MG/0.05 MG

## PAMELOR

**NORTRIPTYLINE HCL**
SANDOZ

10 MG

25 MG

50 MG

75 MG

## PANCREASE

**PANCRELIPASE**
MCNEIL

## PARAFON FORTE DSC

**CHLORZOXAZONE**
MCNEIL

500 MG

## PARLODEL

**BROMOCRIPTINE MESYLATE**
SANDOZ

2.5 MG

5 MG

## PATHOCIL

**DICLOXACILLIN SODIUM**
WYETH-AYERST

250 MG

500 MG

## PAXIL

**PAROXETINE HCL**
SMITHKLINE BEECHAM

20 MG

30 MG

## PCE

**ERYTHROMYCIN**
ABBOTT

333 MG

500 MG

## PENETREX

**ENOXACIN**
RHONE-POULENC RORER

200 MG

400 MG

## PENTASA

**MESALAMINE**
HOECHST MARION ROUSSEL

250 MG
CONTROLLED RELEASE CAPSULE

## PEN-VEE K

**PENICILLIN V POTASSIUM**
WYETH-AYERST

250 MG      500 MG

## PEPCID

**FAMOTIDINE**
MERCK

20 MG      40 MG

## PERCOCET

**OXYCODONE HCL/
ACETAMINOPHEN**
DUPONT

5 MG / 325 MG

## PERIACTIN

**CYPROHEPTADINE HCL**
MERCK

4 MG

## PERSANTINE

**DIPYRIDAMOLE**
BOEHRINGER INGELHEIM

25MG      50 MG

75 MG

## PHENAPHEN W/CODEINE NO. 3

**ACETAMINOPHEN/ CODEINE
PHOSPHATE**
A. H. ROBINS

325 MG / 30 MG

## PHENERGAN

**PROMETHAZINE HCL**
WYETH-AYERST

12.5 MG      25 MG

50 MG

## PLAQUENIL

**HYDROXCHLOROQUINE
SULFATE**
SANOFI WINTHROP

200 MG

## PLENDIL

**FELODIPINE**
ASTRA MERCK

2.5 MG

5 MG

10 MG

## POLY-VI-FLOR

**SODIUM FLUORIDE/
MULTIVITAMINS**
MEAD JOHNSON

0.5 MG
CHEWABLE

1 MG
CHEWABLE

## PONSTEL KAPSEALS

**MEFENAMIC ACID**
PARKE-DAVIS

250 MG

## PRAVACHOL

**PRAVASTATIN SODIUM**
BRISTOL-MYERS SQUIBB

10 MG

20 MG

40 MG

## PREMARIN

**CONJUGATED ESTROGENS**
WYETH-AYERST

0.3 MG     0.625 MG

0.9 MG

1.25 MG

2.5 MG

## PREMPRO

**CONJUGATED ESTROGENS /
MEDROXYPROGESTERONE
ACETATE**
WYETH-AYERST

0.625 MG / 2.5 MG

## PREMPHASE

**CONJUGATED ESTROGENS /
MEDROXYPROGESTERONE
ACETATE**
WYETH-AYERST

0.625 MG / 5.0 MG

## PRILOSEC

**OMEPRAZOLE**
ASTRA MERCK

10 MG

20 MG

## PRINCIPEN

**AMPICILLIN**
APOTHECON

250 MG

500 MG

---

## PRINIVIL

**LISINOPRIL**
MERCK

2.5 MG     5 MG

10 MG     20 MG

40 MG

## PRINZIDE

**LISINOPRIL/
HYDROCHLOROTHIAZIDE**
MERCK

10 MG / 12.5 MG

20 MG / 12.5 MG

20 MG / 25 MG

## PROCAN SR

**PROCAINAMIDE HCL**
PARKE-DAVIS

500 MG

750 MG

1000 MG

## PROCARDIA

**NIFEDIPINE**
PRATT

10 MG

20 MG

---

## PROCARDIA XL

**NIFEDIPINE**
PRATT

30 MG     60 MG

90 MG

## PRONESTYL

**PROCAINAMIDE HCL**
APOTHECON

250 MG

500 MG

## PRONESTYL-SR

**PROCAINAMIDE HCL**
APOTHECON

500 MG

## PROPULSID

**CISAPRIDE**
JANSSEN

10 MG

20 MG

## PROSCAR

**FINASTERIDE**
MERCK

5 MG

## PROSOM

**ESTAZOLAM**
ABBOTT

1 MG     2 MG

---

## PROTOSTAT

**METRONIDAZOLE**
ORTHO

250 MG

500 MG

## PROVENTIL

**ALBUTEROL SULFATE**
SCHERING

2 MG     4 MG

4 MG
REPETABS

## PROVERA

**MEDROXYPROGESTERONE
ACETATE**
UPJOHN

2.5 MG     10 MG

5 MG

## PROZAC

**FLUOXETINE HCL**
DISTA

10 MG

20 MG

## PYRIDIUM

**PHENAZOPYRIDINE HCL**
PARKE-DAVIS

100 MG

200 MG

---

## QUINIDEX EXTENTABS

**QUINIDINE SULFATE**
A. H. ROBINS

300 MG

## REGLAN

**METOCLOPRAMIDE HCL**
A. H. ROBINS

5 MG

10 MG

## RELAFEN

**NABUMETONE**
SMITHKLINE BEECHAM

500 MG

750 MG

## RESTORIL

**TEMAZEPAM**
SANDOZ

7.5 MG

15 MG

30 MG

## RETROVIR

**ZIDOVUDINE**
BURROUGHS WELLCOME

100 MG

## REVIA

**NALTREXONE HCL**
DUPONT

50 MG

## RIDAURA

**AURANOFIN**
SMITHKLINE BEECHAM

3 MG

## RIFATER

**ISONIAZID/ RIFAMPIN/ PYRAZINAMIDE**
HOECHST MARION ROUSSEL

50 MG / 120 MG / 300 MG

## RISPERDAL

**RISPERIDONE**
JANSSEN

1 MG          2 MG

3 MG

4 MG

## RITALIN

**METHYLPHENIDATE HCL**
CIBAGENEVA

5 MG          10 MG

20 MG

## RITALIN-SR

**METHYLPHENIDATE HCL**
CIBAGENEVA

20 MG

## ROBAXIN

**METHOCARBAMOL**
A. H. ROBINS

500 MG

750 MG

## ROCALTROL

**CALCITRIOL**
ROCHE

0.25 MCG     0.5 MCG

## RONDEC

**CARBINOXAMINE MALEATE/ PSEUDOEPHEDRINE HCL**
ROSS

4 MG / 60 MG

## ROXICET

**ACETAMINOPHEN/ OXYCODONE HCL**
ROXANE

325 MG / 5 MG

## RUFEN

**IBUPROFEN**
KNOLL

400 MG

## RU-TUSS

**PHENYLEPHRINE/ PHENYLPROPANOLAMINE/ CHLORPHENIRAMINE/ BELLADONNA ALKALOIDS**
KNOLL

## RYNATAN

**PHENYLEPHRINE/ CHLORPHENIRAMINE/ PYRILAMINE TANNATES**
WALLACE

25 MG / 8 MG / 25 MG

## RYTHMOL

**PROPAFENONE HCL**
KNOLL

150 MG        225 MG

300 MG

## SANDIMMUNE

**CYCLOSPORINE**
SANDOZ

25 MG

50 MG

100 MG

## SECTRAL

**ACEBUTOLOL HCL**
WYETH-AYERST

200 MG

400 MG

## SELDANE

**TERFENADINE**
HOECHST MARION ROUSSEL

60 MG

## SELDANE-D

**TERFENADINE / PSEUDOEPHEDRINE HCL**
HOECHST MARION ROUSSEL

60 MG / 120 MG

## SEMPREX D

**ACRIVASTINE/ PSEUDOEPHEDRINE HCL**
GLAXO WELLCOME

8 MG / 60 MG

## SEPTRA

**SULFAMETHOXAZOLE/ TRIMETHOPRIM**
BURROUGHS WELLCOME

400 MG / 80 MG

## SEPTRA DS

**SULFAMETHOXAZOLE/ TRIMETHOPRIM**
GLAXO WELLCOME

800 MG / 160 MG

## SER-AP-ES

**RESERPINE/HYDRALAZINE HCl/ HYDROCHLOROTHIAZIDE**
CIBAGENEVA

0.1 MG / 25 MG / 15 MG

## SERAX

**OXAZEPAM**
WYETH-AYERST

10 MG

15 MG

15 MG

30 MG

## SERZONE

**NEFAZODONE HCL**
BRISTOL-MYERS SQUIBB

100 MG

150 MG

200 MG

250 MG

## SINEMET

**CARBIDOPA-LEVODOPA**
DUPONT

10 MG / 100 MG

25 MG / 100 MG

25 MG / 250 MG

## SINEMET CR

**CARBIDOPA-LEVODOPA**
DUPONT

25 MG / 100 MG
SUSTAINED RELEASE

50 MG / 200 MG
SUSTAINED RELEASE

## SINEQUAN

**DOXEPIN HCL**
ROERIG

10 MG

25 MG

50 MG

75 MG

100 MG

150 MG

## SLO-BID GYROCAPS

**THEOPHYLLINE**
RHONE-POULENC RORER

100 MG

200 MG

300 MG

## SLO-PHYLLIN

**THEOPHYLLINE**
RHONE-POULENC RORER

100 MG    200 MG

## SLOW-K

**POTASSIUM CHLORIDE**
CIBAGENEVA

8 MEQ

## SOMA

**CARISOPRODOL**
WALLACE

350 MG

## SORBITRATE

**ISOSORBIDE DINITRATE**
ZENECA

10 MG

5 MG
CHEWABLE

5 MG
SUBLINGUAL

## SPORANOX

**ITRACONAZOLE**
JANSSEN

100 MG

## STELAZINE

**TRIFLUOPERAZINE HCL**
SMITHKLINE BEECHAM

1 MG    2 MG

## STUARTNATAL PLUS

**VITAMINS, PRENATAL**
WYETH-AYERST

WYETH
792

## SUPRAX

**CEFIXIME**
LEDERLE

200 MG

400 MG

## SURMONTIL

**TRIMIPRAMINE MALEATE**
WYETH-AYERST

WYETH 4132
25 MG

WYETH 4133
50 MG

WYETH 4158
100 MG

## SYNALGOS-DC

**DIHYDROCODEINE
BITARTRATE/ASPIRIN/
CAFFEINE**
WYETH-AYERST

WYETH 4191
16 MG / 356.4 MG / 30 MG

## SYNTHROID

**LEVOTHYROXINE SODIUM**
KNOLL

0.025 MG    0.05 MG

0.075 MG    0.088 MG

0.1 MG    0.112 MG

0.125 MG    0.15 MG

0.175 MG    0.2 MG

0.3 MG

## T-PHYL

**THEOPHYLLINE**
PURDUE FREDERICK

U 200
200 MG

## TAGAMET

**CIMETIDINE**
SMITHKLINE BEECHAM

200 MG    300 MG

400 MG

800 MG

## TAMBOCOR

**FLECAINIDE ACETATE**
3M PHARMACEUTICALS

50 MG    100 MG

TR 150
150 MG

## TAVIST

**CLEMASTINE FUMARATE**
SANDOZ

2.68 MG

## TEGRETOL

**CARBAMAZEPINE**
CIBAGENEVA

200 MG

100 MG
CHEWABLE

## TENEX

**GUANFACINE HCL**
A. H. ROBINS

1 MG    2 MG

## TENORETIC

**ATENOLOL /
CHLORTHALIDONE**
ZENECA

50 MG/    100 MG/
25 MG     25 MG

## TENORMIN

**ATENOLOL**
ZENECA

107
25 MG

50 MG

100 MG

## TENUATE

**DIETHYLPROPION HCL**
HOECHST MARION ROUSSEL

25 MG

75 MG
SUSTAINED RELEASE

## TESSALON PERLES

**BENZONATATE**
FOREST

100 MG

## THEOCHRON

**THEOPHYLLINE**
INWOOD

100 MG

200 MG

300 MG

## THEO-DUR

**THEOPHYLLINE**
KEY

100 MG

200 MG

300 MG

450 MG

50 MG

75 MG

125 MG

200 MG

## THEOLAIR

**THEOPHYLLINE**
3M

342
125 MG

250 MG

## THEOLAIR-SR

**THEOPHYLLINE**
3M

250 MG

300 MG

## THORAZINE

**CHLORPROMAZINE HCL**
SMITHKLINE BEECHAM

25 MG    50 MG

75 MG
SUSTAINED RELEASE

## THYROLAR-1/2

**LIOTRIX**
FOREST

30 MG

## THYROLAR-1

**LIOTRIX**
FOREST

60 MG

## TIGAN

**TRIMETHOBENZAMIDE HCL**
SMITHKLINE BEECHAM

100 MG

250 MG

## TOFRANIL

**IMIPRAMINE HCL**
CIBAGENEVA

10 MG    25 MG

50 MG

## TOLECTIN

**TOLMETIN SODIUM**
MCNEIL

200 MG

400 MG

600 MG

## TONOCARD

**TOCAINIDE HCL**
MERCK

400 MG

600 MG

## TORADOL

**KETOROLAC TROMETHAMINE**
SYNTEX

10 MG

## TRANDATE

**LABETALOL HCL**
ALLEN & HANBURYS

100 MG

200 MG

300 MG

## TRANXENE

**CLORAZEPATE DIPOTASSIUM**
ABBOTT

11.25 MG    22.5 MG

3.75 MG    7.5 MG

15 MG

## TRENTAL

**PENTOXIFYLLINE**
HOECHST MARION ROUSSEL

400 MG

## TRILISATE

**CHOLINE MAGNESIUM TRISALICYLATE**
PURDUE FREDERICK

500 MG

750 MG

1000 MG

## TRIMOX

**AMOXICILLIN**
APOTHECON

250 MG

500 MG

## TRINALIN REPETABS

**AZATADINE MALEATE/ PSEUDOEPHEDRINE SULFATE**
KEY

1 MG / 120 MG

## TRIPHASIL

**LEVONORGESTREL / ETHINYL ESTRADIOL**
WYETH-AYERST LABS

0.050 MG / 0.030 MG

0.075 MG / 0.040 MG

0.125 MG / 0.030 MG

## TYLENOL W/CODEINE

**ACETAMINOPHEN/ CODEINE PHOSPHATE**
MCNEIL

300 MG / 15 MG    300 MG / 30 MG

300 MG / 60 MG

## TYLOX

**OXYCODONE HCL/ ACETAMINOPHEN**
MCNEIL

5 MG / 500 MG

## ULTRASE

**PANCRELIPASE**
SCANDIPHARM

## UNIPHYL

**THEOPHYLLINE**
PURDUE FREDERICK

400 MG

## URISED

**ATROPINE SULFATE/ BENZOIC ACID/ HYOSCYAMINE/ METHENAMINE/ METHYLENE BLUE/ PHENYL SALICYLATE**
POLYMEDICA

0.03 MG / 4.5 MG / 0.03 MG / 40.8 MG / 5.4 MG / 18.1 MG

## URISPAS

**FLAVOXATE HCL**
SMITHKLINE BEECHAM

100 MG

## VALIUM

**DIAZEPAM**
ROCHE

2 MG    5 MG

10 MG

## VASERETIC

**ENALAPRIL MALEATE/ HYDROCHLOROTHIAZIDE**
MERCK

5 MG / 12.5 MG    10 MG / 25 MG

## VASOTEC

**ENALAPRIL MALEATE**
MERCK

2.5 MG    5 MG

10 MG    20 MG

## V-CILLIN K

**PENICILLIN V POTASSIUM**
ELI LILLY

125 MG

250 MG

500 MG

## VEETIDS

**PENICILLIN V POTASSIUM**
APOTHECON

250 MG

## VENTOLIN

**ALBUTEROL SULFATE**
GLAXO WELLCOME

2 MG    4 MG

**VERELAN**

VERAPAMIL HCL
LEDERLE

120 MG

180 MG

240 MG

**VIBRAMYCIN**

DOXYCYCLINE HYCLATE
PFIZER

50 MG

100 MG

**VIBRA-TABS**

DOXYCYCLINE HYCLATE
PFIZER

100 MG

**VICODIN**

HYDROCODONE
BITARTRATE/
ACETAMINOPHEN
KNOLL

5 MG / 500 MG

**VIOKASE**

PANCRELIPASE
A. H. ROBINS

**VISKEN**

PINDOLOL
SANDOZ

5 MG     10 MG

**VISTARIL**

HYDROXYZINE PAMOATE
PFIZER LABS

25 MG

50 MG

100 MG

**VOLTAREN**

DICLOFENAC SODIUM
CIBAGENEVA

25 MG     50 MG

75 MG

**WELLBUTRIN**

BUPROPION HCL
GLAXO WELLCOME

75 MG     100 MG

**WYMOX**

AMOXICILLIN
WYETH-AYERST

250 MG

500 MG

**WYTENSIN**

GUANABENZ ACETATE
WYETH-AYERST

4 MG     8 MG

**XANAX**

ALPRAZOLAM
UPJOHN

0.25 MG     0.5 MG

1 MG

2 MG

**YOCON**

YOHIMBINE HCL
PALISADES

5.4 MG

**YOHIMEX**

YOHIMBINE HCL
KRAMER

5.4 MG

**ZANTAC**

RANITIDINE HCL
GLAXO

150 MG

300 MG

**ZAROXOLYN**

METOLAZONE
FISONS

2.5 MG     5 MG

10 MG

**ZERIT**

STAVUDINE
BRISTOL-MYERS ONCOLOGY

BMS
1964   15

15 MG

BMS
1965   20

20 MG

BMS
1966   30

30 MG

BMS
1967   40

40 MG

**ZESTORETIC**

LISINOPRIL/
HYDROCHLOROTHIAZIDE
ZENECA

10 MG/12.5 MG

20 MG/12.5 MG

20 MG/25 MG

**ZESTRIL**

LISINOPRIL
ZENECA

5 MG     5 MG

20 MG

40 MG

**ZITHROMAX**

AZITHROMYCIN DIHYDRATE
PFIZER

PFIZER   PFIZER
305      305

250 MG

**ZOCOR**

SIMVASTATIN
MERCK

5 MG

10 MG

20 MG

40 MG

**ZOFRAN**

ONDANSETRON HCL
CERENEX

4 MG

8 MG

**ZOLOFT**

SERTRALINE HCL
ROERIG

50 MG

100 MG

**ZOVIRAX**

ACYCLOVIR
GLAXO WELLCOME

200 MG

400 MG

800 MG

**ZYDONE**

HYDROCODONE BITARTRATE/
ACETAMINOPHEN
DUPONT

5 MG/500 MG

**ZYLOPRIM**

ALLOPURINOL
BURROUGHS WELLCOME

100 MG     300 MG

Generic name:

# Acarbose

See Precose, page 428.

Brand name:

# Accupril

Pronounced: AK-you-prill
Generic name: Quinapril hydrochloride

## Why is this drug prescribed?

Accupril is used in the treatment of high blood pressure. It can be taken alone or in combination with a thiazide type of diuretic such as Hydro-DIURIL. Accupril is in a family of drugs known as "ACE inhibitors." It works by preventing a chemical in your blood called angiotensin I from converting into a more potent form that increases salt and water retention in your body. Accupril also enhances blood flow throughout your blood vessels. Drugs such as Accupril are sometimes prescribed in the treatment of congestive heart failure.

## Most important fact about this drug

You must take Accupril regularly for it to be effective. Since blood pressure declines gradually, it may be several weeks before you get the full benefit of Accupril; and you must continue taking it even if you are feeling well. Accupril does not cure high blood pressure; it merely keeps it under control.

## How should you take this medication?

You can take Accupril with or without meals.

Alcohol may increase the effect of Accupril, and could cause dizziness or fainting. Avoid alcohol until you have checked with your doctor.

Take Accupril exactly as prescribed, and see your doctor regularly to make sure the drug is working properly without unwanted side effects. Do not stop taking this drug without first consulting your doctor.

■ *If you miss a dose...*
Take the forgotten dose as soon as you remember. However, if it is almost time for your next dose, skip the one you missed and go back to your regular schedule. Never try to "catch up" by doubling the dose.

■ *Storage instructions...*
Accupril can be stored at room temperature. Protect from light.

## What side effects may occur?

Side effects cannot be anticipated. If any develop or change in intensity, inform your doctor as soon as possible. Only your doctor can determine if it is safe for you to continue taking Accupril.

■ *More common side effects may include:*
Dizziness, headache
■ *Less common side effects may include:*
Abdominal pain, coughing, fatigue, nausea, vomiting
■ *Rare side effects may include:*
Angina (severe chest pain), back pain, bleeding in the stomach or intestines, bronchitis, changes in heart rhythm, constipation, depression, dimmed vision, dizziness when first standing up, dry mouth or throat, extremely high blood pressure, fainting, heart attack, heart failure, high potassium, increased blood pressure, increased sweating, inflammation of the pancreas, inflammation of the sinuses, itching, kidney failure, nervousness, palpitations, rapid heartbeat, sensitivity to light, severe allergic reactions, skin peeling, sleepiness, sore throat, stroke, swelling of the mouth and throat, vague feeling of illness, vertigo

## Why should this drug not be prescribed?

If you are sensitive to or have ever had an allergic reaction to Accupril or similar drugs, such as Capoten and Vasotec, you should not take this medication. Make sure your doctor is aware of any drug reactions you have experienced.

## Special warnings about this medication

If you develop swelling of the face, lips, tongue, or throat, or of your arms and legs, or have difficulty swallowing or breathing, you should contact your doctor immediately. You may need emergency treatment.

You may feel light-headed, especially during the first few days of Accupril therapy. If this occurs, notify your doctor. If you actually faint, stop taking the medication until you have consulted with your doctor.

Vomiting, diarrhea, and heavy perspiration can all deplete your body fluid; and dehydration can cause your blood pressure to drop. If this leads to light-headedness or fainting, you should check with your doctor.

Inform your doctor or dentist that you are taking Accupril before undergoing surgery or anesthesia.

Do not use potassium supplements or salt substitutes containing potassium without consulting your doctor.

If you develop a sore throat or fever contact your doctor immediately. It could indicate a more serious illness.

If you are taking Accupril, your doctor will do a complete assessment of your kidney function and will watch it closely as long as you are taking this drug.

If you notice a yellow tinge to your skin and the whites of your eyes, stop taking the drug and notify your doctor immediately. This could be a sign of liver damage.

### Possible food and drug interactions when taking this medication

If Accupril is taken with certain other drugs, the effects of either could be increased, decreased, or altered. It is especially important to check with your doctor before combining Accupril with the following:

Diuretics such as Lasix
Lithium (Eskalith, Lithobid)
Potassium-sparing diuretics such as Aldactone, Dyazide, and Moduretic
Potassium supplements such as Slow-K and K-Dur
Salt substitutes containing potassium
Tetracycline (Sumycin)

### Special information if you are pregnant or breastfeeding

ACE inhibitors such as Accupril have been shown to cause injury and even death to the unborn child when used in pregnancy during the second and third trimesters. If you are pregnant, your doctor should discontinue Accupril as soon as possible. If you plan to become pregnant, make sure your doctor knows you are taking this medication. Accupril may appear in breast milk and could affect a nursing infant. If this medication is essential to your health, your doctor may advise you to discontinue breastfeeding until your treatment is finished.

### Recommended dosage

#### ADULTS

The usual starting dose for high blood pressure is 10 milligrams taken once a day. If you have any problems with your kidneys or if you are also taking a diuretic, your starting dose may be lower. Depending on how your blood pressure responds, your doctor may increase your dose up to a total of 80 milligrams a day taken once a day or divided into two doses.

#### CHILDREN

The safety and effectiveness of Accupril in children have not been established.

### Overdosage

Any medication taken in excess can have serious consequences. If you suspect an overdose, seek medical attention immediately.

A severe drop in blood pressure is the primary sign of an Accupril overdose.

*Brand name:*

# Accutane

Pronounced: ACC-u-tane
Generic name: Isotretinoin

### Why is this drug prescribed?

Accutane, a chemical cousin of vitamin A, is prescribed for the treatment of severe, disfiguring cystic acne that has not cleared up in response to milder medications such as antibiotics. It works on the oil glands within the skin, shrinking them and diminishing their output. You take Accutane by mouth every day for several months, then stop. The antiacne effect can last even after you have finished your course of medication.

### Most important fact about this drug

Because Accutane can cause severe birth defects, including mental retardation and physical malformations, a woman *must not* become pregnant while taking it. If you are a woman of childbearing age, your doctor will ask you to sign a detailed consent form before you start taking Accutane. If you accidentally become pregnant while taking the medication, you should immediately consult your doctor.

### How should you take this medication?

Take Accutane with food. Follow your doctor's instructions carefully.

Depending on your reaction to Accutane, your doctor may need to adjust the dosage upward or downward. If you respond quickly and very well, your doctor may take you off Accutane even before the 15 or 20 weeks are up.

After you finish taking Accutane, there should be at least a 2-month "rest period" during which you are off the drug. This is because your acne may continue to get better even though you are no longer taking the medication. Once the 2 months are up, if your acne is still severe, your doctor may want to give you a second course of Accutane.

Avoid consumption of alcoholic beverages.

Read the patient information leaflet available with the product.

Do not crush the capsules.

■ *If you miss a dose...*
Take the forgotten dose as soon as you remember. If it is almost time for your next dose, skip the one you missed and go back to your regular schedule. Do not take 2 doses at the same time.

■ *Storage instructions...*
Store at room temperature, away from light.

## What side effects may occur?
Side effects cannot be anticipated. If any develop or change in intensity, inform your doctor as soon as possible. Only your doctor can determine if it is safe for you to continue taking Accutane.

■ *More common side effects may include:*
Conjunctivitis ("pinkeye"), dry or fragile skin, dry or cracked lips, dry mouth, dry nose, itching, joint pains, nosebleed

■ *Less common side effects may include:*
Bowel inflammation and pain, chest pain, decreased night vision, decreased tolerance to contact lenses, delay in wound healing, depression, fatigue, headache, nausea, peeling palms or soles, rash, skin infections, stomach and intestinal discomfort, sunburn-sensitive skin, thinning hair, urinary discomfort, vision problems, vomiting

## Why should this drug not be prescribed?
You should not take Accutane if you are sensitive to or have ever had an allergic reaction to parabens, the preservative used in the capsules.

If you are a woman of childbearing age, you should not take Accutane if you are pregnant, if you think there is a possibility you might get pregnant during the treatment, or if you are unable to keep coming back to the doctor for monthly checkups, including pregnancy testing.

## Special warnings about this medication
When you first start taking Accutane, it is possible that your acne will get worse before it starts to get better.

If you are a woman of childbearing age and you are considering taking Accutane, you will be given both spoken and written warnings about the importance of avoiding pregnancy during the treatment. You will be asked to sign a consent form noting that:

■ Accutane is a powerful, "last resort" medication for severe acne;
■ You must not take Accutane if you are pregnant or may become pregnant during treatment;
■ If you get pregnant while taking Accutane, your baby will be at high risk for birth defects;
■ If you take Accutane, you must use effective birth control from 1 month before the start of treatment through 1 month after the end of treatment;
■ You must test negative for pregnancy within 2 weeks before starting Accutane, and you must start Accutane on the second or third day of your menstrual period;
■ You may participate in a program that includes an initial free pregnancy test and birth control counseling session;
■ If you become pregnant, you must immediately stop taking Accutane and see your doctor;
■ You have read and understood the Accutane patient brochure and asked your doctor any questions you had;
■ You are not currently pregnant and do not plan to become pregnant for at least 30 days after you finish taking Accutane;
■ You have been invited to participate in a survey of women being treated with Accutane.

Some people taking Accutane, including some who simultaneously took tetracycline, have experienced headache, nausea, and visual disturbances caused by increased pressure within the skull. See a doctor immediately if you have these symptoms; if the doctor finds swelling of the optic nerve at the back of your eye, you must stop taking Accutane at once and see a neurologist for further care.

Be careful driving at night. Some people have experienced a sudden decrease in night vision.

Some people taking Accutane have had problems regulating their blood sugar level.

You may not be able to tolerate your contact lenses during and after your therapy with Accutane.

You should stop taking Accutane immediately if you have abdominal pain, bleeding from the rectum, or severe diarrhea. You may have an inflammatory disease of the bowel.

You should not donate blood during your therapy with Accutane and for a month after you stop taking it.

### Possible food and drug interactions when taking this medication

While taking Accutane, do not take vitamin supplements containing vitamin A. Accutane and vitamin A are chemically related; taking them together is like taking an overdose of vitamin A.

### Special information if you are pregnant or breastfeeding

Accutane causes birth defects; do not use it while pregnant. Nursing mothers should not take Accutane because of the possibility of passing the drug on to the baby via breast milk.

### Recommended dosage

The recommended dosage range for Accutane is 0.5 to 2 milligrams per 2.2 pounds of body weight, divided into 2 doses daily, for 15 to 20 weeks. The usual starting dose is 0.5 to 1 milligram per 2.2 pounds per day.

People whose disease is very severe or is primarily on the body may have to take up to the maximum recommended dose.

If after a period of 2 months or more off therapy, severe cystic acne persists, your doctor may prescribe a second course of therapy.

### Overdosage

Any medication taken in excess can have serious consequences. If you suspect an overdose of Accutane, seek medical attention immediately.

■ *Overdosage of Accutane, like overdosage of vitamin A, can cause:*
Abdominal pain, dizziness, dry or cracked lips, facial flushing, incoordination and clumsiness, headache, vomiting

*Generic name:*

# Acebutolol

See Sectral, page 489.

*Generic name:*

# Acetaminophen

See Tylenol, page 571.

*Generic name:*

# Acetaminophen with Codeine

See Tylenol with Codeine, page 572.

*Generic name:*

# Acetaminophen with Oxycodone

See Percocet, page 407.

*Generic name:*

# Acetazolamide

See Diamox, page 157.

*Brand name:*

# Aclovate

Pronounced: AK-low-vait
Generic name: Alclometasone dipropionate

### Why is this drug prescribed?

Aclovate, a synthetic steroid medication of the cortisone family, is spread on the skin to relieve certain types of itchy rashes, including psoriasis.

### Most important fact about this drug

When you use Aclovate, you inevitably absorb some of the medication through your skin and into the bloodstream. Too much absorption can lead to unwanted side effects elsewhere in the body. To keep this problem to a minimum, avoid using large amounts of Aclovate over large areas, and do not cover it with airtight dressings such as plastic wrap or adhesive bandages unless specifically told to by your doctor.

### How should you use this medication?

Use Aclovate exactly as prescribed by your doctor and only to treat the condition for which your doctor prescribed it. The usual procedure is to spread a thin film of Aclovate cream or ointment over the rash and massage gently until the medication disappears. Do this 2 or 3 times a day.

For areas of deep-seated, persistent rash, your doctor may recommend a thick layer of Aclovate cream or ointment topped with waterproof bandaging, to be left in place for 1 to 4 days. If necessary, this procedure may be repeated 3 or 4 times. Do not use bandaging at all, however, unless your doctor so advises.

Aclovate is for use only on the skin. Be careful to keep it out of your eyes.

■ *If you miss a dose...*

Apply it as soon as you remember. If it is almost time for the next dose, skip the one you missed and go back to your regular schedule.

■ *Storage instructions...*

Store at room temperature.

## What side effects may occur?

Side effects cannot be anticipated. If any develop or change in intensity, inform your doctor as soon as possible. Only your doctor can determine if it is safe for you to continue taking Aclovate.

■ *Side effects may include:*

Abnormally excessive growth of hair, acne-like pimples, allergic rash, burning, dryness, infection, irritation, itching, maceration (sponginess), pale (depigmented) spots, prickly heat, rash around the mouth, redness, skin inflammation, stretch marks on skin

## Why should this drug not be prescribed?

Do not use Aclovate if you are sensitive to or have ever had an allergic reaction to alclometasone dipropionate (the active ingredient) or other corticosteroids, or to any of the oils, waxes, alcohols, or other chemicals in the cream or ointment.

## Special warnings about this medication

Aclovate is for external use only. Do not let the cream or ointment get into your eyes.

Avoid covering a treated area with waterproof diapers or plastic pants. They can increase unwanted absorption of Aclovate.

If you use Aclovate over large areas of skin for prolonged periods of time, the amount of hormone absorbed into your bloodstream may eventually lead to Cushing's syndrome: a moon-faced appearance, fattened neck and trunk, and purplish streaks on the skin. Children, because of their relatively larger ratio of skin surface to body weight, are particularly susceptible to overabsorption of hormone from Aclovate.

## Possible food and drug interactions when taking this medication

Check with your doctor before combining Aclovate with other more potent steroids, since this could lead to undesirably large amounts of hormone circulating in your bloodstream.

## Special information
## if you are pregnant or breastfeeding

Drug absorbed from Aclovate cream or ointment into the bloodstream may find its way into an unborn child's blood, or may seep into breast milk. To avoid any possible harm to your child, use Aclovate very sparingly—and only with your doctor's permission—if you are pregnant or nursing a baby.

## Recommended dosage

Apply a thin film of Aclovate cream or ointment to the affected skin areas 2 or 3 times daily; massage gently until the medication disappears.

Bandages that block out air may be used to control psoriasis and other severe skin rashes, if your doctor recommends them. Apply as follows:

1. Cover the affected area with a thick layer of Aclovate cream or ointment and a light gauze dressing, then cover the area with a pliable plastic film.
2. Seal the edges to the normal skin by adhesive tape or other means.
3. Leave the dressing in place 1 to 4 days and repeat the procedure 3 or 4 times as needed.

With this method of treatment, marked improvement is often seen in a few days. If an infection develops, the use of airtight bandages should be discontinued. Your doctor will recommend an alternative treatment.

## Overdosage

Any medication taken in excess can have serious consequences. If you suspect an overdose, seek medical attention immediately.

In a child, an overdose of Aclovate may cause increased pressure within the skull leading to bulging soft spots (in an infant's head), headache, and nausea or vomiting. If this happens, see a doctor without delay.

Over the long term, overuse of Aclovate can interfere with a child's normal growth and development.

*Generic name:*

# Acrivastine with Pseudoephedrine

*See Semprex-D, page 492.*

*Brand name:*

# Actigall

*Pronounced: AK-ti-gawl*
*Generic name: Ursodiol*

## Why is this drug prescribed?

Actigall is used to help dissolve certain kinds of gallstones. If you suffer from gallstones but do not want to undergo surgery to remove them, or if age, infirmity, or a poor reaction to anesthesia makes you a poor candidate for surgery, Actigall treatment may be a good alternative.

## Most important fact about this drug

Actigall is not a quick remedy. It takes months of Actigall therapy to dissolve gallstones; and there is a possibility of incomplete dissolution and recurrence of stones. Your doctor will weigh Actigall against alternative treatments and recommend the best one for you.

Actigall is most effective if your gallstones are small or "floatable" (i.e., high cholesterol content). In addition, your gallbladder must still be functioning properly.

## How should you take this medication?

Actigall should be taken exactly as prescribed by your doctor; otherwise the gallstones may dissolve slowly or not dissolve at all. During treatment, your doctor will do periodic ultrasound exams to see if your stones are dissolving.

■ *If you miss a dose...*
Take it as soon as you remember, or at the same time as the next dose.
■ *Storage instructions...*
Store at room temperature in a tightly closed container.

## What side effects may occur?

Side effects cannot be anticipated. If any develop or change in intensity, inform your doctor as soon as possible. Only your doctor can determine if it is safe for you to continue taking Actigall.

■ *Side effects may include:*
Abdominal pain, anxiety, back pain, constipation, cough, depression, dry skin, fatigue, gas, hair thinning, headache, hives, indigestion, inflammation of the mouth or nose, itching, metallic taste, mild temporary diarrhea, muscle and joint pain, nausea, rash, severe pain in the upper right side of the abdomen, sleep disorders, sweating, vomiting

## Why should this drug not be prescribed?

Do not take this medication if you are sensitive to or have ever had an allergic reaction to ursodiol (ursodeoxycholic acid) or to other bile acids.

Actigall will not dissolve certain types of gallstones. If your doctor tells you that your gallstones are calcified cholesterol stones, radio-opaque stones, or radiolucent bile pigment stones, you are not a candidate for treatment with Actigall.

Also, if you have biliary tract (liver, gallbladder, bile duct) problems or certain liver and pancreas diseases, your doctor may not be able to prescribe Actigall for you.

## Special warnings about this medication

Although Actigall is not known to cause liver damage, it is theoretically possible in some people. Your doctor may check the levels of liver enzymes in your blood before you start to take Actigall and again while you are taking it.

## Possible food and drug interactions when taking this medication

If Actigall is taken with certain other drugs, the effects of either could be increased, decreased, or altered. It is especially important to check with your doctor before combining Actigall with the following:

Aluminum-based antacid medications (Alu-Cap, Alu-Tab, Rolaids, others)
Certain cholesterol-lowering medications, such as Questran and Colestid
Estrogens, such as Premarin
Lipid-lowering medications, such as Lopid and Mevacor
Oral contraceptives

## Special information if you are pregnant or breastfeeding

If you are pregnant or plan to become pregnant, inform your doctor immediately. So far, there is no evidence that Actigall can harm an unborn baby; but to be safe, the medication is not recommended during pregnancy. Caution is needed during breastfeeding; it is not known whether Actigall taken by a nursing mother passes into her breast milk.

## Recommended dosage

The recommended dose for Actigall treatment of radiolucent gallbladder stones is 8 to 10 milligrams per 2.2 pounds of body weight per day divided into 2 or 3 doses.

## Overdosage

Although there have been no reports of overdose with Actigall, the most likely symptom of severe overdose would be diarrhea. Since any medication taken in excess can have serious consequences, you should seek medical attention immediately if you suspect an Actigall overdose.

*Generic name:*

# Acyclovir

*See Zovirax, page 612.*

*Brand name:*

# Adalat

*See Procardia, page 438.*

*Brand name:*

# Advil

*See Motrin, page 337.*

*Brand name:*

# AeroBid

*Pronounced: AIR-oh-bid*
*Generic name: Flunisolide*
*Other brand names: AeroBid-M, Nasalide*

## Why is this drug prescribed?

AeroBid is prescribed for people who need long-term treatment to control the symptoms of bronchial asthma. It contains an anti-inflammatory steroid type of medication. A nasal-spray form of the drug (Nasalide) is available for relief of hay fever.

## Most important fact about this drug

AeroBid helps to reduce the likelihood of an asthma attack, but will not relieve one that has already started. To be effective as a preventive measure, it must be taken every day at regularly spaced intervals. It may be several weeks before you receive its full benefit.

## How should you take this medication?

Take this medication at regular intervals, exactly as prescribed by your doctor. Taking doses higher than your doctor has prescribed may impair the function of your adrenal glands.

*Administration technique:*
1. Remove the cap and hold inhaler upright.
2. Shake the inhaler thoroughly.
3. Take a drink of water to moisten the throat.
4. Tilt your head slightly and breathe out.
5. While activating the inhaler, take a slow deep breath for 3 to 5 seconds, hold the breath for about 10 seconds, then breathe out slowly.
6. Allow at least 1 minute between inhalations.

If you are also using a bronchodilator inhalant, it should be used before the AeroBid inhalant to derive the best effects from this drug. Use of the two inhalers should be separated by several minutes.

To help reduce hoarseness, throat irritation, and mouth infection, rinse out with water after each use.

Illustrated instructions for use are available with the product.

■ *If you miss a dose...*
Use it as soon as you remember. If it is almost time for your next dose, skip the one you missed and go back to your regular schedule. Do not take 2 doses at the same time.
■ *Storage instructions...*
Store away from heat or cold and light. Keep away from open flames.

## What side effects may occur?

Side effects cannot be anticipated. If any develop or change in intensity, inform your doctor as soon as possible. Only your doctor can determine if it is safe for you to continue taking AeroBid.

■ *More common side effects may include:*
Cold symptoms, diarrhea, flu, headache, infection of the upper respiratory tract, nasal congestion, nausea, sore throat, unpleasant taste, upset stomach, vomiting
■ *Less common side effects may include:*
Abdominal pain, chest congestion, chest pain, cough, decreased appetite, dizziness, ear infection, eczema (inflamed skin with sores and crust-

ing), fever, heartburn, hoarseness, inflamed lining of the nose, irritability, itching, loss of smell or taste, menstrual disturbances, nervousness, phlegm, rapid, fluttering heartbeat, rash, runny nose, shakiness, sinus congestion, sinus drainage, sinus infection, sinus inflammation, sneezing, swelling due to fluid retention, wheezing, yeastlike fungal infection of the mouth and throat

■ *Rare side effects may include:*
Acne, anxiety, blurred vision, bronchitis, chest tightness, chills, constipation, depression, difficult or labored breathing, dry throat, earache, excessive restlessness, eye discomfort, eye infection, faintness, fatigue, gas, general feeling of illness, head stuffiness, high blood pressure, hives, inability to fall or stay asleep, increased appetite, indigestion, inflammation of the tongue, laryngitis, moodiness, mouth irritation, nasal irritation, nosebleed, numbness, pneumonia, rapid heart rate, sinus discomfort, sluggishness, sweating, swelling of the arms and legs, throat irritation, vertigo, weakness, weight gain

### Why should this drug not be prescribed?
AeroBid should not be used if your asthma can be controlled with bronchodilators and other nonsteroid medications.

This medication should not be used if you require only occasional corticosteroid treatment for asthma. It is not for treatment of prolonged, severe asthma attacks where more intensive measures are required.

AeroBid should not be used for the treatment of nonasthmatic bronchitis.

If you are allergic or sensitive to AeroBid or other steroid drugs, advise your doctor before using this medication.

### Special warnings about this medication
Your asthma should be reasonably stable before treatment with AeroBid Inhaler is started. AeroBid should be started in combination with your usual dose of an oral steroid medication. After approximately 1 week, your doctor will start to withdraw gradually the oral steroid by reducing the daily or alternate daily dose. A slow rate of reduction is very important, as some people have experienced withdrawal symptoms such as joint and/or muscular pain, fatigue, and depression. Tell your doctor if

you lose weight or feel light-headed. You may need to take more oral corticosteroid temporarily.

This medication is not useful when you need rapid relief of asthma symptoms.

Transferring from steroid tablet therapy to AeroBid Inhaler may produce allergic conditions that were previously controlled by the steroid tablet therapy. These include rhinitis (inflammation of the mucous membrane of the nose), conjunctivitis (pinkeye), and eczema.

Contact your doctor immediately if you have an asthma attack that isn't controlled by a bronchodilator while you are being treated with AeroBid. You may need an oral steroid drug.

While you are being treated with AeroBid, particularly at higher doses, your doctor will carefully observe you for any evidence of side effects such as the suppression of glandular function and diminished bone growth in children. If you have just had surgery or are under extreme stress, your doctor will also closely monitor you.

The use of AeroBid may cause a yeastlike fungal infection of the mouth, pharynx (throat), or larynx (voice box). If you suspect a fungal infection, notify your doctor. Treatment with antifungal medication may be necessary.

Since the contents of this inhalant are under pressure, do not puncture the container and do not use or store the medication near heat or an open flame. Exposure to temperatures above 120 degrees may cause the container to explode.

People taking drugs such as AeroBid that suppress the immune system are more open to infection. Take extra care to avoid exposure to measles and chickenpox if you've never had them or never had shots. Such diseases can be serious or even fatal when your immune system is below par. If you are exposed, tell your doctor immediately.

### Possible food and drug interactions when taking this medication
No interactions have been reported.

### Special information if you are pregnant or breastfeeding
The effects of AeroBid during pregnancy have not been adequately studied. If you are pregnant or plan to become pregnant, inform your doctor immediately. It is not known whether AeroBid appears in breast milk. If this medication is essential to your health, your doctor may advise you to discontinue

breastfeeding your baby until your treatment with this medication is finished.

## Recommended dosage

The AeroBid Inhaler system is for oral inhalation only.

### ADULTS

The recommended starting dose is 2 inhalations twice daily, in the morning and evening, for a total daily dose of 1 milligram. The daily dose should not exceed 4 inhalations twice a day, for a total daily dose of 2 milligrams.

### CHILDREN

For children 6 to 15 years of age, 2 inhalations may be used twice daily, for a total daily dose of 1 milligram.

The safety and effectiveness of this drug have not been established in children under 6 years of age.

## Overdosage

Any medication taken in excess can have serious consequences. If you suspect an overdose, seek emergency medical treatment immediately.

Brand name:

# Aktob

See Tobrex, page 548.

Generic name:

# Albuterol

See Proventil, page 446.

Generic name:

# Alclometasone

See Aclovate, page 4.

Brand name:

# Aldactazide

Pronounced: al-DAK-tah-zide
Generic ingredients: Spironolactone, Hydrochlorothiazide
Other brand name: Spirozide

## Why is this drug prescribed?

Aldactazide is used in the treatment of high blood pressure and other conditions that require the elimi-

nation of excess fluid from the body. These conditions include congestive heart failure, cirrhosis of the liver, and kidney disease. Aldactazide combines two diuretic drugs that help your body produce and eliminate more urine. Spironolactone, one of the ingredients, helps to minimize the potassium loss that can be caused by the hydrochlorothiazide component.

## Most important fact about this drug

If you have high blood pressure, you must take Aldactazide regularly for it to be effective. Since blood pressure declines gradually, it may be several weeks before you get the full benefit of Aldactazide; and you must continue taking it even if you are feeling well. Aldactazide does not cure high blood pressure; it merely keeps it under control.

## How should you take this medication?

Take Aldactazide exactly as prescribed. Stopping Aldactazide suddenly could cause your condition to worsen.

■ *If you miss a dose...*
Take it as soon as you remember. If it is almost time for your next dose, skip the one you missed and go back to your regular schedule. Never take 2 doses at the same time.
■ *Storage instructions...*
Store at room temperature.

## What side effects may occur?

Side effects cannot be anticipated. If any develop or change in intensity, inform your doctor as soon as possible. Only your doctor can determine if it is safe for you to continue taking Aldactazide.

■ *Side effects may include:*
Abdominal cramps, breast development in males, change in potassium levels (leading to such symptoms as dry mouth, excessive thirst, weak or irregular heartbeat, and muscle pain or cramps), deepening of the voice, diarrhea, dizziness, dizziness on rising, drowsiness, excessive hairiness, fever, headache, hives, inflammation of blood vessels or lymph vessels, inflammation of the pancreas, irregular menstruation, lack of coordination, loss of appetite, mental confusion, muscle spasms, nausea, postmenopausal bleeding, rash, red or purple spots on skin, restless-

ness, sensitivity to light, sexual dysfunction, sluggishness, stomach bleeding, stomach inflammation, stomach ulcers, tingling or pins and needles, vertigo, vomiting, weakness, yellow eyes and skin, yellow vision

### Why should this drug not be prescribed?

Aldactazide should not be used if you have acute kidney disease or liver failure, have difficulty urinating or are unable to urinate, or have high potassium levels in your blood.

If you are sensitive to or have ever had an allergic reaction to spironolactone, hydrochlorothiazide, or similar drugs, or if you are sensitive to sulfa drugs, you should not take this medication. Make sure your doctor is aware of any drug reactions you may have experienced.

### Special warnings about this medication

This medication should be used only if your doctor has determined that the precise amount of each ingredient in Aldactazide meets your specific needs.

Potassium supplements (including salt substitutes) or diuretics that leave high levels of potassium in your body should not be used while taking Aldactazide, unless specifically recommended by your doctor.

If you are taking an ACE-inhibitor type of blood pressure medication such as Vasotec, this drug should be used with extreme caution.

If you have liver disease or lupus erythematosus (a disease that causes skin eruptions), Aldactazide should be used with caution.

Excessive sweating, dehydration, severe diarrhea, or vomiting could cause you to lose too much water and cause your blood pressure to become too low. Be careful when exercising and in hot weather.

Notify your doctor or dentist that you are taking Aldactazide if you have a medical emergency, and before you have surgery or dental treatment.

### Possible food and drug interactions when taking this medication

If Aldactazide is taken with certain other drugs, the effects of either could be increased, decreased, or altered. It is especially important to check with your doctor before combining Aldactazide with the following:

ACE-inhibitor blood pressure drugs such as Vasotec
Antigout medications such as Zyloprim
Digoxin (Lanoxin)
Diuretics such as Lasix and Midamor
Indomethacin (Indocin)
Insulin or oral antidiabetic drugs such as Micronase
Lithium (Lithonate)
Norepinephrine (Levophed)
Potassium supplements such as Slow-K
Steroids such as prednisone

### Special information
### if you are pregnant or breastfeeding

The effects of Aldactazide during pregnancy have not been adequately studied. If you are pregnant or plan to become pregnant, inform your doctor immediately. Aldactazide appears in breast milk and could affect a nursing infant. If this medication is essential to your health, your doctor may advise you to discontinue breastfeeding until your treatment is finished.

### Recommended dosage

ADULTS

*Congestive Heart Failure, Cirrhosis,
Nephrotic Syndrome (kidney disorder)*
The usual dosage is 100 milligrams each of spironolactone and hydrochlorothiazide daily, taken as a single dose or in divided doses. Dosage may range from 25 milligrams to 200 milligrams of each ingredient daily, depending on your individual needs.

*High Blood Pressure*
The usual dose is 50 milligrams to 100 milligrams each of spironolactone and hydrochlorothiazide daily, in a single dose divided into smaller doses.

CHILDREN

The usual dose of Aldactazide should provide 0.75 milligram to 1.5 milligrams of spironolactone per pound of body weight.

### Overdosage

Although there is no information on specific signs of Aldactazide overdose, any medication taken in excess can have serious consequences. If you suspect an overdose, seek medical attention immediately.

*Brand name:*

# Aldactone

*Pronounced: al-DAK-tone*
*Generic name: Spironolactone*

## Why is this drug prescribed?

Aldactone is a diuretic and high blood pressure medication. It is used in the diagnosis and treatment of hyperaldosteronism, a condition in which the adrenal gland secretes too much aldosterone (a hormone that regulates the body's salt and potassium levels). It is also used in treating other conditions that require the elimination of excess fluid from the body. These conditions include congestive heart failure, high blood pressure, cirrhosis of the liver, kidney disease, and unusually low potassium levels in the blood. When used for high blood pressure, Aldactone can be used alone or with other high blood pressure medications. Aldactone causes increased amounts of sodium and water to be eliminated, without potassium loss.

## Most important fact about this drug

If you have high blood pressure, you must take Aldactone regularly for it to be effective. Since blood pressure declines gradually, it may be several weeks before you get the full benefit of Aldactone; and you must continue taking it even if you are feeling well. Aldactone does not cure high blood pressure; it merely keeps it under control.

## How should you take this medication?

Take Aldactone exactly as prescribed by your doctor. Stopping Aldactone suddenly could cause your condition to worsen.

■ *If you miss a dose...*
Take it as soon as you remember. If it is almost time for your next dose, skip the one you missed and go back to your regular schedule. Never take 2 doses at the same time.

■ *Storage instructions...*
Store at room temperature.

## What side effects may occur?

Side effects cannot be anticipated. If any develop or change in intensity, inform your doctor as soon as possible. Only your doctor can determine if it is safe for you to continue taking Aldactone.

■ *Side effects may include:*
Abdominal cramps, breast development in males, change in potassium levels (leading to such symptoms as dry mouth, excessive thirst, weak or irregular heartbeat, and muscle pain or cramps), deepening of voice, diarrhea, drowsiness, excessive hairiness, fever, headache, hives, irregular menstruation, lack of coordination, lethargy, mental confusion, postmenopausal bleeding, sexual dysfunction, skin eruptions, stomach bleeding, stomach inflammation, ulcers, vomiting

## Why should this drug not be prescribed?

You should not take Aldactone if you have kidney disease, an inability to urinate, difficulty urinating, or high potassium levels in your blood.

## Special warnings about this medication

Potassium supplements or other diuretics that leave your potassium levels high, such as Maxzide, should not be used while taking Aldactone, unless specifically indicated by your doctor.

ACE inhibitors (Vasotec, Capoten), used for blood pressure and heart failure, should not be taken while using Aldactone.

If you are taking Aldactone, your kidney function should be given a complete assessment and should continue to be monitored.

If you have liver disease, your doctor will be cautious about using this medication.

Excessive sweating, dehydration, severe diarrhea, or vomiting could cause you to lose too much water and cause your blood pressure to become too low. Be careful when exercising and in hot weather.

Notify your doctor or dentist that you are taking Aldactone if you have a medical emergency, and before you have surgery or dental treatment.

## Possible food and drug interactions when taking this medication

If Aldactone is taken with certain other drugs, the effects of either could be increased, decreased, or altered. It is especially important to check with your doctor before combining Aldactone with the following:

ACE inhibitors such as Vasotec and Capoten
Digoxin (Lanoxin)
Indomethacin (Indocin)
Norepinephrine (Levophed)

Other diuretics such as Lasix and HydroDIURIL

Other high blood pressure medications such as Aldomet and Procardia XL

**Special information
if you are pregnant or breastfeeding**

The effects of Aldactone during pregnancy have not been adequately studied. If you are pregnant or plan to become pregnant, inform your doctor immediately. Aldactone appears in breast milk and could affect a nursing infant. If this medication is essential to your health, your doctor may advise you to discontinue breastfeeding until your treatment with this medication is finished.

**Recommended dosage**

ADULTS

*Primary Hyperaldosteronism*

Initial dosages of this medication are used to determine the presence of primary hyperaldosteronism (too much secretion of the adrenal hormone aldosterone). People can be tested with this medication over either a long or a short period of time.

In the long test, you take 400 milligrams per day for 3 to 4 weeks. If your potassium levels and blood pressure are corrected with this dosage in this time period, your physician may assume you have this condition.

In the short test, you receive 400 milligrams per day for 4 days. A laboratory test compares potassium levels while on Aldactone and after the medication is stopped. Your doctor may then make a diagnosis.

After the diagnosis of primary hyperaldosteronism is made and confirmed by more tests, the usual dose is 100 to 400 milligrams per day, prior to surgery. In those who are not good candidates for surgery, this drug is given over the long term at the lowest effective dose.

*Adult Edema (Congestive Heart Failure, Cirrhosis of the Liver, or Kidney Disorders)*

The usual starting dosage is 100 milligrams daily either in a single dose or divided into smaller doses. However, your doctor may have you take daily doses as low as 25 milligrams or as high as 200 milligrams.

Your doctor may choose to adjust your dosage after an initial 5-day trial period or add another diuretic medication to this one.

*Essential Hypertension (High Blood Pressure)*

The usual starting dosage is 50 to 100 milligrams daily in a single dose or divided into smaller doses. This medication may be given with another diuretic or with other high blood pressure medications.

It may take up to 2 weeks before the full effect of this medication is seen. Your doctor can then adjust the dosage according to your response.

*Hypokalemia (Potassium Loss)*

Your doctor may have you take daily dosages of 25 milligrams to 100 milligrams when potassium loss caused by the effects of a diuretic cannot be treated by a potassium supplement.

CHILDREN

*Edema (Swelling Due to Water Retention)*

The usual starting dosage is 1.5 milligrams per pound of body weight daily in a single dose or divided into smaller doses.

**Overdosage**

Although no specific information on signs of Aldactone overdose is available, any medication taken in excess can have serious consequences. If you suspect an overdose, seek medical attention immediately.

*Brand name:*

# Aldomet

*Pronounced: AL-doe-met*
*Generic name: Methyldopa*

**Why is this drug prescribed?**

Aldomet is used to treat high blood pressure. It is effective when used alone or with other high blood pressure medications.

**Most important fact about this drug**

You must take Aldomet regularly for it to be effective. Since blood pressure declines gradually, it may be several weeks before you get the full benefit of Aldomet; and you must continue taking it even if you are feeling well. Aldomet does not cure high blood pressure; it merely keeps it under control.

**How should you take this medication?**

Take this medication exactly as prescribed. Try not to miss any doses. Do not stop taking the drug without your doctor's knowledge.

Drowsiness may occur when dosage is increased. If your doctor increases the amount of Aldomet you take, start the new dosage in the evening.

■ *If you miss a dose...*
Take it as soon as you remember. If it is almost time for your next dose, skip the one you missed and go back to your regular schedule. Never take 2 doses at the same time.

■ *Storage instructions...*
Keep Aldomet in the container it came in, tightly closed. Store Aldomet tablets at room temperature. Keep oral suspension in the refrigerator. Protect from light.

## What side effects may occur?
Side effects cannot be anticipated. If any develop or change in intensity, inform your doctor as soon as possible. Only your doctor can determine if it is safe for you to continue taking Aldomet.

■ *More common side effects may include:*
Drowsiness during the first few weeks of therapy, fluid retention or weight gain, headache, weakness

■ *Less common or rare side effects may include:*
Anemia, Bell's palsy (paralysis of the face, making it look distorted), bloating, blood disorders, breast development in males, breast enlargement, changes in menstruation, chest pain, congestive heart failure, constipation, decreased mental ability, decreased sex drive, depression, diarrhea, dizziness when standing up, dry mouth, fever, gas, hepatitis, impotence, inflammation of the large intestine, inflammation of the pancreas, inflammation of the salivary glands, involuntary movements, joint pain, lightheadedness, liver disorders, milk production, muscle pain, nasal stuffiness, nausea, nightmares, parkinsonism (tremors, shuffling walk, stooped posture, muscle weakness), rash, slow heartbeat, sore or "black" tongue, tingling or pins and needles, vomiting, yellow eyes and skin

## Why should this drug not be prescribed?
If you have liver disease or cirrhosis, or if you have taken Aldomet before and developed liver disease, do not take this medication.

If you are sensitive to or have ever had an allergic reaction to Aldomet, or if you have been prescribed the oral suspension form of Aldomet and have ever had an allergic reaction to sulfites, you should not take this medication.

If you are taking drugs known as monoamine oxidase (MAO) inhibitors, you should not take Aldomet.

## Special warnings about this medication
Before you begin taking Aldomet, your doctor should perform a complete study of your liver tion, and it should be monitored periodically thereafter.

Aldomet can cause liver disorders. You may develop a fever, jaundice (yellow eyes and skin), or both, usually within the first 2 to 3 months of therapy. If either of these symptoms occurs, stop taking Aldomet and contact your doctor immediately. If the fever and/or jaundice were caused by the medication, your liver function should gradually return to normal.

If you have a history of liver disease, this medication should be used with caution.

Hemolytic anemia, a blood disorder in which red blood cells are destroyed, can develop with long-term use of Aldomet; your doctor will do periodic blood counts to check for this problem.

Aldomet can cause water retention or weight gain in some people. A diuretic will usually relieve these symptoms.

If you have asthma and are taking the liquid form of Aldomet, you could have an allergic reaction to the sulfite component of the liquid.

If you are on dialysis and are taking Aldomet for high blood pressure, your blood pressure may rise after your dialysis treatments.

Aldomet can cause you to become drowsy or less alert, especially during the first few weeks of therapy or when dosage levels are increased. If it affects you this way, driving or operating heavy machinery or participating in any hazardous activity that requires full mental alertness is not recommended.

Notify your doctor or dentist that you are taking Aldomet if you have a medical emergency and before you have surgery or dental treatment.

## Possible food and drug interactions when taking this medication
If Aldomet is taken with certain other drugs, the effects of either could be increased, decreased, or altered. It is especially important to check with your doctor before combining Aldomet with the following:

Antidepressants known as MAO inhibitors, including
Nardil and Parnate
Dextroamphetamine (Dexedrine)
Imipramine (Tofranil)
Iron-containing products such as Feosol
Lithium (Lithonate)
Other blood pressure medications such as Catapres and Calan
Phenylpropanolamine (a decongestant used in common cold remedies such as Dimetapp, Entex LA, and others)
Propranolol (Inderal)
Tolbutamide (Orinase)

### Special information
### if you are pregnant or breastfeeding

The use of Aldomet during pregnancy appears to be relatively safe. However, if you are pregnant or plan to become pregnant, inform your doctor immediately. Aldomet appears in breast milk and could affect a nursing infant. If this medication is essential to your health, your doctor may advise you to discontinue breastfeeding until your treatment is finished.

### Recommended dosage

ADULTS

The usual starting dose is 250 milligrams, 2 or 3 times per day in the first 48 hours of treatment. Your doctor may increase or decrease your dose over the next few days to achieve the correct blood pressure.

To reduce the effect of any sedation the medication may cause, dosage increases will usually be given in the evening.

The usual maintenance dosage is 500 milligrams to 2 grams per day divided into 2 to 4 doses. The maximum dose is usually 3 grams.

Your doctor will also adjust your dosage of Aldomet when it is taken in combination with certain other high blood pressure drugs.

If you take Aldomet with a non-thiazide high blood pressure medicine, your doctor will limit the initial dosage to 500 milligrams daily divided into small doses.

Dosages will be adjusted, and other high blood pressure drugs may be added, during the first few months of treatment with Aldomet. Those with reduced kidney function may require smaller doses. Older people who are prone to fainting spells due to arterial disease may also require smaller doses.

CHILDREN

The usual starting dose is 10 milligrams per 2.2 pounds of body weight daily, divided into 2 to 4 doses. Doses will be adjusted until blood pressure is normal. The maximum daily dose is usually 65 milligrams per 2.2 pounds of body weight or 3 grams, whichever is less.

OLDER ADULTS

Dosages of this drug are adjusted to each individual's needs. Lower doses may be prescribed by your doctor.

### Overdosage

Any medication taken in excess can have serious consequences. If you suspect an overdose, seek medical attention immediately.

■ *Symptoms of Aldomet overdose may include:*
Bloating, constipation, diarrhea, dizziness, extreme drowsiness, gas, light-headedness, nausea, severely low blood pressure, slow heartbeat, vomiting, weakness

---

*Generic name:*

# Alendronate

*See Fosamax, page 221.*

---

*Brand name:*

# Aleve

*See Anaprox, page 26.*

---

*Generic name:*

# Allopurinol

*See Zyloprim, page 613.*

---

*Generic name:*

# Alprazolam

*See Xanax, page 595.*

*Generic name:*

# Alprostadil

*See Caverject, page 84.*

*Brand name:*

# Altace

*Pronounced: AL-tayce*
*Generic name: Ramipril*

## Why is this drug prescribed?

Altace is used in the treatment of high blood pressure. It is effective when used alone or in combination with other high blood pressure medications, especially thiazide-type diuretics. Altace works by preventing the conversion of a chemical in your blood called angiotensin I into a more potent substance that increases salt and water retention in your body. It also enhances blood flow in your circulatory system. It is a member of the group of drugs called ACE inhibitors.

## Most important fact about this drug

You must take Altace regularly for it to be effective. Since blood pressure declines gradually, it may be several weeks before you get the full benefit of Altace; and you must continue taking it even if you are feeling well. Altace does not cure high blood pressure; it merely keeps it under control.

## How should you take this medication?

Take this medication exactly as prescribed by your doctor. If you have difficulty swallowing the capsule, you can sprinkle the contents on a small amount (about 4 ounces) of apple sauce, or mix the contents with 4 ounces of water or apple juice. Be sure to eat or drink the entire mixture so that you get the full dose of the drug. You can prepare the mixture ahead of time; it will keep for 24 hours at room temperature or 48 hours in the refrigerator.

■ *If you miss a dose...*
If you forget to take a dose, take it as soon as you remember. If it is almost time for your next dose, skip the one you missed and go back to your regular schedule. Never take 2 doses at the same time.

■ *Storage instructions...*
Store Altace at room temperature in a tightly closed container.

## What side effects may occur?

Side effects cannot be anticipated. If any develop or change in intensity, inform your doctor as soon as possible. Only your doctor can determine if it is safe for you to continue taking Altace.

■ *More common side effects may include:*
Cough, headache
■ *Less common or rare side effects may include:*
Abdominal pain, anemia, angina pectoris (chest pain), anxiety, arthritis, bruises, change in taste, constipation, convulsions, depression, diarrhea, difficulty swallowing, dizziness, dry mouth, fainting, fatigue, feeling of general discomfort, fluid retention, hearing loss, heart attack, impotence, inability to sleep, increased salivation, indigestion, inflammation of the stomach and intestines, irregular heartbeat, itching, joint pain or inflammation, labored breathing, light-headedness, loss of appetite, low blood pressure, memory loss, muscle pain, nausea, nerve pain, nervousness, nosebleed, rash, ringing in ears, skin inflammation, skin sensitivity to light, sleepiness, sudden loss of strength, sweating, tingling or pins and needles, tremors, vertigo, very rapid heartbeat, vision changes, vomiting, weakness, weight gain

## Why should this drug not be prescribed?

If you are sensitive to or have ever had an allergic reaction to Altace or similar drugs such as Capoten, Vasotec and Zestril, or if you have a history of swelling of the face, tongue, or throat while taking these drugs, you should not take this medication. Make sure that your doctor is aware of any drug reactions that you have experienced.

## Special warnings about this medication

If you develop chest pain, palpitations or other heart effects, swelling of the face around your lips, tongue, or throat or difficulty swallowing, difficulty breathing, swelling of arms and legs or infection, sore throat, and fever, you should contact your doctor immediately. You may have a serious side effect of the drug and need emergency treatment.

If you are taking Altace, your kidney function should be given a complete assessment and should continue to be monitored.

If you notice your skin or the whites of your eyes turning yellow, notify your doctor. Your liver may be affected, and you may have to stop taking Altace. Your doctor should routinely test your liver function while you are on this drug.

Altace should be used with caution if you have liver disease, diabetes, or a disease of the connective tissue such as lupus erythematosus or scleroderma.

If you are taking high doses of diuretics and Altace, you may develop excessively low blood pressure.

Do not use salt substitutes containing potassium without consulting your doctor.

Altace may cause you to become drowsy or less alert, especially if you are also taking a water pill (diuretic) at the same time. If it has this effect on you, driving or operating dangerous machinery or participating in any hazardous activity that requires full mental alertness is not recommended.

Light-headedness can occur when taking Altace, especially during the first days of therapy, and should be reported to your doctor. If fainting occurs, stop taking the medication and notify your doctor immediately.

Dehydration, excessive sweating, severe diarrhea or vomiting could deplete your body's fluids, causing your blood pressure to drop dangerously.

### Possible food and drug interactions when taking this medication

If Altace is taken with certain other drugs, the effects of either could be increased, decreased, or altered. It is especially important to check with your doctor before combining Altace with the following:

Alcohol
Diuretics such as hydrochlorothiazide (found in many blood pressure medicines) and furosemide (Lasix)
Lithium (Lithonate, Eskalith)
Potassium-sparing diuretics (found in Dyazide, Maxzide, Moduretic, and others)
Spironolactone (Aldactone)
Potassium supplements such as K-lyte and K-Tab
Potassium-containing salt substitutes

### Special information if you are pregnant or breastfeeding

Altace can cause birth defects, prematurity and death to developing and newborn babies. If you are pregnant or plan to become pregnant and are taking Altace, contact your doctor immediately. Altace

may appear in breast milk and could affect a nursing infant. If this medication is essential to your health, your doctor may advise you to discontinue breastfeeding until your treatment is finished.

### Recommended dosage

ADULTS

For patients not on diuretics, the usual starting dose is 2.5 milligrams, taken once daily. After blood pressure is under control, the dosage will range from 2.5 to 20 milligrams a day in a single dose or divided into 2 equal doses.

Diuretic use should, if possible, be stopped before using Altace. If not, your physician may give you an initial dose of Altace under his supervision before any further medication is prescribed.

If you have kidney problems, your doctor may prescribe a lower than normal dose.

CHILDREN

The safety and effectiveness of Altace in children have not been established.

OLDER ADULTS

Dosage varies according to the individual's response.

### Overdosage

Any medication taken in excess can have serious consequences. If you suspect an overdose, seek medical attention immediately.

A sudden drop in blood pressure is likely to be the primary sign of an Altace overdose.

*Brand name:*

# Alupent

*Pronounced: AL-yew-pent*
*Generic name: Metaproterenol sulfate*
*Other brand name: Metaprel*

### Why is this drug prescribed?

Alupent is a bronchodilator prescribed for the prevention and relief of bronchial asthma and bronchial spasms (wheezing) associated with bronchitis and emphysema. Alupent Inhalation Solution is also used to treat acute asthmatic attacks in children 6 years of age and older.

## Most important fact about this drug

Alupent's effects last up to 6 hours. It should not be used more frequently than your doctor recommends.

Increasing the number of doses can be dangerous and may actually make symptoms of asthma worse. Fatalities have occurred with excessive use of this medication.

If the dose your doctor recommends does not provide relief of your symptoms, if your symptoms become worse, or if side effects occur, seek medical attention immediately.

## How should you take this medication?

Take this medication exactly as prescribed by your doctor.

■ *If you miss a dose...*
Take the dose as soon as you remember. Take any remaining doses for the day at equal intervals thereafter. Do not increase the total for the day or take 2 doses at the same time.

■ *Storage instructions...*
Store at room temperature. Protect from light and excessive humidity. Keep out of reach of children.

## What side effects may occur?

Side effects cannot be anticipated. If any develop or change in intensity, inform your doctor as soon as possible. Only your doctor can determine if it is safe for you to continue taking Alupent.

■ *Side effects may include:*
Bad taste in mouth, cough, diarrhea, dizziness, fatigue, headache, high blood pressure, insomnia, nausea, nervousness, rapid or throbbing heartbeat, stomach and intestinal upset, throat irritation, tremors, vomiting, worsening or aggravation of asthma

Side effects can occur when a new aerosol container is used, even though you have had no trouble with the medication in the past. Replacing the container may solve the problem.

## Why should this drug not be prescribed?

If you are sensitive to or have ever had an allergic reaction to Alupent or similar drugs, such as Proventil, you should not take this medication. Make sure your doctor is aware of any drug reactions you have experienced.

Unless you are directed to do so by your doctor, do not take this medication if you have an irregular, rapid heart rate.

## Special warnings about this medication

When taking Alupent, you should not use other inhaled medications (called sympathomimetics) before checking with your doctor. Only your doctor can determine the sufficient amount of time between inhaled medications.

A single dose of nebulized Alupent used to treat an acute attack of asthma may temporarily relieve symptoms but not completely stop the attack.

Consult your doctor before using this medication if you have a heart condition or convulsive disorder (e.g., epilepsy), high blood pressure, hyperthyroidism, or diabetes mellitus. Alupent can cause significant changes in blood pressure.

## Possible food and drug interactions when taking this medication

If Alupent is taken with certain other drugs, the effects of either could be increased, decreased, or altered. It is especially important to check with your doctor before combining Alupent with the following:

MAO inhibitors (antidepressant drugs such as Nardil and Parnate)
Bronchodilators such as Ventolin and Proventil inhalers
Tricyclic antidepressants such as Elavil and Tofranil

## Special information if you are pregnant or breastfeeding

The effects of Alupent during pregnancy have not been adequately studied. If you are pregnant or plan to become pregnant, inform your doctor immediately. It is not known whether Alupent appears in breast milk. If this medication is essential to your health, your doctor may advise you to stop nursing your baby until your treatment is finished.

## Recommended dosage

ADULTS

*Inhalation Aerosol*
The usual single dose is 2 to 3 inhalations. Inhalation should usually not be repeated more often than about every 3 to 4 hours. Total dosage per day should not exceed 12 inhalations.

*Inhalation Solution 5%*
Treatment usually need not be repeated more often than every 4 hours to relieve acute attacks of bronchospasm.

As part of a total treatment program for chronic breathing disorders, the inhalation solution may be taken 3 to 4 times per day, as determined by your doctor.

Inhalation solution is given by oral inhalation with the aid of a nebulizer or an intermittent positive pressure breathing (IPPB) apparatus.

The usual single dose with the nebulizer is 10 inhalations. However, a single dose of 5 to 15 inhalations can be taken, as determined by your doctor. The usual single daily dose with the IPPB is 0.3 milliliter diluted in approximately 2.5 milliliters of saline solution. The dosage range is 0.2 to 0.3 milliliter, as determined by your doctor.

*Inhalation Solution 0.4% and 0.6% Unit-Dose Vials*
The inhalation solution unit-dose vial is administered by oral inhalation using an intermittent positive pressure breathing (IPPB) apparatus. The usual adult dose is 1 vial per treatment. You usually should not need to repeat the treatment more often than every 4 hours for severe attacks of wheezing. You can use the unit-dose vials 3 to 4 times a day.

*Syrup*
The usual dose is 2 teaspoonfuls, 3 or 4 times a day.

*Tablets*
The usual dose is 20 milligrams, 3 or 4 times per day.

CHILDREN

*Inhalation Aerosol*
Alupent Inhalation Aerosol is not recommended for use in children under 12 years of age.

*Inhalation Solution 5%*
For children aged 6 to 12 years, the usual single dose is 0.1 milliliter, given by oral inhalation with a nebulizer. Dosage can be increased to 0.2 milliliter 3 to 4 times a day.

The unit-dose vial is not recommended for children under 12 years of age.

*Syrup*
The usual dose for children 6 to 9 years of age or weighing under 60 pounds is 1 teaspoonful, 3 or 4 times a day.

The usual dose for children 9 years of age or weighing over 60 pounds is 2 teaspoonfuls, 3 or 4 times a day.

*Tablets*
The usual dose for children 6 to 9 years of age or weighing under 60 pounds is 10 milligrams, 3 or 4 times a day.

The usual dose for children over 9 years of age or weighing over 60 pounds is 20 milligrams, 3 or 4 times a day.

Tablets are not recommended for use in children under 6 years of age.

### Overdosage
Any medication taken in excess can have serious consequences.

If you suspect an overdose, seek medical attention immediately.

■ *Symptoms of Alupent overdose may include:*
Dizziness, dry mouth, fatigue, general feeling of bodily discomfort, headache, high or low blood pressure, inability to fall or stay asleep, irregular heartbeat, nausea, nervousness, rapid, fluttery heartbeat, severe, suffocating chest pain, tremors

*Brand name:*

# Amaryl

*Pronounced: AM-a-ril*
*Generic name: Glimepiride*

### Why is this drug prescribed?
Amaryl is an oral medication used to treat Type II (non-insulin-dependent) diabetes when diet and exercise alone fail to control abnormally high levels of blood sugar. Like other diabetes drugs classified as sulfonylureas, Amaryl lowers blood sugar by stimulating the pancreas to produce more insulin. Amaryl may also be used along with insulin and other diabetes drugs.

### Most important fact about this drug
Always remember that Amaryl is an aid to, not a substitute for, good diet and exercise. Failure to follow a sound diet and exercise plan may diminish the results of Amaryl and can lead to serious complications such as dangerously high or low blood sugar levels. Remember, too, that Amaryl is not an oral form of insulin, and cannot be used in place of insulin.

### How should you take this medication?
Do not take more or less of this medication than directed by your doctor. Amaryl should be taken with breakfast or the first main meal.

■ *If you miss a dose...*

Take it as soon as you remember. If it is almost time for the next dose, skip the one you missed and go back to your regular schedule. Do not take 2 doses at the same time.

■ *Storage instructions...*

Amaryl should be stored at room temperature in a well-closed container.

## What side effects may occur?

Side effects cannot be anticipated. If any develop or change in intensity, tell your doctor as soon as possible. Only your doctor can determine if it is safe for you to continue taking Amaryl.

■ *Less common or rare side effects may include:*

Anemia and other blood disorders, blurred vision, diarrhea, dizziness, headache, itching, muscle weakness, nausea, sensitivity to light, skin rash and eruptions, stomach and intestinal pain, vomiting, yellow eyes and skin

Amaryl, like all oral antidiabetics, can result in hypoglycemia (low blood sugar). The risk of hypoglycemia can be increased by missed meals, alcohol, other medications, fever, injury, infection, surgery, and excessive exercise. To avoid hypoglycemia, closely follow the dietary and exercise regimen suggested by your doctor.

■ *Symptoms of mild low blood sugar may include:*

Blurred vision, cold sweats, dizziness, fast heartbeat, fatigue, headache, hunger, light-headedness, nausea, nervousness

■ *Symptoms of more severe low blood sugar may include:*

Coma, disorientation, pale skin, seizures, shallow breathing

Ask your doctor what steps you should take if you experience mild hypoglycemia. If symptoms of severe low blood sugar occur, contact your doctor immediately; severe hypoglycemia is a medical emergency.

## Why should this drug not be prescribed?

Avoid Amaryl if you have ever had an allergic reaction to it.

Do not take Amaryl to correct diabetic keto^acidosis (a life-threatening medical emergency caused by insufficient insulin and marked by excessive thirst, nausea, fatigue, and fruity breath). This condition should be treated with insulin.

## Special warnings about this medication

It's possible that drugs such as Amaryl may lead to more heart problems than diet treatment alone, or treatment with diet and insulin. If you have a heart condition, you may want to discuss this with your doctor.

When taking Amaryl, you should check your blood and urine regularly for abnormally high sugar (glucose) levels. The effectiveness of any oral antidiabetic, including Amaryl, may decrease with time. This may occur because of either a diminished responsiveness to the medication or a worsening of the diabetes.

Even people with well-controlled diabetes may find that stress such as injury, infection, surgery, or fever triggers a loss of control. If this happens, your doctor may recommend that you add insulin to your treatment with Amaryl or that you temporarily stop taking Amaryl and use insulin instead.

## Possible food and drug interactions when taking this medication

If Amaryl is taken with certain other drugs, the effects of either could be increased, decreased, or altered. It is especially important to check with your doctor before combining Amaryl with the following:

Airway-opening drugs such as Proventil and Ventolin

Aspirin and other salicylate medications

Chloramphenicol (Chloromycetin)

Corticosteroids such as prednisone (Deltasone)

Diuretics such as hydrochlorothiazide (HydroDIURIL) and chlorothiazide (Diuril)

Estrogens such as Premarin

Heart and blood pressure medications called beta blockers, including

Tenormin, Inderal, and Lopressor

Isoniazid (Nydrazid)

Major tranquilizers such as Mellaril and Thorazine

MAO inhibitors (antidepressants such as Nardil and Parnate)

Miconazole (Monistat)

Nicotinic acid (Nicobid)

Nonsteroidal anti-inflammatory drugs such as Advil, Motrin,

Naprosyn, Nuprin, Ponstel, and Voltaren

Oral contraceptives

Phenytoin (Dilantin)
Probenecid (Benemid)
Sulfa drugs such as Bactrim DS, Septra DS
Thyroid medications such as Synthroid
Warfarin (Coumadin)

Use alcohol with care; excessive alcohol intake can cause low blood sugar.

## Special information
## if you are pregnant or breastfeeding

Do not take Amaryl while pregnant. Since studies suggest the importance of maintaining normal blood sugar levels during pregnancy, your doctor may prescribe injected insulin instead. Drugs similar to Amaryl do appear in breast milk and may cause low blood sugar in nursing infants. You should not take Amaryl while nursing. If diet alone does not control your sugar levels, your doctor may prescribe injected insulin.

## Recommended dosage

### ADULTS

The usual starting dose is 1 to 2 milligrams taken once daily with breakfast or the first main meal. The maximum starting dose is 2 milligrams.

If necessary, your doctor will gradually increase the dose 1 or 2 milligrams at a time every 1 or 2 weeks. Your diabetes will probably be controlled on 1 to 4 milligrams a day; the most you should take in a day is 8 milligrams.

Weakened or malnourished people and those with adrenal, pituitary, kidney, or liver disorders are particularly sensitive to hypoglycemic drugs such as Amaryl and should start at 1 milligram once daily. Your doctor will increase your medication based on your response to the drug.

### CHILDREN

Safety and effectiveness in children have not been established.

## Overdosage

An overdose of Amaryl can cause low blood sugar (see "What side effects may occur?" for symptoms).

Eating sugar or a sugar-based product will often correct mild hypoglycemia. For severe hypoglycemia, seek medical attention immediately.

*Brand name:*

# Ambien

*Pronounced: AM-bee-en*
*Generic name: Zolpidem tartrate*

## Why is this drug prescribed?

Ambien is used for short-term treatment of insomnia (difficulty falling asleep or staying asleep, or early awakening). A relatively new drug, it is chemically different from other common sleep medications such as Halcion and Dalmane.

## Most important fact about this drug

Sleep problems are usually temporary and require medication for a week or two at most. Insomnia that lasts longer could be a sign of another medical problem. If you find that you need this medicine for more than 7 to 10 days, be sure to check with your doctor.

## How should you take this medication?

Ambien works very quickly. Take it just before going to bed. Take only the prescribed dose, exactly as instructed by your doctor.

■ *If you miss a dose...*
Take Ambien only as needed. Never double the dose.
■ *Storage instructions...*
Store at room temperature. Protect from extreme heat.

## What side effects may occur?

Side effects cannot be anticipated. If any develop or change in intensity, tell your doctor immediately. Only your doctor can determine whether it is safe to continue taking Ambien.

■ *More common side effects may include:*
Allergy, daytime drowsiness, dizziness, drugged feeling, headache, indigestion, nausea
■ *Less common side effects may include:*
Abdominal pain, abnormal dreams, abnormal vision, agitation, amnesia, anxiety, arthritis, back pain, bronchitis, burning sensation, chest pain, confusion, constipation, coughing, daytime sleeping, decreased mental alertness, depression, diarrhea, difficulty breathing, difficulty concentrating, difficulty swallowing, diminished sensitivity to touch, dizziness on standing, double vision, dry mouth, emotional instability, exagger-

ated feeling of well-being, eye irritation, falling, fatigue, fever, flu-like symptoms, gas, general discomfort, hallucination, hiccup, high blood pressure, high blood sugar, increased sweating, infection, insomnia, joint pain, lack of bladder control, lack of coordination, lethargy, light-headedness, loss of appetite, menstrual disorder, migraine, muscle pain, nasal inflammation, nervousness, numbness, paleness, prickling or tingling sensation, rapid heartbeat, rash, ringing in the ears, sinus inflammation, sleep disorder, speech difficulties, swelling due to fluid retention, taste abnormalities, throat inflammation, throbbing heartbeat, tremor, unconsciousness, upper respiratory infection, urinary tract infection, vertigo, vomiting, weakness

■ *Rare side effects may include:*
Abnormal tears or tearing, abscess, acne, aggravation of allergies, aggravation of high blood pressure, aggression, allergic reaction, altered production of saliva, anemia, belching, blisters, blood clot in lung, boils, breast pain, breast problems, breast tumors, bruising, chill with high temperature, followed by heat and perspiration, decreased sex drive, delusion, difficulties with blood circulation, difficulty urinating, excess hemoglobin in the blood, excessive urine production, eye pain, facial swelling due to fluid retention, fainting, false perceptions, feeling intoxicated, feeling strange, flushing, frequent urination, glaucoma, gout, heart attack, hemorrhoids, herpes infection, high cholesterol, hives, hot flashes, impotence, inability to urinate, increased appetite, increased tolerance to the drug, intestinal blockage, irregular heartbeat, joint degeneration, kidney failure, kidney pain, laryngitis, leg cramps, loss of reality, low blood pressure, mental deterioration, muscle spasms in arms and legs, muscle weakness, nosebleed, pain, painful urination, panic attacks, paralysis, pneumonia, rectal bleeding, rigidity, sciatica (lower back pain), sensation of seeing flashes of lights or sparks, sensitivity to light, sleepwalking, speech difficulties, swelling of the eye, thinking abnormalities, thirst, tooth decay, uncontrolled leg movements, urge to go to the bathroom, varicose veins, weight loss, yawning

## Why should this drug not be prescribed?
There are no known situations in which Ambien cannot be used.

## Special warnings about this medication
When sleep medications are used every night for more than a few weeks, some may lose their effectiveness. Remember, too, that you can become dependent on some sleep medications if you use them for a long time or at high doses.

Some people using Ambien have experienced unusual changes in their thinking and/or behavior. Alert your doctor if you notice a change.

Ambien and other sleep medicines can cause a special type of memory loss. It should not be taken on an overnight airplane flight of less than 7 to 8 hours, since "traveler's amnesia" may occur.

When you first start taking Ambien, until you know whether the medication will have any "carry over" effect the next day, use extreme care while doing anything that requires complete alertness, such as driving a car or operating machinery.

Use Ambien cautiously if you have liver problems. It will take longer for its effects to wear off.

If you take Ambien for more than 1 or 2 weeks, consult your doctor before stopping. Sudden discontinuation of a sleep medicine can bring on withdrawal symptoms ranging from unpleasant feelings to vomiting and cramps.

When taking Ambien, do *not* drink alcohol. It can increase the drug's side effects.

If you have breathing problems, they may become worse when you use Ambien.

## Possible food and drug interactions when taking this medication
If Ambien is used with certain other drugs, the effects of either drug could be increased, decreased, or altered. It is especially important to check with your doctor before combining Ambien with the following:

The major tranquilizer, chlorpromazine (Thorazine)
The antidepressant drug, imipramine (Tofranil)
Other drugs that depress the central nervous system, including Valium, Percocet, and Benadryl

## Special information if you are pregnant or breastfeeding
If you are pregnant or plan to become pregnant, inform your doctor immediately. Babies whose mothers take some sedative/hypnotic drugs may

have withdrawal symptoms after birth and may seem limp and flaccid. Ambien is not recommended for use by nursing mothers.

## Recommended dosage

### ADULTS

The recommended dosage for adults is 10 milligrams right before bedtime. Your doctor will prescribe a smaller dose if you are likely to be sensitive to the drug or have a liver problem. Never take more than 10 milligrams of Ambien per day.

### CHILDREN

Safety and effectiveness have not been established in children below the age of 18.

### OLDER ADULTS

Because older people and those in a weakened condition may be more sensitive to Ambien's effects, the recommended starting dosage is 5 milligrams just before bedtime.

## Overdosage

People who take too much Ambien may become excessively sleepy or even go into a light coma. The symptoms of overdose are more severe if the person is also taking other drugs that depress the central nervous system. Some cases of multiple overdose have been fatal.

If you suspect an overdose, seek medical attention immediately.

*Generic name:*

# Amcinonide

See Cyclocort, page 124.

*Generic name:*

# Amiloride with Hydrochlorothiazide

See Moduretic, page 332.

*Generic name:*

# Amitriptyline

See Elavil, page 187.

*Generic name:*

# Amitriptyline with Perphenazine

See Triavil, page 561.

*Generic name:*

# Amlodipine

See Norvasc, page 375.

*Generic name:*

# Amlodipine and Benazepril

See Lotrel, page 298.

*Generic name:*

# Amoxicillin

See Amoxil, page 22.

*Generic name:*

# Amoxicillin with Clavulanate

See Augmentin, page 42.

*Brand name:*

# Amoxil

Pronounced: a-MOX-il
Generic name: Amoxicillin
Other brand names: Trimox, Wymox

## Why is this drug prescribed?

Amoxil, an antibiotic, is used to treat a wide variety of infections, including: gonorrhea, middle ear infections, skin infections, upper and lower respiratory tract infections, and infections of genital and urinary tract.

## Most important fact about this drug

If you are allergic to either penicillin or cephalosporin antibiotics in any form, consult your doctor before taking Amoxil. There is a possibility that you are allergic to both types of medication; and if a reaction occurs, it could be extremely severe. If you take the drug and feel signs of a reaction, seek medical attention immediately.

## How should you take this medication?

Amoxil can be taken with or without food. If you are using Amoxil suspension, shake it well before using.

■ *If you miss a dose...*

Take it as soon as you remember. If it is almost time for the next dose, and you take 2 doses a day, take the one you missed and the next dose 5 to 6 hours later. If you take 3 or more doses a day, take the one you missed and the next dose 2 to 4 hours later. Then go back to your regular schedule.

■ *Storage instructions...*

Amoxil suspension and pediatric drops should be stored in a tightly closed bottle. Discard any unused medication after 14 days. Refrigeration is preferable.

## What side effects may occur?

Side effects cannot be anticipated. If any develop or change in intensity, inform your doctor as soon as possible. Only your doctor can determine if it is safe for you to continue taking Amoxil.

■ *Side effects may include:*

Agitation, anemia, anxiety, changes in behavior, confusion, diarrhea, dizziness, hives, hyperactivity, insomnia, nausea, rash, vomiting

## Why should this drug not be prescribed?

You should not use Amoxil if you are allergic to penicillin or cephalosporin antibiotics (for example, Ceclor).

## Special warnings about this medication

If you have ever had asthma, hives, hay fever, or other allergies, consult with your doctor before taking Amoxil.

You should stop using Amoxil if you experience reactions such as bruising, fever, skin rash, itching, joint pain, swollen lymph nodes, and/or sores on the genitals. If these reactions occur, stop taking Amoxil unless your doctor advises you to continue.

For infections such as strep throat, it is important to take Amoxil for the entire amount of time your doctor has prescribed. Even if you feel better, you need to continue taking Amoxil. If you stop taking Amoxil before your treatment time is complete, you may get other infections, such as glomerulonephritis (a kidney infection) or rheumatic fever.

If you are diabetic, be aware that Amoxil may cause a *false positive* Clinitest (urine glucose test) result to occur. You should consult with your doctor about using different tests while taking Amoxil.

Before taking Amoxil, tell your doctor if you have ever had asthma, colitis (inflammatory bowel disease), diabetes, or kidney or liver disease.

## Possible food and drug interactions when taking this medication

If Amoxil is taken with certain other drugs, the effects of either could be increased, decreased, or altered. It is especially important to check with your doctor before combining Amoxil with the following:

Chloramphenicol (Chloromycetin)
Erythromycin (E.E.S., PCE, others)
Oral contraceptives
Probenecid (Benemid)
Tetracycline (Achromycin V, others)

## Special information if you are pregnant or breastfeeding

Amoxil should be used during pregnancy only when clearly needed. If you are pregnant or plan to become pregnant, inform your doctor immediately. Since Amoxil may appear in breast milk, you should consult your doctor if you plan to breastfeed your baby.

## Recommended dosage

Dosages will be determined by the type of infection being treated.

ADULTS

*Ear, Nose, Throat, Skin, Genital, and Urinary Tract Infections*
The usual dosage is 250 milligrams, taken every 8 hours.

*Infections of the Lower Respiratory Tract*
The usual dosage is 500 milligrams, taken every 8 hours.

*Gonorrhea*
The usual dosage is 3 grams in a single oral dose.

*Gonococcal Infections Such as Acute, Uncomplicated Anogenital and Urethral Infections*
3 grams as a single oral dose.

### CHILDREN

Children weighing 44 pounds and over should follow the recommended adult dose schedule.

Children weighing under 44 pounds will have their dosage determined by their weight.

*Dosage of Pediatric Drops:*
Use the dropper provided with the medication to measure all doses.

*All Infections Except Those of the Lower Respiratory Tract*
Under 13 pounds:
0.75 milliliter every 8 hours.
13 to 15 pounds:
1 milliliter every 8 hours.
16 to 18 pounds:
1.25 milliliters every 8 hours.

*Infections of the Lower Respiratory Tract*
Under 13 pounds:
1.25 milliliters every 8 hours.
13 to 15 pounds:
1.75 milliliters every 8 hours.
16 to 18 pounds:
2.25 milliliters every 8 hours.

Children weighing more than 18 pounds should take the oral liquid. The required amount of suspension should be placed directly on the child's tongue for swallowing. It can also be added to formula, milk, fruit juice, water, ginger ale, or cold drinks. The preparation should be taken immediately. To be certain the child is getting the full dose of medication, make sure he or she drinks the entire preparation.

### Overdosage

Any medication taken in excess can have serious consequences. If you suspect an overdose, seek medical attention immediately.

■ *Symptoms of Amoxil overdose may include:*
Diarrhea, nausea, stomach cramps, vomiting

*Generic name:*

# Ampicillin

*See Omnipen, page 381.*

*Brand name:*

# Anafranil

*Pronounced: an-AF-ran-il*
*Generic name: Clomipramine hydrochloride*

### Why is this drug prescribed?

Anafranil, a chemical cousin of tricyclic antidepressant medications such as Tofranil and Elavil, is used to treat people who suffer from obsessions and compulsions.

An obsession is a persistent, disturbing idea, image, or urge that keeps coming to mind despite the person's efforts to ignore or forget it—for example, a preoccupation with avoiding contamination.

A compulsion is an irrational action that the person knows is senseless but feels driven to repeat again and again—for example, hand-washing perhaps dozens or even scores of times throughout the day.

### Most important fact about this drug

Serious, even fatal, reactions have been known to occur when drugs such as Anafranil are taken along with the antidepressant drugs known as MAO inhibitors. Drugs in this category include Nardil and Parnate. Never take Anafranil with one of these drugs.

### How should you take this medication?

Take Anafranil with meals, at first, to avoid stomach upset. After your regular dosage has been established, you can take 1 dose at bedtime to avoid sleepiness during the day. Always take it exactly as prescribed.

This medicine may cause dry mouth. Hard candy, chewing gum, or bits of ice may relieve this problem

■ *If you miss a dose...*
If you take 1 dose at bedtime, consult your doctor. Do not take the missed dose in the morning. If you take 2 or more doses a day, take the missed dose as soon as you remember. If it is almost time for your next dose, skip the one you missed and go back to your regular schedule. Do not take 2 doses at the same time.
■ *Storage instructions...*
Store at room temperature in a tightly closed container, away from moisture.

## What side effects may occur?

Side effects cannot be anticipated. If any develop or change in intensity, inform your doctor as soon as possible. Only your doctor can determine if it is safe for you to continue taking Anafranil.

The most significant risk is that of seizures (convulsions). Headache, fatigue, and nausea can be a problem. Men are likely to experience problems with sexual function. Unwanted weight gain is a potential problem for many people who take Anafranil, although a small number actually lose weight.

■ *More common side effects may include:*
Abdominal pain, abnormal dreaming, abnormal tearing, abnormal milk secretion, agitation, allergy, anxiety, appetite loss, back pain, chest pain, confusion, constipation, coughing, depression, diarrhea, dizziness, dry mouth, extreme sleepiness, failure to ejaculate, fast heartbeat, fatigue, fever, flushing, fluttery heartbeat, frequent urination, gas, headache, hot flushes, impotence, inability to concentrate, increased appetite, increased sweating, indigestion, inflamed lining of nose or sinuses, itching, joint pain, light-headedness on standing up, memory problems, menstrual pain and disorders, middle ear infection (children), migraine, muscle pain or tension, nausea, nervousness, pain, rash, red or purple areas on the skin, ringing in the ears, sex-drive changes, sleeplessness, sleep disturbances, sore throat, speech disturbances, taste changes, tingling or pins and needles, tooth disorder, tremor, twitching, urinary problems, urinary tract infection, vision problems, vomiting, weight gain, weight loss (children), yawning

■ *Less common side effects may include:*
Abnormal skin odor (children), acne, aggression (children), eye allergy (children), anemia (children), bad breath (children), belching (children), breast enlargement, breast pain, chills, conjunctivitis (pinkeye), difficult or labored breathing (children), difficulty swallowing, difficulty or pain in urinating, dilated pupils, dry skin, emotional instability, eye twitching (children), fainting (children), hearing disorder (children), hives, irritability, lack of menstruation, loss of sense of identity, mouth inflammation (children), muscle weakness, nosebleed, panic, paralysis (children), skin inflammation, sore throat (children), stomach and intestinal problems, swelling due to fluid retention, thirst, unequal size of pupils of the eye (children), vaginal inflammation, weakness (children), wheezing, white or yellow vaginal discharge

## Why should this drug not be prescribed?

Do not take this medication if you are sensitive to or have ever had an allergic reaction to a tricyclic antidepressant such as Tofranil and Elavil.

Be sure to avoid Anafranil if you are taking, or have taken within the past 14 days, an MAO inhibitor antidepressant such as Parnate or Nardil. Combining Anafranil with one of these medications could lead to fever, seizures, coma, and even death.

Do not take Anafranil if you have recently had a heart attack.

## Special warnings about this medication

If you have narrow-angle glaucoma (increased pressure in the eye) or are having difficulty urinating, Anafranil could make these conditions worse. Use Anafranil with caution if your kidney function is not normal.

If you have a tumor of the adrenal gland, this medication could cause your blood pressure to rise suddenly and dangerously.

Because Anafranil poses a possible risk of seizures, and because it may impair mental or physical ability to perform complicated tasks, your doctor will probably warn you to take special precautions if you need to drive a car, operate complicated machinery, or take part in activities such as swimming or climbing, in which suddenly losing consciousness could be dangerous. Note that your risk of seizures is increased:

■ If you have ever had a seizure
■ If you have a history of brain damage or alcoholism
■ If you are taking another medication that might predispose you to seizures

As with Tofranil, Elavil, and other tricyclic antidepressants, an overdose of Anafranil can be fatal. Do not be surprised if your doctor prescribes only a small quantity of Anafranil at a time. This is standard procedure to minimize the risk of overdose.

Anafranil may cause your skin to become more sensitive to sunlight. Avoid prolonged exposure to sunlight.

Before having any kind of surgery involving the use of general anesthesia, tell your doctor or dentist that you are taking Anafranil. You may be advised to discontinue the drug temporarily.

When it is time to stop taking Anafranil, do not stop abruptly. Your doctor will have you taper off gradually to avoid withdrawal symptoms such as dizziness, fever, general feeling of illness, headache, high fever, irritability or worsening emotional or mental problems, nausea, sleep problems, vomiting.

### Possible food and drug interactions when taking this medication

Avoid alcoholic beverages while taking Anafranil.

If Anafranil is taken with certain other drugs, the effects of either could be increased, decreased, or altered. It is especially important to check with your doctor before combining Anafranil with the following:

Antispasmodic drugs such as Donnatal, Cogentin, and Bentyl
Barbiturates such as phenobarbital
Certain blood pressure drugs such as Ismelin and Catapres-TTS
Cimetidine (Tagamet)
Digoxin (Lanoxin)
Fluoxetine (Prozac)
Haloperidol (Haldol)
Methylphenidate (Ritalin)
Major tranquilizers such as Thorazine
MAO inhibitors such as Nardil and Parnate
Phenytoin (Dilantin)
Thyroid medications such as Synthroid
Tranquilizers such as Xanax and Valium
Warfarin (Coumadin)

### Special information if you are pregnant or breastfeeding

If you are pregnant or plan to become pregnant, inform your doctor immediately. Anafranil should not be used during pregnancy unless absolutely necessary; some babies born to women who took Anafranil have had withdrawal symptoms such as jitteriness, tremors, and seizures. Anafranil appears in breast milk. Your doctor may advise you to stop breastfeeding while you are taking Anafranil.

### Recommended dosage

ADULTS

The usual recommended initial dose is 25 milligrams daily. Your doctor may gradually increase this dosage to 100 milligrams during the first 2 weeks. During this period you will be asked to take this drug, divided into smaller doses, with meals. The maximum daily dosage is 250 milligrams. After the dose has been determined, your doctor may direct you to take a single dose at bedtime, to avoid sleepiness during the day.

CHILDREN

The usual recommended initial dose is 25 milligrams daily, divided into smaller doses and taken with meals. Your doctor may gradually increase the dose to a maximum of 100 milligrams or 3 milligrams per 2.2 pounds of body weight per day, whichever is smaller. The maximum dose is 200 milligrams or 3 milligrams per 2.2 pounds of body weight, whichever is smaller. Once the dose has been determined, the child can take it in a single dose at bedtime.

### Overdosage

An overdose of Anafranil can be fatal. If you suspect an overdose, seek medical attention immediately.

■ *Early signs and symptoms of Anafranil overdose may include:*
Agitation, coma, convulsions, delirium, drowsiness, grimacing, exaggerated reflexes, loss of coordination, restlessness, rigid muscles, staggering gait, stupor, sweating, twitching, writhing
■ *Other signs and symptoms of overdosage may include:*
Bluish skin color, dilated pupils, excessive perspiration, fever, irregular heartbeat, little or no urine, low blood pressure, rapid heartbeat, shallow breathing, shock, vomiting

There is a danger of heart malfunction and even, in rare cases, cardiac arrest.

*Brand name:*

# Anaprox

*Pronounced: AN-uh-procks*
*Generic name: Naproxen sodium*
*Other brand name: Aleve*

### Why is this drug prescribed?

Anaprox, a nonsteroidal anti-inflammatory drug, is used to relieve mild to moderate pain and menstrual cramps. It is also prescribed for relief of the inflammation, swelling, stiffness, and joint pain associated with rheumatoid arthritis and osteoarthritis (the most common form of arthritis), and for juvenile arthritis, ankylosing spondylitis (spinal arthritis), tendinitis, bursitis, acute gout, and other conditions.

The over-the-counter form of naproxen, Aleve, is used for temporary relief of minor aches and pains, and to reduce fever.

## Most important fact about this drug

You should have frequent checkups with your doctor if you take Anaprox regularly. Ulcers or internal bleeding can occur without warning.

## How should you take this medication?

Your doctor may ask you to take Anaprox with food or an antacid to avoid stomach upset. Take Aleve with a full glass of water.

Take this medication exactly as prescribed by your doctor.

If you are using Anaprox for arthritis, it should be taken regularly.

■ *If you miss a dose...*
Take the forgotten dose as soon as you remember. If it is almost time for your next dose, skip the one you missed and go back to your regular schedule. Never take 2 doses at the same time.

■ *Storage instructions...*
Store at room temperature in a tightly closed container.

## What side effects may occur?

Side effects cannot be anticipated. If any develop or change in intensity, inform your doctor as soon as possible. Only your doctor can determine if it is safe for you to continue taking Anaprox.

■ *More common side effects may include:*
Abdominal pain, bruising, constipation, diarrhea, difficult or labored breathing, dizziness, drowsiness, headache, hearing changes, heartburn, indigestion, inflammation of the mouth, itching, light-headedness, nausea, rapid, fluttery heartbeat, red or purple spots on the skin, ringing in the ears, skin eruptions, sweating, swelling due to fluid retention, thirst, vertigo, vision changes

■ *Less common or rare side effects may include:*
Abdominal bleeding, black stools, blood in the urine, change in dream patterns, changes in hearing, chills and fever, colitis (inflammation of the large intestine), congestive heart failure,

depression, general feeling of illness, hair loss, inability to concentrate, inability to sleep, inflammation of the lungs, kidney disease or failure, menstrual problems, muscle weakness and/or pain, peptic ulcer, severe allergic reactions, skin inflammation due to sensitivity to light, skin rashes, vomiting, vomiting blood, yellow skin and eyes

## Why should this drug not be prescribed?

If you are sensitive to or have ever had an allergic reaction to Anaprox, aspirin, or similar drugs such as Motrin, or if you have had asthma attacks caused by aspirin or other drugs of this type, you should not take this medication. Make sure your doctor is aware of any drug reactions you have experienced.

## Special warnings about this medication

Remember that peptic ulcers and bleeding can occur without warning.

This drug should be used with caution if you have kidney or liver disease. It can cause liver inflammation in some people.

Do not take aspirin or any other anti-inflammatory medications while taking Anaprox, unless your doctor tells you to do so.

Anaprox contains sodium. If you are on a low sodium diet, discuss this with your doctor.

Use with caution if you have heart disease or high blood pressure. This drug can increase water retention.

Anaprox may cause vision problems. If you experience any changes in your vision, inform your doctor.

Anaprox may cause you to become drowsy or less alert; therefore, driving or operating dangerous machinery or participating in any hazardous activity that requires full mental alertness is not recommended.

Do not take Aleve for more than 10 days for pain or 3 days for fever. Contact your doctor if pain or fever persists or gets worse, if the painful area becomes red or swollen, or if you develop more than a mild digestive upset.

## Possible food and drug interactions when taking this medication

If Anaprox is taken with certain other drugs, the effects of either could be increased, decreased, or altered. It is especially important to check with your doctor before combining Anaprox with the following:

Antiseizure drugs such as Dilantin
Aspirin
Beta blockers, including blood pressure drugs such
   as Inderal
Blood thinners such as Coumadin
Lithium (Lithonate)
Loop diuretics such as Lasix
Methotrexate
Naproxen in other forms such as Naprosyn
Oral diabetes drugs such as Micronase
Other pain relievers such as aspirin, acetaminophen
   (Tylenol), and ibuprofen (Motrin)
Probenecid (Benemid)

If you have more than 3 alcoholic drinks per day,
check with your doctor before using painkillers.

**Special information
if you are pregnant or breastfeeding**
The effects of Anaprox during pregnancy have not
been adequately studied. If you are pregnant or plan
to become pregnant, inform your doctor immediately. Avoid Anaprox and Aleve during the last 3
months of pregnancy. Anaprox appears in breast
milk and could affect a nursing infant. If this medication is essential to your health, your doctor may
advise you to discontinue breastfeeding until your
treatment with this medication is finished.

**Recommended dosage**
ANAPROX: ADULTS

*Mild to Moderate Pain, Menstrual Cramps,
Acute Tendinitis and Bursitis*
The starting dose is 550 milligrams, followed by
275 milligrams every 6 to 8 hours or 550 milligrams every 12 hours. You should not take more
than 1,375 milligrams a day to start, or 1,100 milligrams a day thereafter.

*Rheumatoid Arthritis, Osteoarthritis, and
Ankylosing Spondylitis*
The starting dose is 275 milligrams or 550 milligrams 2 times a day (morning and evening). Your
physician can adjust the doses for maximum benefit. Symptoms should improve within 2 to 4 weeks.

*Acute Gout*
The starting dose is 825 milligrams, followed by 275
milligrams every 8 hours, until symptoms subside.

ANAPROX: CHILDREN

*Juvenile Arthritis*
The usual daily dosage is a total of 10 milligrams
per 2.2 pounds of body weight, divided into 2

doses. Dosage should not exceed 15 milligrams per
2.2 pounds per day.
   The safety and effectiveness of Anaprox have
not been established in children under 2 years of age.

ANAPROX: OLDER ADULTS

Your doctor will determine the dosage based on
your particular needs. Adjustments in the normal
adult dosage may be needed.

ALEVE

1 tablet or caplet every 8 to 12 hours, to a
maximum of 3 per day. For those over age 65, no
more than 1 tablet or caplet every 12 hours. Not
recommended for children under 12.

**Overdosage**
Any medication taken in excess can cause symp-
toms of overdose. If you suspect an overdose of
Anaprox, seek medical attention immediately.

■ *The symptoms of Anaprox overdose may include:*
   Drowsiness, heartburn, indigestion, nausea,
   vomiting

Brand name:
# Anaspaz
See Levsin, page 278.

Brand name:
# Anexsia
See Vicodin, page 587.

Brand name:
# Anolor 300
See Fioricet, page 209.

Brand name:
# Ansaid

*Pronounced: AN-sed*
*Generic name: Flurbiprofen*

**Why is this drug prescribed?**
Ansaid, a nonsteroidal anti-inflammatory drug, is
used to relieve the inflammation, swelling, stiff-

ness, and joint pain associated with rheumatoid arthritis and osteoarthritis (the most common form of arthritis).

## Most important fact about this drug

You should have frequent checkups with your doctor if you take Ansaid regularly. Ulcers or internal bleeding can occur without warning.

## How should you take this medication?

Your doctor may ask you to take Ansaid with food or an antacid.

Take this medication exactly as prescribed by your doctor.

If you are using Ansaid for arthritis, it should be taken regularly.

■ *If you miss a dose...*
Take the forgotten dose as soon as you remember. If it is almost time for your next dose, skip the one you missed and go back to your regular schedule. Never take 2 doses at the same time.

■ *Storage instructions...*
Store at room temperature.

## What side effects may occur?

Side effects cannot be anticipated. If any develop or change in intensity, inform your doctor as soon as possible. Only your doctor can determine if it is safe for you to continue taking Ansaid.

■ *More common side effects may include:*
Abdominal pain, diarrhea, general feeling of illness, headache, indigestion, nausea, swelling due to fluid retention, urinary tract infection

■ *Less common or rare side effects may include:*
Altered sense of smell, anemia, anxiety, asthma, blood in the urine, bloody diarrhea, bruising, chills and fever, confusion, conjunctivitis (pinkeye), constipation, depression, dizziness, feeling of illness, gas, heart failure, hepatitis, high blood pressure, hives, inflammation of the nose or mouth, inflammation of the stomach, insomnia, itching, kidney failure, lack of coordination, memory loss, nervousness, nosebleed, peptic ulcer, pins and needles, rash, ringing in the ears, sensitivity of skin to light, severe allergic reaction, skin inflammation with or without sores and crusting, sleepiness, stomach and intestinal bleeding, swelling of throat, tremor, twitching,

vision changes, vomiting, vomiting blood, weakness, weight changes, welts, yellow eyes and skin

## Why should this drug not be prescribed?

If you are sensitive to or have ever had an allergic reaction to Ansaid, aspirin, or similar drugs such as Motrin, or if you have had asthma attacks caused by aspirin or other drugs of this type, you should not take this medication. Fatal attacks have occurred in people allergic to this drug. Make sure your doctor is aware of any drug reactions you have experienced.

## Special warnings about this medication

This drug should be used with caution if you have kidney or liver disease. Kidney problems are most likely to develop in such people, as well as in those with heart failure, those taking diuretics (water pills), and older adults.

If you have asthma, take Ansaid with extra caution. Do not take aspirin or similar drugs while taking Ansaid, unless your doctor tells you to do so.

Ansaid can cause vision problems. If you experience a change in your vision, inform your doctor. Blurred and/or decreased vision has occurred while taking this medication.

Ansaid prolongs bleeding time. If you are taking blood-thinning medication, this drug should be taken with caution.

This drug can increase water retention. If you have heart disease or high blood pressure, use with caution.

If you want to take Ansaid for pain less serious than that of arthritis, be sure to discuss the risks of using this drug with your doctor.

## Possible food and drug interactions when taking this medication

If Ansaid is taken with certain other drugs, the effects of either could be increased, decreased, or altered. It is especially important to check with your doctor before combining Ansaid with the following:

Antacids
Aspirin
Beta blockers such as Inderal and Tenormin
Blood thinners such as Coumadin
Cimetidine (Tagamet)

Diuretics such as Lasix and Bumex
Methotrexate (Rheumatrex)
Oral diabetes drugs such as Micronase
Ranitidine (Zantac)

### Special information
### if you are pregnant or breastfeeding
The effects of Ansaid during pregnancy have not been adequately studied. If you are pregnant or plan to become pregnant, inform your doctor immediately. In particular, you should not use Ansaid in late pregnancy, as it can affect the developing baby's circulatory system. Ansaid appears in breast milk and could affect a nursing infant. If this medication is essential to your health, your doctor may advise you to discontinue breastfeeding until your treatment is finished.

### Recommended dosage
ADULTS

*Rheumatoid Arthritis or Osteoarthritis:*
The usual starting dosage is a total of 200 to 300 milligrams a day, divided into 2, 3, or 4 smaller doses (usually 3 or 4 for rheumatoid arthritis). Your doctor will tailor the dose to suit your needs, but you should not take more than 100 milligrams at any one time or more than 300 milligrams in a day.

CHILDREN

The safety and effectiveness of Ansaid have not been established in children.

OLDER ADULTS

Older people are among those most apt to develop kidney problems while taking this drug.

Your doctor will determine the dosage according to your needs.

### Overdosage
Any medication taken in excess can cause symptoms of overdose. If you suspect an overdose of Ansaid, seek medical attention immediately.

■ *The symptoms of Ansaid overdose may include:*
Agitation, change in pupil size, coma, disorientation, dizziness, double vision, drowsiness, headache, nausea, semiconsciousness, shallow breathing, stomach pain

*Category:*
# Antacids

*Brand names: Gaviscon, Gelusil, Maalox, Mylanta, Rolaids, Tums*

### Why is this drug prescribed?
Available under a number of brand names, antacids are used to relieve the uncomfortable symptoms of acid indigestion, heartburn, gas, and sour stomach.

### Most important fact about this drug
Do not take antacids for longer than 2 weeks or in larger than recommended doses unless directed by your doctor. If your symptoms persist, contact your doctor. Antacids should be used only for occasional relief of stomach upset.

### How should you take this medication?
If you take a chewable antacid tablet, chew thoroughly before swallowing so that the medicine can work faster and be more effective. Allow Mylanta Soothing Lozenges to completely dissolve in your mouth. Shake liquids well before using.

■ *If you miss a dose...*
Take this medication only as needed or as instructed by your doctor.
■ *Storage instructions...*
Store at room temperature. Keep liquids tightly closed and protect from freezing.

### What side effects may occur?
When taken as recommended, antacids are relatively free of side effects. Occasionally, one of the following symptoms may develop.

■ *Side effects may include:*
Chalky taste, constipation, diarrhea, increased thirst, stomach cramps

### Why should this drug not be prescribed?
Do not take antacids if you have signs of appendicitis or an inflamed bowel; symptoms include stomach or lower abdominal pain, cramping, bloating, soreness, nausea, or vomiting.

If you are sensitive to or have ever had an allergic reaction to aluminum, calcium, magnesium, or simethicone, do not take an antacid containing these ingredients. If you are elderly and have bone problems or if you are taking care of an elderly person with Alzheimer's disease, do not use an antacid containing aluminum.

## Special warnings about this medication

If you are taking any prescription drug, check with your doctor before you take an antacid. Also, tell your doctor or pharmacist about any drug allergies or medical conditions you have.

If you have kidney disease, do not take an antacid containing aluminum or magnesium. If you are on a sodium-restricted diet, do not take Gaviscon without checking first with your doctor or pharmacist.

## Possible food and drug interactions when taking this medication

If antacids are taken with certain other medications, the effects of either could be increased, decreased, or altered. It is especially important to check with your doctor before combining antacids with the following:

Cellulose sodium phosphate (Calcibind)
Isoniazid (Rifamate)
Ketoconazole (Nizoral)
Mecamylamine (Inversine)
Methenamine (Mandelamine)
Sodium polystyrene sulfonate resin (Kayexalate)
Tetracycline antibiotics (Achromycin, Minocin)

## Special information if you are pregnant or breastfeeding

As with all medications, ask your doctor or health care professional whether it is safe for you to use antacids while you are pregnant or breastfeeding.

## Recommended dosage

ADULTS

Take antacids according to the following schedules, or as directed by your doctor.

*Gaviscon and Gaviscon Extra Strength Relief Formula Chewable Tablets*
Chew 2 to 4 tablets 4 times a day after meals and at bedtime or as needed. Follow with half a glass of water or other liquid. Do not swallow the tablets whole.

*Gaviscon Extra Strength Relief Formula Liquid*
Take 2 to 4 teaspoonfuls 4 times a day after meals and at bedtime. Follow with half a glass of water or other liquid.

*Gaviscon Liquid*
Take 1 or 2 tablespoonfuls 4 times a day after meals and at bedtime. Follow with half a glass of water.

*Gelusil Liquid and Chewable Tablets*
Take 2 or more teaspoonfuls or tablets 1 hour after meals and at bedtime. The tablets should be chewed.

*Maalox Antacid Caplets*
Take 1 caplet as needed. Swallow the tablets whole; do not chew them.

*Maalox Heartburn Relief Chewable Tablets*
Chew 2 to 4 tablets after meals and at bedtime. Follow with half a glass of water or other liquid.

*Maalox Heartburn Relief Suspension, Maalox Magnesia and Alumina Oral Suspension, and Extra Strength Maalox Antacid Plus Anti-Gas Suspension*
Take 2 to 4 teaspoonfuls 4 times a day, 20 minutes to 1 hour after meals and at bedtime.

*Maalox Plus Chewable Tablets*
Chew 1 to 4 tablets 4 times a day, 20 minutes to 1 hour after meals and at bedtime.

*Extra Strength Maalox Antacid Plus Anti-Gas Chewable Tablets*
Chew 1 to 3 tablets 20 minutes to 1 hour after meals and at bedtime.

*Mylanta and Mylanta Double Strength Liquid and Chewable Tablets Antacid/Anti-Gas*
Take 2 to 4 teaspoonfuls of liquid or chew 2 to 4 tablets between meals and at bedtime.

*Mylanta Gelcaps*
Take 2 to 4 gelcaps as needed.

*Mylanta Soothing Lozenges*
Dissolve 1 lozenge in your mouth. If needed, follow with a second. Repeat as needed.

*Rolaids, Calcium-Rich/Sodium Free Rolaids, and Extra Strength Rolaids*
Chew 1 or 2 tablets as symptoms occur. Repeat hourly if symptoms return.

*Tums, Tums E-X, and Tums Anti-Gas Formula*
Chew 1 or 2 tablets as symptoms occur. Repeat hourly if symptoms return. You may also hold the tablet between your gum and cheek and let it dissolve gradually.

CHILDREN

Do not give to children under 6 years of age, unless directed by your doctor.

### Overdosage

Any medication taken in excess can have serious consequences. If you suspect an overdose, seek medical attention immediately.

■ *Symptoms of antacid overdose may include:*
  *For aluminum-containing antacids (Gaviscon, Gelusil, Maalox, Mylanta)*
  Bone pain, constipation (severe and continuing), feeling of discomfort (continuing), loss of appetite (continuing), mood or mental changes, muscle weakness, swelling of wrists or ankles, weight loss (unusual)

  *For calcium-containing antacids (Mylanta, Rolaids, Tums)*
  Constipation (severe and continuing), difficult or painful urination, frequent urge to urinate, headache (continuing), loss of appetite (continuing), mood or mental changes, muscle pain or twitching, nausea or vomiting, nervousness or restlessness, slow breathing, unpleasant taste, unusual tiredness or weakness

  *For magnesium-containing antacids (Gaviscon, Gelusil, Maalox, Mylanta)*
  Difficult or painful urination, dizziness or light-headedness, irregular heartbeat, mood or mental changes, unusual tiredness or weakness

*Generic name:*

# Antipyrine, Benzocaine, and Glycerin

*See Auralgan, page 44.*

*Brand name:*

# Antivert

*Pronounced: AN-tee-vert*
*Generic name: Meclizine hydrochloride*
*Other brand names: Bonine*

### Why is this drug prescribed?

Antivert, an antihistamine, is prescribed for the management of nausea, vomiting, and dizziness associated with motion sickness.

Antivert may also be prescribed for the management of vertigo (a spinning sensation or a feeling that the ground is tilted) due to diseases affecting the vestibular system (the bony labyrinth of the ear, which contains the sensors that control your balance).

### Most important fact about this drug

Antivert may cause you to become drowsy or less alert; therefore, driving a car or operating dangerous machinery is not recommended.

### How should you take this medication?

Take this medication exactly as prescribed by your doctor.

■ *If you miss a dose...*
  Take it as soon as you remember. If it is almost time for your next dose, skip the one you missed and go back to your regular schedule. Do not take 2 doses at the same time.
■ *Storage instructions...*
  Store away from heat, light, and moisture.

### What side effects may occur?

Side effects cannot be anticipated. If any develop or change in intensity, inform your doctor as soon as possible. Only your doctor can determine if it is safe for you to continue taking Antivert.

■ *More common side effects may include:*
  Drowsiness, dry mouth
■ *Rare side effects may include:*
  Blurred vision

### Why should this drug not be prescribed?

If you are sensitive to or have ever had an allergic reaction to Antivert or similar drugs, do not take this drug. Make sure that your doctor is aware of any drug reactions you have experienced.

### Special warnings about this medication

If you have asthma, glaucoma, or an enlarged prostate gland, check with your doctor before using Antivert.

### Possible food and drug interactions when taking this medication

Antivert may intensify the effects of alcohol. Do not drink alcohol while taking this medication.

### Special information if you are pregnant or breastfeeding

Studies regarding the use of Antivert in pregnant women do not indicate that this drug increases the risk of abnormalities. However, if you are pregnant or plan to become pregnant, inform your doctor before using Antivert. Check with him, too, if you are breastfeeding your baby.

## Recommended dosage

ADULTS AND CHILDREN 12 AND OVER

*Motion Sickness:*

For protection against motion sickness, take 25 to 50 milligrams 1 hour before traveling. You may repeat the dose every 24 hours for the duration of the journey.

*Vertigo:*

The recommended dosage is 25 to 100 milligrams per day, divided into equal, smaller doses as determined by your doctor.

CHILDREN

The safety and effectiveness of Antivert have not been established in children under 12 years of age.

## Overdosage

Any medication taken in excess can have serious consequences. If you suspect an overdose of Antivert, seek emergency medical treatment immediately.

*Brand name:*

# Anusol-HC

*Pronounced: AN-yoo-sol AICH-SEE*
*Generic name: Hydrocortisone*
*Other brand names: Hytone, ProctoCream-HC*

## Why is this drug prescribed?

Anusol is a steroid cream for use on the skin. It is prescribed to treat certain itchy rashes and other inflammatory skin conditions.

## Most important fact about this drug

When you use Anusol-HC, you inevitably absorb some of the medication through your skin and into the bloodstream. Too much absorption can lead to unwanted side effects elsewhere in the body. To keep this problem to a minimum, avoid using large amounts of Anusol-HC over extensive areas, and do not cover it with airtight dressings such as plastic wrap or adhesive bandages unless specifically told to by your doctor.

## How should you use this medication?

Use Anusol-HC exactly as directed, and only to treat the condition for which your doctor prescribed it.

Anusol-HC is for use only on the skin. Be careful to keep it out of your eyes.

Apply the medication directly to the affected area.

If you are using Anusol-HC for psoriasis or a condition that has been difficult to cure, your doctor may advise you to use a bandage or covering over the affected area. If an infection develops, remove the bandage and contact your doctor.

■ *If you miss a dose...*
Apply it as soon as you remember. If it is almost time for the next dose, skip the one you missed and go back to your regular schedule.
■ *Storage instructions...*
Keep the container tightly closed, and store it at room temperature, away from heat. Protect from freezing.

## What side effects may occur?

Side effects cannot be anticipated. If any develop or change in intensity, inform your doctor as soon as possible. Only your doctor can determine if it is safe for you to continue using Anusol-HC.

■ *Side effects may include:*
Acne-like skin eruptions, burning, dryness, growth of excessive hair, inflammation of the hair follicles, inflammation around the mouth, irritation, itching, peeling skin, prickly heat, secondary infection, skin inflammation, skin softening, stretch marks, unusual lack of skin color

## Why should this drug not be prescribed?

Do not use Anusol-HC if you are sensitive to or have ever had an allergic reaction to any of its ingredients.

## Special warnings about this medication

Avoid covering a treated area with waterproof diapers or plastic pants. They can increase unwanted absorption of Anusol-HC.

If you use this medication over large areas of skin for prolonged periods of time—or cover the treated area—the amount of the hormone absorbed into your bloodstream may eventually lead to Cushing's syndrome: a moon-faced appearance, fattened neck and trunk, and purplish streaks on the skin. You can also develop glandular problems or high blood sugar, or show sugar in your urine. Children, because of their relatively larger ratio of skin surface area to body weight, are particularly susceptible to overabsorption of hormone from Anusol-HC.

Long-term treatment of children with steroids such as Anusol-HC may interfere with growth and development.

If an irritation develops, stop using the medication and contact your doctor.

### Possible food and drug interactions when using this medication

No interactions have been reported.

### Special information if you are pregnant or breastfeeding

The effects of Anusol-HC during pregnancy have not been adequately studied. If you are pregnant or plan to become pregnant, inform your doctor immediately. It is not known whether this medication appears in breast milk in sufficient amounts to affect a nursing baby. To avoid any possible harm to your baby, use Anusol-HC sparingly, and only with your doctor's permission, when breastfeeding.

### Recommended dosage

ADULTS

Apply Anusol-HC to the affected area 2 to 4 times a day, depending on the severity of the condition.

CHILDREN

Limit use to the least amount necessary, as directed by your doctor.

### Overdosage

Extensive or long-term use can cause Cushing's syndrome (see "Special warnings about this medication"), glandular problems, higher than normal amounts of sugar in the blood, and high amounts of sugar in the urine. If you suspect an overdose of Anusol-HC, seek medical treatment immediately.

*Brand name:*

# Armour Thyroid

*Pronounced: ARE-more THIGH-roid*
*Generic name: Natural thyroid hormones TC and TD*

### Why is this drug prescribed?

Armour Thyroid is prescribed when your thyroid gland is unable to produce enough hormone. It is also used to treat or prevent goiter (enlargement of the thyroid gland), and is given in a "suppression test" to diagnose an overactive thyroid.

### Most important fact about this drug

Although Armour Thyroid will speed up your metabolism, it is not effective as a weight-loss drug and should not be used for that purpose. Too much Armour Thyroid may cause severe side effects, especially if you are also taking appetite suppressants.

### How should you take this medication?

Take Armour Thyroid exactly as prescribed by your doctor. There is no "typical" dosage; the amount you need to take will depend on how much thyroid hormone your body is able to produce. Take no more or less than the amount your doctor prescribes. Take your dose at the same time every day for consistent effect.

Do not change brands of medication without consulting your doctor.

If you are taking Armour Thyroid to compensate for an underactive thyroid gland, you will probably need to take the medication indefinitely.

■ *If you miss a dose...*
Take it as soon as you remember. If it is almost time for your next dose, skip the one you missed and go back to your regular schedule. Do not take 2 doses at the same time. If you miss 2 or more doses in a row, consult your doctor.

■ *Storage instructions...*
Store at room temperature in a tightly closed container.

### What side effects may occur?

Side effects are rare when Armour Thyroid is taken at the correct dosage. However, taking too much medication or increasing the dosage too quickly may lead to overstimulation of the thyroid gland.

*Symptoms of overstimulation may include:*
Changes in appetite, diarrhea, fever, headache, increased heart rate, irritability, nausea, nervousness, sleeplessness, sweating, weight loss

Although children treated with Armour Thyroid may initially lose some hair, the hair loss is temporary.

### Why should this drug not be prescribed?

You should not take Armour Thyroid if you have ever had an allergic reaction to this drug; your thyroid gland is overactive; or your adrenal glands are not making enough corticosteroid hormone.

## Special warnings about this medication

If you are elderly, particularly if you suffer from angina (chest pain due to a heart condition), you should take Armour Thyroid at a lower dosage, and your doctor should schedule frequent checkups.

Armour Thyroid tends to aggravate symptoms of diabetes and underactive adrenal glands. If you take medication to treat one of these disorders, your dosage of that medication will probably need to be adjusted once you start taking Armour Thyroid.

## Possible food and drug interactions when taking this medication

If you take Armour Thyroid with certain other drugs, the effect of either drug could be increased, decreased, or altered. It is especially important to check with your doctor before combining Armour Thyroid with the following:

Asthma medications such as Theo-Dur
Blood thinners such as Coumadin
Cholestyramine (Questran)
Colestipol (Colestid)
Estrogen preparations (including some birth control pills such as Ortho-Novum and Premarin)
Insulin
Oral diabetes drugs such as Diabinese and Glucotrol)

## Special information if you are pregnant or breastfeeding

If you need to take Armour Thyroid because of a thyroid hormone deficiency, you may continue using the medication during pregnancy, but your doctor will test you regularly and may change your dosage. Once your baby is born, you may breastfeed while continuing treatment with Armour Thyroid.

## Recommended dosage

ADULTS

Your doctor will tailor the dosage of Armour Thyroid to meet your individual requirements, taking into consideration the status of your thyroid gland and any other medical conditions you may have.

## Overdosage

An overdose of Armour Thyroid will speed up all of the body's vital processes, causing physical and mental hyperactivity, increased appetite, excessive sweating, chest pain, increased pulse rate, palpitations, nervousness, intolerance to heat, and possibly tremors or a rapid heartbeat.

*Brand name:*

# Artane

*Pronounced: AR-tane*
*Generic name: Trihexyphenidyl hydrochloride*

## Why is this drug prescribed?

Artane is used, in conjunction with other drugs, for the relief of certain symptoms of Parkinson's disease, a brain disorder that causes muscle tremor, stiffness, and weakness. It is also used to control certain side effects induced by antipsychotic drugs such as Thorazine and Haldol. Artane works by correcting the chemical imbalance that causes Parkinson's disease.

## Most important fact about this drug

Artane is not a cure for Parkinson's disease; it merely minimizes and reduces the frequency of symptoms such as tremors.

## How should you take this medication?

You may take Artane either before meals or after meals, whichever you find more convenient. Your doctor will probably start you on a small amount and increase the dosage gradually. Take Artane exactly as prescribed.

If the medication makes your mouth feel dry, try chewing gum, sucking mints, or simply sipping water.

Artane comes in tablet and liquid form. With either, you will probably need to take 3 or 4 doses a day.

Once you have reached the dosage that is best for you, your doctor may switch you to sustained-release capsules ("Sequels") which are to be taken only once or twice a day. Do not open or crush the sequels. Always swallow them whole.

■ *If you miss a dose...*
  Take it as soon as you remember. If it is within 2 hours or your next dose, skip the one you missed and go back to your regular schedule. Do not take 2 doses at the same time.
■ *Storage instructions...*
  Store at room temperature. Do not allow the liquid to freeze.

## What side effects may occur?

Side effects cannot be anticipated. If any develop or change in intensity, inform your doctor as soon as possible. Only your doctor can determine if it is safe for you to continue taking Artane.

■ *Common side effects may include:*
  Blurred vision, dry mouth, nausea, nervousness

These side effects, which appear in 30% to 50% of all people who take Artane, tend to be mild. They may disappear as your body gets used to the drug; if they persist, your doctor may want to lower your dosage slightly.

■ *Other potential side effects include:*
  Agitation, bowel obstruction, confusion, constipation, delusions, difficulty urinating, dilated pupils, disturbed behavior, drowsiness, hallucinations, headache, pressure in the eye, rapid heartbeat, rash, vomiting, weakness

### Why should this drug not be prescribed?
Do not take Artane if you are known to be sensitive to it or if you have ever had an allergic reaction to it or to other antiparkinson medications of this type.

### Special warnings about this medication
The elderly are highly sensitive to drugs such as Artane and should use it with caution.

Artane can reduce the body's ability to perspire, one of the key ways your body prevents overheating. Avoid excess sun or exercise that also cause you to become overheated.

If you have any of the following conditions, make sure your doctor knows about them, since Artane could make them worse:

Enlarged prostate
Glaucoma
Stomach/intestinal obstructive disease
Urinary tract obstructive disease

It is important to stick to the prescribed dosage; taking larger amounts "for kicks" could lead to an overdose.

Your doctor should watch you carefully if you have heart, liver, or kidney disease or high blood pressure, and should check your eyes frequently. You should also be watched for the development of any allergic reactions.

### Possible food and drug interactions when taking this medication
If you take Artane along with any of the drugs listed below, your doctor may need to adjust the dosage of Artane, the other medication, or possibly both.

Amantadine (Symmetrel)
Amitriptyline (Elavil)
Chlorpromazine (Thorazine)
Doxepin (Sinequan)
Haloperidol (Haldol)

### Special information if you are pregnant or breastfeeding
No specific information is available concerning the use of Artane during pregnancy or breastfeeding. If you are pregnant or plan to become pregnant while taking Artane, inform your doctor immediately.

### Recommended dosage
Your doctor will individualize the dose to your needs, starting with a low dose and then increasing it gradually, especially if you are over 60 years of age.

ADULTS

*Parkinson's Disease:*
The usual starting dose, in tablet or liquid form, is 1 milligram on the first day.

After the first day, your doctor may increase the dose by 2 milligrams at intervals of 3 to 5 days, until you are taking a total of 6 to 10 milligrams a day.

Your total daily dose will depend upon what is found to be the most effective level. For many people, 6 to 10 milligrams is most effective. Some, however, may require a total daily dose of 12 to 15 milligrams.

*Drug-Induced Parkinsonism:*
Your doctor will have to determine by trial and error the size and frequency of the dose of Artane needed to control the tremors and muscle rigidity that sometimes result from commonly used tranquilizers.

The total daily dosage usually ranges between 5 and 15 milligrams, although, in some cases, symptoms have been satisfactorily controlled on as little as 1 milligram daily.

Your doctor may start you on 1 milligram of Artane a day. If your symptoms are not controlled in a few hours, he or she may slowly increase the dose until satisfactory control is achieved.

*Use of Artane with Levodopa:*
When Artane is used at the same time as levodopa, the usual dose of each may need to be reduced. Your doctor will adjust the dosages carefully,

depending on the side effects and the degree of symptom control. Artane dosage of 3 to 6 milligrams daily, divided into equal doses, is usually adequate.

*Artane Tablets and Liquid:*
You will be able to handle the total daily intake of Artane tablets or liquid best if the medication is divided into 3 doses and taken at mealtimes. If you are taking high doses (more than 10 milligrams daily), your doctor may divide them into 4 parts, so that you take 3 doses at mealtimes and the fourth at bedtime.

## Overdosage
Overdosage with Artane may cause agitation, delirium, disorientation, hallucinations, or psychotic episodes.

■ *Other symptoms may include:*
Clumsiness or unsteadiness, fast heartbeat, flushing of skin, seizures, severe drowsiness, shortness of breath or troubled breathing, trouble sleeping, unusual warmth

If you suspect an overdose of Artane, seek medical attention immediately.

*Brand name:*

# Asacol

*See Rowasa, page 480.*

*Generic name:*

# Aspirin

*Pronounced: ASS-per-in*
*Brand names: Empirin, Ecotrin, Genuine Bayer, Halfprin*

## Why is this drug prescribed?
Aspirin is an anti-inflammatory pain medication (analgesic) that is used to relieve headaches, toothaches, and minor aches and pains, and to reduce fever. It also temporarily relieves the minor aches and pains of arthritis, muscle aches, colds, flu, and menstrual discomfort. In some patients, a small daily dose of aspirin may be used to ensure sufficient blood flow to the brain and prevent stroke. Aspirin may also be taken to decrease recurrence of a heart attack or other heart problems.

## Most important fact about this drug
Aspirin should not be used during the last 3 months of pregnancy unless specifically prescribed by a doctor. It may cause problems in the unborn child or complications during delivery.

## How should you take this medication?
Do not take more than the recommended dose.

Do not use aspirin if it has a strong, vinegar-like odor.

If aspirin upsets your stomach, use of a coated or buffered brand may reduce the problem.

Do not chew or crush sustained-release brands, such as Bayer time-release aspirin, or pills coated to delay breakdown of the drug, such as Ecotrin. To make them easier to swallow, take them with a full glass of water.

■ *If you miss a dose...*
Take it as soon as you remember. If it is almost time for your next dose, skip the one you missed and go back to your regular schedule. Never take 2 doses at the same time.
■ *Storage instructions...*
Store at room temperature.

## What side effects may occur?
Side effects cannot be anticipated. If any develop or change in intensity, inform your doctor as soon as possible. Only your doctor can determine if it is safe for you to continue using aspirin.

■ *Side effects may include:*
Heartburn, nausea and/or vomiting, possible involvement in formation of stomach ulcers and bleeding, small amounts of blood in stool, stomach pain, stomach upset

## Why should this drug not be prescribed?
Do not take aspirin if you are allergic to it, if you have asthma, ulcers or ulcer symptoms, or if you are taking a medication that affects the clotting of your blood, unless specifically told to do so by your doctor.

## Special warnings about this medication
Aspirin should not be given to children or teenagers for flu symptoms or chickenpox. Aspirin has been associated with the development of Reye's syndrome, a dangerous disorder characterized by disorientation, and lethargy leading to coma.

If you have a continuous or high fever, or a severe or persistent sore throat, especially with a high fever, vomiting and nausea, consult your doctor. It could indicate a more serious illness.

If pain persists for more than 10 days or if redness or swelling appears at the site of inflammation, consult your doctor immediately.

If you experience ringing in the ears, hearing loss, upset stomach, or dizziness, consult your doctor before taking more aspirin.

Check with your doctor before giving aspirin for arthritis or rheumatism to a child under 12.

### Possible food and drug interactions when taking this medication

If aspirin is taken with certain other drugs, the effects of either could be increased, decreased, or altered. It is especially important to check with your doctor before combining aspirin with the following:

Acetazolamide (Diamox)
ACE-inhibitor-type blood pressure medications such as Capoten
Anti-gout medications such as Zyloprim
Arthritis medications such as Motrin and Indocin
Blood thinners such as Coumadin
Certain diuretics such as Lasix
Diabetes medications such as DiaBeta and Micronase
Diltiazem (Cardizem)
Dipyridamole (Persantine)
Insulin
Seizure medications such as Depakene
Steroids such as prednisone

### Special information if you are pregnant or breastfeeding

The use of aspirin during pregnancy should be discussed with your doctor. Aspirin should not be used during the last 3 months of pregnancy unless specifically indicated by your doctor. It may cause problems in the fetus and complications during delivery. Aspirin may appear in breast milk and could affect a nursing infant. Ask your doctor whether it is safe to take aspirin while you are breastfeeding.

### Recommended dosage

ADULTS

*Treatment of Minor Pain and Fever*
The usual dose is 1 or 2 tablets every 3 to 4 hours up to 6 times a day.

*Prevention of Stroke*
The usual dose is 1 tablet 4 times daily or 2 tablets 2 times a day.

*Prevention of Heart Attack*
The usual dose is 1 tablet daily. Your physician may suggest that you take a larger dose, however. If you use Halfprin low-strength tablets (162 milligrams), adjust dosage accordingly.

CHILDREN

Consult your doctor.

### Overdosage

Any medication used in excess can have serious consequences. If you suspect symptoms of an aspirin overdose, seek medical treatment immediately.

*Brand name:*

# Aspirin Free Anacin

*See Tylenol, page 571.*

*Generic name:*

# Aspirin with Codeine

*See Empirin with Codeine, page 192.*

*Generic name:*

# Astemizole

*See Hismanal, page 237.*

*Brand name:*

# Atarax

*Pronounced: AT-a-raks*
*Generic name: Hydroxyzine hydrochloride*
*Other brand name: Vistaril*

### Why is this drug prescribed?

Atarax is an antihistamine used to relieve the symptoms of common anxiety and tension and, in combination with other medications, to treat anxiety that results from physical illness. It also relieves itching from allergic reactions and can be used as a sedative before and after general anesthesia. Antihistamines work by decreasing the effects of histamine, a chemical the body releases that narrows air passages in the lungs and contributes to inflammation. Antihistamines reduce itching and swelling and dry up secretions from the nose, eyes, and throat.

## Most important fact about this drug

Atarax is not intended for long-term use (more than 4 months). Your doctor should re-evaluate the prescription periodically.

## How should you take this medication?

Take this medication exactly as prescribed by your doctor.

■ *If you miss a dose...*
Take it as soon as you remember. If it is almost time for your next dose, skip the one you missed and go back to your regular schedule. Do not take 2 doses at once.

■ *Storage instructions...*
Store tablets and syrup away from heat, light, and moisture. Keep the syrup from freezing.

## What side effects may occur?

Side effects cannot be anticipated. If any develop or change in intensity, inform your doctor as soon as possible. Only your doctor can determine if it is safe for you to continue taking Atarax.

Drowsiness, the most common side effect of Atarax, is usually temporary and may disappear in a few days or when dosage is reduced. Other side effects include dry mouth, twitches, tremors, and convulsions. The last two usually occur with higher than recommended doses of Atarax.

## Why should this drug not be prescribed?

Atarax should not be taken in early pregnancy or if you are sensitive to or have ever had an allergic reaction to it. Make sure your doctor is aware of any drug reactions you have experienced.

## Special warnings about this medication

Atarax increases the effects of drugs that depress the activity of the central nervous system. If you are taking narcotics, non-narcotic analgesics, or barbiturates in combination with Atarax, their dosage should be reduced.

This medication can cause drowsiness. Driving or operating dangerous machinery or participating in any hazardous activity that requires full mental alertness is not recommended until you know how you react to Atarax.

## Possible food and drug interactions when taking this medication

Atarax may increase the effects of alcohol. Avoid alcohol while taking this medication.

If Atarax is taken with certain other drugs, the effects of either could be increased, decreased, or altered. It is especially important to check with your doctor before combining Atarax with the following:

Barbiturates such as Seconal and Phenobarbital
Narcotics such as Demerol and Percocet
Non-narcotic analgesics such as Motrin and Tylenol

## Special information if you are pregnant or breastfeeding

Although the effects of Atarax during pregnancy have not been adequately studied in humans, birth defects have appeared in animal studies with this medication. You should not take Atarax in early pregnancy. If you are pregnant or plan to become pregnant, inform your doctor immediately. Atarax may appear in breast milk and could affect a nursing infant. If this medication is essential to your health, your doctor may advise you to discontinue breastfeeding until your treatment is finished.

## Recommended dosage

When treatment begins with injections, it can be continued in tablet form.

Your doctor will adjust your dosage based on your response to the drug.

### FOR ANXIETY AND TENSION

*Adults*
The usual dose is 50 to 100 milligrams 4 times per day.

*Children under Age 6*
The total dose is 50 milligrams daily, divided into several smaller doses.

*Children over Age 6*
The total dose is 50 to 100 milligrams daily, divided into several smaller doses.

### FOR ITCHING DUE TO ALLERGIC CONDITIONS

*Adults*
The usual dose is 25 milligrams 3 or 4 times a day.

*Children under Age 6*
The total dose is 50 milligrams daily, divided into several smaller doses.

*Children over Age 6*
The total dose is 50 to 100 milligrams daily, divided into several smaller doses.

BEFORE AND AFTER GENERAL ANESTHESIA

*Adults*
The usual dose is 50 to 100 milligrams.

*Children*
The usual dose is 0.6 milligram per 2.2 pounds of body weight.

### Overdosage

Any medication taken in excess can have serious consequences. If you suspect an overdose of Atarax, seek medical attention immediately.

The most common symptom of Atarax overdose is excessive calm; your blood pressure may drop, although it is not likely.

*Generic name:*

# Atenolol

See Tenormin, page 531.

*Generic name:*

# Atenolol with Chlorthalidone

See Tenoretic, page 530.

*Brand name:*

# Ativan

*Pronounced: AT-i-van*
*Generic name: Lorazepam*

### Why is this drug prescribed?

Ativan is used in the treatment of anxiety disorders and for short-term (up to 4 months) relief of the symptoms of anxiety. It belongs to a class of drugs known as benzodiazepines.

### Most important fact about this drug

Tolerance and dependence can develop with the use of Ativan. You may experience withdrawal symptoms if you stop using it abruptly. Only your doctor should advise you to discontinue or change your dose.

### How should you take this drug?

Take this medication exactly as prescribed by your doctor.

■ *If you miss a dose...*
If it is within an hour or so of the scheduled time, take the forgotten dose as soon as you remember. Otherwise, skip the dose and go back to your regular schedule. Do not take 2 doses at once.
■ *Storage instructions...*
Store at room temperature in a tightly closed container, away from light.

### What side effects may occur?

Side effects cannot be anticipated. If any develop or change in intensity, inform your doctor as soon as possible. Only your doctor can determine if it is safe for you to continue taking Ativan.

If you experience any side effects, it will usually be at the beginning of your treatment; they will probably disappear as you continue to take the drug, or if your dosage is reduced.

■ *More common side effects may include:*
Dizziness, sedation (excessive calm), unsteadiness, weakness
■ *Less common or rare side effects may include:*
Agitation, change in appetite, depression, eye function disorders, headache, memory impairment, mental disorientation, nausea, skin problems, sleep disturbance, stomach and intestinal disorders
■ *Side effects due to rapid decrease or abrupt withdrawal of Ativan:*
Abdominal and muscle cramps, convulsions, depressed mood, inability to fall or stay asleep, sweating, tremors, vomiting

### Why should this drug not be prescribed?

If you are sensitive to or have ever had an allergic reaction to Ativan or similar drugs such as Valium, you should not take this medication.

Also avoid Ativan if you have the eye disease, acute narrow-angle glaucoma.

Anxiety or tension related to everyday stress usually does not require treatment with Ativan. Discuss your symptoms thoroughly with your doctor.

### Special warnings about this medication

Ativan may cause you to become drowsy or less alert; therefore, driving or operating dangerous machinery or participating in any hazardous activity that requires full mental alertness is not recommended.

If you are severely depressed or have suffered from severe depression, consult with your doctor before taking this medication.

If you have decreased kidney or liver function, use of this drug should be discussed with your doctor.

If you are an older person or if you have been using Ativan for a prolonged period of time, your doctor will watch you closely for stomach and upper intestinal problems.

### Possible food and drug interactions when taking this medication

Ativan may intensify the effects of alcohol. Avoid alcohol while taking this medication.

If Ativan is taken with certain other drugs, the effects of either could be increased, decreased, or altered. It is especially important to check with your doctor before combining Ativan with barbiturates (phenobarbital, Seconal, Amytal) or sedative-type medications such as Valium and Halcion.

### Special information if you are pregnant or breastfeeding

Do not take Ativan if you are pregnant or planning to become pregnant. There is an increased risk of birth defects. It is not known whether Ativan appears in breast milk. If this medication is essential to your health, your doctor may advise you to discontinue breastfeeding until your treatment is finished.

### Recommended dosage

ADULTS

The usual recommended dosage is a total of 2 to 6 milligrams per day divided into smaller doses. The largest dose should be taken at bedtime. The daily dose may vary from 1 to 10 milligrams.

*Anxiety*
The usual starting dose is a total of 2 to 3 milligrams per day taken in 2 or 3 smaller doses.

*Insomnia Due to Anxiety*
A single daily dose of 2 to 4 milligrams may be taken, usually at bedtime.

CHILDREN

The safety and effectiveness of Ativan have not been established in children under 12 years of age.

OLDER ADULTS

The usual starting dosage for older adults and those in a weakened condition should not exceed a total of 1 to 2 milligrams per day, divided into smaller doses, to avoid oversedation. This dose can be adjusted by your doctor as needed.

### Overdosage

Any medication taken in excess can have serious consequences. An overdose of Ativan can be fatal, though this is rare. If you suspect an overdose, seek medical attention immediately.

■ *The symptoms of Ativan overdose may include:*
Coma, confusion, drowsiness, hypnotic state, lack of coordination, low blood pressure, sluggishness

*Brand name:*

# Atretol

*See Tegretol, page 525.*

*Brand name:*

# Atrovent

*Pronounced: AT-row-vent*
*Generic name: Ipratropium bromide*

### Why is this drug prescribed?

Atrovent is a bronchodilator prescribed for long-term treatment of bronchial spasms (wheezing) associated with chronic obstructive pulmonary disease, including chronic bronchitis and emphysema. A bronchodilator improves the passage of air into the lungs.

### Most important fact about this drug

This medication is not for initial use in acute attacks of bronchial spasm when fast action is needed.

### How should you take this medication?

Atrovent is not intended for occasional use. To get the most benefit from this drug, you must use it consistently throughout your course of treatment, as prescribed by your doctor.

■ *If you miss a dose...*
Take it as soon as you remember. If it is almost time for your next dose, skip the one you missed and go back to your regular schedule. Do not take 2 doses at once.
■ *Storage instructions...*
Store at room temperature. Protect from excess humidity.

## What side effects may occur?

Side effects cannot be anticipated. If any develop or change in intensity, inform your doctor as soon as possible. Only your doctor can determine if it is safe for you to continue taking Atrovent.

■ *More common side effects may include:*
Blurred vision, cough, dizziness, dry mouth, fluttering heartbeat, headache, irritation from aerosol, nausea, nervousness, rash, stomach and intestinal upset, worsening of symptoms

■ *Less common or rare side effects may include:*
Allergic reactions, constipation, coordination difficulty, difficulty in urinating, drowsiness, fatigue, flushing, hives, hoarseness, inability to fall or stay asleep, increased heart rate, itching, low blood pressure, loss of hair, mouth sores, sharp eye pain, swelling of the tongue, lips, and face, tightening of the throat, tingling sensation, tremors

## Why should this drug not be prescribed?

If you are sensitive to or have ever had an allergic reaction to Atrovent or any of its ingredients, or to soybeans, soy lecithin, or peanuts, you should not take this medication.

You should also avoid Atrovent if you are allergic to drugs based on atropine. Make sure your doctor is aware of any drug reactions you have experienced.

## Special warnings about this medication

Unless you are directed to do so by your doctor, do not take this medication if you have the eye condition called narrow-angle glaucoma, an enlarged prostate, or obstruction in the neck of the bladder.

Your vision may be temporarily blurred if you accidentally spray the aerosol in your eyes.

## Possible food and drug interactions when taking this medication

No interactions have been reported.

## Special information if you are pregnant or breastfeeding

The effects of Atrovent during pregnancy have not been adequately studied. If you are pregnant or plan to become pregnant, inform your doctor immediately. It is not known whether Atrovent may appear in breast milk. If this drug is essential to your health, your doctor may advise you to stop nursing your baby until your treatment is finished.

## Recommended dosage

### ADULTS

The usual starting dose is 2 inhalations, 4 times per day. Additional inhalations may be taken, but the total should not exceed 12 in 24 hours.

### CHILDREN

Safety and effectiveness have not been established in children below 12 years of age.

## Overdosage

There is no information on specific symptoms of Atrovent overdose. However, any drug taken in excess can have serious consequences. If you suspect an overdose of Atrovent, seek medical attention immediately.

*Brand name:*

# A/T/S

*See Erythromycin, Topical, page 198.*

*Brand name:*

# Augmentin

*Pronounced: awg-MENT-in*
*Generic ingredients: Amoxicillin, Clavulanate potassium*

## Why is this drug prescribed?

Augmentin is used in the treatment of lower respiratory, middle ear, sinus, skin, and urinary tract infections that are caused by certain specific bacteria. These bacteria produce a chemical enzyme called beta lactamase that makes some infections particularly difficult to treat.

## Most important fact about this drug

If you are allergic to either penicillin or cephalosporin antibiotics in any form, consult your doctor *before taking Augmentin.* There is a possibility that you are allergic to both types of medication and if a reaction occurs, it could be extremely severe. If you take the drug and feel signs of a reaction, seek medical attention immediately.

## How should you take this medication?

Augmentin may be taken with or without food.
Shake the suspension well before using.

■ *If you miss a dose...*
Take it as soon as you remember. If it is almost time for the next dose, and you take 2 doses a day, take the one you missed and the next dose 5 to 6 hours later. If you take 3 or more doses a day, take the one you missed and the next dose 2 to 4 hours later. Then go back to your regular schedule.

■ *Storage instructions...*
Store the suspension under refrigeration and discard after 10 days. Store tablets away from heat, light, and moisture.

## What side effects may occur?

Side effects cannot be anticipated. If any develop or change in intensity, inform your doctor as soon as possible. Only your doctor can determine if it is safe for you to continue taking Augmentin.

■ *More common side effects may include:*
Diarrhea/loose stools, nausea, skin rashes and hives

■ *Less common side effects may include:*
Abdominal discomfort, anemia, arthritis, black "hairy" tongue, blood disorders, fever, gas, headache, indigestion, intestinal inflammation, itching, itching or burning of the vagina, joint pain, muscle pain, skin inflammation, skin peeling, sores and inflammation in the mouth and on the tongue and gums, stomach inflammation, vomiting, yeast infection

■ *Rare side effects may include:*
Agitation, anxiety, behavioral changes, blood in the urine, change in liver function, confusion, dizziness, hyperactivity, insomnia, kidney problems

## Why should this drug not be prescribed?

If you are sensitive to or have ever had an allergic reaction to any penicillin medication, do not take this drug.

Also avoid taking Augmentin if it has ever given you liver problems or yellowing of the skin and eyes.

## Special warnings about this medication

Augmentin and other penicillin-like medicines are generally safe; however, anyone with liver, kidney, or blood disorders is at increased risk when using this drug. Alternative choices may be available to your doctor.

If you have diabetes and test your urine for the presence of sugar, you should ask your doctor or pharmacist if this medication will interfere with the type of test you use.

Allergic reactions to this medication can be serious and possibly fatal. Let your doctor know about previous allergic reactions to medicines, food, or other substances before using Augmentin. If you experience a reaction, report it to your doctor immediately and seek medical treatment.

If you develop diarrhea while taking Augmentin, inform your doctor. It could be a sign of a potentially dangerous form of bowel inflammation.

## Possible food and drug interactions when taking this medication

Augmentin may react with the antigout medication Benemid, resulting in changes in blood levels. A reaction with another antigout drug, Zyloprim, may cause rashes. Notify your doctor if you are taking either of these drugs.

Do not take Augmentin when using Antabuse (disulfiram).

## Special information if you are pregnant or breastfeeding

The effects of Augmentin during pregnancy have not been adequately studied. Because there may be risk to the developing baby, doctors usually recommend Augmentin to pregnant women only when the benefits of therapy outweigh any potential danger. Augmentin appears in breast milk and could affect a nursing infant. If Augmentin is essential to your health, your doctor may advise you to stop nursing your baby until your treatment with this drug is finished.

## Recommended dosage

ADULTS

The usual adult dose is one 250-milligram tablet every 8 hours. For more severe infections and infections of the respiratory tract, the dose should be one 500-milligram tablet every 8 hours. It is essential that you take this medicine according to your doctor's directions.

CHILDREN

The usual total daily dosage is 20 milligrams per 2.2 pounds of body weight per day, divided into 4 doses and taken every 8 hours. For middle ear infections, sinus infections, and lower respiratory infections, the dose should be 40 milligrams per 2.2 pounds per day, divided into smaller doses and taken every 8 hours. Severe infections should be treated with the higher recommended dose. Children weighing 88 pounds or more will take the adult dosage.

### Overdosage

Augmentin is generally safe; however, large amounts may cause overdose symptoms, including exaggerated side effects listed above. Suspected overdoses of Augmentin must be treated immediately; contact your physician or an emergency room.

Brand name:

# Auralgan

Pronounced: Aw-RAL-gan
Generic ingredients: Antipyrine, Benzocaine, Glycerin
Other brand name: Auroto Otic

### Why is this drug prescribed?

Auralgan is prescribed to reduce the inflammation and congestion and relieve the pain and discomfort of severe middle ear infections. This drug may be used in combination with an antibiotic for curing the infection.

Auralgan is also used to remove excessive or impacted earwax.

### Most important fact about this drug

Discard this product 6 months after the dropper is first placed in the drug solution.

### How should you use this medication?

Use this medication exactly as prescribed. Administer as follows:

1. Warm the drops to body temperature by holding the bottle in your hand for a few minutes.
2. Shake the bottle.
3. Lie on your side or tilt the affected ear up.
4. Gently pull the ear lobe up.
5. Administer the prescribed number of drops.
6. Avoid touching the dropper to the ear.
7. Keep the ear tilted up for about 5 to 7 minutes.

Do not rinse the dropper; replace it in the bottle after each use. Hold the dropper assembly by the screw cap and, without squeezing the rubber bulb, insert the dropper into the bottle and screw down tightly.

■ *If you miss a dose...*
Use it as soon as you remember. If it is almost time for your next dose, skip the one you missed and go back to your regular schedule.
■ *Storage instructions...*
Store at room temperature.

### What side effects may occur?

Side effects cannot be anticipated. If any develop or change in intensity, inform your doctor as soon as possible. For Auralgan, no specific side effects have been reported.

### Why should this drug not be prescribed?

If you are sensitive to or allergic to any of the ingredients contained in Auralgan or similar drugs, you should not take this medication. Make sure your doctor is aware of any drug reactions you have experienced.

Unless directed to do so by your doctor, do not use this medication if you have a punctured eardrum.

### Special warnings about this medication

Notify your doctor if irritation occurs or if you develop an allergic reaction to this medication.

### Possible food and drug interactions when taking this medication

No food or drug interactions have been reported.

### Special information if you are pregnant or breastfeeding

The effects of Auralgan during pregnancy have not been adequately studied. If you are pregnant or plan to become pregnant, notify your doctor immediately. It is not known whether Auralgan appears in breast milk. If this medication is essential to your health, your doctor may advise you to discontinue breastfeeding until your treatment is finished.

### Recommended dosage

ADULTS AND CHILDREN

*Acute Otitis Media (Severe Middle Ear Infection):*
Apply the medication drop by drop into the ear, permitting the solution to run along the wall of the ear canal until it is filled. Avoid touching the ear with the dropper. Then moisten a piece of cotton dressing material, such as gauze, with Auralgan and insert it into the opening of the ear. Repeat every 1 to 2 hours until pain and congestion are relieved.

*Removal of Earwax:*

Apply Auralgan drop by drop into the ear 3 times daily for 2 or 3 days to help detach and remove earwax from the wall of the ear canal.

After the wax has been removed, Auralgan is useful for drying out the canal or relieving discomfort.

Before and after the removal of earwax, cotton dressing material such as gauze should be moistened with Auralgan and inserted into the opening of the ear following use of the medication.

## Overdosage

No information on overdosage with Auralgan is available.

Generic name:

# Auranofin

*See Ridaura, page 469.*

Brand name:

# Auroto Otic

*See Auralgan, page 44.*

Brand name:

# Aventyl

*See Pamelor, page 390.*

Brand name:

# Axid

*Pronounced: AK-sid*
*Generic name: Nizatidine*

## Why is this drug prescribed?

Axid is prescribed for the treatment of duodenal ulcers and noncancerous stomach ulcers. Full-dose therapy for these problems lasts no longer than 8 weeks. However, your doctor may prescribe Axid at a reduced dosage after a duodenal ulcer has healed. The drug is also prescribed for the heartburn and the inflammation that result when acid stomach contents flow backward into the esophagus. Axid belongs to a class of drugs known as histamine $H_2$ blockers.

## Most important fact about this drug

Although Axid can be used for up to 8-12 weeks, most ulcers are healed within 4 weeks of therapy.

## How should you take this medication?

Take this medication exactly as prescribed by your doctor.

■ *If you miss a dose...*
Take it as soon as you remember. If it is almost time for your next dose, skip the one you missed and go back to your regular schedule. Do not take 2 doses at once.
■ *Storage instructions...*
Store at room temperature.

## What side effects may occur?

Side effects cannot be anticipated. If any develop or change in intensity, inform your doctor as soon as possible. Only your doctor can determine if it is safe for you to continue taking Axid.

■ *More common side effects may include:*
Abdominal pain, diarrhea, dizziness, gas, headache, indigestion, inflammation of the nose, nausea, pain, sore throat, vomiting, weakness
■ *Less common or rare side effects may include:*
Abnormal dreams, anxiety, back pain, chest pain, constipation, dimmed vision, dry mouth, fever, inability to sleep, increased cough, infection, itching, loss of appetite, muscle pain, nervousness, rash, sleepiness, stomach/intestinal problems, tooth problems

## Why should this drug not be prescribed?

If you are sensitive to or have ever had an allergic reaction to Axid or similar drugs such as Zantac, you should not take this medication. Make sure your doctor is aware of any drug reactions you have experienced.

## Special warnings about this medication

Axid could mask a stomach malignancy. If you continue to have any problems, notify your doctor.

If you have moderate to severe kidney disease, your doctor will reduce your dosage.

## Possible food and drug interactions when taking this medication

If Axid is taken with certain other drugs, the effects of either could be increased, decreased, or altered. It is especially important to check with your doctor before combining Axid with aspirin, especially in high doses.

## Special information
## if you are pregnant or breastfeeding

The effects of Axid during pregnancy have not been adequately studied. If you are pregnant or plan to become pregnant, inform your doctor immediately. Axid appears in breast milk and could affect a nursing infant. If this medication is essential to your health, your doctor may advise you to discontinue breastfeeding until your treatment with this medication is finished.

## Recommended dosage

ADULTS

*Active Duodenal Ulcer:*
The usual dose is 300 milligrams once a day at bedtime, but your doctor may have you take 150 milligrams twice a day.

*Active Noncancerous Stomach Ulcer:*
The usual dose is 150 milligrams twice a day or 300 milligrams once a day at bedtime.

*Maintenance of a Healed Duodenal Ulcer:*
The usual dose is 150 milligrams once a day at bedtime.

If you have moderate to severe kidney disease, your doctor will prescribe a lower dose.

CHILDREN

The safety and effectiveness of Axid have not been established in children.

## Overdosage

No specific information on Axid overdose is available. However, any medication taken in excess can have serious consequences. If you suspect an overdose of Axid, seek medical attention immediately.

*Generic name:*

# Azatadine with Pseudoephedrine

*See Trinalin Repetabs, page 566.*

*Generic name:*

# Azithromycin

*See Zithromax, page 606.*

*Brand name:*

# Azmacort

*Pronounced: AZ-ma-court*
*Generic name: Triamcinolone acetonide*
*Other brand name: Nasacort*

## Why is this drug prescribed?

Azmacort and Nasacort are metered-dose inhalers containing the anti-inflammatory steroid medication, triamcinolone acetonide. Azmacort is used as long-term therapy to control bronchial asthma attacks. Nasacort is prescribed to relieve the symptoms of hay fever and other nasal allergies. Nasacort is also used in the treatment of nasal polyps (projecting masses of tissue in the nose).

## Most important fact about this drug

Azmacort does not provide rapid relief in an asthma attack. Instead, it reduces the frequency and severity of attacks when taken on a regular basis. For quick relief, you must still use airway-opening medications.

## How should you take this medication?

Take these drugs on a regular daily basis, exactly as prescribed.

Shake the canister before each use. Do not use an Azmacort inhaler more than 240 times. Discard the Nasacort canister after 100 inhalations.

If the drug irritates your throat, gargling and rinsing your mouth with water after each dose can help to relieve the problem.

If you are using a bronchodilator inhalant, it should be used before the Azmacort inhalant to derive the best effects from this drug. Use of the two inhalers should be separated by several minutes.

Illustrated instructions for use are available with the product.

■ *If you miss a dose...*
Use it as soon as you remember. If it is almost time for your next dose, skip the one you missed and go back to your regular schedule. Do not take 2 doses at once.
■ *Storage instructions...*
Store at room temperature.

Since the contents of this inhalant are under pressure, do not puncture the container and do not use or store the medication near heat or open flame. Exposure to temperatures above 120 degrees F may cause the container to explode.

## What side effects may occur?

Side effects cannot be anticipated. If any develop or change in intensity, inform your doctor as soon as possible. Only your doctor can determine if it is safe for you to continue taking these medications.

■ *More common side effects of Azmacort may include:*
Dry mouth, dry throat, hoarseness, irritated throat
■ *Less common side effects of Azmacort may include:*
Facial swelling, increased wheezing and cough, mouth and throat infections
■ *More common side effects of Nasacort may include:*
Headache
■ *Less common side effects of Nasacort may include:*
Dryness of the membranes lining the nose, mouth, and throat, nasal irritation, nasal and sinus congestion, nosebleeds, sneezing, throat discomfort

## Why should this drug not be prescribed?

Do not use either of these medications if you are allergic to or sensitive to any of the ingredients.
Do not use Azmacort if:

your asthma can be controlled with airway openers and other non-steroid medications.
you require only occasional steroid treatment for asthma. (Azmacort is not for treatment of prolonged, severe asthma attacks where fast-acting measures are required.)
you have bronchitis not associated with asthma.

## Special warnings about this medication

Your doctor will see that your asthma is reasonably under control before starting you on Azmacort Inhaler. For about a week, he or she will have you take Azmacort along with your usual dose of oral steroid. After that, you will gradually take less and less of the oral drug. If you develop joint or muscular pain, weariness, and depression, contact your doctor immediately. If you feel light-headed or find that you are losing weight, also tell your doctor.

If you are using Azmacort and your airway-opening medication is not effective during an asthma attack, contact your doctor immediately.

The use of triamcinolone acetonide may cause a yeast-like fungal infection in the mouth and throat (Azmacort) or nose and throat (Nasacort). If you

suspect a fungal infection, notify your doctor. Treatment with antifungal medication may be necessary.

Children using steroid medications such as these are more susceptible to infection. Chickenpox and measles, for example, can be far more serious for these children and for adults who have not had them. Try to avoid exposure, but if you are exposed, inform your doctor. Medication may be needed.

Switching from steroid tablet therapy to Azmacort Inhaler may allow allergic conditions to surface that were previously controlled by the tablets. These include rhinitis (inflammation of the inside of the nose), conjunctivitis (pinkeye), and eczema.

If your child is using Azmacort, your doctor will watch to be sure he or she is growing properly. If you have just had an operation, or if you are experiencing extreme stress, your doctor will watch you closely.

Use these medications with extreme caution if you have tuberculosis, untreated fungal, bacterial, or systemic viral infections, or herpes infections of the eye.

Use Nasacort with caution if you have not fully healed from nasal ulcers, or an injury to your nose. Steroids can slow wound healing, and there have been rare cases of perforation inside the nose caused by inhaled steroids.

If you are using Nasacort, contact your doctor if your symptoms don't improve after 3 weeks or if they get worse. Also notify your doctor if you have nasal irritation, burning, or stinging after you use the spray.

## Possible food and drug interactions while taking this medication

Inhaled steroids such as Azmacort and Nasacort are not recommended for long-term use with alternate-day prednisone treatment.

## Special information if you are pregnant or breastfeeding

The effects of triamcinolone acetonide during pregnancy have not been adequately studied. If you are pregnant or plan to become pregnant, inform your doctor immediately. It is not known whether triamcinolone acetonide appears in breast milk. If this medication is essential to your health, your doctor may advise you to discontinue breastfeeding until your treatment with this medication is finished.

## Recommended dosage

AZMACORT

The Azmacort Inhaler unit is for oral inhalation only.

### Adults

The usual dose is 2 inhalations (about 200 micrograms), taken 3 or 4 times a day. The daily dose should not exceed 16 inhalations.

### Children 6 to 12 Years of Age

The usual dose is 1 or 2 inhalations (100 to 200 micrograms), taken 3 or 4 times a day. The daily dose should not exceed 12 inhalations.

### Children Under 6 Years of Age

The safety and effectiveness of this drug have not been established in children under 6 years of age.

NASACORT

### Adults and Children Aged 12 and Older

The usual starting dose is 220 micrograms a day, taken as 2 sprays in each nostril once a day. (One spray is 55 micrograms.) If necessary, your doctor may increase the dose up to 440 micrograms a day, taken all at once, twice a day, or 4 times a day. Once Nasacort has started to work, your doctor may decrease the dose to 110 micrograms a day.

### Children Under 12 Years of Age

The safety and effectiveness of Nasacort in children under 12 years of age have not been established.

## Overdosage

Any medication taken in excess can have serious consequences. If you suspect an overdose, seek emergency medical treatment immediately. An overdose is likely to be signaled by an increase in side effects. Accidentally getting the contents of the canister on your skin would most likely irritate your nose and give you a headache.

*Brand name:*

# Azulfidine

*Pronounced: A-ZUL-fi-deen*
*Generic name: Sulfasalazine*

## Why is this drug prescribed?

Azulfidine, an anti-inflammatory medicine, is prescribed for the treatment of mild to moderate ulcerative colitis (a long-term, progressive bowel disease) and as an added treatment in severe ulcerative colitis (chronic inflammation and ulceration of the lining of large bowel and rectum, the main symptom of which is bloody diarrhea). This medication is also prescribed to decrease severe attacks of ulcerative colitis.

Azulfidine EN-tabs are prescribed for people who cannot take the regular Azulfidine tablet because of symptoms of stomach and intestinal irritation such as nausea and vomiting when taking the first few doses of the drug, or for those in whom a reduction in dosage does not lessen the stomach or intestinal side effects.

## Most important fact about this drug

Although ulcerative colitis rarely disappears completely, the risk of recurrence can be substantially reduced by the continued use of this drug.

## How should you take this medication?

Take this medication in evenly spaced, equal doses, as determined by your doctor, preferably after meals or with food to avoid stomach upset.

It is important that you drink plenty of fluids while taking this medication to avoid kidney stones.

■ *If you miss a dose...*
Take it as soon as you remember. If it is almost time for your next dose, skip the one you missed and go back to your regular schedule. Do not take 2 doses at once.
■ *Storage instructions...*
Store at room temperature.

## What side effects may occur?

Side effects cannot be anticipated. If any develop or change in intensity, inform your doctor as soon as possible. Only your doctor can determine if it is safe for you to continue taking Azulfidine.

■ *More common side effects may include:*
Headache, lack or loss of appetite, nausea, stomach distress, vomiting
■ *Less common side effects may include:*
Anemia, bluish discoloration of the skin, fever, hives, itching, skin rash
■ *Rare side effects may include:*
Abdominal pain, blood disorders, blood in the urine, bloody diarrhea, convulsions, diarrhea, drowsiness, hallucinations, hearing loss, hepatitis, inability to fall or stay asleep, inflammation of the mouth, intestinal inflammation, itchy skin eruptions, joint pain, kidney disorders, lack of

muscle coordination, loss of hair, mental depression, red, raised rash, ringing in the ears, sensitivity to light, severe allergic reaction, skin discoloration, skin disorders, spinal cord defects, swelling around the eye, urine discoloration, vertigo

## Why should this drug not be prescribed?

If you are sensitive to or have ever had an allergic reaction to Azulfidine, salicylates (aspirin), or other sulfa drugs, you should not take this medication. Make sure your doctor is aware of any drug reactions you have experienced.

Unless you are directed to do so by your doctor, do not take Azulfidine if you have an intestinal or urinary obstruction or if you have porphyria (an inherited disorder involving the substance that gives color to the skin and iris of the eyes).

## Special warnings about this medication

If you have kidney or liver damage or any blood disease, your doctor will check you very carefully before prescribing Azulfidine. Deaths have been reported from allergic reactions, blood diseases, kidney or liver damage, changes in nerve and muscle impulses, and fibrosing alveolitis (inflammation of the lungs due to a thickening or scarring of tissue). Signs such as sore throat, fever, abnormal paleness of the skin, purple or red spots on the skin, or jaundice (yellowing of the skin) may be an indication of a serious blood disorder. Your doctor will do frequent blood counts and urine tests. Use caution taking Azulfidine if you have a severe allergy or bronchial asthma.

If Azulfidine EN-tabs are eliminated un^disintegrated, stop taking the drug and notify your doctor immediately. (You may lack the intestinal enzymes necessary to dissolve this medication.)

Men taking Azulfidine may experience temporary infertility and a low sperm count.

Skin and urine may become yellow-orange in color while taking Azulfidine.

In addition, prolonged exposure to the sun should be avoided.

## Possible food and drug interactions when taking this medication

If Azulfidine is taken with certain other drugs, the effects of either could be increased, decreased, or altered. It is especially important to check with your doctor before combining Azulfidine with the following:

Digoxin (Lanoxin)
Folic acid (a B-complex vitamin)

## Special information if you are pregnant or breastfeeding

The effects of Azulfidine during pregnancy have not been adequately studied. If you are pregnant or plan to become pregnant, inform your doctor immediately. Azulfidine is secreted in breast milk and could affect a nursing infant. If this medication is essential to your health, your doctor may advise you to discontinue breastfeeding until your treatment is finished.

## Recommended dosage

Your doctor will carefully individualize your dosage and monitor your response periodically.

ADULTS

The usual recommended initial dose is 3 to 4 grams daily divided into smaller doses (intervals between nighttime doses should not exceed 8 hours). In some cases the initial dosage is 1 to 2 grams daily to lessen side effects.

*Maintenance Therapy*
The usual maintenance dose is 2 grams daily.

CHILDREN AGED 2 AND OLDER

The usual recommended initial dose is 40 to 60 milligrams per 2.2 pounds of body weight in each 24-hour period, divided into 3 to 6 doses.

*Maintenance Therapy*
The usual maintenance dose is 30 milligrams per 2.2 pounds of body weight in each 24-hour period, divided into 4 doses.

## Overdosage

Any medication taken in excess can have serious consequences. If you suspect an Azulfidine overdose, seek emergency medical attention immediately.

■ *Symptoms of Azulfidine overdose may include:*
Abdominal pain, convulsions, drowsiness, nausea, stomach upset, vomiting

*Brand name:*

# Bacticort

*See Cortisporin Ophthalmic Suspension, page 115.*

*Brand name:*

# Bactrim

*Pronounced: BAC-trim*
*Generic ingredients: Trimethoprim,*
  *Sulfamethoxazole*
*Other brand names: Cotrim, Septra*

## Why is this drug prescribed?

Bactrim, an antibacterial combination drug, is pre-scribed for the treatment of certain urinary tract infections, severe middle ear infections in children, long-lasting or frequently recurring bronchitis in adults that has increased in seriousness, inflamma-tion of the intestine due to a severe bacterial infec-tion, pneumonia in patients who have a suppressed immune system (*Pneumocystis carinii* pneumonia) and for travelers' diarrhea in adults.

## Most important fact about this drug

Sulfamethoxazole, an ingredient in Bactrim, is one of a group of drugs called sulfonamides, which prevent the growth of bacteria in the body. Rare but sometimes fatal reactions have occurred with use of sulfonamides. These reactions include Stevens-Johnson syndrome (severe eruptions around the mouth, anus, or eyes), progressive disintegration of the outer layer of the skin, sudden and severe liver damage, a severe blood disorder (agranulocytosis), and a lack of red and white blood cells because of a bone marrow disorder.

Notify your doctor at the first sign of an adverse reaction such as skin rash, sore throat, fever, joint pain, cough, shortness of breath, abnormal skin paleness, reddish or purplish skin spots, or yellow-ing of the skin or whites of the eyes.

Frequent blood counts by a doctor are recom-mended for patients taking sulfonamide drugs.

## How should you take this medication?

It is important that you drink plenty of fluids while taking this medication in order to prevent sediment in the urine and the formation of stones.

Bactrim works best when there is a constant amount in the blood. Take Bactrim exactly as pre-scribed; try not to miss any doses. It is best to take doses at evenly spaced times day and night.

If you are taking Bactrim suspension, ask your pharmacist for a specially marked measuring spoon that delivers accurate doses.

■ *If you miss a dose...*
Take the forgotten dose as soon as you remem-ber. If it is almost time for your next dose, skip the one you missed and go back to your regular schedule. Do not take 2 doses at once.

■ *Storage instructions...*
Store tablets and suspension at room temperature and protect from light. Keep tablets in a dry place. Protect the suspension from freezing.

## What side effects may occur?

Side effects cannot be anticipated. If any develop or change in intensity, inform your doctor as soon as possible. Only your doctor can determine if it is safe for you to continue taking Bactrim.

■ *More common side effects may include:*
Hives, lack or loss of appetite, nausea, skin rash, vomiting

■ *Less common or rare side effects may include:*
Abdominal pain, allergic reactions, anemia, chills, convulsions, depression, diarrhea, eye irri-tation, fatigue, fever, hallucinations, headache, hepatitis, inability to fall or stay asleep, inability to urinate, increased urination, inflammation of heart muscle, inflammation of the mouth and/or tongue, itching, joint pain, kidney failure, lack of feeling or concern, lack of muscle coordination, loss of appetite, low blood sugar, meningitis (inflammation of the brain or spinal cord), muscle pain, nausea, nervousness, red, raised rash, redness and swelling of the tongue, ringing in the ears, scaling of dead skin due to inflamma-tion, sensitivity to light, severe skin welts or swelling, skin eruptions, skin peeling, vertigo, weakness, yellowing of eyes and skin

## Why should this drug not be prescribed?

If you are sensitive to or have ever had an allergic reaction to trimethoprim, sulfamethoxazole, or other sulfa drugs such as Septra, you should not take this medication. Make sure that your doctor is aware of any drug reactions that you have experienced.

Unless you are directed to do so by your doctor, do not take this medication if you have been diag-nosed as having megaloblastic anemia, which is a blood disorder due to a deficiency of folic acid.

This drug should not be prescribed for infants less than 2 months of age.

Bactrim is not recommended for preventative or prolonged use in middle ear infections and should not be used in the treatment of streptococcal pharyngitis (inflammation or infection of the pharynx due to streptococcus bacteria).

You should not take Bactrim if you are pregnant or nursing a baby.

## Special warnings about this medication

Make sure your doctor knows if you have impaired kidney or liver function, have a folic acid deficiency, are a chronic alcoholic, are taking anticonvulsants, have been diagnosed as having malabsorption syndrome (abnormal intestinal absorption), are in a state of poor nutrition, or have severe allergies or bronchial asthma. Bactrim should be used cautiously under these conditions.

If you have AIDS (acquired immunodeficiency syndrome) and are being treated for *Pneumocystis carinii* pneumonia, you will experience more side effects than will someone without AIDS.

## Possible food and drug interactions when taking this medication

If Bactrim is taken with certain other drugs, the effects of either could be increased, decreased, or altered. It is especially important to check with your doctor before combining Bactrim with the following:

Amantadine (Symmetrel)
Anticonvulsants such as Dilantin
Blood thinners such as Coumadin
Diuretics (in the elderly) such as HydroDIURIL
Methotrexate (Rheumatrex)
Oral diabetes medications such as Micronase

## Special information if you are pregnant or breastfeeding

Bactrim should not be taken during pregnancy. If you are pregnant or plan to become pregnant, notify your doctor immediately. Bactrim does appear in breast milk and could affect a nursing infant. It should not be taken while breastfeeding.

## Recommended dosage

ADULTS

### Urinary Tract Infections and Intestinal Inflammation

The usual adult dosage in the treatment of urinary tract infection is 1 Bactrim DS (double strength tablet) or 2 Bactrim tablets, or 4 teaspoonfuls (20

milliliters) of Bactrim Pediatric Suspension every 12 hours for 10 to 14 days. The dosage for inflammation of the intestine is the same but is taken for 5 days.

### Worsening of Chronic Bronchitis

The usual recommended dosage is 1 Bactrim DS (double strength tablet), 2 Bactrim tablets, or 4 teaspoonfuls (20 milliliters) of Bactrim Pediatric Suspension every 12 hours for 14 days.

### Pneumocystis Carinii Pneumonia

The recommended dosage is 20 milligrams of trimethoprim and 100 milligrams of sulfamethoxazole per 2.2 pounds of body weight per 24 hours divided into equal doses every 6 hours for 14 days.

### Travelers' Diarrhea

The usual recommended dosage is 1 Bactrim DS (double strength tablet), 2 Bactrim tablets, or 4 teaspoonfuls (20 milliliters) of Bactrim Pediatric Suspension every 12 hours for 5 days.

CHILDREN

### Urinary Tract Infections or Middle Ear Infections

The recommended dose for children 2 months of age or older, given every 12 hours for 10 days, is determined by weight. The following table is a guideline for this dosage:

22 pounds, 1 teaspoonful (5 milliliters)
44 pounds, 2 teaspoonfuls (10 milliliters) or
  1 tablet
66 pounds, 3 teaspoonfuls (15 milliliters) or
  1-and-a-half tablets
88 pounds, 4 teaspoonfuls (20 milliliters) or
  2 tablets or 1 DS tablet

### Intestinal Inflammation

The recommended dose is identical to the dosage recommended for urinary tract and middle ear infections; however, it should be taken for 5 days.

### Pneumocystis Carinii Pneumonia

The recommended dose, taken every 6 hours for 14 days, is determined by weight. The following table is a guideline for this dosage:

18 pounds, 1 teaspoonful (5 milliliters)
35 pounds, 2 teaspoonfuls (10 milliliters) or
  1 tablet
53 pounds, 3 teaspoonfuls (15 milliliters) or
  1-and-a-half tablets

70 pounds, 4 teaspoonfuls (20 milliliters) or
2 tablets or 1 DS tablet

The safety of repeated use of Bactrim in children under 2 years of age has not been established.

## OLDER ADULTS

There may be an increased risk of severe side effects when Bactrim is taken by older people, especially in those who have impaired kidney and/or liver function or who are taking other medication. Consult with your doctor before taking Bactrim.

### Overdosage

If you suspect an overdose of Bactrim, seek emergency medical attention immediately.

■ *Symptoms of an overdose of Bactrim include:*
Blood or sediment in the urine, colic, confusion, dizziness, drowsiness, fever, headache, lack or loss of appetite, mental depression, nausea, unconsciousness, vomiting, yellowed eyes and skin

*Brand name:*

# Bactroban

*Pronounced: BAC-tro-ban*
*Generic name: Mupirocin*

### Why is this drug prescribed?

Bactroban is prescribed for the treatment of impetigo, a bacterial infection of the skin.

### Most important fact about this drug

If the use of Bactroban does not clear your skin infection within 3 to 5 days, or if the infection becomes worse, notify your doctor.

### How should you use this medication?

This drug is for external use only.

■ *If you miss a dose...*
Apply it as soon as you remember. If it is almost time for the next dose, skip the one you missed and go back to your regular schedule.
■ *Storage instructions...*
Store at room temperature.

### What side effects may occur?

Side effects cannot be anticipated. If any develop or change in intensity, inform your doctor as soon as possible. Only your doctor can determine if it is safe for you to continue using Bactroban.

■ *More common side effects may include:*
Burning, pain, stinging
■ *Less common side effects may include:*
Itching
■ *Rare side effects may include:*
Abnormal redness, dry skin, inflammation of the skin, nausea, oozing, skin rash, swelling, tenderness

### Why should this drug not be prescribed?

If you are sensitive to or have ever had an allergic reaction to Bactroban or similar drugs, you should not use this medication. Make sure your doctor is aware of any drug reactions you have experienced.

### Special warnings about this medication

Continued or prolonged use of Bactroban may result in the growth of bacteria that do not respond to this medication and can cause a secondary infection.

This drug is not intended for use in the eyes.

If your skin shows signs of an allergic reaction or irritation, stop using Bactroban and consult your doctor.

### Possible food and drug interactions when taking this medication

There are no known interactions.

### Special information if you are pregnant or breastfeeding

The effects of Bactroban during pregnancy have not been adequately studied. If you are pregnant or plan to become pregnant, inform your doctor immediately. Bactroban may appear in breast milk and could affect a nursing infant. Your doctor may advise you to discontinue breastfeeding until your treatment with this medication is finished.

### Recommended dosage

Apply a small amount of this medication to the affected area 3 times a day. Cover the treated area with gauze if you want.

### Overdosage

There is no information available on overdosage.

*Generic name:*

# Beclomethasone Dipropionate

*Pronounced: BECK-low-METH-ah-sone dye-PRO-pee-uh-nate*

*Brand names: Beclovent Inhalation Aerosol, Beconase AQ Nasal Spray, Beconase Inhalation Aerosol, Vancenase AQ Nasal Spray, Vancenase Nasal Inhaler, Vanceril Inhaler*

## Why is this drug prescribed?

Beclomethasone is a type of steroid used for respiratory problems. Beclovent and Vanceril are prescribed for the treatment of recurring symptoms of bronchial asthma.

Beconase and Vancenase are used for the symptomatic relief of hay fever and for the prevention of the recurrence of nasal polyps following surgical removal.

## Most important fact about this drug

Beclomethasone is not a bronchodilator medication (it does not quickly open the airways); and it should not be used for relief of asthma when bronchodilators and other nonsteroid drugs prove effective. Do not expect immediate relief from beclomethasone, and do not take higher doses in an attempt to make it work. It is not intended for rapid relief, but it will help control symptoms when taken routinely.

## How should you take this medication?

Beclomethasone is prescribed in an oral inhalant or a nasal spray form. Use this medication only as preventive therapy exactly as prescribed by your doctor. Many people will require additional drugs to control asthma symptoms fully, but this drug may allow other drugs to be used in smaller doses.

If you are also using a bronchodilator inhalant, take it before inhaling beclomethasone. This will improve the effect of the second drug. Take the two inhalations several minutes apart.

*To use the inhaler:*

1. Remove the cap and hold inhaler upright.
2. Shake the inhaler thoroughly.
3. Take a drink of water to moisten the throat.
4. Tilt your head slightly and breathe out.
5. While activating the inhaler, take a slow deep breath for 3 to 5 seconds, hold the breath for about 10 seconds, then breathe out slowly.
6. Allow at least 1 minute between inhalations.

Gargling and rinsing your mouth with water after each dose may help prevent hoarseness and throat irritation. Do not swallow the water after you rinse.

This medication comes with directions. Read them carefully before using this medicine.

■ *If you miss a dose...*
Take it as soon as you remember and take the remaining doses for that day at evenly spaced intervals. If it is time for your next dose, skip the one you missed. Never take 2 doses at the same time.

■ *Storage instructions...*
Store at room temperature, away from heat and cold. Do not puncture the container, store it near open flame, or dispose of it in a fire or incinerator.

## What side effects may occur?

Side effects cannot be anticipated. If any develop or change in intensity, inform your doctor as soon as possible. Only your doctor can determine if it is safe for you to continue taking this medication.

■ *Side effects may include:*
Dry mouth, fluid retention, hives, hoarseness, increased pressure within the eye (glaucoma), skin rash, wheezing

■ *When using a nasal spray, other possible side effects are:*
Headache, light-headedness, nasal burning, nasal irritation, nausea, nose and throat infections, nosebleed, runny nose, sneezing, stuffy nose, tearing eyes

## Why should this drug not be prescribed?

Your doctor will prescribe beclomethasone only if your asthma cannot be controlled with bronchodilators and other non-steroid medications.

Beclomethasone is not used for the treatment of non-asthmatic bronchitis, or for intermittent asthma therapy.

If you are sensitive to or have ever had an allergic reaction to beclomethasone or other steroid drugs, you should not take this medication. Make sure that your doctor is aware of any drug reactions that you have experienced.

## Special warnings about this medication

When steroid drugs are taken by mouth they substitute for and decrease the body's normal ability to make its own steroids as well as its ability to respond to stress.

There is a risk of causing a serious condition called "adrenal insufficiency" when people change from steroid tablets taken by mouth to aerosol beclomethasone dipropionate. Although the aerosol may provide adequate control of asthma during the changeover period, it does not provide the normal amount of steroid the body needs during acute stress situations. If you are being transferred from steroid tablets to beclomethasone and you experience a period of stress or a severe asthma attack, your doctor may prescribe additional treatment with steroid tablets.

Transfer from steroid tablet therapy to beclomethasone dipropionate aerosol may reactivate allergic conditions that were previously suppressed by the steroid tablet therapy, such as runny nose, inflamed eyelids, and eczema. Inform your doctor if you experience any of these symptoms.

High doses of steroids can suppress your immune system. Take extra care to avoid exposure to measles or chickenpox if you have never had them or never had shots. These infections can be serious or even fatal if your immune system is below par. If you are exposed, seek medical advice immediately.

Symptoms such as mental disturbances, increased bruising, weight gain, facial swelling (moon-faced), and reduced growth in children may occur with orally inhaled corticosteroids such as Beclovent. If you experience any of these symptoms, notify your doctor immediately.

### Recommended dosage
ADULTS

*Beclomethasone Oral Inhalant*
The usual recommended dose for adults and children 12 years of age and over is 2 inhalations given 2 to 4 times a day. Four inhalations given twice daily have been shown to be effective in some people. If you have severe asthma, your doctor may advise you to start with 12 to 16 inhalations a day. Daily intake should not exceed 20 inhalations.

*Beclomethasone Nasal Spray*
The usual dosage is 1 or 2 inhalations in each nostril 2 to 4 times a day for adults and children 12 years of age and over.

CHILDREN

*Beclomethasone Oral Inhalant*
Children 6 to 12 years of age: The usual recommended dose is 1 or 2 inhalations given 3 or 4 times a day. Four inhalations given twice daily have been effective for some children. Daily intake should not exceed 10 inhalations.

*Beclomethasone Nasal Spray*
Children 6 to 12 years of age: The usual dosage is 1 inhalation in each nostril 3 times daily.

Beclomethasone should not be given to children under the age of 6 unless advised by your doctor.

### Overdosage
Any medication taken in excess can have serious consequences. If you suspect an overdose, seek medical attention immediately.

*Brand name:*

# Beclovent

*See Beclomethasone, page 53.*

*Brand name:*

# Beconase

*See Beclomethasone, page 53.*

*Brand name:*

# Beepen-VK

*See Penicillin V Potassium, page 403.*

*Brand name:*

# Bellatal

*See Donnatal, page 174.*

*Brand name:*

# Benadryl

*Pronounced: BEN-ah-dril*
*Generic name: Diphenhydramine hydrochloride*

### Why is this drug prescribed?
Benadryl is an antihistamine with drying and sedative effects. It relieves red, inflamed eyes caused by food allergies and the itching, swelling, and redness from hives and other rashes that are caused by mild allergic reactions. It also relieves the sneezing, coughing, runny or stuffy nose, and red, teary,

itching eyes caused by seasonal allergies (hay fever) and the common cold. Antihistamines work by decreasing the effects of histamine, a chemical released in the body that narrows air passages in the lungs and contributes to inflammation. Antihistamines reduce itching and swelling and dry up secretions from the nose, eyes, and throat.

Benadryl is also used to treat allergic reactions to blood transfusions, to prevent and treat motion sickness, and, with other drugs, to treat anaphylactic shock (severe allergic reaction) and Parkinson's disease, a nerve disorder characterized by tremors, stooped posture, shuffling walk, muscle weakness, drooling, and emotional instability.

### Most important fact about this drug
Antihistamines may produce excitability in children. In the elderly they may cause dizziness, excessive calm, or low blood pressure.

### How should you take this medication?
Benadryl should be taken exactly as prescribed, or follow instructions on the label.

■ *If you miss a dose...*
Take it as soon as you remember. If it is almost time for your next dose, skip the one you missed and go back to your regular schedule. Do not take 2 doses at once.
■ *Storage instructions...*
Store at room temperature. Protect from moisture.

### What side effects may occur?
Side effects cannot be anticipated. If any develop or change in intensity, inform your doctor as soon as possible. Only your doctor can determine if it is safe for you to continue taking Benadryl.

■ *More common side effects may include:*
Disturbed coordination, dizziness, excessive calm, increased chest congestion, sleepiness, stomach upset
■ *Less common or rare side effects may include:*
Anaphylactic shock (extreme allergic reaction), anemia, blurred vision, chills, confusion, constipation, convulsions, diarrhea, difficulty sleeping, double vision, dry mouth, nose, throat, early menstruation, excessive perspiration, excitation, fast, fluttery heartbeat, fatigue, frequent or difficult urination, headache, hives, inability to urinate, increased sensitivity to light, irregular

heartbeat, irritability, loss of appetite, low blood pressure, nausea, nervousness, rapid heartbeat, rash, restlessness, ringing in the ears, stuffy nose, tightness of chest and wheezing, tingling or pins and needles, tremor, unreal or exaggerated sense of well-being, vertigo, vomiting

### Why should this drug not be prescribed?
Benadryl should not be used in newborn or premature infants, or if you are breastfeeding your infant.

Do not take this medication if you are sensitive to or have ever had an allergic reaction to diphenhydramine hydrochloride or other antihistamines.

### Special warnings about this medication
In general, you should use antihistamines very cautiously if you have the eye condition called narrow-angle glaucoma, narrowing of the stomach or intestine because of peptic ulcer or other stomach problems, intestinal blockage, symptoms of an enlarged prostate, or difficulty urinating due to obstruction in the bladder.

Antihistamines can make adults and children less alert and, in young children, may cause excitability.

Elderly people (60 years or older) are more likely to experience dizziness, extreme calm, and low blood pressure.

Use Benadryl cautiously if you have a history of asthma or other chronic lung disease, an over-active thyroid, high blood pressure, or heart disease.

This medication can cause drowsiness. Driving or operating dangerous machinery or participating in any hazardous activity that requires full mental alertness is not recommended until you know how you react to Benadryl.

### Possible food and drug interactions when taking this medication
Benadryl may increase the effects of alcohol, and alcohol may increase the sedative effects of Benadryl. Do not drink alcohol while taking this medication.

If Benadryl is taken with certain other drugs, the effects of either could be increased, decreased, or altered. It is especially important to check with your doctor before combining Benadryl with the following:

Antidepressant drugs known as MAO inhibitors, such as Parnate and Nardil

Sedative/hypnotics such as Halcion, Nembutal, and
  Seconal
Tranquilizers such as Xanax and Valium

### Special information
### if you are pregnant or breastfeeding
The effects of Benadryl during pregnancy have not
been adequately studied. If you are pregnant or plan
to become pregnant, inform your doctor immediately. Benadryl should be used during pregnancy
only if clearly needed. Antihistamine therapy is not
advised for nursing mothers. If this medication is
essential to your health, your doctor may advise
you to discontinue breastfeeding until your treatment with Benadryl is finished.

### Recommended dosage
Your doctor will tailor the dosage to suit your
needs. Benadryl reaches its peak effect in 1 hour,
and 1 dose will continue to work for 4 to 6 hours.

ADULTS

The usual recommended dose is 25 to 50 milligrams 3 or 4 times daily. The sleep-aid dosage is
50 milligrams at bedtime.

*Motion Sickness*
For prevention of motion sickness, take the first
dose 30 minutes before exposure to motion; take
the other doses before meals and at bedtime for as
long as the motion continues.

CHILDREN (OVER 20 POUNDS)

The usual dose is 12.5 to 25 milligrams, 3 to 4
times daily. A child should not take more than 300
milligrams a day.

This medication should not be used as a sleep
aid for children under age 12.

Your physician will determine the best use of
the drug in response to its effects on the child.

### Overdosage
Any medication taken in excess can have serious
consequences. If you suspect an overdose, seek
medical attention immediately. Antihistamine overdose has caused hallucinations, convulsions, and
death in children.

■ *Symptoms of Benadryl overdose may include:*
  Central nervous system depression or stimulation, especially in children, dry mouth, fixed,
  dilated pupils, flushing, stomach and intestinal
  symptoms

*Generic name:*

# Benazepril

See Lotensin, page 296.

*Brand name:*

# Bentyl

*Pronounced: BEN-til*
*Generic name: Dicyclomine hydrochloride*

### Why is this drug prescribed?
Bentyl is prescribed for the treatment of functional
bowel/irritable bowel syndrome (abdominal pain,
accompanied by diarrhea and constipation associated with stress).

### Most important fact about this drug
Heat prostration (fever and heat stroke due to
decreased sweating) can occur with use of this drug
in hot weather. If symptoms occur, stop taking the
drug and notify your doctor immediately.

### How should you take this medication?
Take this medication exactly as prescribed.

■ *If you miss a dose...*
  Take it as soon as you remember. If it is almost
  time for your next dose, skip the one you missed
  and go back to your regular schedule. Do not
  take 2 doses at once.

■ *Storage instructions...*
  Store at room temperature. Keep tablets out of
  direct sunlight. Keep syrup away from excessive heat.

### What side effects may occur?
Side effects cannot be anticipated. If any develop or
change in intensity, inform your doctor as soon as
possible. Only your doctor can determine if it is
safe for you to continue taking Bentyl.

■ *Side effects may include:*
  Blurred vision, dizziness, drowsiness, dry mouth,
  light-headedness, nausea, nervousness, weakness

Not all of the following side effects have been
reported with dicyclomine hydrochloride, but they
have been reported for similar drugs with antispasmodic action; contact your doctor if they occur.

  Abdominal pain, bloated feeling, constipation,
  decreased sweating, difficulty in urinating,

double vision, enlargement of the pupil of the eye, eye paralysis, fainting, headache, hives, impotence, inability to urinate, increased pressure in the eyes, itching, labored, difficult breathing, lack of coordination, lack or loss of appetite, nasal stuffiness or congestion, numbness, rapid heartbeat, rash, severe allergic reaction, sluggishness, sneezing, suffocation, suppression of breast milk, taste loss, temporary cessation of breathing, throat congestion, tingling, vomiting

## Why should this drug not be prescribed?

If you are sensitive to or have ever had an allergic reaction to Bentyl, you should not take this medication. Make sure your doctor is aware of any drug reactions you have experienced.

Unless you are directed to do so by your doctor, do not take this drug if you have a blockage of the urinary tract, stomach, or intestines; severe ulcerative colitis (inflammatory disease of the large intestine); reflux esophagitis (inflammation of the esophagus usually caused by the backflow of acid stomach contents); glaucoma; or myasthenia gravis (a disease characterized by long-lasting fatigue and muscle weakness).

This drug should not be given to infants less than 6 months of age or used by women who are nursing an infant.

## Special warnings about this medication

Bentyl may produce drowsiness or blurred vision. Therefore, driving a car, operating machinery, or participating in any activity that requires full mental alertness is not recommended.

Diarrhea may be an early symptom of a partial intestinal blockage, especially in people who have had bowel removals and an ileostomy or colostomy. If this occurs, notify your doctor immediately.

You should use this medication with caution if you have autonomic neuropathy (a nerve disorder); liver or kidney disease; hyperthyroidism; high blood pressure; coronary heart disease; congestive heart failure; rapid, irregular heartbeat; hiatal hernia (protrusion of part of the stomach through the diaphragm); or enlargement of the prostate gland.

## Possible food and drug interactions
## when taking this medication

If Bentyl is taken with certain other drugs, the effects of either could be increased, decreased, or altered. It is especially important to check with your doctor before combining Bentyl with the following:

Airway-opening drugs such as Proventil and Ventolin

Amantadine (Symmetrel)

Antacids such as Maalox

Antiarrhythmics such as quinidine (Quinidex)

Antiglaucoma drugs such as Pilopine

Antihistamines such as Tavist

Benzodiazepines (tranquilizers) such as Valium and Xanax

Corticosteroids such as prednisone (Deltasone)

Digoxin (the heart failure medication Lanoxin)

Major tranquilizers such as Mellaril and Thorazine

MAO inhibitors (antidepressants such as Nardil and Parnate)

Metoclopramide (the gastrointestinal stimulant Reglan)

Narcotic analgesics (pain relievers such as Demerol)

Nitrates and nitrites (heart medications such as nitroglycerin)

Tricyclic antidepressant drugs such as Elavil and Tofranil

## Special information
## if you are pregnant or breastfeeding

The effects of Bentyl during pregnancy have not been adequately studied. If you are pregnant or plan to become pregnant, notify your doctor. Bentyl does appear in breast milk and could affect a nursing infant. Do not use it when breastfeeding.

## Recommended dosage

ADULTS

The usual dosage is 160 milligrams per day divided into 4 equal doses. Since this dose is associated with a significant incidence of side effects, your doctor may recommend a starting dose of 80 milligrams per day divided into 4 equal doses. If no side effects appear, the doctor will then increase the dose.

If this drug is not effective within 2 weeks or side effects require doses below 80 milligrams per day, your doctor may discontinue it.

## Overdosage

Any medication taken in excess can have serious consequences. If you suspect an overdose, seek medical attention immediately.

■ *Symptoms of a Bentyl overdose include:*
Blurred vision, difficulty in swallowing, dilated pupils, dizziness, dryness of the mouth, headache, hot, dry skin, nausea, nerve blockage causing weakness and possible paralysis, vomiting

*Brand name:*

# Benzac W

*See Desquam-E, page 150.*

*Brand name:*

# Benzagel

*See Desquam-E, page 150.*

*Brand name:*

# Benzamycin

*Pronounced: BEN-za-MI-sin*
*Generic ingredients: Erythromycin, Benzoyl peroxide*

### Why is this drug prescribed?
A combination of the antibiotic erythromycin and the antibacterial agent benzoyl peroxide, Benzamycin is effective in stopping the bacteria that cause acne and in reducing acne infection.

### Most important fact about this drug
If you experience excessive irritation or dryness, stop using Benzamycin and notify your doctor.

### How should you use this medication?
Use Benzamycin 2 times per day, once in the morning and once in the evening, or as directed by your doctor. Apply to the affected areas after thoroughly washing, rinsing with warm water, and then gently patting dry.

■ *If you miss a dose...*
Apply it as soon as you remember. If it is almost time for your next dose, skip the one you missed and go back to your regular schedule.
■ *Storage instructions...*
This medication should be stored in your refrigerator in a tightly closed container and discarded after 3 months. Do not freeze.

### What side effects may occur?
Very few side effects have been reported with the use of Benzamycin. However, those reported include abnormal redness of the skin, dryness, and itching.

If any develop or change in intensity, inform your doctor as soon as possible. Only your doctor can determine if it is safe for you to continue taking Benzamycin.

### Why should this drug not be prescribed?
If you are sensitive to or have ever had an allergic reaction to erythromycin or benzoyl peroxide, or any other ingredients in Benzamycin, you should not take this medication. Make sure your doctor is aware of any drug reactions you have experienced.

### Special warnings about this medication
Benzamycin Topical Gel is for external use only. Avoid contact with your eyes and mucous membranes.

Benzamycin may bleach hair or colored fabric. Avoid contact with scalp and clothes.

As you use this antibiotic, organisms that are resistant to it may start to grow. Your doctor will have you stop taking Benzamycin and will give you a medication to fight the new bacteria.

### Possible food and drug interactions when using this medication
If Benzamycin is used with other acne medications, the effects of either could be increased, decreased, or altered. Always check with your doctor before combining any other prescription or over-the-counter acne remedy with Benzamycin.

### Special information if you are pregnant or breastfeeding
The effects of Benzamycin during pregnancy have not been adequately studied. If you are pregnant or plan to become pregnant, inform your doctor immediately. It is not known whether Benzamycin appears in breast milk. If this medication is essential to your health, your doctor may advise you to discontinue breastfeeding your baby until your treatment with this medication is finished.

### Recommended dosage
ADULTS

Apply to affected areas twice daily, once in the morning and once in the evening.

CHILDREN

The safety and effectiveness of Benzamycin have not been established in children under 12 years of age.

## Overdosage

There is no information available on overdosage.

*Brand name:*

# BenzaShave

See Desquam-E, page 150.

*Generic name:*

# Benzonatate

See Tessalon, page 536.

*Generic name:*

# Benzoyl peroxide

See Desquam-E, page 150.

*Generic name:*

# Benztropine

See Cogentin, page 104.

*Brand name:*

# Betagan

*Pronounced: BAIT-ah-gan*
*Generic name: Levobunolol hydrochloride*

## Why is this drug prescribed?

Betagan eyedrops are given to treat chronic open-angle glaucoma (increased pressure inside the eye). This medication is a beta blocker. It works by lowering pressure within the eyeball.

## Most important fact about this drug

Although Betagan eyedrops are applied to the eye, the medication is absorbed and may have effects in other parts of the body. If you have diabetes, asthma or other respiratory diseases, or decreased heart function, make sure your doctor is aware of the problem.

## How should you use this medication?

Use Betagan eyedrops exactly as prescribed. Some people also need to use eyedrops that constrict their pupils.

Administer Betagan eyedrops as follows:

1. Wash your hands thoroughly.
2. Gently pull your lower eyelid down to form a pocket between your eye and eyelid.
3. Hold the bottle on the bridge of your nose or on your forehead.
4. Do not touch the applicator tip to any surface, including your eye.
5. Tilt your head back and squeeze the medication into your eye.
6. Close your eyes gently.
7. Keep your eyes closed for 1 to 2 minutes.
8. Wait 5 to 10 minutes before using any other eyedrops.
9. Do not rinse the dropper.

■ *If you miss a dose...*
If you take Betagan once a day, use it as soon as you remember. If you do not remember until the next day, skip the dose you missed and go back to your regular schedule. Do not take 2 doses at once. If you take Betagan 2 or more times a day, use it as soon as you remember. If it is almost time for your next dose, skip the one you missed and go back to your regular schedule. Do not take 2 doses at once.
■ *Storage instructions...*
Store at room temperature, away from light.

## What side effects may occur?

Side effects from Betagan cannot be anticipated. If any develop or change in intensity, inform your doctor. Only your doctor can determine whether it is safe for you to continue using this medication. You may feel a momentary burning and stinging when you place the drops in your eyes. More rarely, you may develop an eye inflammation.

Beta blockers may cause muscle weakness; weakened muscles around the eyes may cause double vision or drooping eyelids.

■ *Other potential side effects include:*
Burning and tingling (pins and needles), chest pain, congestive heart failure, depression, diarrhea, difficult or labored breathing, dizziness, fainting, headache, heart palpitations, hives, low

blood pressure, nasal congestion, nausea, rash, slow or irregular heartbeat, stroke, temporary heart stoppage, vision problems, weakness, wheezing

### Why should this drug not be prescribed?

Do not use Betagan if you have ever had an allergic reaction to it or are sensitive to it.

*You should not use Betagan if you have any of the following conditions:*
Asthma
Cardiogenic shock (shock due to insufficient heart action)
Certain heart irregularities
Heart failure
Severe chronic obstructive lung disease
Slow heartbeat (sinus bradycardia)

### Special warnings about this medication

Betagan contains a sulfite preservative. In a few people, sulfites can cause an allergic reaction, which may be life-threatening. If you suffer from asthma, you are at increased risk for sulfite allergy.

Betagan may be absorbed into your bloodstream. If too much of the drug is absorbed, this may worsen asthma or other lung diseases or lead to heart failure, which sometimes happens with oral beta-blocker medications.

Beta blockers may increase the risks of anesthesia. If you are facing elective surgery, your doctor may want you to taper off Betagan prior to your operation.

Use Betagan cautiously if you have diminished lung function.

Since beta blockers may mask some signs and symptoms of low blood sugar (hypoglycemia), you should use Betagan very carefully if you have low blood sugar, or if you have diabetes and are taking insulin or an oral antidiabetic medication.

If your body tends to produce too much thyroid hormone, you should taper off Betagan very gradually rather than stopping the drug all at once. Abrupt withdrawal of any beta blocker may provoke a rush of thyroid hormone ("thyroid storm").

Do not use 2 or more beta-blocker eye medications at the same time.

### Possible food and drug interactions when taking this medication

If Betagan is used with certain other drugs, the effects of either could be increased, decreased, or altered. It is especially important to check with your doctor before combining Betagan with the following:

Calcium-blocking blood pressure medications such as Calan and Cardizem
Digitalis (the heart medication Lanoxin)
Epinephrine (Epifrin)
Oral beta blockers such as Inderal and Tenormin
Reserpine (Serpasil)

### Special information if you are pregnant or breastfeeding

The use of Betagan in pregnancy has not been adequately studied. If you are pregnant or plan to become pregnant, notify your doctor immediately. Betagan eyedrops should be used during pregnancy only if the benefit justifies the potential risk to the unborn child. Since other beta blocker medications are known to appear in breast milk, use Betagan eyedrops with caution if you are breastfeeding.

### Recommended dosage

ADULTS

The recommended starting dose is 1 or 2 drops of Betagan 0.5% in the affected eye(s) once a day.

The typical dose of Betagan 0.25% is 1 or 2 drops twice daily.

For more severe glaucoma, your doctor may have you use Betagan 0.5% twice a day.

### Overdosage

Overuse of Betagan eyedrops may produce symptoms of beta blocker overdosage—slowed heartbeat, low blood pressure, breathing difficulty, and/or heart failure. Any medication taken in excess can have serious consequences. If you suspect an overdose of Betagan, seek medical attention immediately.

*Generic name:*

# Betamethasone

*See Diprolene, page 167.*

*Generic name:*

# Betaxolol

*See Betoptic, page 61.*

*Brand name:*

# Betimol

See Timoptic, page 546.

*Brand name:*

# Betoptic

Pronounced: bet-OP-tick
Generic name: Betaxolol hydrochloride

### Why is this drug prescribed?

Betoptic Ophthalmic Solution and Betoptic S Ophthalmic Suspension contain a medication that lowers internal eye pressure and is used to treat open-angle glaucoma (high pressure of the fluid in the eye).

### Most important fact about this drug

Although Betoptic, a type of drug called a beta blocker, is applied directly to the eye, it may be absorbed into the bloodstream. Because it may have effects in other parts of the body, you should use Betoptic cautiously if you have diabetes, asthma or other respiratory diseases, or decreased heart function.

### How should you use this medication?

Use this medication exactly as prescribed. You may need to use other medications at the same time.

Betoptic S Suspension should be shaken well before each dose.

Administer Betoptic as follows:

1. Wash your hands thoroughly.
2. Gently pull your lower eyelid down to form a pocket between your eye and eyelid.
3. Hold the bottle on the bridge of your nose or on your forehead.
4. Do not touch the applicator tip to any surface, including your eye.
5. Tilt your head back and squeeze the medication into your eye.
6. Close your eyes gently.
7. Keep your eyes closed for 1 to 2 minutes.
8. Wait for 5 to 10 minutes before using any other eyedrops.
9. Do not rinse the dropper.

■ *If you miss a dose...*
Use it as soon as you remember. If it is almost time for your next dose, skip the one you missed and go back to your regular schedule. Do not use 2 doses at once.

■ *Storage instructions...*
Store at room temperature.

### What side effects may occur?

Side effects cannot be anticipated. If any develop or change in intensity, inform your doctor as soon as possible. Only your doctor can determine if it is safe for you to continue using Betoptic.

■ *More common side effects may include:*
Temporary eye discomfort

■ *Less common or rare side effects may include:*
Allergic reactions, asthma, changes in taste or smell, congestive heart failure, decreased corneal sensitivity, dead skin, depression, difficulty breathing, difficulty sleeping or drowsiness, dizziness, hair loss, headache, hives, inflammation of the cornea, inflammation of the tongue, intolerance to light, itching, peeling skin, pupils of different sizes, red eyes and skin, slow heartbeat, sluggishness, tearing, thickening chest secretions, vertigo, wheezing

### Why should this drug not be prescribed?

Do not use Betoptic if you are sensitive to or have ever had an allergic reaction to it.

People with certain heart conditions should not use Betoptic.

### Special warnings about this medication

Before you use Betoptic, tell your doctor if you have any of the following:

Asthma
Diabetes
Heart disease
Thyroid disease

If you are having surgery, your doctor may advise you to gradually stop using Betoptic before you undergo general anesthesia.

This drug may lose some of its effectiveness for glaucoma after you have been taking it a long time.

### Possible food and drug interactions when using this medication

If Betoptic is used with certain other drugs, the effects of either could be increased, decreased, or altered. It is especially important to check with your doctor before combining Betoptic with the following:

Drugs that alter mood, such as Nardil and Elavil
Oral beta blockers such as Inderal and Tenormin
Reserpine (Serpasil)

### Special information
### if you are pregnant or breastfeeding

The effects of Betoptic during pregnancy have not been adequately studied. If you are pregnant or plan to become pregnant, inform your doctor immediately. Betoptic may appear in breast milk and could affect a nursing infant. If this medication is essential to your health, your doctor may advise you to stop breastfeeding until your treatment with Betoptic is finished.

### Recommended dosage

Your doctor may have you take another medication with Betoptic or Betoptic-S.

ADULTS

*Betoptic*
The usual recommended dose is 1 to 2 drops of Betoptic in the affected eye(s) twice daily.

*Betoptic S*
The usual recommended dose is 1 to 2 drops of Betoptic S in the affected eye(s) twice daily.

### Overdosage

Any medication used in excess can have serious consequences. If you suspect an overdose of Betoptic, seek medical attention immediately.

*With an oral beta blocker, symptoms of overdose might include:*
Heart failure, low blood pressure, slow heartbeat

Brand name:

# Biaxin

*Pronounced: buy-AX-in*
*Generic name: Clarithromycin*

### Why is this drug prescribed?

Biaxin, an antibiotic chemically related to erythromycin, is used to treat certain bacterial infections of the respiratory tract, including:

Strep throat
Pneumonia
Sinusitis (inflammation of sinuses due to infection)
Tonsillitis (inflammation of tonsils due to infection)
Acute middle ear infections
It is also used to treat infections of the skin.

### Most important fact about this drug

Biaxin, like any other antibiotic, works best when there is a constant amount of drug in the blood. To keep the amount constant, try not to miss any doses.

### How should you take this medication?

You may take Biaxin with or without food. Take it exactly as prescribed; continue taking it for the full course of treatment.

■ *If you miss a dose...*
Take it as soon as you remember. If it is almost time for your next dose, take the one you missed and take the next one 5 to 6 hours later. Then go back to your regular schedule.

■ *Storage instructions...*
Store at room temperature in a tightly closed container, away from light. Do not refrigerate the suspension.

### What side effects may occur?

Side effects cannot be anticipated. If any side effects develop or change in intensity, tell your doctor immediately. Only your doctor can determine whether it is safe for you to continue taking Biaxin.

■ *Side effects may include:*
Abdominal pain/discomfort, altered sense of taste, diarrhea, headache, indigestion, nausea

### Why should this drug not be prescribed?

Do not take Biaxin if you have ever had an allergic reaction to it, or if you are sensitive to it or erythromycin, or similar antibiotics such as Tao and Zithromax. Also avoid Biaxin if you have a heart condition or an imbalance in the body's water and minerals. Do not take Biaxin while taking Seldane.

### Special warnings about this medication

If you have severe kidney disease, the doctor may need to prescribe a smaller dose of Biaxin. Make sure the doctor is aware of any kidney problems you may have.

Like other antibiotics, Biaxin may cause a potentially life-threatening form of diarrhea that signals a condition called pseudomembranous colitis (inflammation of the large intestine). Mild diarrhea, a fairly common Biaxin side effect, may disappear as your body gets used to the drug. However, if Biaxin gives you prolonged or severe diarrhea, stop taking the drug and call your doctor immediately.

### Possible food and drug interactions when taking this medication

If Biaxin is taken with certain other drugs, the effects of either can be increased, decreased, or altered. It is especially important to check with your doctor before combining Biaxin with the following:

Carbamazepine (Tegretol)
Terfenadine (Seldane)
Theophylline (Slo-Phyllin, Theo-Dur, others)
Zidovudine (Retrovir)

Biaxin is chemically related to erythromycin. It is possible that other drugs reported to interact with erythromycin could also interact with Biaxin. They include:

Astemizole (Hismanal)
Blood thinners such as Coumadin
Bromocriptine (Parlodel)
Cisapride (Propulsid)
Cyclosporine (Sandimmune, Neoral)
Digoxin (Lanoxin)
Disopyramide (Norpace)
Ergotamine (Cafergot)
Hexobarbital
Lovastatin (Mevacor)
Phenytoin (Dilantin)
Pimozide (Orap)
Triazolam (Halcion)
Valproate (Depakene, Depakote)

### Special information if you are pregnant or breastfeeding

If you are pregnant or plan to become pregnant, notify your doctor immediately. Since Biaxin may have the potential to produce birth defects, it is prescribed during pregnancy only when there is no alternative. Caution is advised when using Biaxin while breastfeeding. Biaxin may appear in breast milk, as does its chemical cousin, erythromycin.

### Recommended dosage

ADULTS

Your doctor will carefully tailor your individual dosage of Biaxin depending upon the type of infection and organism causing it.

The usual dose varies from 250 to 500 milligrams every 12 hours for 7 to 14 days.

CHILDREN

Biaxin is not recommended for children under 6 months of age.

The dose for children older than 6 months depends on how much the child weighs. Biaxin is usually given twice a day for 10 days.

### Overdosage

Although no specific information is available, any medication taken in excess can have serious consequences. If you suspect an overdose of Biaxin, seek medical attention immediately.

*Brand name:*

# Bleph-10

*See Sodium Sulamyd, page 504.*

*Brand name:*

# Bonine

*See Antivert, page 32.*

*Brand name:*

# Brethaire

*See Brethine, page 63.*

*Brand name:*

# Brethine

*Pronounced: Breath-EEN*
*Generic name: Terbutaline sulfate*
*Other brand names: Bricanyl, Brethaire*

### Why is this drug prescribed?

Brethine is a bronchodilator (a medication that opens the bronchial tubes), prescribed for the prevention and relief of bronchial spasms in asthma. This medication is also used for the relief of bronchial spasm associated with bronchitis and emphysema.

## Most important fact about this drug

If you experience an immediate allergic reaction and a worsening of a bronchial spasm, notify your doctor immediately.

## How should you take this medication?

Take this drug exactly as prescribed by your doctor.

The action of Brethine may last up to 8 hours. Do not use it more frequently than recommended.

■ *If you miss a dose...*
Take it as soon as you remember. Then take the rest of your medication for that day in evenly spaced doses. Do not take 2 doses at once.

■ *Storage instructions...*
Store at room temperature in a tightly closed container, away from light.

## What side effects may occur?

Side effects cannot be anticipated. If any develop or change in intensity, inform your doctor as soon as possible. Only your doctor can determine if it is safe for you to continue taking Brethine.

■ *More common side effects may include:*
Chest discomfort, difficulty in breathing, dizziness, drowsiness, fast, fluttery heartbeat, flushed feeling, headache, increased heart rate, nausea, nervousness, pain at injection site, rapid heartbeat, sweating, tremors, vomiting, weakness

■ *Less common side effects may include:*
Anxiety, dry mouth, muscle cramps

■ *Rare side effects may include:*
Inflamed blood vessels

## Why should this drug not be prescribed?

If you are sensitive to or have ever had an allergic reaction to Brethine or similar drugs such as Ventolin, you should not take this medication. Make sure your doctor is aware of any drug reactions you have experienced.

## Special warnings about this medication

When taking Brethine, you should not use other asthma medications before checking with your doctor. Only your doctor can determine what is a sufficient amount of time between doses.

Consult with your doctor before using this medication if you have diabetes, high blood pressure, or an overactive thyroid gland, or if you have had seizures at any time.

Unless you are directed to do so by your doctor, do not take this medication if you have heart disease, especially if you also have an irregular heart rate.

## Possible food and drug interactions when taking this medication

If Brethine is taken with certain other drugs, the effects of either could be increased, decreased, or altered. It is especially important to check with your doctor before combining Brethine with the following:

Antidepressant drugs known as MAO inhibitors (Nardil, Parnate, others)
Beta blockers (blood pressure medications such as Inderal and Tenormin)
Other bronchodilators such as Proventil and Ventolin
Tricyclic antidepressant drugs such as Elavil and Tofranil

## Special information if you are pregnant or breastfeeding

The effects of Brethine during pregnancy have not been adequately studied. If you are pregnant or plan to become pregnant, inform your doctor immediately. It is not known whether Brethine appears in breast milk. If this drug is essential to your health, your doctor may advise you to stop nursing your baby until your treatment is finished.

## Recommended dosage

FOR BRETHINE

*Adults*

The usual tablet dose is 5 milligrams taken at approximately 6-hour intervals, 3 times per day during waking hours. If side effects are excessive, your doctor may reduce your dose to 2.5 milligrams, 3 times per day.

Do not take more than 15 milligrams in a 24-hour period.

*Children*

This medication is not recommended for use in children below 12 years of age.

For children 12 to 15 years of age, the usual dose is 2.5 milligrams, 3 times per day, not to exceed a total of 7.5 milligrams in a 24-hour period.

FOR BRETHAIRE

The usual dosage for adults and children 12 years and older is 2 inhalations separated by a 60-second interval, repeated every 4 to 6 hours.

## Overdosage

Any drug taken or used in excess can have serious consequences. Signs of a Brethine overdose are the same as the side effects. If you suspect an overdose, seek medical attention immediately.

Brand name:

# Brevicon

See Oral Contraceptives, page 382.

Brand name:

# Bricanyl

See Brethine, page 63.

Generic name:

# Bromocriptine

See Parlodel, page 395.

Generic name:

# Brompheniramine, Phenylpropanolamine, and Codeine

See Dimetane-DC, page 165.

Brand name:

# Brontex

See Tussi-Organidin NR, page 569.

Generic name:

# Budesonide

See Rhinocort, page 468.

Generic name:

# Bumetanide

See Bumex, page 65.

Brand name:

# Bumex

Pronounced: BYOO-meks
Generic name: Bumetanide

## Why is this drug prescribed?

Bumex is used to lower the amount of excess salt and water in your body by increasing the output of urine. It is prescribed in the treatment of edema, or fluid retention, associated with congestive heart failure and liver or kidney disease. It is also occasionally prescribed, along with other drugs, to treat high blood pressure.

## Most important fact about this drug

Bumex is a powerful drug. If taken in excessive amounts, it can severely decrease the levels of water and minerals, especially potassium, your body needs to function. Therefore, your doctor should monitor your dose carefully.

## How should you take this medication?

Bumex can increase the frequency of urination and may cause loss of sleep if taken at night. Therefore, if you are taking a single dose of Bumex daily, it should be taken in the morning after breakfast. If you take more than one dose a day, take the last dose no later than 6:00 PM.

■ *If you miss a dose...*
Take the forgotten dose as soon as you remember. If it is almost time for your next dose, skip the one you missed and go back to your regular schedule. Never take 2 doses at the same time.

■ *Storage instructions...*
Store at room temperature.

## What side effects may occur?

Side effects cannot be anticipated. If any develop or change in intensity, inform your doctor as soon as possible. Only your doctor can determine if it is safe for you to continue taking Bumex.

■ *More common side effects may include:*
Dizziness, headache, low blood pressure, muscle cramps, nausea

■ *Signs of too much potassium loss are:*
Dry mouth, irregular heartbeat, muscle cramps or
pains, unusual tiredness or weakness

■ *Less common or rare side effects may include:*
Abdominal pain, black stools, chest pain, dehydration, diarrhea, dry mouth, ear discomfort,
fatigue, hearing loss, itching, joint pain, kidney
failure, muscle and bone pain, nipple tenderness,
premature ejaculation and difficulty maintaining
erection, rapid breathing, skin rash or hives,
sweating, upset stomach, vertigo, vomiting,
weakness

### Why should this drug not be prescribed?
Bumex should not be used if you are unable to
urinate or if you are dehydrated.

If you are sensitive to or have ever had an allergic reaction to Bumex or similar drugs such as
Lasix, you should not take this medication. Make
sure your doctor is aware of any drug reactions you
have experienced.

### Special warnings about this medication
If you are allergic to sulfur-containing drugs such
as sulfonamides (antibacterial drugs), check with
your doctor before taking Bumex.

Bumex can decrease the number of platelets in
your blood. Your doctor should monitor your blood
status regularly.

Bumex can cause a loss of potassium from the
body. Your doctor may recommend foods or fluids
high in potassium or may want you to take a potassium supplement to help prevent this. Follow your
doctor's recommendation carefully.

While taking this medication you may feel dizzy
or light-headed or actually faint when getting up
from a lying or sitting position. If getting up slowly
does not help or if this problem continues, notify
your doctor.

### Possible food and drug interactions
### when taking this medication
If Bumex is taken with certain other drugs, the effects of either could be increased, decreased, or altered. It is especially important to check with your
doctor before combining Bumex with the following:

Blood pressure medications such as Vasotec and
    Tenormin
Indomethacin (Indocin) and other nonsteroidal anti-
    inflammatory drugs
Probenecid (Benemid)

The combination of Bumex and certain antibiotics
or cisplatin (Platinol) may increase the risk of
hearing loss.

Because Bumex can lower potassium levels, the
combination of Bumex and digitalis or digoxin
(Lanoxin) may increase the risk of changes in
heartbeat.

The combination of Bumex and lithium
(Lithonate) may increase the levels of lithium in the
body, causing it to become poisonous.

### Special information
### if you are pregnant or breastfeeding
The effects of Bumex during pregnancy have not
been adequately studied. If you are pregnant or plan
to become pregnant, inform your doctor immediately. It is not known if this medication appears in
breast milk. Your doctor may advise you to discontinue breastfeeding your baby until your treatment
with Bumex is finished.

### Recommended dosage
ADULTS

The usual total daily dose is 0.5 to 2.0 milligrams a
day. For most people, this is taken as a single dose.
However, if the initial dose is not adequate, your
doctor may have you take a second and, possibly, a
third dose at 4- to 5-hour intervals, up to a
maximum daily dose of 10 milligrams.

For the continuing control of edema, your doctor
may tell you to take Bumex on alternate days or for
3 to 4 days at a time with rest periods of 1 to 2 days
in between.

If you have liver failure, your dose will be kept
to a minimum and increased very carefully.

CHILDREN

The safety and effectiveness of Bumex have not
been established in children below the age of 18.

### Overdosage
An overdose of Bumex can lead to severe dehydration, reduction of blood volume, and severe problems with the circulatory system.

■ *The signs of an overdose include:*
Cramps, dizziness, lethargy (sluggishness), loss
or lack of appetite, mental confusion, vomiting,
weakness

If you suspect an overdose, get medical attention
immediately.

Generic name:

# Bupropion

See Wellbutrin, page 592.

Brand name:

# BuSpar

Pronounced: BYOO-spar
Generic name: Buspirone hydrochloride

## Why is this drug prescribed?
BuSpar is used in the treatment of anxiety disorders and for short-term relief of the symptoms of anxiety.

## Most important fact about this drug
BuSpar should not be used with antidepressant drugs known as monoamine oxidase (MAO) inhibitors. Brands include Nardil and Parnate.

## How should you take this medication?
Take BuSpar exactly as prescribed. Do not be discouraged if you feel no immediate effect. The full benefit of this drug may not be seen for 1 to 2 weeks after you start to take it.

■ If you miss a dose...
Take the forgotten dose as soon as you remember. If it is almost time for your next dose, skip the one you missed and go back to your regular schedule. Never take 2 doses at the same time.
■ Storage instructions...
Store at room temperature in a tightly closed container, away from light.

## What side effects may occur?
Side effects cannot be anticipated. If any develop or change in intensity, inform your doctor as soon as possible. Only your doctor can determine if it is safe for you to continue taking BuSpar.

■ More common side effects may include:
Dizziness, dry mouth, fatigue, headache, lightheadedness, nausea, nervousness, unusual excitement
■ Less common or rare side effects may include:
Anger/hostility, blurred vision, bone aches/pain, confusion, constipation, decreased concentration, depression, diarrhea, fast, fluttery heartbeat, incoordination, muscle pain/aches, numbness, pain or weakness in hands or feet, rapid heart-

beat, rash, restlessness, stomach and abdominal upset, sweating/clamminess, tingling or pins and needles, tremor, urinary incontinence, vomiting, weakness

## Why should this drug not be prescribed?
If you are sensitive to or have ever had an allergic reaction to BuSpar or similar mood-altering drugs, you should not take this medication. Make sure your doctor is aware of any drug reactions you have experienced.

Anxiety or tension related to everyday stress usually does not require treatment with BuSpar. Discuss your symptoms thoroughly with your doctor.

The use of BuSpar is not recommended if you have severe kidney or liver damage.

## Special warnings about this medication
The effects of BuSpar on the central nervous system (brain and spinal cord) are unpredictable. Therefore, you should not drive or operate dangerous machinery or participate in any hazardous activity that requires full mental alertness while you are taking BuSpar.

## Possible food and drug interactions when taking this medication
Although BuSpar does not intensify the effects of alcohol, it is best to avoid alcohol while taking this medication.

If BuSpar is taken with certain other drugs, the effects of either can be increased, decreased, or altered. It is especially important to check with your doctor before combining BuSpar with the following:

The blood-thinning drug Coumadin
Haloperidol (Haldol)
MAO inhibitors (antidepressant drugs such as Nardil and Parnate)
Trazodone (Desyrel)

## Special information if you are pregnant or breastfeeding
The effects of BuSpar during pregnancy have not been adequately studied. If you are pregnant or plan to become pregnant, inform your doctor immediately. It is not known whether BuSpar appears in breast milk. If this medication is essential to your health, your doctor may advise you to discontinue breastfeeding until your treatment is finished.

## Recommended dosage

ADULTS

The recommended starting dose is a total of 15 milligrams per day divided into smaller doses, usually 5 milligrams 3 times a day. Every 2 to 3 days, your doctor may increase the dosage 5 milligrams per day as needed. The daily dose should not exceed 60 milligrams.

CHILDREN

The safety and effectiveness of BuSpar have not been established in children under 18 years of age.

## Overdosage

Any medication taken in excess can have serious consequences. If you suspect an overdose of BuSpar, seek medical attention immediately.

■ *The symptoms of BuSpar overdose may include:*
 Dizziness, drowsiness, nausea or vomiting, severe stomach upset, unusually small pupils

*Generic name:*

# Buspirone

See *BuSpar*, page 67.

*Generic name:*

# Butalbital, Acetaminophen, and Caffeine

See *Fioricet*, page 209.

*Generic name:*

# Butalbital, Aspirin, and Caffeine

See *Fiorinal*, page 210.

*Generic name:*

# Butalbital, Codeine, Aspirin, and Caffeine

See *Fiorinal with Codeine*, page 212.

*Generic name:*

# Butoconazole

See *Femstat*, page 208.

*Brand name:*

# Cafergot

*Pronounced: KAF-er-got*
*Generic ingredients: Ergotamine tartrate, Caffeine*

## Why is this drug prescribed?

Cafergot is prescribed for the relief or prevention of vascular headaches—for example, migraine, migraine variants, or cluster headaches.

## Most important fact about this drug

The excessive use of Cafergot can lead to ergot poisoning resulting in symptoms such as headache, pain in the legs when walking, muscle pain, numbness, coldness, and abnormal paleness of the fingers and toes. If this condition is not treated, it can lead to gangrene (tissue death due to decreased blood supply).

## How should you take this medication?

Cafergot is available in both tablet and suppository form. Be sure to take it exactly as prescribed, remaining within the limits of your recommended dosage.

   Cafergot works best if you use it at the first sign of a migraine attack. If you get warning signals of a coming migraine, take the drug before the headache actually starts.

   Lie down and relax in a quiet, dark room for at least a couple of hours or until you feel better.

   Avoid exposure to cold.

   To use the suppositories, follow these steps:

1. If the suppository feels too soft, leave it in the refrigerator for about 30 minutes or put it, still wrapped, in ice water until it hardens.
2. Remove the foil wrapper and dip the tip of the suppository in water.
3. Lie down on your side and with a finger insert the suppository into the rectum. Hold it in place for a few moments.

■ *If you miss a dose...*
 Take this medication only when threatened with an attack.
■ *Storage instructions...*
 Store at room temperature in a tightly closed container away from light. Keep suppositories away from heat.

## What side effects may occur?

Side effects cannot be anticipated. If any develop or change in intensity, inform your doctor as soon as possible. Only your doctor can determine if it is safe for you to continue taking Cafergot.

■ *Side effects may include:*
Fluid retention, high blood pressure, itching, nausea, numbness, rapid heart rate, slow heartbeat, tingling or pins and needles, vertigo, vomiting, weakness

■ *Complications caused by constriction of the blood vessels can be serious. They include:*
Bluish tinge to the skin, chest pain, cold arms and legs, gangrene, muscle pains

Although these symptoms occur most commonly with long-term therapy at relatively high doses, they have been reported with short-term or normal doses. A few people on long-term therapy have developed heart valve problems.

## Why should this drug not be prescribed?

If you are sensitive to or have ever had an allergic reaction to ergotamine tartrate, caffeine, or similar drugs, you should not take this medication. Make sure your doctor is aware of any drug reactions you have experienced.

Unless directed to do so by your doctor, do not take this medication if you have coronary heart disease, circulatory problems, high blood pressure, impaired liver or kidney function, or an infection, or if you are pregnant.

## Special warnings about this medication

It is extremely important that you do not exceed your recommended dosage, especially when Cafergot is used over long periods. There have been reports of psychological dependence in people who have abused this drug over long periods of time. Discontinuance of the drug may produce withdrawal symptoms such as sudden, severe headaches.

If you experience excessive nausea and vomiting during attacks, making it impossible for you to retain oral medication, your doctor will probably tell you to use rectal suppositories.

This drug is effective only for migraine and migraine-type headaches. Do not use it for any other kind of headache.

## Possible food and drug interactions when taking this medication

If Cafergot is taken with certain other drugs, the effects of either could be increased, decreased, or altered. It is especially important to check with your doctor before combining Cafergot with the following:

Beta-blocker drugs (blood pressure medications such as Inderal and Tenormin)
Drugs that constrict the blood vessels, such as EpiPen and the oral decongestant Sudafed
Macrolide antibiotics such as PCE, E.E.S., and Biaxin
Nicotine (Nicoderm, Habitrol, others)

## Special information if you are pregnant or breastfeeding

Do not take Cafergot if you are pregnant. Cafergot appears in breast milk and may have serious effects in your baby. If this medication is essential for your health, your doctor may advise you to discontinue breastfeeding.

## Recommended dosage

Dosage should start at the first sign of an attack.

ADULTS

*Orally*
The total dose for any single attack should not exceed 6 tablets.

*Rectally*
The maximum dose for an individual attack is 2 suppositories.

The total weekly dosage should not exceed 10 tablets or 5 suppositories.

A preventive, short-term dose may be given at bedtime to certain people, but only as prescribed by a doctor.

## Overdosage

If you suspect an overdose of Cafergot, seek emergency medical treatment immediately.

■ *Symptoms of Cafergot overdose include:*
Coma, convulsions, diminished or absent pulses, drowsiness, high or low blood pressure, numbness, shock, stupor, tingling, pain and bluish discoloration of the limbs, unresponsiveness, vomiting

*Brand name:*

# Calan

*Pronounced: CAL-an*
*Generic name: Verapamil hydrochloride*
*Other brand names: Calan SR, Isoptin, Isoptin SR,*
*Verelan*

### Why is this drug prescribed?

Verapamil, the active ingredient in Calan, Isoptin, and Verelan, is prescribed for the treatment of various types of angina (chest pain, often accompanied by a feeling of choking, usually caused by lack of oxygen to the heart due to clogged arteries). It is also used for irregular heartbeat and for high blood pressure. The sustained release formulas (SR and Verelan) are used only for the treatment of high blood pressure. Verapamil is a type of medication called a calcium channel blocker. It eases the heart's workload by slowing down the passage of nerve impulses through it, and hence the contractions of the heart muscle. This improves blood flow through the heart and throughout the body, reduces blood pressure, corrects irregular heartbeat, and helps prevent angina pain.

Some doctors also prescribe verapamil to prevent migraine headache and asthma and to treat manic depression and panic attacks.

### Most important fact about this drug

If you have high blood pressure, you must take verapamil regularly for it to be effective. Since blood pressure declines gradually, it may be several weeks before you get the full benefit of verapamil; and you must continue taking it even if you are feeling well. Verapamil does not cure high blood pressure; it merely keeps it under control.

### How should you take this medication?

Calan, Isoptin, and Verelan can be taken with or without food. Calan SR and Isoptin SR should be taken with food.

Calan SR, Isoptin SR, and Verelan must be swallowed whole and should not be crushed or chewed.

You may open Verelan capsules and sprinkle the pellets on a spoonful of cool applesauce. Swallow all of the mixture immediately, and then drink a glass of cool water.

Take this medication exactly as prescribed, even if you are feeling well. Try not to miss any doses. If the drug is not taken regularly, your condition can get worse.

Check with your doctor before you stop taking this drug; a slow reduction in the dose may be required.

■ *If you miss a dose...*
Take it as soon as you remember. If it is almost time for your next dose, skip the one you missed and go back to your regular schedule. Never take 2 doses at the same time.

■ *Storage instructions...*
Store at room temperature away from heat, light, and moisture.

### What side effects may occur?

Side effects cannot be anticipated. If any develop or change in intensity, inform your doctor as soon as possible. Only your doctor can determine if it is safe for you to continue taking verapamil.

■ *More common side effects may include:*
Congestive heart failure, constipation, dizziness, fatigue, fluid retention, headache, low blood pressure, nausea, rash, shortness of breath, slow heartbeat

■ *Less common or rare side effects may include:*
Angina, blurred vision, breast development in males, bruising, chest pain, confusion, diarrhea, difficulty sleeping, drowsiness, dry mouth, excessive milk secretion, fainting, fatigue, fever and rash, flushing, hair loss, heart attack, hives, impotence, increased urination, indigestion, intestinal blockage, joint pain, limping, loss of balance, muscle cramps, pounding heartbeat, rash, shakiness, skin peeling, sleepiness, spotty menstruation, sweating, tingling or pins and needles, upset stomach

### Why should this drug not be prescribed?

If you have low blood pressure or certain types of heart disease or heartbeat irregularities, you should not take verapamil. Make sure the doctor is aware of any cardiac problems you may have.

If you are sensitive to or have ever had an allergic reaction to Calan or any other brands of verapamil, or other calcium channel blockers, do not take this medication.

### Special warnings about this medication

Verapamil can reduce or eliminate angina pain caused by exertion or exercise. Be sure to discuss with your doctor how much exertion is safe for you.

Verapamil may cause your blood pressure to become too low. If you experience dizziness or light-headedness, notify your doctor.

Congestive heart failure and fluid in the lungs have occurred in people taking verapamil together with other heart drugs known as beta blockers. Make sure your doctor is aware of all medications you are taking.

If you have a heart condition, liver disease, kidney disease, or Duchenne's dystrophy (the most common type of muscular dystrophy), make certain your doctor knows about it. Verapamil should be used with caution.

### Possible food and drug interactions when taking this medication

If verapamil is taken with certain other drugs, the effects of either could be increased, decreased, or altered. It is especially important to check with your doctor before combining verapamil with the following:

Alcohol
ACE inhibitor-type blood pressure drugs such as
  Capoten and Vasotec
Amiodarone (Cordarone)
Beta-blocker-type blood pressure drugs such as
  Lopressor, Tenormin, and Inderal
Carbamazepine (Tegretol)
Chloroquine (Aralen)
Cimetidine (Tagamet)
Cyclosporine (Sandimmune, Neoral)
Dantrolene (Dantrium)
Digitalis (Lanoxin)
Disopyramide (Norpace)
Diuretics such as Lasix and HydroDIURIL
Flecainide (Tambocor)
Glipizide (Glucotrol)
Imipramine (Tofranil)
Lithium (Lithonate)
Nitrates such as Transderm Nitro and Isordil
Phenobarbital
Phenytoin (Dilantin)
Quinidine (Quinidex)
Rifampin (Rifadin)
Theophylline (Theo-Dur)
Vasodilator-type blood pressure drugs such
  as Loniten
Other high blood pressure drugs such as Minipress

### Special information
### if you are pregnant or breastfeeding

The effects of verapamil during pregnancy have not been adequately studied. If you are pregnant or plan to become pregnant, inform your doctor immediately. The drug appears in breast milk and could affect a nursing infant. If this medication is essential to your health, your doctor may advise you to discontinue breastfeeding until your treatment is finished.

### Recommended dosage
FOR CALAN AND ISOPTIN

Dosages of this medication must be adjusted to meet individual needs. In general, dosages of this medication should not exceed 480 milligrams per day. Your doctor will closely monitor your response to this drug, usually within 8 hours of the first dose.

Safety and effectiveness of this drug in children have not been established.

*Angina*

The usual initial dose is 80 to 120 milligrams, 3 times a day. Lower doses of 40 milligrams 3 times a day may be used by people who have a stronger response to this medication, such as the elderly or those with decreased liver function. The dosage may be increased by your doctor either daily or weekly until the desired response is seen.

*Irregular Heartbeat*

The usual dose in people who are also on digitalis ranges from 240 to 320 milligrams per day divided into 3 or 4 doses.

In those not on digitalis, doses range from a total of 240 to 480 milligrams per day divided into 3 or 4 doses.

Maximum effects of this drug should be seen in the first 48 hours of use.

*High Blood Pressure*

Effects of this drug on blood pressure should be seen within the first week of use. Any adjustment of this medication to a higher dose will be based on its effectiveness as determined by your doctor.

The usual dose of this drug, when used alone for high blood pressure, is 80 milligrams, 3 times per day. Total daily doses of 360 milligrams and 480 milligrams may be used. Smaller doses of 40 milligrams 3 times per day may be taken by smaller individuals and the elderly.

FOR CALAN SR, ISOPTIN SR, AND VERELAN

Dosages for high blood pressure should be adjusted to meet each individual's needs.

### Adults

The usual starting dose of Calan SR and Isoptin SR is 180 milligrams taken in the morning. For Verelan, it is 240 milligrams. A lower starting dose of 120 milligrams may be taken if the person is smaller. Your doctor will monitor your response to this drug and may adjust it each week. In addition, your doctor may increase the dose and add evening doses to the morning dose, based on the effectiveness of the drug.

You should see results from the drug within a week.

### Children

The safety and effectiveness of this drug in children under age 18 have not been established.

### Older Adults

Your doctor may start you at a lower dose of 120 milligrams and then adjust it according to your response.

### Overdosage

Any medication taken in excess can have serious consequences. If you suspect an overdose, seek medical attention immediately.

An overdose of Calan can cause dangerously low blood pressure and life-threatening heart problems. After treatment for an overdose, you should remain under observation in the hospital for at least 48 hours, especially if you have taken the sustained-release form of the drug.

*Brand name:*

# Calcimar

See Miacalcin, page 321.

*Generic name:*

# Calcitonin-salmon

See Miacalcin, page 321.

*Generic name:*

# Calcitriol

See Rocaltrol, page 477.

*Brand name:*

# Capoten

Pronounced: KAP-o-ten
Generic name: Captopril

### Why is this drug prescribed?

Capoten is used in the treatment of high blood pressure and congestive heart failure. When prescribed for high blood pressure, it is effective used alone or combined with diuretics. If it is prescribed for congestive heart failure, it is used in combination with digitalis and diuretics. Capoten is in a family of drugs known as "ACE (angiotensin converting enzyme) inhibitors." It works by preventing a chemical in your blood called angiotensin I from converting into a more potent form that increases salt and water retention in your body. Capoten also enhances blood flow throughout your blood vessels.

In addition, Capoten is used to improve survival in certain people who have suffered heart attacks and to treat kidney disease in diabetics.

Some doctors also prescribe Capoten for angina pectoris (crushing chest pain), Raynaud's phenomenon (a disorder of the blood vessels that causes the fingers to turn white when exposed to cold), and rheumatoid arthritis.

### Most important fact about this drug

If you have high blood pressure, you must take Capoten regularly for it to be effective. Since blood pressure declines gradually, it may be several weeks before you get the full benefit of Capoten; you must continue taking it even if you are feeling well. Capoten does not cure high blood pressure; it merely keeps it under control.

### How should you take this medication?

Capoten should be taken 1 hour before meals. If you are taking an antacid such as Mylanta, take it 2 hours prior to Capoten.

Take this medication exactly as prescribed. Stopping Capoten suddenly could cause your blood pressure to increase.

■ *If you miss a dose...*
Take it as soon as you remember. If it is almost time for your next dose, skip the one you missed and go back to your regular schedule. Never take two doses at the same time.

■ *Storage instructions...*
Store Capoten at room temperature, away from moisture, in a tightly closed container.

## What side effects may occur?

Side effects cannot be anticipated. If any develop or change in intensity, inform your doctor as soon as possible. Only your doctor can determine if it is safe for you to continue taking Capoten.

■ *More common side effects may include:*
Itching, loss of taste, low blood pressure, rash

■ *Less common or rare side effects may include:*
Abdominal pain, anemia, angina pectoris (severe chest pain), blisters, blurred vision, breast development in males, cardiac arrest, changes in heart rhythm, chest pain, confusion, constipation, cough, depression, diarrhea, difficulty swallowing, dizziness, dry mouth, fatigue, fever and chills, flushing, general feeling of ill health, hair loss, headache, heart attack, heart failure, impotence, inability to sleep, indigestion, inflammation of the nose, inflammation of the tongue, labored breathing, lack of coordination, loss of appetite, lung inflammation, muscle pain and/or weakness, nausea, nervousness, pallor, palpitations, peptic ulcer, rapid heartbeat, sensitivity to light, skin inflammation, skin peeling, sleepiness, sore throat, stomach irritation, stroke, sudden fainting or loss of strength, swelling of face, lips, tongue, throat, or arms and legs, tingling or pins and needles, vomiting, weakness, wheezing, yellow eyes and skin

## Why should this drug not be prescribed?

If you are sensitive to or have ever had an allergic reaction to Capoten or similar drugs such as Vasotec, you should not take this medication. Make sure that your doctor is aware of any drug reactions that you have experienced.

## Special warnings about this medication

If you develop swelling of the face around your lips, tongue or throat (or of your arms and legs) or have difficulty swallowing, you should stop taking Capoten and contact your doctor immediately. You may need emergency treatment.

If you are receiving bee or wasp venom to prevent an allergic reaction to stings, use of Capoten at the same time may cause a severe allergic reaction.

If you are taking Capoten, a complete assessment of your kidney function should be done; and your kidney function should continue to be monitored. If you have kidney disease, Capoten should be used only if you have taken other blood pressure medications and your doctor has determined that the results were unsatisfactory.

Some people taking Capoten have had a severe allergic reaction during kidney dialysis.

If you are taking Capoten for your heart, be careful not to increase physical activity too quickly. Check with your doctor as to how much exercise is safe for you.

If you are taking Capoten for congestive heart failure, your blood pressure may drop temporarily after the first few doses and you may feel lightheaded for a time. Your doctor should monitor you closely when you start taking the medication or when your dosage is increased.

If you are taking high doses of diuretics and Capoten, you may develop excessively low blood pressure. Your doctor may reduce your diuretic dose so that your blood pressure doesn't drop too far.

If you notice a yellow coloring to your skin or the whites of your eyes, stop taking the drug and notify your doctor immediately. You could be developing a liver problem.

Capoten may cause you to become drowsy or less alert, especially if you are also taking a diuretic at the same time. If it has this effect on you, driving or participating in any potentially hazardous activity is not recommended.

Dehydration may cause a drop in blood pressure. If you experience symptoms such as excessive perspiration, vomiting, and/or diarrhea, notify your doctor immediately.

If you develop a sore throat or fever you should contact your doctor immediately. It could indicate a more serious illness.

If you develop a persistent, dry cough, tell your doctor. It may be due to the medication and, if so, will disappear if you stop taking Capoten.

## Possible food and drug interactions when taking this medication

If Capoten is taken with certain other drugs, the effects of either could be increased, decreased, or altered. It is especially important to check with your doctor before combining Capoten with the following:

Allopurinol (Zyloprim)

Aspirin

Blood pressure drugs known as beta blockers, such as Inderal and Tenormin

Cyclosporine (Sandimmune)

Digoxin (Lanoxin)

Diuretics such as HydroDIURIL

Lithium (Lithonate)

Nitroglycerin and similar heart medicines (Nitro-Dur, Transderm-Nitro, others)

Nonsteroidal anti-inflammatory drugs such as Indocin and Feldene

Potassium preparations such as Micro-K and Slow-K

Potassium-sparing diuretics such as Aldactone and Midamor

Do not use potassium-containing salt substitutes while taking Capoten.

### Special information
### if you are pregnant or breastfeeding

ACE inhibitors such as Capoten have been shown to cause injury and even death to the developing baby when used in pregnancy during the second and third trimesters. If you are pregnant or plan to become pregnant, contact your doctor immediately. Capoten appears in breast milk and could affect a nursing infant. If this medication is essential to your health, your doctor may advise you to discontinue breastfeeding until your treatment is finished.

### Recommended dosage

ADULTS

#### High Blood Pressure

The usual starting dose is 25 milligrams taken 2 or 3 times a day. If you have any problems with your kidneys or suffer from other major health problems, your starting dose may be lower. Depending on how your blood pressure responds, your doctor may increase your dose later, up to a total of 150 milligrams 2 or 3 times a day. The maximum recommended daily dose is 450 milligrams.

#### Heart Failure

For most people, the usual dose is 25 milligrams taken 3 times a day. A daily dosage of 450 milligrams should not be exceeded.

#### After a Heart Attack

The usual starting dose is 6.25 milligrams, taken once, followed by 12.5 milligrams 3 times a day.

Your doctor will increase the dose over the next several days to 25 milligrams taken 3 times a day and then, over the next several weeks, to 50 milligrams 3 times a day.

#### Kidney Disease in Diabetes

The usual dose is 25 milligrams taken 3 times a day.

CHILDREN

The safety and effectiveness of Capoten in children have not been established.

### Overdosage

Any medication taken in excess can cause symptoms of overdose. If you suspect an overdose of Capoten, seek medical attention immediately.

Light-headedness or dizziness due to a sudden drop in blood pressure is the primary effect of a Capoten overdose.

*Brand name:*

# Capozide

*Pronounced: KAP-oh-zide*
*Generic ingredients: Captopril, Hydrochlorothiazide*

### Why is this drug prescribed?

Capozide is used in the treatment of high blood pressure. It combines an ACE inhibitor with a thiazide diuretic. Captopril, the ACE inhibitor, works by preventing a chemical in your blood called angiotensin I from converting into a more potent form that increases salt and water retention in your body. Captopril also enhances blood flow throughout your blood vessels. Hydrochlorothiazide, the diuretic, helps your body produce and eliminate more urine, which helps in lowering blood pressure.

### Most important fact about this drug

You must take Capozide regularly for it to be effective. Since blood pressure declines gradually, it may be several weeks before you get the full benefit of Capozide; and you must continue taking it even if you are feeling well. Capozide does not cure high blood pressure; it merely keeps it under control.

### How should you take this medication?

Capozide should be taken 1 hour before meals. Take it exactly as prescribed. Stopping Capozide suddenly could cause your blood pressure to increase.

■ *If you miss a dose...*
Take it as soon as you remember. If it is almost time for your next dose, skip the one you missed and go back to your regular schedule. Never take 2 doses at the same time.

■ *Storage instructions...*
Capozide should be stored at room temperature in a tightly closed container away from moisture.

## What side effects may occur?
Side effects cannot be anticipated. If any develop or change in intensity, inform your doctor as soon as possible. Only your doctor can determine if it is safe for you to continue taking Capozide.

■ *More common side effects may include:*
Itching, loss of taste, low blood pressure, rash

■ *Less common or rare side effects may include:*
Abdominal pain, anemia, angina pectoris (severe chest pain), angioedema (swelling of the arms and legs, face, lips, tongue, or throat), blurred vision, breast development in males, bronchitis, bronchospasm, changes in heart rhythm, chest pain, confusion, constipation, cough, cramping, depression, diarrhea, dizziness, dizziness upon standing up, dry mouth, fainting, fatigue, fever, flushing, general feeling of ill health, hair loss, headache, heart attack, heart failure, hepatitis, hives, inability to sleep, indigestion, impotence, inflammation of nose, inflammation of tongue, labored breathing, lack of coordination, loss of appetite, low potassium levels leading to symptoms such as dry mouth, excessive thirst, weak or irregular heartbeat, muscle pain or cramps, muscle weakness, muscle spasm, nausea, nervousness, pallor, peptic ulcer, rapid heartbeat, Raynaud's Syndrome (circulatory disorder), restlessness, sensitivity to light, severe allergic reactions, skin inflammation and/or peeling, sleepiness, stomach irritation, stroke, tingling or pins and needles, vomiting, vertigo, weakness, wheezing, yellow eyes and skin

## Why should this drug not be prescribed?
If you are sensitive to or have ever had an allergic reaction to captopril, hydrochlorothiazide, other ACE inhibitors such as Vasotec, or other thiazide diuretics such as Diuril, or if you are sensitive to other sulfonamide-derived drugs, you should not take this medication. If you have a history of angioedema (swelling of face, extremities, and throat) or inability to urinate, you should not take this medication.

## Special warnings about this medication
If you develop swelling of your face around your lips, tongue, or throat, or in your arms and legs, or if you begin to have difficulty swallowing, you should contact your doctor immediately. You may need emergency treatment.

If you develop a sore throat or fever you should contact your doctor immediately. It could indicate a more serious illness.

If you are taking Capozide, your doctor will make a complete assessment of your kidney function and will continue to monitor it.

If you have impaired kidney function, Capozide should be used only if you have taken other blood pressure medications and your doctor has determined that the results were unsatisfactory.

If you have liver disease or a disease of the connective tissue called lupus erythematosus, Capozide should be used with caution. Tell your doctor immediately if you notice a yellowish color in your skin or the whites of your eyes.

If you have congestive heart failure, you should be carefully watched for low blood pressure. You should not increase your physical activity too quickly.

Excessive sweating, dehydration, severe diarrhea, or vomiting could deplete your fluids and cause your blood pressure to become too low. Be careful when exercising and in hot weather.

This drug should be used with caution if you are on dialysis. There have been reports of extreme allergic reactions during dialysis in people taking ACE-inhibitor medications such as Capozide. Your odds of an allergic reaction also increase if you are being desensitized with bee venom while you are taking Capozide.

While taking Capozide, do not use potassium-sparing diuretics (such as Moduretic), potassium supplements, or salt substitutes containing potassium without talking to your doctor first.

## Possible food and drug interactions when taking this medication
Capozide may intensify the effects of alcohol. Do not drink alcohol while taking this medication.

If Capozide is taken with certain other drugs, the effects of either could be increased, decreased, or altered. It is especially important to check with your doctor before combining Capozide with the following:

Antigout drugs such as Zyloprim
Barbiturates such as phenobarbital or Seconal
Calcium
Cardiac glycosides such as Lanoxin
Cholestyramine (Questran)
Colestipol (Colestid)
Corticosteroids such as prednisone (Deltasone)
Diabetes medications such as Micronase
    and Insulin
Diazoxide (Proglycem)
Heart medications such as Lanoxin
Lithium (Lithonate)
MAO inhibitors (antidepressants such
    as Nardil)
Methenamine (Mandelamine)
Narcotics such as Percocet
Nitroglycerin or other nitrates such as
    Transderm-Nitro
Nonsteroidal anti-inflammatory drugs such
    as Naprosyn
Norepinephrine (Levophed)
Oral blood thinners such as Coumadin
Other blood pressure drugs such as Hytrin
    and Minipress
Potassium-sparing diuretics such as Moduretic
Potassium supplements such as Slow K
Probenecid (Benemid)
Salt substitutes containing potassium
Sulfinpyrazone (Anturane)

## Special information
## if you are pregnant or breastfeeding

ACE inhibitors such as Capozide have been shown to cause injury and even death to the developing baby when used in pregnancy during the second or third trimesters. If you are pregnant your doctor should discontinue your use of this medication as soon as possible. If you plan to become pregnant and are taking Capozide, contact your doctor immediately to discuss the potential hazard to your unborn child. Capozide appears in breast milk and could affect a nursing infant. If this medication is essential to your health, your doctor may advise you to discontinue breastfeeding until your treatment is finished.

## Recommended dosage

### ADULTS

Dosages of this drug are always individualized, and your doctor will determine what combination works best for you. This medication can be used in conjunction with other blood pressure medications such as beta blockers. Dosages are also adjusted for people with decreased kidney function.

The initial dose is one 25 milligram/15 milligram tablet, once a day. If this is not effective, your doctor may adjust the dosage upward every 6 weeks. In general, the daily dose of captopril should not exceed 150 milligrams. The maximum recommended daily dose of hydrochlorothiazide is 50 milligrams.

### CHILDREN

The safety and effectiveness of Capozide in children have not been established. Capozide should be used in children only if other measures for controlling blood pressure have not been effective.

### OLDER ADULTS

Your doctor will determine the dosage according to your particular needs.

## Overdosage

Any medication taken in excess can have serious consequences. If you suspect an overdose, seek medical attention immediately.

■ *The symptoms of Capozide overdose may include:* Coma, lethargy, low blood pressure, sluggishness, stomach and intestinal irritation and hyperactivity

*Generic name:*

# Captopril

*See Capoten, page 72.*

*Generic name:*

# Captopril with Hydrochlorothiazide

*See Capozide, page 74.*

*Brand name:*

# Carafate

*Pronounced: CARE-uh-fate*
*Generic name: Sucralfate*

## Why is this drug prescribed?
Carafate Tablets and Suspension are used for the short-term treatment (up to 8 weeks) of an active duodenal ulcer; Carafate Tablets are also used for longer-term therapy at a reduced dosage after a duodenal ulcer has healed.

Carafate helps ulcers heal by forming a protective coating over them.

Some doctors also prescribe Carafate for ulcers in the mouth and esophagus that develop during cancer therapy, for digestive tract irritation caused by drugs, for long-term treatment of stomach ulcers, and to relieve pain following tonsil removal.

## Most important fact about this drug
A duodenal ulcer is a recurring illness. While Carafate can cure an acute ulcer, it cannot prevent other ulcers from developing or lessen their severity.

## How should you take this medication?
Carafate works best when taken on an empty stomach. If you take an antacid to relieve pain, avoid doing it within one-half hour before or after you take Carafate. Always take Carafate exactly as prescribed.

■ *If you miss a dose...*
Take it as soon as you remember. If it is almost time for your next dose, skip the one you missed and go back to your regular schedule. Never take 2 doses at the same time.
■ *Storage instructions...*
Store at room temperature. Protect the suspension from freezing.

## What side effects may occur?
Side effects cannot be anticipated. If any develop or change in intensity, inform your doctor as soon as possible. Only your doctor can determine if it is safe for you to continue taking Carafate.

■ *More common side effects may include:*
Constipation
■ *Less common or rare side effects may include:*
Back pain, diarrhea, dizziness, dry mouth, gas, headache, indigestion, insomnia, itching, nausea, possible allergic reactions, including hives and breathing difficulty, rash, sleepiness, stomach upset, vertigo, vomiting

## Why should this drug not be prescribed?
There are no restrictions on the use of this drug.

## Special warnings about this medication
If you have kidney failure or are on dialysis, the doctor will be cautious about prescribing this drug. Use of Carafate while taking aluminum-containing antacids may increase the possibility of aluminum poisoning in those with kidney failure.

## Possible food and drug interactions when taking this medication
If Carafate is taken with certain other drugs, the effects of either could be increased, decreased, or altered. It is especially important to check with your doctor before combining Carafate with the following:

Antacids such as Mylanta and Maalox
Blood-thinning drugs such as Coumadin
Cimetidine (Tagamet)
Digoxin (Lanoxin)
Drugs for controlling spasms, such as Bentyl
Ketoconazole (Nizoral)
Levothyroxine (Synthroid)
Phenytoin (Dilantin)
Quinidine (Quinidex)
Quinolone antibiotics such as Cipro and Floxin
Ranitidine (Zantac)
Tetracycline (Sumycin)
Theophylline (Theo-Dur)

## Special information if you are pregnant or breastfeeding
The effects of Carafate during pregnancy have not been adequately studied. If you are pregnant or plan to become pregnant, inform your doctor immediately. Carafate may appear in breast milk and could affect a nursing infant. If this medication is essential to your health, your doctor may advise you to discontinue breastfeeding until your treatment with this medication is finished.

## Recommended dosage
ADULTS

*Active Duodenal Ulcer:*
The usual dose is 1 gram (1 tablet or 2 teaspoonfuls of suspension) 4 times a day on an empty stomach.

Although your ulcer may heal during the first 2 weeks of therapy, Carafate should be continued for 4 to 8 weeks.

*Maintenance Therapy:*
The usual dose is 1 gram (1 tablet) 2 times a day.

CHILDREN

The safety and effectiveness of Carafate in children have not been established.

### Overdosage
Although the risk of overdose with Carafate is low, any medication taken in excess can have serious consequences. If you suspect an overdose, seek medical attention immediately.

■ *Symptoms of overdose may include:*
  Abdominal pain, indigestion, nausea, vomiting

---

*Generic name:*

# Carbamazepine

*See Tegretol, page 525.*

---

*Generic name:*

# Carbidopa with Levodopa

*See Sinemet CR, page 500.*

---

*Brand name:*

# Cardene

*Pronounced: CAR-deen*
*Generic name: Nicardipine hydrochloride*

### Why is this drug prescribed?
Cardene, a type of medication called a calcium channel blocker, is prescribed for the treatment of chronic stable angina (chest pain usually caused by lack of oxygen to the heart resulting from clogged arteries, brought on by exertion) and for high blood pressure. When used to treat angina, Cardene is effective alone or in combination with beta-blocking medications such as Tenormin or Inderal. If it is used to treat high blood pressure, Cardene is effective alone or in combination with other high blood pressure medications. Calcium channel blockers ease the workload of the heart by slowing down its muscle contractions and the passage of nerve impulses through it. This improves blood flow through the heart and throughout the body, reducing blood pressure.

Cardene SR, a long-acting form of the drug, is prescribed only for high blood pressure.

Some doctors also prescribe Cardene to prevent migraine headache and to treat congestive heart failure. In combination with other drugs, such as Amicar, Cardene is also prescribed to manage neurological problems following certain kinds of stroke.

### Most important fact about this drug
If you have high blood pressure, you must take Cardene regularly for it to be effective. Since blood pressure declines gradually, it may be several weeks before you get the full benefit of Cardene and you must continue taking it even if you are feeling well. Cardene does not cure high blood pressure; it merely keeps it under control.

### How should you take this medication?
Take this medication exactly as prescribed, even if your symptoms have disappeared.

If you are taking Cardene SR, swallow the capsule whole; do not chew, crush, or divide it.

Try not to miss any doses. If Cardene is not taken regularly, your condition may worsen.

■ *If you miss a dose...*
  Take it as soon as you remember. If it is almost time for the next dose, skip the one you missed and go back to your regular schedule. Do not take 2 doses at the same time.
■ *Storage instructions...*
  Store at room temperature, away from light and moisture.

### What side effects may occur?
Side effects cannot be anticipated. If any develop or change in intensity, inform your doctor as soon as possible. Only your doctor can determine if it is safe for you to continue taking Cardene.

■ *More common side effects may include:*
  Dizziness, flushing, headache, increased chest pain (angina), indigestion, nausea, pounding or rapid heartbeat, sleepiness, swelling of feet, weakness
■ *Less common side effects may include:*
  Abnormal dreaming, constipation, difficulty sleeping, drowsiness, dry mouth, excessive night-

time urination, fainting, fluid retention, muscle pain, nervousness, rash, shortness of breath, tingling or pins and needles, tremors, vomiting, vague feeling of bodily discomfort

■ *Rare side effects may include:*
Allergic reactions, anxiety, blurred vision, confusion, dizziness when standing, depression, hot flashes, increased movements, infection, inflammation of the nose, inflammation of the sinuses, impotence, joint pain, low blood pressure, more frequent urination, ringing in ears, sore throat, unusual chest pain, vertigo, vision changes

## Why should this drug not be prescribed?

If you have advanced aortic stenosis (a narrowing of the aorta that causes obstruction of blood flow from the heart to the body), you should not take this medication.

If you are sensitive to or have ever had an allergic reaction to Cardene, you should not take this medication. Make sure your doctor is aware of any drug reactions you may have experienced.

## Special warnings about this medication

Cardene can reduce or eliminate chest (angina) pain caused by exertion or exercise. Be sure to discuss with your doctor how much exercise or exertion is safe for you.

If you experience increased chest pain when you start taking Cardene or when your dosage is increased, contact your doctor immediately.

Your doctor will monitor your progress especially carefully if you have congestive heart failure, particularly if you are also taking a beta-blocking medication such as Tenormin or Inderal.

Cardene can cause your blood pressure to become too low, making you feel light-headed or faint. Your doctor should check your blood pressure when you start taking Cardene and continue to monitor it while your dosage is being adjusted.

If you have liver disease or decreased liver function, use this drug with caution.

## Possible food and drug interactions when taking this medication

If Cardene is taken with certain other drugs, the effects of either could be increased, decreased, or altered. It is especially important to check with your doctor before combining Cardene with the following:

Amiodarone (Cordarone)
Cimetidine (Tagamet)
Cyclosporine (Sandimmune)
Digoxin (Lanoxin)
Phenytoin (Dilantin)
Propranolol (Inderal)

## Special information
## if you are pregnant or breastfeeding

The effects of Cardene during pregnancy have not been adequately studied. If you are pregnant or plan to become pregnant, inform your doctor immediately. Cardene may appear in breast milk and could affect a nursing infant. If this medication is essential to your health, your doctor may advise you to discontinue breastfeeding until your treatment with Cardene is finished.

## Recommended dosage

ADULTS

*Angina*
Your doctor will adjust the dosage according to your needs, usually beginning with 20 milligrams, 3 times a day. The usual regular dose is 20 to 40 milligrams, 3 times a day. Your physician may monitor your condition for at least 3 days before adjusting your dose.

*High Blood Pressure*
Your doctor will adjust the dosage to suit your needs. The starting dose of Cardene is usually 20 milligrams 3 times a day. The regular dose ranges from 20 to 40 milligrams 3 times a day.

The starting dose of Cardene SR is usually 30 milligrams 2 times a day. The regular dose ranges from 30 to 60 milligrams 2 times a day.

Your doctor may monitor your response to this medication for a few hours after the first dose, and will check your condition for at least 3 days before adjusting your dose.

CHILDREN

The safety and effectiveness of this drug in children under age 18 have not been established.

## Overdosage

■ *The symptoms of overdose may include:*
Confusion, drowsiness, severe low blood pressure, slow heartbeat, slurred speech

If you suspect a Cardene overdose, seek medical attention immediately.

*Brand name:*

# Cardizem

*Pronounced: CAR-di-zem*
*Generic name: Diltiazem hydrochloride*

### Why is this drug prescribed?

Cardizem and Cardizem CD (a controlled release form of diltiazem) are used in the treatment of angina pectoris (chest pain usually caused by lack of oxygen to the heart due to clogged arteries) and chronic stable angina (caused by exertion). Cardizem CD is also used to treat high blood pressure. Another controlled release form, Cardizem SR, is used only in the treatment of high blood pressure. Cardizem, a calcium channel blocker, dilates blood vessels and slows the heart to reduce blood pressure and the pain of angina.

Doctors sometimes prescribe Cardizem for loss of circulation in the fingers and toes (Raynaud's Syndrome), for involuntary movements (tardive dyskinesia), and to prevent heart attack.

### Most important fact about this drug

If you are taking Cardizem for high blood pressure, remember that it does not cure the problem; it merely controls it. You may need to take a blood pressure medication for the rest of your life.

If you are taking Cardizem for angina, do not stop suddenly. This can lead to an increase in your attacks.

### How should you take this medication?

Cardizem should be taken before meals and at bedtime. Cardizem CD and Cardizem SR should be swallowed whole; do not chew, crush, or divide.

Take this medication exactly as prescribed by your doctor, even if your symptoms have disappeared.

■ *If you miss a dose...*
If you forget to take a dose, take it as soon as you remember. If it's almost time for your next dose, skip the missed dose and go back to your regular schedule. Never take 2 doses at the same time.

■ *Storage instructions...*
Cardizem should be stored at room temperature.

### What side effects may occur?

Side effects cannot be anticipated. If any develop or change in intensity, inform your doctor as soon as possible. Only your doctor can determine if it is safe for you to continue taking Cardizem.

■ *More common side effects may include:*
Abnormally slow heartbeat (more common with Cardizem SR and Cardizem CD), dizziness, fluid retention, flushing (more common with Cardizem SR and Cardizem CD), headache, nausea, rash, weakness

■ *Less common or rare side effects may include:*
Abnormal dreams, amnesia, anemia, angina (severe chest pain), blood disorders, congestive heart failure, constipation, depression, diarrhea, difficulty sleeping, drowsiness, dry mouth, excessive urination at night, eye irritation, fainting, hair loss, hallucinations, heart attack, high blood sugar, hives, impotence, increased output of pale urine, indigestion, insomnia, irregular heartbeat, itching, joint pain, labored breathing, loss of appetite, low blood pressure, low blood sugar, muscle cramps, nasal congestion, nervousness, nosebleed, palpitations, personality change, rapid heartbeat, reddish or purplish spots on skin, ringing in ears, sexual difficulties, skin peeling, sensitivity to light, sleepiness, taste alteration, thirst, tingling or pins and needles, tremor, unusual gait, vision changes, vomiting, welts, weight increase

### Why should this drug not be prescribed?

If you suffer from "sick sinus" syndrome or second- or third-degree heart block (various types of irregular heartbeat), you should not take this drug unless you have a ventricular pacemaker.

Do not take Cardizem if you have low blood pressure or an allergy to the drug.

### Special warnings about this medication

If you have congestive heart failure or suffer from kidney or liver disease, use Cardizem with caution.

This medication may cause your heart rate to become too slow. You should check your pulse regularly.

### Possible food and drug interactions when taking this medication

If Cardizem is taken with certain other drugs, the effects of either could be increased, decreased, or altered. It is especially important to check with your doctor before combining Cardizem with the following:

Beta-blockers (heart and blood pressure drugs such as Tenormin and Inderal)
Carbamazepine (Tegretol)

Cimetidine (Tagamet)
Cyclosporine (Sandimmune, Neoral)
Digoxin (Lanoxin)

## Special information
## if you are pregnant or breastfeeding

The effects of Cardizem during pregnancy have not been adequately studied. If you are pregnant or plan to become pregnant, inform your doctor immediately. Cardizem appears in breast milk and could affect a nursing infant. If this medication is essential to your health, your doctor may advise you to discontinue breastfeeding until your treatment with this medication is finished.

## Recommended dosage

### ADULTS

Dosage levels are determined by each individual's needs. However, the average daily dosage is between 180 milligrams and 360 milligrams, divided into 3 or 4 smaller doses.

The recommended starting dosage for Cardizem SR is 60 to 120 milligrams 2 times a day to be increased to 240 to 360 milligrams a day. Cardizem CD is a once-a-day form of this drug. For hypertension, starting doses of Cardizem CD range from 180 to 240 milligrams; for angina, 120 to 180 milligrams.

### CHILDREN

Safety and effectiveness in children have not been established.

## Overdosage

Any medication taken in excess can cause overdose. If you suspect an overdose of Cardizem, seek medical attention immediately.

■ *The symptoms of Cardizem overdose may include:*
Fainting, dizziness, and irregular pulse, heart failure, low blood pressure, very slow heartbeat

*Brand name:*

# Cardura

*Pronounced: car-DUHR-uh*
*Generic name: Doxazosin mesylate*

## Why is this drug prescribed?

Cardura is used in the treatment of benign prostatic hyperplasia, a condition in which the prostate gland grows larger, pressing on the urethra and threatening to block the flow of urine from the bladder. The drug relieves symptoms such as a weak stream, dribbling, incomplete emptying of the bladder, frequent urination, and burning during urination.

Cardura is also used in the treatment of high blood pressure. It is effective when used alone or in combination with diuretics or beta-blocking medications.

Doctors also prescribe Cardura, along with other drugs such as digitalis and diuretics, for treatment of congestive heart failure.

## Most important fact about this drug

If you have high blood pressure, you must take Cardura regularly for it to be effective. Since blood pressure declines gradually, it may be several weeks before you get the full benefit of Cardura; and you must continue taking it even if you are feeling well. Cardura does not cure high blood pressure; it merely keeps it under control.

## How should you take this medication?

This medication can be taken with or without food.

Cardura should be taken exactly as prescribed, even if your symptoms have disappeared. Try not to miss any doses. If this medication is not taken regularly, your condition may worsen.

■ *If you miss a dose...*
Take it as soon as you remember. If it is almost time for your next dose, skip the one you missed and go back to your regular schedule. Never take 2 doses at the same time.
■ *Storage instructions...*
Store at room temperature.

## What side effects may occur?

Side effects cannot be anticipated. If any develop or change in intensity, inform your doctor as soon as possible. Only your doctor can determine if it is safe for you to continue taking Cardura.

■ *More common side effects may include:*
Dizziness, drowsiness, fatigue, headache
■ *Less common side effects may include:*
Arthritis, constipation, depression, difficulty sleeping, eye pain, flushing, gas, inability to hold urine or other urination problems, indigestion, inflammation of conjunctiva (pinkeye), itching, joint pain, lack of muscle coordination, low blood pressure, motion disorders, muscle cramps,

muscle pain, muscle weakness, nausea, nervousness, nosebleeds, rash, ringing in ears, shortness of breath, tingling or pins and needles, weakness

■ *Rare side effects may include:*
Abnormal thinking, abnormal vision, agitation, altered sense of smell, amnesia, back pain, breast pain, changeable emotions, changes in taste, chest pain, confusion, coughing, decreased sense of touch, diarrhea, dizziness when standing up, dry mouth, dry skin, earache, excessive urination, fainting, fecal incontinence, fever, fluid retention, flu-like symptoms, gout, hair loss, heart attack, hot flushes, inability to concentrate, inability to tolerate light, increased appetite, increased sweating, increased thirst, infection, inflammation of the nose, loss of appetite, loss of sense of personal identity, migraine headache, morbid dreams, nausea, nervousness, pain, pallor, rapid pounding heartbeat, sexual problems, sinus inflammation, slight or partial paralysis, sore throat, tremors, twitching, vertigo, weight gain, weight loss, wheezing

## Why should this drug not be prescribed?

Cardura should not be taken if you are sensitive to or have ever had an allergic reaction to Cardura or such drugs as Minipress or Hytrin. Make sure your doctor is aware of any drug reactions you may have experienced.

## Special warnings about this medication

Cardura can cause low blood pressure, especially when you first start taking the medication and when dosage is increased. This can cause you to become faint, dizzy, or light-headed, particularly when first standing up. You should avoid driving or any hazardous tasks where injury could occur for 24 hours after taking the first dose, after your dose has been increased, or if Cardura has been stopped and then restarted.

If you have liver disease or are taking other medications that alter liver function, your doctor will monitor you closely when you take Cardura.

Cardura may lower blood counts. Your doctor will most likely monitor your blood counts while you are taking this medication.

This medication may cause you to become drowsy or sleepy. For this reason, too, driving or operating dangerous machinery or participating in any hazardous activity that requires full mental alertness is not recommended.

Prostate cancer has some of the same symptoms as benign prostatic hyperplasia; your doctor will want to make sure you do not have cancer before starting you on Cardura.

## Possible food and drug interactions when taking this medication

No significant interactions have been reported.

## Special information if you are pregnant or breastfeeding

The effects of Cardura during pregnancy have not been adequately studied. If you are pregnant or plan to become pregnant, inform your doctor immediately. Cardura may appear in breast milk and could affect a nursing infant. If this medication is essential to your health, your doctor may advise you to discontinue breastfeeding until your treatment with this medication is finished.

## Recommended dosage

ADULTS

Your doctor will adjust the dosage to fit your needs.

The usual starting dose is 1 milligram taken once a day. To minimize the potential for dizziness or fainting associated with Cardura, which may occur between 2 and 6 hours after a dose, your doctor will monitor your blood pressure during this period and afterwards.

After the effects of the starting dose are measured, your doctor may increase the daily dose to 2 milligrams and then, if necessary, to 4 milligrams, 8 milligrams, or, in people with high blood pressure only, up to 16 milligrams. As the dose increases, the potential for side effects such as dizziness, vertigo, light-headedness, and fainting also increases.

CHILDREN

The safety and effectiveness of this drug in children have not been established.

## Overdosage

Any medication taken in excess can have serious consequences. Although no specific information is available, low blood pressure is the most likely symptom of an overdose of Cardura.

If you suspect an overdose, seek medical attention immediately.

*Generic name:*

# Carisoprodol

*See Soma, page 505.*

*Brand name:*

# Cataflam

*See Voltaren, page 590.*

*Brand name:*

# Catapres

Pronounced: KAT-uh-press
Generic name: Clonidine hydrochloride

## Why is this drug prescribed?

Catapres is prescribed for high blood pressure. It is effective when used alone or with other high blood pressure medications.

Doctors also prescribe Catapres for alcohol, nicotine, or benzodiazepine (tranquilizer) withdrawal; migraine headaches; smoking cessation programs; Tourette's syndrome (tics and uncontrollable utterances); narcotic/methadone detoxification; premenstrual tension; and diabetic diarrhea.

## Most important fact about this drug

If you have high blood pressure, you must take Catapres regularly for it to be effective. Since blood pressure declines gradually, it may be several weeks before you get the full benefit of Catapres; and you must continue taking it even if you are feeling well. Catapres does not cure high blood pressure; it merely keeps it under control.

## How should you take this medication?

Take this medication exactly as prescribed, even if you are feeling well.

Try not to miss any doses. If Catapres is not taken regularly, your condition may worsen.

■ *If you miss a dose...*
  Take it as soon as you remember, then go back to your regular schedule. If you forget to take the medication 2 or more times in a row, or if you forget to change the transdermal patch for 3 or more days, contact your doctor.
■ *Storage instructions...*
  Store at room temperature in a tightly closed container away from light.

## What side effects may occur?

Side effects cannot be anticipated. If any develop or change in intensity, inform your doctor as soon as possible. Only your doctor can determine if it is safe for you to continue taking Catapres.

■ *More common side effects may include:*
  Constipation, dizziness, drowsiness, dry mouth, sedation (calm), skin reactions (Catapres-TTS)
■ *Less common side effects may include:*
  Agitation, breast development in males, changes in heartbeat, changes in taste, decreased sexual activity, difficulty sleeping, difficulty urinating, dizziness on standing up, excessive nighttime urination, fatigue, fluid retention, hair loss, headache, hives, impotence, itching, joint pain, leg cramps, loss of appetite, loss of sexual drive, mental depression, muscle pain, nausea, nervousness, rash, retention of urine, sluggishness, vague bodily discomfort, vomiting, weakness, weight gain
■ *Rare side effects may include:*
  Anxiety, behavior changes, blurred vision, burning eyes, congestive heart failure, delirium, dry eyes, dry nasal passages, fever, greater sensitivity to alcohol, hallucinations, hepatitis, pallor, restlessness, vivid dreams or nightmares

## Why should this drug not be prescribed?

Do not take this medication if you have ever had an allergic reaction to Catapres or to any of the components of the adhesive layer of the transdermal patch.

## Special warnings about this medication

Catapres should not be stopped suddenly. Headache, nervousness, agitation, and rapid rise in blood pressure can occur. Severe reactions such as disruption of brain functions and death have also been reported. Your doctor should therefore gradually reduce your dosage over several days to avoid withdrawal symptoms.

If your doctor has switched you to oral Catapres (tablet) because you had an allergic reaction, such as a rash or hives, to the transdermal skin patch, be aware that you may have a similar reaction to the Catapres tablet.

If you have severe heart or kidney disease, are recovering from a heart attack, or have a disease of the blood vessels of the brain, your doctor will prescribe Catapres with caution.

If you are taking Catapres and a beta blocker such as Inderal or Tenormin, and your doctor wants to stop your medication, the beta blocker should be stopped several days before the gradual withdrawal of Catapres.

Catapres may cause you to become drowsy or less alert; therefore, you should avoid driving, operating dangerous machinery, or participating in any hazardous activity that requires full mental alertness.

### Possible food and drug interactions when taking this medication

Catapres may increase the effects of alcohol. Do not drink alcohol while taking this medication.

If Catapres is taken with certain other drugs, the effects of either could be increased, decreased, or altered. It is especially important to check with your doctor before combining Catapres with the following:

Barbiturates such as Nembutal and Seconal
Sedatives such as Valium, Xanax, and Halcion
Tricyclic antidepressants such as Elavil and Tofranil

### Special information if you are pregnant or breastfeeding

The effects of Catapres during pregnancy have not been adequately studied. If you are pregnant or plan to become pregnant, inform your doctor immediately. Catapres appears in breast milk and could affect a nursing infant. If this medication is essential to your health, your doctor may advise you to discontinue breastfeeding until your treatment with this medication is finished.

### Recommended dosage

ADULTS

The dosage will be adjusted to your individual needs.

The usual starting dose is 0.1 milligram, twice a day (usually in the morning and at bedtime).

The regular dose of Catapres is determined by increasing the starting dose by 0.1 milligram per day until the desired response is achieved. A larger portion of the increased dose can be taken at bedtime to reduce potential side effects of drowsiness and dry mouth that may appear when you begin taking this drug.

The most common effective dosages range from 0.2 milligram to 0.6 milligram per day divided into smaller doses. The maximum effective dose is 2.4 milligrams per day; however, this dose is not usually prescribed.

*Transdermal Patch*
The patch comes in different strengths, and your doctor will determine which is best for you based on your blood pressure response.

People who are using another high blood pressure medication should not stop taking it abruptly when they begin using the patch, because the medication in the patch may take a few days to work. The other medication should be discontinued slowly as the patch begins to work.

The Catapres-TTS patch should be put on a hairless, clean area of the upper arm or body. Normally, a new one is applied every 7 days to a new area of the skin. If the patch becomes loose, use some adhesive tape or an adhesive bandage to keep it in place.

CHILDREN

Safety and effectiveness of Catapres in children have not been established. Safety of Catapres-TTS has not been established in children under 12.

OLDER ADULTS

Dosages are generally as above; however, the initial dosage for an older person may be lower than the regular starting dose.

### Overdosage

■ *Symptoms of Catapres overdose may include:*
Changes in heart function, constriction of pupils of the eye, high blood pressure, irritability, low blood pressure, reduced rate of breathing, seizures, sleepiness, slow heartbeat, slowed reflexes, sluggishness, temporary failure to breathe, vomiting, weakness

If you suspect symptoms of a Catapres overdose, seek medical attention immediately.

*Brand name:*

# Caverject

*Pronounced: CA-vur-jekt*
*Generic name: Alprostadil*

### Why is this drug prescribed?

Caverject is used to treat male impotence. Your doctor also may use Caverject to help diagnose the exact nature of your impotence.

## Most important fact about this drug

Caverject is known to have caused extremely long-lasting erections. Serious harm can occur from such a prolonged erection, so call your doctor or seek other professional help if an erection lasts more than 6 hours. Usually the erection should last about 1 hour.

## How should you use this medication?

Caverject is injected into a specific area of the penis and produces an erection within 5 to 20 minutes. Do not use Caverject more than 3 times a week. Wait at least 24 hours between use.

The first injections are performed by your doctor in the doctor's office in order to determine the proper dosage. Afterwards, you can inject Caverject yourself as needed. Your doctor will train you in the proper technique for injecting Caverject and you'll be given complete printed instructions. Follow these directions exactly and do not change the dose your doctor has determined.

Do not use a Caverject solution that appears cloudy or colored or that contains particles. Do not shake the vial.

Wash your hands thoroughly and do not touch the needle. Carefully choose the injection site as instructed by your doctor, always avoiding visible veins. Cleanse the site with an alcohol swab. With each use, alternate the side of the penis and the site of the injection.

Use the needle/syringe and vial only once, then discard them properly. Do not share needles or allow anyone else to use your medication.

Caverject comes in both 10 microgram and 20 microgram strengths. Make sure you are using a vial with the correct strength.

■ *Storage instructions...*
Store unused packs of Caverject at room temperature for up to 3 months. Protect from freezing or from overheating.

Once the Caverject solution is mixed, you must use it immediately or discard it.

When traveling, take care to prevent exposing Caverject to freezing or excessive heat. Do not store Caverject in checked luggage or leave it in a closed car.

## What side effects may occur?

Side effects cannot be anticipated. If any develop or change in intensity, inform your doctor as soon as possible. Only your doctor can determine if it is safe for you to continue using Caverject.

The most common side effect is mild to moderate pain in the penis after injection, reported by about one-third of users. A small amount of bleeding may occur at the injection site. Notify your doctor if you have a condition or are taking a medication that interferes with blood clotting. As with any injection, the site can become infected. Call your doctor if you notice any redness, lumps, swelling, tenderness, or curving of the erect penis.

Your doctor should examine your penis regularly if you use Caverject. Use of Caverject may result in formation of fibrous (hardened) tissue in the penis or erections at an unusual angle. If those side effects occur, inform your doctor and stop using Caverject.

■ *More common side effects may include:*
Blood-filled swelling at the site of injection, disorder of the penis (such as discoloration of the head, strange feeling, tearing of the skin), hardened tissue in the penis, pain in the penis, prolonged erection, upper respiratory infection

■ *Less common side effects may include:*
Back pain, bruising at the injection site, cough, dizziness, flu symptoms, headache, high blood pressure, inflamed or enlarged prostate, injuries/fractures/abrasions/lacerations/dislocations, nasal congestion, pain, sinus inflammation

■ *Rare side effects may include:*
Abnormal ejaculation, bleeding at the urethra, blood in the urine, dry mouth, extreme dilation of the pupils, fluid retention at the injection site, frequent or urgent urination, hemorrhage at the injection site, impaired urination, inflammation, irritation, itching, lack of sensation, leg cramps, low blood pressure, nausea, numbness, painful erection, pelvic pain, profuse sweating, rash on the penis, redness, sensitivity, swelling at the injection site, swelling of the head of the penis, swelling of the scrotum, testicular pain, tightness of the foreskin, warmth, weakness, yeast infection

## Why should this drug not be prescribed?

Do not use Caverject if you have a condition that might result in long-lasting erections, such as sickle cell anemia, leukemia, and tumor of the bone marrow.

Men with penile implants or an unusually formed penis should not use Caverject. The drug is not for use in women, children, or men whose doctors have advised them not to have sex.

Do not use Caverject if it causes an allergic reaction.

### Special warnings about this medication

Caverject offers no protection from the transmission of sexually transmitted diseases, such as HIV, the virus that causes AIDS. Small amounts of bleeding at the injection site can increase the risk of transmission of blood-borne diseases such as HIV.

### Possible food and drug interactions when using this medication

No interactions have been reported, but Caverject should not be used with other drugs that act on blood vessels.

You may have some bleeding at the site of injection. If you are taking anticoagulants, you may bleed more after you inject Caverject.

### Recommended dosage

The correct dose of Caverject must be carefully determined by your doctor. Each man will need a different dose of Caverject, but the usual starting dosage is 1.25 or 2.5 micrograms, which is then increased gradually. Your doctor will adjust the dosage, particularly if it produces erections lasting longer than 1 hour.

Do not change your dosage of Caverject without your doctor's approval.

See your doctor every 3 months for a checkup.

### Overdosage

No overdose of Caverject has been reported. However, any medication taken in excess can have serious consequences. If you suspect an overdose, seek medical attention immediately.

---

*Brand name:*

# Ceclor

*Pronounced: SEE-klor*
*Generic name: Cefaclor*

### Why is this drug prescribed?

Ceclor, a cephalosporin antibiotic, is used in the treatment of ear, nose, throat, respiratory tract, urinary tract, and skin infections caused by specific

bacteria, including staph, strep, and *E. coli*. Uses include treatment of sore or strep throat, pneumonia, and tonsillitis.

### Most important fact about this drug

If you are allergic to either penicillin or cephalosporin antibiotics in any form, consult your doctor *before taking* Ceclor. There is a possibility that you are allergic to both types of medication; and if a reaction occurs, it could be extremely severe. If you take the drug and feel signs of a reaction, seek medical attention immediately.

### How should you take this medication?

Take this medication exactly as prescribed. It is important that you finish taking all of this medication to obtain the maximum benefit.

This medication works fastest when taken on an empty stomach. However, your doctor may ask you to take this drug with food to avoid stomach upset.

Ceclor suspension should be shaken well before using.

■ *If you miss a dose...*
Take it as soon as you remember. If it is almost time for your next dose, skip the one you missed and go back to your regular schedule. Never take 2 doses at the same time.

■ *Storage instructions...*
Keep Ceclor capsules in the container they came in, tightly closed. Store at room temperature.

Refrigerate Ceclor suspension. Discard any unused portion after 14 days.

### What side effects may occur?

Side effects cannot be anticipated. If any develop or change in intensity, inform your doctor as soon as possible. Only your doctor can determine if it is safe for you to continue taking Ceclor.

■ *More common side effects may include:*
Diarrhea, hives, itching

■ *Less common or rare side effects may include:*
Blood disorders (an increase in certain types of white blood cells), liver disorders, nausea, severe allergic reactions (including swelling, weakness, breathing difficulty, or fainting), skin rashes accompanied by joint pain, vaginal inflammation, vomiting

Other problems have been reported in patients taking Ceclor, although it is not known whether the drug was the cause. Check with your doctor if you suspect a side effect.

## Why should this drug not be prescribed?

If you are sensitive to or have ever had an allergic reaction to Ceclor or any other cephalosporin antibiotic, you should not take this medication. Make sure your doctor is aware of any drug reactions you have experienced.

Unless you are directed to do so by your doctor, do not take this medication if you have a history of gastrointestinal problems, particularly bowel inflammation (colitis). You may be at increased risk for side effects.

## Special warnings about this medication

Ceclor may cause a false positive result with some urine sugar tests for diabetics. Your doctor can advise you of any adjustments you may need to make in your medication or diet.

Ceclor occasionally causes diarrhea. Some diarrhea medications can make this diarrhea worse. Check with your doctor before taking any diarrhea remedy.

Oral contraceptives may not work properly while you are taking Ceclor. For greater certainty, use other measures while taking Ceclor.

## Possible food and drug interactions when taking this medication

If Ceclor is taken with certain other drugs, the effects of either could be increased, decreased, or altered. It is especially important to check with your doctor before combining Ceclor with the following:

Certain antibiotics such as Amikin
Certain potent diuretics such as Edecrin and Lasix
Probenecid (Benemid)

## Special information if you are pregnant or breastfeeding

The effects of Ceclor during pregnancy have not been adequately studied. If you are pregnant or plan to become pregnant, this drug should be used only when prescribed by your doctor. Ceclor appears in breast milk and could affect a nursing infant. If this medication is essential to your health, your doctor may advise you to stop nursing your baby until your treatment with Ceclor is finished.

## Recommended dosage

### ADULTS

The usual adult dose is 250 milligrams every 8 hours. For more severe infections (such as pneumonia), your doctor may increase the dosage.

### CHILDREN

The usual daily dosage is 20 milligrams per 2.2 pounds of body weight per day divided into smaller doses and taken every 8 hours. In more serious infections, such as middle ear infection, the usual dose is 40 milligrams per 2.2 pounds of body weight per day divided into smaller doses. The total daily dose should not exceed 1 gram.

## Overdosage

■ *Symptoms of Ceclor overdose may include:*
Diarrhea, nausea, stomach upset, vomiting

If other symptoms are present, they may be related to an allergic reaction or other underlying disease. In any case, you should contact your doctor or an emergency room immediately.

*Generic name:*

# Cefaclor

*See Ceclor, page 86.*

*Generic name:*

# Cefadroxil

*See Duricef, page 179.*

*Generic name:*

# Cefixime

*See Suprax, page 512.*

*Generic name:*

# Cefprozil

*See Cefzil, page 89.*

*Brand name:*

# Ceftin

*Pronounced: SEF-tin*
*Generic name: Cefuroxime axetil*

## Why is this drug prescribed?

Ceftin, a cephalosporin antibiotic, is prescribed for mild to moderately severe bacterial infections of the throat, lungs, ears, skin, and urinary tract, and for gonorrhea.

## Most important fact about this drug

If you are allergic to either penicillin or cephalosporin antibiotics such as Ceclor, Cefzil, or Keflex, consult your doctor *before taking* Ceftin. There is a possibility that you are allergic to both types of medication; if a reaction occurs, it could be extremely severe. If you take the drug and develop shortness of breath, a pounding heartbeat, a skin rash, or hives, seek medical attention immediately.

## How should you take this medication?

Ceftin tablets can be taken on a full or empty stomach. However, this drug enters the bloodstream and works faster when taken after meals. Ceftin oral suspension must be taken with food. Shake the suspension well before each use.

Take this medication exactly as prescribed: It is important that you finish taking all of this medication to obtain the maximum benefit.

The crushed tablet has a strong, persistent, bitter taste. Children who cannot swallow the tablet whole should take the oral suspension. Shake the oral suspension well before each use.

■ *If you miss a dose...*
Take it as soon as you remember. If it is almost time for your next dose skip the one you missed and go back to the regular schedule. Do not take 2 doses at once.

■ *Storage instructions...*
Store tablets at room temperature in a tightly closed container. Protect from moisture. The oral suspension may be stored either in the refrigerator or at room temperature. Replace the cap securely after each use. Discard any unused suspension after 10 days.

## What side effects may occur?

Side effects cannot be anticipated. If any develop or change in intensity, inform your doctor as soon as possible. Only your doctor can determine if it is safe for you to continue taking Ceftin.

■ *More common side effects may include:*
Diaper rash in infants, diarrhea, nausea, vomiting
■ *Rare side effects of the tablets include:*
Abdominal pain or cramps, chest pain, chills, gas, headache, hives, indigestion, itch, loss of appetite, mouth ulcers, rash, shortness of breath, sleepiness, swollen tongue, thirst, urinary problems, vaginitis
■ *Rare side effects of the oral suspension include:*
Abdominal pain, cough, drooling, fever, gas, gastrointestinal infection, hyperactivity, inflamed sinuses, irritability, joint pain and swelling, rash, upper respiratory infection, urinary infection, vaginal irritation, virus infection, yeast infection

## Why should this drug not be prescribed?

Ceftin should not be prescribed if you have a known allergy to cephalosporin antibiotics.

## Special warnings about this medication

Inflammation of the bowel (colitis) has been reported with the use of Ceftin; therefore, if you develop diarrhea while taking this medication, notify your doctor.

Continued or prolonged use of Ceftin may result in an overgrowth of bacteria that do not respond to this medication and can cause a second infection. You should take this drug only when it is prescribed by your doctor, even if you have symptoms like those of a previous infection. Tell your doctor if you have any kidney problems. Your dosage may need to be lowered.

If you are allergic to Penicillin you may also be allergic to Ceftin. Make sure your doctor is aware of any allergies you have.

## Possible food and drug interactions when taking this medication

It is important to consult your doctor before taking this drug with probenecid, (Benemid), a gout medication.

If diarrhea occurs while taking Ceftin, consult your doctor before taking an antidiarrhea medication. Certain drugs, such as Lomotil, may cause your diarrhea to become worse.

Be cautious if you are taking potent water pills (diuretics) such as Lasix while on Ceftin. The combination could affect your kidneys.

## Special information if you are pregnant or breastfeeding

The effects of Ceftin during pregnancy have not been adequately studied. If you are pregnant or plan to become pregnant, inform your doctor immediately. Ceftin appears in breast milk and could affect a nursing infant. If this medication is essential to your health, your doctor may advise you to discontinue breastfeeding until your treatment with this medication is finished.

### Recommended dosage

ADULTS

The usual dose for adults and children 13 years and older is 250 milligrams, 2 times a day for 10 days. For more severe infections the dose may be increased to 500 milligrams, 2 times a day.

The usual dose for urinary tract infection is 125 milligrams, 2 times a day for 7 to 10 days. This dose may be increased to 250 milligrams 2 times a day for severe infection.

The usual dosage for gonorrhea is a single dose of 1 gram.

CHILDREN

Ceftin oral suspension may be given to children ranging in age from 3 months to 12 years.

Your doctor will determine the dosage based on your child's weight and the type of infection being treated. Ceftin oral suspension is given twice a day for 10 days. The maximum daily dose ranges from 500 to 1000 milligrams.

### Overdosage

Any medication taken in excess can have serious consequences. Overdosage with cephalosporin antibiotics can cause brain irritation leading to convulsions. If you suspect an overdose, seek medical attention immediately.

*Generic name:*

# Cefuroxime

*See Ceftin, page 87.*

*Brand name:*

# Cefzil

*Pronounced: SEFF-zil*
*Generic name: Cefprozil*

### Why is this drug prescribed?

Cefzil, a cephalosporin antibiotic, is prescribed for mild to moderately severe bacterial infections of the throat, ear, respiratory tract, and skin. Among these infections are strep throat, tonsillitis, bronchitis, and pneumonia.

### Most important fact about this drug

If you are allergic to either penicillin or cephalosporin antibiotics in any form, consult your doctor *before taking* Cefzil. There is a possibility that you are allergic to both types of medication; and if a reaction occurs, it could be extremely severe. If you take the drug and feel signs of a reaction, seek medical attention immediately.

### How should you use this medication?

Take this medication exactly as prescribed. It is important that you finish all of the medication to obtain the maximum benefit.

Cefzil works fastest when taken on an empty stomach, but can be taken with food to avoid stomach upset.

Cefzil oral suspension should be shaken well before using.

■ *If you miss a dose...*
Take it as soon as you remember. If it is almost time for your next dose, skip the one you missed and go back to your regular schedule. Never take 2 doses at the same time.

■ *Storage instructions...*
Store Cefzil tablets at room temperature. Keep the oral suspension in the refrigerator; discard any unused portion after 14 days.

### What side effects may occur?

Side effects cannot be anticipated. If any develop or change in intensity, notify your doctor as soon as possible. Only your doctor can determine whether it is safe for you to continue taking Cefzil.

The most common side effect is nausea.

■ *Less common or rare side effects may include:*
Abdominal pain, confusion, diaper rash, diarrhea, difficulty sleeping, dizziness, genital itching, headache, hives, hyperactivity, nervousness, rash, sleepiness, superinfection (additional infection), vaginal inflammation, vomiting, yellow eyes and skin

Although not reported for Cefzil, similar antibiotics have been known occasionally to have severe side effects such as anaphylaxis (a severe allergic reaction), skin rash with blisters, Stevens-Johnson syndrome (a rare skin condition characterized by severe blisters and bleeding in the lips, eyes, mouth, nose, and genitals), and "serum-sickness" (itchy rash, fever, and pain in the joints).

### Why should this drug not be prescribed?

If you are sensitive to or have ever had an allergic reaction to Cefzil or other cephalosporin antibiotics, do not take this medication. Make sure your doctor is aware of any drug reactions you have experienced.

### Special warnings about this medication

Cefzil occasionally causes colitis (inflammation of the bowel) leading to diarrhea. Some diarrhea medications can make this diarrhea worse. Check with your doctor before taking any diarrhea remedy.

Oral contraceptives may not work properly while you are taking Cefzil. For greater certainty, use other measures while taking Cefzil.

Your doctor will check your kidney function before and during your treatment with this medication.

Use Cefzil with caution if you are taking a strong diuretic, or if you have ever had stomach and intestinal disease, particularly colitis.

If new infections (called superinfections) occur, talk to your doctor. You may need to be treated with a different antibiotic.

Cefzil may alter the results of some urine sugar tests for diabetics. Your doctor can advise you of any adjustments you may need to make in your medication or diet.

### Possible food and drug interactions when taking this medication

When Cefzil is taken with certain other drugs, the effects of either could be increased, decreased, or altered. It is especially important to check with your doctor before combining Cefzil with the following:

Certain other antibiotics such as Amikin
Certain potent diuretics such as Edecrin and Lasix
Oral contraceptives
Probenecid (Benemid)
Propantheline (Pro-Banthine)

### Special information if you are pregnant or breastfeeding

The effects of Cefzil during pregnancy have not been adequately studied. If you are pregnant or plan to become pregnant, inform your doctor immediately. Cefzil may appear in breast milk and could affect a nursing infant. If this medication is essential to your health, your doctor may advise you to stop breastfeeding until your treatment with this medication is finished.

### Recommended dosage

ADULTS

*Throat and Respiratory Tract Infections*
The usual dose is 500 milligrams, taken once or twice a day for 10 days.

*Skin Infections*
The dosage is usually either 250 milligrams taken 2 times a day, or 500 milligrams taken once or twice a day for 10 days.

CHILDREN 2 TO 12 YEARS OF AGE

*Throat Infections and Tonsillitis*
The usual dose is 7.5 milligrams for each 2.2 pounds of body weight, taken 2 times a day for 10 days.

INFANTS AND CHILDREN 6 MONTHS TO 12 YEARS OF AGE

*Ear Infections*
The usual dose is 15 milligrams for each 2.2 pounds of body weight, taken 2 times a day for 10 days.

INFANTS UNDER 6 MONTHS OF AGE

The safety and effectiveness of Cefzil in children below the age of 6 months have not been established.

### Overdosage

Although no specific information is available, any medication taken in excess can have serious consequences. If you suspect an overdose of Cefzil, seek medical attention immediately.

*Brand name:*

# Centrum

*See Multivitamins, page 341.*

*Generic name:*

# Cephalexin

*See Keflex, page 266.*

Generic name:
# Chlordiazepoxide
*See Librium, page 282.*

Generic name:
# Chlordiazepoxide with Clidinium
*See Librax, page 280.*

Generic name:
# Chlorhexidine
*See Peridex, page 410.*

Generic name:
# Chlorothiazide
*See Diuril, page 171.*

Generic name:
# Chlorpheniramine with Pseudoephedrine
*See Deconamine, page 141.*

Generic name:
# Chlorpromazine
*See Thorazine, page 541.*

Generic name:
# Chlorpropamide
*See Diabinese, page 155.*

Generic name:
# Chlorthalidone
*See Hygroton, page 242.*

Generic name:
# Chlorzoxazone
*See Parafon Forte DSC, page 394.*

Generic name:
# Cholestyramine
*See Questran, page 454.*

Generic name:
# Choline magnesium trisalicylate
*See Trilisate, page 564.*

Brand name:
# Chronulac Syrup

*Pronounced: KRON-yoo-lak*
*Generic name: Lactulose*
*Other brand name: Duphalac*

### Why is this drug prescribed?
Chronulac treats constipation. In people who are chronically constipated, Chronulac increases the number and frequency of bowel movements.

### Most important fact about this drug
It may take 24 to 48 hours to produce a normal bowel movement.

### How should you take this medication?
Take this medication exactly as prescribed. If you find the taste of Chronulac unpleasant, it can be taken with water, fruit juice, or milk.

■ *If you miss a dose...*
  Take the forgotten dose as soon as you remember; but do not try to "catch up" by taking a double dose.
■ *Storage instructions...*
  Store at room temperature. Avoid excessive heat or direct light. The liquid may darken in color, which is normal.

### What side effects may occur?
Side effects cannot be anticipated. If any develop or change in intensity, inform your doctor as soon as possible. Only your doctor can determine if it is safe for you to continue taking Chronulac.

■ *Side effects may include:*
  Diarrhea, gas (temporary, at the beginning of use), intestinal cramps (temporary, at the beginning of use), nausea, potassium and fluid loss, vomiting

### Why should this drug not be prescribed?

Chronulac contains galactose, a simple sugar. If you are on a low-galactose diet, do not take this medication.

### Special warnings about this medication

Because of its sugar content, this medication should be used with caution if you have diabetes.

If unusual diarrhea occurs, contact your doctor.

### Possible food and drug interactions when taking this medication

If Chronulac is taken with certain other drugs, the effects of either could be increased, decreased, or altered. It is especially important to check with your doctor before combining Chronulac with non-absorbable antacids such as Maalox and Mylanta.

### Special information if you are pregnant or breastfeeding

The effects of Chronulac during pregnancy have not been adequately studied. If you are pregnant or plan to become pregnant, inform your doctor immediately. Chronulac may appear in breast milk and could affect a nursing infant. If this medication is essential to your health, your doctor may advise you to stop breastfeeding until your treatment is finished.

### Recommended dosage

The usual dose is 1 to 2 tablespoonfuls (15 to 30 milliliters) daily. Your doctor may increase the dose to 60 milliliters a day, if necessary.

### Overdosage

Any medication taken in excess can have serious consequences. If you suspect an overdose, seek medical treatment immediately.

■ *Symptoms of Chronulac overdose may include:*
  Abdominal cramps, diarrhea

*Brand name:*

# Cibalith-S

See Lithonate, page 285.

*Generic name:*

# Ciclopirox

See Loprox, page 293.

*Generic name:*

# Cimetidine

See Tagamet, page 518.

*Brand name:*

# Cipro

*Pronounced: SIP-roh*
*Generic name: Ciprofloxacin hydrochloride*

### Why is this drug prescribed?

Cipro is used to treat infections of the lower respiratory tract, the skin, the bones and joints, and the urinary tract. It is also prescribed for infectious diarrhea, typhoid fever, and some sexually transmitted diseases; some doctors also prescribe Cipro for certain serious ear infections, tuberculosis, and some of the infections common in people with AIDS.

Because Cipro is effective only for certain types of bacterial infections, before beginning treatment your doctor may perform tests to identify the specific organisms causing your infection.

### Most important fact about this drug

Cipro kills a variety of bacteria, and is frequently used to treat infections in many parts of the body. However, be sure to notify your doctor immediately at the first sign of a skin rash or any other allergic reaction. Although quite rare, serious and occasionally fatal allergic reactions—some following the first dose—have been reported in people receiving this type of antibacterial drug. Some reactions have been accompanied by collapse of the circulatory system, loss of consciousness, swelling of the face and throat, shortness of breath, tingling, itching, and hives.

### How should you take this medication?

Cipro may be taken with or without meals but is best tolerated when taken 2 hours after a meal.

Drink plenty of fluids while taking this medication.

Cipro, like other antibiotics, works best when there is a constant amount in the blood and urine. To help keep the level constant, try not to miss any doses, and take them at evenly spaced intervals around the clock.

■ *If you miss a dose...*
Take it as soon as you remember. If it is almost time for your next dose, skip the one you missed and go back to your regular schedule. Never take 2 doses at the same time.

■ *Storage instructions...*
Cipro should be stored at room temperature.

## What side effects may occur?

Side effects cannot be anticipated. If any develop or change in intensity, inform your doctor as soon as possible. Only your doctor can determine if it is safe for you to continue taking Cipro.

■ *Most common side effect:*
Nausea

■ *Less common side effects may include:*
Abdominal pain/discomfort, diarrhea, headache, rash, restlessness, vomiting

■ *Rare side effects may include:*
Abnormal dread or fear, achiness, bleeding in the stomach and/or intestines, blood clots in the lungs, blurred vision, change in color perception, chills, confusion, constipation, convulsions, coughing up blood, decreased vision, depression, difficulty in swallowing, dizziness, double vision, drowsiness, eye pain, fainting, fever, flushing, gas, gout flare up, hallucinations, hearing loss, heart attack, hiccups, high blood pressure, hives, inability to fall or stay asleep, inability to urinate, indigestion, intestinal inflammation, involuntary eye movement, irregular heartbeat, irritability, itching, joint or back pain, joint stiffness, kidney failure, labored breathing, lack of muscle coordination, lack or loss of appetite, large volumes of urine, light-headedness, loss of sense of identity, loss of sense of smell, mouth sores, neck pain, nightmares, nosebleed, pounding heartbeat, ringing in the ears, seizures, sensitivity to light, severe allergic reaction, skin peeling, redness, sluggishness, speech difficulties, swelling of the face, neck, lips, eyes, or hands, swelling of the throat, tender, red bumps on skin, tingling sensation, tremors, unpleasant taste, unusual darkening of the skin, vaginal inflammation, vague feeling of illness, weakness, yellowed eyes and skin

## Why should this drug not be prescribed?

If you are sensitive to or have ever had an allergic reaction to Cipro or certain other antibiotics of this type, you should not take this medication. Make sure that your doctor is aware of any drug reactions that you have experienced.

## Special warnings about this medication

Cipro may cause you to become dizzy or lightheaded; therefore, you should not drive a car, operate dangerous machinery, or participate in any hazardous activity that requires full mental alertness until you know how the drug affects you.

Continued or prolonged use of this drug may result in a growth of bacteria that do not respond to this medication and can cause a secondary infection. Therefore, it is important that your doctor monitor your condition on a regular basis.

Convulsions have been reported in people receiving Cipro. If you experience a seizure or convulsion, notify your doctor immediately.

This medication may stimulate the central nervous system, which may lead to tremors, restlessness, light-headedness, confusion, and hallucinations. If these reactions occur, consult your doctor at once.

If you have a known or suspected central nervous system disorder such as epilepsy or hardening of the arteries in the brain, make sure your doctor knows about it when prescribing Cipro.

You may become more sensitive to light while taking this drug. Try to stay out of the sun as much as possible.

If you must take Cipro for an extended period of time, your doctor will probably order blood tests and tests for urine, kidney, and liver function.

## Possible food and drug interactions when taking this medication

Serious and fatal reactions have occurred when Cipro was taken in combination with theophylline (Theo-Dur). These reactions have included cardiac arrest, seizures, status epilepticus (continuous attacks of epilepsy with no periods of consciousness), and respiratory failure.

Products containing iron, multi-vitamins containing zinc, or antacids containing magnesium, aluminum, or calcium, when taken in combination with Cipro, may interfere with absorption of this medication.

Cipro may increase the effects of caffeine.

If Cipro is taken with certain other drugs, the effects of either could be increased, decreased, or altered. These drugs include:

Cyclophosphamide (Cytoxan)
Cyclosporine (Sandimmune, Neoral)
Glyburide (DiaBeta, Glynase, Micronase)
Metoprolol (Lopressor)
Phenytoin (Dilantin)
Probenecid (Benemid)
Sucralfate (Carafate)
Theophylline (Theo-Dur)
Warfarin (Coumadin)

### Special information
### if you are pregnant or breastfeeding

The effects of Cipro during pregnancy have not been adequately studied. If you are pregnant or plan to become pregnant, notify your doctor immediately. Cipro does appear in breast milk and could affect a nursing infant. If this medication is essential to your health, your doctor may advise you to discontinue breastfeeding your baby until your treatment is finished.

### Recommended dosage

ADULTS

The length of treatment with Cipro depends upon the severity of infection. Generally, Cipro should be continued for at least 2 days after the signs and symptoms of infection have disappeared. The usual length of time is 7 to 14 days; however, for severe and complicated infections, treatment may be prolonged.

Bone and joint infections may require treatment for 4 to 6 weeks or longer.

Infectious diarrhea may be treated for 5 to 7 days.

Typhoid fever should be treated for 10 days.

*Urinary Tract Infections*
The usual adult dosage is 250 milligrams taken every 12 hours. Complicated infections, as determined by your doctor, may require 500 milligrams taken every 12 hours.

*Lower Respiratory Tract, Skin, Bone, and Joint Infections*
The usual recommended dosage is 500 milligrams taken every 12 hours. Complicated infections, as determined by your doctor, may require a dosage of 750 milligrams taken every 12 hours.

*Infectious Diarrhea, Typhoid Fever*
The recommended dosage is 500 milligrams taken every 12 hours.

*Uncomplicated Urethral and Cervical Gonococcal Infections*
For these sexually transmitted diseases, a single 250-milligram dose is the usual treatment.

CHILDREN

Safety and effectiveness have not been established in children and adolescents under 18 years of age.

### Overdosage

Any medication taken in excess can have serious consequences. If you suspect an overdose, seek medical attention immediately.

*Generic name:*
# Ciprofloxacin

*See Cipro, page 92.*

*Generic name:*
# Cisapride

*See Propulsid, page 442.*

*Generic name:*
# Clarithromycin

*See Biaxin, page 62.*

*Brand name:*
# Claritin

*Pronounced: CLAR-i-tin*
*Generic name: Loratadine*

### Why is this drug prescribed?

Claritin is an antihistamine that relieves the sneezing, runny nose, stuffiness, itching, and tearing eyes caused by hay fever.

### Most important fact about this drug

If you have liver or kidney disease, your doctor should prescribe a lower starting dose of Claritin.

### How should you take this medication?

Take Claritin exactly as prescribed by your doctor.

■ *If you miss a dose...*
Take the forgotten dose as soon as you remember. If it is almost time for your next dose, skip

the one you missed. Never take two doses at the same time.

■ *Storage instructions...*
Claritin can be stored at room temperature.

## What side effects may occur?

Side effects cannot be anticipated. If any develop or change in intensity, inform your doctor as soon as possible. Only your doctor can determine if it is safe for you to continue taking Claritin.

■ *More common side effects may include:*
Dry mouth, fatigue, headache, sleepiness

■ *Less common or rare side effects may include:*
Abdominal discomfort or pain, abnormal dreams, agitation, anxiety, back pain, blurred vision, breast enlargement, breast pain, bronchitis, change in salivation, change in taste, chest pain, chills and fever, confusion, conjunctivitis (pink-eye), constipation, coughing up blood, coughing, decreased sensitivity to touch, decreased sex drive, depression, diarrhea, difficult or labored breathing, difficulty concentrating, difficulty speaking, discoloration of urine, dizziness, dry hair, dry skin, earache, eye pain, fainting, fever, flushing, gas, general feeling of illness, hair loss, hepatitis, high blood pressure, hives, hyperactivity, impotence, increased appetite, increased or decreased eye tearing, increased sweating, indigestion, inflammation of the mouth, insomnia, itching, joint pain, laryngitis, leg cramps, loss of appetite, low blood pressure, memory loss, menstrual changes, migraine, muscle pain, nasal congestion or dryness, nausea, nervousness, nosebleeds, palpitations, rapid heartbeat, rash, ringing in ears, seizures, sensitivity to light, sinus inflammation, skin inflammation, sneezing, sore throat, stomach inflammation, swelling, thirst, tingling, toothache, tremor, twitching of the eye, upper respiratory infection, urinary changes, vaginal inflammation, vertigo, vomiting, weakness, weight gain, wheezing, yellow eyes and skin

## Why should this drug not be prescribed?

Do not take Claritin if you are sensitive to or have ever had an allergic reaction to it. Make sure your doctor is aware of any drug reactions that you have experienced.

## Special warnings about this medication

This medication may cause excessive sleepiness in people with liver or kidney disease, or the elderly, and should be used with caution.

## Possible food and drug interactions when taking this medication

Although no harmful interactions with Claritin have been reported, there is a theoretical possibility of an interaction with the following drugs:

Antibiotics such as erythromycin and Biaxin
Cimetidine (Tagamet)
Ketoconazole (Nizoral)
Ranitidine (Zantac)
Theophylline (Theo-Dur)

## Special information if you are pregnant or breastfeeding

The effects of Claritin during pregnancy have not been adequately studied. If you are pregnant or plan to become pregnant, inform your doctor immediately. Claritin appears in breast milk and could affect a nursing infant. If this medication is essential to your health, your doctor may advise you to discontinue breastfeeding until your treatment with Claritin is finished.

## Recommended dosage

ADULTS AND CHILDREN 12 YEARS OF AGE AND OVER

The usual dose is one 10-milligram tablet taken once a day. In people with liver or kidney disease, the usual dose is one 10-milligram tablet taken every other day.

## Overdosage

Any medication taken in excess can have serious consequences. If you suspect an overdose, seek medical attention immediately.

■ *Symptoms of Claritin overdose may include:*
Headache, rapid heartbeat, sleepiness

*Brand name:*

# Claritin-D

*Pronounced: CLAR-i-tin dee*
*Generic ingredients: Loratadine, Pseudoephedrine sulfate*

## Why is this drug prescribed?

Claritin-D is an antihistamine and decongestant that relieves the sneezing, runny nose, stuffiness, and itchy, tearing eyes caused by hay fever.

## Most important fact about this drug

If you have liver disease, make sure the doctor is aware of it. Claritin-D is not recommended in this situation.

## How should you take this medication?

Take Claritin-D on an empty stomach. Take it exactly as prescribed by your doctor. Do not break or chew the tablet.

■ *If you miss a dose...*
Take it as soon as you remember. If it is almost time for your next dose, skip the one you missed. Never take 2 doses at the same time.

■ *Storage instructions...*
Store at room temperature.

## What side effects may occur?

Side effects cannot be anticipated. If any develop or change in intensity, inform your doctor as soon as possible. Only your doctor can determine if it is safe for you to continue taking Claritin-D.

■ *More common side effects may include:*
Dry mouth, insomnia

■ *Less common or rare side effects may include:*
Dizziness, fatigue, headache, indigestion, insomnia, nausea, nervousness, sleepiness, sore throat

## Why should this drug not be prescribed?

Do not take Claritin-D if you have ever had an allergic reaction to any of its ingredients.

Avoid Claritin-D if you have the eye condition called narrow-angle glaucoma, very high blood pressure, or coronary artery disease; and do not take the drug if you have difficulty urinating. Also avoid taking Claritin-D within 14 days of taking any antidepressant drug classified as an MAO inhibitor, including Nardil and Parnate.

## Special warnings about this medication

If you are taking Claritin-D and experience insomnia, dizziness, weakness, tremor, or unusual heartbeats, tell your doctor; you may be having an allergic reaction.

You must be careful using Claritin-D if you have diabetes, heart disease, an overactive thyroid gland, kidney or liver problems, or an enlarged prostate gland.

Do not use Claritin-D with over-the-counter antihistamines and decongestants.

## Possible food and drug interactions when taking this medication

Check with your doctor before combining Claritin-D with any of the following:

Antidepressant drugs classified as MAO inhibitors, including Nardil and Parnate
Blood pressure medications classified as beta blockers, such as Inderal and Tenormin
Digoxin (Lanoxin)
Mecamylamine (Inversine)
Methyldopa (Aldomet)
Reserpine

## Special information if you are pregnant or breastfeeding

The effects of Claritin-D during pregnancy have not been adequately studied. If you are pregnant or plan to become pregnant, inform your doctor immediately. Claritin-D may appear in breast milk. If this medication is essential to your health, your doctor may advise you not to breastfeed until your treatment is finished.

## Recommended dosage

ADULTS AND CHILDREN 12 YEARS OF AGE AND OVER

The usual dose is 1 tablet every 12 hours. If you have kidney trouble, your doctor will start you on 1 tablet a day.

## Overdosage

Any medication taken in excess can have serious consequences. If you suspect an overdose, seek medical attention immediately.

■ *Symptoms of Claritin-D overdose may include:*
Anxiety, breathing difficulty, chest pain, coma, convulsions, delusions, difficulty urinating, fast, fluttery heartbeat, giddiness, hallucinations, headache, insomnia, irregular heartbeat, nausea, rapid heartbeat, restlessness, sleepiness, sweating, tension, thirst, vomiting, weakness

*Generic name:*

# Clemastine

*See Tavist, page 523.*

*Brand name:*

# Cleocin T

*Pronounced: KLEE-oh-sin tee*
*Generic name: Clindamycin phosphate*

## Why is this drug prescribed?

Cleocin T is an antibiotic used to treat acne.

## Most important fact about this drug

Although applied only to the skin, some of this medication could be absorbed into the bloodstream; and it has been known to cause severe—sometimes even fatal—colitis (an inflammation of the lower bowel) when taken internally. Symptoms, which can occur a few days, weeks, or months after beginning treatment with this drug, include severe diarrhea, severe abdominal cramps, and the possibility of the passage of blood.

## How should you take this medication?

Use this medication exactly as prescribed. Excessive use of Cleocin T can cause your skin to become too dry or irritated.

■ *If you miss a dose...*
Apply it as soon as you remember. If it is almost time for your next dose, skip the one you missed and go back to your regular schedule.

■ *Storage instructions...*
Store at room temperature. Keep from freezing. Store liquids in tightly closed containers.

## What side effects may occur?

Side effects cannot be anticipated. If any develop or change in intensity, inform your doctor as soon as possible. Only your doctor can determine if it is safe for you to continue taking Cleocin T.

■ *More common side effects may include:*
Burning, itching, peeling skin, reddened skin, skin dryness

■ *Less common or rare side effects may include:*
Abdominal pain, bloody diarrhea, colitis, diarrhea, oily skin, skin inflammation and irritation, stomach and intestinal disturbances

## Why should this drug not be prescribed?

If you are sensitive to or have ever had an allergic reaction to Cleocin T or similar drugs, such as Lincocin, you should not use this medication. Make sure your doctor is aware of any drug reactions you have experienced.

Unless you are directed to do so by your doctor, do not take this medication if you have ever had an intestinal inflammation, ulcerative colitis, or antibiotic-associated colitis.

## Special warnings about this medication

Cleocin T contains an alcohol base, which can cause burning and irritation of the eyes. It also has an unpleasant taste. Use caution when applying this medication so as not to get it in the eyes, nose, mouth, or skin abrasions. In the event of accidental contact, rinse the affected area with cool water.

Use with caution if you have hay fever, asthma, or eczema.

## Possible food and drug interactions when taking this medication

If you have diarrhea while taking Cleocin T, check with your doctor before taking an antidiarrhea medication, as certain drugs may cause your diarrhea to become worse.

The diarrhea should not be treated with the commonly used drugs that slow movement through the intestinal tract, such as Lomotil or products containing paregoric.

## Special information if you are pregnant or breastfeeding

The effects of Cleocin T during pregnancy have not been adequately studied. If you are pregnant or plan to become pregnant, inform your doctor immediately. Cleocin T may appear in breast milk and could affect a nursing infant. If this medication is essential to your health, your doctor may advise you to discontinue breastfeeding your baby until your treatment with this medication is finished.

## Recommended dosage

ADULTS

Apply a thin film of gel, solution, or lotion to the affected area 2 times a day, or use a solution pledget (application pad). Discard a pledget after you have used it once; you may use more than 1 pledget for a treatment. Do not remove the pledget from its foil container until you are ready to use it.

If you are using the lotion, shake it well immediately before using.

CHILDREN

The safety and effectiveness of Cleocin T have not been established in children under 12 years of age.

## Overdosage

Cleocin T can be absorbed through the skin and produce side effects in the body. If you suspect an overdose, seek medical attention immediately.

Brand name:

# Climara

See Estraderm, page 199.

Generic name:

# Clindamycin

See Cleocin T, page 97.

Brand name:

# Clindex

See Librax, page 280.

Brand name:

# Clinoril

Pronounced: CLIN-or-il
Generic name: Sulindac

## Why is this drug prescribed?

Clinoril, a nonsteroidal anti-inflammatory drug, is used to relieve the inflammation, swelling, stiffness, and joint pain associated with rheumatoid arthritis, osteoarthritis (the most common form of arthritis), and ankylosing spondylitis (stiffness and progressive arthritis of the spine). It is also used to treat bursitis, tendinitis, acute gouty arthritis, and other types of pain.

The safety and effectiveness of this medication in the treatment of people with rheumatoid arthritis who are incapacitated, almost or completely bedridden, in wheelchairs, or unable to care for themselves, have not been established.

## Most important fact about this drug

You should have frequent checkups with your doctor if you take Clinoril regularly. Ulcers or internal bleeding can occur without warning.

## How should you take this medication?

Take this medication exactly as prescribed by your doctor.

If you are using Clinoril for arthritis, it should be taken regularly.

■ *If you miss a dose...*
Take it as soon as you remember. If it is almost time for your next dose, skip the one you missed and go back to your regular schedule. Never take two doses at the same time.

■ *Storage instructions...*
Do not store in damp places like the bathroom.

## What side effects may occur?

Side effects cannot be anticipated. If any develop or change in intensity, inform your doctor as soon as possible. Only your doctor can determine if it is safe for you to continue taking Clinoril.

■ *More common side effects may include:*
Abdominal pain, constipation, diarrhea, dizziness, gas, headache, indigestion, itching, loss of appetite, nausea, nervousness, rash, ringing in ears, stomach cramps, swelling due to fluid retention, vomiting

■ *Less common or rare side effects may include:*
Abdominal bleeding, abdominal inflammation, anemia, appetite change, bloody diarrhea, blurred vision, change in color of urine, chest pain, colitis, congestive heart failure, depression, fever, hair loss, hearing loss, hepatitis, high blood pressure, inability to sleep, inflammation of lips and tongue, kidney failure, liver failure, loss of sense of taste, low blood pressure, muscle and joint pain, nosebleed, painful urination, pancreatitis, peptic ulcer, sensitivity to light, shortness of breath, skin eruptions, sleepiness, Stevens-Johnson syndrome (blisters in the mouth and eyes), vaginal bleeding, weakness, yellow eyes and skin

## Why should this drug not be prescribed?

If you are sensitive to or have ever had an allergic reaction to Clinoril, aspirin, or similar drugs, or if you have had asthma attacks caused by aspirin or other drugs of this type, you should not take this medication. Make sure that your doctor is aware of any drug reactions that you have experienced.

## Special warnings about this medication

Peptic ulcers and bleeding can occur without warning.

This drug should be used with caution if you have kidney or liver disease; it can cause liver inflammation in some people.

Do not take aspirin or any other anti-inflammatory medications while taking Clinoril, unless your doctor tells you to do so.

Nonsteroidal anti-inflammatory drugs such as Clinoril can hide the signs and symptoms of an infection. Be sure your doctor knows about any infection you may have.

Clinoril can cause vision problems. If you experience a change in your vision, inform your doctor.

If you have heart disease or high blood pressure, this drug can increase water retention. Use with caution.

If you develop pancreatitis (inflammation of the pancreas), Clinoril should be stopped immediately and not restarted.

Clinoril may cause you to become drowsy or less alert. If this happens, driving or operating dangerous machinery or participating in any hazardous activity that requires full mental alertness is not recommended.

### Possible food and drug interactions when taking this medication

If Clinoril is taken with certain other drugs, the effects of either could be increased, decreased, or altered. It is especially important to check with your doctor before combining Clinoril with the following:

Aspirin
Blood thinners such as Coumadin
Cyclosporine (Sandimmune)
Diflunisal (Dolobid)
Dimethyl sulfoxide (DMSO)
Lithium
Loop diuretics such as Lasix
Methotrexate
Oral diabetes medications
The anti-gout medication Benemid

### Special information if you are pregnant or breastfeeding

The effects of Clinoril during pregnancy have not been adequately studied; drugs of this class are known to cause birth defects. If you are pregnant or plan to become pregnant, inform your doctor immediately. Clinoril may appear in breast milk and could affect a nursing infant. If this medication is essential to your health, your doctor may advise you to discontinue breastfeeding until your treatment with Clinoril is finished.

### Recommended dosage

ADULTS

*Osteoarthritis, Rheumatoid Arthritis, Ankylosing Spondylitis*
Starting dosage is 150 milligrams 2 times a day. Take with food. Doses should not exceed 400 milligrams per day.

*Acute Gouty Arthritis or Arthritic Shoulder and Joint Condition*
400 milligrams daily taken in doses of 200 milligrams 2 times a day.

For acute painful shoulder, therapy lasting 7 to 14 days is usually adequate.

For acute gouty arthritis, therapy lasting 7 days is usually adequate.

The lowest dose that proves beneficial should be used.

CHILDREN

The safety and effectiveness of Clinoril have not been established in children.

### Overdosage

Any medication taken in excess can cause symptoms of overdose. If you suspect an overdose, seek medical attention immediately.

■ *Symptoms of Clinoril overdose may include:*
Coma, low blood pressure, reduced output of urine, stupor

*Generic name:*

# Clobetasol

*See Temovate, page 527.*

*Brand name:*

# Clomid

*See Clomiphene Citrate, page 99.*

*Generic name:*

# Clomiphene Citrate

*Pronounced: KLAHM-if-een SIT-rate*
*Brand names: Clomid, Serophene*

### Why is this drug prescribed?

Clomiphene is prescribed for the treatment of ovulatory failure in women who wish to become pregnant and whose husbands are fertile and potent.

## Most important fact about this drug

Properly timed sexual intercourse is very important to increase the chances of conception. The likelihood of conception diminishes with each succeeding course of treatment. Your doctor will determine the need for continuing therapy after the first course. If you do not become pregnant after 3 courses, your doctor will stop the therapy.

## How should you take this medication?

Take this medication exactly as prescribed by your doctor.

■ *If you miss a dose...*
Take it as soon as you remember. If it is time for your next dose, take the 2 doses together and go back to your regular schedule. If you miss more than 1 dose, contact your doctor.

■ *Storage instructions...*
Store at room temperature in a tightly closed container, away from light, moisture, and excessive heat.

## What side effects may occur?

Side effects occur infrequently and generally do not interfere with treatment at the recommended dosage of clomiphene. They tend to occur more frequently at higher doses and during long-term treatment.

■ *More common side effects include:*
Abdominal discomfort, enlargement of the ovaries, hot flushes

■ *Less common side effects include:*
Abnormal uterine bleeding, breast tenderness, depression, dizziness, fatigue, hair loss, headache, hives, inability to fall or stay asleep, increased urination, inflammation of the skin, light-headedness, nausea, nervousness, ovarian cysts, visual disturbances, vomiting, weight gain

## Why should this drug not be prescribed?

If you are pregnant or think you may be, do not take this drug.

Unless directed to do so by your doctor, do not use this medication if you have an uncontrolled thyroid or adrenal gland disorder, an abnormality of the brain such as a pituitary gland tumor, a liver disease or a history of liver problems, abnormal uterine bleeding of undetermined origin, ovarian cysts, or enlargement of the ovaries not caused by polycystic ovarian syndrome (a hormonal disorder causing lack of ovulation).

## Special warnings about this medication

Your doctor will evaluate you for normal liver function and normal estrogen levels before considering you for treatment with clomiphene.

Your doctor will also examine you for pregnancy, ovarian enlargement, or cyst formation prior to treatment with this drug and between each treatment cycle. He or she will do a complete pelvic examination before each course of this medication.

Clomiphene treatment increases the possibility of multiple births; also, birth defects have been reported following treatment to induce ovulation with clomiphene, although no direct effects of the drug on the unborn child have been established.

Because blurring and other visual symptoms may occur occasionally with clomiphene treatment, you should be cautious about driving a car or operating dangerous machinery, especially under conditions of variable lighting.

If you experience visual disturbances, notify your doctor immediately. Symptoms of visual disturbance may include blurring, spots or flashes, double vision, intolerance to light, decreased visual sharpness, loss of peripheral vision, and distortion of space. Your doctor may recommend a complete evaluation by an eye specialist.

Ovarian hyperstimulation syndrome (or OHSS, enlargement of the ovary) has occurred in women receiving treatment with clomiphene. OHSS may progress rapidly and become serious. The early warning signs are severe pelvic pain, nausea, vomiting, and weight gain. Symptoms include abdominal pain, abdominal enlargement, nausea, vomiting, diarrhea, weight gain, difficult or labored breathing, and less urine production. If you experience any of these warning signs or symptoms, notify your doctor immediately.

To lessen the risks associated with abnormal ovarian enlargement during treatment with clomiphene, the lowest effective dose should be prescribed. Women with the hormonal disorder, polycystic ovarian syndrome, may be unusually sensitive to certain hormones and may respond abnormally to usual doses of this drug. If you experience pelvic pain, notify your doctor. He may discontinue your use of clomiphene until the ovaries return to pretreatment size.

Because the safety of long-term treatment with clomiphene has not been established, your doctor will not prescribe more than 3 courses of therapy. Prolonged use may increase the risk of a tumor in the ovaries.

### Possible food and drug interactions when taking this medication
No food or drug interactions have been reported with clomiphene therapy.

### Special information if you are pregnant or breastfeeding
If you become pregnant, notify your doctor immediately. You should not be taking this drug while you are pregnant.

### Recommended dosage
The recommended dosage for the first course of treatment is 50 milligrams (1 tablet) daily for 5 days. If ovulation does not appear to have occurred, your doctor may prescribe up to 2 more courses of treatment.

### Overdosage
Taking any medication in excess can have serious consequences. If you suspect an overdose of clomiphene, contact your doctor immediately.

*Generic name:*

# Clomipramine

*See Anafranil, page 24.*

*Generic name:*

# Clonazepam

*See Klonopin, page 268.*

*Generic name:*

# Clonidine

*See Catapres, page 83.*

*Generic name:*

# Clorazepate

*See Tranxene, page 558.*

*Generic name:*

# Clotrimazole

*See Gyne-Lotrimin, page 232.*

*Generic name:*

# Clotrimazole with Betamethasone

*See Lotrisone, page 300.*

*Generic name:*

# Clozapine

*See Clozaril, page 101.*

*Brand name:*

# Clozaril

*Pronounced: KLOH-zah-ril*
*Generic name: Clozapine*

### Why is this drug prescribed?
Clozaril is given to help people with severe schizophrenia who have failed to respond to standard treatments. Clozaril is not a cure, but it can help some people return to more normal lives.

### Most important fact about this drug
Even though it does not produce some of the disturbing side effects of other antipsychotic medications, Clozaril may cause agranulocytosis, a potentially lethal disorder of the white blood cells. Because of the risk of agranulocytosis, anyone who takes Clozaril is required to have a blood test once a week. The drug is carefully controlled so that those taking it must get their weekly blood test before receiving the following week's supply of medication. Anyone whose blood test results are abnormal will be taken off Clozaril either temporarily or permanently, depending on the results of an additional 4 weeks of testing.

### How should you take this medication?
Take Clozaril exactly as directed by your doctor. Because of the significant risk of serious side effects associated with this drug, your doctor will periodically reassess the need for continued Clozaril therapy. Clozaril is distributed *only*

through the Clozaril Patient Management System, which ensures weekly white blood cell testing, monitoring, and pharmacy services prior to delivery of the next week's supply.

Clozaril may be taken with or without food.

■ *If you miss a dose...*
Take it as soon as you remember. If it is almost time for your next dose, skip the one you missed and go back to your regular schedule. Do not take 2 doses at once.

If you stop taking Clozaril for more than 2 days, do not start taking it again without consulting your physician.

■ *Storage instructions...*
Store at room temperature.

## What side effects may occur?
Side effects cannot be anticipated. If any develop or change in intensity, inform your doctor as soon as possible. Only your doctor can determine if it is safe for you to continue taking Clozaril.

The most feared side effect is agranulocytosis, a dangerous drop in the number of a certain kind of white blood cell. Symptoms include fever, lethargy, sore throat, and weakness. If not caught in time, agranulocytosis can be fatal. That is why all people who take Clozaril must have a blood test every week. About 1 percent develop agranulocytosis and must stop taking the drug.

Seizures are another potential side effect, occurring in some 5 percent of people who take Clozaril. The higher the dosage, the greater the risk of seizures.

■ *More common side effects may include:*
Abdominal discomfort, agitation, confusion, constipation, disturbed sleep, dizziness, drowsiness, dry mouth, fainting, fever, headache, heartburn, high blood pressure, inability to sit down, loss or slowness of muscle movement, low blood pressure, nausea, nightmares, rapid heartbeat and other heart conditions, restlessness, rigidity, salivation, sedation, sweating, tremors, vertigo, vision problems, vomiting, weight gain
■ *Less common side effects may include:*
Abdominal distention, abnormal stools, anemia, angina (severe, crushing chest pain), anxiety, appetite increase, belching, bitter taste, blood clots, bloodshot eyes, bluish tinge in the skin, breast pain or discomfort, bronchitis, bruising, chest pain, chills or chills and fever, constant involuntary eye movement, coughing, delusions, depression, diarrhea, difficult or labored breathing, dilated pupils, disorientation, dry throat, ear disorders, ejaculation problems, excessive movement, eyelid disorder, fast, fluttery heartbeat, fatigue, fluid retention, frequent urination, hallucinations, heart problems, hives, hot flashes, impotence, inability to fall asleep or stay asleep, inability to hold urine, inability to urinate, increase or decrease in sex drive, inflamed stomach and intestines, involuntary movement, irritability, itching, jerky movements, joint pain, lack of coordination, laryngitis, lethargy, lightheadedness (especially when rising quickly from a seated or lying position), loss of appetite, loss of speech, low body temperature, memory loss, muscle pain or ache, muscle spasm, muscle weakness, nervous stomach, nosebleed, numbness, pain in back, neck, or legs, painful menstruation, pallor, paranoia, pneumonia or pneumonia-like symptoms, poor coordination, rapid breathing, rash, rectal bleeding, runny nose, shakiness, shortness of breath, skin inflammation, redness, scaling, slow heartbeat, slurred speech, sneezing, sore or numb tongue, speech difficulty, stomach pain, stomach ulcer, stuffy nose, stupor, stuttering, thirst, throat discomfort, tics, twitching, urination problems, vaginal infection, vaginal itch, a vague feeling of being sick, vomiting blood, weakness, wheezing

## Why should this drug not be prescribed?
Clozaril is considered a somewhat risky medication because of its potential to cause agranulocytosis and seizures. It should be taken only by people whose condition is serious, and who have not been helped by more traditional antipsychotic medications such as Haldol or Mellaril.

You should not take Clozaril if:

■ You have a bone marrow disease or disorder;
■ You have epilepsy that is not controlled;
■ You ever developed an abnormal white blood cell count while taking Clozaril;
■ You are currently taking some other drug, such as Tegretol, that could cause a decrease in white blood cell count or a drug that could affect the bone marrow.

## Special warnings about this medication

Clozaril can cause drowsiness, especially at the start of treatment. For this reason, and also because of the potential for seizures, you should not drive, swim, climb, or operate dangerous machinery while you are taking this medication, at least in the early stages of treatment.

Even though you will have weekly blood tests while taking Clozaril, you should stay alert for early symptoms of agranulocytosis: weakness, lethargy, fever, sore throat, a general feeling of illness, a flu-like feeling, or ulcers of the lips, mouth, or other mucous membranes. If any such symptoms develop, tell your doctor immediately.

Especially during the first 3 weeks of treatment, you may develop a fever. If you do, notify your doctor.

While taking Clozaril, do not drink alcohol or use drugs of any kind, including over-the-counter medicines, without first checking with your doctor.

If you take Clozaril, you must be monitored especially closely if you have either the eye condition called narrow-angle glaucoma or an enlarged prostate; Clozaril could make these conditions worse.

On rare occasions, Clozaril can cause intestinal problems—constipation, impaction, or blockage—that can, in extreme cases, be fatal.

Especially when you begin taking Clozaril, you may feel light-headed upon standing up, to the point where you pass out.

If you have kidney, liver, lung or heart disease, or a history of seizures or prostate problems, you should discuss these with your doctor before taking Clozaril.

Drugs such as Clozaril can sometimes cause a set of symptoms called Neuroleptic Malignant Syndrome. Symptoms include high fever, muscle rigidity, irregular pulse or blood pressure, rapid heartbeat, excessive perspiration, and changes in heart rhythm. Your doctor will have you stop taking Clozaril while this condition is being treated.

There is also a risk of developing tardive dyskinesia, a condition of involuntary, slow, rhythmical movements. It happens more often in the elderly, especially elderly women.

## Possible food and drug interactions when taking this medication

If Clozaril is taken with certain other drugs, the effects of either could be increased, decreased, or altered. It is especially important to check with your doctor before combining Clozaril with the following:

Alcohol
Antidepressants such as Prozac and Zoloft
Antipsychotic drugs such as Thorazine and Mellaril
Blood pressure medication such as Aldomet and Hytrin
Cimetidine (Tagamet)
Digitoxin (Crystodigin)
Digoxin (Lanoxin)
Drugs that depress the central nervous system such as phenobarbital and Seconal
Drugs that contain atropine such as Donnatal and Levsin
Epilepsy drugs such as Tegretol and Dilantin
Epinephrine (EpiPen)
Heart rhythm stabilizers such as Quinidex and Tambocor
Tranquilizers such as Valium and Xanax
Warfarin (Coumadin and Panwarfin)

## Special information if you are pregnant or breastfeeding

The effects of Clozaril during pregnancy have not been adequately studied. If you are pregnant or plan to become pregnant, inform your doctor immediately. Clozaril treatment should be continued during pregnancy only if absolutely necessary. You should not breastfeed if you are taking Clozaril, since the drug may appear in breast milk.

## Recommended dosage

ADULTS

Your doctor will carefully individualize your dosage and monitor your response weekly.

The usual recommended initial dose is half of a 25-milligram tablet (12.5 milligrams) 1 or 2 times daily. Your doctor may increase the dosage in increments of 25 to 50 milligrams a day to achieve a daily dose of 300 to 450 milligrams by the end of 2 weeks. Dosage increases after that will be only once or twice a week and will be no more than 100 milligrams each time. The most you can take is 900 milligrams a day divided into 2 or 3 doses.

Your doctor will determine long-term dosage depending upon your response and results of the weekly blood test.

CHILDREN

Safety and efficacy have not been established for children up to 16 years of age.

## Overdosage

Any medication taken in excess can have serious consequences. If you suspect an overdose, seek emergency medical attention immediately.

■ *Symptoms of overdose with Clozaril may include:*
Coma, delirium, drowsiness, excess salivation, low blood pressure, faintness, pneumonia, rapid heartbeat, seizures, shallow breathing or absence of breathing

*Brand name:*

# Cogentin

*Pronounced: co-JEN-tin*
*Generic name: Benztropine mesylate*

## Why is this drug prescribed?

Cogentin is given to help relieve the symptoms of "parkinsonism": the muscle rigidity, tremors, and difficulties with posture and balance that occur in Parkinson's disease and that sometimes develop as unwanted side effects of antipsychotic drugs such as Haldol and Thorazine.

Cogentin is an "anticholinergic" medication, a drug that controls spasms. It reduces the symptoms of parkinsonism, but it is not a cure.

## Most important fact about this drug

When starting Cogentin, you may not feel its effect for 2 or 3 days. Symptoms caused by drugs such as Haldol and Thorazine are often temporary, so if drug-induced parkinsonism is your problem, you may need to take Cogentin for only a couple of weeks.

## How should you take this medication?

Take Cogentin exactly as prescribed. Unlike some of the other antiparkinsonian medications, Cogentin acts over a long period of time. It is thus particularly suitable as a bedtime medication because it lasts through the night. Taken at bedtime, it may help a person regain enough muscle control to move and roll over during sleep and to arise unaided in the morning.

Cogentin causes dry mouth. Sucking on sugarless hard candy or sipping water can relieve this problem.

Cogentin can reduce the ability to sweat, one of the key ways your body prevents overheating. Avoid excess sun or exercise that may cause overheating.

■ *If you miss a dose...*
Take it as soon as you remember. If it is within 2 hours of your next dose, skip the one you missed and go back to your regular schedule. Do not take 2 doses at once.

■ *Storage instructions...*
Store away from heat, light, and moisture.

## What side effects may occur?

Side effects cannot be anticipated. If any develop or change in intensity, inform your doctor as soon as possible. Only your doctor can determine if it is safe for you to continue taking Cogentin.

■ *Side effects may include:*
Blurred vision, bowel blockage, confusion, constipation, depression, dilated pupils, disorientation, dry mouth, fever, hallucinations, heat stroke, impaired memory, inability to urinate, listlessness, nausea, nervousness, numbness in fingers, painful urination, rapid heartbeat, rash, vomiting

## Why should this drug not be prescribed?

Do not take Cogentin if you are sensitive to it or if you have ever had an allergic reaction to it or to any similar antispasmodic medication.

Do not take Cogentin if you have an eye condition called angle-closure glaucoma.

Some people who take certain antipsychotic medications develop tardive dyskinesia, a syndrome of involuntary movements of the mouth, jaw, arms, and legs. Cogentin should not be given to treat tardive dyskinesia; it will not help, and it may make the condition worse.

Cogentin should not be given to children under the age of 3; it should be used with caution in older children.

## Special warnings about this medication

Do not drive or operate dangerous machinery while taking Cogentin, since the drug may impair your mental or physical abilities.

Be sure to tell your doctor if you have ever had tachycardia (excessively rapid heartbeats) or if you have an enlarged prostate; you will require especially close monitoring while taking Cogentin in these cases.

Tell your doctor if Cogentin produces weakness in particular muscle groups. For example, if you have been suffering from neck rigidity and Cogentin suddenly causes your neck to relax so much that it feels weak, you may be taking more Cogentin than you need.

If you have been taking another antiparkinsonism drug, do not stop taking it abruptly when you start taking Cogentin. If you are to stop taking the other drug, your doctor will have you taper off gradually.

Cogentin has a drying effect on the mouth and other moist tissues. If you take it along with another drug that also has a drying effect, you are at risk for anhidrosis (inability to sweat), heat stroke, and even death from hyperthermia (high fever). Chronic illness, alcoholism, central nervous system (brain and spinal cord) disease, or heavy manual labor in a hot environment can increase this risk. In hot weather, your doctor may lower your dosage of Cogentin.

## Possible food and drug interactions when taking this medication

When taken simultaneously with an antipsychotic medication (Thorazine, Stelazine, Haldol, others) or a tricyclic antidepressant medication (Elavil, Norpramin, Tofranil, others), Cogentin has occasionally caused bowel blockage or heat stroke that proved dangerous or even fatal. If you are taking Cogentin along with an antipsychotic or with a tricyclic antidepressant, tell your doctor immediately if you begin to have any stomach or bowel complaint, fever, or heat intolerance.

Antacids, such as Tums, Maalox, and Mylanta, may decrease the effects of Cogentin. Do not take them within 1 hour of taking Cogentin.

Certain other drugs may also interact with Cogentin. Consult your doctor before combining Cogentin with any of the following:

Amantadine (Symmetrel)
Doxepin (Sinequan)
Antihistamines such as Benadryl and Tavist
Other anticholinergic agents such as Bentyl

## Special information if you are pregnant or breastfeeding

If you are pregnant or plan to become pregnant, inform your doctor immediately. No information is available about the safety of taking Cogentin during pregnancy or while you are breastfeeding.

## Recommended dosage

Your doctor will individualize the dose of Cogentin, taking into consideration your age and weight, the condition being treated, the presence of other diseases, and any physical disorder.

In general, the usual oral dose is 1 to 2 milligrams a day, but it can range from 0.5 to 6 milligrams a day.

## Overdosage

Any medication taken in excess can have serious consequences. If you suspect symptoms of an overdose of Cogentin, seek medical attention immediately. Symptoms of overdose may include any of those listed in the "side effects section" (see above) or any of the following:

Blurred vision, confusion, coma, constipation, convulsions, delirium, difficulty swallowing or breathing, dilated pupils, dizziness, dry mouth, flushed, dry skin, glaucoma, hallucinations, headache, high blood pressure, high body temperature, inability to sweat, listlessness, muscle weakness, nausea, nervousness, numb fingers, painful urination, palpitations, rapid heartbeat, rash, shock, uncoordinated movements, vomiting

*Brand name:*

# Co-Gesic

*See Vicodin, page 587.*

*Brand name:*

# Cognex

*Pronounced: COG-necks*
*Generic name: Tacrine hydrochloride*

## Why is this drug prescribed?

Cognex is used for the treatment of mild to moderate Alzheimer's disease. This progressive, degenerative disorder causes physical changes in the brain that disrupt the flow of information and affect memory, thinking, and behavior. As someone caring for a person with Alzheimer's, you should be aware that Cognex is not a cure, but has helped some people.

## Most important fact about this drug

Do not abruptly stop Cognex treatment, or reduce the dosage, without consulting the doctor. A sudden reduction can cause the person you are caring for to become more disturbed and forgetful. Taking more Cognex than the doctor advises can also cause serious problems. Do not change the dosage of Cognex unless instructed by the doctor.

## How should you take this medication?

This medication will work better if taken at regular intervals, usually 4 times a day. Cognex is best taken between meals; however, if it is irritating to the stomach, the doctor may advise taking it with meals. If Cognex is not taken regularly, as the doctor directs, the condition may get worse.

■ *If you miss a dose...*
Give the forgotten dose as soon as possible. If it is within 2 hours of the next dose, skip the missed dose and go back to the regular schedule. Do not double the doses.

■ *Storage instructions...*
Store at room temperature away from moisture.

## What side effects may occur?

Side effects cannot be anticipated. If any develop or change in intensity, tell the doctor as soon as possible. Only the doctor can determine if it is safe to continue giving Cognex.

■ *More common side effects may include:*
Abdominal pain, abnormal thinking, agitation, anxiety, chest pain, clumsiness or unsteadiness, confusion, constipation, coughing, depression, diarrhea, dizziness, fatigue, flushing, frequent urination, gas, headache, inflamed nasal passages, insomnia, indigestion, liver function disorders, loss of appetite, muscle pain, nausea, rash, sleepiness, upper respiratory infection, urinary tract infection, vomiting, weight loss

■ *Less common side effects may include:*
Back pain, hallucinations, hostile attitude, purple or red spots on the skin, skin discoloration, tremor, weakness

Be sure to report any symptoms that develop while on Cognex therapy. You should alert the doctor if the person you are caring for develops nausea, vomiting, loose stools, or diarrhea at the start of therapy or when the dosage is increased. Later in therapy, be on the lookout for rash or fever, yellowing of the eyes and skin, or changes in the color of the stool.

## Why should this drug not be prescribed?

People who are sensitive to or have ever had an allergic reaction to Cognex should not take this medication. Before starting treatment with Cognex, it is important to discuss any medical problems with the doctor. If during previous Cognex therapy the person you are caring for developed jaundice (yellow skin and eyes), which signals that something is wrong with the liver, Cognex should not be used again.

## Special warnings about this medication

Use Cognex with caution if the person you are caring for has a history of liver disease, certain heart disorders, stomach ulcers, or asthma.

Because of the risk of liver problems when taking Cognex, the doctor will schedule blood tests every other week to monitor liver function for the first 16 weeks of treatment. After 16 weeks, blood tests will be given monthly for 2 months and every 3 months after that. If the person you are caring for develops any liver problems, the doctor may temporarily discontinue Cognex treatment until further testing shows that the liver has returned to normal. If the doctor resumes Cognex treatment, regular blood tests will be conducted again. Blood tests should be performed every other week for at least the first 16 weeks at the beginning of Cognex treatment in order to monitor liver function. If no significant changes in liver function have been observed, monitoring may be decreased to monthly for 2 months and every 3 months thereafter.

Before having any surgery, including dental surgery, tell the doctor that the person is being treated with Cognex.

Cognex can cause seizures, and may cause difficulty urinating.

## Possible food and drug interactions when taking this medication

If Cognex is taken with certain other drugs, the effects of either could be increased, decreased, or altered. It is especially important that you check with your doctor before combining Cognex with the following:

Antispasmodic drugs such as Bentyl and Cogentin
Bethanechol chloride (Urecholine)
Cimetidine (Tagamet)
Theophylline (Theo-Dur)

## Special information
## if you are pregnant or breastfeeding

The effects of Cognex during pregnancy have not been studied; and it is not known whether Cognex appears in breast milk.

## Recommended dosage

### ADULTS

The usual starting dose is 10 milligrams 4 times a day, for at least 6 weeks. Do not increase the dose during this 6-week period unless directed by your doctor. The doctor may then increase the dosage to 20 milligrams 4 times a day.

### CHILDREN

The safety and effectiveness of Cognex have not been established in children.

## Overdosage

Any medication taken in excess can have serious consequences. If you suspect an overdose, seek medical attention immediately.

■ *Symptoms of Cognex overdose include:*
Collapse, convulsions, extreme muscle weakness, possibly ending in death (if breathing muscles are affected), low blood pressure, nausea, salivation, slowed heart rate, sweating, vomiting.

*Brand name:*

# Colace

*Pronounced: KOH-lace*
*Generic name: Docusate sodium*
*Other brand name: Sof-Lax*

## Why is this drug prescribed?

Colace, a stool softener, promotes easy bowel movements without straining. It softens the stool by mixing in fat and water. Colace is helpful for people who have had recent rectal surgery, people with heart problems, high blood pressure, hemorrhoids, or hernias, and women who have just had babies.

## Most important fact about this drug

Colace is for short-term relief only, unless your doctor directs otherwise. It usually takes a day or two for the drug to achieve its laxative effect; some people may need to wait 4 or 5 days. Sof-Lax Overnight works in 6 to 12 hours.

## How should you take this medication?

To conceal the drug's bitter taste, take Colace liquid in half a glass of milk or fruit juice; it can be given in infant formula. The proper dosage of this medication may also be added to a retention or flushing enema.

■ *If you miss a dose...*
Take this medication only as needed.
■ *Storage instructions...*
Store at room temperature. Keep from freezing.

## What side effects may occur?

Side effects are unlikely. The main ones reported are bitter taste, throat irritation, and nausea (mainly associated with use of the syrup and liquid). Rash has occurred.

## Why should this drug not be prescribed?

There are no known reasons this drug should not be prescribed.

## Special warnings about this medication

Do not use this product if you have any abdominal pain, nausea, or vomiting, unless your doctor advises it. Do not take this product if you are taking mineral oil. If you have noticed a change in your bowel habits that has lasted for 2 weeks, ask your doctor before you use this product. If you bleed from the rectum or you do not have a bowel movement after using this product, stop using it and call your doctor; you may have a more serious condition.

## Possible food and drug interactions
## when taking this medication

No interactions have been reported with Colace.

## Special information
## if you are pregnant or breastfeeding

If you are pregnant, plan to become pregnant, or are breastfeeding your baby, notify your doctor before using this medication.

## Recommended dosage

Your doctor will adjust the dosage according to your needs.

You will be using higher doses at the start of treatment with Colace. You should see an effect on stools 1 to 3 days after the first dose.

### ADULTS AND CHILDREN 12 AND OLDER

The suggested daily dosage is 50 to 200 milligrams.

In enemas, add 50 to 100 milligrams of Colace or 5 to 10 milliliters of Colace liquid to a retention or flushing enema, as prescribed by your doctor.

## CHILDREN UNDER 12

The suggested daily dosage for children 6 to 12 years of age is 40 to 120 milligrams; for children 3 to 6 years of age, it is 20 to 60 milligrams; for children under 3 years of age, it is 10 to 40 milligrams.

### Overdosage

Overdose is unlikely with normal use of Colace. If you or your child should accidentally take too much, call your doctor or a Poison Control Center.

*Brand name:*

# Colestid

*Pronounced: Koh-LESS-tid*
*Generic name: Colestipol hydrochloride*

### Why is this drug prescribed?

Colestid, in conjunction with diet, is used to help lower high levels of cholesterol in the blood. It is available in plain and orange-flavored granules and in tablet form.

### Most important fact about this drug

Accidentally inhaling Colestid granules may cause serious effects. To avoid this, NEVER take them in their dry form. Colestid granules should always be mixed with water or other liquids BEFORE you take them.

### How should you take this medication?

Colestid granules should be mixed with liquids such as:

Carbonated beverages (may cause stomach or intestinal discomfort)
Flavored drinks
Milk
Orange juice
Pineapple juice
Tomato juice
Water
Colestid may also be mixed with:
Milk used on breakfast cereals
Pulpy fruit (such as crushed peaches, pears, or pineapple) or fruit cocktail
Soups with a high liquid content (such as chicken noodle or tomato)

To take Colestid granules with beverages:

1. Measure at least 3 ounces of liquid into a glass.
2. Add the prescribed dose of Colestid to the liquid.
3. Stir until Colestid is completely mixed (it will not dissolve) and then drink the mixture.
4. Pour a small amount of the beverage into the glass, swish it around, and drink it. This will help make sure you have taken all the medication.

Swallow Colestid tablets whole—do not cut, chew, or crush them. You can take the tablets with water or another liquid.

■ *If you miss a dose...*
Take the forgotten dose as soon as you remember. If it is almost time for the next dose, skip the one you missed and go back to your regular schedule. Never try to "catch up" by doubling the dose.

■ *Storage instructions...*
Store Colestid granules and tablets at room temperature.

### What side effects may occur?

Side effects cannot be anticipated. If any develop or change in intensity, inform your doctor as soon as possible. Only your doctor can determine if it is safe for you to continue taking Colestid.

■ *Most common side effects:*
Constipation, worsening of hemorrhoids
■ *Less common or rare side effects may include:*
Abdominal bloating or distention/ cramping/pain, arthritis, diarrhea, dizziness, fatigue, gas, headache, hives, joint pain, loss of appetite, muscle pain, nausea, shortness of breath, skin inflammation, vomiting, weakness
■ *Additional side effects from regular Colestid granules may include:*
Anxiety, belching, drowsiness, vertigo
■ *Additional side effects from Flavored Colestid granules or Colestid tablets may include:*
Aches and pains in arms and legs, angina (crushing chest pain), backache, bleeding hemorrhoids, blood in the stool, bone pain, chest pain, heartburn, indigestion, insomnia, light-headedness, loose stools, migraine, rapid heartbeat, rash, sinus headache, swelling of hands or feet

## Why should this drug not be prescribed?

You should not be using Colestid if you are allergic to it or any of its components.

## Special warnings about this medication

Before starting treatment with Colestid, you should:

■ Be tested (and treated) for diseases that may contribute to increased blood cholesterol, such as an underactive thyroid gland, diabetes, nephrotic syndrome (a kidney disease), dysproteinemia (a blood disease), obstructive liver disease, and alcoholism.

■ Be on a diet plan (approved by your doctor) that stresses low-cholesterol foods and weight loss (if necessary).

Because certain medications may increase cholesterol, you should tell your doctor all of the medications you use.

Colestid may prevent the absorption of vitamins such as A, D, and K. Long-term use of Colestid may be connected to increased bleeding from a lack of vitamin K. Taking vitamin $K_1$ will help relieve this condition and prevent it in the future.

Your cholesterol and triglyceride levels should be checked regularly while you are taking Colestid.

Colestid may cause or worsen constipation. Dosages should be adjusted by your doctor. You may need to increase your intake of fiber and fluid. A stool softener also may be needed occasionally. People with coronary artery disease should be especially careful to avoid constipation. Hemorrhoids may be worsened by constipation related to Colestid.

If you have phenylketonuria (a hereditary disease caused by your body's inability to handle the amino acid phenylalanine), be aware that Flavored Colestid granules contain phenylalanine.

## Possible food and drug interactions when taking this medication

Colestid may delay or reduce the absorption of other drugs. The time period between taking Colestid and taking other medications should be as long as possible. Other drugs should be taken at least 1 hour before or 4 hours after taking Colestid.

If Colestid is taken with certain other drugs, the effects of either could be increased, decreased, or altered. It is especially important to check with your doctor before combining Colestid with the following:

Chlorothiazide (Diuril)
Digitalis (Lanoxin)
Furosemide (Lasix)
Gemfibrozil (Lopid)
Hydrochlorothiazide (HydroDIURIL)
Penicillin G, including brands such as Pentids
Phosphate supplements
Propranolol (Inderal)
Tetracycline drugs such as Sumycin
Vitamins such as A, D, and K

## Special information if you are pregnant or breastfeeding

The effects of Colestid during pregnancy have not been adequately studied. If you are pregnant or planning to become pregnant, or plan to breastfeed, check with your doctor. Since Colestid interferes with the absorption of fat soluble vitamins A, D, and K it may affect both the mother and the nursing infant.

## Recommended dosage

ADULTS

One packet or 1 level scoopful of Flavored Colestid granules contains 5 grams of Colestipol.

The usual starting dose is 1 packet or 1 level scoopful once or twice a day. Your doctor may increase this by 1 dose a day every month or every other month, up to 6 packets or 6 level scoopfuls taken once a day or divided into smaller doses.

If you are taking Colestid tablets, the usual starting dose is 2 grams (2 tablets) once or twice a day. Your doctor may increase the dose every month or every other month, to a maximum of 16 grams a day, taken once a day or divided into smaller doses.

CHILDREN

The safety and effectiveness of Colestid have not been established for children.

## Overdosage

Overdoses of Colestid have not been reported. If an overdose occurred, the most likely harmful effect would be obstruction of the stomach and/or intestines. If you suspect an overdose, seek medical help immediately.

*Generic name:*

# Colestipol

*See Colestid, page 108.*

*Generic name:*

# Colistin, Neomycin, Hydrocortisone, and Thonzonium

*See Coly-Mycin S Otic, page 110.*

*Brand name:*

# Coly-Mycin S Otic

*Pronounced: KOH-lee-MY-sin ESS OH-tic*
*Generic ingredients: Colistin sulfate, Neomycin*
*sulfate, Hydrocortisone acetate, Thonzonium*
*bromide*

## Why is this drug prescribed?

Coly-Mycin S Otic is a liquid suspension used to treat ear infections. Colistin sulfate and neomycin sulfate are antibiotics used to treat the bacterial infection itself, while hydrocortisone acetate is a steroid that helps reduce the inflammation, swelling, itching, and other skin reactions associated with an ear infection; thonzonium bromide facilitates the drug's effects.

## Most important fact about this drug

As with other antibiotics, long-term treatment may encourage other infections. Therefore, if your ear infection does not improve within a week, your physician may want to change your medication.

## How should you use this medication?

Use Coly-Mycin S for the full course of treatment (but no more than 10 days) even if you start to feel better in a few days.

Shake well before using.

The external ear canal should be thoroughly cleaned and dried with a sterile cotton swab (applicator). The person should lie with the infected ear facing up. Pull the earlobe down and back (for children) or up and back (for adults) to straighten the ear canal. Drop the suspension into the ear. The person should lie in this position for 5 minutes to help the drops penetrate into the ear. If necessary, this procedure should be repeated for the other ear. To keep the medicine from leaking out, you can gently insert a sterile cotton plug.

If you prefer, a sterile cotton wick or plug may be inserted into the ear canal and then soaked with the Coly-Mycin S Otic suspension. This cotton wick should be moistened every 4 hours with more suspension and replaced at least once every 24 hours.

Avoid touching the dropper to the ear or other surfaces.

■ *If you miss a dose...*
Apply it as soon as you remember. If it is almost time for your next dose, skip the one you missed and go back to your regular schedule.
■ *Storage instructions...*
Store at room temperature; avoid prolonged exposure to high temperatures.

## What side effects may occur?

No specific side effects have been reported; however, neomycin (an ingredient in Coly-Mycin S Otic) may be associated with an increased risk of allergic skin reaction.

## Why should this drug not be prescribed?

You should not take this drug if you have had an allergic reaction to any of the ingredients, or if you suffer from herpes simplex, vaccinia (cowpox), or varicella (chickenpox).

## Special warnings about this medication

Treatment should not continue for more than 10 days.

If you warm Coly-Mycin S Otic before applying, do not heat the suspension to above body temperature, since this will lessen its potency. Warm the drops by holding the bottle in your hand for a few minutes.

If an allergic reaction occurs, you should stop using Coly-Mycin S Otic immediately. Your doctor may also recommend that future treatment with kanamycin, paromomycin, streptomycin, and possibly gentamicin be avoided, since you may also be allergic to these medications.

Use Coly-Mycin S Otic with care if you have a perforated eardrum or chronic otitis media (inflammation of the middle ear).

## Possible food and drug interactions when using this medication

No interactions have been reported.

## Special information if you are pregnant or breastfeeding

The effects of Coly-Mycin S Otic during pregnancy have not been adequately studied. If you are pregnant or plan to become pregnant, inform your doctor immediately. Coly-Mycin S Otic may appear in breast milk and could affect a nursing infant. If this medication is essential to your health, your doctor may advise you to stop breastfeeding until your treatment is finished.

## Recommended dosage

### ADULTS

The usual dose is 5 drops (when using the supplied measured dropper) or 4 drops (when using the dropper-bottle container) in the affected ear, 3 or 4 times daily.

### INFANTS AND CHILDREN

The usual dose is 4 drops (when using the supplied measured dropper) or 3 drops (when using the dropper-bottle container) in the affected ear 3 or 4 times daily.

Please see the "How should you use this medication?" section above for more information on applying Coly-Mycin S Otic.

## Overdosage

Although no specific information is available, any medication taken in excess can have serious consequences. If you suspect an overdose of Coly-Mycin S Otic, seek medical treatment immediately.

*Brand name:*

# Compazine

*Pronounced: KOMP-ah-zeen*
*Generic name: Prochlorperazine*

## Why is this drug prescribed?

Compazine is used to control severe nausea and vomiting. It is also used to treat symptoms of mental disorders such as schizophrenia, and is occasionally prescribed for anxiety.

## Most important fact about this drug

Compazine may cause tardive dyskinesia—involuntary muscle spasms and twitches in the face and body. This condition may be permanent. It appears to be most common among the elderly, especially women. Ask your doctor for information about this possible risk.

## How should you take this medication?

Never take more Compazine than prescribed. It can increase the risk of serious side effects.

If you are using the suppository form of Compazine and find it is too soft to insert, you can chill it in the refrigerator for about 30 minutes or run cold water over it before removing the wrapper.

To insert a suppository, first remove the wrapper and moisten the suppository with cold water. Then lie down on your side and use a finger to push the suppository well up into the rectum.

■ *If you miss a dose...*
Take the forgotten dose as soon as you remember. If it is almost time for the next dose, skip the one you missed and go back to your regular schedule. Never try to "catch up" by doubling the dose.

■ *Storage instructions...*
Store at room temperature. Protect from heat and light.

## What side effects may occur?

Side effects cannot be anticipated. If any develop or change in intensity, inform your doctor as soon as possible. Only your doctor can determine if it is safe for you to continue taking Compazine.

■ *Side effects may include:*
Abnormal muscle rigidity, abnormal secretion of milk, abnormal sugar in urine, abnormalities of posture and movement, agitation, anemia, appetite changes, asthma, blurred vision, breast development in males, chewing movements, constipation, convulsions, difficulty swallowing, discolored skin tone, dizziness, drooling, drowsiness, dry mouth, ejaculation problems, exaggerated reflexes, fever, fluid retention, head arched backward, headache, heart attack, heels bent back on legs, high or low blood sugar, hives, impotence, inability to urinate, increased psychotic symptoms, increased weight, infection, insomnia, intestinal obstruction, involuntary movements of arms, hands, legs, and feet, involuntary movements of face, tongue, and jaw, irregular movements, jerky movements, jitteriness, light sensitivity, low blood pressure, mask-like face, menstrual irregularities, narrowed or dilated pupils, nasal congestion, nausea, pain in the shoulder and neck area, painful muscle spasm, parkinsonism-like symptoms, persistent, painful erections, pill-rolling motion, protruding tongue, puckering of the mouth, puffing of the cheeks, rigid arms, feet, head, and muscles, rota-

tion of eyeballs or state of fixed gaze, shock, shuffling gait, skin peeling, rash and inflammation, sore throat, mouth, and gums, spasms in back, feet and ankles, jaw, and neck, swelling and itching skin, swelling in throat, tremors, yellowed eyes and skin

### Why should this drug not be prescribed?

Do not take Compazine if you are sensitive to or have ever had an allergic reaction to prochlorperazine or other phenothiazine drugs such as Thorazine, Prolixin, Triavil, Mellaril, or Stelazine.

### Special warnings about this medication

Never take large amounts of alcohol, barbiturates, or narcotics when taking Compazine. Serious problems can result.

If you suddenly stop taking Compazine, you may experience a change in appetite, dizziness, nausea, vomiting, and tremors. Follow your doctor's instructions closely when discontinuing this drug.

Make sure the doctor knows if you are being treated for a brain tumor, intestinal blockage, heart disease, glaucoma, or an abnormal blood condition such as leukemia, or if you are exposed to extreme heat or pesticides.

This drug may impair your ability to drive a car or operate potentially dangerous machinery. Do not participate in any activities that require full alertness if you are unsure about your ability.

While taking Compazine, try to stay out of the sun. Use sun block and wear protective clothing. Your eyes may become more sensitive to sunlight, too, so keep sunglasses handy.

Compazine interferes with your ability to shed extra heat. Be cautious in hot weather.

Compazine may cause false-positive pregnancy tests.

### Possible food and drug interactions when taking this medication

If Compazine is taken with certain other drugs, the effects of either could be increased, decreased, or altered. It is especially important to check with your doctor before combining Compazine with the following:

Antiseizure drugs such as Dilantin and Tegretol
Anticoagulants such as Coumadin
Guanethidine (Ismelin)
Lithium (Lithobid, Eskalith)

Narcotic painkillers such as Demerol and Tylenol with Codeine
Other central nervous system depressants such as Xanax, Valium, Seconal, Halcion
Propranolol (Inderal)
Thiazide diuretics such as Dyazide

### Special information if you are pregnant or breastfeeding

Compazine is not usually recommended for pregnant women. However, your doctor may prescribe it for severe nausea and vomiting if the potential benefits of the drug outweigh the potential risks. Compazine appears in breast milk and may affect a nursing infant. If this drug is essential to your health, your doctor may recommend that you stop breastfeeding until your treatment is finished.

### Recommended dosage

ADULTS

*To Control Severe Nausea and Vomiting*

Tablets: The usual dosage is one 5-milligram or 10-milligram tablet 3 or 4 times a day.

"Spansule" Capsules: The usual starting dose is one 15-milligram capsule on getting out of bed or one 10-milligram capsule every 12 hours.

The usual rectal dosage (suppository) is 25 milligrams, taken 2 times a day.

*For Non-psychotic Anxiety*

Tablets: The usual dose is 5 milligrams, taken 3 or 4 times a day.

"Spansule" capsule: The usual starting dose is one 15-milligram capsule on getting up or one 10-milligram capsule every 12 hours.

Treatment should not continue for longer than 12 weeks, and daily doses should not exceed 20 milligrams.

*Relatively Mild Psychotic Disorders*

The usual dose is 5 or 10 milligrams, taken 3 or 4 times daily.

*Moderate to Severe Psychotic Disorders*

Dosages usually start at 10 milligrams, taken 3 or 4 times a day. If needed, dosage may be gradually increased; 50 to 75 milligrams daily has been helpful for some people.

*More Severe Psychotic Disorders*

Dosages may range from 100 to 150 milligrams per day.

CHILDREN

Children under 2 years of age or weighing less than 20 pounds should not be given Compazine. If a child becomes restless or excited after taking Compazine, do not give the child another dose.

*For Severe Nausea and Vomiting*
An oral or rectal dose of Compazine is usually not needed for more than 1 day.

*Children 20 to 29 Pounds*
The usual dose is 2$^1/_2$ milligrams 1 or 2 times daily. Total daily amount should not exceed 7.5 milligrams.

*Children 30 to 39 Pounds*
The usual dose is 2$^1/_2$ milligrams 2 or 3 times daily. Total daily amount should not exceed 10 milligrams.

*Children 40 to 85 Pounds*
The usual dose is 2$^1/_2$ milligrams 3 times daily, or 5 milligrams 2 times daily.

Total daily amount should not exceed 15 milligrams.

*For Psychotic Disorders*
*Children 2 to 5 Years Old*
The starting oral or rectal dose is 2$^1/_2$ milligrams 2 or 3 times daily. Do not exceed 10 milligrams the first day and 20 milligrams thereafter.

*Children 6 to 12 Years Old*
The starting oral or rectal dose is 2$^1/_2$ milligrams 2 or 3 times daily. Do not exceed 10 milligrams the first day and 25 milligrams thereafter.

OLDER ADULTS

In general, older people take lower dosages of Compazine. Because they may develop low blood pressure while taking the drug, the doctor should monitor them closely. Older people (especially women) may be more susceptible to tardive dyskinesia—a possibly permanent condition. Tardive dyskinesia causes involuntary muscle spasms and twitches in the face and body. Consult your doctor for more information about these potential risks.

### Overdosage

An overdose of Compazine can be fatal. If you suspect an overdose, seek medical help immediately.

■ *Symptoms of Compazine overdose may include:*
Agitation, coma, convulsions, dry mouth, extreme sleepiness, fever, intestinal blockage, irregular heart rate, restlessness

*Generic name:*
# Conjugated estrogens
*See Premarin, page 431.*

*Brand name:*
# Corgard
*Pronounced: CORE-guard*
*Generic name: Nadolol*

### Why is this drug prescribed?
Corgard is used in the treatment of angina pectoris (chest pain, usually caused by lack of oxygen to the heart due to clogged arteries) and to reduce high blood pressure.

When prescribed for high blood pressure, it is effective when used alone or in combination with other high blood pressure medications. Corgard is a type of drug known as a beta blocker. It decreases the force and rate of heart contractions, reducing the heart's demand for oxygen and lowering blood pressure.

### Most important fact about this drug
If you have high blood pressure, you must take Corgard regularly for it to be effective. Since blood pressure declines gradually, it may be several weeks before you get the full benefit of Corgard; and you must continue taking it even if you are feeling well. Corgard does not cure high blood pressure; it merely keeps it under control.

### How should you take this medication?
Corgard can be taken with or without food. Take it exactly as prescribed even if your symptoms have disappeared.

Try not to miss any doses. Corgard is taken once a day. If it is not taken regularly, your condition may worsen.

■ *If you miss a dose...*
Take it as soon as you remember. If it is within 8 hours of your next scheduled dose, skip the one you missed and go back to your regular schedule. Never take 2 doses at the same time.

■ *Storage instructions...*
Store at room temperature, away from light and heat, in a tightly closed container.

## What side effects may occur?

Side effects cannot be anticipated. If any develop or change in intensity, inform your doctor as soon as possible. Only your doctor can determine if it is safe for you to continue taking Corgard.

■ *More common side effects may include:*
Change in behavior, changes in heartbeat, dizziness or light-headedness, mild drowsiness, slow heartbeat, weakness or tiredness

■ *Less common or rare side effects may include:*
Abdominal discomfort, asthma-like symptoms, bloating, confusion, constipation, cough, decreased sex drive, diarrhea, dry eyes, dry mouth, dry skin, facial swelling, gas, headache, heart failure, impotence, indigestion, itching, loss of appetite, low blood pressure, nasal stuffiness, nausea, rash, ringing in ears, slurred speech, vision changes, vomiting, weight gain

## Why should this drug not be prescribed?

If you have a slow heartbeat, bronchial asthma, certain types of heartbeat irregularity, cardiogenic shock (shock due to inadequate blood supply from the heart), or active heart failure, you should not take this medication.

## Special warnings about this medication

If you have a history of congestive heart failure, your doctor will prescribe Corgard with caution.

Corgard should not be stopped suddenly. This can cause increased chest pain and even a heart attack. Dosage should be gradually reduced.

If you suffer from asthma, chronic bronchitis, emphysema, seasonal allergies or other bronchial conditions, or kidney or liver disease, this medication should be used with caution.

Ask your doctor if you should check your pulse while taking Corgard. It can cause your heartbeat to become too slow.

This medication may mask the symptoms of low blood sugar or alter blood sugar levels. If you are diabetic, discuss this with your doctor.

This medication may cause you to become drowsy or less alert; therefore, driving or operating dangerous machinery or participating in any hazardous activity that requires full mental alertness is not recommended until you know how you respond to this medication.

Notify your doctor or dentist that you are taking Corgard if you have a medical emergency or before you have surgery or dental treatment.

## Possible food and drug interactions when taking this medication

If Corgard is taken with certain other drugs, the effects of either could be increased, decreased, or altered. It is especially important to check with your doctor before combining Corgard with the following:

Antidiabetic drugs, including insulin and oral drugs such as Micronase
Certain blood pressure drugs such as Diupres and Ser-Ap-Es
Epinephrine (EpiPen)

## Special information if you are pregnant or breastfeeding

The effects of Corgard during pregnancy have not been adequately studied. If you are pregnant or plan to become pregnant, inform your doctor immediately. Corgard appears in breast milk and could affect a nursing infant. If this medication is essential to your health, your doctor may advise you to discontinue breastfeeding until your treatment with this medication is finished.

## Recommended dosage

ADULTS

Dosage is tailored to each individual's needs.

*Angina Pectoris*
The usual starting dose is 40 milligrams once daily. The usual long-term dose is 40 or 80 milligrams, once a day. Doses up to 160 or 240 milligrams, once a day, may be needed.

*High Blood Pressure*
The usual starting dose is 40 milligrams once daily.

The usual long-term dose is 40 or 80 milligrams, once a day. Doses up to 240 or 320 milligrams, once a day, may be needed.

CHILDREN

The safety and effectiveness of Corgard have not been established in children.

## Overdosage

Any medication taken in excess can have serious consequences. If you suspect an overdose, seek medical attention immediately.

■ *The symptoms of Corgard overdose may include:*
Difficulty in breathing, heart failure, low blood pressure, slow heartbeat

*Brand name:*

# Cortisporin Ophthalmic Suspension

*Pronounced: KORE-ti-SPORE-in*
*Generic ingredients: Polymyxin B sulfate,*
*Neomycin sulfate, Hydrocortisone*
*Other brand name: Bacticort*

## Why is this drug prescribed?

Cortisporin Ophthalmic Suspension is a combination of the steroid drug, hydrocortisone, and two antibiotics. It is prescribed to relieve inflammatory conditions such as irritation, swelling, redness, and general eye discomfort, and to treat superficial bacterial infections of the eye.

## Most important fact about this drug

Prolonged use of this medication may increase pressure within the eye, leading to potential damage to the optic nerve and visual problems. Prolonged use also may suppress your immune response and thus increase the hazard of secondary eye infections. Your doctor should measure your eye pressure periodically if you are using this product for 10 days or longer.

## How should you use this medication?

To help clear up your infection completely, use this medication exactly as prescribed for the full time of treatment, even if your symptoms have disappeared.
  Administer the eyedrops as follows:

1. Shake the dropper bottle well.
2. Wash your hands thoroughly.
3. Gently pull your lower eyelid down to form a pocket between your eye and eyelid.
4. Hold the bottle on the bridge of your nose or on your forehead.
5. Tilt your head back and squeeze the medication into your eye.

6. Do not touch the applicator tip to any surface, including your eye.
7. Close your eyes gently, and keep them closed for 1 to 2 minutes.
8. Do not rinse the dropper.
9. Wait 5 to 10 minutes before using any other eyedrops.

If you do not improve after 2 days, your doctor should re-evaluate your case.
  Do not share this medication with anyone else; you may spread the infection.

■ *If you miss a dose...*
Apply it as soon as you remember. If it is almost time for your next dose, skip the one you missed and go back to your regular schedule.

■ *Storage instructions...*
Store at room temperature. Keep tightly closed and protect from freezing.

## What side effects may occur?

Side effects cannot be anticipated. If any develop or change in intensity, inform your doctor as soon as possible. Only your doctor can determine if it is safe for you to continue using Cortisporin.

■ *Side effects may include:*
Cataract formation (results in blurred vision), delayed wound healing, increased eye pressure (with possible development of glaucoma and, infrequently, optic nerve damage), irritation when drops are instilled, local allergic reactions (itching, swelling, redness), other infections (particularly fungal infections of the cornea and bacterial eye infections), severe allergic reactions

## Why should this drug not be prescribed?

Cortisporin should not be used if you have certain viral or fungal diseases of the eye, including inflammation of the cornea caused by herpes simplex, chickenpox, or cowpox, or if you are sensitive to or have ever had an allergic reaction to any of its ingredients.

## Special warnings about this medication

Remember that steroids such as hydrocortisone may hide the existence of an infection or worsen an existing one.
  If you are using this medication for more than 10 days, your doctor should routinely check your eye pressure. If you already have high pressure within the eye (glaucoma), use this medication cautiously.

Neomycin, one of the ingredients in Cortisporin, may cause an allergic reaction—usually itching, redness, and swelling—or failure to heal. If you develop any of these signs, stop using Cortisporin; the symptoms should quickly subside. If the condition persists or gets worse, or if a rash or allergic reaction develops, call your doctor immediately. You are more likely to be sensitive to neomycin if you are sensitive to the following antibiotics: kanamycin, paromomycin, streptomycin, and possibly gentamicin.

The use of steroids in the eye can prolong and worsen many viral infections of the eye, including herpes simplex. Use this medication with extreme caution if you have this infection.

If you develop a sensitivity to Cortisporin, avoid other topical medications that contain neomycin.

Eye products that are not handled properly can become contaminated with bacteria that cause eye infections. If you use a contaminated product, you can seriously damage your eyes, even to the point of blindness.

### Possible food and drug interactions when taking this medication
No interactions have been reported.

### Special information if you are pregnant or breastfeeding
Although the effects of Cortisporin during pregnancy have not been adequately studied, steroids should be used during pregnancy only if the benefits outweigh the dangers to the fetus. If you are pregnant or plan to become pregnant, inform your doctor immediately. Hydrocortisone, when taken orally, appears in breast milk. Since medication may be absorbed into the bloodstream when it is applied to the eye, your doctor may advise you to stop breastfeeding until your treatment with Cortisporin is finished.

### Recommended dosage
ADULTS

The usual recommended dose is 1 or 2 drops in the affected eye every 3 or 4 hours, depending on the severity of the condition. Cortisporin may be used more often if necessary.

### Overdosage
Any medication used in excess can have serious consequences. If you suspect an overdose of Cortisporin Ophthalmic Suspension, seek medical treatment immediately.

*Brand name:*

# Corzide

*Pronounced: CORE-zide*
*Generic ingredients: Nadolol, Bendroflumethiazide*

### Why is this drug prescribed?
Corzide is a combination drug used in the treatment of high blood pressure. It combines a beta blocker and a thiazide diuretic. Nadolol, the beta blocker, decreases the force and rate of heart contractions thereby reducing blood pressure. Bendroflumethiazide, the diuretic, helps your body produce and eliminate more urine, which also helps in lowering blood pressure.

### Most important fact about this drug
You must take Corzide regularly for it to be effective. Since blood pressure declines gradually, it may be several weeks before you get the full benefit of Corzide; and you must continue taking it even if you are feeling well. Corzide does not cure high blood pressure; it merely keeps it under control.

### How should you take this medication?
Corzide may be taken with or without food. Take it exactly as prescribed, even if your symptoms have disappeared.

Try not to miss any doses. Corzide is taken once a day. If this medication is not taken regularly, your condition may worsen.

■ *If you miss a dose...*
Take it as soon as you remember. If it's within 8 hours of your next scheduled dose, skip the one you missed and go back to your regular schedule. Never take 2 doses at the same time.

■ *Storage instructions...*
Store at room temperature, away from heat, in a tightly closed container.

### What side effects may occur?
Side effects cannot be anticipated. If any develop or change in intensity, inform your doctor as soon as possible. Only your doctor can determine if it is safe for you to continue taking Corzide.

■ *More common side effects may include:*
Asthma-like symptoms, changes in heart rhythm, cold hands and feet, dizziness, fatigue, low blood pressure, low potassium levels (symptoms

include dry mouth, excessive thirst, weak or irregular heartbeat, muscle pain or cramps), slow heartbeat

■ *Less common or rare side effects may include:*
Abdominal discomfort, anemia, bloating, blurred vision, certain types of irregular heartbeat, change in behavior, constipation, cough, diarrhea, dry mouth, eyes, or skin, facial swelling, gas, headache, heart failure, hepatitis, impotence, indigestion, inflammation of the pancreas, itching, loss of appetite, lowered sex drive, muscle spasm, nasal stuffiness, nausea, rash, ringing in ears, sedation, sensitivity to light, slurred speech, sweating, tingling or pins and needles, vertigo, vomiting, weakness, weight gain, wheezing, yellowed eyes and skin

## Why should this drug not be prescribed?

If you have bronchial asthma, slow heartbeat, certain heartbeat irregularities (heart block), inadequate blood supply to the circulatory system (cardiogenic shock), active congestive heart failure, inability to urinate, or if you are sensitive to or have ever had an allergic reaction to Corzide, its ingredients, or similar drugs, you should not take this medication.

## Special warnings about this medication

If you have a history of congestive heart failure, your doctor will prescribe Corzide with caution.

Corzide should not be stopped suddenly. This can cause increased chest pain and even a heart attack. Dosage should be gradually reduced.

If you suffer from asthma, seasonal allergies, emphysema or other bronchial conditions, or kidney or liver disease, this medication should be used with caution.

Ask your doctor if you should check your pulse while taking Corzide. It can cause your heartbeat to become too slow.

Corzide may mask the symptoms of low blood sugar or alter blood sugar levels. If you are diabetic, discuss this with your doctor.

This medication can cause you to become drowsy or less alert; therefore, activity that requires full mental alertness is not recommended until you know how you respond to this medication.

Notify your doctor or dentist that you are taking Corzide if you have a medical emergency, or before you have surgery or dental treatment.

## Possible food and drug interactions when taking this medication

Corzide may intensify the effects of alcohol. Do not drink alcohol while taking this medication.

If Corzide is taken with any other drug, the effects of either could be increased, decreased, or altered. It is especially important to check with your doctor before combining Corzide with the following:

Amphotericin B
Antidepressant drugs known as MAO inhibitors, such as Nardil and Parnate
Antidiabetic drugs, including insulin and oral drugs such as Micronase
Antigout drugs such as Benemid
Barbiturates such as phenobarbital
Blood thinners such as Coumadin
Calcium salt
Certain blood pressure drugs such as Diupres and Ser-Ap-Es
Cholestyramine (Questran)
Colestipol (Colestid)
Diazoxide (Proglycem)
Digitalis medications such as Lanoxin
Lithium (Lithonate)
Methenamine (Mandelamine)
Narcotics such as Percocet
Nonsteroidal anti-inflammatory drugs, such as Motrin, Naprosyn, and Nuprin
Other antihypertensives such as Vasotec
Steroid medications such as prednisone
Sulfinpyrazone (Anturane)

## Special information if you are pregnant or breastfeeding

The effects of Corzide during pregnancy have not been adequately studied. If you are pregnant or plan to become pregnant, inform your doctor immediately. Corzide appears in breast milk and could affect a nursing infant. If this medication is essential to your health, your doctor may advise you to discontinue breastfeeding until your treatment with Corzide is finished.

## Recommended dosage

ADULTS

Dosages of this drug are always tailored to the individual's needs.

The usual dose is 1 Corzide 40/5 milligram tablet per day or, if necessary, 1 Corzide 80/5 milligram tablet per day. Your doctor may gradually add another high blood pressure medication to this drug.

### CHILDREN

The safety and effectiveness of Corzide have not been established in children.

### Overdosage

Any medication taken in excess can have serious consequences. If you suspect an overdose, seek medical attention immediately.

■ *The symptoms of Corzide overdose may include:*
Abdominal irritation, central nervous system depression, coma, extremely slow heartbeat, heart failure, lethargy, low blood pressure, wheezing

*Brand name:*

# Cotrim

*See Bactrim, page 50.*

*Brand name:*

# Coumadin

*Pronounced: COO-muh-din*
*Generic name: Warfarin sodium*

### Why is this drug prescribed?

Coumadin is an anticoagulant (blood thinner). It is prescribed to:

Prevent and/or treat a blood clot that has formed within a blood vessel or in the lungs.

Prevent and/or treat blood clots associated with certain heart conditions or replacement of a heart valve.

Aid in the prevention of blood clots that may form in blood vessels anywhere in the body after a heart attack.

Reduce the risk of death, another heart attack, or stroke after a heart attack.

### Most important fact about this drug

The most serious risks associated with Coumadin treatment are hemorrhage (severe bleeding resulting in the loss of a large amount of blood) in any tissue or organ and, less frequently, the destruction of skin tissue cells (necrosis) or gangrene. The risk

of hemorrhage usually depends on the dosage and length of treatment with this drug.

Hemorrhage and necrosis have been reported to result in death or permanent disability. Severe necrosis can lead to the removal of damaged tissue or amputation of a limb. Necrosis appears to be associated with blood clots located in the area of tissue damage and usually occurs within a few days of starting Coumadin treatment.

### How should you take this medication?

The objective of treatment with a blood-thinner is to control the blood-clotting process without causing severe bleeding, so that a clot does not form and cut off the blood supply necessary for normal body function. Therefore, it is very important that you take this medication exactly as prescribed by your doctor and that your doctor monitor your condition on a regular basis. Be especially careful to stick to the exact dosage schedule your doctor prescribes.

Effective treatment with minimal complications depends on your cooperation and communication with the doctor.

Do not take or discontinue any other medication unless directed to do so by your doctor. Avoid alcohol, salicylates such as aspirin, larger than usual amounts of foods rich in vitamin K (including liver, vegetable oil, egg yolks, and green leafy vegetables), which can counteract the effect of Coumadin, or any other drastic change in diet.

Note that Coumadin often turns urine reddish-orange.

You should carry an identification card that indicates you are taking Coumadin.

■ *If you miss a dose...*
Take the forgotten dose as soon as you remember, then go back to your regular schedule. If you do not remember until the next day, skip the dose. Never try to "catch up" by doubling the dose. Keep a record for your doctor of any doses you miss.
■ *Storage instructions...*
Coumadin can be stored at room temperature. Close the container tightly and protect from light.

### What side effects may occur?

Side effects cannot be anticipated. If any develop or change in intensity, inform your doctor as soon as possible. Only your doctor can determine if it is safe for you to continue taking Coumadin.

■ *More common side effects may include:*

Hemorrhage: Signs of severe bleeding resulting in the loss of large amounts of blood depend upon the location and extent of bleeding. Symptoms include: chest, abdomen, joint, or other pain, difficult breathing or swallowing, dizziness, headache, low blood pressure, numbness and tingling, paralysis, shortness of breath, unexplained shock, unexplained swelling, weakness

■ *Less common side effects may include:*

Abdominal cramping, allergic reactions, diarrhea, fever, hepatitis, hives, itching, liver damage, loss of hair, nausea, necrosis (gangrene), purple toes, severe or long-lasting inflammation of the skin, vomiting, yellowed skin and eyes

## Why should this drug not be prescribed?

This drug should not be used for any condition where the danger of hemorrhage may be greater than the potential benefits of treatment. Unless directed to do so by your doctor, do not take this medication if one of the following conditions or situations applies to you:

A tendency to hemorrhage

Alcoholism

An abnormal blood condition

Aneurysm (balloon-like swelling of a blood vessel) in the brain or heart

Bleeding tendencies associated with: ulceration or bleeding of the stomach, intestines, respiratory tract, or the genital or urinary system

Eclampsia (a rare and serious pregnancy disorder producing life-threatening convulsions), or preeclampsia (a toxic condition—including headache, high blood pressure, and swelling of the legs and feet—that can lead to eclampsia)

Excessive bleeding of brain blood vessels

Inflammation, due to bacterial infection, of the membrane that lines the inside of the heart

Inflammation of the sac that surrounds the heart or an escape of fluid from the heart sac

Malignant hypertension (extremely elevated blood pressure that damages the inner linings of blood vessels, the heart, spleen, kidneys, and brain)

Pregnancy

Recent or contemplated surgery of the central nervous system

(brain and spinal cord) or eye

Spinal puncture or any procedure that can cause uncontrollable bleeding

Threatened miscarriage

## Special warnings about this medication

Treatment with blood thinners may increase the risk that fatty plaque will break away from the wall of an artery and lodge at another point, causing the blockage of a blood vessel. If you notice any of the following symptoms, contact your doctor immediately:

Abdominal pain; abrupt and intense pain in the leg, foot, or toes; blood in the urine; bluish mottling of the skin of the legs and hands; foot ulcers; gangrene; high blood pressure; muscle pain; "purple toes syndrome" (see below); rash; or thigh or back pain.

If you have any of the following conditions, tell your doctor. He or she will have to consider the risks against the benefits before giving you Coumadin.

An infectious disease or intestinal disorder

A history of recurrent blood clot disorders in you or your family

An implanted catheter

Dental procedures

Inflammation of a blood vessel

Moderate to severe high blood pressure

Moderate to severe kidney or liver dysfunction

Polycythemia vera (blood disorder)

Severe diabetes

Surgery or injury that leaves large raw surfaces

Trauma or injury that may result in internal bleeding

Purple toes syndrome can occur when taking Coumadin, usually 3 to 10 weeks after the start of anti-coagulation therapy. Symptoms include dark purplish or mottled color of the toes that turns white when pressure is applied and fades when you elevate your legs, pain and tenderness of the toes, and change in intensity of the color over a period of time. If any of these symptoms develop, notify your doctor immediately.

If you are taking Coumadin, your doctor should periodically check the time it takes for your blood to start the clotting process (prothrombin time). Numerous factors such as travel and changes in diet, environment, physical state, and medication may alter your response to treatment with an anticoagulant. Clotting time should also be monitored after your release from the hospital and whenever other medications are started, discontinued, or taken haphazardly.

If you have congestive heart failure, you may become more sensitive to Coumadin and may need to have your dosage reduced. Your doctor will have you tested regularly.

Notify your doctor if any illness, such as diarrhea, infection, or fever develops; if any unusual symptoms, such as pain, swelling, or discomfort, appear; or if you see prolonged bleeding from cuts, increased menstrual flow, vaginal bleeding, nosebleeds, bleeding of gums from brushing, unusual bleeding or bruising, red or dark brown urine, red or tarry black stool, or diarrhea.

### Possible food and drug interactions when taking this medication
Coumadin can interact with a very wide variety of drugs, both prescription and over-the-counter. Check with your doctor before taking ANY other medication or vitamin product.

### Special information if you are pregnant or breastfeeding
Coumadin should not be taken by women who are or may become pregnant since the drug may cause fatal hemorrhage in the developing baby. There have also been reports of birth malformations in children born to mothers who have been treated with Coumadin during pregnancy. Spontaneous abortions and stillbirths are also known to occur. If you become pregnant while taking this drug, inform your doctor immediately. Coumadin may appear in breast milk and could affect a nursing infant. If this medication is essential to your health, your doctor may advise you to stop nursing your baby until your treatment with this drug is finished.

### Recommended dosage
ADULTS

The administration and dosage of Coumadin must be individualized by your doctor according to your sensitivity to the drug.

A common starting dosage of Coumadin tablets for adults is 2 to 5 milligrams per day. Individualized daily dosage adjustments are based on the results of tests that determine the amount of time it takes for the blood clotting process to begin.

A maintenance dose of 2 to 10 milligrams per day is satisfactory for most people. The duration of treatment will be determined by your physician.

CHILDREN

Safety and effectiveness have not been established in children below the age of 18.

### Overdosage
Signs and symptoms of Coumadin overdose reflect abnormal bleeding. They include:

Blood in stools or urine, excessive menstrual bleeding, black stools, reddish or purplish spots on skin, excessive bruising, persistent bleeding from superficial injuries

If you suspect an overdose, seek emergency medical treatment immediately.

*Brand name:*

# Cozaar

*Pronounced: CO-zahr*
*Generic name: Losartan Potassium*

### Why is this drug prescribed?
Cozaar is used in the treatment of high blood pressure. It is effective when used alone or with other high blood pressure medications, such as diuretics that help the body get rid of water.

Cozaar is the first of a new class of blood pressure medications called angiotensin-II receptor antagonists. Cozaar works, in part, by preventing the hormone angiotensin II from constricting the blood vessels, which tends to raise blood pressure.

### Most important fact about this drug
You must take Cozaar regularly for it to be effective. Since blood pressure declines gradually, it may be several weeks before you get the full benefit of Cozaar, and you must continue taking it even if you are feeling well. Cozaar does not cure high blood pressure; it merely keeps it under control.

### How should you take this medication?
Cozaar can be taken with or without food.

Take it at the same time each day. For example, if you take the medication every morning before or after breakfast, you will establish a regular routine and be less likely to forget your dose.

■ *If you miss a dose...*
Take it as soon as possible. If it is almost time for your next dose, skip the missed dose and go back to your regular schedule.

■ *Storage instructions...*
Store at room temperature. Keep in a tightly closed container, away from light.

### What side effects may occur?
Side effects cannot be anticipated. If any develop or change in intensity, tell your doctor as soon as possible. Only your doctor can determine if it is safe for you to continue taking Cozaar.

■ *More common side effects may include:*
Cough, dizziness, upper respiratory infection
■ *Less common side effects may include:*
Back and leg pain, diarrhea, indigestion, insomnia, muscle cramps or pain, nasal congestion, sinus problems

### Why should this drug not be prescribed?
Do not take Cozaar when you are pregnant. Avoid it if you have ever had an allergic reaction to it.

### Special warnings about this medication
Cozaar can cause low blood pressure, especially if you are also taking a diuretic. You may feel lightheaded or faint, especially during the first few days of therapy. If these symptoms occur, contact your doctor. Your dosage may need to be adjusted or discontinued. Be sure you know how you react to Cozaar before you drive or operate machinery.

Excessive sweating, dehydration, severe diarrhea, or vomiting could make you lose too much water, causing a severe drop in blood pressure. Call your doctor if you experience any of these symptoms. Be sure to tell your doctor about any medical conditions you have, especially liver or kidney disease.

### Possible food and drug interactions when taking this medication
If Cozaar is taken with certain other drugs, the effects of either could be increased, decreased, or altered. It is especially important to check with your doctor before taking Cozaar with the following:

Ketoconazole (Nizoral)
Troleandomycin (Tao)

### Special information if you are pregnant or breastfeeding
Drugs such as Cozaar can cause injury or even death to the unborn child when used in the second or third trimester of pregnancy. Stop taking Cozaar as soon as you know you are pregnant. If you are pregnant or plan to become pregnant, tell your doctor before taking Cozaar. Cozaar may appear in breast milk and could affect the nursing infant. If this medication is essential to your health, your doctor may advise you to stop breastfeeding while you are taking Cozaar.

### Recommended dosage
ADULTS

The usual starting dose is 50 milligrams once daily. However, Cozaar can also be taken twice daily, with total daily doses ranging from 25 milligrams to 100 milligrams. If your blood pressure does not respond, your doctor may increase your dose or add a low-dose diuretic to your regimen.

*People taking diuretics and people with liver impairment*
The usual starting dose is 25 milligrams daily. Your doctor may adjust your dosage according to your response.

CHILDREN

The safety and effectiveness of Cozaar in children have not been studied.

### Overdosage
Any medication taken in excess can have serious consequences. If you suspect an overdose, seek medical attention immediately. Information concerning Cozaar overdosage is limited. However, hypotension (low blood pressure) and abnormally rapid or slow heartbeat may be signs of an overdose.

*Brand name:*

# Creon

*See Pancrease, page 392.*

*Brand name:*

# Crixivan

*Pronounced: CRIX-i-van*
*Generic name: Indinavir sulfate*

### Why is this drug prescribed?
Crixivan is used in the treatment of human immunodeficiency virus (HIV) infection. HIV causes the immune system to break down so that it can no

longer fight off other infections. This leads to the fatal disease known as acquired immune deficiency syndrome (AIDS).

HIV thrives by taking over the immune system's vital CD4 cells (white blood cells) and using their inner workings to make additional copies of itself. Crixivan belongs to a new class of HIV drugs called protease inhibitors, which work by interfering with an important step in the virus's reproductive cycle. Although Crixivan cannot eliminate HIV already present in the body, it can reduce the amount of virus available to infect other cells.

Crixivan can be taken alone or in combination with other HIV drugs such as Retrovir. Because Crixivan and Retrovir attack the virus in different ways, the combination is likely to be more effective than either drug alone.

### Most important fact about this drug

It is important that you drink at least 48 ounces (4 soda-can sized glasses) of liquid daily while taking Crixivan. If you do not get enough liquid, you may develop kidney stones and have to temporarily stop taking Crixivan or even discontinue it altogether.

### How should you take this medication?

Take this medication exactly as prescribed by your doctor. Do not share this medication with anyone and do not take more than your recommended dosage.

To ensure maximum absorption, do not take Crixivan with food. Instead, take it with water 1 hour before or 2 hours after a meal. (Crixivan may also be taken with liquids such as skim milk, juice, coffee, or tea, or even with a light meal such as dry toast with jelly, juice, and coffee with skim milk and sugar, or corn flakes with skim milk and sugar.)

■ *If you miss a dose...*
Skip it and take the next dose at the regularly scheduled time. Do not double the dose.
■ *Storage instructions...*
Crixivan capsules are sensitive to moisture. Store Crixivan at room temperature in the original container and leave the drying agent in the bottle to keep the medication dry. Keep the container tightly closed.

### What side effects may occur?

Side effects cannot be anticipated. If any develop or change in intensity, inform your doctor as soon as possible. Only your doctor can determine if it is safe for you to continue taking Crixivan.

■ *Possible side effects may include:*
Abdominal pain, back pain, blood in the urine, changes in taste, diarrhea, dizziness, drowsiness, dry skin and mouth, fatigue, general feeling of illness, headache, indigestion, insomnia, loss of appetite, nausea, pain in the side, rash, sore throat, upper respiratory infection, vomiting, weakness, yellow skin or eyes

### Why should this drug not be prescribed?

If you suffer a severe allergic reaction to Crixivan or any of its ingredients, you should not take this medication.

### Special warnings about this medication

Although Crixivan reduces the amount of HIV in the blood and increases the white blood cell count, its long-term effect on survival is still unknown. The virus remains in the body, and you will continue to face the possibility of complications, including opportunistic infections (rare infections that develop when the immune system falters) such as certain types of pneumonia, tuberculosis, and fungal infection. Therefore, it is important that you remain under the care of a doctor and keep all your follow-up appointments.

Crixivan is not a cure for HIV infection, and it does not reduce the risk of transmission of HIV to others through sexual contact or blood contamination. Therefore, you should continue to avoid practices that could spread HIV.

Check with your doctor if you have liver disease, particularly cirrhosis of the liver, before using Crixivan. Because there is little information concerning the use of this drug in people with kidney disease or severe liver disease, be sure to tell your doctor if you have either condition.

### Possible food and drug interactions when taking this medication

Do not take Crixivan with the following medications. The combination may cause serious or life-threatening effects.

Astemizole (Hismanal)
Cisapride (Propulsid)
Midazolam (Versed)
Terfenadine (Seldane)
Triazolam (Halcion)

Crixivan may also interact with certain other drugs, and the effects of either could be increased, decreased, or altered. It is especially important to check with your doctor before combining Crixivan with the following:

Clarithromycin (Biaxin)
Didanosine (Videx)
Fluconazole (Diflucan)
Isoniazid (Nydrazid)
Ketoconazole (Nizoral)
Ortho-Novum
Quinidine (Quinidex)
Rifabutin (Mycobutin)
Rifampin (Rifadin)
Trimethoprim (Bactrim, Trimpex, Septra)

Avoid drinking grapefruit juice while taking Crixivan. This kind of juice can reduce the drug's effectiveness.

Be sure to tell your doctor and pharmacist about all medications you are taking, both prescription and over-the-counter. Alert them, too, when you *stop* taking a medication.

### Special information
### if you are pregnant or breastfeeding
The effects of Crixivan during pregnancy have not been adequately studied. If you are pregnant or plan to become pregnant, tell your doctor immediately. Do not breastfeed your baby. HIV appears in breast milk and can infect a nursing infant.

### Recommended dosage
ADULTS

The recommended dose of Crixivan is 800 milligrams (two 400-milligram capsules) every 8 hours. Your doctor may lower the dose to 600 milligrams every 8 hours if you have mild-to-moderate liver problems due to cirrhosis. If you have been prescribed another HIV drug along with Crixivan, take it as directed.

CHILDREN

The safety and effectiveness of Crixivan for use in children have not been established.

### Overdosage
There is no information presently available on Crixivan overdose. However, any medication taken in excess can have serious consequences. If you suspect an overdose, seek emergency medical treatment immediately.

*Brand name:*

# Crolom

*Pronounced: CROW-lum*
*Generic name: Cromolyn sodium*

### Why is this drug prescribed?
Crolom is an eyedrop that relieves the itching, tearing, discharge, and redness caused by seasonal and chronic allergies. The drug works by preventing certain cells in the body from releasing histamine and other substances that can cause an allergic reaction.

### Most important fact about this drug
In order for Crolom to work properly, you must continue to use it every day at regular intervals even if your symptoms have disappeared. It can take up to 6 weeks for your condition to clear up.

### How should you use this medication?
Use Crolom exactly as directed by your doctor. Do not use more or less than required and apply it only when scheduled. To administer Crolom, follow these steps:

1. Wash your hands thoroughly.
2. Gently pull your lower eyelid down to form a pocket between your eye and the lid.
3. Drop the medicine into this pocket. Let go of the eyelid and gently close the eye. Do not blink. Keep your eyes closed for a minute or two.
4. Do not touch the applicator tip to your eye or any other surface. This could lead to infection.
5. Do not rinse the dropper.

■ *If you miss a dose...*
  Use it as soon as possible. Then go back to your regular schedule.
■ *Storage instructions...*
  Keep the container tightly closed and away from light. Store at room temperature.

### What side effects may occur?
You may experience temporary burning or stinging in the eye after you apply Crolom.

■ *Rare side effects may include:*
  Dryness around the eye, eye irritation, inflammation of the eyelids, itchy eyes, puffy eyes, styes, watery eyes

### Why should this drug not be prescribed?
If you have ever had an allergic reaction to cromolyn sodium, avoid this medication.

## Special warnings about this medication

Do not wear soft contact lenses while you are using Crolom.

If your symptoms do not begin to improve, alert your doctor.

## Possible food and drug interactions with the medication

No interactions have been reported.

## Special information if you are pregnant or breastfeeding

There are no studies on use of Crolom with pregnant women. If you are pregnant or plan to become pregnant, tell your doctor. Crolom should be used during pregnancy only if clearly needed. It is not known whether Crolom appears in human breast milk. If you are nursing and need to use Crolom, use it with caution.

## Recommended dosage

ADULTS AND CHILDREN

Put 1 or 2 drops into each eye 4 to 6 times a day at evenly spaced intervals.

It is not known whether Crolom is safe and effective for children under 4 years.

## Overdosage

Although there is no information on Crolom overdose, any medication taken in excess can have serious consequences. If you suspect an overdose, seek medical attention immediately.

*Generic name:*

# Cromolyn, inhaled

*See Intal, page 261.*

*Generic name:*

# Cromolyn, ocular

*See Crolom, page 123.*

*Generic name:*

# Cyclobenzaprine

*See Flexeril, page 216.*

*Brand name:*

# Cyclocort

*Pronounced: SIKE-low-court*
*Generic name: Amcinonide*

## Why is this drug prescribed?

Cyclocort is prescribed for the relief of the inflammatory and itchy symptoms of skin disorders that are responsive to corticosteroid treatment.

## Most important fact about this drug

When you use Cyclocort, you inevitably absorb some of the medication through your skin and into the bloodstream. Too much absorption can lead to unwanted side effects elsewhere in the body. To keep this problem to a minimum, avoid using large amounts of Cyclocort over large areas, and do not cover it with airtight dressings such as plastic wrap or adhesive bandages unless specifically told to by your doctor.

## How should you use this medication?

Use this medication exactly as prescribed by your doctor. It is for use only on the skin. Be careful to keep it out of your eyes.

Apply Cyclocort sparingly. Rub it in gently.

■ *If you miss a dose...*
Apply the forgotten dose as soon as you remember. Use the remaining doses for that day at evenly spaced intervals. Never try to "catch up" by doubling the amount applied.

■ *Storage instructions...*
Cyclocort can be stored at room temperature. Protect from freezing.

## What side effects may occur?

Side effects cannot be anticipated. If any develop or change in intensity, inform your doctor as soon as possible. Only your doctor can determine if it is safe for you to continue taking Cyclocort.

■ *More common side effects may include:*
Burning, itching, soreness, stinging
■ *Less common or rare side effects may include:*
Dryness, excessive growth of hair, infection, inflammation of hair follicles, inflammation of the skin around the mouth, irritation, prickly heat, skin eruptions resembling acne, softening of the skin, stretch marks

## Why should this drug not be prescribed?

If you are sensitive to or have ever had an allergic reaction to amcinonide or other steroid medications, you should not use Cyclocort. Make sure your doctor is aware of any drug reactions you have experienced.

## Special warnings about this medication

Do not use this drug for any disorder other than the one for which it was prescribed.

The use of tight-fitting diapers or plastic pants is not recommended for a child being treated in the diaper area. These garments may act as airtight dressings or bandages.

The treated skin area should not be bandaged, covered, or wrapped unless you have been directed to do so by your doctor.

If an irritation or allergic reaction develops while you are using Cyclocort, notify your doctor.

## Possible food and drug interactions when taking this medication

No interactions with food or other drugs have been reported.

## Special information if you are pregnant or breastfeeding

The effects of Cyclocort during pregnancy have not been adequately studied. If you are pregnant or plan to become pregnant, inform your doctor immediately. It is not known whether this medication appears in breast milk. If this drug is essential to your health, your doctor may advise you to discontinue breastfeeding until your treatment is finished.

## Recommended dosage

### ADULTS

Apply a thin film of Cyclocort to the affected area 2 or 3 times a day, depending on the severity of the condition.

Cyclocort lotion may be applied to the affected areas, particularly hairy areas, 2 times per day. The lotion should be rubbed in completely, and the area should not be washed and should be protected from clothing until the lotion has dried.

Your doctor may recommend airtight bandages or dressings if you are being treated for psoriasis (a skin disorder characterized by patches of red, dry, scale-covered skin) or other stubborn skin conditions. If an infection develops, stop bandaging the area.

### CHILDREN

Topical use of Cyclocort on children should be limited to the smallest amount that is effective. Long-term treatment may interfere with children's growth and development.

## Overdosage

A severe overdosage is unlikely with the use of Cyclocort; however, long-term or prolonged use can produce side effects throughout the body (see "Most important fact about this drug").

*Generic name:*

# Cyclophosphamide

*See Cytoxan, page 128.*

*Generic name:*

# Cyclosporine

*See Sandimmune, page 486.*

*Brand name:*

# Cycrin

*See Provera, page 448.*

*Brand name:*

# Cylert

*Pronounced: SIGH-lert*
*Generic name: Pemoline*

## Why is this drug prescribed?

Cylert is used to help treat children who have attention deficit disorder with hyperactivity. However, this condition does not always require drug treatment. Drugs such as Cylert should be taken as part of a comprehensive treatment plan offering psychological and educational support to help the child become more stable.

Children who have attention deficit disorder with hyperactivity may show signs of:

Emotional mood swings
Hyperactivity
Impulsive actions
Moderate to severe distractibility
Short attention span

### Most important fact about this drug

Because long-term use of drugs such as Cylert may affect a child's growth, your doctor will monitor your child carefully if he or she is taking this drug for an extended period.

### How should you take this medication?

Cylert should be taken once a day, in the morning.

■ *If you miss a dose...*
Have your child take it as soon as you remember, then go back to the regular schedule. If you do not remember it until the next day, skip the missed dose and go back to the regular schedule. Do not give 2 doses at once.

■ *Storage instructions...*
Store at room temperature.

### What side effects may occur?

Side effects cannot be anticipated. If any develop or change in intensity, inform your doctor as soon as possible. Only your doctor can determine if it is safe for your child to continue taking Cylert.

■ *More common side effects may include:*
Insomnia

■ *Less common side effects may include:*
Dizziness, drowsiness, hallucinations, headache, hepatitis and other liver problems, increased irritability, involuntary, fragmented movements of the face, eyes, lips, tongue, arms, and legs, loss of appetite, mild depression, nausea, seizures, skin rash, stomachache, suppressed growth (in children), uncontrolled vocal outbursts (such as grunts, shouts, and obscene language), weight loss, yellowing of skin or eyes

■ *Rare side effects may include:*
A rare form of anemia with symptoms such as bleeding gums, bruising, chest pain, fatigue, headache, nosebleeds, and abnormal paleness

### Why should this drug not be prescribed?

Your child should not be using Cylert if he or she is allergic to it or if he or she has liver problems.

### Special warnings about this medication

Cylert may cause dizziness. Warn your child to be careful climbing stairs or participating in activities that require mental alertness.

Although there have been no reports that Cylert is physically addictive, it is chemically similar to a class of drugs that are potentially addictive.

Therefore, anyone who has a history of drug or alcohol abuse should use Cylert cautiously.

Remember that children who take this drug on a long-term basis should be carefully monitored for signs of stunted growth.

Use Cylert cautiously if your child has kidney problems.

Psychotic children who take Cylert may experience increasingly disordered thoughts and behavioral disturbances.

### Possible food and drug interactions when taking this medication

If Cylert is taken with certain other drugs, the effects of either could be increased, decreased, or altered. It is especially important to check with your doctor before combining Cylert with the following:

Antiepileptic medications such as Tegretol
Other drugs that affect the central nervous system (brain and spinal cord) such as Ritalin

### Special information if you are pregnant or breastfeeding

This drug is for use only in children, and its effects in pregnancy have not been adequately studied. Cylert should be used during pregnancy only if it is clearly necessary. The drug may appear in breast milk and affect the baby.

### Recommended dosage

The recommended beginning dose is 37.5 milligrams daily. Dosages may be gradually increased if needed. Most children take doses ranging from 56.25 to 75 milligrams a day. The maximum recommended daily dose of Cylert is 112.5 milligrams. Significant improvement is gradual and may not be apparent until the third or fourth week of treatment with Cylert.

Your doctor may occasionally stop treatment with Cylert to see whether behavioral problems return and whether further treatment with Cylert is necessary.

### Overdosage

Any medication taken in excess can have serious consequences. If you suspect an overdose, seek medical help immediately.

■ *Symptoms of Cylert overdose may include:*
Agitation, coma, confusion, convulsions, delirium, dilated pupils, exaggerated feeling of well-

being, extremely high temperature, flushing, hallucinations, headache, high blood pressure, increased heart rate, increased reflex reactions, muscle twitches, sweating, tremors, vomiting

*Generic name:*

# Cyproheptadine

*See Periactin, page 408.*

*Brand name:*

# Cytotec

Pronounced: SITE-oh-tek
Generic name: Misoprostol

### Why is this drug prescribed?

Cytotec, a synthetic prostaglandin (hormone-like substance), reduces the production of stomach acid and protects the stomach lining. People who take nonsteroidal anti-inflammatory drugs (NSAIDs) may be given Cytotec tablets to help prevent stomach ulcers.

Aspirin and other NSAIDs such as Motrin, Naprosyn, Feldene, and others, which are widely used to control the pain and inflammation of arthritis, are generally hard on the stomach. If you must take an NSAID for a prolonged period of time, and if you are elderly or have ever had a stomach ulcer, your doctor may want you to take Cytotec for as long as you take the NSAID.

### Most important fact about this drug

You must not become pregnant while using Cytotec. This drug causes uterine contractions that could lead to a miscarriage. If you do have a miscarriage, there is a risk that it might be incomplete. This could lead to bleeding, hospitalization, surgery, infertility, or even death. It is vitally important to use reliable contraception while taking Cytotec.

### How should you take this medication?

Take Cytotec with meals, exactly as prescribed.

Take Cytotec for the full course of NSAID treatment, even if you notice no stomach problems.

Take the final dosage at bedtime.

■ *If you miss a dose...*
    Take it as soon as you remember. If it is almost time for your next dose, skip the one you missed

and go back to your regular schedule. Do not take 2 doses at once.

■ *Storage instructions...*
    Store at room temperature in a dry place.

### What side effects may occur?

Cytotec may cause abdominal cramps, diarrhea, and/or nausea, especially during the first few weeks of treatment. These symptoms may disappear as your body gets used to the drug. Taking Cytotec with food can help minimize diarrhea. If you have prolonged difficulty (more than 8 days), or if you have severe diarrhea, cramping, or nausea, call your doctor.

■ *Other side effects may include:*
    Constipation, gas, indigestion, headache, heavy menstrual bleeding, menstrual disorder, menstrual pain or cramps, paleness, spotting (light bleeding between menstrual periods), stomach or intestinal bleeding, vomiting

Cytotec may cause uterine bleeding even if you have gone through menopause. However, postmenopausal bleeding could be a sign of some other gynecological problem. If you experience any such bleeding while taking Cytotec, notify your doctor at once.

### Why should this drug not be prescribed?

Do not take Cytotec if you are sensitive to or have ever had an allergic reaction to it or to another prostaglandin medication.

Do not take Cytotec if you are pregnant or might become pregnant while taking it.

### Special warnings about this medication

Since Cytotec may cause diarrhea, you should use this drug very cautiously if you have inflammatory bowel disease or any other condition in which the loss of fluid caused by diarrhea would be particularly dangerous.

To reduce the risk of diarrhea, take Cytotec with food and avoid taking it with a magnesium-containing antacid, such as Di-Gel, Gelusil, Maalox, Mylanta, and others. Have frequent medical checkups.

Never give Cytotec to anyone else; the dosage might be wrong, and if the other person is pregnant, the drug might harm the unborn baby or cause a miscarriage.

### Possible food and drug interactions when taking this medication

Cytotec does not interfere with arthritis medications such as aspirin and ibuprofen.

### Special information if you are pregnant or breastfeeding

If you are pregnant or plan to become pregnant, inform your doctor immediately. Because Cytotec can cause miscarriage, it should not be taken during pregnancy. If you are a woman of childbearing age, you should not take Cytotec unless you have thoroughly discussed the risks with your doctor and believe you are able to take effective contraceptive measures.

You will need to take a pregnancy test about 2 weeks before starting to take Cytotec. To be sure you are not pregnant at the start of Cytotec treatment, your doctor will have you take your first dose on the second or third day of your menstrual period.

Even the most scrupulous contraceptive measures sometimes fail. If you believe you may have become pregnant while taking Cytotec, stop taking the drug and contact your doctor immediately.

It is not known if Cytotec appears in breast milk. Because of the potential for severe diarrhea in a nursing infant, your doctor may have you stop breastfeeding until your treatment is finished.

### Recommended dosage

ADULTS

The recommended oral dose of Cytotec for the prevention of NSAID-induced stomach ulcers is 200 micrograms 4 times daily with food. Take the last dose of the day at bedtime.

If you cannot tolerate this dosage, your doctor can prescribe a dose of 100 micrograms.

Your should take Cytotec for the duration of NSAID therapy, as prescribed by your doctor.

*For People with Kidney Impairment*

You will not normally need an adjustment in the dosing schedule, but your doctor can reduce the dosage if you have trouble handling the usual dose.

### Overdosage

Any medication taken in excess can have serious consequences. If you suspect symptoms of an overdose of Cytotec, seek medical attention immediately.

■ *Symptoms of Cytotec overdose may include:*

Abdominal pain, breathing difficulty, convulsions, diarrhea, fever, heart palpitations, low blood pressure, sedation (extreme drowsiness), slowed heartbeat, stomach or intestinal discomfort, tremors

*Brand name:*

# Cytoxan

*Pronounced: sigh-TOKS-an*
*Generic name: Cyclophosphamide*

### Why is this drug prescribed?

Cytoxan, an anticancer drug, works by interfering with the growth of malignant cells. It may be used alone but is often given with other anticancer medications.

Cytoxan is used in the treatment of the following types of cancer:

Breast cancer
Leukemias (cancers affecting the white blood cells)
Malignant lymphomas (Hodgkin's disease or cancer of the lymph nodes)
Multiple myeloma (a malignant condition or cancer of the plasma cells)
Advanced mycosis fungoides (cancer of the skin and lymph nodes)
Neuroblastoma (a malignant tumor of the adrenal gland or sympathetic nervous system)
Ovarian cancer (adenocarcinoma)
Retinoblastoma (a malignant tumor of the retina)

In addition, Cytoxan may sometimes be given to children who have "minimal change" nephrotic syndrome (kidney damage resulting in loss of protein in the urine) and who have not responded well to treatment with steroid medications.

### Most important fact about this drug

Cytoxan may cause bladder damage, probably from toxic byproducts of the drug that are excreted in the urine. Potential problems include bladder infection with bleeding and fibrosis of the bladder.

While you are being treated with Cytoxan, drink 3 or 4 liters of fluid a day to help prevent bladder problems. The extra fluid will dilute your urine and make you urinate frequently, thus minimizing the Cytoxan byproducts' contact with your bladder.

## How should you take this medication?

Take Cytoxan exactly as prescribed. You will undergo frequent blood tests, and the doctor will adjust your dosage depending on the evolution of your white blood cell count; a dosage reduction is necessary if the count drops below a certain level. You will also have frequent urine tests to check for blood in the urine, a sign of bladder damage.

Take Cytoxan on an empty stomach. If you have severe stomach upset, then you may take it with food.

If you are unable to swallow the tablet form, you may be given an oral solution made from the injectable form of Cytoxan and Aromatic Elixir. This solution should be used within 14 days.

■ *If you miss a dose...*
Do not take the dose you missed. Go back to your regular schedule and contact your doctor. Do not take 2 doses at once.

■ *Storage instructions...*
Store tablets at room temperature. Store the oral solution in the refrigerator.

## What side effects may occur?

Side effects cannot be anticipated. If any develop or change in intensity, inform your doctor immediately. Only your doctor can determine if it is safe for you to continue using Cytoxan.

One possible Cytoxan side effect is the development of a secondary cancer, typically of the bladder, lymph nodes, or bone marrow. A secondary cancer may occur up to several years after the drug is given.

Cytoxan can lower the activity of your immune system, making you more vulnerable to infection.

Noncancerous bladder problems may occur during Cytoxan therapy (see "Most important fact about this drug" section, above).

■ *More common side effects may include:*
Loss of appetite, nausea and vomiting, temporary hair loss

■ *Less common or rare side effects may include:*
Abdominal pain, anemia, bleeding, inflamed colon, darkening of skin and changes in fingernails, decreased sperm count, diarrhea, fever, impaired wound healing, mouth sores, new tumor growth, prolonged impairment of fertility or temporary sterility in men, rash, severe allergic reaction, temporary failure to menstruate, yellowing of eyes and skin

## Why should this drug not be prescribed?

Do not take this medication if you have ever had an allergic reaction to it.

Also, tell your doctor if you have ever had an allergic reaction to another alkylating anticancer drug such as Alkeran, CeeNU, Emcyt, Leukeran, Myleran, or Zanosar.

In adults, Cytoxan should not be given for "minimal change" nephrotic syndrome or any other kidney disease.

Also, Cytoxan should not be given to anyone who is unable to produce normal blood cells because the bone marrow—where blood cells are made—is not functioning well.

## Special warnings about this medication

You are at increased risk for toxic side effects from Cytoxan if you have any of the following conditions:

Blood disorder (low white blood cell or platelet count)
Bone marrow tumors
Kidney disorder
Liver disorder
Past anticancer therapy
Past X-ray therapy

## Possible food and drug interactions when taking this medication

If Cytoxan is taken with certain other drugs, the effects of either could be increased, decreased, or altered. It is especially important to check with your doctor before combining Cytoxan with the following:

Anticancer drugs such as Adriamycin
Allopurinol (the gout medicine Zyloprim)
Phenobarbital

If you take adrenal steroid hormones because you have had your adrenal glands removed, you are at increased risk for toxic effects from Cytoxan; your dosage of both steroids and Cytoxan may need to be modified.

## Special information if you are pregnant or breastfeeding

If you are pregnant or plan to become pregnant, inform your doctor immediately. When taken during pregnancy, Cytoxan can cause defects in the unborn baby. Women taking Cytoxan should use effective contraception. Cytoxan does appear in breast milk. A new mother will need to choose between taking this drug and nursing her baby.

## Recommended dosage

ADULTS AND CHILDREN

*Malignant Diseases*
Your doctor will tailor your dosage according to your condition and other drugs taken with Cytoxan.

The recommended oral dosage range is 1 to 5 milligrams per 2.2 pounds of body weight per day.

CHILDREN

*"Minimal Change" Nephrotic Syndrome*
The recommended oral dosage is 2.5 to 3 milligrams per 2.2 pounds of body weight per day for a period of 60 to 90 days.

## Overdosage

Although there is no specific information on Cytoxan overdose, any medication taken in excess can have serious consequences. If you suspect an overdose of Cytoxan, seek medical attention immediately.

Brand name:

# Dalmane

*Pronounced: DAL-main*
*Generic name: Flurazepam hydrochloride*

## Why is this drug prescribed?

Dalmane is used for the relief of insomnia, defined as difficulty falling asleep, waking up frequently at night, or waking up early in the morning. It can be used by people whose insomnia keeps coming back and in those who have poor sleeping habits. It belongs to a class of drugs known as benzodiazepines.

## Most important fact about this drug

Tolerance and dependence can occur with the use of Dalmane. You may experience withdrawal symptoms if you stop using this drug abruptly. Discontinue or change your dose only in consultation with your doctor.

## How should you take this medication?

Take this medication exactly as prescribed.

■ *If you miss a dose...*
Take the dose you missed as soon as you remember, if it is within an hour or so of the scheduled time. If you do not remember it until later, skip the dose you missed and go back to your regular schedule. Do not take 2 doses at once.

■ *Storage instructions...*
Store away from heat, light, and moisture.

## What side effects may occur?

Side effects cannot be anticipated. If any develop or change in intensity, inform your doctor as soon as possible. Only your doctor can determine if it is safe for you to continue taking Dalmane.

■ *More common side effects may include:*
Dizziness, drowsiness, falling, lack of muscular coordination, light-headedness, staggering

■ *Less common or rare side effects may include:*
Apprehension, bitter taste, blurred vision, body and joint pain, burning eyes, chest pains, confusion, constipation, depression, diarrhea, difficulty in focusing, dry mouth, exaggerated feeling of well-being, excessive salivation, excitement, faintness, flushes, genital and urinary tract disorders, hallucinations, headache, heartburn, hyperactivity, irritability, itching, loss of appetite, low blood pressure, nausea, nervousness, rapid, fluttery heartbeat, restlessness, shortness of breath, skin rash, slurred speech, stimulation, stomach and intestinal pain, stomach upset, sweating, talkativeness, vomiting, weakness

■ *Side effects due to rapid decrease or abrupt withdrawal from Dalmane:*
Abdominal and muscle cramps, convulsions, depressed mood, inability to fall asleep or stay asleep, sweating, tremors, vomiting

## Why should this drug not be prescribed?

If you are sensitive to or have had an allergic reaction to Dalmane or similar drugs such as Valium, you should not take this medication. Make sure your doctor is aware of any drug reactions you have experienced.

## Special warnings about this medication

Dalmane will cause you to become drowsy or less alert; therefore, you should not drive or operate dangerous machinery or participate in any hazardous activity that requires full mental alertness after taking Dalmane.

If you are severely depressed or have suffered from severe depression, consult with your doctor before taking this medication.

If you have decreased kidney or liver function or chronic respiratory or lung disease, discuss use of this drug with your doctor.

## Possible food and drug interactions when taking this medication

Alcohol intensifies the effects of Dalmane. Do not drink alcohol while taking this medication.

If Dalmane is taken with certain other drugs, the effects of either could be increased, decreased, or altered. It is especially important to check with your doctor before combining Dalmane with the following:

Antidepressants such as Elavil and Tofranil
Antihistamines such as Benadryl and Tavist
Barbiturates such as Seconal and phenobarbital
Major tranquilizers such as Mellaril and
 Thorazine
Narcotic painkillers such as Demerol and Tylenol
 with Codeine
Sedatives such as Xanax and Halcion
Tranquilizers such as Librium and Valium

## Special information if you are pregnant or breastfeeding

Do not take Dalmane if you are pregnant or planning to become pregnant. There is an increased risk of birth defects. This drug may appear in breast milk and could affect a nursing infant. If this medication is essential to your health, your doctor may advise you to discontinue breastfeeding until your treatment with Dalmane is finished.

## Recommended dosage

### ADULTS

The usual recommended dose is 30 milligrams at bedtime; however 15 milligrams may be all that is necessary. Your doctor will adjust the dose to your needs.

### CHILDREN

Safety and effectiveness of Dalmane have not been established in children under 15 years of age.

### OLDER ADULTS

Your doctor will limit the dosage to the smallest effective amount to avoid oversedation, dizziness, confusion, or lack of muscle coordination. The usual starting dose is 15 milligrams.

## Overdosage

Any medication taken in excess can cause symptoms of overdose. If you suspect an overdose of Dalmane, seek medical attention immediately.

■ *The symptoms of Dalmane overdose may include:*
 Coma, confusion, low blood pressure, sleepiness

*Brand name:*

# Darvocet-N

*Pronounced: DAR-voe-set en*
*Generic ingredients: Propoxyphene napsylate,*
 *Acetaminophen*
*Other brand names: Darvon-N (propoxyphene*
 *napsylate), Darvon (propoxyphene*
 *hydrochloride), Darvon Compound-65*
 *(propoxyphene hydrochloride, aspirin, and*
 *caffeine)*

## Why is this drug prescribed?

Darvocet-N and Darvon Compound-65 are mild narcotic analgesics prescribed for the relief of mild to moderate pain, with or without fever.

Darvon-N and Darvon are prescribed for the relief of mild to moderate pain.

## Most important fact about this drug

You can build up tolerance to, and become dependent on, these drugs if you take them in higher than recommended doses over long periods of time.

## How should you take this medication?

Take these drugs exactly as prescribed. Do not increase the amount you take without your doctor's approval. Do not take them for any reason other than those for which they are prescribed. Do not give them to others who may have similar symptoms.

■ *If you miss a dose...*
 Take it as soon as you remember. If it is almost time for your next dose, skip the one you missed and go back to your regular schedule. Do not take 2 doses at once.
■ *Storage instructions...*
 Store at room temperature.

## What side effects may occur?

Side effects cannot be anticipated. If any develop or change in intensity, inform your doctor as soon as possible. Only your doctor can determine if it is safe for you to continue taking one of these medications.

■ *More common side effects may include:*
Drowsiness, dizziness, nausea, sedation, vomiting

If these side effects occur, it may help if you lie down after taking the medication.

■ *Less common side effects may include:*
Abdominal pain, constipation, feelings of elation or depression, hallucinations, headache, kidney problems, light-headedness, liver problems, minor visual disturbances, skin rashes, weakness, yellowed eyes and skin

### Why should this drug not be prescribed?
If you are sensitive to or have ever had an allergic reaction to propoxyphene, any of the other ingredients in these drugs, or other pain relievers of this type, you should not take this medication. Make sure your doctor is aware of any drug reactions you have experienced.

### Special warnings about this medication
These medicines may cause you to become drowsy or less alert; therefore, you should not drive or operate dangerous machinery or participate in any hazardous activity that requires full mental alertness until you know how the drug affects you.

If you have a kidney or liver disorder, consult your doctor before taking Darvocet-N.

Darvon Compound-65 contains aspirin and caffeine. If you have an ulcer or a blood clotting problem, consult your doctor before taking this medication. Aspirin may irritate the stomach lining and could cause bleeding.

Because there is a possible association between aspirin and the severe neurological disorder known as Reye's syndrome, children and teenagers with chickenpox or flu should not take Darvon Compound-65 unless prescribed by a doctor.

Aspirin may cause asthma attacks. If you have had an asthma attack while taking aspirin, consult your doctor before you take Darvon Compound-65.

### Possible food and drug interactions when taking this medication
The propoxyphene in these drugs slows down the central nervous system and intensifies the effects of alcohol. Heavy use of alcohol with this drug may cause overdose symptoms. Therefore, limit or avoid use of alcohol while you are taking this medication.

If these medications are taken with certain other drugs, the effects of either could be increased, decreased, or altered. It is especially important to check with your doctor before combining them with the following:

Antiseizure medications such as Tegretol
Antidepressant drugs such as Elavil
Antihistamines such as Benadryl
Muscle relaxants such as Flexeril
Narcotic pain relievers such as Demerol
Sleep aids such as Halcion
Tranquilizers such as Xanax and Valium
Warfarin-like drugs such as Coumadin

The use of these drugs with propoxyphene can lead to potentially fatal overdose symptoms.

Severe neurologic disorders, including coma, have occurred with the use of propoxyphene in combination with Tegretol.

The use of anticoagulants (blood thinners such as Coumadin) in combination with Darvon Compound-65 may cause bleeding. If you are taking an anticoagulant, consult your doctor before taking this drug.

The use of aspirin with drugs for gout may alter the effects of the antigout medication. Consult your doctor before taking Darvon Compound-65.

### Special information if you are pregnant or breastfeeding
Do not take these medications if you are pregnant or planning to become pregnant unless you are directed to do so by your doctor. Temporary drug dependence may occur in newborns when the mother has taken this drug consistently in the weeks before delivery. The use of Darvon Compound-65 (which contains aspirin) during pregnancy may cause problems in the developing baby or complications during delivery. Do not take it during the last 3 months of pregnancy. Darvocet-N does appear in breast milk. However, no adverse effects have been found in nursing infants.

### Recommended dosage
ADULTS

These medicines may be taken every 4 hours as needed for pain. The usual doses are:

Darvocet-N 50: 2 tablets
Darvocet-N 100: 1 tablet
Darvon: 1 capsule
Darvon Compound-65: 1 capsule

Your doctor may lower the total daily dosage if you have kidney or liver problems.

The most you should take of Darvon or Darvon Compound-65 is 6 capsules a day.

### CHILDREN

The safety and effectiveness of Darvocet-N have not been established in children.

### OLDER ADULTS

Your doctor may lengthen the time between doses.

## Overdosage

Any medication taken in excess can have serious consequences. If you suspect an overdose, seek medical attention immediately.

■ *Symptoms of a propoxyphene overdose may include:*
  Bluish tinge to the skin, coma, convulsions, decreased or difficult breathing to the point of temporary stoppage, decreased heart function, extreme sleepiness, irregular heartbeat, low blood pressure, pinpoint pupils becoming dilated later, stupor

■ *Additional symptoms of overdose with Darvocet-N:*
  Abdominal pain, excessive sweating, general feeling of illness, kidney failure, liver problems, loss of appetite, nausea, vomiting

■ *Additional symptoms of overdose with Darvon Compound-65:*
  Confusion, deafness, excessive perspiration, headache, mental dullness, nausea, rapid breathing, rapid pulse, ringing in the ears, vertigo, vomiting

Extreme overdosage may lead to unconsciousness and death.

*Brand name:*

# Darvon

*See Darvocet-N, page 131.*

*Brand name:*

# Darvon Compound-65

*See Darvocet-N, page 131.*

*Brand name:*

# Darvon-N

*See Darvocet-N, page 131.*

*Brand name:*

# Daypro

*Pronounced: DAY-pro*
*Generic name: Oxaprozin*

### Why is this drug prescribed?

Daypro is a nonsteroidal anti-inflammatory drug used to relieve the inflammation, swelling, stiffness, and joint pain associated with rheumatoid arthritis and osteoarthritis (the most common kind of arthritis).

### Most important fact about this drug

You should have frequent check-ups with your doctor if you take Daypro regularly. Ulcers and internal bleeding can occur without warning.

### How should you take this medication?

Take Daypro with a full glass of water. If the drug upsets your stomach, your doctor may recommend taking Daypro with food, milk, or an antacid, even though food may delay onset of relief.

It will also help to prevent irritation in your upper digestive tract if you avoid lying down for about 20 minutes after taking Daypro.

Take this medication exactly as prescribed.

■ *If you miss a dose...*
  Try to take Daypro at the same time each day, for example, after breakfast. If you forget to take a dose and remember later in the day, you can still take it. If you completely forget to take your medication, do *not* double the dose the next day to make up for the missed dose. You should get back on your normal schedule as soon as possible.

■ *Storage instructions...*
  Store at room temperature in a tightly closed container, away from light.

### What side effects may occur?

Side effects cannot be anticipated. If any develop or change in intensity, tell your doctor as soon as possible. Only your doctor can decide if it is safe for you to continue taking Daypro.

■ *More common side effects may include:*
Constipation, diarrhea, indigestion, nausea, rash
■ *Less common side effects may include:*
Abdominal pain, confusion, depression, frequent or painful urination, gas, loss of appetite, ringing in the ears, sleep disturbances, sleepiness vomiting
■ *Rare side effects may include:*
Anaphylaxis (a severe allergic reaction), anemia, blood in the urine, blood pressure changes, blurred vision, bruising, changes in kidney and liver function, decreased menstrual flow, fluid retention, general feeling of illness, hemorrhoidal or rectal bleeding, hepatitis, hives, inflammation of the mouth, inflammation of the pancreas, irritated eyes, itching, peptic ulcerations, respiratory infection, sensitivity to light, stomach and intestinal bleeding, weight gain or loss, weakness

### Why should this drug not be prescribed?

If you are sensitive to or have ever had an allergic reaction to Daypro, or if you have ever developed asthma, nasal tumors, or other allergic reactions due to aspirin or other nonsteroidal anti-inflammatory drugs, you should not take this medication. Make sure your doctor is aware of any drug reactions you have experienced.

### Special warnings about this medication

Use Daypro with caution if you have kidney or liver disease.

Do not take aspirin or any other anti-inflammatory medications while taking Daypro, unless your doctor tells you to do so.

Daypro can increase water retention. Use with caution if you have heart disease or high blood pressure.

If you are taking Daypro for an extended period, your doctor should check your blood for anemia.

Daypro can prolong bleeding time. If you are taking a blood-thinning medication, use Daypro with caution.

Daypro may cause sensitivity to sunlight. Avoid prolonged exposure to the sun. Use sunscreens and wear protective clothing.

Do not use Daypro if you are planning to have surgery in the immediate future.

### Possible food and drug interactions when taking this medication

If you take Daypro with certain other drugs, the effects of either medication could be increased, decreased, or altered. It is especially important to check with your doctor before combining Daypro with the following medications:

Aspirin
Beta-blocking blood pressure medications such as Inderal
and Tenormin
Blood thinners such as Coumadin
Digitalis and digoxin (Lanoxin)
Diuretics such as Lasix and Midamor
Lithium (Lithonate)
Ulcer drugs such as Tagamet and Zantac
Avoid alcoholic beverages while taking Daypro.

### Special information
### if you are pregnant or breastfeeding

The effects of Daypro during pregnancy have not been adequately studied. If you are pregnant or plan to become pregnant, tell your doctor immediately. Since the effects of Daypro on nursing infants are not known, tell your doctor if you are nursing or plan to nurse. If Daypro treatment is necessary for your health, your doctor may tell you to discontinue nursing until your treatment is finished.

### Recommended dosage

ADULTS

Your doctor will adjust the dose based on your needs.

RHEUMATOID ARTHRITIS

The usual daily dose is 1200 milligrams (two 600-milligram caplets) once a day.

OSTEOARTHRITIS

The usual starting dose for moderate to severe osteoarthritis is 1200 milligrams (two 600-milligram caplets) once a day.

The most you should take in a day is 1800 milligrams divided into smaller doses, or 26 milligrams per 2.2 pounds of body weight, whichever is lower.

CHILDREN

The safety and efficacy of Daypro in children have not been determined.

### Overdosage

If you take too much of any medication, it can have serious consequences. If you suspect an overdose, seek medical attention immediately.

■ *Symptoms of Daypro overdose may include:*
Coma, drowsiness, fatigue, nausea, pain in the stomach, stomach and intestinal bleeding, vomiting

Acute kidney failure, high blood pressure, and a slow down in breathing have occurred rarely.

*Brand name:*

# DDAVP

*Pronounced: dee-dee-ai-vee-pee*
*Generic name: Desmopressin acetate*
*Other brand name: Stimate*

## Why is this drug prescribed?

DDAVP is given to prevent or control the frequent urination and loss of water associated with diabetes insipidus (a rare condition characterized by very large quantities of diluted urine and excessive thirst). It is also used to treat frequent passage of urine and increased thirst in people with certain brain injuries, and those who have undergone surgery in the pituitary region of the brain. It is prescribed to help stop some types of bedwetting.

Stimate nasal spray is used to stop bleeding in certain types of hemophilia (failure of the blood to clot).

DDAVP is available as a nasal spray in a pump bottle, or as nose drops to be taken using a soft plastic tube. An injectable form of DDAVP is also available.

## Most important fact about this drug

When taking DDAVP, elderly and young people in particular should limit their fluid intake to no more than what satisfies thirst. Although extremely rare, there is a possibility of water intoxication, in which reduced sodium levels in the blood can lead to seizures.

## How should you use this medication?

Use DDAVP exactly as prescribed. The spray and drops are for nasal use only; never swallow the medication or allow the liquid to run into your mouth.

Your doctor may increase or decrease your dosage, depending on how you respond to DDAVP. Your response will be judged by how long you are able to sleep without having to get up to urinate and how much urine your kidneys produce.

The DDAVP nasal spray pump bottle accurately delivers 50 doses of the medication. After the 50th dose, the amount of medication that comes out with each spray will no longer be a full dose. When this happens, throw the bottle away even if it is not completely empty. Stimate nasal spray delivers 25 doses; the same instructions apply. The Stimate nasal spray pump must be primed before you use it for the first time: Press down 4 times.

Since the DDAVP spray bottle delivers only a standard-sized dose, those who need more or less medication should use the nose drops instead of the spray.

If nasal congestion, scars, or swelling inside the nose make it difficult to absorb DDAVP, your doctor may temporarily stop the drug or give you an injectable form.

■ *If you miss a dose...*
Take the forgotten dose as soon as you remember. If you take 1 dose a day and don't remember until the next day, skip the dose. If you take DDAVP more than once a day and it is almost time for the next dose, skip the one you missed and go back to your regular schedule. Never try to "catch up" by doubling the dose.

■ *Storage instructions...*
Both spray and drops should be stored in the refrigerator. If you are traveling, they will stay fresh at room temperature for up to 3 weeks.

## What side effects may occur?

Too high a dosage of DDAVP may produce headache, nausea, mild abdominal cramps, stuffy nose, irritation of the nose, or flushing. These symptoms will probably disappear when the dosage is reduced. Some people have complained of nosebleed, sore throat, cough, or a cold or other upper respiratory infections after taking DDAVP.

■ *Other potential side effects include:*
Abdominal pain, chills, conjunctivitis (pinkeye), depression, dizziness, inability to produce tears, leg rash, nostril pain, rash, stomach or intestinal upset, swelling around the eyes, weakness

■ *Side effects of Stimate nasal spray may include:*
Agitation, chest pain, chills, dizziness, fast, fluttery heartbeat, fluid retention and swelling, indigestion, inflammation of the penis, insomnia, itchy or light-sensitive eyes, pain, rapid heartbeat, sleepiness, vomiting, warm feeling

### Why should this drug not be prescribed?

Do not use DDAVP if you are sensitive to or have ever had an allergic reaction to any of its ingredients.

### Special warnings about this medication

If you have cystic fibrosis or any other condition in which there is fluid and electrolyte imbalance, you should use DDAVP with extreme caution.

Because DDAVP may cause a rise in blood pressure, use this medication cautiously if you have high blood pressure and/or coronary artery disease. Your blood pressure could also fall temporarily. If you continue to experience bleeding after using Stimate nasal spray, contact your doctor.

### Possible food and drug interactions when taking this medication

If DDAVP is taken with certain other drugs, the effects of either could be increased, decreased, or altered. It is especially important to check with your doctor before combining DDAVP with the following:

Any drug used to increase blood pressure
Clofibrate (Atromid-S)
Glyburide (Micronase)
Epinephrine (EpiPen)

### Special information if you are pregnant or breastfeeding

If you are pregnant or plan to become pregnant, inform your doctor immediately. Although DDAVP is not known to cause birth defects, it should be used with caution. DDAVP should be taken during pregnancy only if clearly needed. DDAVP is not believed to appear in breast milk. However, check with your doctor before using the drug while breastfeeding.

### Recommended dosage

Your doctor will carefully tailor your dosage to meet your individual needs.

CENTRAL CRANIAL DIABETES INSIPIDUS

*Adults*
The usual recommended dosage range is 0.1 to 0.4 milliliter daily, either as a single dose or divided into 2 or 3 doses. Most adults require 0.2 milliliter per day divided into 2 doses.

*Children*
The usual dosage range for children aged 3 months to 12 years is 0.05 to 0.3 milliliter daily, either as a single dose or divided into 2 doses.

PRIMARY NOCTURNAL ENURESIS
(BED-WETTING)

*Children 6 Years of Age and Older*
The usual recommended dose is 20 micrograms or 0.2 milliliter at bedtime. Dosage requirements range from 10 to 40 micrograms. One-half the dose should be taken in each nostril.

*To stop bleeding in some types of hemophilia*
The usual dose is one 150-microgram spray in each nostril. If you use the spray more frequently than every 48 hours, you may find you are not responding as well as you should to the drug.

### Overdosage

An overdose of DDAVP may cause abdominal cramps, flushing, headache, or nausea. If you suspect an overdose of DDAVP, seek medical attention immediately.

*Brand name:*

# Decadron Tablets

*Pronounced: DECK-uh-drohn*
*Generic name: Dexamethasone*

### Why is this drug prescribed?

Decadron, a corticosteroid drug, is used to reduce inflammation and relieve symptoms in a variety of disorders, including rheumatoid arthritis and severe cases of asthma. It may be given to people to treat primary or secondary adrenal cortex insufficiency (lack of sufficient adrenal hormone). It is also given to help treat the following disorders:

Severe allergic conditions such as drug-induced
    allergies
Blood disorders such as various anemias
Certain cancers (along with other drugs)
Skin diseases such as severe psoriasis
Collagen (connective tissue) diseases such as
    systemic lupus erythematosus
Digestive tract disease such as ulcerative colitis
High serum levels of calcium associated
    with cancer

Fluid retention due to nephrotic syndrome
(a condition in which damage to the kidneys
causes the body to lose protein in the urine)
Eye diseases such as allergic conjunctivitis
Lung diseases such as tuberculosis (along with
other drugs)

## Most important fact about this drug

Decadron lowers your resistance to infections and
can make them harder to treat. Decadron may also
mask some of the signs of an infection, making it
difficult for your doctor to diagnose the actual
problem.

## How should you take this medication?

Decadron should be taken exactly as prescribed by
your doctor.

If you are taking large doses, your doctor may
advise you to take Decadron with meals and to take
antacids between meals, to prevent a peptic ulcer
from developing.

Check with your doctor before stopping
Decadron abruptly. If you have been taking the
drug for a long time, you may need to reduce your
dose gradually over a period of days or weeks.

The lowest possible dose should always be used,
and as symptoms subside, dosage should be
reduced gradually.

■ *If you miss a dose...*
Take the forgotten dose as soon as you remember. If it is almost time for the next dose, skip the
one you missed and go back to your regular
schedule. Never try to "catch up" by doubling
the dose.

■ *Storage instructions...*
There are no special storage requirements.

## What side effects may occur?

Side effects cannot be anticipated. If any develop or
change in intensity, inform your doctor as soon as
possible. Only your doctor can determine if it is
safe for you to continue taking Decadron.

■ *Side effects may include:*
Abdominal distention, allergic reactions, blood
clots, bone fractures and degeneration, bruises,
cataracts, congestive heart failure, convulsions,
"cushingoid" symptoms (moon face, weight gain,
high blood pressure emotional disturbances,
growth of facial hair in women), emotional disturbances, excessive hairiness, fluid and salt

retention, general feeling of illness, glaucoma,
headache, hiccups, high blood pressure, hives,
increased appetite, increased eye pressure,
increased pressure in head, increased sweating,
increases in amounts of insulin or hypoglycemic
medications needed in diabetes, inflammation of
the esophagus, inflammation of the pancreas,
irregular menstruation, loss of muscle mass, low
potassium levels in blood (leading to symptoms
such as dry mouth, excessive thirst, weak or
irregular heartbeat, and muscle pain or cramps),
muscle weakness, nausea, osteoporosis, peptic
ulcer, perforated small and large bowel, poor
healing of wounds, protruding eyeballs, ruptured
tendons, suppression of growth in children, thin
skin, tiny red or purplish spots on the skin,
vertigo, weight gain

## Why should this drug not be prescribed?

Decadron should not be used if you have a fungal
infection, or if you are sensitive or allergic to any
of its ingredients.

## Special warnings about this medication

Decadron can alter the way your body responds to
unusual stress. If you are injured, need surgery, or
develop an acute illness, inform your doctor. Your
dosage may need to be increased.

Corticosteroids such as Decadron can lower
your resistance to infection. Diseases such as
measles and chickenpox can be serious and even
fatal in adults. If you are taking Decadron and are
exposed to chickenpox or measles, notify your
doctor immediately.

Do not get a smallpox vaccination or any other
immunizations while taking Decadron, especially in
high doses. The vaccination might not take, and
could do harm to the nervous system.

Decadron may reactivate a dormant case of
tuberculosis. If you have inactive tuberculosis and
must take Decadron for an extended period, your
doctor will prescribe anti-TB medication as
well.

When you stop taking Decadron after long-term
therapy, you may develop withdrawal symptoms
such as fever, muscle or joint pain, and a feeling of
illness.

Long-term use of Decadron may cause cataracts,
glaucoma, and eye infections.

If you have any of the following conditions,
make sure your doctor knows about it:

Allergy to any cortisone-like drug
Cirrhosis
Diabetes
Diverticulitis
Eye infection (herpes simplex)
Glaucoma
High blood pressure
Impaired thyroid function
Kidney disease (impaired kidney function)
Myasthenia gravis (a muscle disorder)
Osteoporosis (brittle bones)
Peptic ulcer
Recent heart attack
Tuberculosis
Ulcerative colitis

Steroids may alter male fertility.

This medication can aggravate existing emotional problems or cause emotional disturbances. Symptoms range from an exaggerated sense of well-being and difficulty sleeping to mood swings and psychotic episodes. If you experience any changes in mood, contact your doctor.

If you have recently been to the tropics or are suffering from diarrhea with no apparent cause, inform your doctor before taking Decadron.

### Possible food and drug interactions when taking this medication

If Decadron is taken with certain other drugs, the effects of either could be increased, decreased, or altered. It is especially important to check with your doctor before combining Decadron with the following:

Aspirin
Blood-thinning medications such as Coumadin
Ephedrine (a decongestant in drugs such as Marax and Rynatuss)
Indomethacin (Indocin)
Phenobarbital
Phenytoin (Dilantin)
Potassium-depleting diuretics such as Hydro-DIURIL
Rifampin (Rifadin, Rimactane)

### Special information if you are pregnant or breastfeeding

The effects of Decadron during pregnancy have not been adequately studied. If you are pregnant or plan to become pregnant, inform your doctor immediately. Infants born to mothers who have taken substantial doses of corticosteroids during pregnancy should be carefully watched for adrenal problems. Corticosteroids appear in breast milk and can suppress growth in infants. If Decadron is essential to your health, your doctor may advise you to stop breastfeeding until your treatment with Decadron is finished.

### Recommended dosage

ADULTS

Your doctor will tailor your individual dose to the condition being treated. Initial doses range from 0.75 milligram to 9 milligrams a day.

After the drug produces a satisfactory response, your doctor will gradually lower the dose to the minimum effective level.

### Overdosage

Reports of overdose with this medication are rare. However, if you suspect an overdose, seek medical treatment immediately.

*Brand name:*

# Decadron Turbinaire and Respihaler

*Pronounced: DECK-ah-drahn tur-bin-AIR and RESS-pi-hail-er*
*Generic name: Dexamethasone sodium phosphate*
*Other brand name: Dexacort*

### Why is this drug prescribed?

Decadron is a synthetic adrenocortical steroid (a hormone created in the laboratory). Decadron Turbinaire is used to treat hay fever and other nasal allergies, and to assist in the treatment of nasal polyps. Decadron Respihaler is prescribed for bronchial asthma in people who need sustained treatment.

### Most important fact about this drug

Decadron lowers your resistance to infections and can make them harder to treat. Decadron may also mask some of the signs of an infection, making it difficult for your doctor to diagnose the actual problem.

### How should you take this medication?

These medications come with directions. Read them carefully before using the medicine. To work, the medications must be used exactly as directed.

If you are using the Decadron Respihaler, gargling and rinsing your mouth with water after each dose may help prevent hoarseness and throat irritation. Do not swallow the water after you rinse.

■ *If you miss a dose...*
Take the forgotten dose as soon as possible and take the remaining doses for that day at evenly spaced intervals. If it is time for your next dose, skip the one you missed. Never take a double dose.

■ *Storage instructions...*
Store Decadron at room temperature. Since the contents are under pressure, keep the container away from fire or extreme heat.

## What side effects may occur?

Side effects cannot be anticipated. If any develop or change in intensity, inform your doctor as soon as possible. Only your doctor can determine whether it is safe to continue using Decadron.

■ *More common side effects of Decadron Turbinaire may include:*
Nasal dryness and irritation

■ *Less common side effects of Decadron Turbinaire may include:*
Bronchial asthma, headache, hives, light-headedness, loss of smell, nausea, nosebleeds, perforated nasal septum (dividing wall of the nose), rebound nasal congestion

■ *Side effects of Decadron Respihaler may include:*
Coughing, fungal infections in the throat, hoarseness, throat irritation

■ *Side effects that may occur when Decadron is absorbed into the bloodstream:*
Abdominal distention, abnormal skin redness, allergic reactions, blood clots, bruising, cataracts, congestive heart failure, convulsions, development of Cushing's syndrome (moon face, emotional disturbances, high blood pressure, weight gain, and growth of facial and body hair in women), diabetes, emotional disturbances, excessive hairiness, fractures of the long bones, fractures of the vertebrae, fragile skin, glaucoma, headache, hiccups, high blood pressure, hives, increased appetite, increased eye pressure, increased pressure in head), increased sweating, loss of muscle mass, menstrual irregularities, muscle weakness, nausea, osteoporosis, perforated small or large bowel, poor wound healing,

potassium loss, protruding eyeballs, reddish or purplish spots on the skin, ruptured tendons, salt and fluid retention, stomach ulcer, ulcer of the esophagus, vague feeling of weakness, vertigo, weight gain

## Why should this drug not be prescribed?

Do not use Decadron if you have a fungal infection or if you have ever had an allergic reaction or are sensitive to any cortisone-like medication such as Beclovent. Decadron Turbinaire should not be used if you have tuberculosis or a nasal condition caused by a virus or a fungus, or if you have herpes simplex infection of the eye. Decadron Respihaler should not be used if tests show that you have a yeast infection (*Candida albicans*).

## Special warnings about this medication

Decadron does not expand the bronchial passages, and should be used for asthma only if bronchodilators and other asthma medications are not effective. Decadron does not provide rapid relief of symptoms, but does help to control asthma when taken routinely.

Decadron can alter the way your body responds to unusual stress. If you are injured, need surgery, or develop an acute illness, tell your doctor. Your dosage may need to be increased.

If you develop an infection of the throat or voice box while using the Decadron Respihaler, stop using the Respihaler and notify your doctor. You will need medication.

Corticosteroids such as Decadron may mask the symptoms of infection and make you more susceptible to infections. Diseases such as chickenpox and measles can be serious and even fatal in adults who have never had these illnesses. If you are using Decadron Turbinaire or Respihaler and are exposed to chickenpox or measles, notify your doctor immediately. Do not get a smallpox vaccination or any other immunizations while taking Decadron, especially in high doses. The vaccination might not take, and could do harm to the nervous system.

Using Decadron for a long time may cause cataracts, glaucoma, and eye infections.

Large doses of Decadron may raise blood pressure and increase salt and water retention. If this happens, your doctor may tell you to restrict salt in your diet.

Decadron should be used with extreme caution if you have dormant tuberculosis or test positive for tuberculosis. Decadron may reactivate the disease.

When you stop taking Decadron after long-term therapy, you may develop withdrawal symptoms such as fever, muscle or joint pain, and weakness.

Decadron should be used with care if you have an underactive thyroid or cirrhosis.

Your doctor will prescribe the lowest possible dose to control your condition, and reduce your dosage of Decadron gradually. Do not suddenly stop taking it.

Decadron may aggravate existing emotional problems or cause emotional disturbances. Symptoms range from euphoria (an exaggerated sense of well-being) and difficulty sleeping to mood swings, personality changes, severe depression, and psychotic episodes. If you experience any changes in mood, call your doctor.

Decadron should be used with care if you have ulcerative colitis, diverticulitis (an inflammation of the digestive tract), peptic ulcer, kidney disease, high blood pressure, osteoporosis, or myasthenia gravis (muscle weakness, especially in the face and neck), or if you have recently had a heart attack.

Long-term therapy with Decadron may affect the growth and development of children and should be carefully checked by your doctor. Decadron Turbinaire is not recommended for children under 6 years of age.

If you have recently been to the tropics or are suffering from diarrhea with no apparent cause, inform your doctor before using Decadron.

### Possible food and drug interactions when taking this medication

If Decadron is taken with certain other drugs, the effects of either could be increased, decreased, or altered. It is especially important to check with your doctor before combining Decadron with the following:

Aspirin
Blood thinners such as Coumadin
Ephedrine
Phenytoin (Dilantin)
Phenobarbital (Bellergal-S, Donnatal, others)
Potassium-depleting diuretics such as Dyazide and
  Esidrix
Rifampin (Rifadin, Rimactane)

### Special information if you are pregnant or breastfeeding

The effects of Decadron during pregnancy have not been adequately studied. If you are pregnant or plan to become pregnant, inform your doctor immediately. Infants born to mothers who have taken substantial doses of steroids during pregnancy may have problems with their adrenal glands. Corticosteroids appear in breast milk and could affect infant growth or cause other damaging effects. Decadron is not recommended for nursing mothers. If Decadron is essential to your health, your doctor may advise you to stop breastfeeding until your treatment with Decadron is finished.

### Recommended dosage

TURBINAIRE

*Adults*
The usual initial dosage is 2 sprays in each nostril, 2 or 3 times a day.

*Children (6 to 12 Years of Age)*
The usual initial dosage is 1 or 2 sprays in each nostril 2 times a day, depending on age.

Dosage should be gradually reduced when improvement occurs. The maximum daily dosage for adults is 12 sprays and for children, 8 sprays. Therapy should be stopped as soon as possible. If symptoms return, your doctor may start the medication again.

RESPIHALER

*Adults*
The recommended initial dose is 3 inhalations, 3 or 4 times a day.

*Children*
The recommended initial dose is 2 inhalations, 3 or 4 times a day.

Dosage should be gradually reduced when improvement occurs. The maximum daily dosage for adults is 3 inhalations per dose, 12 inhalations per day; and for children, 2 inhalations per dose, 8 inhalations per day.

### Overdosage

There have been rare reports of toxicity (poisoning) and death following steroid overdose. If you suspect Decadron overdose, seek medical treatment immediately.

*Brand name:*

# Deconamine

*Pronounced: dee-CON-uh-meen*
*Generic ingredients: Chlorpheniramine maleate,*
  *d-Pseudoephedrine hydrochloride*

## Why is this drug prescribed?

Deconamine is an antihistamine and decongestant used for the temporary relief of persistent runny nose, sneezing, and nasal congestion caused by upper respiratory infections (the common cold), sinus inflammation, or hay fever. It is also used to help clear nasal passages and shrink swollen membranes and to drain the sinuses and relieve sinus pressure.

## Most important fact about this drug

Deconamine may cause you to become drowsy or less alert. You should not drive or operate machinery or participate in any activity that requires full mental alertness until you know how you react to Deconamine.

## How should you take this medication?

If Deconamine makes you nervous or restless, or you have trouble sleeping, take the last dose of the day a few hours before you go to bed. Take Deconamine exactly as prescribed.

Antihistamines can make your mouth and throat dry. It may help to suck on hard candy, chew gum, or melt bits of ice in your mouth.

■ *If you miss a dose...*
  Take it as soon as you remember. If it is almost time for your next dose, skip the one you missed and go back to your regular schedule. Never take 2 doses at once.
■ *Storage instructions...*
  Store at room temperature.

## What side effects may occur?

Side effects cannot be anticipated. If any develop or change in intensity, inform your doctor as soon as possible. Only your doctor can determine if it is safe for you to continue taking Deconamine.

The most common side effect is mild to moderate drowsiness.

■ *Less common or rare side effects may include:*
  Anaphylactic shock (extreme allergic reaction), anemia, anxiety, blurred vision, breathing difficulty, chills, confusion, constipation, convulsion, diarrhea, difficulty sleeping, difficulty in carrying out movements, disturbed coordination, dizziness, double vision, dry mouth, nose, and throat, early menstruation, exaggerated sense of well being, excessive perspiration, excitation, fatigue, extreme calm (sedation), fear, frequent or difficult urination, hallucinations, headache, hives, hysteria, increased chest congestion, irregular heartbeat, irritability, light-headedness, loss of appetite, low blood pressure, nausea, nervousness, painful urination, pallor, pounding heartbeat, rapid heartbeat, restlessness, ringing in ears, sensitivity to light, skin rash, stomach upset or pain, stuffy nose, tenseness, tightness of chest, tingling or numbness, tremor, unusual bleeding or bruising, vertigo, vomiting, weakness, wheezing

## Why should this drug not be prescribed?

Do not use Deconamine if you have severe high blood pressure or severe heart disease, are taking an antidepressant drug known as an MAO inhibitor (Nardil, Parnate, others), or are sensitive to or have ever had an allergic reaction to antihistamines or decongestants.

## Special warnings about this medication

Use Deconamine with extreme caution if you have the eye condition called glaucoma, peptic ulcer or stomach obstructions, an enlarged prostate, or difficulty urinating.

Also use caution if you have bronchial asthma, emphysema, chronic lung disease, high blood pressure, heart disease, diabetes, or an overactive thyroid.

Deconamine may cause excitability, especially in children.

## Possible food and drug interactions when taking this medication

Alcohol increases the sedative effect of Deconamine. Avoid it while taking this medication.

If Deconamine is taken with certain other drugs, the effects of either may be increased, decreased, or altered. It is especially important to check with your doctor before combining Deconamine with the following:

Antidepressant drugs such as the MAO inhibitors Nardil and Parnate
Asthma medications such as Ventolin and Proventil
Bromocriptine (Parlodel)

Mecamylamine (Inversine)
Methyldopa (Aldomet)
Narcotic pain killers such as Demerol and Percocet
Phenytoin (Dilantin)
Reserpine (Ser-Ap-Es, others)
Sleep aids such as Halcion and Seconal
Tranquilizers such as Valium and Xanax

### Special information
### if you are pregnant or breastfeeding

The effects of Deconamine during pregnancy have not been adequately studied. If you are pregnant or plan to become pregnant, notify your doctor immediately. Deconamine appears in breast milk and could affect a nursing infant. If this medication is essential to your health, your doctor may advise you to discontinue breastfeeding until your treatment with Deconamine is finished.

### Recommended dosage
DECONAMINE TABLETS

*Adults and Children over 12 Years*
The usual dosage is 1 tablet 3 or 4 times daily.

*Children under 12 Years*
Use Deconamine Syrup or Chewable Tablets instead of the tablets.

DECONAMINE SYRUP

*Adults and Children over 12 Years*
The usual dose is 1 to 2 teaspoonfuls (5 to 10 milliliters) 3 or 4 times daily.

*Children 6 to 12 Years*
The usual dose is 1/2 to 1 teaspoonful (2.5 to 5 milliliters) 3 or 4 times daily, not to exceed 4 teaspoonfuls in 24 hours.

*Children 2 to 6 Years*
The usual dose is 1/2 teaspoonful (2.5 milliliters) 3 or 4 times daily, not to exceed 2 teaspoonfuls in 24 hours.

*Children under 2 Years*
Use as directed by your doctor.

DECONAMINE SR CAPSULES

*Adults and Children over 12 Years*
The usual dose is 1 capsule every 12 hours.

*Children under 12 Years*
Use Deconamine Syrup or Chewable Tablets instead of the capsules.

DECONAMINE CHEWABLE TABLETS

*Adults*
The usual dose is 2 tablets 3 or 4 times a day.

*Children 6 to 12 Years*
The usual dose is 1 tablet 3 or 4 times a day.

*Children 2 to 6 Years*
The usual dose is 1/2 tablet 3 or 4 times a day.

### Overdosage

Any medication taken in excess can have serious consequences. If you suspect an overdose, seek medical attention immediately.

■ *Symptoms of Deconamine overdose include:*
Convulsions, diminished alertness, hallucinations, severe drowsiness, severe dryness of mouth, nose, and throat, shortness of breath/difficulty breathing, sleep problems, slow or rapid heartbeat, tremors

*Brand name:*

# Deltasone

*Pronounced: DELL-tuh-zone*
*Generic name: Prednisone*
*Other brand name: Orasone*

### Why is this drug prescribed?

Deltasone, a steroid drug, is used to reduce inflammation and alleviate symptoms in a variety of disorders, including rheumatoid arthritis and severe cases of asthma. It may be given to treat primary or secondary adrenal cortex insufficiency (lack of sufficient adrenal hormone in the body). It is used in treating all of the following:

Abnormal adrenal gland development
Allergic conditions (severe)
Blood disorders
Certain cancers (along with other drugs)
Diseases of the connective tissue including systemic lupus
erythematosus
Eye diseases of various kinds
Flare-ups of multiple sclerosis
Fluid retention due to "nephrotic syndrome" (a condition in which damage to the kidneys causes protein to be lost in the urine)
Lung diseases, including tuberculosis
Meningitis (inflamed membranes around the brain)

Prevention of organ rejection
Rheumatoid arthritis and related disorders
Severe flare-ups of ulcerative colitis or enteritis
(inflammation of the intestines)
Skin diseases
Thyroid gland inflammation
Trichinosis (with complications)

## Most important fact about this drug

Deltasone lowers your resistance to infections and can make them harder to treat. Deltasone may also mask some of the signs of an infection, making it difficult for your doctor to diagnose the actual problem.

## How should you take this medication?

Take Deltasone exactly as prescribed. Dosages are kept to an absolute minimum.

If you need long-term Deltasone treatment, your doctor may prescribe alternate-day therapy, in which you take the medication only every other morning. The "resting day" gives your adrenal glands a chance to produce some hormone naturally so they will not lose the ability.

If you have been taking Deltasone for a period of time, you will probably need an increased dosage of the medication before, during, and after any stressful situation. Always consult your doctor if you are anticipating stress and think you may need a temporary dosage increase.

When stopping Deltasone treatment, tapering off is better than quitting abruptly. Your doctor will probably have you decrease the dosage very gradually over a period of days or weeks.

You should take Deltasone with food to avoid stomach upset.

If you are on alternate-day therapy or have been prescribed a single daily dose, take Deltasone in the morning with breakfast (about 8 AM). If you have been prescribed several doses per day, take them at evenly spaced intervals around the clock.

Patients on long-term Deltasone therapy should wear or carry identification.

■ *If you miss a dose...*
  If you take your dose once a day, take it as soon as you remember. If you don't remember until the next day, skip the one you missed.

  If you take several doses a day, take the forgotten dose as soon as you remember and then go back to your regular schedule. If you don't remember until your next dose, double the dose you take.

If you take your dose every other day, and you remember it the same morning, take it as soon as you remember, then go back to your regular schedule. If you don't remember until the afternoon, do not take a dose until the following morning, then skip a day.

■ *Storage instructions...*
  Store at room temperature.

## What side effects may occur?

Side effects cannot be anticipated. If any develop or change in intensity, inform your doctor as soon as possible. Only your doctor can determine if it is safe for you to continue taking Deltasone.

Deltasone may cause euphoria, insomnia, mood changes, personality changes, psychotic behavior, or severe depression. It may worsen any existing emotional instability.

At a high dosage, Deltasone may cause fluid retention and high blood pressure. If this happens, you may need a low-salt diet and a potassium supplement.

With prolonged Deltasone treatment, eye problems may develop (e.g., a viral or fungal eye infection, cataracts, or glaucoma).

If you take Deltasone over the long term, the buildup of adrenal hormones in your body may cause a condition called Cushing's syndrome, marked by weight gain, a "moon-faced" appearance, thin, fragile skin, muscle weakness, brittle bones, and purplish stripe marks on the skin. Women are more vulnerable to this problem than men. Alternate-day therapy may help prevent its development.

■ *Other potential side effects from Deltasone include:*
  Bone fractures, bruising, bulging eyes, congestive heart failure, convulsions, distended abdomen, face redness, glaucoma, headache, hives and other allergic-type reactions, increased pressure inside eyes or skull, inflamed esophagus or pancreas, irregular menstrual periods, muscle weakness or disease, osteoporosis, peptic ulcer, poor healing of wounds, stunted growth (in children), sweating, thin, fragile skin, vertigo

## Why should this drug not be prescribed?

Do not take Deltasone if you have ever had an allergic reaction to it.

You should not be treated with Deltasone if you have a body-wide fungus infection, such as candidiasis or cryptococcosis.

### Special warnings about this medication

Do not get a smallpox vaccination or any other immunization while you are taking Deltasone. The vaccination might not "take," and could do harm to the nervous system.

Deltasone may reactivate a dormant case of tuberculosis. If you have inactive TB and must take Deltasone for an extended time, you should be given anti-TB medication as well.

If you have an underactive thyroid gland or cirrhosis of the liver, your doctor will probably need to prescribe Deltasone for you at a lower-than-average dosage.

If you have an eye infection caused by the herpes simplex virus, Deltasone should be used with great caution; there is a potential danger that the cornea will become perforated.

A few people taking Deltasone develop Kaposi's sarcoma, a form of cancer; it may disappear when the drug is stopped.

Deltasone should also be taken with caution if you have any of the following conditions:

Diverticulitis or other disorder of the intestine
High blood pressure
Kidney disorder
Myasthenia gravis (a muscle-weakness disorder)
Osteoporosis (brittle bones)
Peptic ulcer
Ulcerative colitis (inflammation of the bowel)

Long-term treatment with Deltasone may stunt growth. If this medication is given to a child, the youngster's growth should be monitored carefully.

Diseases such as chickenpox or measles can be very serious or even fatal in both children and adults who are taking this drug. Try to avoid exposure to these diseases.

### Possible food and drug interactions when taking this medication

Deltasone may decrease your carbohydrate tolerance or activate a latent case of diabetes. If you are already taking insulin or oral medication for diabetes, make sure your doctor knows this; you may need an increased dosage while you are being treated with Deltasone.

If you have a blood-clotting disorder caused by a vitamin K deficiency and are taking Deltasone, check with your doctor before you use aspirin.

You may be at risk of convulsions if you take the immunosuppressant drug cyclosporine (Sandimmune) while being treated with Deltasone.

If Deltasone is taken with certain other drugs, the effects of either could be increased, decreased, or altered. Check with your doctor before combining Deltasone with any of the following:

Amphotericin B (Fungizone)
Blood thinners such as Coumadin
Carbamazepine (Tegretol)
Estrogen drugs such as Premarin
Ketoconazole (Nizoral)
Oral contraceptives
Phenobarbital (Donnatal, others)
Phenytoin (Dilantin)
Potent diuretics such as Lasix
Rifampin (Rifadin)
Troleandomycin (Tao)

### Special information
### if you are pregnant or breastfeeding

If you are pregnant or plan to become pregnant, inform your doctor immediately. Deltasone should be taken during pregnancy or while breastfeeding only if clearly needed and only if the benefit outweighs the potential risks to the child.

### Recommended dosage

Dosage is determined by the condition being treated and your response to the drug. Typical starting doses can range from 5 milligrams to 60 milligrams a day. Once you respond to the drug, your doctor will lower the dose gradually to the minimum effective amount. For treatment of acute attacks of multiple sclerosis, doses of as much as 200 milligrams per day may be given for a week, followed by 80 mg every other day for a month.

### Overdosage

Long-term high doses of Deltasone may produce Cushing's syndrome (see "side effects" section). Although no specific information is available regarding short-term overdosage, any medication taken in excess can have serious consequences. If you suspect an overdose of Deltasone, seek medical attention immediately.

*Brand name:*

# Demerol

*Pronounced: DEM-er-awl*
*Generic name: Meperidine hydrochloride*

## Why is this drug prescribed?

Demerol, a narcotic analgesic, is prescribed for the relief of moderate to severe pain.

## Most important fact about this drug

Do not take Demerol if you are currently taking antidepressant drugs known as MAO inhibitors or have used them in the previous 2 weeks. Drugs in this category include Nardil and Parnate. When taken with Demerol, they can cause unpredictable, severe, and occasionally fatal reactions.

## How should you take this medication?

Take Demerol exactly as prescribed. Do not increase the amount or length of time you take this drug without your doctor's approval.

If you are using Demerol in syrup form, take each dose in a half glass of water.

■ *If you miss a dose...*
Take it as soon as you remember. If it is almost time for your next dose, skip the one you missed and go back to your regular schedule. Never take 2 doses at once.
■ *Storage instructions...*
Store away from heat, light, and moisture.

## What side effects may occur?

Side effects cannot be anticipated. If any develop or change in intensity, inform your doctor as soon as possible. Only your doctor can determine if it is safe for you to continue taking Demerol.

■ *More common side effects may include:*
Dizziness, light-headedness, nausea, sedation, sweating, vomiting

If any of these side effects occur, it may help if you lie down after taking the medication.

■ *Less common or rare side effects may include:*
Agitation, constipation, difficulty urinating, disorientation, dry mouth, fainting, fast heartbeat, feeling of elation or depression, flushing of the face, hallucinations, headache, hives, impairment of physical performance, itching, low blood pressure, mental sluggishness or clouding, palpitations, rashes, restlessness, severe convulsions, slow heartbeat, tremors, troubled and slowed breathing, uncoordinated muscle movements, visual disturbances, weakness

## Why should this drug not be prescribed?

If you are sensitive to or have ever had an allergic reaction to Demerol or other narcotic painkillers, you should not use this medication. Make sure your doctor is aware of any drug reactions you have experienced.

Do not take Demerol with MAO inhibitors such as Nardil and Parnate.

## Special warnings about this medication

Demerol may affect you both mentally and physically. You should not drive a car, operate machinery, or perform any other potentially hazardous activities until you know how the drug affects you.

You can build up tolerance to, and both mental and physical dependence on, Demerol if you take it repeatedly. If you have ever had a problem with drug abuse, consult with your doctor before taking this drug.

Use Demerol with caution if you have a severe liver or kidney disorder, hypothyroidism (underactive thyroid gland), Addison's disease (adrenal gland failure), an enlarged prostate, a urethral stricture (narrowing of the tube leading from the bladder), a head injury, a severe abdominal condition, or an irregular heartbeat, or if you have ever had convulsions.

Be very careful taking this drug if you are having a severe asthma attack, if you have frequently recurring lung disease, if you are unable to inhale or exhale extra air when needed, or if you have any pre-existing breathing difficulties.

Because Demerol may cause unusually slow or troubled breathing and may increase the pressure from fluid surrounding the brain and spinal cord, this drug should be used by people with head injury only if the doctor considers it absolutely necessary.

Demerol may make you feel light-headed or dizzy when you get up from lying down.

Before having surgery, make sure the doctor knows you are taking Demerol.

## Possible food and drug interactions when taking this medication

Demerol slows brain activity and intensifies the effects of alcohol. Do not drink alcohol while taking this medication.

If Demerol is taken with certain other drugs, the effects of either could be increased, decreased, or altered. It is especially important to check with your doctor before combining Demerol with the following:

Antidepressant drugs such as Elavil, Tofranil

Antihistamines such as Benadryl

Cimetidine (Tagamet)

Major tranquilizers such as Mellaril and Thorazine

MAO inhibitors such as Nardil and Parnate

Other narcotic painkillers such as Percocet and Tylenol with Codeine

Phenytoin (Dilantin)

Sedatives such as Halcion and Restoril

Tranquilizers such as Xanax and Valium

### Special information
### if you are pregnant or breastfeeding

Do not take Demerol if you are pregnant or planning to become pregnant unless you are directed to do so by your doctor. Demerol appears in breast milk and could affect a nursing infant. If this medication is essential to your health, your doctor may advise you to discontinue breastfeeding your baby until your treatment is finished.

### Recommended dosage

ADULTS

The usual dosage of Demerol is 50 milligrams to 150 milligrams every 3 or 4 hours, determined according to your response and the severity of the pain.

CHILDREN

The usual dosage is 0.5 milligram to 0.8 milligram per pound of body weight, taken every 3 or 4 hours, as determined by your doctor.

OLDER ADULTS

Your doctor may reduce the dosage.

### Overdosage

■ *Symptoms of Demerol overdose include:*
Bluish discoloration of the skin, cold and clammy skin, coma or extreme sleepiness, limp, weak muscles, low blood pressure, slow heartbeat, troubled or slowed breathing

With severe overdose, a person may stop breathing, have a heart attack, and even die.

If you suspect an overdose, seek emergency medical treatment immediately.

*Brand name:*

# Demulen

See Oral Contraceptives, page 382.

*Brand name:*

# Depakene

*Pronounced: DEP-uh-keen*
*Generic name: Valproic acid*

### Why is this drug prescribed?

Depakene, an epilepsy medicine, is used to treat certain types of seizures and convulsions. It may be prescribed alone or with other anticonvulsant medications.

### Most important fact about this drug

Depakene can cause serious liver damage, especially during the first 6 months of treatment. Children under 2 years of age are the most vulnerable, especially if they are also taking other anticonvulsant medicines and have certain other disorders such as mental retardation. The risk of liver damage decreases with age; but you should always be alert for the following symptoms: loss of seizure control, weakness, dizziness, drowsiness, a general feeling of ill health, facial swelling, loss of appetite, vomiting, and yellowing of the skin and eyes. If you suspect a liver problem, call your doctor immediately.

### How should you take this medication?

If Depakene irritates your digestive system, take it with food. To avoid irritating your mouth and throat, swallow Depakene capsules whole; do not chew them.

■ *If you miss a dose...*
If you take 1 dose a day, take the dose you missed as soon as you remember. If you do not remember until the next day, skip the dose you missed and go back to your regular schedule.

If you take more than 1 dose a day and you remember the missed dose within 6 hours of the scheduled time, take it immediately. Take the rest of the doses for that day at equally spaced intervals. Never take 2 doses at once.

■ *Storage instructions...*
Store at room temperature.

## What side effects may occur?

Side effects cannot be anticipated. If any develop or change in intensity, inform your doctor as soon as possible. Only your doctor can determine if it is safe for you to continue taking Depakene.

■ *More common side effects may include:*
Indigestion, nausea, vomiting

■ *Less common or rare side effects may include:*
Abdominal cramps, aggression, anemia, bleeding, blood disorders, breast enlargement, breast milk not associated with pregnancy or nursing, bruising, changes in behavior, coma, constipation, depression, diarrhea, difficulty in speaking, dizziness, double vision, drowsiness, emotional upset, excessive urination (mainly children), fever, growth failure in children, hair loss (temporary), hallucinations, headache, involuntary eye movements, involuntary jerking or tremors, irregular menstrual periods, itching, lack of coordination, liver disease, loss of bladder control, loss of or increased appetite, overactivity, rash, rickets (mainly children), sedation, sensitivity to light, skin eruptions or peeling, spots before the eyes, swelling of the arms and legs due to fluid retention, swollen glands, weakness, weight loss or gain

## Why should this drug not be prescribed?

You should not take this drug if you have liver disease or your liver is not functioning properly, or if you have had an allergic reaction to it.

## Special warnings about this medication

Remember that liver failure is possible when taking Depakene (see "Most important fact about this drug"). Your doctor should test your liver function at regular intervals.

Because of the potential for side effects involving blood disorders, your doctor will probably test your blood before prescribing Depakene and at regular intervals while you are taking it. Bruising, hemorrhaging, or clotting disorders usually mean the dosage should be reduced or the drug should be stopped altogether.

Since Depakene may cause drowsiness, you should not drive a car, operate heavy machinery, or engage in hazardous activity until you know how you react to the drug.

Do not abruptly stop taking this medicine without first consulting your doctor. A gradual reduction in dosage is usually required.

This drug can also increase the effect of painkillers and anesthetics. Before any surgery or dental procedure, make sure the doctor knows you are taking Depakene.

## Possible food and drug interactions when taking this medication

If Depakene is taken with certain other drugs, the effects of either could be increased, decreased, or altered. It is especially important to check with your doctor before combining Depakene with the following:

Aspirin
Barbiturates such as phenobarbital and Seconal
Blood-thinning drugs such as Coumadin
   and Dicumarol
Carbamazepine (Tegretol)
Clonazepam (Klonopin)
Felbamate (Felbatol)
Oral contraceptives
Phenytoin (Dilantin)
Primidone (Mysoline)

Extreme drowsiness and other serious effects may occur if Depakene is taken with alcohol or other central nervous system depressants such as Halcion, Restoril, or Xanax.

## Special information if you are pregnant or breastfeeding

If taken during pregnancy, Depakene may harm the baby. The drug is not recommended for pregnant women unless the benefits of therapy clearly outweigh the risks. In fact, women in their childbearing years should take Depakene only if it has been shown to be essential in the control of seizures. Since Depakene appears in breast milk, nursing mothers should use it only with caution.

## Recommended dosage

The usual starting dose is 15 milligrams per 2.2 pounds of body weight per day. Your doctor may increase the dose at weekly intervals by 5 to 10 milligrams per 2.2 pounds per day until seizures are controlled or side effects become too severe. The daily dose should not exceed 60 milligrams per 2.2 pounds per day.

## Overdosage

Any medication taken in excess can have serious consequences. An overdose of Depakene can be fatal. If you suspect an overdose, seek medical help immediately.

■ *Symptoms of Depakene overdose may include:*
 Coma, extreme drowsiness, heart problems

*Brand name:*

# Depakote

*Pronounced: DEP-uh-coat*
*Generic name: Divalproex sodium (Valproic acid)*

### Why is this drug prescribed?
Depakote, an epilepsy medicine, is used to treat certain types of seizures and convulsions. It may be prescribed alone or with other anticonvulsant medications.

### Most important fact about this drug
Depakote can cause serious liver damage, especially during the first 6 months of treatment. Children under 2 years of age are the most vulnerable, especially if they are also taking other anticonvulsant medicines and have certain other disorders such as mental retardation. The risk of liver damage decreases with age; but you should always be alert for the following symptoms: loss of seizure control, weakness, dizziness, drowsiness, a general feeling of ill health, facial swelling, loss of appetite, vomiting, and yellowing of the skin and eyes. If you suspect a liver problem, call your doctor immediately.

### How should you take this medication?
Take the tablet with water and swallow it whole (don't chew it or crush it). It has a special coating to avoid upsetting your stomach.

  If you are taking the sprinkle capsule, you can swallow it whole or open it and sprinkle the contents on a teaspoon of soft food such as applesauce or pudding. Swallow it immediately, without chewing. The sprinkle capsules are large enough to be opened easily.

  Depakote can be taken with meals or snacks to avoid stomach upset. Take it exactly as prescribed.

■ *If you miss a dose...*
 If you take Depakote once a day, take your dose as soon as you remember. If you don't remember until the next day, skip the missed dose and return to your regular schedule. Never take 2 doses at the same time.

  If you take more than one dose a day, take your dose right away if it's within 6 hours of the sched-uled time, and take the rest of the day's doses at equal intervals during the day. Never take 2 doses at the same time.

■ *Storage instructions...*
 Store at room temperature.

### What side effects may occur?
Side effects cannot be anticipated. If any develop or change in intensity, inform your doctor as soon as possible. Because Depakote is often used with other antiseizure drugs, it may not be possible to determine whether a side effect is due to Depakote alone. Only your doctor can determine if it is safe for you to continue taking Depakote.

■ *More common side effects may include:*
 Indigestion, nausea, vomiting
■ *Less common or rare side effects may include:*
 Abdominal cramps, abnormal milk secretion, aggression, anemia, behavior problems, bleeding, blood disorders, breast enlargement, bruising, coma, constipation, depression, diarrhea, dizziness, double vision, drowsiness, emotional upset, excessive urination (mainly children), fever, growth failure in children, hallucinations, headache, increased appetite, involuntary rapid movement of eyeball, irregular menstruation, itching, jerky movements, lack of muscular coordination, liver problems, loss of appetite, loss of bladder control, overactivity, rickets (mainly children), sedation, seeing "spots before your eyes", sensitivity to light, skin eruptions or peeling, skin rash, speech difficulties, swelling of arms and legs due to fluid retention, swollen glands, temporary hair loss, tremor, weakness, weight loss or gain

### Why should this drug not be prescribed?
You should not take this medication if you have liver disease or your liver is not functioning well.

  If you are sensitive to or have ever had an allergic reaction to Depakote, you should not take this medication.

### Special warnings about this medication
This medication can severely damage the liver (see "Most important fact about this drug").

  Depakote causes some people to become drowsy or less alert. You should not drive or operate dangerous machinery or participate in any hazardous activity that requires full mental alertness until you are certain the drug does not have this effect on you.

Do not abruptly stop taking this medicine without first consulting your doctor. A gradual reduction in dosage is usually required.

Depakote prolongs the time it takes blood to clot, which increases your chances of serious bleeding.

This drug can also increase the effect of painkillers and anesthetics. Before any surgery or dental procedure, make sure the doctor knows you are taking Depakote.

### Possible food and drug interactions when taking this medication

Depakote depresses activity of the central nervous system, and may increase the effects of alcohol. Do not drink alcohol while taking this medication.

If Depakote is taken with certain other drugs, the effects of either could be increased, decreased, or altered. It is especially important to check with your doctor before combining Depakote with the following:

Aspirin
Barbiturates such as phenobarbital and Seconal
Blood thinners such as Coumadin
Cyclosporine (Sandimmune, Neoral)
Oral contraceptives
Other seizure medications, including carba-
    mazepine (Tegretol), clonazepam (Klonopin),
    ethosuximide (Zarontin), felbamate (Felbatol),
    phenytoin (Dilantin), and Primidone (Mysoline)
Sleep aids such as Halcion
Tranquilizers such as Valium and Xanax

### Special information if you are pregnant or breastfeeding

Depakote may produce birth defects if it is taken during pregnancy. If you are pregnant or plan to become pregnant, inform your doctor immediately. Depakote appears in breast milk and could affect a nursing infant. If Depakote is essential to your health, your doctor may advise you to discontinue breastfeeding until your treatment with this medication is finished.

### Recommended dosage

ADULTS AND CHILDREN

Dosage is determined by your body weight. The usual recommended starting dose is 15 milligrams per 2.2 pounds per day; your doctor may increase the dose at 1-week intervals by 5 to 10 milligrams per 2.2 pounds per day until your seizures are controlled or the side effects become too severe. The most you should take is 60 milligrams per 2.2 pounds per day. If your total dosage is more than 250 milligrams a day, your doctor will divide it into smaller individual doses.

### Overdosage

Any medication taken in excess can have serious consequences. An overdose of Depakote can be fatal. If you suspect an overdose, seek medical attention immediately.

■ *Symptoms of Depakote overdose may include:*
    Coma, extreme sleepiness, heart problems

---

*Brand name:*

# Dermacin

*See Lidex, page 283.*

---

*Generic name:*

# Desipramine

*See Norpramin, page 373.*

---

*Generic name:*

# Desmopressin

*See DDAVP, page 135.*

---

*Brand name:*

# Desogen

*See Oral Contraceptives, page 382.*

---

*Generic name:*

# Desonide

*See Tridesilon, page 563.*

---

*Brand name:*

# DesOwen

*See Tridesilon, page 563.*

*Generic name:*

# Desoximetasone

*See Topicort, page 555.*

*Brand name:*

# Desquam-E

*Pronounced: DES-kwam ee*
*Generic name: Benzoyl peroxide*
*Other brand names: Benzac W, Benzagel,*
  *BenzaShave, Theroxide, Triaz*

## Why is this drug prescribed?

Desquam-E gel is used to treat various types of acne. It can be used alone or with other treatments, including antibiotics and products that contain retinoic acid, sulfur, or salicylic acid.

## Most important fact about this drug

Significant clearing of the skin should occur after 2 to 3 weeks of treatment with Desquam-E.

## How should you use this medication?

Cleanse the affected area thoroughly before applying the medication. Desquam-E should then be gently rubbed in.

■ *If you miss a dose...*
  Apply it as soon as you remember. Then go back to your regular schedule.
■ *Storage instructions...*
  Store at room temperature.

## What side effects may occur?

Side effects cannot be anticipated. If any develop or change in intensity, notify your doctor as soon as possible. Only your doctor can determine whether it is safe for you to continue using Desquam-E.

■ *Side effects may include:*
  Allergic reaction (itching, rash in area where the medication was applied), excessive drying (red and peeling skin and possible swelling)

## Why should this drug not be prescribed?

Do not use Desquam-E if you are sensitive to or allergic to benzoyl peroxide or any other components of the drug.

## Special warnings about this medication

Desquam-E is for external use only. Avoid contact with your eyes, nose, lips, or throat. If the drug does touch these areas accidentally, rinse with water.

If you are sensitive to medications derived from benzoic acid (including certain topical anesthetics) or to cinnamon, you may also be sensitive to Desquam-E.

If your skin becomes severely irritated, stop using the drug and call your doctor.

Desquam-E can bleach or discolor hair or colored fabric.

Stay out of the sun as much as possible, and use a sunscreen.

## Possible food and drug interactions when using this medication

When used with sunscreens containing PABA (para-aminobenzoic acid), Desquam-E may cause temporary skin discoloration.

## Special information if you are pregnant or breastfeeding

The effects of Desquam-E during pregnancy have not been adequately studied. It should be used only if clearly needed. If you are pregnant or plan to become pregnant, inform your doctor immediately. This medication may appear in breast milk and could affect a nursing infant. If this medication is essential to your health, your doctor may advise you to stop breastfeeding until your treatment with Desquam-E is finished.

## Recommended dosage

ADULTS AND CHILDREN 12 YEARS AND OVER

Gently rub Desquam-E gel into all affected areas once or twice a day. If you are fair-skinned or live in an excessively dry climate, you should probably start with one application a day. You can continue to use Desquam-E for as long as your doctor thinks it is necessary.

## Overdosage

Overdosage of Desquam-E can result in excessive scaling of the skin, reddening skin, or swelling due to fluid retention. Any medication taken in excess can have serious consequences. If you suspect an overdose, seek medical attention.

*Brand name:*

# Desyrel

*Pronounced: DES-ee-rel*
*Generic name: Trazodone hydrochloride*

## Why is this drug prescribed?

Desyrel is prescribed for the treatment of depression.

## Most important fact about this drug

Desyrel does not provide immediate relief. It may take up to 4 weeks before you begin to feel better, although most patients notice improvement within 2 weeks.

## How should you take this medication?

Take Desyrel shortly after a meal or light snack. You may be more apt to feel dizzy or light-headed if you take the drug before you have eaten.

Desyrel may cause dry mouth. Sucking on a hard candy, chewing gum, or melting bits of ice in your mouth can relieve the problem.

■ *If you miss a dose...*
Take it as soon as you remember. If it is within 4 hours of your next dose, skip the one you missed and go back to your regular schedule. Never take 2 doses at once.

■ *Storage instructions...*
Store at room temperature in a tightly closed container away from light and excessive heat.

## What side effects may occur?

Side effects cannot be anticipated. If any develop or change in intensity, inform your doctor as soon as possible. Only your doctor can determine if it is safe for you to continue taking Desyrel.

■ *More common side effects may include:*
Abdominal or stomach disorder, aches or pains in muscles and bones, anger or hostility, blurred vision, brief loss of consciousness, confusion, constipation, decreased appetite, diarrhea, dizziness or light-headedness, drowsiness, dry mouth, excitement, fainting, fast or fluttery heartbeat, fatigue, fluid retention and swelling, headache, inability to fall or stay asleep, low blood pressure, nasal or sinus congestion, nausea, nervousness, nightmares or vivid dreams, tremors, uncoordinated movements, vomiting, weight gain or loss

■ *Less common or rare side effects may include:*
Allergic reactions, anemia, bad taste in mouth, blood in the urine, chest pain, delayed urine flow, decreased concentration, decreased sex drive, disorientation, ejaculation problems, excess salivation, gas, general feeling of illness, hallucinations or delusions, high blood pressure, impaired memory, impaired speech, impotence, increased appetite, increased sex drive, menstrual problems, more frequent urination, muscle twitches, numbness, prolonged erections, red, tired, itchy eyes, restlessness, ringing in the ears, shortness of breath, sweating or clammy skin, tingling or pins and needles

## Why should this drug not be prescribed?

If you are sensitive to or have ever had an allergic reaction to Desyrel or similar drugs, you should not take this medication. Make sure your doctor is aware of any drug reactions you have experienced.

## Special warnings about this medication

Desyrel may cause you to become drowsy or less alert and may affect your judgment. Therefore, you should not drive or operate dangerous machinery or participate in any hazardous activity that requires full mental alertness until you know how this drug affects you.

Desyrel has been associated with priapism, a persistent, painful erection of the penis. Men who experience prolonged or inappropriate erections should stop taking this drug and consult their doctor.

Notify your doctor or dentist that you are taking this drug if you have a medical emergency, and before you have surgery or dental treatment. Your doctor will ask you to stop using the drug if you are going to have elective surgery.

Be careful taking this drug if you have heart disease. Desyrel can cause irregular heartbeats.

## Possible food and drug interactions when taking this medication

Desyrel may intensify the effects of alcohol. Do not drink alcohol while taking this medication.

If Desyrel is taken with certain other drugs, the effects of either could be increased, decreased, or altered. It is especially important to check with your doctor before combining Desyrel with the following:

Antidepressant drugs known as MAO inhibitors, including Nardil and Parnate
Barbiturates such as Seconal
Central nervous system depressants such as Demerol and Halcion
Chlorpromazine (Thorazine)
Digoxin (Lanoxin)

Drugs for high blood pressure such as Catapres and Wytensin

Other antidepressants such as Prozac and Norpramin

Phenytoin (Dilantin)

Warfarin (Coumadin)

### Special information
### if you are pregnant or breastfeeding

The effects of Desyrel during pregnancy have not been adequately studied. If you are pregnant or planning to become pregnant, inform your doctor immediately. This medication may appear in breast milk. If treatment with this drug is essential to your health, your doctor may advise you to discontinue breastfeeding your baby until your treatment is finished.

### Recommended dosage

ADULTS

The usual starting dosage is a total of 150 milligrams per day, divided into 2 or more smaller doses. Your doctor may increase your dose by 50 milligrams per day every 3 or 4 days. Total dosage should not exceed 400 milligrams per day, divided into smaller doses. Once you have responded well to the drug, your doctor may gradually reduce your dose. Because this medication makes you drowsy, your doctor may tell you to take the largest dose at bedtime.

CHILDREN

The safety and effectiveness of Desyrel have not been established in children below 18 years of age.

### Overdosage

Any medication taken in excess can have serious consequences. An overdose of Desyrel in combination with other drugs can be fatal.

■ *Symptoms of a Desyrel overdose may include:*
Breathing failure, drowsiness, irregular heartbeat, prolonged, painful erection, seizures, vomiting

If you suspect an overdose, seek medical attention immediately.

*Brand name:*

# Dexacort

*See Decadron Turbinaire and Respihaler, page 138.*

*Generic name:*

# Dexamethasone

*See Decadron Tablets, page 136.*

*Generic name:*

# Dexamethasone sodium phosphate

*See Decadron Turbinaire and Respihaler, page 138.*

*Generic name:*

# Dexamethasone with Neomycin

*See Neodecadron Ophthalmic Ointment and Solution, page 352.*

*Brand name:*

# Dexedrine

*Pronounced: DEX-eh-dreen*
*Generic name: Dextroamphetamine sulfate*

### Why is this drug prescribed?

Dexedrine, a stimulant drug available in tablet or sustained-release capsule form, is prescribed to help treat the following conditions:

1. Narcolepsy (recurrent "sleep attacks")
2. Attention deficit disorder with hyperactivity. (The total treatment program should include social, psychological, and educational guidance along with Dexedrine.)
3. Short-term treatment of obesity (along with a behavioral modification program).

### Most important fact about this drug

Because it is a stimulant, this drug has high abuse potential. The stimulant effect may give way to a letdown period of depression and fatigue. Although the letdown can be relieved by taking another dose, this soon becomes a vicious circle.

If you habitually take Dexedrine in doses higher than recommended, or if you take it over a long period of time, you may eventually become dependent on the drug and suffer from withdrawal symptoms when it is unavailable.

## How should you take this medication?

Take Dexedrine exactly as prescribed. If it is prescribed in tablet form, you may need up to 3 doses a day. Take the first dose when you wake up; take the next 1 or 2 doses at intervals of 4 to 6 hours. You can take the sustained-release capsules only once a day.

Do not take Dexedrine late in the day, since this could cause insomnia. If you experience insomnia or an unwanted loss of appetite while taking this drug, notify your doctor; you may need a lower dosage.

It is likely that your doctor will periodically take you off Dexedrine to determine whether you still need it.

Do not chew or crush the sustained release form, Dexedrine Spansules.

Do not increase the dosage, except on your doctor's advice.

Do not use Dexedrine to improve mental alertness or stay awake. Do not share it with others.

■ *If you miss a dose...*
  If you take 1 dose a day, take it as soon as you remember, but not within 6 hours of going to bed. If you do not remember until the next day, skip the dose you missed and go back to your regular schedule.

  If you take 2 or 3 doses a day, take the dose you missed if it is within an hour or so of the scheduled time. Otherwise, skip the dose and go back to your regular schedule. Never take 2 doses at once.

■ *Storage instructions...*
  Store at room temperature in a tightly closed container, away from light.

## What side effects may occur?

Side effects cannot be anticipated. If any develop or change in intensity, inform your doctor as soon as possible. Only your doctor can determine if it is safe for you to continue taking Dexedrine.

■ *More common side effects may include:*
  Excessive restlessness, overstimulation
■ *Other side effects may include:*
  Changes in sex drive, constipation, diarrhea, dizziness, dry mouth, exaggerated feeling of well-being or depression, headache, heart palpitations, high blood pressure, hives, impotence, rapid heartbeat, sleeplessness, stomach and intestinal disturbances, tremors, uncontrollable twitching or jerking, unpleasant taste in the mouth

Unless you are being treated for obesity, you may find appetite suppression and weight loss to be unwanted side effects.

■ *Effects of chronic heavy abuse of Dexedrine may include:*
  Hyperactivity, irritability, personality changes, schizophrenia-like thoughts and behavior, severe insomnia, severe skin disease

## Why should this drug not be prescribed?

Do not take Dexedrine if you are sensitive to or have ever had an allergic reaction to it.

Do not take Dexedrine for at least 14 days after taking a monoamine oxidase inhibitor (MAO inhibitor) type of antidepressant such as Nardil or Parnate. Dexedrine and MAO inhibitor antidepressants may interact to cause a sharp, potentially life-threatening rise in blood pressure.

Your doctor will not prescribe Dexedrine for you if you suffer from any of the following conditions:

Agitation
Cardiovascular disease
Glaucoma
Hardening of the arteries
High blood pressure
Overactive thyroid gland
Substance abuse

## Special warnings about this medication

In the treatment of obesity, only a short course of Dexedrine should be prescribed. When the drug's appetite-suppressing effect no longer seems to work, it is time to stop taking Dexedrine—not take more of it. Increasing the dosage will lead to drug dependence.

Be aware that one of the inactive ingredients in Dexedrine is a yellow food coloring called tartrazine (Yellow No. 5). In a few people, particularly those who are allergic to aspirin, tartrazine can cause a severe allergic reaction.

Dexedrine may impair judgment or coordination. Do not drive or operate dangerous machinery until you know how you react to the medication.

There is some concern that Dexedrine may stunt a child's growth. For the sake of safety, any child who takes Dexedrine should have his or her growth monitored.

## Possible food and drug interactions when taking this medication

If Dexedrine is taken with certain foods or drugs, the effects of either could be increased, decreased, or altered. It is especially important to check with your doctor before combining Dexedrine with the following:

*Substances that dampen the effects of Dexedrine:*
Ammonium chloride
Chlorpromazine (Thorazine)
Fruit juices
Glutamic acid hydrochloride
Guanethidine (Ismelin)
Haloperidol (Haldol)
Lithium carbonate (Lithonate)
Methenamine (Urised)
Reserpine (Diupres)
Sodium acid phosphate
Vitamin C (as ascorbic acid)

*Substances that boost the effects of Dexedrine:*
Acetazolamide (Diamox)
MAO-inhibitor antidepressants such as Nardil
    and Parnate
Propoxyphene (Darvon)
Sodium bicarbonate (baking soda)
Thiazide diuretics such as Diuril

*Substances that have decreased effect when taken with Dexedrine:*
Antihistamines such as Benadryl
Blood pressure medications such as Catapres,
    Hytrin, and Minipress
Ethosuximide (Zarontin)
Veratrum alkaloids (found in certain blood
    pressure drugs)

*Substances that have increased effect when taken with Dexedrine:*
Antidepressants such as Norpramin and Vivactil
Meperidine (Demerol)
Norepinephrine (Levophed)
Phenobarbital
Phenytoin (Dilantin)

## Special information if you are pregnant or breastfeeding

The effects of Dexedrine during pregnancy have not been adequately studied. If you are pregnant or plan to become pregnant, inform your doctor immediately. Babies born to women taking Dexedrine may be premature or have low birth weight. They may also be depressed, agitated, or apathetic due to withdrawal symptoms. Since Dexedrine appears in breast milk, it should not be taken by a nursing mother.

## Recommended dosage

Regardless of what the drug is to be used for, take no more Dexedrine than your doctor prescribes. Intake should be kept to the lowest level that proves effective.

NARCOLEPSY

*Adults*
The usual dose is 5 to 60 milligrams per day, divided into smaller, equal doses.

*Children*
Narcolepsy seldom occurs in children under 12 years of age; however, when it does, Dexedrine may be used.

The suggested initial dose for children between 6 and 12 years of age is 5 milligrams per day. Your doctor may increase the daily dose in increments of 5 milligrams at weekly intervals until it becomes effective.

Children 12 years of age and older will be started with 10 milligrams daily. The daily dosage may be raised in increments of 10 milligrams at weekly intervals until effective. If side effects such as insomnia or anorexia appear, the dosage will probably be reduced.

ATTENTION DEFICIT DISORDER WITH HYPERACTIVITY

This drug is not recommended for children under 3 years of age.

*Children from 3 to 5 Years of Age*
The usual starting dose is 2.5 milligrams daily, in tablet form. Your doctor may raise the daily dosage by 2.5 milligrams at weekly intervals until the drug becomes effective.

*Children 6 Years of Age and Older*
The usual starting dose is 5 milligrams once or twice a day. Your doctor may raise the dose by 5 milligrams at weekly intervals until he or she is satisfied with the response. Only in rare cases will the child take more than 40 milligrams per day.

The doctor may prescribe "Spansule" capsules for your child. They are taken once a day.

Your child should take the first dose when he or she wakes up; the remaining 1 or 2 doses are taken at intervals of 4 to 6 hours. Your doctor may interrupt the schedule occasionally to see if behavioral symptoms come back enough to require continued therapy.

OBESITY

The usual dosage is one 10- or 15-milligram "Spansule" capsule daily, taken in the morning, or up to 30 milligrams daily as tablets divided into doses of 5 to 10 milligrams taken 30 to 60 minutes before meals.

Dexedrine is not recommended for this use in children under 12 years of age.

## Overdosage

An overdose of Dexedrine can be fatal. If you suspect an overdose, seek medical attention immediately.

■ *Symptoms of an acute Dexedrine overdose may include:*
Abdominal cramps, assaultiveness, coma, confusion, convulsions, depression, diarrhea, fatigue, hallucinations, high fever, heightened reflexes, high or low blood pressure, irregular heartbeat, nausea, panic, rapid breathing, restlessness, tremor, vomiting

*Generic name:*

# Dextroamphetamine

*See Dexedrine, page 152.*

*Brand name:*

# DiaBeta

*See Micronase, page 324.*

*Brand name:*

# Diabinese

*Pronounced: dye-AB-in-eez*
*Generic name: Chlorpropamide*

## Why is this drug prescribed?

Diabinese is an oral antidiabetic medication used to treat Type II (non-insulin-dependent) diabetes. Diabetes occurs when the body fails to produce enough insulin or is unable to use it properly. Insulin is believed to work by helping sugar penetrate the cell wall so it can be used by the cell.

There are two forms of diabetes: Type I insulin-dependent and Type II non-insulin-dependent. Type I usually requires insulin injection for life, while Type II diabetes can usually be treated by dietary changes and oral antidiabetic medications such as Diabinese. Apparently, Diabinese controls diabetes by stimulating the pancreas to secrete more insulin. Occasionally, Type II diabetics must take insulin injections on a temporary basis, especially during stressful periods or times of illness.

## Most important fact about this drug

Always remember that Diabinese is an aid to, not a substitute for, good diet and exercise. Failure to follow a sound diet and exercise plan can lead to serious complications, such as dangerously high or low blood sugar levels. Remember, too, that Diabinese is *not* an oral form of insulin, and cannot be used in place of insulin.

## How should you take this medication?

Ordinarily, your doctor will ask you to take a single daily dose of Diabinese each morning with breakfast. However, if this upsets your stomach, he or she may ask you to take Diabinese in smaller doses throughout the day.

To prevent low blood sugar levels (hypoglycemia):

■ You should understand the symptoms of hypoglycemia
■ Know how exercise affects your blood sugar levels
■ Maintain an adequate diet
■ Keep a source of quick-acting sugar with you all the time

■ *If you miss a dose...*
Take it as soon as you remember. If it is almost time for the next dose, skip the one you missed and go back to your regular schedule. Do not take 2 doses at the same time.
■ *Storage instructions...*
Store at room temperature.

## What side effects may occur?

Side effects cannot be anticipated. If any develop or change in intensity, inform your doctor as soon as possible. Only your doctor can determine if it is safe for you to continue taking Diabinese.

Side effects from Diabinese are rare and seldom require discontinuation of the medication.

■ *More common side effects include:*
Diarrhea, hunger, itching, loss of appetite, nausea, stomach upset, vomiting
■ *Less common or rare side effects may include:*
Anemia and other blood disorders, hives, inflammation of the rectum and colon, sensitivity to light, yellowing of the skin and eyes

Diabinese, like all oral antidiabetics, can cause hypoglycemia (low blood sugar). The risk of hypoglycemia is increased by missed meals, alcohol, other medications, and excessive exercise. To avoid hypoglycemia, closely follow the dietary and exercise regimen suggested by your physician.

■ *Symptoms of mild hypoglycemia may include:*
Cold sweat, drowsiness, fast heartbeat, headache, nausea, nervousness
■ *Symptoms of more severe hypoglycemia may include:*
Coma, pale skin, seizures, shallow breathing

Contact your doctor immediately if these symptoms of severe low blood sugar occur.

### Why should this drug not be prescribed?
You should not take Diabinese if you have ever had an allergic reaction to it.

Do not take Diabinese if you are suffering from diabetic ketoacidosis (a life-threatening medical emergency caused by insufficient insulin and marked by excessive thirst, nausea, fatigue, pain below the breastbone, and a fruity breath).

### Special warnings about this medication
It's possible that drugs such as Diabinese may lead to more heart problems than diet treatment alone, or diet plus insulin. If you have a heart condition, you may want to discuss this with your doctor.

If you are taking Diabinese, you should check your blood and urine periodically for the presence of abnormal sugar levels.

Remember that it is important that you closely follow the diet and exercise regimen established by your doctor.

Even people with well-controlled diabetes may find that stress, illness, surgery, or fever results in a loss of control. If this happens, your doctor may recommend that Diabinese be discontinued temporarily and insulin used instead.

In addition, the effectiveness of any oral antidiabetic, including Diabinese, may decrease with time. This may occur because of either a diminished responsiveness to the medication or a worsening of the diabetes.

### Possible food and drug interactions when taking this medication
When you take Diabinese with certain other drugs, the effects of either could be increased, decreased, or altered. It is important that you consult with your doctor before taking Diabinese with the following:

Anabolic steroids
Aspirin in large doses
Barbiturates such as Seconal
Beta-blocking blood pressure medications such as Inderal and Tenormin
Calcium-blocking blood pressure medications such as Cardizem and Procardia
Chloramphenicol (Chloromycetin)
Coumarin (Coumadin)
Diuretics such as Diuril and HydroDIURIL
Epinephrine (EpiPen)
Estrogen medications such as Premarin
Isoniazid (Nydrazid)
Major tranquilizers such as Mellaril and Thorazine
MAO inhibitor-type antidepressants such as Nardil and Parnate
Nicotinic acid (Nicobid, Nicolar)
Nonsteroidal anti-inflammatory agents such as Advil, Motrin, Naprosyn, and Nuprin
Oral contraceptives
Phenothiazines
Phenylbutazone
Phenytoin (Dilantin)
Probenecid (Benemid, ColBENEMID)
Steroids such as prednisone
Sulfa drugs such as Bactrim and Septra
Thyroid medications such as Synthroid

Avoid alcohol since excessive alcohol consumption can cause low blood sugar, breathlessness, and facial flushing.

### Special information if you are pregnant or breastfeeding
The effects of Diabinese during pregnancy have not been adequately established. If you are pregnant or plan to become pregnant you should inform your doctor immediately. Since studies suggest the importance of maintaining normal blood sugar

(glucose) levels during pregnancy, your physician may prescribe injected insulin.

To minimize the risk of low blood sugar (hypoglycemia) in newborn babies, Diabinese, if prescribed during pregnancy, should be discontinued at least 1 month before the expected delivery date.

Since Diabinese appears in breast milk, it is not recommended for nursing mothers. If diet alone does not control glucose levels, then insulin should be considered.

## Recommended dosage

Dosage levels are determined by each individual's needs.

### ADULTS

Usually, an initial daily dose of 250 milligrams is recommended for stable, middle-aged, non-insulin-dependent diabetics. After 5 to 7 days, your doctor may adjust this dosage in increments of 50 to 125 milligrams every 3 to 5 days to achieve the best benefit. People with mild diabetes may respond well to daily doses of 100 milligrams or less of Diabinese, while those with severe diabetes may require 500 milligrams daily. Maintenance doses above 750 milligrams are not recommended.

### OLDER ADULTS

People who are old, malnourished, or debilitated and those with impaired kidney and liver function usually take an initial dose of 100 to 125 milligrams.

### CHILDREN

Safety and effectiveness have not been established.

## Overdosage

An overdose of Diabinese can cause low blood sugar (see "What side effects may occur?" for symptoms).

Eating sugar or a sugar-based product will often correct the condition. If you suspect an overdose, seek medical attention immediately.

*Brand name:*

# Diamox

*Pronounced: DYE-uh-mocks*
*Generic name: Acetazolamide*

## Why is this drug prescribed?

Diamox controls fluid secretion. It is used in the treatment of glaucoma (excessive pressure in the eyes), epilepsy (for both brief and unlocalized seizures), and fluid retention due to congestive heart failure or drugs. It is also used to prevent or relieve the symptoms of acute mountain sickness in climbers attempting a rapid climb and those who feel sick even though they are making a gradual climb.

## Most important fact about this drug

This drug is considered to be a sulfa drug because of its chemical properties. Although rare, severe reactions have been reported with sulfa drugs. If you develop a rash, bruises, sore throat, or fever contact your doctor immediately.

## How should you take this medication?

Take this medication exactly as prescribed by your doctor.

■ *If you miss a dose...*
  Take it as soon as you remember. If it is almost time for your next dose, skip the one you missed and go back to your regular schedule. Never take 2 doses at the same time.
■ *Storage instructions...*
  Store at room temperature.

## What side effects may occur?

Side effects cannot be anticipated. If any develop or change in intensity, inform your doctor as soon as possible. Only your doctor can determine if it is safe for you to continue taking Diamox.

■ *More common side effects may include:*
  Change in taste, diarrhea, increase in amount or frequency of urination, loss of appetite, nausea, ringing in the ears, tingling or pins and needles in hands or feet, vomiting
■ *Less common or rare side effects may include:*
  Anemia, black or bloody stools, blood in urine, confusion, convulsions, drowsiness, fever, hives, liver dysfunction, nearsightedness, paralysis, rash, sensitivity to light, severe allergic reaction, skin peeling

## Why should this drug not be prescribed?

Your doctor will not prescribe this medication for you if your sodium or potassium levels are low, or if you have kidney or liver disease, including cirrhosis.

Diamox should not be used as a long-term treatment for the type of glaucoma called chronic non-congestive angle-closure glaucoma.

### Special warnings about this medication

Be very careful about taking high doses of aspirin if you are also taking Diamox. Effects of this combination can range from loss of appetite, sluggishness, and rapid breathing to unresponsiveness; the combination can be fatal.

If you have emphysema or other breathing disorders, use this drug with caution.

If you are taking Diamox to help in rapid ascent of a mountain, you must still come down promptly if you show signs of severe mountain sickness.

### Possible food and drug interactions when taking this medication

If Diamox is taken with certain other drugs, the effects of either could be increased, decreased, or altered. It is especially important to check with your doctor before combining Diamox with the following:

Amitriptyline (Elavil)
Amphetamines such as Dexedrine
Aspirin
Cyclosporine (Sandimmune)
Lithium (Lithonate)
Methenamine (Urex)
Oral diabetes drugs such as Micronase
Quinidine (Quinidex)

### Special information if you are pregnant or breastfeeding

The effects of Diamox during pregnancy have not been adequately studied. If you are pregnant or plan to become pregnant, inform your doctor immediately. Diamox may appear in breast milk and could affect a nursing infant. If this medication is essential to your health, your doctor may advise you to discontinue breastfeeding until your treatment with Diamox is finished.

### Recommended dosage

ADULTS

This medication is available in both oral and injectable form. Dosages are for the oral form only.

*Glaucoma*

This medication is used as an addition to regular glaucoma treatment. Dosages for open-angle glaucoma range from 250 milligrams to 1 gram per 24 hours in 2 or more smaller doses. Your doctor will supervise your dosage and watch the effect of this medication carefully if you are using it for glaucoma. In secondary glaucoma and before surgery in acute congestive (closed-angle) glaucoma, the usual dosage is 250 milligrams every 4 hours or, in some cases, 250 milligrams twice a day. Some people may take 500 milligrams to start, and then 125 or 250 milligrams every 4 hours. The injectable form of this drug is occasionally used in acute cases.

The usual dosage of Diamox Sequels (sustained-release capsules) is 1 capsule (500 milligrams) twice a day, usually in the morning and evening.

Your doctor may adjust the dosage, as needed.

*Epilepsy*

The daily dosage is 8 to 30 milligrams per 2.2 pounds of body weight in 2 or more doses. Typical dosage may range from 375 to 1,000 milligrams per day. Your doctor will adjust the dosage to suit your needs; Diamox can be used with other anticonvulsant medication.

*Congestive Heart Failure*

The usual starting dosage to reduce fluid retention in people with congestive heart failure is 250 milligrams to 375 milligrams per day or 5 milligrams per 2.2 pounds of body weight, taken in the morning. Diamox works best when it is taken every other day—or 2 days on, 1 day off—for this condition.

*Edema Due to Medication*

The usual dose is 250 milligrams to 375 milligrams daily for 1 or 2 days, alternating with a day of rest.

*Acute Mountain Sickness*

The usual dose is 500 milligrams to 1,000 milligrams a day in 2 or more doses, using either tablets or sustained-release capsules. Doses of this medication are often begun 1 or 2 days before attempting to reach high altitudes.

CHILDREN

The safety and effectiveness of Diamox in children have not been established. However, doses of 8 milligrams to 30 milligrams per 2.2 pounds of body weight have been used in children with various forms of epilepsy.

## Overdosage

There is no specific information available on Diamox overdose, but any medication taken in excess can have serious consequences. If you suspect an overdose, seek medical attention immediately.

*Generic name:*

# Diazepam

*See Valium, page 580.*

*Generic name:*

# Diclofenac

*See Voltaren, page 590.*

*Generic name:*

# Dicyclomine

*See Bentyl, page 56.*

*Generic name:*

# Diethylpropion

*See Tenuate, page 533.*

*Generic name:*

# Diflorasone

*See Psorcon, page 452.*

*Brand name:*

# Diflucan

*Pronounced: Dye-FLEW-can*
*Generic name: Fluconazole*

## Why is this drug prescribed?

Diflucan is used to treat fungal infections called candidiasis (also known as thrush or yeast infections). These include vaginal infections, throat infections, and fungal infections elsewhere in the body, such as infections of the urinary tract, peritonitis (inflammation of the lining of the abdomen), and pneumonia. Diflucan is also prescribed to guard against candidiasis in some people receiving bone marrow transplants. It is also used to treat meningitis (brain or spinal cord inflammation) caused by another type of fungus.

In addition, Diflucan is now being prescribed for fungal infections in kidney and liver transplant patients, and fungal infections in patients with AIDS.

## Most important fact about this drug

Strong allergic reactions to Diflucan, although rare, have been reported. Symptoms may include hives, itching, swelling, sudden drop in blood pressure, difficulty breathing or swallowing, diarrhea, or abdominal pain. If you experience any of these symptoms, notify your doctor immediately.

## How should you take this medication?

You can take Diflucan with or without meals.

Take this medication exactly as prescribed, and continue taking it for as long as your doctor instructs. You may begin to feel better after the first few days; but it takes weeks or even months of treatment to completely cure certain fungal infections.

■ *If you miss a dose...*
Take the forgotten dose as soon as you remember. However, if it is almost time for your next dose, skip the one you missed and return to your regular schedule. Do not take double doses.
■ *Storage instructions...*
Diflucan tablets should be stored at normal room temperature. Avoid exposing them to temperatures above 86°F.

## What side effects may occur?

Side effects cannot be anticipated. If any develop or change in intensity, inform your doctor as soon as possible. Only your doctor can determine if it is safe for you to continue taking Diflucan.

The most common side effect for people taking more than one dose is nausea.

For women taking a single dose to treat vaginal infection, the most common side effects are abdominal pain, diarrhea, headache, and nausea; changes in taste, dizziness, and indigestion may occur less often.

■ *Less common side effects may include:*
Abdominal pain, diarrhea, headache, skin rash, vomiting

## Why should this drug not be prescribed?

Do not take Diflucan if you are sensitive to any of its ingredients or have ever had an allergic reaction to similar drugs, such as Nizoral. Make sure your doctor is aware of any drug reactions you have experienced.

## Special warnings about this medication

Your doctor will watch your liver function carefully while you are taking Diflucan.

If your immunity is low and you develop a rash, your doctor should monitor your condition closely. You may have to stop taking Diflucan if the rash gets worse.

## Possible food and drug interactions when taking this medication

If Diflucan is taken with certain other drugs, the effects of either could be increased, decreased, or altered. It is especially important to check with your doctor before combining Diflucan with the following:

Anticoagulants (Coumadin)
Antidiabetic drugs such as Orinase, DiaBeta and Glucotrol
Certain antihistamines, such as Hismanal
Cyclosporine (Sandimmune, Neoral)
Hydrochlorothiazide (HydroDIURIL)
Phenytoin (Dilantin)
Rifampin (Rifadin)
Ulcer medications such as Tagamet

## Special information if you are pregnant or breastfeeding

The effects of Diflucan during pregnancy have not been adequately studied. If you are pregnant or plan to become pregnant, inform your doctor immediately. Diflucan appears in breast milk and could affect a nursing infant. If this medication is essential to your health, your doctor may advise you to stop breastfeeding until your treatment with Diflucan is finished.

## Recommended dosage

ADULTS

*For vaginal infections*
The usual treatment is a single 150-milligram dose.

*For throat infections*
The usual dose for candidiasis of the mouth and throat is 200 milligrams on the first day, followed by 100 milligrams once a day. Treatment should continue for at least 2 weeks to avoid a relapse. For candidiasis of the esophagus (gullet) the usual dose is 200 milligrams on the first day, followed by 100 milligrams once a day. Treatment should continue for a minimum of 3 weeks and for at least 2 weeks after symptoms have stopped.

*For systemic (bodywide) infections*
Doses of up to 400 milligrams per day are sometimes prescribed.

*For cryptococcal meningitis*
The usual dose is 400 milligrams on the first day, followed by 200 milligrams once a day. Treatment should continue for 10 to 12 weeks once tests of spinal fluid come back negative. For AIDS patients, a 200-milligram dose taken once a day is recommended to prevent relapse.

*Prevention of candidiasis during bone marrow transplantation*
The usual dose is 400 milligrams once a day.

If you have kidney disease, your doctor may have to reduce your dosage.

CHILDREN

*For throat infections*
The usual dose for candidiasis of the mouth and throat is 6 milligrams for each 2.2 pounds of the child's weight on the first day, and 3 milligrams per 2.2 pounds once a day after that.

The duration of treatment is the same as that for adults.

*For systemic (bodywide) infections*
The drug has been given at 6 to 12 milligrams per 2.2 pounds of weight per day.

*For cryptococcal meningitis*
The usual dose is 12 milligrams per 2.2 pounds of body weight per day on the first day, and 6 milligrams per 2.2 pounds per day after that. Treatment will last 10 to 12 weeks after the fungus disappears.

## Overdosage

Any medication taken in excess can have serious consequences. If you suspect an overdose, seek medical treatment immediately.

■ *Symptoms of Diflucan overdose may include:*
Hallucinations, paranoia

Generic name:

# Diflunisal

See Dolobid, page 173.

Generic name:

# Digoxin

See Lanoxin, page 273.

Generic name:

# Dihydrocodeine, Aspirin, and Caffeine

See Synalgos-DC, page 515.

Brand name:

# Dilantin

Pronounced: dye-LAN-tin
Generic name: Phenytoin sodium

## Why is this drug prescribed?

Dilantin is an antiepileptic drug, prescribed to control grand mal seizures (a type of seizure in which the individual experiences a sudden loss of consciousness immediately followed by generalized convulsions) and temporal lobe seizures (a type of seizure caused by disease in the cortex of the temporal [side] lobe of the brain affecting smell, taste, sight, hearing, memory, and movement).

Dilantin may also be used to prevent and treat seizures occurring during and after neurosurgery (surgery of the brain and spinal cord).

## Most important fact about this drug

If you have been taking Dilantin regularly, do not stop abruptly. This may precipitate prolonged or repeated epileptic seizures without any recovery of consciousness between attacks—a condition called status epilepticus that can be fatal if not treated promptly.

## How should you take this medication?

It is important that you strictly follow the prescribed dosage regimen and tell your doctor about any condition that makes it impossible for you to take Dilantin as prescribed.

If you are given Dilantin Oral Suspension, shake it well before using. Use the specially marked measuring spoon, a plastic syringe, or a small measuring cup to measure each dose accurately.

Swallow Dilantin Kapseals whole. Dilantin Infatabs can be either chewed thoroughly and then swallowed, or swallowed whole. The Infatabs are not to be used for once-a-day dosing.

Do not change from one form of Dilantin to another without consulting your doctor. Different products may not work the same way.

Depending on the type of seizure disorder, your doctor may give you another drug with Dilantin.

■ *If you miss a dose...*
If you take one dose a day, take the dose you missed as soon as you remember. If you do not remember until the next day, skip the missed dose and go back to your regular schedule. Do not take 2 doses at once.

If you take more than 1 dose a day, take the missed dose as soon as possible. If it is within 4 hours of your next dose, skip the one you missed and go back to your regular schedule. Do not take 2 doses at once.

If you forget to take your medication 2 or more days in a row, check with your doctor.

■ *Storage instructions...*
Store at room temperature away from light and moisture.

## What side effects may occur?

Side effects cannot be anticipated. If any develop or change in intensity, inform your doctor as soon as possible. Only your doctor can determine whether it is safe for you to continue taking Dilantin.

■ *More common side effects may include:*
Decreased coordination, involuntary eye movement, mental confusion, slurred speech
■ *Other side effects may include:*
Abnormal hair growth, abnormal muscle tone, blood disorders, coarsening of facial features, constipation, dizziness, enlargement of lips, fever, headache, inability to fall asleep or stay asleep, joint pain, nausea, nervousness, overgrowth of gum tissue, Peyronie's disease (a disorder of the penis that causes the penis to bend on an angle during erection, often making intercourse painful or difficult), rapid and spastic

involuntary movement, skin peeling or scaling, skin rash, tremors, twitching, vomiting, yellowing of skin and eyes

## Why should this drug not be prescribed?

If you have ever had an allergic reaction to or are sensitive to phenytoin or similar epilepsy medications such as Peganone or Mesantoin, do not take Dilantin. Make sure your doctor is aware of any drug reactions you have experienced.

## Special warnings about this medication

Tell your doctor if you develop a skin rash. If the rash is scale-like, characterized by reddish or purplish spots, or consists of (fluid-filled) blisters, your doctor may stop Dilantin and prescribe an alternative treatment. If the rash is more like measles, your doctor may have you stop taking Dilantin until the rash is completely gone.

Because Dilantin is processed by the liver, people with impaired liver function, the elderly, and those who are seriously ill may show early signs of drug poisoning.

Practicing good dental hygiene minimizes the development of gingival hyperplasia (excessive formation of the gums over the teeth) and its complications.

Avoid drinking alcoholic beverages while taking Dilantin.

## Possible food and drug interactions when taking this medication

If Dilantin is taken with certain other drugs, the effects of either could be increased, decreased, or altered. It is especially important to check with your doctor before combining Dilantin with the following:

Alcohol
Amiodarone (Cordarone)
Antacids containing calcium
Blood-thinning drugs such as Coumadin
Chloramphenicol (Chloromycetin)
Chlordiazepoxide (Librium)
Diazepam (Valium)
Dicumarol
Digitoxin (Crystodigin)
Disulfiram (Antabuse)
Doxycycline (Vibramycin)
Estrogens such as Premarin
Felbamate (Felbatol)
Fluoxetine (Prozac)

Furosemide (Lasix)
Isoniazid (Nydrazid)
Major tranquilizers such as Mellaril and Thorazine
Methylphenidate (Ritalin)
Molindone hydrochloride (Moban)
Oral contraceptives
Phenobarbital
Quinidine (Quinidex)
Reserpine (Diupres)
Rifampin (Rifadin)
Salicylates such as aspirin
Seizure medications such as Depakene, Depakote, Tegretol, and Zarontin
Steroid drugs such as prednisone (Deltasone)
Sucralfate (Carafate)
Sulfa drugs such as Gantrisin
Theophylline (Theo-Dur, others)
Tolbutamide (Orinase)
Trazodone (Desyrel)
Ulcer medications such as Tagamet and Zantac

Tricyclic antidepressants (such as Elavil, Norpramin, and others) may cause seizures in susceptible people, making a dosage adjustment of Dilantin necessary.

Hyperglycemia (high blood sugar) may occur in people taking Dilantin, which blocks the release of insulin. People with diabetes may experience increased blood sugar levels due to Dilantin.

Abnormal softening of the bones may occur in people taking Dilantin because of Dilantin's interference with vitamin D metabolism.

## Special information if you are pregnant or breastfeeding

If you are pregnant or plan to become pregnant, inform your doctor immediately. Because of the possibility of birth defects with antiepileptic drugs such as Dilantin, you may need to discontinue the drug. Do not, however, stop taking it without first consulting your doctor. Dilantin appears in breast milk; breastfeeding is not recommended during treatment with this drug.

## Recommended dosage

Dosage is tailored to each individual's needs. Your doctor will monitor blood levels of the drug closely, particularly when switching you from one drug to another.

ADULTS

*Standard Daily Dosage*

If you have not had any previous treatment, your doctor will have you take one 100-milligram Dilantin capsule 3 times daily to start.

On a continuing basis, most adults need 1 capsule 3 to 4 times a day. Your doctor may increase that dosage to 2 capsules 3 times a day, if necessary.

*Once-A-Day Dosage*

If your seizures are controlled on 100-milligram Dilantin capsules 3 times daily, your doctor may allow you to take the entire 300 milligrams as a single dose once daily.

CHILDREN

The starting dose is 5 milligrams per 2.2 pounds of body weight per day, divided into 2 or 3 equal doses; the most a child should take is 300 milligrams a day. The regular daily dosage is usually 4 to 8 milligrams per 2.2 pounds. Children over 6 years of age may need the minimum adult dose (300 milligrams per day).

## Overdosage

An overdose of Dilantin can be fatal. If you suspect an overdose, seek medical attention immediately.

■ *Symptoms of Dilantin overdose may include:*
Coma, difficulty in pronouncing words correctly, involuntary eye movement, lack of muscle coordination, low blood pressure, nausea, sluggishness, slurred speech, tremors, vomiting

*Brand name:*

# Dilaudid

*Pronounced: Dye-LAW-did*
*Generic name: Hydromorphone hydrochloride*

## Why is this drug prescribed?

Dilaudid, a narcotic analgesic, is prescribed for the relief of moderate to severe pain such as that due to:

Biliary colic (pain caused by an obstruction in the gallbladder or bile duct)
Burns
Cancer
Heart attack
Injury (soft tissue and bone)

Renal colic (sharp lower back and groin pain usually caused by the passage of a stone through the ureter)
Surgery

## Most important fact about this drug

High dose tolerance leading to mental and physical dependence can occur with the use of Dilaudid when it is taken repeatedly. Physical dependence (need for continual doses to prevent withdrawal symptoms) can occur after only a few days of narcotic use, although it usually takes several weeks.

## How should you take this medication?

Take Dilaudid exactly as prescribed by your doctor. Never increase the amount you take without your doctor's approval.

■ *If you miss a dose...*
Take the forgotten dose as soon as you remember. If it is almost time for the next dose, skip the one you missed and go back to your regular schedule. Never try to "catch up" by doubling the dose.

■ *Storage instructions...*
Tablets and liquid should be stored at room temperature. Protect from light and extreme cold or heat. Suppositories should be stored in the refrigerator.

## What side effects may occur?

Side effects cannot be anticipated. If any develop or change in intensity, inform your doctor as soon as possible. Only your doctor can determine if it is safe for you to continue taking Dilaudid.

■ *More common side effects may include:*
Anxiety, constipation, dizziness, drowsiness, fear, impairment of mental and physical performance, inability to urinate, mental clouding, mood changes, nausea, restlessness, sedation, sluggishness, troubled and slowed breathing, vomiting

■ *Less common side effects may include:*
Agitation, blurred vision, chills, cramps, diarrhea, difficulty urinating, disorientation, double vision, dry mouth, exaggerated feelings of depression or well-being, failure of breathing or heartbeat, faintness/fainting, flushing, hallucinations, headache, increased pressure in the head, insomnia, involuntary eye movements, itching, light-headedness, loss of appetite, low or high

blood pressure, muscle rigidity or tremor, muscle spasms of the throat or air passages, palpitations, rashes, shock, slow or rapid heartbeat, small pupils, sudden dizziness on standing, sweating, taste changes, tingling and/or numbness, tremor, uncoordinated muscle movements, visual disturbances, weakness

## Why should this drug not be prescribed?

If you are sensitive to or have ever had an allergic reaction to Dilaudid or narcotic pain killers you should not take this medication. Make sure that your doctor is aware of any drug reactions that you have experienced.

## Special warnings about this medication

Dilaudid may impair the mental and/or physical abilities required for the performance of potentially hazardous tasks such as driving a car or operating machinery.

Dilaudid should be used with caution if you are in a weakened condition or if you have a severe liver or kidney disorder, hypothyroidism (underactive thyroid gland), Addison's disease (adrenal gland failure), an enlarged prostate, a urethral stricture (narrowing of the urethra), low blood pressure or a head injury.

Dilaudid suppresses the cough reflex; therefore, the doctor will be cautious about prescribing Dilaudid after an operation or for patients with a lung disease.

High doses of Dilaudid may produce labored or slowed breathing. This drug also affects centers that control breathing rhythm and may produce irregular breathing. People who already have breathing difficulties should be very careful about taking Dilaudid.

Narcotics such as Dilaudid may mask or hide the symptoms of sudden or severe abdominal conditions, making diagnosis and treatment difficult.

If you are prone to convulsions, your doctor may not prescribe Dilaudid. It can make seizures worse.

## Possible food and drug interactions when taking this medication

Dilaudid is a central nervous system depressant and intensifies the effects of alcohol. Do not drink alcohol while taking this medication.

If Dilaudid is taken with certain other drugs, the effects of either could be increased, decreased, or altered. It is especially important to check with your doctor before combining Dilaudid with the following:

Antiemetics (drugs that prevent or lessen nausea and vomiting such as Compazine and Phenergan)
Antihistamines such as Benadryl
General anesthetics
Other central nervous system depressants such as Nembutal,
Restoril
Other narcotic analgesics such as Demerol and Percocet
Phenothiazines such as Thorazine
Sedative/hypnotics such as Valium, Halcion
Tranquilizers such as Xanax
Tricyclic antidepressants such as Elavil and Tofranil

## Special information
## if you are pregnant or breastfeeding

Do not take Dilaudid if you are pregnant or plan to become pregnant unless you are directed to do so by your doctor. Drug dependence occurs in newborns when the mother has taken narcotic drugs regularly during pregnancy. Withdrawal signs include irritability and excessive crying, tremors, overactive reflexes, increased breathing rate, increased stools, sneezing, yawning, vomiting, and fever. Dilaudid may appear in breast milk and could affect a nursing infant. If this medication is essential to your health, your doctor may advise you to discontinue breastfeeding your baby until your treatment is finished.

## Recommended dosage

ADULTS

*Tablets*

The usual starting dose of Dilaudid tablets is 2 to 4 milligrams every 4 to 6 hours as determined by your doctor. Severity of pain, your individual response, and your size are used to determine your exact dosage.

*Liquid*

The usual dose of Dilaudid liquid is 1/2 to 2 teaspoonfuls every 3 to 6 hours. In some cases, the dosage may be higher.

*Suppositories*

Dilaudid suppositories (3 milligrams) may provide relief for a longer period of time. The usual adult dose is 1 suppository inserted rectally every 6 to 8 hours or as directed by your doctor.

CHILDREN

The safety and effectiveness of Dilaudid have not been established in children.

OLDER ADULTS

Be very careful when using Dilaudid. Your doctor will prescribe a dose individualized to suit your needs.

## Overdosage

■ *Symptoms of Dilaudid overdose include:*
Bluish tinge to skin, cold and clammy skin, constricted pupils, coma, extreme sleepiness progressing to a state of unresponsiveness, labored or slowed breathing, limp, weak muscles, low blood pressure, slow heart rate

In severe overdosage, the patient may stop breathing. Shock, heart attack, and death can occur.
If you suspect an overdose, seek emergency medical treatment immediately.

*Generic name:*

# Diltiazem

*See Cardizem, page 80.*

*Brand name:*

# Dimetane-DC

*Pronounced: DYE-meh-tayne DEE SEE*
*Generic ingredients: Brompheniramine maleate,*
*Phenylpropanolamine hydrochloride, Codeine*
*phosphate*

## Why is this drug prescribed?

Dimetane-DC cough syrup is an antihistamine/ decongestant/cough suppressant combination that relieves coughs and nasal congestion caused by allergies and the common cold. Brompheniramine, the antihistamine, reduces itching and dries up secretions from the nose, eyes, and throat. Phenylpropanolamine, the decongestant, clears nasal stuffiness and makes breathing easier. Codeine calms a cough.

## Most important fact about this drug

Dimetane-DC may cause you to become drowsy or less alert. You should not drive or operate dangerous machinery or participate in any hazardous activity that requires full mental alertness until you know how you react to Dimetane-DC.

## How should you take this medication?

Take this medication exactly as prescribed.
Do not exceed the directed dosage.

■ *If you miss a dose...*
Take it as soon as you remember. If it is almost time for your next dose, skip the one you missed and go back to your regular schedule. Do not take 2 doses at once.
■ *Storage instructions...*
Store at room temperature in a tightly closed container, away from light.

## What side effects may occur?

Side effects cannot be anticipated. If any side effects develop or change in intensity, tell your doctor as soon as possible. Only your doctor can determine whether it is safe for you to continue taking Dimetane-DC.

■ *More common side effects may include:*
Dizziness/light-headedness, drowsiness, dry mouth, nose, and throat, sedation, thickening of phlegm
■ *Less common or rare side effects may include:*
Anemia, constipation, convulsions, diarrhea, difficulty sleeping, difficulty urinating, disturbed coordination, exaggerated sense of well-being or depression, frequent urination, headache, high blood pressure, hives, increased sensitivity to light, irregular heartbeat, irritability, itching, loss of appetite, low blood pressure, nausea, nervousness, rash, shortness of breath, stomach upset, tightness in chest, tremor, vision changes, vomiting, weakness, wheezing

## Why should this drug not be prescribed?

This medication should not be given to children under 2 years of age or used by nursing mothers.
Do not take Dimetane-DC if you have severe high blood pressure or heart disease, or if you are taking antidepressant drugs known as MAO inhibitors (Nardil, Parnate). Dimetane-DC is not for treatment of asthma or other breathing disorders. Avoid Dimetane-DC if you have ever had an allergic reaction to it or are sensitive to any of its ingredients.

## Special warnings about this medication

Use Dimetane-DC cautiously if you have, or have ever had, bronchial asthma, the eye condition called narrow-angle glaucoma, stomach, intestinal, or bladder obstruction, diabetes, high blood pressure, heart disease, or thyroid disease.

Codeine can cause drug dependence and tolerance with continued use; your doctor will monitor your use of this drug carefully.

Antihistamines can make young children excited.

## Possible food and drug interactions when taking this medication

Dimetane-DC may increase the effects of alcohol. Do not drink alcohol while taking this medication.

If Dimetane-DC is taken with certain other drugs, the effects of either drug could be increased, decreased, or altered. It is especially important to check with your doctor before combining Dimetane-DC with the following:

MAO inhibitor-type antidepressant drugs such as Nardil and Parnate

Medications for high blood pressure such as Aldomet

Sedatives/hypnotics such as phenobarbital, Halcion, and Seconal

Tranquilizers such as Xanax, BuSpar, Librium, and Valium

## Special information if you are pregnant or breastfeeding

No information is available about the safety of Dimetane-DC during pregnancy. If you are pregnant or plan to become pregnant, inform your doctor immediately.

Dimetane-DC should not be taken if you are breastfeeding. If Dimetane-DC is essential to your health, your doctor may advise you to stop breastfeeding until your treatment is finished.

## Recommended dosage

Do not take more than 6 doses in 24 hours.

ADULTS AND CHILDREN 12 YEARS OLD AND OVER

The recommended dosage is 2 teaspoonfuls every 4 hours.

CHILDREN 6 TO UNDER 12 YEARS OLD

The usual dosage is 1 teaspoonful every 4 hours.

CHILDREN 2 TO UNDER 6 YEARS OLD

The dosage is one-half teaspoonful every 4 hours.

## Overdosage

An overdose of antihistamines may cause hallucinations, convulsions, and death, especially in infants and small children. If you suspect an overdose, seek medical treatment immediately.

■ *Symptoms of Dimetane-DC overdose may include:* Anxiety, breathing difficulty, convulsions, delirium, depression, dilated pupils, excessive excitement or stimulation, extreme sleepiness leading to loss of consciousness, hallucinations, heart attack, high blood pressure, irregular heartbeat, rapid heartbeat, restlessness, tremors

*Brand name:*

# Dipentum

*Pronounced: dye-PENT-um*
*Generic name: Olsalazine sodium*

## Why is this drug prescribed?

Dipentum is an anti-inflammatory drug used to maintain long-term freedom from symptoms of ulcerative colitis (chronic inflammation and ulceration of the large intestine and rectum). It is prescribed for people who cannot take sulfasalazine (Azulfidine).

## Most important fact about this drug

If you have kidney disease, Dipentum could cause further damage. You'll need regular checks on your kidney function, so be sure to keep all regular appointments with your doctor.

## How should you take this medication?

Take Dipentum for as long as your doctor has directed, even if you feel better.

Take Dipentum with food.

■ *If you miss a dose...*
Take it as soon as you remember. If it is almost time for your next dose, skip the one you missed and go back to your regular schedule. Do not take 2 doses at once.

■ *Storage instructions...*
Store at room temperature.

## What side effects may occur?

Side effects cannot be anticipated. If any develop or change in intensity, inform your doctor as soon as

possible. Only your doctor can determine if it is safe for you to continue taking Dipentum.

Diarrhea or loose stools are the most common side effects.

■ *Other side effects may include:*
Abdominal pain/cramping, bloating, depression, dizziness, drowsiness, headache, heartburn, indigestion, inflammation of the mouth, insomnia, joint pain, light-headedness, loss of appetite, nausea, rectal bleeding, skin itching, skin rash, sluggishness, upper respiratory infection, vertigo, vomiting

Rare cases of hepatitis have been reported in people taking Dipentum. Symptoms may include aching muscles, chills, fever, headache, joint pain, loss of appetite, vomiting, and yellowish skin.

### Why should this drug not be prescribed?
You should not be using Dipentum if you are allergic to salicylates such as aspirin.

### Special warnings about this medication
If diarrhea occurs, contact your doctor.

### Possible food and drug interactions when taking this medication
If Dipentum is taken with certain other drugs, the effects of either could be increased, decreased, or altered. It is especially important to check with your doctor before combining Dipentum with warfarin (Coumadin).

### Special information if you are pregnant or breastfeeding
The effects of Dipentum in pregnancy have not been adequately studied. Pregnant women should use Dipentum only if the possible gains warrant the possible risks to the unborn child. Women who breastfeed an infant should use Dipentum cautiously, because it is not known whether this drug appears in breast milk and what effect it might have on a nursing infant.

### Recommended dosage
ADULTS

The usual dose is a total of 1 gram per day, divided into 2 equal doses.

CHILDREN

Safety and effectiveness have not been established in children.

### Overdosage
There have been no reports of Dipentum overdose. However, should you suspect one, seek medical help immediately.

*Generic name:*
# Diphenhydramine
*See Benadryl, page 54.*

*Generic name:*
# Diphenoxylate with Atropine
*See Lomotil, page 288.*

*Generic name:*
# Dipivefrin
*See Propine, page 441.*

*Brand name:*
# Diprolene

Pronounced: dye-PROH-leen
*Generic name: Betamethasone dipropionate*

### Why is this drug prescribed?
Diprolene, a synthetic cortisone-like steroid available in cream, gel, lotion, or ointment form, is used to treat certain itchy rashes and other inflammatory skin conditions.

### Most important fact about this drug
When you use Diprolene, you inevitably absorb some of the medication through your skin and into the bloodstream. Too much absorption can lead to unwanted side effects elsewhere in the body. To keep this problem to a minimum, avoid using large amounts of Diprolene over large areas, and do not cover it with airtight dressings such as plastic wrap or adhesive bandages.

### How should you use this medication?
Apply Diprolene in a thin film, exactly as prescribed by your doctor. A typical regimen is 1 or 2 applications per day. Do not use the medication for longer than prescribed.

Diprolene is for use only on the skin. Be careful to keep it out of your eyes.

Once you have applied Diprolene, never cover the skin with an airtight bandage or other tight dressing.

For a fungal or bacterial skin infection, you will need antifungal or antibacterial medication in addition to Diprolene. If improvement is not prompt, you should stop using Diprolene until the infection is visibly clearing.

■ *If you miss a dose...*
Apply it as soon as you remember. If it is almost time for the next dose, skip the one you missed and go back to your regular schedule.
■ *Storage instructions...*
Store at room temperature.

## What side effects may occur?
Side effects cannot be anticipated. A possible side effect of Diprolene is stinging or burning of the skin where the medication is applied.

■ *Other side effects on the skin may include:*
Acne-like eruptions, atrophy, "broken" capillaries (fine reddish lines), cracking or tightening, dryness, infected hair follicles, irritation, itching, prickly heat, rash, redness, sensitivity

Using too much Diprolene, or using Diprolene for too long, may produce side effects elsewhere in the body; see the "Overdosage" section below.

## Why should this drug not be prescribed?
Do not use Diprolene if you are sensitive to it or have ever had an allergic reaction to it.

## Special warnings about this medication
Do not use Diprolene to treat any condition other than the one for which it was prescribed.

## Possible food and drug interactions when using this medication
No interactions have been reported.

## Special information if you are pregnant or breastfeeding
It is not known whether Diprolene, when applied to skin, causes any problem during pregnancy or while breastfeeding. Nevertheless, let your doctor know if you are pregnant or are planning to become pregnant.

## Recommended dosage
ADULTS

Diprolene products are not to be used with airtight dressings.

*Cream or ointment*
Apply a thin film to the affected skin areas once or twice daily. Treatment should be limited to 45 grams per week.

*Lotion*
Apply a few drops of Diprolene Lotion to the affected area once or twice daily and massage lightly until the lotion disappears.

Treatment must be limited to 14 days; do not use any more than 50 milliliters per week.

*Gel*
Apply a thin layer of Diprolene Gel to the affected area once or twice daily and rub in gently and completely.

Treatment must be limited to 14 days; do not use any more than 50 grams per week.

CHILDREN

Use of Diprolene Gel, Lotion, Ointment, and AF Cream is not recommended for children under 12 years of age.

## Overdosage
With copious or prolonged use of Diprolene, hormone absorbed into the bloodstream may cause high blood sugar, sugar in the urine, and a group of symptoms called Cushing's syndrome.

■ *Symptoms of Cushing's syndrome may include:*
Acne, depression, high blood pressure, humped upper back, insomnia, moonfaced appearance, muscle weakness, obese trunk, paranoia, stretch marks, susceptibility to bruising, fractures, infections, retardation of growth, delayed weight gain, wasted limbs

Cushing's syndrome may also trigger the development of diabetes mellitus. Left uncorrected, the syndrome may become serious. If you suspect your use of Diprolene has led to this problem, seek medical attention immediately.

*Generic name:*

# Dipyridamole

*See Persantine, page 411.*

*Brand name:*

# Disalcid

*Pronounced: dye-SAL-sid*
*Generic name: Salsalate*

## Why is this drug prescribed?
Disalcid, a nonsteroidal anti-inflammatory drug, is used to relieve the symptoms of rheumatoid arthri-

tis, osteoarthritis (the most common form of arthritis), and other rheumatic disorders (conditions that involve pain and inflammation in joints and the tissues around them).

## Most important fact about this drug

Disalcid contains salicylate, an ingredient that may be associated with the development of Reye's syndrome (a disorder that causes abnormal brain and liver function). It occurs mostly in children who have taken aspirin or other medications containing salicylate to relieve symptoms of the flu or chickenpox. Do not take Disalcid if you have flu symptoms or chickenpox.

## How should you take this medication?

Take Disalcid exactly as prescribed. Food may slow its absorption. However, your doctor may ask you to take Disalcid with food in order to avoid stomach upset.

■ *If you miss a dose...*
   Take it as soon as you remember. If it is almost time for your next dose, skip the one you missed and go back to your regular schedule. Never take two doses at once.
■ *Storage instructions...*
   Store at room temperature. Keep out of the reach of children.

## What side effects may occur?

Side effects cannot be anticipated. If any develop or change in intensity, inform your doctor as soon as possible. Only your doctor can determine if it is safe for you to continue taking Disalcid.

■ *Side effects may include:*
   Hearing impairment, nausea, rash, ringing in the ears, vertigo

## Why should this drug not be prescribed?

Disalcid should not be taken if you are sensitive to or have ever had an allergic reaction to salsalate.

## Special warnings about this medication

Use Disalcid with extreme caution if you have chronic kidney disease or a peptic ulcer.

Salicylates occasionally cause asthma in people who are sensitive to aspirin. Although Disalcid contains a salicylate, it is less likely than aspirin to cause this reaction.

## Possible food and drug interactions when taking this medication

If Disalcid is taken with certain other drugs, the effects of either could be increased, decreased, or altered. It is especially important to check with your doctor before combining Disalcid with the following:

ACE inhibitor-type blood pressure drugs such as Capoten and Vasotec
Acetazolamide (Diamox)
Aspirin and other drugs containing salicylates such as Bufferin and Empirin
Blood-thinning medications such as Coumadin
Medications for gout such as Zyloprim and Benemid
Methotrexate (Rheumatrex)
Naproxen (Anaprox, Naprosyn)
Oral diabetes drugs such as Glucotrol and Tolinase
Penicillin (Pen-Vee K)
Phenytoin (Dilantin)
Steroids such as Deltasone and Decadron
Sulfinpyrazone (Anturane)
Thyroid medications such as Synthroid

## Special information if you are pregnant or breastfeeding

The effects of Disalcid during pregnancy have not been adequately studied. If you are pregnant or plan to become pregnant, inform your doctor immediately. Disalcid may appear in breast milk and could affect a nursing infant. If this medication is essential to your health, your doctor may advise you to stop breastfeeding until your treatment with Disalcid is finished.

## Recommended dosage

You may not feel the full benefit of this medication for 3 to 4 days.

ADULTS

The usual dosage is 3,000 milligrams daily, divided into smaller doses as follows:

(1) 2 doses of two 750-milligram tablets
(2) 2 doses of three 500-milligram tablets or capsules
(3) 3 doses of two 500-milligram tablets or capsules

CHILDREN

Safety and effectiveness of Disalcid use in children have not been established.

## OLDER ADULTS

A lower dosage may be sufficient to achieve desired blood levels without the more common side effects.

### Overdosage

Any medication taken in excess can have serious consequences. Deaths have occurred from salicylate overdose. If you suspect an overdose, seek medical treatment immediately.

■ *Symptoms of Disalcid overdose may include:*
Confusion, dehydration, diarrhea, drowsiness, headache, high body temperature, hyperventilation, ringing in the ears, sweating, vertigo, vomiting

*Generic name:*

# Disopyramide

*See Norpace, page 371.*

*Brand name:*

# Ditropan

*Pronounced: DYE-tro-pan*
*Generic name: Oxybutynin chloride*

### Why is this drug prescribed?

Ditropan relaxes the bladder muscle and reduces spasms. It is used to treat the urgency, frequency, leakage, incontinence, and painful or difficult urination caused by a neurogenic bladder (altered bladder function due to a nervous system abnormality).

### Most important fact about this drug

Ditropan can cause heat prostration (fever and heat stroke due to decreased sweating) in high temperatures. If you live in a hot climate or will be exposed to high temperatures, take appropriate precautions.

### How should you take this medication?

Take this medication exactly as prescribed.

Ditropan can make your mouth dry. Sucking hard candies or melting bits of ice in your mouth can remedy the problem.

■ *If you miss a dose...*
Take the forgotten dose as soon as you remember. If it is almost time for your next dose, skip the one you missed and go back to your regular schedule. Never take 2 doses at once.

■ *Storage...*
Keep this medication in a tightly closed container and store it at room temperature. Protect the syrup from direct light.

### What side effects may occur?

Side effects cannot be anticipated. If any develop or change in intensity, inform your doctor as soon as possible. Only your doctor can determine if it is safe for you to continue taking Ditropan.

■ *Side effects may include:*
Constipation, decreased production of tears, decreased sweating, difficulty falling or staying asleep, dilation of the pupil of the eye, dim vision, dizziness, drowsiness, dry mouth, eye paralysis, hallucinations, impotence, inability to urinate, nausea, palpitations, rapid heartbeat, rash, restlessness, suppression of milk production, weakness

### Why should this drug not be prescribed?

You should not take Ditropan if you have certain types of untreated glaucoma (excessive pressure in the eye), partial or complete blockage of the gastrointestinal tract, or paralytic ileus (obstructed bowel). Ditropan should also be avoided if you have severe colitis (inflamed colon), myasthenia gravis (abnormal muscle weakness), or urinary tract obstruction. This drug is usually not prescribed for the elderly or debilitated.

Do not take this medication if you are sensitive or have ever had an allergic reaction to it. Make sure your doctor is aware of any allergic reactions you have experienced.

### Special warnings about this medication

If you have an ileostomy or colostomy (an artificial opening to the bowel) and develop diarrhea while taking Ditropan, inform your doctor immediately.

Ditropan may cause drowsiness or blurred vision. Driving or operating dangerous machinery or participating in any hazardous activity that requires full mental alertness is not recommended until you know how this medication affects you.

Your doctor will prescribe Ditropan with caution if you have liver disease, kidney disease, or a nervous system disorder.

Ditropan may aggravate the symptoms of overactive thyroid, heart disease or congestive heart failure, irregular or rapid heartbeat, high blood pressure, or enlarged prostate.

## Possible food and drug interactions when taking this medication

If Ditropan is taken with certain other drugs, the effects of either may be increased, decreased or altered. It is especially important to check with your doctor before combining Ditropan with alcohol or sedatives such as Halcion or Restoril because increased drowsiness may occur.

## Special information if you are pregnant or breastfeeding

The effects of Ditropan during pregnancy have not been adequately studied. If you are pregnant or plan to become pregnant, inform your doctor immediately. Ditropan may appear in breast milk and could affect a nursing infant. If this medication is essential to your health, your doctor may advise you to stop breastfeeding until your treatment is finished.

## Recommended dosage

ADULTS

*Tablets*

The usual dose is one 5 milligram tablet taken 2 to 3 times a day. You should not take more than 4 tablets a day.

*Syrup*

The usual dose is one teaspoonful 2 to 3 times a day, but not more than 4 times a day.

CHILDREN OVER 5 YEARS OF AGE

*Tablets*

The usual dose is one 5 milligram tablet taken twice a day. The most a child should take is 3 tablets a day.

*Syrup*

The usual dose is one teaspoonful 2 times a day, but not more than 3 times a day.

Ditropan is not recommended for children under 5 years of age.

## Overdosage

Any medication taken in excess can have serious consequences. If you suspect an overdose, seek medical attention immediately.

■ *Symptoms of Ditropan overdose may include:*
Coma, convulsions, delirium, difficulty breathing, fever, flushing, hallucinations, irritability, low or high blood pressure, nausea, paralysis, rapid heartbeat, restlessness, tremor, vomiting

*Brand name:*

# Diuril

*Pronounced: DYE-your-il*
*Generic name: Chlorothiazide*

## Why is this drug prescribed?

Diuril is used in the treatment of high blood pressure and other conditions that require the elimination of excess fluid (water) from the body. These conditions include congestive heart failure, cirrhosis of the liver, corticosteroid and estrogen therapy, and kidney disease. When used for high blood pressure, Diuril can be used alone or with other high blood pressure medications. Diuril contains a form of thiazide, a diuretic that prompts your body to eliminate more fluid, which helps lower blood pressure.

## Most important fact about this drug

If you have high blood pressure, you must take Diuril regularly for it to be effective. Since blood pressure declines gradually, it may be several weeks before you get the full benefit of Diuril; and you must continue taking it even if you are feeling well. Diuril does not cure high blood pressure; it merely keeps it under control.

## How should you take this medication?

Take Diuril exactly as prescribed. Stopping Diuril suddenly could cause your condition to worsen.

■ *If you miss a dose...*
Take it as soon as you remember. If it is almost time for your next dose, skip the one you missed and go back to your regular schedule. Never take 2 doses at the same time.

■ *Storage instructions...*
Store at room temperature in a tightly closed container. Protect from moisture and freezing.

## What side effects may occur?

Side effects cannot be anticipated. If any develop or change in intensity, inform your doctor as soon as possible. Only your doctor can determine if it is safe for you to continue taking Diuril.

■ *Side effects may include:*
Abdominal cramps, anemia, changes in blood sugar, constipation, diarrhea, difficulty breathing, dizziness, dizziness on standing up, fever, fluid in lungs, hair loss, headache, high levels of sugar in urine, hives, hypersensitivity reactions, impo-

tence, inflammation of the pancreas, inflammation of the salivary glands, light-headedness, loss of appetite, low blood pressure, low potassium (leading to symptoms such as dry mouth, excessive thirst, weak or irregular heartbeat, muscle pain or cramps), lung inflammation, muscle spasms, nausea, rash, reddish or purplish spots on skin, restlessness, sensitivity to light, Stevens-Johnson syndrome, stomach irritation, stomach upset, tingling or pins and needles, vertigo, vision changes, vomiting, weakness, yellow eyes and skin

### Why should this drug not be prescribed?

If you are unable to urinate, you should not take this medication. If you are sensitive to or have ever had an allergic reaction to Diuril or other thiazide-type diuretics, or if you are sensitive to sulfa drugs, you should not take this medication.

### Special warnings about this medication

Diuretics can cause your body to lose too much potassium. Signs of an excessively low potassium level include muscle weakness and rapid or irregular heartbeat. To boost your potassium level, your doctor may recommend eating potassium-rich foods or taking a potassium supplement.

If you are taking Diuril, your doctor will do a complete assessment of your kidney function and continue to monitor it. Use with caution if you have severe kidney disease.

If you have liver disease, diabetes, gout, or the connective tissue disease lupus erythematosus, your doctor will prescribe Diuril cautiously.

If you have bronchial asthma or a history of allergies you may be at greater risk for an allergic reaction to this medication.

Dehydration, excessive sweating, severe diarrhea, or vomiting could deplete your body's fluids and lower your blood pressure too much. Be careful when exercising and in hot weather.

Notify your doctor or dentist that you are taking Diuril if you have a medical emergency, and before you have surgery or dental treatment.

### Possible food and drug interactions when taking this medication

Diuril may increase the effects of alcohol. Do not drink alcohol while taking this medication.

If Diuril is taken with certain other drugs, the effects of either may be increased, decreased, or altered. It is especially important to check with your doctor before combining Diuril with the following:

Barbiturates such as phenobarbital and Seconal
Cholesterol-lowering drugs such as Questran and Colestid
Drugs to treat diabetes such as insulin and Micronase
Lithium (Lithonate)
Narcotic painkillers such as Percocet
Nonsteroidal anti-inflammatory drugs such as Naprosyn and Motrin
Norepinephrine (Levophed)
Other drugs for high blood pressure such as Capoten and Procardia XL
Steroids such as prednisone

### Special information
### if you are pregnant or breastfeeding

The effects of Diuril during pregnancy have not been adequately studied. If you are pregnant or plan to become pregnant, inform your doctor immediately. Diuril appears in breast milk and could affect a nursing infant. If this medication is essential to your health, your doctor may advise you to discontinue breastfeeding until your treatment is finished.

### Recommended dosage

ADULTS

Diuril comes in tablets, an oral suspension, and an intravenous preparation, reserved for emergencies. Dosages below are for the oral preparations.

*Swelling due to excess water*
The usual dose is 0.5 gram to 1 gram 1 or 2 times per day. Your doctor may have you take this medication on alternate days or on some other on-off schedule.

*High Blood Pressure*
The starting dose is 0.5 gram to 1 gram per day, taken as one dose or two or more smaller doses. Your doctor will adjust the dosage to suit your needs.

CHILDREN

Dosages for children are adjusted according to weight, generally 10 milligrams per pound of body weight daily in 2 doses.

*Under 6 months*
Dosage may be up to 15 milligrams per pound of body weight per day in 2 doses.

*Under 2 years*
The usual dosage is 125 milligrams to 375 milligrams per day in 2 doses. The liquid form of this drug may be used in children under 2 years of age at $1/2$ to $1^1/2$ teaspoons (2.5 to 7.5 milliliters) per day.

*2 to 12 years*
The usual dosage is 375 milligrams to 1 gram daily in 2 doses. The liquid form of this medication may be used in children 2 to 12 years at $1^1/2$ to 4 teaspoons (7.5 milliliters to 20 milliliters) per day.

### Overdosage

Any medication taken in excess can have serious consequences. If you suspect an overdose, seek medical attention immediately.

■ *Signs of Diuril overdose may include:*
Dehydration and symptoms of low potassium (dry mouth, excessive thirst, weak or irregular heartbeat, muscle pain or cramps)

*Generic name:*

# Divalproex sodium

*See Depakote, page 148.*

*Generic name:*

# Docusate

*See Colace, page 107.*

*Brand name:*

# Dolobid

*Pronounced: DOLL-oh-bid*
*Generic name: Diflunisal*

### Why is this drug prescribed?

Dolobid, a nonsteroidal anti-inflammatory drug, is used to treat mild to moderate pain and relieve the inflammation, swelling, stiffness, and joint pain associated with rheumatoid arthritis and osteoarthritis (the most common form of arthritis).

### Most important fact about this drug

You should have frequent check-ups with your doctor if you take Dolobid regularly. Ulcers or internal bleeding can occur without warning.

### How should you take this medication?

Dolobid should be taken with food or food together with an antacid, and with a full glass of water or milk. Never take it on an empty stomach.

Tablets should be swallowed whole, not chewed or crushed.

Take this medication exactly as prescribed by your doctor. If you are using Dolobid for arthritis, it should be taken regularly.

■ *If you miss a dose...*
Take it as soon as you remember. If it is almost time for your next dose, skip the one you missed and go back to your regular schedule. Never take two doses at the same time.
■ *Storage instructions...*
Do not store in damp places, like the bathroom.

### What side effects may occur?

Side effects cannot be anticipated. If any develop or change in intensity, inform your doctor as soon as possible. Only your doctor can determine if it is safe for you to continue taking Dolobid.

■ *More common side effects may include:*
Abdominal pain, constipation, diarrhea, dizziness, fatigue, gas, headache, inability to sleep, indigestion, nausea, rash, ringing in ears, sleepiness, vomiting
■ *Less common or rare side effects may include:*
Abdominal bleeding, anemia, blurred vision, confusion, depression, disorientation, dry mouth and nose, fluid retention, flushing, hepatitis, hives, inflammation of lips and tongue, itching, kidney failure, light-headedness, loss of appetite, nervousness, painful urination, peptic ulcer, pins and needles, protein or blood in urine, rash, sensitivity to light, skin eruptions, Stevens-Johnson syndrome, vertigo, weakness, yellow eyes and skin

### Why should this drug not be prescribed?

If you are sensitive to or have had an allergic reaction to Dolobid, aspirin, or similar drugs, or if you have had asthma attacks caused by aspirin or other drugs of this type, you should not take this medication. Make sure that your doctor is aware of any drug reactions that you have experienced.

## Special warnings about this medication

Peptic ulcers and bleeding can occur without warning.

This drug should be used with caution if you have kidney or liver disease; and it can cause liver inflammation in some people.

Do not take aspirin or any other anti-inflammatory medications while taking Dolobid, unless your doctor tells you to do so.

Nonsteroidal anti-inflammatory drugs such as Dolobid can hide the signs and symptoms of infection. Be sure your doctor knows about any infection you may have.

Dolobid can cause vision problems. If you experience any changes in your vision, inform your doctor.

Dolobid may prolong bleeding time. If you are taking blood-thinning medication, take Dolobid with caution.

If you have heart disease or high blood pressure, use Dolobid with caution. It can increase water retention.

Dolobid may cause you to become drowsy or less alert; therefore, driving or operating dangerous machinery or participating in any hazardous activity that requires full mental alertness is not recommended.

## Possible food and drug interactions when taking this medication

If Dolobid is taken with certain other drugs, the effects of either could be increased, decreased, or altered. It is especially important to check with your doctor before combining Dolobid with the following:

Acetaminophen (Tylenol)
Antacids taken regularly
Aspirin
Cyclosporine (Sandimmune)
Methotrexate (Rheumatrex)
Naproxen (Naprosyn)
Oral anticoagulants (blood thinners)
The arthritis medication sulindac (Clinoril)
The diuretic hydrochlorothiazide

## Special information if you are pregnant or breastfeeding

The effects of Dolobid during pregnancy have not been adequately studied. If you are pregnant or plan to become pregnant, inform your doctor immediately. Dolobid appears in breast milk and could affect a nursing infant. If this medication is essential to your health, your doctor may advise you to discontinue breastfeeding until your treatment with Dolobid is finished.

## Recommended dosage

ADULTS

*Mild to Moderate Pain*
Starting dose is 1,000 milligrams, followed by 500 milligrams every 8 to 12 hours, depending on the individual. Your physician may adjust your dosage according to your age and weight, and the severity of your symptoms.

*Osteoarthritis and Rheumatoid Arthritis*
The usual dose is 500 to 1,000 milligrams per day in 2 doses of 250 milligrams or 500 milligrams.

The lowest dose that proves beneficial should be used.

The maximum recommended dosage is 1,500 milligrams per day.

CHILDREN

Safety and effectiveness of Dolobid have not been established in children under 12 years of age. However, your doctor may decide that the benefits of this medication may outweigh the potential risks.

## Overdosage

Any medication taken in excess can cause symptoms of overdose. If you suspect an overdose, seek medical attention immediately.

■ *Symptoms of Dolobid overdose may include:*
Abnormally rapid heartbeat, coma, diarrhea, disorientation, drowsiness, hyperventilation, nausea, ringing in the ears, stupor, sweating, vomiting

*Brand name:*

# Donnatal

*Pronounced: DON-nuh-tal*
*Generic ingredients: Phenobarbital, Hyoscyamine*
*  sulfate, Atropine sulfate, Scopolamine*
*  hydrobromide*
*Other brand name: Bellatal*

## Why is this drug prescribed?

Donnatal is a mild antispasmodic medication; it has been used with other drugs for relief of cramps and pain associated with various stomach, intestinal, and bowel disorders, including irritable bowel syndrome, acute colitis, and duodenal ulcer.

One of its ingredients, phenobarbital, is a mild sedative.

## Most important fact about this drug

Phenobarbital, one of the ingredients of Donnatal, can be habit-forming. If you have ever been dependent on drugs, do not take Donnatal.

## How should you take this medication?

Take Donnatal one-half hour to 1 hour before meals. Use it exactly as prescribed.

■ *If you miss a dose...*
Take it as soon as you remember. If it is almost time for your next dose, skip the one you missed and go back to your regular schedule. Never take 2 doses at the same time.

■ *Storage instructions...*
Store at room temperature in a tightly closed container. Protect from light.

## What side effects may occur?

Side effects cannot be anticipated. If any develop or change in intensity, inform your doctor as soon as possible. Only your doctor can determine if it is safe for you to continue taking Donnatal.

■ *Side effects may include:*
Agitation, allergic reaction, bloated feeling, blurred vision, constipation, decreased sweating, difficulty sleeping, difficulty urinating, dilation of the pupil of the eye, dizziness, drowsiness, dry mouth, excitement, fast or fluttery heartbeat, headache, hives, impotence, muscular and bone pain, nausea, nervousness, rash, reduced sense of taste, suppression of lactation, vomiting, weakness

## Why should this drug not be prescribed?

Do not take Donnatal if you suffer from the eye condition called glaucoma, diseases that block the urinary or gastrointestinal tracts, or myasthenia gravis, a condition in which the muscles become progressively paralyzed. Also, you should not use Donnatal if you have intestinal atony (loss of strength in the intestinal muscles), unstable cardiovascular status, severe ulcerative colitis (chronic inflammation and ulceration of the bowel), or hiatal hernia (a rupture in the diaphragm above the stomach). You should also avoid Donnatal if you

have acute intermittent porphyria—a disorder of the metabolism in which there is severe abdominal pain and sensitivity to light.

If you are sensitive to or have ever had an allergic reaction to Donnatal, its ingredients, or similar drugs, you should not take this medication. Also avoid Donnatal if phenobarbital makes you excited or restless, instead of calming you down. Make sure your doctor is aware of any drug reactions you have experienced.

## Special warnings about this medication

Be cautious in using Donnatal if you suffer from high blood pressure, overactive thyroid (hyperthyroidism), irregular or rapid heartbeat, or heart, kidney, or liver disease.

Donnatal can decrease sweating. If you are exercising or are subjected to high temperatures, be alert for heat prostration.

If you develop diarrhea, especially if you have an ileostomy or colostomy (artificial openings to the bowel), check with your doctor.

If you have a gastric ulcer, use this medication with caution.

Donnatal may cause you to become drowsy or less alert. You should not drive or operate dangerous machinery or participate in any hazardous activity that requires full mental alertness until you know how this drug affects you.

## Possible food and drug interactions when taking this medication

Donnatal may intensify the effects of alcohol. Check with your doctor before using alcohol with this medication.

Avoid taking antacids within 1 hour of a dose of Donnatal; they may reduce its effectiveness.

If Donnatal is taken with certain other drugs, the effects of either could be increased, decreased, or altered. It is especially important to check with your doctor before combining Donnatal with the following:

Antidepressants such as Elavil and Tofranil
Antidepressants known as MAO inhibitors, including
 Nardil and Parnate
Antihistamines such as Benadryl
Antispasmodic drugs such as Bentyl and Cogentin
Barbiturates such as Seconal
Blood-thinning drugs such as Coumadin

Diarrhea medications containing Kaolin or attapulgite

Digitalis (Lanoxin)

Narcotics such as Percocet

Potassium (Slow-K, K-Dur, others)

Steroids such as Medrol and Deltasone

Tranquilizers such as Valium

## Special information if you are pregnant or breastfeeding

The effects of Donnatal during pregnancy have not been adequately studied. If you are pregnant or plan to become pregnant, this drug should be used only when prescribed by your doctor. It is not known whether Donnatal appears in breast milk. If this medication is essential to your health, your doctor may advise you to discontinue breastfeeding until your treatment is finished.

## Recommended dosage

ADULTS

Your doctor will adjust the dosage to your needs.

*Tablets or Capsules*
The usual dosage is 1 or 2 tablets or capsules, 3 or 4 times a day.

*Liquid*
The usual dosage is 1 or 2 teaspoonfuls, 3 or 4 times a day.

*Donnatal Extentabs*
The usual dosage is 1 tablet every 12 hours. Your doctor may tell you to take 1 tablet every 8 hours, if necessary.

CHILDREN

Dosage of the elixir is determined by body weight; it can be given every 4 to 6 hours. Follow your doctor's instructions carefully when giving this medication to a child.

## Overdosage

Any medication taken in excess can cause symptoms of overdose. If you suspect an overdose, seek medical attention immediately.

■ *The symptoms of Donnatal overdose may include:*
Blurred vision, central nervous system stimulation, difficulty swallowing, dilated pupils, dizziness, dry mouth, headache, hot and dry skin, nausea, vomiting

*Brand name:*

# Doral

*Pronounced: DOHR-al*
*Generic name: Quazepam*

## Why is this drug prescribed?

Doral, a sleeping medication available in tablet form, is taken as short-term treatment for insomnia. Symptoms of insomnia may include difficulty falling asleep, frequent awakenings throughout the night, or very early morning awakening.

## Most important fact about this drug

Doral is a chemical cousin of Valium and is potentially addictive. Over time, your body will get used to the prescribed dosage of Doral, and you will no longer derive any benefit from it. If you were to increase the dosage against medical advice, the drug would again work as a sleeping pill—but only until your body adjusted to the higher dosage. This is a vicious circle that can lead to addiction. To avoid this danger, use Doral only as prescribed.

## How should you take this medication?

Take Doral exactly as prescribed by your doctor— one dose per day, at bedtime. Keep in touch with your doctor; if you respond very well, it may be possible to cut your dosage in half after the first few nights. The older or more run-down you are, the more desirable it is to try for this early dosage reduction.

If you have been taking Doral regularly for 6 weeks or so, you may experience withdrawal symptoms if you stop suddenly, or even if you reduce the dosage without specific instructions on how to do it. Always follow your doctor's advice for tapering off gradually from Doral.

■ *If you miss a dose...*
Take this medication only if needed.
■ *Storage instructions...*
Store at room temperature, away from moisture.

## What side effects may occur?

Side effects cannot be anticipated. If any develop or change in intensity, inform your doctor as soon as possible. Only your doctor can determine if it is safe for you to continue taking Doral.

■ *More common side effects may include:*
Drowsiness during the day, headache

■ *Less common side effects may include:*
Changes in sex drive, dizziness, dry mouth, fatigue, inability to urinate, incontinence, indigestion, irregular menstrual periods, irritability, muscle spasms, slurred or otherwise abnormal speech, yellowed eyes and skin

In rare instances, Doral produces agitation, sleep disturbances, hallucinations, or stimulation—exactly the opposite of the desired effect. If this should happen to you, tell your doctor; he or she will take you off the medication.

## Why should this drug not be prescribed?
Do not take Doral if you are sensitive to it, or if you have ever had an allergic reaction to it or to another Valium-type medication.

You should not take Doral if you know or suspect that you have sleep apnea (short periods of interrupted breathing that occur during sleep).

You should not take Doral if you are pregnant.

## Special warnings about this medication
Because Doral may decrease your daytime alertness, do not drive, climb, or operate dangerous machinery until you find out how the drug affects you. In some cases, Doral's sedative effect may last for several days after the last dose.

If you are suffering from depression, Doral may make your depression worse.

If you have ever abused alcohol or drugs, you are at special risk for addiction to Doral.

Never increase the dosage of Doral on your own. Tell your doctor right away if the medication no longer seems to be working.

## Possible food and drug interactions when taking this medication
If Doral is taken with certain other drugs, the effects of either could be increased, decreased, or altered. It is especially important to check with your doctor before combining Doral with the following:

Antihistamines such as Benadryl
Antiseizure medications such as Dilantin and Tegretol
Mood-altering medications such as Thorazine and Clozaril
Other central nervous system depressants such as Xanax and Valium
Do not drink alcohol while taking Doral; it can increase the drug's effects.

## Special information
## if you are pregnant or breastfeeding
Because Doral may cause harm to the unborn child, it should not be taken during pregnancy. If you want to have a baby, tell your doctor, and plan to discontinue taking Doral before getting pregnant.

Babies whose mothers are taking Doral at the time of birth may experience withdrawal symptoms from the drug. Such babies may be "floppy" (flaccid) instead of having normal muscle tone.

Since Doral does appear in breast milk, you should not take this medication if you are nursing a baby.

## Recommended dosage
ADULTS

The recommended initial dose is 15 milligrams daily. Your doctor may later reduce this dosage to 7.5 milligrams.

CHILDREN

Safety and efficacy of Doral in children under 18 years old have not been established.

OLDER ADULTS

You may be more sensitive to this drug, and the doctor may reduce the dosage after only 1 or 2 nights.

## Overdosage
Any medication taken in excess can have serious consequences. If you suspect an overdose of Doral, seek medical attention immediately.

■ *Symptoms of an overdose of Doral may include:*
Coma, confusion, extreme sleepiness

*Brand name:*
# Doryx

*Pronounced: DORE-icks*
*Generic name: Doxycycline hyclate*
*Other brand names: Vibramycin, Vibra-Tabs*

## Why is this drug prescribed?
Doxycycline is a broad-spectrum tetracycline antibiotic used against a wide variety of bacterial infections, including Rocky Mountain spotted fever and other fevers caused by ticks, fleas, and lice; urinary tract infections; trachoma (chronic infections of the eye); and some gonococcal infections in

adults. It is also used with other medications to treat severe acne and amoebic dysentery (diarrhea caused by severe parasitic infection of the intestines).

Doxycycline may also be taken for the prevention of malaria on foreign trips of less than 4 months' duration.

Occasionally doctors prescribe doxycycline to treat early Lyme disease and to prevent "traveler's diarrhea." These are not yet officially approved uses for this drug.

### Most important fact about this drug
Children under 8 years old and women in the last half of pregnancy should not take this medication. It may cause developing teeth to become permanently discolored (yellow-gray-brown).

### How should you take this medication?
Take doxycycline with a full glass of water or other liquid to avoid irritating your throat or stomach. Doxycycline can be taken with or without food. However, if the medicine does upset your stomach, you may wish to take it with a glass of milk or after you have eaten. Doxycycline tablets should be swallowed whole.

Take this medication exactly as prescribed by your doctor, even if your symptoms have disappeared.

If you are taking an oral suspension form of doxycycline, shake the bottle well before using. Do not use outdated doxycycline.

■ *If you miss a dose...*
Take the forgotten dose as soon as you remember. If it is almost time for the next dose, put it off for several hours after taking the missed dose. Specifically, if you are taking one dose a day, take the next one 10 to 12 hours after the missed dose. If you are taking two doses a day, take the next one 5 to 6 hours after the missed dose. If you are taking three doses a day, take the next one 2 to 4 hours after the missed dose. Then return to your regular schedule.

■ *Storage instructions...*
Doxycycline can be stored at room temperature. Protect from light and excessive heat.

### What side effects may occur?
Side effects cannot be anticipated. If any develop or change in intensity, inform your doctor as soon as possible. Only your doctor can determine if it is safe for you to continue taking doxycycline.

■ *More common side effects may include:*
Angioedema (chest pain; swelling of face, around lips, tongue and throat, arms and legs; difficulty swallowing), bulging foreheads in infants, diarrhea, difficulty swallowing, discolored teeth in infants and children (more common during long-term use of tetracycline), inflammation of the tongue, loss of appetite, nausea, rash, rectal or genital itching, severe allergic reaction (hives, itching, and swelling), skin sensitivity to light, vomiting

■ *Less common or rare side effects may include:*
Aggravation of lupus erythematosus (disease of the connective tissue), skin inflammation and peeling, throat inflammation and ulcerations

### Why should this drug not be prescribed?
If you are sensitive to or have ever had an allergic reaction to doxycycline or drugs of this type, you should not take this medication. Make sure your doctor is aware of any drug reactions that you have experienced.

### Special warnings about this medication
As with other antibiotics, treatment with doxycycline may result in a growth of bacteria that do not respond to this medication and can cause a secondary infection.

Bulging foreheads in infants and headaches in adults have occurred. These symptoms disappeared when doxycycline was discontinued.

You may become more sensitive to sunlight while taking doxycycline. Be careful if you are going out in the sun or using a sunlamp. If you develop a skin rash, notify your doctor immediately.

Birth control pills that contain estrogen may not be as effective while you are taking tetracycline drugs. Ask your doctor or pharmacist if you should use another form of birth control while taking doxycycline.

Doxycycline syrup (Vibramycin) contains a sulfite that may cause allergic reactions in certain people. This reaction happens more frequently to people with asthma.

### Possible food and drug interactions when taking this medication
If doxycycline is taken with certain other drugs, the effects of either could be increased, decreased, or altered. It is especially important to check with your doctor before combining doxycycline with the following:

Antacids containing aluminum, calcium, or magnesium, and iron-containing
preparations such as Maalox, Mylanta, and others
Barbiturates such as phenobarbital
Bismuth subsalicylate (Pepto-Bismol)
Blood-thinning medications such as Coumadin
Carbamazepine (Tegretol)
Oral contraceptives
Penicillin (V-Cillin K, Pen-vee K, others)
Phenytoin (Dilantin)
Sodium bicarbonate

### Special information
### if you are pregnant or breastfeeding

Doxycycline should not be used during pregnancy. Tetracycline can damage developing teeth during the last half of pregnancy. If you are pregnant or plan to become pregnant, inform your doctor immediately. Tetracyclines such as doxycycline appear in breast milk and can affect a nursing infant. If this medication is essential to your health, your doctor may advise you to discontinue breastfeeding until your treatment is finished.

### Recommended dosage

ADULTS

The usual dose of oral doxycycline is 200 milligrams on the first day of treatment (100 milligrams every 12 hours) followed by a maintenance dose of 100 milligrams per day. The maintenance dose may be taken as a single dose or as 50 milligrams every 12 hours.

Your doctor may prescribe 100 milligrams every 12 hours for severe infections such as chronic urinary tract infection.

*For Uncomplicated Gonorrhea (Except Anorectal Infections in Men)*
The usual dose is 100 milligrams by mouth, twice a day for 7 days. An alternate, single-day treatment is 300 milligrams, followed in 1 hour by a second 300-milligram dose.

*For Primary and Secondary Syphilis*
The usual dose is 200 milligrams a day, divided into smaller, equal doses for 14 days.

*For Prevention of Malaria*
The usual dose is 100 milligrams a day. Treatment should begin 1 to 2 days before travel to the area where malaria is found, then continue daily during travel in the area and 4 weeks after leaving.

CHILDREN

For children above 8 years of age, the recommended dosage schedule for those weighing 100 pounds or less is 2 milligrams per pound of body weight, divided into 2 doses, on the first day of treatment, followed by 1 milligram per pound of body weight given as a single daily dose or divided into 2 doses on subsequent days.

For more severe infections, up to 2 milligrams per pound of body weight may be used.

For prevention of malaria, the recommended dose is 2 milligrams per 2.2 pounds of body weight up to 100 milligrams.

For children over 100 pounds, the usual adult dose should be used.

### Overdosage

Any medication taken in excess can have serious consequences. If you suspect an overdose, seek medical treatment immediately.

*Generic name:*
# Doxazosin

*See Cardura, page 81.*

*Generic name:*
# Doxepin

*See Sinequan, page 502.*

*Generic name:*
# Doxycycline

*See Doryx, page 177.*

*Brand name:*
# Duphalac

*See Chronulac Syrup, page 91.*

*Brand name:*
# Duricef

*Pronounced: DUHR-i-sef*
*Generic name: Cefadroxil monohydrate*
*Other brand name: Ultracef*

### Why is this drug prescribed?

Duricef, a cephalosporin antibiotic, is used in the treatment of nose, throat, urinary tract, and skin infections that are caused by specific bacteria, including staph, strep, and *E. coli*.

### Most important fact about this drug
If you are allergic to either penicillin or cephalosporin antibiotics in any form, consult your doctor *before taking* Duricef. There is a possibility that you are allergic to both types of medication and if a reaction occurs, it could be extremely severe. If you take the drug and feel signs of a reaction, seek medical attention immediately.

### How should you take this medication?
Take this medication exactly as prescribed. It is important that you finish all of it to obtain the maximum benefit.

■ *If you miss a dose...*
Take it as soon as you remember. If it is almost time for the next dose, and you take it once a day, take the one you missed and the next dose 10 to 12 hours later. If you take 2 doses a day, take the one you missed and the next dose 5 to 6 hours later. If you take it 3 or more times a day, take the one you missed and the next dose 2 to 4 hours later. Then go back to your regular schedule.

■ *Storage information...*
Store at room temperature.

### What side effects may occur?
Side effects cannot be anticipated. If any develop or change in intensity, inform your doctor as soon as possible. Only your doctor can determine if it is safe for you to continue taking Duricef.

■ *More common side effects may include:*
Diarrhea
■ *Less common or rare side effects may include:*
Inflammation of the bowel (colitis), nausea, redness and swelling of skin, skin rash and itching, vaginal inflammation, vomiting

### Why should this drug not be prescribed?
If you are sensitive to or have ever had an allergic reaction to a cephalosporin antibiotic, you should not take Duricef.

### Special warnings about this medication
If you have allergies, particularly to drugs, or often develop diarrhea when taking other antibiotics, you should tell your doctor before taking Duricef.

Use with caution if you have a history of gastrointestinal disease, particularly inflammation of the bowel (colitis).

Continued or prolonged use of Duricef may result in a growth of bacteria that do not respond to this medication and can cause a second infection.

### Possible food and drug interactions when taking this medication
No significant interactions have been reported.

### Special information if you are pregnant or breastfeeding
The effects of Duricef during pregnancy have not been adequately studied. If you are pregnant or plan to become pregnant, inform your doctor immediately. Duricef may appear in breast milk and could affect a nursing infant. If this medication is essential to your health, your doctor may advise you to stop nursing your baby until your treatment time with Duricef is finished.

### Recommended dosage
ADULTS

*Urinary Tract Infections*
The usual dosage for uncomplicated infections is a total of 1 to 2 grams per day in a single dose or 2 smaller doses. For all other urinary tract infections, the usual dosage is a total of 2 grams per day taken in 2 doses.

*Skin and Skin Structure Infections*
The usual dose is a total of 1 gram per day in a single dose or 2 smaller doses.

*Throat Infections—Strep Throat and Tonsillitis:*
The usual dosage is a total of 1 gram per day in a single dose or 2 smaller doses for 10 days.

CHILDREN

For urinary tract and skin infections, the usual dose is 30 milligrams per 2.2 pounds of body weight per day, divided into 2 doses and taken every 12 hours. For throat infections, the recommended dose per day is 30 milligrams per 2.2 pounds of body weight in a single dose or 2 smaller doses. In the treatment of strep throat, the dose should be taken for at least 10 days.

OLDER ADULTS

Your dose may be reduced by your doctor.

### Overdosage
Duricef is generally safe. However, large amounts may cause seizures or the side effects listed above.

If you suspect an overdose of Duricef, seek medical attention immediately.

*Brand name:*

# Dyazide

*Pronounced: DYE-uh-zide*
*Generic ingredients: Hydrochlorothiazide,*
*Triamterene*

## Why is this drug prescribed?

Dyazide is a combination of diuretic drugs used in the treatment of high blood pressure and other conditions that require the elimination of excess fluid from the body. When used for high blood pressure, Dyazide can be taken alone or with other high blood pressure medications. Diuretics help your body produce and eliminate more urine, which helps lower blood pressure. Triamterene, one of the ingredients of Dyazide, helps to minimize the potassium loss that can be caused by the other component, hydrochlorothiazide.

## Most important fact about this drug

If you have high blood pressure, you must take Dyazide regularly for it to be effective. Since blood pressure declines gradually, it may be several weeks before you get the full benefit of Dyazide; and you must continue taking it even if you are feeling well. Dyazide does not cure high blood pressure; it merely keeps it under control.

## How should you take this medication?

Dyazide should be taken early in the day. To avoid stomach upset, take it with food.

■ *If you miss a dose...*
  Take it as soon as you remember. If it is almost time for the next dose, skip the one you missed and go back to your regular schedule. Do not take 2 doses at the same time.
■ *Storage instructions...*
  Store at room temperature, away from light.

## What side effects may occur?

Side effects cannot be anticipated. If any occur or change in intensity, inform your doctor as soon as possible. Only your doctor can determine if it is safe for you to continue taking Dyazide.

■ *Side effects may include:*
  Abdominal pain, anemia, breathing difficulty, change in potassium level (causing symptoms such as numbness, tingling, muscle weakness, slow heart rate, shock), constipation, diabetes, diarrhea, dizziness, dizziness when standing up, dry mouth, fatigue, headache, hives, impotence, irregular heartbeat, kidney stones, muscle cramps, nausea, rash, sensitivity to light, strong allergic reaction (localized hives, itching, and swelling or, in severe cases, shock), vomiting, weakness, yellow eyes and skin

## Why should this drug not be prescribed?

If you are unable to urinate or have any serious kidney disease, if you have high potassium levels in your blood, or if you are taking other drugs that prevent loss of potassium, you should not take Dyazide.

If you are sensitive to or have ever had an allergic reaction to triamterene (Dyrenium), hydrochlorothiazide (Oretic), or sulfa drugs such as Gantrisin you should not take this medication.

## Special warnings about this medication

When taking Dyazide, do not use potassium-containing salt substitutes. Take potassium supplements only if specifically directed to by your doctor. Your potassium level should be checked frequently.

If you are taking Dyazide and have kidney disease, your doctor should monitor your kidney function closely.

If you have liver disease, diabetes, cirrhosis of the liver, heart failure, or kidney stones, this medication should be used with care.

## Possible food and drug interactions when taking this medication

Dyazide should be used with caution if you are taking a type of blood pressure medication called an ACE inhibitor, such as Vasotec or Capoten.

If Dyazide is taken with certain other drugs, the effects of either could be increased, decreased, or altered. It is especially important to check with your doctor before combining Dyazide with the following:

Blood-thinning medications such as Coumadin
Corticosteroids such as Deltasone
Drugs for diabetes such as Micronase
Gout medications such as Zyloprim
Laxatives
Lithium (Lithonate)
Methenamine (Urised)

Nonsteroidal anti-inflammatory drugs such as Indocin and Dolobid

Other drugs that minimize potassium loss or contain potassium

Other high blood pressure medications such as Minipress

Salt substitutes containing potassium

Sodium polystyrene sulfonate (Kayexalate)

### Special information
### if you are pregnant or breastfeeding

The effects of Dyazide during pregnancy have not been adequately studied. If you are pregnant or plan to become pregnant, inform your doctor immediately. Dyazide appears in breast milk and could affect a nursing infant. If this medication is essential to your health, your doctor may advise you to discontinue breastfeeding until your treatment is finished.

### Recommended dosage

ADULTS

The usual dose of Dyazide is 1 or 2 capsules once daily, with appropriate monitoring of blood potassium levels by your doctor.

CHILDREN

Safety and effectiveness in children have not been established.

### Overdosage

Any medication taken in excess can have serious consequences. If you suspect an overdose, seek medical treatment immediately.

■ *Symptoms of Dyazide overdose may include:*
Fever, flushed face, nausea, production of large amounts of pale urine, vomiting, weakness, weariness

*Brand name:*

# Dynacin

*See Minocin, page 330.*

*Brand name:*

# DynaCirc

*Pronounced: DYE-na-serk*
*Generic name: Isradipine*

### Why is this drug prescribed?

DynaCirc, a type of medication called a calcium channel blocker, is prescribed for the treatment of high blood pressure. It is effective when used alone or with a thiazide-type diuretic. Calcium channel blockers ease the workload of the heart by slowing down the passage of nerve impulses through the heart muscle, thereby slowing the beat. This improves blood flow through the heart and throughout the body and reduces blood pressure.

### Most important fact about this drug

You must take DynaCirc regularly for it to be effective. Since blood pressure declines gradually, it may be several weeks before you get the full benefit of DynaCirc; and you must continue taking it even if you are feeling well. DynaCirc does not cure high blood pressure; it merely keeps it under control.

### How should you take this medication?

Take this medication exactly as prescribed, even if your symptoms have disappeared. Try not to miss any doses. If DynaCirc is not taken regularly, your condition may worsen.

Swallow the capsule whole, without crushing or chewing it.

■ *If you miss a dose...*
Take it as soon as you remember. If it is almost time for your next dose, skip the one you missed and go back to your regular schedule. Never take 2 doses at the same time.

■ *Storage instructions...*
Store at room temperature, away from light, in a tightly closed container.

### What side effects may occur?

Side effects cannot be anticipated. If any develop or change in intensity, inform your doctor as soon as possible. Only your doctor can determine if it is safe for you to continue taking DynaCirc.

■ *More common side effects may include:*
Dizziness, fluid retention, flushing, headache, pounding heartbeat

■ *Less common side effects may include:*
Chest pain, diarrhea, fatigue, nausea, rapid heartbeat, rash, shortness of breath, stomach upset, unusually frequent urination, vomiting, weakness

■ *Rare side effects may include:*
Constipation, cough, decreased sex drive, depression, difficulty sleeping, drowsiness, dry mouth, excessive sweating, fainting, changes in heart-

beat, heart attack, heart failure, hives, impotence, itching, leg and foot cramps, low blood pressure, nervousness, numbness, severe dizziness, sluggishness, stroke, throat discomfort, tingling or pins and needles, vision changes

## Why should this drug not be prescribed?

If you are sensitive to or have ever had an allergic reaction to DynaCirc or other calcium channel blockers such as Vascor and Procardia, you should not take this medication. Tell your doctor about any drug reactions you have experienced.

## Special warnings about this medication

DynaCirc can cause your blood pressure to become too low. If you feel light-headed or faint, contact your doctor.

This medication should be carefully monitored if you have congestive heart failure, especially if you are also taking a beta-blocking medication such as Tenormin or Inderal.

Before having surgery, including dental surgery, tell the doctor that you are taking DynaCirc.

## Possible food and drug interactions when taking this medication

If DynaCirc is taken with certain other drugs, the effects of either could be increased, decreased, or altered. It is especially important to check with your doctor before combining DynaCirc with the following:

Beta-blocking blood pressure drugs such as
   Tenormin, Inderal, and Lopressor
Cimetidine (Tagamet)
Rifampin (Rifadin)

## Special information if you are pregnant or breastfeeding

The effects of DynaCirc during pregnancy have not been adequately studied. If you are pregnant or plan to become pregnant, consult your doctor immediately. DynaCirc may appear in breast milk and could affect a nursing infant. If this medication is essential to your health, your doctor may advise you to discontinue breastfeeding until your treatment with DynaCirc is finished.

## Recommended dosage

ADULTS

Your dosage will be adjusted to meet your individual needs.

The usual starting dose is 2.5 milligrams, 2 times a day, either alone or in combination with a thiazide diuretic drug. DynaCirc may lower blood pressure 2 to 3 hours after taking the first dose, but the full effect of the drug may not take place for 2 to 4 weeks.

After a 2- to 4-week trial, your doctor may increase the dosage by 5 milligrams per day every 2 to 4 weeks until a maximum dose of 20 milligrams per day is reached. Side effects may increase or become more common after a 10-milligram dose.

If you have kidney or liver disease, you should still begin treatment with a 2.5-milligram dose 2 times per day; however, your doctor will monitor you closely, since your condition may alter the effects of this drug.

OLDER ADULTS

This drug's effects may be stronger in older people. The usual starting dose should still be 2.5 milligrams 2 times per day.

## Overdosage

Although there is little information on DynaCirc, overdose has resulted in sluggishness, low blood pressure, and rapid heartbeat. The symptoms of overdose with other calcium channel blockers include drowsiness, severe low blood pressure, and rapid heartbeat.

If you suspect a DynaCirc overdose, seek medical attention immediately.

*Generic name:*

# Echothiophate

*See Phospholine Iodide, page 418.*

*Brand name:*

# EC-Naprosyn

*See Naprosyn, page 346.*

*Generic name:*

# Econazole

*See Spectazole Cream, page 506.*

*Brand name:*

# Ecotrin

*See Aspirin, page 37.*

*Brand name:*

# E.E.S.

*See Erythromycin, Oral, page 196.*

*Brand name:*

# Effexor

*Pronounced: ef-ecks-OR*
*Generic name: Venlafaxine hydrochloride*

### Why is this drug prescribed?

Effexor is prescribed for the treatment of depression—that is, a continuing depression that interferes with daily functioning. The symptoms usually include changes in appetite, sleep habits, and mind/body coordination, decreased sex drive, increased fatigue, feelings of guilt or worthlessness, difficulty concentrating, slowed thinking, and suicidal thoughts.

### Most important fact about this drug

Serious, sometimes fatal reactions have occurred when Effexor is used in combination with other antidepressant drugs known as MAO inhibitors, including Nardil and Parnate. Never take Effexor with one of these drugs; and do not begin therapy with Effexor within 14 days of discontinuing treatment with one of them. Also, allow at least 7 days between the last dose of Effexor and the first dose of an MAO inhibitor.

### How should you take this medication?

Take Effexor with food, exactly as prescribed. It may take several weeks before you begin to feel better. Your doctor should check your progress periodically.

■ *If you miss a dose...*
It is not necessary to make it up. Skip the missed dose and continue with your next scheduled dose. Do not take 2 doses at once.
■ *Storage instructions...*
Store in a tightly closed container at room temperature. Protect from excessive heat and moisture.

### What side effects may occur?

Side effects cannot be anticipated. If any develop or change in intensity, tell your doctor as soon as possible. Only your doctor can determine if it is safe for you to continue taking Effexor.

■ *More common side effects may include:*
Abnormal dreams, abnormal ejaculation/orgasm, anxiety, blurred vision, chills, constipation, diarrhea, dizziness, dry mouth, extreme muscle tension, flushing, frequent urination, gas, headache, impotence, inability to sleep, indigestion, loss of appetite, nausea, nervousness, prickling or burning sensation, rash, sleepiness, sweating, tremor, vomiting, weakness, yawning
■ *Less common side effects may include:*
Abnormal thinking, abnormal vision, accidental injury, agitation, belching, blood in the urine, bronchitis, bruising, changeable emotions, chest pain, confusion, decreased sex drive, depression, difficult or painful urination, difficulty in breathing, difficulty swallowing, dilated pupils, ear pain, high or low blood pressure, inflammation of the vagina, injury, itching, lack of orgasm, light-headedness on standing up, lockjaw, loss of touch with reality, menstrual problems, migraine headache, neck pain, orgasm disturbance, rapid heartbeat, ringing in the ears, taste changes, twitching, uterine bleeding between menstrual periods, vague feeling of illness, vertigo, weight loss or gain
■ *Rare side effects may include:*
Abnormally slow movements, abnormal movements, abnormal sensitivity to sound, abnormal speech, abortion, abuse of alcohol, acne, alcohol intolerance, allergic reaction, anemia, angina pectoris (crushing chest pain), apathy, appendicitis, arthritis, asthma, bad breath, black stools, bleeding gums, blocked intestine, blood clots, blood clots in the lungs, blood disorders, bluish color to the skin, body odor, bone disease and/or pain (including osteoporosis), breast enlargement or swelling, breast pain, brittle nails, bulging eyes, cancerous growth, cataracts, changed sense of smell, chest congestion, cold hands and feet, colitis (inflamed bowel), confusion, conjunctivitis ("pinkeye"), coughing up blood, deafness, delusions, depression, diabetes, double vision, drug withdrawal symptoms, dry eyes, dry skin, ear infection, eczema, enlarged abdomen,

enlarged thyroid gland, exaggerated feeling of well-being, excessive hair growth, excessive menstrual flow, eye disorders, eye pain, fainting, fungus infection, gallstones, glaucoma, gout, hair discoloration, hair loss, hallucinations, hangover effect, heart disorders, hemorrhoids, hepatitis, herpes infections, high cholesterol, hives, hostility, hyperventilation (fast, deep breathing), inability to communicate, increased mucus, increased physical activity, increased salivation, increased sensitivity to touch, increased sex drive, inflammation of the stomach, intestines, anus and rectum, gums, tongue, eyelid, or inner ear, intolerance to light, involuntary eye movements, irregular or slow heartbeat, kidney disorders, lack of menstruation, large amounts of urine, laryngitis, loss of consciousness, loss of muscle movement, low or high blood sugar, menstrual problems, middle ear infection, mouth fungus, mouth sores, muscle spasms, muscle weakness, nosebleeds, over- and underactive thyroid gland, overdose, paranoia, pelvic pain, pinpoint pupils, "pins and needles" around the mouth, pneumonia, prolonged erection, psoriasis, rectal hemorrhage, reduced menstrual flow, restlessness, secretion of milk, sensitivity to light, skin disorders, skin eruptions or hemorrhage, skin inflammation, sleep disturbance, soft stools, stiff neck, stomach or peptic ulcer, stroke, stupor, sugar in the urine, swelling due to fluid retention, swollen or discolored tongue, taste loss, temporary failure to breathe, thirst, twisted neck, ulcer, unconsciousness, uncoordinated movements, urgent need to urinate, urination at night, uterine and vaginal hemorrhage, varicose veins, voice changes, vomiting blood, yellowed eyes and skin

## Why should this drug not be prescribed?

Never take Effexor while taking other antidepressants known as MAO inhibitors. (See "Most important fact about this drug.") Also avoid this drug if it has ever given you an allergic reaction.

## Special warnings about this medication

Your doctor will prescribe Effexor with caution if you have high blood pressure, heart, liver, or kidney disease or a history of seizures or mania (extreme agitation or excitability). You should discuss all of your medical problems with your doctor before taking Effexor.

Effexor may cause you to feel drowsy or less alert and may affect your judgment. Therefore, avoid driving or operating dangerous machinery or participating in any hazardous activity that requires full mental alertness until you know how this drug affects you.

If you have ever been addicted to drugs, tell your doctor before you start taking Effexor.

If you develop a skin rash or hives while taking Effexor, notify your doctor.

Do not stop taking the drug without consulting your doctor. If you stop suddenly, you may have withdrawal symptoms, even though this drug does not seem to be habit-forming. Your doctor will have you taper off gradually.

## Possible food and drug interactions when taking this medication

Combining Effexor with MAO inhibitors could cause a fatal reaction. (See "Most important fact about this drug.")

Although Effexor does not interact with alcohol, the manufacturer recommends avoiding alcohol while taking this medication.

If you have high blood pressure or liver disease, or are elderly, check with your doctor before combining Effexor with cimetidine (Tagamet).

Effexor does not interact with Lithium or Valium. However, you should consult your doctor before combining Effexor with other drugs that affect the central nervous system, including narcotic painkillers, sleep aids, tranquilizers, and other antidepressants.

## Special information if you are pregnant or breastfeeding

The effects of Effexor during pregnancy have not been adequately studied. If you are pregnant or are planning to become pregnant, tell your doctor immediately. Effexor should be used during pregnancy only if clearly needed. Effexor may appear in breast milk. If this medication is essential to your health, your doctor may tell you to discontinue breastfeeding your baby until your treatment with Effexor is finished.

## Recommended dosage

ADULTS

The usual starting dose is 75 milligrams a day, divided into 2 or 3 smaller doses, and taken with food. If needed, your doctor may gradually increase your daily dose in steps of no more than 75 milligrams at a time up to a maximum of 375 milligrams per day.

If you have kidney or liver disease or are taking other medications, your doctor will adjust your dosage accordingly.

CHILDREN

The safety and effectiveness of Effexor have not been established in children under 18 years of age.

## Overdosage

Any medication taken in excess can have serious consequences. If you suspect an overdose, seek medical attention immediately.

■ *Symptoms of Effexor overdose include:*
Convulsions, rapid heartbeat, sleepiness

*Brand name:*

# Efudex

*Pronounced: EFF-you-decks*
*Generic name: Fluorouracil*

## Why is this drug prescribed?

Efudex is prescribed for the treatment of actinic or solar keratoses (small red horny growths or flesh-colored wartlike growths caused by overexposure to ultraviolet radiation or the sun). Such growths may develop into skin cancer. When conventional methods are impractical—as when the affected sites are hard to get at—Efudex is useful in the treatment of superficial basal cell carcinomas, or slow-growing malignant tumors of the face usually found at the edge of the nostrils, eyelids, or lips. Efudex is available in cream and solution forms.

## Most important fact about this drug

If you use an airtight dressing to cover the skin being treated, there may be inflammatory reactions in the normal skin around the treated area. If it is necessary to cover the treated area, use a porous gauze dressing to avoid skin reactions.

## How should you take this medication?

Use care when applying Efudex around the eyes, nose, and mouth. Wash your hands immediately after applying this medication.

■ *If you miss a dose...*
Apply it as soon as you remember. If more than a few hours have passed, skip the dose you missed

and go back to your regular schedule. If you miss more than 1 dose, contact your doctor.

■ *Storage instructions...*
Store away from heat, light, and moisture.

## What side effects may occur?

Side effects cannot be anticipated. If any develop or change in intensity, inform your doctor as soon as possible. Only your doctor can determine if it is safe for you to continue using Efudex.

■ *More common side effects may include:*
Burning, discoloration of the skin, itching, pain
■ *Less common side effects may include:*
Allergic skin inflammation, pus, scaling, scarring, soreness, swelling, tenderness

## Why should this drug not be prescribed?

If you are sensitive to or have ever had an allergic reaction to Efudex or similar drugs, you should not take this medication. Make sure your doctor is aware of any drug reactions you have experienced.

## Special warnings about this medication

Avoid prolonged exposure to ultraviolet rays while you are under treatment with Efudex.

Skin may be unsightly during treatment with this drug and, in some cases, for several weeks after treatment has ended.

If your solar keratoses do not clear up with use of this drug, your doctor will probably order a biopsy (removal of a small amount of tissue to be examined under a microscope) to confirm the skin disease.

Your doctor will perform follow-up biopsies if you are being treated for superficial basal cell carcinoma.

## Possible food and drug interactions when taking this medication

There are no reported food or drug interactions.

## Special information if you are pregnant or breastfeeding

The effects of Efudex during pregnancy have not been adequately studied. If you are pregnant, plan to become pregnant, or are breastfeeding your baby, consult your doctor immediately.

## Recommended dosage

When Efudex is applied to affected skin, the skin becomes abnormally red, blisters form, and the surface skin wears away. A lesion or sore forms at the affected site, and the diseased or cancerous skin cells die before a new layer of skin forms.

ADULTS

### Actinic or Solar Keratosis

Apply cream or solution 2 times a day in an amount sufficient to cover the affected area. Continue using the medication until the inflammatory response reaches the stage where the skin wears away, a sore or lesion forms, and the skin cells die; your doctor will then have you stop using the medication. The usual length of treatment is from 2 to 4 weeks. You may not see complete healing of the affected area for 1 to 2 months after ending the treatment.

### Superficial Basal Cell Carcinomas

You should use only the 5% strength of this medication. Twice a day, apply enough cream or solution to cover the affected area. Continue the treatment for at least 3 to 6 weeks; it may take 10 to 12 weeks of application before the lesions are gone.

Your doctor will want to monitor your condition to make sure it has been cured.

### Overdosage

Although no specific information is available on Efudex overdosage, any medication used in excess can have serious consequences. If you suspect an overdosage, seek medical attention immediately.

Brand name:

# Elavil

Pronounced: ELL-uh-vil
Generic name: Amitriptyline hydrochloride
Other brand name: Endep

### Why is this drug prescribed?

Elavil is prescribed for the relief of symptoms of mental depression. It is a member of the group of drugs called tricyclic antidepressants. Some doctors also prescribe Elavil to treat bulimia (an eating disorder), to control chronic pain, to prevent migraine headaches, and to treat a pathological weeping and laughing syndrome associated with multiple sclerosis.

### Most important fact about this drug

You may need to take Elavil regularly for several weeks before it becomes fully effective. Do not skip doses, even if they seem to make no difference or you feel you don't need them.

### How should you take this medication?

Take Elavil exactly as prescribed. You may experience side effects, such as mild drowsiness, early in therapy. However, they usually disappear after a few days.

Elavil may cause dry mouth. Sucking a hard candy, chewing gum, or melting bits of ice in your mouth can provide relief.

■ *If you miss a dose...*
Take it as soon as you remember. If it is almost time for your next dose, skip the one you missed and go back to your regular schedule. Never take 2 doses at the same time.

If you take a single daily dose at bedtime, do not make up for it in the morning. It may cause side effects during the day.

■ *Storage instructions...*
Keep Elavil in a tightly closed container. Store at room temperature. Protect from light and excessive heat.

### What side effects may occur?

Side effects cannot be anticipated. If any develop or change in intensity, inform your doctor as soon as possible. Only your doctor can determine if it is safe for you to continue taking Elavil.

■ *Side effects may include:*
Abnormal movements, anxiety, black tongue, blurred vision, breast development in males, breast enlargement, coma, confusion, constipation, delusions, diarrhea, difficult or frequent urination, difficulty in speech, dilation of pupils, disorientation, disturbed concentration, dizziness on getting up, dizziness or light-headedness, drowsiness, dry mouth, excessive or spontaneous flow of milk, excitement, fatigue, fluid retention, hair loss, hallucinations, headache, heart attack, hepatitis, high blood pressure, high fever, high or low blood sugar, hives, impotence, inability to sleep, increased or decreased sex drive, increased perspiration, increased pressure within the eye, inflammation of the mouth, intestinal obstruction, irregular heartbeat, lack or loss of coordination, loss of appetite, low blood pressure, nausea, nightmares, numbness, rapid and/or fast, fluttery heartbeat, rash, red or purple spots on skin, restlessness, ringing in the ears, seizures, sensitivity to light, stomach upset, strange taste, stroke,

swelling due to fluid retention in the face and tongue, swelling of testicles, swollen glands, tingling and pins and needles in the arms and legs, tremors, vomiting, weakness, weight gain or loss, yellowed eyes and skin

■ *Side effects due to rapid decrease or abrupt withdrawal from Elavil include:*
Headache, nausea, vague feeling of bodily discomfort
■ *Side effects due to gradual dosage reduction may include:*
Dream and sleep disturbances, irritability, restlessness

These side effects do not signify an addiction to the drug.

### Why should this drug not be prescribed?
If you are sensitive to or have ever had an allergic reaction to Elavil or similar drugs such as Norpramin and Tofranil, you should not take this medication. Make sure your doctor is aware of any drug reactions you have experienced.

Do not take Elavil while taking other antidepressants known as MAO inhibitors. Drugs in this category include Nardil and Parnate.

Unless you are directed to do so by your doctor, do not take this medication if you are recovering from a heart attack.

### Special warnings about this medication
Do not stop taking Elavil abruptly, especially if you have been taking large doses for a long time. Your doctor probably will want to decrease your dosage gradually. This will help prevent a possible relapse and will reduce the possibility of withdrawal symptoms.

Elavil may make your skin more sensitive to sunlight. Try to stay out of the sun, wear protective clothing, and apply a sun block.

Elavil may cause you to become drowsy or less alert; therefore, you should not drive or operate dangerous machinery or participate in any hazardous activity that requires full mental alertness until you know how this drug affects you.

While taking this medication, you may feel dizzy or light-headed or actually faint when getting up from a lying or sitting position. If getting up slowly doesn't help or if this problem continues, notify your doctor.

Use Elavil with caution if you have ever had seizures, urinary retention, glaucoma or other chronic eye conditions, a heart or circulatory system disorder, or liver problems. Be cautious, too, if you are receiving thyroid medication. You should discuss all of your medical problems with your doctor before starting Elavil therapy.

Before having surgery, dental treatment, or any diagnostic procedure, tell the doctor that you are taking Elavil. Certain drugs used during surgery, such as anesthetics and muscle relaxants, and drugs used in certain diagnostic procedures may react badly with Elavil.

### Possible food and drug interactions when taking this medication
Elavil may intensify the effects of alcohol. Do not drink alcohol while taking this medication.

If Elavil is taken with certain other drugs, the effects of either could be increased, decreased, or altered. It is especially important that you consult with your doctor before taking Elavil in combination with the following:

Airway-opening drugs such as Sudafed and Proventil
Antidepressants that raise serotonin levels, such as Paxil, Prozac, and Zoloft
Antidepressants classified as MAO inhibitors, such as Nardil and Parnate
Other antidepressants, such as Asendin
Antihistamines such as Benadryl and Tavist
Barbiturates such as phenobarbital
Certain blood pressure medicines such as Catapres and Ismelin
Cimetidine (Tagamet)
Disulfiram (Antabuse)
Drugs that control spasms such as Bentyl and Donnatal
Estrogen drugs such as Premarin and oral contraceptives
Ethchlorvynol (Placidyl)
Major tranquilizers such as Mellaril and Thorazine
Medications for irregular heartbeat, such as Tambocor and Rythmol
Painkillers such as Demerol and Percocet
Parkinsonism drugs such as Cogentin and Larodopa
Quinidine (Quinidex)
Seizure medications such as Tegretol and Dilantin
Sleep medicines such as Halcion and Dalmane

Thyroid hormones (Synthroid)
Tranquilizers such as Librium and Xanax
Warfarin (Coumadin)

## Special information
## if you are pregnant or breastfeeding

The effects of Elavil during pregnancy have not
been adequately studied. If you are pregnant or
planning to become pregnant, inform your doctor
immediately. This medication appears in breast
milk. If Elavil is essential to your health, your
doctor may advise you to discontinue breastfeeding
until your treatment is finished.

## Recommended dosage
ADULTS

The usual starting dosage is 75 milligrams per day
divided into 2 or more smaller doses. Your doctor
may gradually increase this dose to 150 milligrams
per day. The total daily dose is generally never
higher than 200 milligrams.

Alternatively, your doctor may want you to start
with 50 milligrams to 100 milligrams at bedtime.
He or she may increase this bedtime dose by 25 or
50 milligrams up to a total of 150 milligrams
a day.

For long-term use, the usual dose ranges from
40 to 100 milligrams taken once daily, usually at
bedtime.

CHILDREN

Use of Elavil is not recommended for children
under 12 years of age.

The usual dose for adolescents 12 years of age
and over is 10 milligrams, 3 times a day, with 20
milligrams taken at bedtime.

OLDER ADULTS

The usual dose is 10 milligrams taken 3 times a
day, with 20 milligrams taken at bedtime.

## Overdosage
An overdose of Elavil can prove fatal.

■ *Symptoms of Elavil overdose may include:*
Abnormally low blood pressure, congestive heart
failure, convulsions, dilated pupils and other eye
problems, drowsiness, rapid or irregular heartbeat, reduced body temperature, stupor, unresponsiveness or coma

■ *Symptoms contrary to the effect of this
medication are:*
Agitation, extremely high body temperature,
rigid muscles, vomiting

If you suspect an overdose, seek medical attention
immediately.

*Brand name:*

# Eldepryl

*Pronounced: ELL-dep-rill*
*Generic name: Selegiline hydrochloride*

## Why is this drug prescribed?
Eldepryl is prescribed along with Sinemet (lev-
odopa/carbidopa) for people with Parkinson's
disease. It is used when Sinemet no longer seems to
be working well. Eldepryl has no effect when taken
by itself; it works only in combination with
Larodopa (levodopa) or Sinemet.

Parkinson's disease, which causes muscle rigidity and difficulty with walking and talking, involves
the progressive degeneration of a particular type of
nerve cell. Early on, Larodopa or Sinemet alone
may alleviate the symptoms of the disease. In time,
however, these medications work less well; their
effectiveness seems to switch on and off at random,
and the individual may begin to experience side
effects such as involuntary movements and "freezing" in mid-motion.

Eldepryl may be prescribed at this stage of the
disease to help restore the effectiveness of Larodopa or Sinemet. When you begin to take Eldepryl,
you may need a reduced dosage of the other
medication.

## Most important fact about this drug
Eldepryl belongs to a class of drugs known as MAO
inhibitors. These drugs can interact with certain
foods—including aged cheeses and meats, pickled
herring, beer, and wine—to cause a life-threatening
surge in blood pressure. At the dose recommended
for Eldepryl, this interaction is not a problem. But
for safety's sake, you may want to watch your diet;
and you should never take more Eldepryl than the
doctor prescribed.

## How should you take this medication?
Take Eldepryl and your other Parkinson's medication exactly as prescribed.

■ *If you miss a dose...*
Take it as soon as you remember. If you do not remember until late afternoon or evening, skip the dose you missed and go back to your regular schedule. Never take 2 doses at once.

■ *Storage instructions...*
Store at room temperature.

## What side effects may occur?
Side effects cannot be anticipated. If any develop or change in intensity, inform your doctor as soon as possible. Only your doctor can determine if it is safe for you to continue taking Eldepryl.

■ *Side effects may include:*
Abdominal pain, abnormal movements, abnormally fast walking, aches, agitation, angina (crushing chest pain), anxiety, apathy, asthma, back pain, behavior or mood changes, bleeding from the rectum, blurred vision, burning lips and mouth or throat, chills, confusion, constipation, delusions, depression, diarrhea, difficulty swallowing, disorientation, dizziness, double vision, drowsiness, dry mouth, excessive urination at night, eyelid spasm, facial grimace, facial hair, fainting, falling down, freezing, frequent urination, general feeling of illness, hair loss, hallucinations, headache, heartburn, heart palpitations, heart rhythm abnormalities, "heavy leg", high blood pressure, hollow feeling, inability to carry out purposeful movements, inability to urinate, increased or excessive sweating, increased tremor, insomnia, involuntary movements, irritability, lack of appetite, leg pain, lethargy, lightheadedness upon standing up, loss of balance, low blood pressure, lower back pain, migraine, muscle cramps, nausea, nervousness, numbness in toes/fingers, overstimulation, pain over the eyes, personality change, poor appetite, rapid heartbeat, rash, restlessness (desire to keep moving), ringing in the ears, sensitivity to light, sexual problems, shortness of breath, sleep disturbance, slow heartbeat, slow urination, slowed body movements, speech problems, stiff neck, stomach and intestinal bleeding, swelling of the ankles or arms and legs, taste disturbance, tension, tiredness, twitching, urinary problems, vertigo, vivid dreams or nightmares, vomiting, weakness, weight loss

## Why should this drug not be prescribed?
Do not take Eldepryl if you are sensitive to or have ever had an allergic reaction to it. Do not take narcotic painkillers such as Demerol while you are taking Eldepryl.

## Special warnings about this medication
Never take Eldepryl at a higher dosage than prescribed; doing so could put you at risk for a dangerous rise in blood pressure. If you develop a severe headache or any other unusual symptoms, contact your doctor immediately.

You may suffer a severe reaction if you combine Eldepryl with tricyclic antidepressants such as Elavil and Tofranil, or with antidepressants that affect serotonin levels, such as Prozac and Paxil. Wait at least 14 days after taking Eldepryl before beginning therapy with any of these drugs. If you have been taking antidepressants such as Prozac and Paxil, you should wait at least *5 weeks* before taking Eldepryl. This much time is needed to clear the antidepressant completely from your system.

## Possible food and drug interactions when taking this medication
If Eldepryl is taken with certain other drugs, the effects of either could be increased, decreased, or altered. It is especially important to check with your doctor before combining Eldepryl with the following:

Antidepressant medications that raise serotonin levels, such as Paxil, Prozac, and Zoloft
Antidepressant medications classified as tricyclics, such as Elavil and Tofranil
Narcotic painkillers such as Demerol, Percocet, and Tylenol with Codeine

Eldepryl may worsen side effects caused by your usual dosage of levodopa.

## Special information if you are pregnant or breastfeeding
The effects of Eldepryl during pregnancy have not been adequately studied. If you are pregnant or plan to become pregnant, inform your doctor immediately. Although Eldepryl is not known to cause specific birth defects, it should not be taken during pregnancy unless it is clearly needed. It is not known whether Eldepryl appears in breast milk. As a general rule, a nursing mother should not take any drug unless it is clearly necessary.

## Recommended dosage

ADULTS

The recommended dose of Eldepryl is 10 milligrams per day divided into 2 smaller doses of 5 milligrams each, taken at breakfast and lunch. There is no evidence of additional benefit from higher doses, and they increase the risk of side effects.

CHILDREN

The use of Eldepryl in children has not been evaluated.

## Overdosage

Although no specific information is available about Eldepryl overdosage, it is assumed, because of chemical similarities, that the symptoms would resemble those of overdose with an MAO inhibitor antidepressant.

■ *Symptoms of MAO inhibitor overdose may include:*
Agitation, chest pain, clammy skin, coma, convulsions, dizziness, drowsiness, extremely high fever, faintness, fast and irregular pulse, hallucinations, headache (severe), high blood pressure, hyperactivity, inability to breathe, irritability, lockjaw, low blood pressure (severe), shallow breathing, spasm of the entire body, sweating

It is important to note that after a large overdose, symptoms may not appear for up to 12 hours and may not reach their full force for 24 hours or more. An overdose can be fatal. If you suspect an Eldepryl overdose, seek medical attention immediately. Hospitalization is recommended, with continuous observation and monitoring for at least 2 days.

*Brand name:*

# Elocon

*Pronounced: ELL-oh-con*
*Generic name: Mometasone furoate*

## Why is this drug prescribed?

Elocon is a cortisone-like steroid available in cream, ointment, and lotion form. It is used to treat certain itchy rashes and other inflammatory skin conditions.

## Most important fact about this drug

When you use Elocon, you inevitably absorb some of the medication through your skin and into the bloodstream. Too much absorption can lead to unwanted side effects elsewhere in the body. To keep this problem to a minimum, avoid using large amounts of Elocon over large areas, and do not cover it with airtight dressings such as plastic wrap or adhesive bandages unless specifically told to by your doctor.

## How should you use this medication?

Apply a thin film of the cream or ointment or a few drops of the lotion to the affected skin once a day. Massage it in until it disappears.

Elocon is for use only on the skin. Be careful to keep it out of your eyes.

For the most effective and economical use of Elocon lotion, hold the tip of the bottle very close to (but not touching) the affected skin and squeeze the bottle gently.

Once you have applied Elocon, never cover the skin with an airtight bandage, a tight diaper, plastic pants, or any other airtight dressing. This could encourage excessive absorption of the medication into your bloodstream.

Be careful not to use Elocon for a longer time than prescribed. If you do, you may disrupt your ability to make your own natural adrenal corticoid hormones (hormones secreted by the outer layer of the adrenal gland).

■ *If you miss a dose...*
Apply it as soon as you remember. If it is almost time for your next dose, skip the one you missed and go back to your regular schedule.

■ *Storage instructions...*
Store at room temperature.

## What side effects may occur?

Side effects cannot be anticipated. If any develop or change in intensity, notify your doctor as soon as possible. Only your doctor can determine if it is safe for you to continue using Elocon.

■ *Side effects may include:*
Acne-like pimples, allergic skin rash, boils, burning, damaged skin, dryness, excessive hairiness, infected hair follicles, infection of the skin, irritation, itching, light colored patches on skin, prickly heat, rash around the mouth, skin atrophy and wasting, softening of the skin, stretch marks, tingling or stinging

### Why should this drug not be prescribed?
Do not use Elocon if you are sensitive to it or have ever had an allergic reaction to it or any other steroid medication.

### Special warnings about this medication
Remember, Elocon is for external use only. Avoid getting it into your eyes. Do not use it to treat anything other than the condition for which it was prescribed.

### Possible food and drug interactions when using this medication
No interactions have been noted.

### Special information
### if you are pregnant or breastfeeding
If you are pregnant or plan to become pregnant, inform your doctor immediately. Elocon should not be used during pregnancy unless the benefit outweighs the potential risk to the unborn child.

You should not use Elocon while breastfeeding, since absorbed hormone could make its way into the breast milk and perhaps harm the nursing baby. If you are a new mother, you should contact your doctor, who will help you decide between breastfeeding and using Elocon.

### Recommended dosage
ADULTS

Apply once daily.

CHILDREN

Use should be limited to the least amount necessary. Use of steroids over a long period of time may interfere with growth and development.

### Overdosage
With extensive or long-term use of Elocon, hormone absorbed into the bloodstream may cause a group of symptoms called Cushing's syndrome.

■ *Symptoms of Cushing's syndrome may include:*
Acne, depression, excessive hair growth, high blood pressure, humped upper back, insomnia, moon-faced appearance, obese trunk, paranoia, stretch marks, wasted limbs, stunted growth (in children), susceptibility to bruising, fractures, and infections

Cushing's syndrome may also trigger diabetes mellitus.

If it is left uncorrected, Cushing's syndrome may become serious. If you suspect your long-term use of Elocon has led to this problem, seek medical attention immediately.

*Brand name:*

# Eltroxin

*See Synthroid, page 516.*

*Brand name:*

# Empirin

*See Aspirin, page 37.*

*Brand name:*

# Empirin with Codeine

*Pronounced: EM-pir-in with KOE-deen*
*Generic ingredients: Aspirin, Codeine phosphate*

### Why is this drug prescribed?
Empirin with Codeine is a narcotic pain reliever and anti-inflammatory medication. It is prescribed for mild, moderate, and moderate to severe pain.

### Most important fact about this drug
Codeine can be habit-forming when taken over a long period of time or in high doses. Do not take more of the drug, or use it for a longer period of time than your doctor has indicated.

### How should you take this medication?
Take Empirin with Codeine with food or a full glass of milk or water to reduce stomach irritation. Take it exactly as prescribed.

■ *If you miss a dose...*
Take it as soon as you remember. If it is almost time for your next dose, skip the one you missed and go back to your regular schedule. Never take 2 doses at once.
■ *Storage instructions...*
Store at room temperature in a dry place; protect from light.

### What side effects may occur?
Side effects cannot be anticipated. If any develop or change in intensity, inform your doctor as soon as possible. Only your doctor can determine if it is safe for you to continue using Empirin with Codeine.

■ *More common side effects may include:*
Constipation, dizziness, drowsiness, light-headedness, nausea, shallow breathing, vomiting

■ *Less common side effects may include:*
Abdominal pain, aggravation of peptic ulcer, anaphylactic shock (severe allergic reaction), asthma, bruising or bleeding, confusion, dizziness, drowsiness, exaggerated sense of well-being or depression, excessive bleeding following injury or surgery, fatigue, headache, hearing problems, heartburn, hives, indigestion, itching, nausea, rapid heartbeat, ringing in ears, runny nose, skin rashes, sweating, thirst, vision problems, vomiting, weakness

## Why should this drug not be prescribed?

Empirin with Codeine should not be used if you: are sensitive or allergic to aspirin or codeine, experience severe bleeding, have a blood clotting disorder or severe vitamin K deficiency, are taking blood-thinning medications, have a peptic ulcer or have liver damage. Children or teenagers with symptoms of chickenpox or the flu should not take Empirin with Codeine because of the danger of contracting Reye's Syndrome, a condition characterized by nausea, vomiting, and lethargy and disorientation deepening to coma.

## Special warnings about this medication

Aspirin can cause severe allergic reactions including anaphylactic shock (difficulty breathing, bluish skin color caused by lack of oxygen, fever, rash or hives, irregular pulse, convulsions, or collapse).

Aspirin can cause bleeding if you have a peptic ulcer, open sores in the stomach or intestines, or a bleeding disorder. It may also prolong bleeding time after an injury or surgery.

Codeine can hide symptoms of serious abdominal conditions.

Use codeine with care if you have a head or brain injury. It can slow your breathing, make you drowsy, and increase pressure in your head.

Be careful taking Empirin with Codeine if you are elderly or in a weakened condition or have severe kidney or liver disease, gallstones or gallbladder disease, a breathing disorder, an irregular heartbeat, an inflamed stomach or intestines, an underactive thyroid gland, Addison's disease (a disorder of the adrenal glands), or an enlarged prostate or narrowing of the urethra.

Use aspirin with care if you have ever had any allergies. Sensitivity reactions are relatively common in people with asthma and nasal polyps (swollen growths in the nose).

Empirin with Codeine may make you drowsy or less alert. Be careful driving, operating machinery, or using appliances that require full mental alertness until you know how you react to this medication.

Remember, this medication can be habit-forming and should be taken exactly as prescribed. Do not take more of the medication, or use it more often, than your doctor has indicated.

## Possible food and drug interactions when taking this medication

The effects of alcohol may be increased if taken with Empirin with Codeine. Avoid using alcohol while taking this medication.

If Empirin with Codeine is taken with certain other drugs, the effects of either could be increased, decreased, or altered. It is especially important to check with your doctor before combining Empirin with Codeine with the following:

Blood thinners such as Coumadin
Furosemide (Lasix)
Insulin
MAO inhibitors such as the antidepressants Parnate and Nardil
Methotrexate (Rheumatrex)
Mercaptopurine
Nonsteroidal anti-inflammatory drugs such as Advil, Motrin, and Indocin
Oral diabetes medications such as Diabinese and Tolinase
Other narcotic analgesics such as Percodan and Tylox
Para-amino salicylic acid
Penicillin
Probenecid (Benemid)
Sedatives such as phenobarbital and Nembutal
Steroids such as Medrol and prednisone
Sulfa drugs such as Azo Gantrisin and Septra
Sulfinpyrazone (Anturane)
Tranquilizers such as Xanax and Valium
Vitamin C

## Special information
## if you are pregnant or breastfeeding

The effects of Empirin with Codeine during pregnancy have not been adequately studied. If you are pregnant or plan to become pregnant, inform your doctor immediately. Aspirin and codeine appear in small amounts in breast milk and may affect a nursing infant. If this medication is essential to your health, your doctor may advise you to stop breastfeeding until your treatment with this medication is finished.

### Recommended dosage

Dosage is determined by the severity of your pain and your response to this medication. Your doctor may prescribe more than the usual recommended dose if your pain is severe or if you are no longer getting enough pain relief from the dose you have been taking.

The usual adult dose for Empirin with Codeine No. 3 is 1 or 2 tablets every 4 hours as needed. The usual adult dose for Empirin with Codeine No. 4 is 1 tablet every 4 hours as required.

### Overdosage

■ *In adults, symptoms of Empirin with Codeine overdose may include:*
Bluish skin color due to lack of oxygen, circulatory collapse, clammy skin, coma, constricted pupils, delirium, delusions, difficult or labored breathing, double vision, excitability, flabby muscles, garbled speech, hallucinations, restlessness, skin eruptions, slow and shallow breathing, stupor, vertigo

■ *In children, symptoms of Empirin with Codeine overdose may include:*
Confusion, convulsions, dehydration, difficulty hearing, dim vision, dizziness, drowsiness, extremely high body temperature, headache, nausea, rapid breathing, ringing in ears, sweating, thirst, vomiting

If you suspect an overdose, seek medical treatment immediately.

*Brand name:*

# E-Mycin

*See Erythromycin, Oral, page 196.*

*Generic name:*

# Enalapril

*See Vasotec, page 584.*

*Generic name:*

# Enalapril with Hydrochlorothiazide

*See Vaseretic, page 582.*

*Brand name:*

# Endep

*See Elavil, page 187.*

*Generic name:*

# Enoxacin

*See Penetrex, page 402.*

*Brand name:*

# Entex LA

*Pronounced: ENN-teks ell ai*
*Generic ingredients: Guaifenesin,*
   *Phenylpropanolamine hydrochloride*
*Other brand name: Exgest LA*

### Why is this drug prescribed?

Entex LA is used to treat bronchitis, the common cold, sinus inflammation, nasal congestion, and sore throat.

Entex LA is a combination of two medications, phenylpropanolamine (a decongestant) and guaifenesin (an expectorant), specially formulated to deliver prolonged action. Phenylpropanolamine helps reduce congestion in the nasal passages, while guaifenesin breaks up mucus in the lower respiratory tract, making it easier to clear the passages.

### Most important fact about this drug

Certain medical conditions can affect your use of Entex LA. If you have heart disease, high blood pressure, or diabetes, make sure the doctor knows about it. The phenylpropanolamine in Entex LA can raise blood pressure and speed up the heart, and can put you at a greater risk of heart or blood-vessel disease if you are diabetic.

### How should you take this medication?

You may break Entex LA tablets in half to make them easier to swallow, but you must not chew or crush them.

■ *If you miss a dose...*
Take it as soon as you remember. If it is almost time for your next dose, skip the one you missed and go back to your regular schedule. Never take 2 doses at once.

■ *Storage instructions...*
Store at room temperature.

## What side effects may occur?
Side effects cannot be anticipated. If any develop or change in intensity, inform your doctor as soon as possible. Only your doctor can determine if it is safe for you to continue taking Entex LA.

■ *Side effects may include:*
Difficulty urinating (in men with an enlarged prostate), headache, inability to sleep or difficulty sleeping, irritated stomach, nausea, nervousness, restlessness

## Why should this drug not be prescribed?
You should not use Entex LA if you have severe high blood pressure, are sensitive to other stimulating drugs such as Dristan Decongestant, or take antidepressant medications known as MAO inhibitors, including Nardil and Parnate.

## Special warnings about this medication
Use Entex LA cautiously if you have any of the following conditions:

Diabetes
Glaucoma (excessive pressure in the eyes)
Heart disease
High blood pressure
Hyperthyroidism (excessive thyroid gland activity)
Prostate enlargement

## Possible food and drug interactions when taking this medication
Do not take Entex LA if you are taking an antidepressant medication classified as an MAO inhibitor including Nardil and Parnate. Avoid other stimulating drugs such as Proventil, Ventolin, and many decongestants. Interactions can also occur with the following:

Bromocriptine (Parlodel)
Methyldopa (Aldomet)

## Special information if you are pregnant or breastfeeding
The effects of Entex LA during pregnancy have not been adequately studied. If you are pregnant or plan to become pregnant, notify your doctor immediately. It is not known whether Entex LA appears in breast milk. If this medication is essential to your health, your doctor may advise you to discontinue breastfeeding until treatment with this drug is finished.

## Recommended dosage
ADULTS AND CHILDREN 12 YEARS AND OLDER

The usual dosage is 1 tablet every 12 hours.

CHILDREN 6 TO 12 YEARS OLD

The usual dosage is one-half tablet every 12 hours.
The safety and effectiveness of Entex LA have not been established in children under the age of 6.

## Overdosage
Any medication taken in excess can have serious consequences. If you suspect an overdose, seek medical help immediately.

■ *Symptoms of Entex LA overdose may include:*
Coma, convulsions, high blood pressure

*Brand name:*

# Epitol

*See Tegretol, page 525.*

*Brand name:*

# Equanil

*See Miltown, page 327.*

*Generic name:*

# Ergoloid mesylates

*See Hydergine, page 238.*

*Generic name:*

# Ergotamine with Caffeine

*See Cafergot, page 68.*

*Brand name:*

# ERYC

*See Erythromycin, Oral, page 196.*

Brand name:

# Erycette

See Erythromycin, Topical, page 198.

Brand name:

# Ery-Tab

See Erythromycin, Oral, page 196.

Brand name:

# Erythrocin

See Erythromycin, Oral, page 196.

Generic name:

# Erythromycin, Oral

Pronounced: er-ITH-row MY-sin
Brand names: E.E.S., E-Mycin, ERYC, Ery-Tab,
   Erythrocin, Ilosone, PCE

## Why is this drug prescribed?

Erythromycin is an antibiotic used to treat many kinds of infections, including:

Acute pelvic inflammatory disease
Gonorrhea
Intestinal parasitic infections
Legionnaires' disease
Pinkeye
Skin infections
Syphilis
Upper and lower respiratory tract infections
Urinary tract infections
Whooping cough

Erythromycin is also prescribed to prevent infections of the heart (rheumatic fever and bacterial endocarditis) in people who are allergic to penicillin and who have congenital or rheumatic heart disease.

## Most important fact about this drug

Erythromycin, like any other antibiotic, works best when there is a constant amount of drug in the blood. To help keep the drug amount constant, it is important not to miss any doses. Also, it is advisable to take the doses at evenly spaced times around the clock.

## How should you take this medication?

Your doctor may advise you to take erythromycin at least 1 hour before or 2 hours after meals. If the drug upsets your stomach, taking it with meals may help. Ask your doctor whether this is advisable for you.

Chewable forms of erythromycin should be crushed or chewed before being swallowed.

Delayed-release brands and tablets and capsules that are coated to slow their breakdown should be swallowed whole. Do not crush or break. If you are not sure about the form of erythromycin you are taking, ask your pharmacist.

The liquid should be shaken well before each use.

■ *If you miss a dose...*
   Take it as soon as you remember. If it is almost time for your next dose, and you take 2 doses a day, space the missed dose and the next dose 5 to 6 hours apart; if you take 3 or more doses a day, space the missed dose and the next one 2 to 4 hours apart. Never take 2 doses at the same time.
■ *Storage instructions...*
   The liquid form of erythromycin should be kept in the refrigerator. Do not freeze. Store tablets and capsules at room temperature.

## What side effects may occur?

Side effects cannot be anticipated. If any develop or change in intensity, inform your doctor as soon as possible. Only your doctor can determine whether it is safe to continue taking this medication.

■ *More common side effects may include:*
   Abdominal pain, diarrhea, loss of appetite, nausea, vomiting
■ *Less common side effects may include:*
   Hives, rash, skin eruptions, yellow eyes and skin
■ *Rare side effects may include:*
   Hearing loss (temporary), inflammation of the large intestine, irregular heartbeat, severe allergic reaction, skin reddening

## Why should this drug not be prescribed?

You should not use erythromycin if you have ever had an allergic reaction to it or are sensitive to it. Erythromycin should not be used with Seldane or Hismanal.

## Special warnings about this medication

If you have ever had liver disease, consult your doctor before taking erythromycin.

If a new infection (called superinfection) develops, talk to your doctor. You may need to be treated with a different antibiotic.

## Possible food and drug interactions when taking this medication

If erythromycin is taken with certain other drugs, the effects of either could be increased, decreased, or altered. It is especially important to check with your doctor before combining erythromycin with the following:

Astemizole (Hismanal)
Blood-thinning drugs such as Coumadin
Bromocriptine (Parlodel)
Carbamazepine (Tegretol)
Cyclosporine (Sandimmune, Neoral)
Digoxin (Lanoxin)
Dihydroergotamine (D.H.E. 45)
Disopyramide (Norpace)
Ergotamine (Cafergot)
Hexobarbital
Lovastatin (Mevacor)
Phenytoin (Dilantin)
Terfenadine (Seldane)
Theophylline (Theo-Dur)
Triazolam (Halcion)

## Special information if you are pregnant or breastfeeding

If you are pregnant or plan to become pregnant, inform your doctor immediately. Erythromycin appears in breast milk and could affect a nursing infant. If this medication is essential to your health, your doctor may advise you to discontinue breastfeeding until your treatment is finished.

## Recommended dosage

Dosage instructions are determined by the type (and severity) of infection being treated and may vary slightly for different brands of erythromycin. The following are recommended dosages for PCE, one of the most commonly prescribed brands.

### ADULTS

*Streptococcal Infections*
The usual dose is 333 milligrams every 8 hours, or 500 milligrams every 12 hours. Depending on the severity of the infection, the dose may be increased to a total of 4 grams a day. However, when the daily dosage is larger than 1 gram, twice-a-day doses are not recommended, and the drug should be taken more often in smaller doses.

To treat streptococcal infections of the upper respiratory tract (tonsillitis or strep throat), erythromycin should be taken for 10 days.

*To Prevent Bacterial Endocarditis (Inflammation and Infection of the Heart Lining and Valves) in Those Allergic to Penicillin*
The oral regimen is 1 gram of erythromycin taken 1 hour before dental surgery or surgical procedures of the upper respiratory tract, followed by 500 milligrams 6 hours later.

*Urinary Tract Infections Due to Chlamydia Trachomatis During Pregnancy*
The usual dosage is 500 milligrams of erythromycin orally 4 times a day or 666 milligrams every 8 hours on an empty stomach for at least 7 days. For women who cannot tolerate this regimen, a decreased dose of 500 milligrams every 12 hours or 333 milligrams every 8 hours a day should be used for at least 14 days.

*For Those with Uncomplicated Urinary, Reproductive Tract, or Rectal Infections Caused by Chlamydia Trachomatis When Tetracycline Cannot Be Taken*
The usual oral dosage is 500 milligrams of erythromycin 4 times a day or 666 milligrams every 8 hours for at least 7 days.

*For Those with Nongonococcal Urethral Infections When Tetracycline Cannot Be Taken*
The usual dosage is 500 milligrams of erythromycin by mouth 4 times a day or 666 milligrams orally every 8 hours for at least 7 days.

*Acute Pelvic Inflammatory Disease Caused by Neisseria Gonorrhoeae*
The usual treatment is three days of intravenous erythromycin followed by 500 milligrams orally every 12 hours or 333 milligrams orally every 8 hours for 7 days.

*Syphilis*
The usual dosage is 30 to 40 grams divided into smaller doses over a period of 10 to 15 days.

*Intestinal Infections*
The usual dosage is 500 milligrams every 12 hours, or 333 milligrams every 8 hours, for 10 to 14 days.

*Legionnaires' Disease*
The usual dosage ranges from 1 to 4 grams daily, divided into smaller doses.

CHILDREN

Age, weight, and severity of the infection determine the correct dosage.

The usual dosage is from 30 to 50 milligrams daily for each 2.2 pounds of body weight, divided into equal doses.

For more severe infections, this dosage may be doubled, but it should not exceed 4 grams per day.

Children weighing over 44 pounds should follow the recommended adult dose schedule.

### Overdosage
Any medication taken in excess can have serious consequences. If you suspect an overdose, seek medical help immediately.

■ *Symptoms of erythromycin overdose may include:*
Diarrhea, nausea, stomach cramps, vomiting

*Generic name:*

# Erythromycin, Topical

*Pronounced: err-rith-ro-MY-sin*
*Brand names: A/T/S, Erycette, T-Stat*

### Why is this drug prescribed?
Topical erythromycin (applied directly to the skin) is used for the treatment of acne.

### Most important fact about this drug
For best results, you should continue the treatment for as long as prescribed, even if your acne begins to clear up. This medicine is not an instant cure.

### How should you use this medication?
Use exactly as prescribed by your doctor.

Thoroughly wash the affected area with soap and water and pat dry before applying medication.

Moisten the applicator or pad with the medication and lightly spread it over the affected area. A/T/S Topical Gel should not be rubbed in.

■ *If you miss a dose...*
Apply the forgotten dose as soon as you remember. If it is almost time for the next application, skip the one you missed and go back to your regular schedule.
■ *Storage instructions...*
This medicine can be stored at room temperature.

### What side effects may occur?
Side effects cannot be anticipated. If any develop or change in intensity, inform your doctor as soon as possible. Only your doctor can determine if it is safe for you to continue using topical erythromycin.

■ *Side effects may include:*
Burning sensation, dryness, hives, irritation of the eyes, itching, oiliness, peeling, scaling, tenderness, unusual redness of the skin

### Why should this drug not be prescribed?
Erythromycin should not be used if you are sensitive to or have ever had an allergic reaction to any of the ingredients.

### Special warnings about this medication
This type of erythromycin is for external use only. Do not use it in the eyes, nose, or mouth.

If the acne does not improve after 6 to 8 weeks of treatment, or if it gets worse, stop using the topical erythromycin preparation and call your doctor.

The use of antibiotics can stimulate the growth of other bacteria that are resistant to the antibiotic you are taking. If new infections (called superinfections) occur, talk to your doctor. You may need to be treated with a different antibiotic drug.

The use of other topical acne medications in combination with topical erythromycin may cause irritation, especially with the use of peeling, scaling, or abrasive medications.

The safety and effectiveness of A/T/S have not been established in children.

### Possible food and drug interactions when using this medication
If topical erythromycin is used with certain other drugs, the effects of either could be increased, decreased, or altered. It is especially important to check with your doctor before combining topical erythromycin with other topical acne medications.

### Special information if you are pregnant or breastfeeding
The effects of topical erythromycin during pregnancy have not been adequately studied. If you are pregnant or plan to become pregnant, inform your doctor immediately. Erythromycin may appear in breast milk and could affect a nursing infant. If this medication is essential to your health, your doctor may advise you to stop breastfeeding until your treatment with erythromycin is finished.

## Recommended dosage

Apply solution to the affected area 2 times a day. Moisten the applicator or a pad, then spread over the affected area. Use additional pads as needed. Apply gel products as a thin film over the affected area once or twice a day.

Make sure the area is thoroughly washed with soap and water and patted dry before applying medication. Thoroughly wash your hands after application of the medication.

Reducing the frequency of applications may reduce peeling and drying.

## Overdosage

Although overdosage is unlikely, any medication used in excess can have serious consequences. If you suspect an overdose, seek medical treatment immediately.

*Generic name:*

# Erythromycin with Benzoyl peroxide

*See Benzamycin, page 58.*

*Generic name:*

# Erythromycin with Sulfisoxazole

*See Pediazole, page 400.*

*Brand name:*

# Esgic

*See Fioricet, page 209.*

*Brand name:*

# Esidrix

*See HydroDIURIL, page 240.*

*Brand name:*

# Eskalith

*See Lithonate, page 285.*

*Generic name:*

# Estazolam

*See ProSom, page 444.*

*Brand name:*

# Estrace

*See Estraderm, page 199.*

*Brand name:*

# Estraderm

Pronounced: ESS-tra-derm
Generic name: Estradiol
Other brand names: Climara, Estrace

## Why is this drug prescribed?

Estraderm is an estrogen replacement drug. It is used to reduce symptoms of menopause, including feelings of warmth in face, neck, and chest, and the sudden intense episodes of heat and sweating known as "hot flashes." It is also used for other conditions caused by lack of estrogen, such as dry, itchy external genitals and vaginal irritation, and may be prescribed for teenagers who fail to mature at the usual rate.

Along with diet, calcium supplements, and exercise, Estraderm is also prescribed to prevent osteoporosis, a condition in which the bones become brittle and easily broken.

In addition, Climara is used to treat abnormal bleeding from the uterus in some cases. Estrace and Climara are also used to treat low levels of estrogen in certain people; Estrace is used to provide relief in breast or prostate cancer.

## Most important fact about this drug

Because estrogens have been linked with increased risk of endometrial cancer (cancer in the lining of the uterus), it is essential to have regular checkups and to report any unusual vaginal bleeding to your doctor immediately.

## How should you take this medication?

Each Estraderm and Climara patch is individually sealed in a protective pouch and is applied directly to the skin.

A stiff protective liner covers the adhesive side of the patch. Remove the liner by sliding it sideways between your thumb and index finger. Holding the patch at one edge, remove the protective liner and discard it. Try to avoid touching the adhesive. Use immediately after removing the liner.

Apply the adhesive side to a clean, dry area of your skin on the trunk of your body (including the buttocks and abdomen). Do not apply to your breasts or waist. Firmly press the patch in place with the palm of your hand for about 10 seconds, to make sure the edges are flat against your skin. Climara is applied only to the abdomen and is pressed in place with the fingers.

Contact with water during bathing, swimming, or showering will not affect the patch.

The application site must be rotated. Allow an interval of at least 1 week between applications to a particular site.

Estrace Tablets are taken orally.

If you are using Estrace vaginal cream, follow these steps to apply:

1. Load the supplied applicator to the fill line.
2. Lie on your back with your knees drawn up.
3. Gently insert the applicator high into the vagina. Release the medicine by pushing the plunger.
4. Withdraw the applicator.
5. Wash the applicator with soap and water.

■ *If you miss a dose...*
If you forget to apply a new patch when you are supposed to, do it as soon as you remember. If it is almost time to change patches anyway, skip the one you missed and go back to your regular schedule. Do not apply more than one patch at a time.

If you miss a dose of the tablets, take it as soon as you remember. If it is almost time for your next dose, skip the one you missed and go back to your regular schedule. Do not take 2 doses at once.

■ *Storage instructions...*
Store Estraderm and Climara at room temperature, in their sealed pouches. Store Estrace at room temperature.

## What side effects may occur?
Side effects cannot be anticipated. If any develop or change in intensity, notify your doctor as soon as possible. Only your doctor can determine if it is safe for you to continue taking Estraderm.

■ *The most common side effect is:*
Skin redness and irritation at the site of the patch.
■ *Less common or rare side effects may include:*
Abdominal cramps, bloating, breakthrough bleeding, breast enlargement, breast tenderness, change in cervical secretions, change in menstrual flow, change in sex drive, change in weight, darkening of skin, dizziness, fluid retention, growth of benign fibroid tumors in the uterus, headache, intolerance to contact lenses, migraine, nausea, rash, severe allergic reaction, spotting, vomiting, yellowing of eyes and skin
■ *Other side effects reported with estradiol include:*
Abnormal withdrawal bleeding, certain cancers, cardiovascular disease, depression, excessive growth of hair, gallbladder disease, hair loss, high blood pressure, reddened skin, skin discoloration, skin eruptions, twitching, vaginal yeast infection

## Why should this drug not be prescribed?
Estraderm should not be used if you are sensitive to or have ever had an allergic reaction to any of its components.

Estrogens should not be used if you have ever had breast or uterine cancer or a tumor promoted by estrogen. Also avoid estrogens if you are pregnant or think you are pregnant, if you have abnormal, undiagnosed genital bleeding, if you have blood clots or a blood clotting disorder, or if you have a history of blood clotting disorders associated with previous estrogen use.

## Special warnings about this medication
The risk of cancer of the uterus increases when estrogen is used for a long time or taken in large doses. There also may be increased risk of breast cancer in women who take estrogen for an extended period of time or in high doses.

Women who take estrogen after menopause are more likely to develop gallbladder disease.

Estrogen also increases the risk of blood clots. These blood clots can cause stroke, heart attack, or other serious disorders.

While taking Estraderm, get in touch with your doctor right away if you notice any of the following:

Abdominal pain, tenderness, or swelling
Abnormal bleeding of the vagina
Breast lumps

Coughing up blood
Pain in your chest or calves
Severe headache, dizziness, or faintness
Sudden shortness of breath
Vision changes
Yellowing of the skin

A complete medical and family history should be taken by your doctor before starting any estrogen therapy.

In general, you should not take estrogen for more than 1 year without another physical examination by your doctor.

Estraderm may cause fluid retention in some people. If you have asthma, epilepsy, migraine, or heart or kidney disease, use this medication cautiously.

Estrogen therapy may cause uterine bleeding or breast pain.

## Possible food and drug interactions when taking this medication

If you take certain other drugs while using Estraderm, the effects of either could be increased, decreased, or altered. It is especially important to check with your doctor before taking the following:

Barbiturates such as phenobarbital and Seconal
Blood thinners such as Coumadin
Dantrolene (Dantrium)
Epilepsy drugs such as Tegretol and Dilantin
Rifampin (Rifadin)
Steroids such as Deltasone
Tricyclic antidepressants such as Elavil and
    Tofranil

## Special information if you are pregnant or breastfeeding

Estrogens should not be used during pregnancy or immediately after childbirth. Use of estrogens during pregnancy has been linked to reproductive tract problems in the children. If you are pregnant or plan to become pregnant, notify your doctor immediately. Estraderm may appear in breast milk and could affect a nursing infant. Estrogens decrease the quantity and quality of breast milk. If this medication is essential to your health, your doctor may advise you to discontinue breastfeeding until your treatment is finished.

## Recommended dosage
### SYMPTOMS OF MENOPAUSE

*Estraderm*
The usual starting dose is one 0.05 milligram patch applied to the skin 2 times a week. Dosage should be decreased at 3- to 6-month intervals.

*Estrace*
The usual starting dose is 1 or 2 milligrams a day; you will take the tablets for 3 weeks and then have 1 week off for each cycle.

*Climara*
The usual starting dose for all uses is one 3.9 milligram patch applied to the skin once a week. You will use the patch for 3 weeks, then have 1 week off. Your doctor will prescribe the lowest effective dose, and try to reduce the dose or discontinue the medication every 3 to 6 months.

### PREVENTION OF OSTEOPOROSIS

*Estraderm*
The usual starting dose is 0.05 milligram per day.

*Estrace*
The usual dose is 0.5 milligram taken every day for 23 days, followed by 5 days off.

### LOW ESTROGEN LEVELS

*Estrace*
The usual starting dose is 1 or 2 milligrams a day.

### RELIEF IN BREAST CANCER

*Estrace*
The usual dose is 10 milligrams 3 times a day for at least 3 months.

### RELIEF IN PROSTATE CANCER

*Estrace*
The usual dose is 1 to 2 milligrams 3 times a day.

### VAGINAL ITCHING AND DRYNESS

*Estrace Vaginal Cream*
The usual dosage is 2 to 4 grams (marked on the applicator) inserted into the vagina once a day, for 1 to 2 weeks. The dosage and frequency may be reduced after your condition improves.

To prevent recurrence, a dosage of 1 gram 1 to 3 times a week is recommended.

### Overdosage

Any medication taken in excess can have serious consequences. If you suspect an overdose, seek medical attention immediately.

■ *Symptoms of Estraderm overdose may include:*
Nausea, vomiting, withdrawal bleeding

---

*Generic name:*

# Estradiol

See Estraderm, page 199.

---

*Generic name:*

# Estropipate

See Ogen, page 379.

---

*Generic name:*

# Etodolac

See Lodine, page 287.

---

*Brand name:*

# Eulexin

*Pronounced: you-LEKS-in*
*Generic name: Flutamide*

### Why is this drug prescribed?

Eulexin is used along with drugs such as Lupron to treat prostate cancer. Eulexin belongs to a class of drugs known as antiandrogens. It blocks the effect of the male hormone testosterone. Giving Eulexin with Lupron, which reduces the body's testosterone levels, is one way of treating prostate cancer.

### Most important fact about this drug

Taking Eulexin and Lupron together is essential in this form of treatment. You should not interrupt their doses or stop taking either of these medications without consulting your doctor.

### How should you take this medication?

Take Eulexin exactly as prescribed. Do not use more or less, and do not take it more often than instructed.

■ *If you miss a dose...*
Take it as soon as you remember. If it is almost time for your next dose, skip the one you missed and go back to your regular schedule. Never take 2 doses at once.
■ *Storage instructions...*
Store at room temperature.

### What side effects may occur?

Side effects cannot be anticipated. If any develop or change in intensity, inform your doctor immediately. Since Eulexin is always given with another antiandrogen drug, when a side effect develops, it is difficult to know which drug is responsible. Only your doctor can determine if it is safe for you to continue taking Eulexin.

■ *More common side effects may include:*
Breast tissue swelling and tenderness, diarrhea, hot flashes, impotence, loss of sex drive, nausea, vomiting
■ *Less common side effects may include:*
Confusion, decreased sexual ability, jaundice and liver damage, rash, sun sensitivity (rashes, blisters upon exposure to sun), urine discoloration (amber or yellow-green)

### Why should this drug not be prescribed?

Do not take Eulexin if you have ever had an allergic reaction to it or are sensitive to it or to any of the colorings or other inactive ingredients in the capsules.

### Special warnings about this medication

Eulexin may cause liver damage in some people. Your doctor will do blood tests to check your liver function before you start treatment with Eulexin, and at regular intervals thereafter. If a liver problem does develop, you may need to take less Eulexin or stop taking the drug altogether. Report any signs or symptoms that might suggest liver damage to your doctor right away. Warning signs include dark urine, itching, flu-like symptoms, jaundice (a yellowing of the skin and eyes), persistent appetite loss, and persistent tenderness on the right side of the upper abdomen.

### Possible food and drug interactions when taking this medication

If you are already taking the anticoagulant drug warfarin (Coumadin), you will need to be monitored especially closely after treatment with Eulexin begins. Your doctor may need to lower your dosage of warfarin.

## Recommended dosage

The recommended adult Eulexin dosage is 2 capsules 3 times a day at 8-hour intervals for a total daily dosage of 750 milligrams.

## Overdosage

You may notice breast development or tenderness with an overdose of Eulexin. Any medication taken in excess can have serious consequences. If you suspect an overdose, seek medical attention immediately.

*Brand name:*

# Exgest LA

*See Entex LA, page 194.*

*Generic name:*

# Famciclovir

*See Famvir, page 203.*

*Generic name:*

# Famotidine

*See Pepcid, page 405.*

*Brand name:*

# Famvir

*Pronounced: FAM-veer*
*Generic name: Famciclovir*

## Why is this drug prescribed?

Famvir tablets are used to treat herpes zoster, commonly referred to as "shingles," in adults. Shingles is a painful rash with raised, red pimples on the trunk of the body, usually the back. Because it is caused by the same virus that causes chickenpox, only people who have had chickenpox can get shingles.

## Most important fact about this drug

Famvir is most effective if started within the first 48 hours after shingles first appears. The effectiveness of Famvir if treatment is begun more than 72 hours after the rash first appears is not known. Thus, it is important to see your doctor as soon as possible after symptoms appear.

## How should you take this medication?

Take this medication exactly as prescribed by your doctor. You may take Famvir with meals or in between.

■ *If you miss a dose...*
Take the forgotten dose as soon as you remember. If it is almost time for your next dose, skip the one you missed and go back to your regular schedule. Never take two doses at the same time.
■ *Storage instructions...*
Store at room temperature.

## What side effects may occur?

Side effects cannot be anticipated. If any develop or change in intensity, inform your doctor as soon as possible. Only your doctor can determine if it is safe for you to continue taking Famvir.

■ *More common side effects may include:*
Constipation, diarrhea, dizziness, fatigue, fever, headache, nausea, vomiting
■ *Less common side effects may include:*
Abdominal pain, back pain, chills and fever, injury, irritated sinuses, itching, joint pain, loss of appetite, pain, prickling or burning sensation of the skin, sleepiness, sore throat

## Why should this drug not be prescribed?

Do not take Famvir if you are sensitive to it or have ever had an allergic reaction to it.

## Special warnings about this medication

Famvir helps relieve the rash associated with shingles, but it is not a cure. Studies of the drug have found that the rash and pimples healed faster with Famvir than they did in people not taking Famvir. If you have any kidney problems, be sure your doctor knows about them before prescribing Famvir for you.

## Possible food and drug interactions when taking this medication

If Famvir is taken with certain other drugs, the effects of either could be increased, decreased, or altered. It is especially important to check with your doctor before combining Famvir with probenecid (Benemid), a drug used to treat gout (a type of arthritis).

## Special information if you are pregnant or breastfeeding

The effects of Famvir during pregnancy have not been adequately studied. If you are pregnant or plan to become pregnant, inform your doctor immediately. Famvir should be used during pregnancy only when the benefit to the mother clearly outweighs the potential risk to the baby. Famvir may appear in breast milk, and could affect a nursing infant. If this drug is essential to your health, your doctor may advise you to discontinue breastfeeding until your treatment with Famvir is finished.

### Recommended dosage
ADULTS

The usual adult dose is 500 milligrams every 8 hours for 7 days.

### Overdosage
There have been no reported cases of Famvir overdose, but any medication taken in excess can have serious consequences. If you suspect an overdose, seek medical attention immediately.

*Brand name:*

# Fastin

*Pronounced: FAS-tin*
*Generic name: Phentermine hydrochloride*
*Other brand names: Ionamin, Oby-Cap*

### Why is this drug prescribed?
Fastin, an appetite suppressant, is prescribed for short-term use (a few weeks) as part of an overall diet plan for weight reduction. Fastin should be used along with a behavior modification program.

### Most important fact about this drug
Always remember that Fastin is an aid to, not a substitute for, good diet and exercise. Take Fastin only as directed by your doctor. Do not take it more often or for a longer time than your doctor has ordered. Fastin can lose its effectiveness after a few weeks.

### How should you take this medication?
Take Fastin about 2 hours after breakfast. Do not take it late in the evening because it may keep you from sleeping.

Take Ionamin before breakfast or 10 to 14 hours before you go to bed. Ionamin capsules should be swallowed whole.

■ *If you miss a dose...*
Skip the missed dose completely; then take the next dose at the regularly scheduled time.

■ *Storage instructions...*
Store at room temperature.

### What side effects may occur?
Side effects cannot be anticipated. If any develop or change in intensity, inform your doctor as soon as possible. Only your doctor can determine if it is safe for you to continue taking this medication.

■ *Side effects may include:*
Changes in sex drive, constipation, diarrhea, dizziness, dry mouth, exaggerated feelings of depression or elation, headache, high blood pressure, hives, impotence, inability to fall or stay asleep, increased heart rate, overstimulation, restlessness, stomach or intestinal problems, throbbing heartbeat, tremors, unpleasant taste

### Why should this drug not be prescribed?
If you are sensitive to or have ever had an allergic reaction to phentermine hydrochloride or other drugs that stimulate the nervous system, you should not take this medication. Make sure your doctor is aware of any drug reactions you have experienced.

Do not take this drug if you have hardening of the arteries, symptoms of heart or blood vessel disease, an overactive thyroid gland, the eye condition known as glaucoma, or moderate to severe high blood pressure. Also avoid this drug if you are agitated, have ever abused drugs, or have taken an MAO inhibitor, including antidepressant drugs such as Nardil and Parnate, within the last 14 days.

### Special warnings about this medication
Fastin may affect your ability to perform potentially hazardous activities. Therefore, you should be extremely careful if you have to drive a car or operate machinery.

You can become psychologically dependent on this drug. Consult your doctor if you rely on this drug to maintain a state of well-being.

If you stop taking Fastin suddenly after you have taken high doses for a long time, you may find you are extremely fatigued or depressed, or that you have trouble sleeping.

If you continually take too much of any appetite suppressant it can cause severe skin disorders, a pronounced inability to fall or stay asleep, irritability, hyperactivity, and personality changes.

Even if your blood pressure is only mildly high, be careful taking this drug.

## Possible food and drug interactions when taking this medication

This drug may react badly with alcohol. Avoid alcoholic beverages while you are taking it.

If Fastin is taken with certain other drugs, the effects of either can be increased, decreased, or altered. It is especially important that you check with your doctor before combining Fastin with the following:

Antidepressants classified as MAO inhibitors, including Nardil and Parnate
Diabetes medications such as insulin and Micronase
High blood pressure medications such as guanethidine (Ismelin)

## Special information if you are pregnant or breastfeeding

The effects of Fastin during pregnancy have not been adequately studied. If you are pregnant, plan to become pregnant, or are breastfeeding, notify your doctor immediately.

## Recommended dosage

ADULTS

*Fastin or Oby-Cap*
The usual dosage is 1 capsule approximately 2 hours after breakfast. One capsule should suppress your appetite for 12 to 14 hours.

*Ionamin*
The usual dose is 1 capsule a day, taken before breakfast or 10 to 14 hours before bedtime.

CHILDREN

This drug is not recommended for use in children under 12 years of age.

## Overdosage

Any medication taken in excess can have serious consequences. An overdose of Fastin can be fatal. If you suspect an overdose, seek emergency medical treatment immediately.

■ *Symptoms of Fastin overdose may include:*
Abdominal cramps, aggressiveness, confusion, diarrhea, exaggerated reflexes, hallucinations, high or low blood pressure, irregular heartbeat, nausea, panic states, rapid breathing, restlessness, tremors, vomiting

Fatigue and depression may follow the stimulant effects of Fastin.

In cases of fatal poisoning, convulsions and coma usually precede death.

*Generic name:*

# Felbamate

See Felbatol, page 205.

*Brand name:*

# Felbatol

Pronounced: FELL-ba-tohl
Generic name: Felbamate

## Why is this drug prescribed?

Felbatol, a relatively new epilepsy medication, is used alone or with other drugs to treat partial seizures with or without generalization (seizures in which consciousness may be retained or lost). It is also used with other medications to treat seizures associated with Lennox-Gastaut syndrome (a childhood condition characterized by brief loss of awareness and muscle tone).

Felbatol is prescribed only when other medications have failed to control severe cases of epilepsy.

## Most important fact about this drug

When taking Felbatol, be alert for signs of a very rare but dangerous side effect called aplastic anemia, in which the red blood cell count declines drastically. Warning signs include weakness, fatigue, and a tendency to easily bruise or bleed. Be on the watch, also, for signs of liver problems such as yellowing of the skin or eyes. There have been reports of fatal cases of liver failure among people taking Felbatol.

## How should you take this medication?

Take this medication exactly as prescribed by your doctor. Felbatol should not be stopped suddenly. This could increase the frequency of your seizures.

If you are taking Felbatol liquid, shake well before using.

■ *If you miss a dose...*
Take the forgotten dose as soon as you remember. If it is almost time for your next dose, skip the one you missed and go back to your regular schedule. Never take a double dose.

■ *Storage instructions...*
Felbatol should be stored in a tightly closed container, at room temperature, away from excessive heat and moisture.

## What side effects may occur?
Side effects cannot be anticipated. If any develop or change in intensity, notify your doctor as soon as possible. Only your doctor can determine if it is safe for you to continue taking Felbatol.

■ *Side effects in adults taking Felbatol alone may include:*
Acne, anxiety, constipation, diarrhea, double vision, ear infection, facial swelling, fatigue, headache, inability to fall or stay asleep, indigestion, loss of appetite, menstrual irregularities, nausea, nasal inflammation, rash, upper respiratory infection, urinary tract infection, vomiting, weight decrease

■ *Side effects in adults taking Felbatol with other medication may include:*
Abdominal pain, abnormal stride, abnormal taste, abnormal vision, anxiety, chest pain, constipation, depression, diarrhea, dizziness, double vision, dry mouth, fatigue, fever, headache, inability to fall or stay asleep, indigestion, lack of muscle coordination, loss of appetite, muscle pain, nausea, nervousness, pins and needles, rash, sinus inflammation, sleepiness, sore throat, stupor, tremor, upper respiratory infection, vomiting

■ *Side effects in children taking Felbatol with other medication may include:*
Abnormal stride, abnormal thinking, abnormally small pupils (pinpoint pupils), constipation, coughing, diarrhea, ear infection, fatigue, fever, headache, hiccups, inability to control urination, inability to fall or stay asleep, indigestion, lack of muscle coordination, loss of appetite, mood changes, nausea, nervousness, pain, rash, red or purple spots on skin, sleepiness, sore throat, taste changes, unstable emotions, upper respiratory infection, vomiting, weight decrease

## Why should this drug not be prescribed?
If you are sensitive to or have ever had an allergic reaction to Felbatol or similar drugs, or if you have ever had any blood abnormalities or liver problems, do not take this medication. Make sure your doctor is aware of any drug reactions you have experienced.

## Special warnings about this medication
Remember to watch for signs of aplastic anemia. (See "Most important fact about this drug.") If you have ever had liver problems, be sure to tell your doctor.

Expect your doctor to monitor your response carefully when you start taking Felbatol and to check your liver function every 1 or 2 weeks.

## Possible food and drug interactions when taking this medication
If you are taking Felbatol with certain other drugs, the effects of either could be increased, decreased, or altered. It is especially important to check with your doctor before combining Felbatol with other epilepsy drugs, such as Dilantin, Depakene, Depakote, and Tegretol.

## Special information if you are pregnant or breastfeeding
The effects of Felbatol during pregnancy have not been adequately studied. If you are pregnant or plan to become pregnant, inform your doctor immediately. Felbatol appears in breast milk and could affect a nursing infant. If this medication is essential to your health, your doctor may advise you to discontinue breastfeeding until your treatment is finished.

## Recommended dosage
ADULTS 14 YEARS OF AGE AND OVER

Whether Felbatol is taken alone or with other antiepileptic drugs, the usual starting dose is 1,200 milligrams per day divided into smaller doses and taken 3 or 4 times daily. Your doctor may gradually increase your daily dose to as much as 3,600 milligrams.

If you are already taking a drug to control your epilepsy, your doctor will reduce its dosage when you add Felbatol.

CHILDREN WITH LENNOX-GASTAUT SYNDROME (2 TO 14 YEARS)

The usual dose is 15 milligrams per 2.2 pounds of body weight per day divided into smaller doses taken 3 or 4 times daily. Your doctor may gradually increase your child's dose to 45 milligrams per 2.2 pounds of body weight per day. The doctor will reduce the amount of any other epilepsy drug your child is taking when starting Felbatol.

## Overdosage

Any medication taken in excess can have serious consequences. If you suspect an overdose, seek medical treatment immediately.

■ *Symptoms of Felbatol overdose may include:*
Mild stomach upset, unusually fast heartbeat

*Brand name:*

# Feldene

*Pronounced: FELL-deen*
*Generic name: Piroxicam*

### Why is this drug prescribed?

Feldene, a nonsteroidal anti-inflammatory drug, is used to relieve the inflammation, swelling, stiffness, and joint pain associated with rheumatoid arthritis and osteoarthritis (the most common form of arthritis). It is prescribed both for sudden flare-ups and for long-term treatment.

### Most important fact about this drug

In a few patients on long-term therapy, Feldene can cause stomach ulcers and bleeding. Warning signs include severe abdominal or stomach cramps, pain or burning in the stomach, and black, tarry stools. Inform your doctor immediately if you develop any of these symptoms.

### How should you take this medication?

To avoid digestive side effects, take Feldene with food or an antacid, and with a full glass of water. Never take it on an empty stomach.

Take this medication exactly as prescribed by your doctor. Avoid alcohol and aspirin while taking this drug.

■ *If you miss a dose...*
If you forget to take a dose, take it as soon as you remember. If it is almost time for your next dose, skip the one you missed and go back to your regular schedule. Never take two doses at the same time.

■ *Storage instructions...*
Store at room temperature. Protect from light and heat.

### What side effects may occur?

Side effects cannot be anticipated. If any develop or change in intensity, inform your doctor as soon as possible. Only your doctor can determine if it is safe for you to continue taking Feldene.

■ *More common side effects may include:*
Abdominal pain or discomfort, anemia, constipation, diarrhea, dizziness, fluid retention, gas, general feeling of ill health, headache, heartburn, indigestion, inflammation inside the mouth, itching, loss of appetite, nausea, rash, ringing in ears, sleepiness, stomach upset, vertigo

■ *Less common or rare side effects may include:*
Abdominal bleeding, severe allergic reactions, angioedema (swelling of lips, face, tongue and throat), black stools, blood in the urine, blurred vision, bruising, colicky pain, congestive heart failure (worsening of), depression, dry mouth, eye irritations, fatigue, fever, flu-like symptoms, hepatitis, high blood pressure, hives, inability to sleep, joint pain, labored breathing, low or high blood sugar, nervousness, nosebleed, serum sickness (fever, painful joints, enlarged lymph nodes, skin rash), skin allergy to sunlight, skin eruptions, Stevens-Johnson syndrome (blisters in the mouth and eyes), sweating, swollen eyes, vomiting, vomiting blood, weight loss or gain, wheezing, worsening of angina, yellow eyes and skin

### Why should this drug not be prescribed?

If you are sensitive to or have ever had an allergic reaction to Feldene, aspirin, or similar drugs, or if you have had asthma attacks caused by aspirin or other drugs of this type, you should not take this medication. Make sure that your doctor is aware of any drug reactions that you have experienced.

### Special warnings about this medication

If you have heart disease, or high blood pressure, or other conditions that cause fluid retention, use this drug with caution. Feldene can increase water retention.

This drug should be used with caution if you have kidney or liver disease; it can cause liver inflammation in some people.

Drugs such as Feldene may cause eye disturbances in some people. If you develop visual problems, notify your eye doctor.

### Possible food and drug interactions when taking this medication

If Feldene is taken with certain other drugs, the effects of either could be increased, decreased, or altered. It is especially important to check with your doctor before combining Feldene with the following:

Anticoagulants (blood thinners such as Coumadin)
Aspirin
Lithium

### Special information if you are pregnant or breastfeeding

Feldene is not recommended for use in nursing mothers or pregnant women. If you are pregnant or plan to become pregnant, inform your doctor immediately.

### Recommended dosage

ADULTS

*Rheumatoid Arthritis and Osteoarthritis:*
The usual dose is 20 milligrams a day in one dose. Your doctor may want you to divide this dose into smaller ones. You will not feel Feldene's full effects for 7 to 12 days, although some relief of symptoms will start to occur soon after you take the medication.

CHILDREN

The safety and effectiveness of Feldene have not been established in children.

### Overdosage

Although there are no specific symptoms of a Feldene overdose, any medication taken in excess can have serious consequences. If you suspect an overdose, seek medical attention immediately.

*Generic name:*

# Felodipine

*See Plendil, page 422.*

*Brand name:*

# Femstat

*Pronounced: FEM-stat*
*Generic name: Butoconazole nitrate*

### Why is this drug prescribed?

Femstat Vaginal Cream is prescribed for the treatment of yeast-like fungal infections of the vulva and vagina.

### Most important fact about this drug

To obtain maximum benefit, it is important that you continue to use Femstat Vaginal Cream during menstruation and that you finish using all of the medication, even if your symptoms have disappeared.

### How should you use this medication?

Use this medication exactly as prescribed. To keep it from getting on your clothing, wear a sanitary napkin. Do not use a tampon; it will absorb the drug. Do not douche unless your doctor tells you to do so.

While using Femstat, wear cotton underwear or pantyhose with a cotton crotch. Avoid synthetic fabrics such as rayon and nylon.

*To apply Femstat:*
1. Fill the applicator that comes with the vaginal cream to the level indicated.
2. Lie on your back with your knees drawn up.
3. Gently insert the applicator high into the vagina and push the plunger.
4. Withdraw the applicator and discard if disposable or wash with soap and water.

To avoid reinfection, refrain from intercourse during treatment or ask your partner to use a condom.

■ *If you miss a dose...*
Insert it as soon as you remember. If it is almost time for your next dose, skip the one you missed and go back to your regular schedule.

■ *Storage instructions...*
Store at room temperature, away from heat. Do not freeze.

### What side effects may occur?

Side effects cannot be anticipated. If any develop or change in intensity, inform your doctor as soon as possible. Only your doctor can determine if it is safe for you to continue using Femstat.

■ *Side effects may include:*
Itching of the fingers, soreness, swelling, vaginal discharge, vulvar itching, vulvar or vaginal burning

### Why should this drug not be prescribed?

If you are sensitive to or have ever had an allergic reaction to butoconazole nitrate or any other ingredients in Femstat Cream, you should not use this medication. Make sure your doctor is aware of any drug reactions you have experienced.

## Special warnings about this medication

If your symptoms persist, or if you become irritated or have an allergic reaction while using this medication, notify your doctor.

## Possible food and drug interactions when taking this medication

No interactions with other drugs have been reported.

## Special information if you are pregnant or breastfeeding

The effects of Femstat Cream during the first trimester (first 3 months) of pregnancy have not been adequately studied. However, women using this cream for 3 to 6 days during the second or third trimester of pregnancy have experienced no adverse effects or complications, nor have their infants. It is not known whether this drug appears in breast milk. If Femstat is essential to your health, your doctor may advise you to discontinue breastfeeding until your treatment is finished.

## Recommended dosage

ADULTS

*Non-pregnant Women*
The recommended dose is 1 applicatorful of cream inserted in the vagina at bedtime for 3 days. Your doctor may extend your treatment for an additional 3 days if necessary.

*Pregnant Women (Second and Third Trimesters Only)*
The recommended dose is 1 applicatorful of cream inserted in the vagina at bedtime for 6 days.

CHILDREN

Safety and effectiveness have not been established in children.

## Overdosage

No overdosage has been reported.

*Generic name:*

# Finasteride

*See Proscar, page 443.*

*Brand name:*

# Fioricet

*Pronounced: fee-OAR-i-set*
*Generic ingredients: Butalbital, Acetaminophen, Caffeine*
*Other brand names: Anolor 300, Esgic, Esgic Plus*

## Why is this drug prescribed?

Fioricet, a strong, nonnarcotic pain reliever and relaxant, is prescribed for the relief of tension headache symptoms caused by muscle contractions in the head, neck, and shoulder area. It combines a sedative barbiturate (butalbital), a non-aspirin pain reliever (acetaminophen), and caffeine.

## Most important fact about this drug

Mental and physical dependence can occur with the use of barbiturates such as butalbital when these drugs are taken in higher than recommended doses over long periods of time.

## How should you take this medication?

Take Fioricet exactly as prescribed. Do not increase the amount you take without your doctor's approval.

■ *If you miss a dose...*
Take it as soon as you remember. If it is almost time for your next dose, skip the one you missed and go back to your regular schedule. Never take 2 doses at the same time.

■ *Storage instructions...*
Store at room temperature in a tight, light-resistant container.

## What side effects may occur?

Side effects cannot be anticipated. If any develop or change in intensity, inform your doctor as soon as possible. Only your doctor can determine if it is safe for you to continue taking Fioricet.

■ *More common side effects may include:*
Abdominal pain, dizziness, drowsiness, intoxicated feeling, light-headedness, nausea, sedation, shortness of breath, vomiting

■ *Less common or rare side effects may include:*
Agitation, allergic reactions, constipation, depression, difficulty swallowing, dry mouth, earache, exaggerated feeling of well-being, excessive sweating, excessive urination, excitement, fainting, fatigue, fever, flatulence, headache, heartburn, heavy eyelids, high energy, hot spells, itching, leg pain, mental confusion, muscle fatigue, numbness, rapid heartbeat, ringing in the

ears, seizure, shaky feeling, skin redness and/or peeling, sluggishness, stuffy nose, tingling

## Why should this drug not be prescribed?

If you are sensitive to or have ever had an allergic reaction to barbiturates, acetaminophen, or caffeine, you should not take this medication. Make sure that your doctor is aware of any drug reactions that you have experienced.

Unless you are directed to do so by your doctor, do not take this medication if you have porphyria (an inherited metabolic disorder affecting the liver or bone marrow).

## Special warnings about this medication

Fioricet may cause you to become drowsy or less alert; therefore, driving or operating dangerous machinery or participating in any hazardous activity that requires full mental alertness is not recommended until you know your response to this drug.

If you are being treated for severe depression or have a history of severe depression or drug abuse, consult with your doctor before taking Fioricet.

Use this drug with caution if you are elderly or in a weakened condition, if you have liver or kidney problems, or if you have severe abdominal trouble.

## Possible food and drug interactions
## when taking this medication

Butalbital is a central nervous system (brain and spinal cord) depressant and intensifies the effects of alcohol and other CNS depressants. Use of alcohol with this drug may also cause overdose symptoms. Therefore, use of alcohol should be avoided.

If Fioricet is taken with certain other drugs, the effects of either could be increased, decreased, or altered. It is especially important to check with your doctor before combining Fioricet with the following:

Antidepressant drugs known as monoamine oxidase inhibitors, including Nardil and Parnate
Antihistamines such as Benadryl
Antipsychotics such as Haldol and Thorazine
Drugs to treat depression such as Elavil
Muscle relaxants such as Flexeril
Narcotic pain relievers such as Darvon
Sleep aids such as Halcion
Tranquilizers such as Xanax and Valium

## Special information
## if you are pregnant or breastfeeding

If you are pregnant or plan to become pregnant, inform your doctor immediately. Fioricet can affect a developing baby. It also appears in breast milk. If

this medication is essential to your health, your doctor may advise you to discontinue breastfeeding your baby until your treatment is finished.

## Recommended dosage

ADULTS

The usual dose of Fioricet is 1 or 2 tablets taken every 4 hours as needed. Do not exceed a total dose of 6 tablets per day.

The usual dose of Esgic-Plus is 1 tablet every 4 hours as needed. Do not take more than 6 tablets a day.

CHILDREN

The safety and effectiveness of Fioricet have not been established in children under 12 years of age.

OLDER ADULTS

Fioricet may cause excitement, depression, and confusion in older people. Therefore, your doctor will prescribe a dose individualized to suit your needs.

## Overdosage

Symptoms of Fioricet overdose can be due to its barbiturate or its acetaminophen component.

■ *Symptoms of barbiturate poisoning may include:*
Coma, confusion, drowsiness, low blood pressure, shock, slow or troubled breathing

Overdose due to the acetaminophen component of Fioricet may cause kidney and liver damage, blood disorders, or coma due to low blood sugar. Massive doses may cause liver failure.

■ *Symptoms of liver damage include:*
Excess perspiration, feeling of bodily discomfort, nausea, vomiting

If you suspect an overdose, seek emergency medical treatment immediately.

*Brand name:*

# Fiorinal

*Pronounced: fee-OR-i-nahl*
*Generic ingredients: Butalbital, Aspirin, Caffeine*
*Other brand name: Isollyl*

## Why is this drug prescribed?

Fiorinal, a strong, non-narcotic pain reliever and muscle relaxant, is prescribed for the relief of tension headache symptoms caused by stress or muscle contraction in the head, neck, and shoulder area. It combines a non-narcotic, sedative barbiturate (butalbital) with a pain reliever (aspirin) and a stimulant (caffeine).

### Most important fact about this drug

Barbiturates such as butalbital can be habit-forming if you take them over long periods of time.

### How should you take this medication?

For best relief, take Fiorinal as soon as a headache begins.

Take the medication with a full glass of water or food to reduce stomach irritation. Do not take this medication if it has a strong odor of vinegar.

Take Fiorinal exactly as prescribed. Do not increase the amount you take without your doctor's approval, or take the drug for longer than prescribed.

■ *If you miss a dose...*
If you take Fiorinal on a regular schedule, take the forgotten dose as soon as you remember. If it is almost time for your next dose, skip the one you missed and go back to your regular schedule. Do not take 2 doses at once.

■ *Storage instructions...*
Store at room temperature. Keep the container tightly closed.

### What side effects may occur?

Side effects cannot be anticipated. If any develop or change in intensity, inform your doctor as soon as possible. Only your doctor can determine if it is safe for you to continue taking Fiorinal.

■ *More common side effects may include:*
Dizziness, drowsiness
■ *Less common or rare side effects may include:*
Gas, light-headedness, nausea, skin problems, vomiting

### Why should this drug not be prescribed?

If you are sensitive to or have ever had an allergic reaction to barbiturates, aspirin, caffeine, or other sedatives and pain relievers, you should not take this medication. The aspirin in Fiorinal, in particular, can cause a severe reaction in someone allergic to it. Make sure your doctor is aware of any drug reactions you have experienced.

Unless you are directed to do so by your doctor, do not take this medication if you have porphyria

(an inherited metabolic disorder affecting the liver or bone marrow).

Because aspirin, when given to children and teenagers suffering from flu or chickenpox, can cause a dangerous neurological disease called Reye's syndrome, do not use Fiorinal under these circumstances.

Fiorinal contains aspirin. If you have a stomach (peptic) ulcer or a disorder affecting the blood clotting process, you should not take Fiorinal. Aspirin may irritate the stomach lining and may cause bleeding.

### Special warnings about this medication

Fiorinal may make you drowsy or less alert; therefore, you should not drive or operate dangerous machinery or participate in any hazardous activity that requires full mental alertness until you know your response to this drug.

If you have chronic (long-lasting or frequently recurring) tension headaches and your prescribed dose of Fiorinal does not relieve the pain, consult your doctor. Taking more of this drug than your doctor has prescribed may cause dependence and symptoms of overdose.

Be especially careful with Fiorinal if you are an older person or in a weakened condition, if you have any kidney, liver, or intestinal problems or an enlarged prostate gland, or if you have had a head injury. Also be cautious if you have a thyroid problem, blood clotting difficulties, or a urinary disorder.

### Possible food and drug interactions when taking this medication

Butalbital decreases the activity of the central nervous system and intensifies the effects of alcohol. Avoid drinking alcohol while you are taking Fiorinal.

If Fiorinal is taken with certain other drugs, the effects of either could be increased, decreased, or altered. It is especially important to check with your doctor before combining Fiorinal with the following:

Acetazolamide (Diamox)
Antidepressant drugs known as MAO inhibitors
  (Nardil, Parnate)
Beta-blocking blood pressure drugs such as Inderal
  and Tenormin
Blood-thinning drugs such as Coumadin
Insulin
Mercaptopurine (Purinethol)

Methotrexate (Rheumatrex)
Narcotic pain relievers such as Darvon and
    Percocet
Nonsteroidal anti-inflammatory drugs such as
    Naprosyn, Motrin
Oral contraceptives
Oral diabetes drugs such as Micronase
Probenecid (Benemid)
Sleep aids such as Halcion and Nembutal
Steroid medications such as prednisone
Sulfinpyrazone (Anturane)
Theophylline (Theo-Dur, others)
Tranquilizers such as Librium, Valium, and Xanax
Valproic acid (Depakene, Depakote)

### Special information
### if you are pregnant or breastfeeding

The effects of Fiorinal during pregnancy have not
been adequately studied. If you are pregnant or plan
to become pregnant, inform your doctor immediately. If you take aspirin late in your pregnancy it
could cause bleeding in you or your baby, or could
delay the baby's birth. Aspirin, butalbital, and caffeine appear in breast milk. If this medication is
essential to your health, your doctor may advise
you to discontinue breastfeeding until your treatment with this medication is finished.

### Recommended dosage
ADULTS

The usual dose of Fiorinal is 1 or 2 tablets or capsules taken every 4 hours. You should not take
more than 6 tablets or capsules in a day.

CHILDREN

The safety and effectiveness of Fiorinal have not
been established in children under 12 years of age.

### Overdosage

Any medication taken in excess can have serious
consequences. If you suspect an overdose, seek
medical attention immediately.

■ *Symptoms of an overdose of Fiorinal are mainly
attributed to its barbiturate component. These
symptoms may include:*
    Coma, confusion, drowsiness, low blood pres-
    sure, shock, slow or troubled breathing
■ *Symptoms attributed to the aspirin and caffeine
components of Fiorinal may include:*
    Abdominal pain, deep, rapid breathing, delirium,
    high fever, inability to fall or stay asleep, rapid or
    irregular heartbeat, restlessness, ringing in the
    ears, seizures, tremor, vomiting

*Brand name:*

# Fiorinal with Codeine

*Pronounced: fee-OR-i-nahl with KO-deen*
*Generic ingredients: Butalbital, Codeine
    phosphate, Aspirin, Caffeine*

### Why is this drug prescribed?

Fiorinal with Codeine, a strong narcotic pain
reliever and muscle relaxant, is prescribed for the
relief of tension headache caused by stress and
muscle contraction in the head, neck, and shoulder
area. It combines a sedative-barbiturate (butalbital),
a narcotic pain reliever and cough suppressant
(codeine), a non-narcotic pain and fever reliever
(aspirin), and a stimulant (caffeine).

### Most important fact about this drug

Barbiturates such as butalbital and narcotics such
as codeine can be habit-forming when taken in
higher than recommended doses over long periods
of time.

### How should you take this medication?

Take Fiorinal with Codeine with a full glass of
water or food to reduce stomach irritation. Do not
take this medication if it has a strong odor of
vinegar.

Take Fiorinal with Codeine exactly as prescribed. Do not increase the amount you take
without your doctor's approval.

Do not take it more frequently than your doctor
has prescribed.

■ *If you miss a dose...*
    If you take the drug on a regular schedule, take
    the forgotten dose as soon as you remember. If it
    is almost time for your next dose, skip the one
    you missed and go back to your regular schedule.
    Do not take 2 doses at once.
■ *Storage instructions...*
    Store at room temperature. Keep the container
    tightly closed.

### What side effects may occur?

Side effects cannot be anticipated. If any develop or
change in intensity, inform your doctor as soon as
possible. Only your doctor can determine if it is
safe for you to continue taking Fiorinal with
Codeine.

■ *More common side effects may include:*
    Abdominal pain, dizziness, drowsiness, nausea

■ *Additional side effects, which can be caused by this drug's components, may include:*

Anemia, blocked air passages, hepatitis, high blood sugar, internal bleeding, intoxicated feeling, irritability, kidney damage, lack of clotting, light-headedness, peptic ulcer, stomach upset, tremors

## Why should this drug not be prescribed?

If you are sensitive to or have ever had an allergic reaction to butalbital, codeine, aspirin, caffeine, or other pain relievers, you should not take this medication. Make sure your doctor is aware of any drug reactions you have experienced.

Unless you are directed to do so by your doctor, do not take this medication if you have: a tendency to bleed too much, severe vitamin K deficiency, severe liver damage, nasal polyps (growths or nodules), asthma due to aspirin or other nonsteroidal anti-inflammatory drugs such as Motrin, swelling due to fluid retention, peptic ulcer, or porphyria (an inherited metabolic disorder affecting the liver and bone marrow).

Because aspirin, when given to children and teenagers with chickenpox or flu, can cause a dangerous neurological disease called Reye's syndrome, do not use Fiorinal with Codeine under these circumstances.

## Special warnings about this medication

Fiorinal with Codeine may make you drowsy or less alert; therefore, you should not drive or operate dangerous machinery or participate in any hazardous activity that requires full mental alertness until you know how this drug affects you.

Codeine may cause unusually slow or troubled breathing and may increase the pressure caused by fluid surrounding the brain and spinal cord in people with head injury. Codeine also affects brain and spinal cord function and makes it hard for the doctor to see how people with head injuries are doing.

If you have chronic (long-lasting or frequently recurring) tension headaches and your prescribed dose of Fiorinal with Codeine does not relieve the pain, consult with your doctor. Taking more of this drug than your doctor has prescribed may cause dependence and symptoms of overdose.

Aspirin can cause internal bleeding in people with ulcers or bleeding disorders.

Codeine can hide signs of severe abdominal problems.

If you have ever developed dependence on a drug, consult with your doctor before taking Fiorinal with Codeine.

If you are being treated for a kidney, liver, or blood clotting disorder, consult with your doctor before taking Fiorinal with Codeine.

If you are older or in a weakened condition, be very careful taking Fiorinal with Codeine. You should also be careful if you have Addison's disease (an adrenal gland disorder), if you have difficulty urinating, if your prostate gland is enlarged, or if your thyroid gland is not working well.

## Possible food and drug interactions when taking this medication

Fiorinal with Codeine reduces the activity of the central nervous system and intensifies the effects of alcohol. Use of alcohol with this drug may also cause overdose symptoms. Therefore, use of alcohol should be avoided.

If Fiorinal with Codeine is taken with certain other drugs, the effects of either could be increased, decreased, or altered. It is especially important to check with your doctor before combining Fiorinal with Codeine with the following:

Acetazolamide (Diamox)
Antidepressant drugs such as Elavil, Nardil, and Parnate
Antigout medications such as Benemid and Anturane
Antihistamines such as Benadryl
Beta-blocking blood pressure drugs such as Inderal and Tenormin
Blood-thinning drugs such as Coumadin
Divalproex (Depakote)
Insulin
6-Mercaptopurine (Purinethol)
Methotrexate (Rheumatrex)
Narcotic pain relievers such as Darvon and Vicodin
Nonsteroidal anti-inflammatory drugs such as Motrin and Indocin
Oral contraceptives
Oral diabetes drugs such as Micronase
Sleep aids such as Nembutal and Halcion
Steroid drugs such as prednisone
Theophylline (Theo-Dur, others)
Tranquilizers such as Librium, Xanax, and Valium
Valproic acid (Depakene)

## Special information
### if you are pregnant or breastfeeding

The effects of Fiorinal with Codeine during pregnancy have not been adequately studied. If you are pregnant or plan to become pregnant, inform your doctor immediately. Butalbital, aspirin, caffeine, and codeine appear in breast milk. If this medication is essential to your health, your doctor may advise you to discontinue breastfeeding until your treatment with this medication is finished.

## Recommended dosage

### ADULTS

The usual dose of Fiorinal with Codeine is 1 or 2 capsules taken every 4 hours. Do not take more than 6 capsules per day.

### CHILDREN

The safety and effectiveness of butalbital have not been established in children under 12 years of age.

## Overdosage

Symptoms of an overdose of Fiorinal with Codeine are mainly attributed to its barbiturate and codeine ingredients.

■ *Symptoms attributed to the barbiturate ingredient of Fiorinal with Codeine may include:*
Coma, confusion, dizziness, drowsiness, low blood pressure, shock, slow or troubled breathing
■ *Symptoms attributed to the codeine ingredient of Fiorinal with Codeine may include:*
Convulsions, loss of consciousness, pinpoint pupils, troubled and slowed breathing
■ *Symptoms attributed to the aspirin ingredient of Fiorinal with Codeine may include:*
Abdominal pain, deep, rapid breathing, delirium, high fever, restlessness, ringing in the ears, seizures, vomiting

Though caffeine poisoning occurs only at very high doses, it can cause delirium, insomnia, irregular heartbeat, rapid heartbeat, restlessness, and tremor.

If you suspect an overdose of Fiorinal with Codeine, seek emergency medical treatment immediately.

*Brand name:*

# Flagyl

*Pronounced: FLAJ-ill*
*Generic name: Metronidazole*
*Other brand name: Protostat*

## Why is this drug prescribed?

Flagyl is an antibacterial drug prescribed for certain vaginal and urinary tract infections in men and women; amebic dysentery and liver abscess; and infections of the abdomen, skin, bones and joints, brain, lungs, and heart caused by certain bacteria.

## Most important fact about this drug

Do not drink alcoholic beverages while taking Flagyl. The combination can cause abdominal cramps, nausea, vomiting, headaches, and flushing. It can also change the taste of the alcoholic beverage. When you have stopped taking Flagyl, wait at least 72 hours (3 days) before consuming any alcohol. Also avoid over-the-counter medications containing alcohol, such as certain cough and cold products.

## How should you take this medication?

Flagyl works best when there is a constant amount in the blood. Take your doses at evenly spaced intervals, day and night, and try to avoid missing any.

If you are being treated for the sexually transmitted genital infection called trichomoniasis, your doctor may want to treat your partner at the same time, even if there are no symptoms. Try to avoid sexual intercourse until the infection is cured. If you do have sex, use a condom.

Flagyl can be taken with or without food. It may cause dry mouth. Hard candy, chewing gum, or bits of ice can help to relieve the problem.

■ *If you miss a dose...*
Take it as soon as you remember. If it is almost time for your next dose skip the one you missed and go back to your regular schedule. Do not take 2 doses at once.
■ *Storage instructions...*
Store at room temperature. Protect from light.

## What side effects may occur?

Side effects cannot be anticipated. If any develop or change in intensity, tell your doctor immediately. Only your doctor can determine whether it is safe for you to continue taking Flagyl.

Two serious side effects that have occurred with Flagyl are seizures and numbness or tingling in the arms, legs, hands, and feet. If you experience either of these symptoms, stop taking the medication and call your doctor immediately.

■ *More common side effects may include:*
Abdominal cramps, constipation, diarrhea, headache, loss of appetite, nausea, upset stomach, vomiting

■ *Less common side effects may include:*
Blood disorders, confusion, dark urine, decreased sex drive, depression, difficulty sleeping, dizziness, dry mouth (or vagina or vulva), fever, flushing, furry tongue, hives, inability to hold urine, increased production of pale urine, inflamed mouth or tongue, inflammation of the rectum, irritability, lack of muscle coordination, metallic taste, occasional joint pain, pain during sexual intercourse, painful or difficult urination, pelvic pressure, rash, stuffy nose, vertigo, weakness, yeast infection (candida) in vagina

## Why should this drug not be prescribed?
Flagyl should not be used during the first 3 months of pregnancy to treat vaginal infections. Do not take Flagyl if you have ever had an allergic reaction to or are sensitive to metronidazole or similar drugs. Tell your doctor about any drug reactions you have experienced.

## Special warnings about this medication
If you experience seizures or numbness or tingling in your arms, legs, hands, or feet, remember that you should stop taking Flagyl and call your doctor immediately.

If you have liver disease, make sure the doctor is aware of it. Flagyl should be used with caution.

Active or undiagnosed yeast infections may appear or worsen when you take Flagyl.

## Possible food and drug interactions when taking this medication
Do not drink alcohol while taking Flagyl and for at least 72 hours after your last dose.

If Flagyl is taken with certain other drugs, the effects of either could be increased, decreased, or altered. It is especially important to check with your doctor before combining Flagyl with any of the following:

Blood thinners such as Coumadin
Cholestyramine (Questran)
Cimetidine (Tagamet)
Disulfiram (Antabuse)
Lithium (Lithonate)
Phenobarbital
Phenytoin (Dilantin)

## Special information if you are pregnant or breastfeeding
The effects of Flagyl in pregnancy have not been adequately studied. If you are pregnant or plan to become pregnant, notify your doctor. This medication should be used during pregnancy only if it is clearly needed. Flagyl appears in breast milk and could affect a nursing infant. If Flagyl is essential to your health, your doctor may advise you to stop breastfeeding until your treatment is finished.

## Recommended dosage
ADULT

*Trichomoniasis*
One-day treatment: 2 grams of Flagyl, taken as a single dose or divided into 2 doses (1 gram each) taken in the same day.

Seven-day course of treatment: 250 milligrams 3 times daily for 7 consecutive days.

*Acute Intestinal Amebiasis (Acute Amebic Dysentery)*
The usual dose is 750 milligrams taken by mouth 3 times daily for 5 to 10 days.

*Amebic Liver Abscess*
The usual dose is 500 milligrams or 750 milligrams taken by mouth 3 times daily for 5 to 10 days.

*Anaerobic Bacterial Infections*
The usual adult oral dosage is 7.5 milligrams per 2.2 pounds of body weight every 6 hours.

CHILDREN

*Amebiasis*
The usual dose is 35 to 50 milligrams for each 2.2 pounds of body weight per day, divided into 3 doses taken for 10 days.

The safety and efficacy of Flagyl for any other condition in children have not been established.

OLDER ADULTS

Your doctor will test to see how much medication is in your blood and will adjust your dosage if necessary.

### Overdosage

Any medication taken in excess can have serious consequences. If you suspect an overdose, seek medical treatment immediately.

■ *Symptoms of Flagyl overdose may include:*
Lack of muscle coordination, nausea, vomiting

*Generic name:*

# Flavoxate

*See Urispas, page 579.*

*Generic name:*

# Flecainide

*See Tambocor, page 522.*

*Brand name:*

# Flexeril

*Pronounced: FLEX-eh-rill*
*Generic name: Cyclobenzaprine hydrochloride*

### Why is this drug prescribed?

Flexeril is a muscle relaxant prescribed to relieve muscle spasms resulting from injuries such as sprains, strains, or pulls. Combined with rest and physical therapy, Flexeril provides relief of muscular stiffness and pain.

### Most important fact about this drug

Flexeril is not a substitute for the physical therapy, rest, or exercise that your doctor orders for proper healing. Although Flexeril relieves the pain of strains and sprains, it is not useful for other types of pain.

### How should you take this medication?

Flexeril may be taken with or without food.

Flexeril should be used only for short periods (no more than 3 weeks). Since the type of injury that Flexeril treats should improve in a few weeks, there is no reason to use it for a longer period.

Flexeril may cause dry mouth. Sucking a hard candy, chewing gum, or melting ice chips in your mouth can provide temporary relief.

■ *If you miss a dose...*
Take it as soon as you remember, if it is within an hour or so of your scheduled time. If you do not remember until later, skip the missed dose and go back to your regular schedule. Do not take 2 doses at once.

■ *Storage instructions...*
Store away from heat, light, and moisture.

### What side effects may occur?

Side effects cannot be anticipated. If any develop or change in intensity, inform your doctor as soon as possible. Only your doctor can determine if it is safe for you to continue taking Flexeril.

■ *More common side effects may include:*
Dizziness, drowsiness, dry mouth

■ *Less common or rare side effects may include:*
Abnormal heartbeats, abnormal sensations, abnormal thoughts or dreams, agitation, anxiety, bloated feeling, blurred vision, confusion, constipation, convulsions, decreased appetite, depressed mood, diarrhea, difficulty falling or staying asleep, difficulty speaking, disorientation, double vision, excitement, fainting, fatigue, fluid retention, gas, hallucinations, headache, heartburn, hepatitis, hives, increased heart rate, indigestion, inflammation of the stomach, itching, lack of coordination, liver diseases, loss of sense of taste, low blood pressure, muscle twitching, nausea, nervousness, palpitations, rash, ringing in the ears, severe allergic reaction, stomach and intestinal pain, sweating, swelling of the tongue or face, thirst, tingling in hands or feet, tremors, unpleasant taste in the mouth, urinating more or less than usual, vague feeling of bodily discomfort, vertigo, vomiting, weakness, yellow eyes and skin

### Why should this drug not be prescribed?

You should not take this drug if you are taking an antidepressant drug known as an MAO inhibitor (such as Nardil or Parnate) or have taken an MAO inhibitor within the last 2 weeks. Also avoid Flexeril if you have ever had an allergic reaction to it, or if your thyroid gland is overactive.

In addition, you should not take Flexeril if you have recently had a heart attack or if you have congestive heart failure, or suffer from irregular heartbeat.

### Special warnings about this medication

Flexeril may cause you to become drowsy or less alert; therefore, you should not drive or operate dangerous machinery or participate in any hazardous activity that requires full mental alertness until you know how this drug affects you.

You should use Flexeril with caution if you have ever been unable to urinate or if you have ever had the eye condition called glaucoma.

### Possible food and drug interactions when taking this medication

Serious, potentially fatal reactions may occur if you take Flexeril with an antidepressant drug known as an MAO inhibitor (such as Nardil, Parnate) or if it has been less than 2 weeks since you last took an MAO inhibitor. You should closely follow your doctor's advice regarding discontinuation of MAO inhibitors before taking Flexeril.

Avoid alcoholic beverages while taking Flexeril.

If Flexeril is taken with certain other drugs, the effects of either could be increased, decreased, or altered. It is especially important to check with your doctor before combining Flexeril with the following:

Antispasmodic drugs such as Donnatal or Bentyl
Barbiturates such as phenobarbital
Guanethidine (Esimil, Ismelin) and other high
  blood pressure drugs
Other drugs that slow the central nervous system,
  such as Halcion and Xanax

### Special information if you are pregnant or breastfeeding

The effects of Flexeril during pregnancy have not been adequately studied. If you are pregnant or plan to become pregnant, inform your doctor immediately. It is not known if Flexeril appears in breast milk. However, cyclobenzaprine is related to tricyclic antidepressants, and some of those drugs do appear in breast milk. If this medication is essential to your health, your doctor may advise you to discontinue breastfeeding your baby until your treatment is finished.

### Recommended dosage

ADULTS

The usual dose is 10 milligrams 3 times a day. You should not take more than 60 milligrams a day.

CHILDREN

Safety and effectiveness of Flexeril have not been established for children under the age of 15.

### Overdosage

Any medication taken in excess can have serious consequences. If you suspect a Flexeril overdose, seek medical attention immediately.

■ *Symptoms of Flexeril overdose may include:*
Agitation, coma, confusion, congestive heart failure, convulsions, dilated pupils, disturbed concentration, drowsiness, hallucinations, high or low temperature, increased heartbeats, irregular heart rhythms, muscle stiffness, overactive reflexes, severe low blood pressure, stupor, vomiting

High doses also may cause any of the conditions listed in "What Side Effects May Occur?"

*Brand name:*

# Floxin

*Pronounced: FLOCKS-in*
*Generic name: Ofloxacin*

### Why is this drug prescribed?

Floxin is an antibiotic. It has been used effectively to treat lower respiratory tract infections, including chronic bronchitis and pneumonia, sexually transmitted diseases (except syphilis), and infections of the urinary tract, prostate gland, and skin.

### Most important fact about this drug

Floxin kills a variety of bacteria, and is frequently used to treat infections in many parts of the body. However, you should stop taking the drug and notify your doctor immediately at the first sign of a skin rash or any other allergic reaction. Although quite rare, serious and occasionally fatal allergic reactions have been reported, some after only one dose. Signs of an impending reaction include swelling of the face and throat, shortness of breath, difficulty swallowing, rapid heartbeat, tingling, itching, and hives.

### How should you take this medication?

You may take Floxin with or without food. Be sure to drink plenty of fluids while taking this medication.

Do not take mineral supplements, vitamins with iron or minerals, or antacids containing calcium, aluminum, or magnesium within 2 hours of taking Floxin.

Take Floxin exactly as prescribed. You need to complete the full course of therapy to obtain best results and decrease the risk of a recurrence of the infection.

■ *If you miss a dose...*
Take it as soon as you remember. If it is almost time for your next dose, skip the one you missed and go back to your regular schedule. Never take 2 doses at the same time.

■ *Storage instructions...*
Store at room temperature in a tightly closed container.

## What side effects may occur?
Side effects cannot be anticipated. If any develop or change in intensity, inform your doctor as soon as possible. Only your doctor can determine if it is safe for you to continue taking Floxin.

■ *More common side effects may include:*
Diarrhea, difficulty sleeping, dizziness, headache, itching of genital area in women, nausea, vaginal inflammation, vomiting

■ *Less common or rare side effects may include:*
Abdominal pain and cramps, aggressiveness or hostility, agitation, anemia, anxiety, asthma, blood in the urine, blurred vision, body pain, bruising, burning or rash of the female genitals, burning sensation in the upper chest, changeable emotions, changes in thinking and perception, chest pain, confusion, conjunctivitis (pinkeye), continual runny nose, constipation, cough, decreased appetite, depression, difficult or labored breathing, disorientation, disturbed dreams, disturbed sense of smell, double vision, dry mouth, exaggerated sense of well-being, excessive perspiration, fainting, fatigue, fear, fever, fluid retention, frequent urination, gas, hallucinations, hearing disturbance or loss, hepatitis, hiccups, high or low blood pressure, high or low blood sugar, hives, inability to urinate, increased urination, indigestion, inflammation of the colon, inflammation or rupture of tendons, intolerance to light, involuntary eye movement, itching, joint pain, kidney problems, lack of coordination, light-headedness, liver problems, menstrual changes, muscle pain, nervousness, nightmares, nosebleed, pain, pain in arms and legs, painful or difficult urination, purple or red areas/spots on the skin, rapid heartbeat, rash, reddened skin, restlessness, ringing in the ears, seizures, sensitivity to light, severe allergic reaction, skin inflammation and flaking or eruptions, sleepiness, sleep problems, sore mouth or throat, speech difficulty, Stevens-Johnson syndrome (severe skin eruptions), stomach and intestinal upset or bleeding, taste distortion, thirst, throbbing or fluttering heartbeat, tingling or pins and needles, tremor, unexplained bleeding from the uterus, vaginal discharge, vaginal yeast infection, vague feeling of illness, vertigo, visual disturbances, weakness, weight loss, yellowing of eyes and skin

## Why should this drug not be prescribed?
Do not take Floxin if you are sensitive to or have ever had an allergic reaction to it or other quinolone antibiotics such as Cipro and Noroxin.

## Special warnings about this medication
Floxin, used in high doses for short periods of time, may hide or delay the symptoms of syphilis, but is not effective in treating syphilis. If you are taking Floxin for gonorrhea, your doctor will test you for syphilis and then perform a follow-up test after 3 months of treatment.

Convulsions, increased pressure in the head, psychosis, tremors, restlessness, light-headedness, nervousness, confusion, depression, nightmares, insomnia, and hallucinations have occasionally been reported with this type of antibiotic. If you experience any of these symptoms, stop taking the drug and contact your doctor immediately.

If you are prone to seizures due to kidney disease, a brain disorder, or epilepsy, make sure your doctor knows about it. Floxin should be used with caution under these conditions.

If you have liver or kidney disease, your doctor will watch you closely while you are taking Floxin.

Avoid being in the sun too much; you can develop sun poisoning while you are taking Floxin.

Floxin may make you feel dizzy or light-headed. Be careful driving, operating machinery, or doing any activity that requires full mental alertness until you know how you react to this medication.

Safety has not been established for children under 18 years of age.

## Possible food and drug interactions when taking this medication
If Floxin is taken with certain other drugs, the effects of either could be increased, decreased, or

altered. It is especially important to check with your doctor before combining Floxin with the following:

Antacids containing calcium, magnesium, or aluminum
Blood thinners such as Coumadin
Calcium supplements such as Caltrate
Cyclosporine (Sandimmune, Neoral)
Insulin
Iron supplements such as Feosol
Multivitamins containing zinc
Nonsteroidal anti-inflammatory drugs such as Motrin and Naprosyn
Oral diabetes drugs such as Diabinese and Micronase
Sucralfate (Carafate)
Theophylline-containing drugs, such as Theo-Dur

## Special information
## if you are pregnant or breastfeeding
The effects of Floxin during pregnancy have not been adequately studied. If you are pregnant or plan to become pregnant, inform your doctor immediately. This medication should not be used during pregnancy unless your doctor has determined that the benefit to you outweighs the risk to the unborn baby. Floxin appears in breast milk and could affect a nursing infant. If this medication is essential to your health, your doctor may advise you to stop breastfeeding until your treatment with Floxin is finished.

## Recommended dosage
LOWER RESPIRATORY TRACT INFECTIONS

*Worsening of Chronic Bronchitis*
The usual dose is 400 milligrams every 12 hours for 10 days, for a total daily dose of 800 milligrams.

*Pneumonia*
The usual dose is 400 milligrams every 12 hours for 10 days, for a total daily dose of 800 milligrams.

SEXUALLY TRANSMITTED DISEASES

*Gonorrhea*
The usual dose is 400 milligrams taken once.

*Infections of the Cervix or Urethra*
The usual dose is 300 milligrams every 12 hours for 7 days, for a total daily dose of 600 milligrams.

MILD TO MODERATE SKIN INFECTIONS

The usual dose is 400 milligrams every 12 hours for 10 days, for a total daily dose of 800 milligrams.

URINARY TRACT INFECTIONS

*Bladder Infections*
The usual dose is 200 milligrams every 12 hours for a total daily dose of 400 milligrams. This dose is taken for 3 days for infections due to *E. coli* or *K. pneumoniae*. For infections due to other microbes, it is taken for 7 days.

*Complicated Urinary Tract Infections*
The usual dose is 200 milligrams every 12 hours for 10 days, for a total daily dose of 400 milligrams.

*Prostatitis*
The usual dose is 300 milligrams every 12 hours for 6 weeks, for a total daily dose of 600 milligrams.

## Overdosage
Although no specific information is available, any medication taken in excess can have serious consequences. If you suspect an overdose, seek medical treatment immediately.

*Generic name:*

# Fluconazole

*See Diflucan, page 159.*

*Generic name:*

# Flunisolide

*See AeroBid, page 7.*

*Generic name:*

# Fluocinonide

*See Lidex, page 283.*

*Generic name:*

# Fluorometholone

*See FML, page 220.*

*Generic name:*

# Fluorouracil

*See Efudex, page 186.*

*Generic name:*

# Fluoxetine

*See Prozac, page 450.*

*Generic name:*

# Flurazepam

*See Dalmane, page 130.*

*Generic name:*

# Flurbiprofen

*See Ansaid, page 28.*

*Generic name:*

# Flutamide

*See Eulexin, page 202.*

*Generic name:*

# Fluvastatin

*See Lescol, page 276.*

*Generic name:*

# Fluvoxamine

*See Luvox, page 304.*

*Brand name:*

# FML

*Generic name: Fluorometholone*

## Why is this drug prescribed?

FML is a steroid (cortisone-like) eye ointment that is used to treat inflammation of the eyelid and the eye itself.

## Most important fact about this drug

Do not use FML more often or for a longer period of time than your doctor orders. Overuse can increase the risk of side effects and lead to eye damage. Also, if your eye problems return, do not use any leftover FML without first consulting your doctor.

## How should you use this medication?

FML may increase the chance of infection from contact lenses. Your doctor may advise you to stop wearing your contacts while using this medication.

Use FML exactly as prescribed. Do not stop until your doctor advises you to do so. To avoid spreading infection, do not let anyone else use your prescription.

To administer FML eyedrops:

1. Wash your hands thoroughly.
2. Shake well before using.
3. Gently pull your lower eyelid down to form a pocket between your eye and eyelid.
4. Hold the eyedrop bottle on the bridge of your nose or on your forehead.
5. Do not touch the applicator tip to any surface, including your eye.
6. Tilt your head back and squeeze the medication into your eye.
7. Close your eyes gently. Keep them closed for 1 to 2 minutes.
8. Do not rinse the dropper.
9. Wait for 5 to 10 minutes before using a second eye medication.

■ *If you miss a dose...*
  Apply it as soon as you remember. If it is almost time for your next dose, skip the one you missed and return to your regular schedule. Do not apply a double dose.

■ *Storage instructions...*
  Store at room temperature. Protect from extreme heat.

## What side effects may occur?

Side effects cannot be anticipated. If any develop or change in intensity, inform your doctor as soon as possible. Only your doctor can determine if it is safe for you to continue using FML.

■ *Side effects may include:*
  Cataract formation, corneal ulcers, dilation of the pupil, drooping eyelids, eye inflammation and infection including pinkeye, glaucoma, increased eye pressure, slow wound healing

## Why should this drug not be prescribed?

Do not use FML if you have ever had an allergic reaction to or are sensitive to fluorometholone or similar drugs (anti-inflammatories and steroids) such as Decadron. Tell your doctor about any drug reactions you have experienced.

FML is not prescribed for patients with certain viral, fungal, and bacterial infections of the eye.

## Special warnings about this medication

Prolonged use of FML may result in glaucoma (elevated pressure in the eye causing optic nerve damage and loss of vision), cataract formation (an eye disorder causing the lens of the eye to cloud up), or the development or worsening of eye infections.

Steroids such as FML have been known to cause punctures when used in the presence of diseases that cause thinning of the cornea or the sclera (tough, opaque covering at the back of the eyeball).

The use of a corticosteroid medication could hide the presence of a severe eye infection or cause the infection to become worse.

Internal pressure of the eye should be checked frequently by your doctor.

This medication should be used with caution after cataract surgery.

If pain or inflammation lasts longer than 48 hours, or becomes worse, discontinue use of FML and notify your doctor.

## Possible food and drug interactions when taking this medication

No interactions with food or other drugs have been reported.

## Special information if you are pregnant or breastfeeding

The effects of FML in pregnancy have not been adequately studied. If you are pregnant or plan to become pregnant, tell your doctor immediately. FML may appear in breast milk and could affect a nursing infant. If using FML is essential to your health, your doctor may advise you to stop breastfeeding until your treatment is finished.

## Recommended dosage

ADULTS

### FML Ointment

Apply a small amount of ointment (a ¹/₂-inch ribbon) between the lower eyelid and eyeball 1 to 3 times a day. During the first 24 to 48 hours, your doctor may increase the dosage to 1 application every 4 hours.

### FML Liquifilm

Place 1 drop of suspension between the lower eyelid and eyeball 2 to 4 times a day. During the first 24 to 48 hours, the dosage may be increased to 1 application every 4 hours.

CHILDREN

The safety and effectiveness of FML have not been established in children under 2 years of age.

## Overdosage

Overdosage with FML will not ordinarily cause severe problems. If FML is accidentally swallowed, drink fluids to dilute the medication.

*Brand name:*

# Fosamax

*Pronounced: FAH-suh-max*
*Generic name: Alendronate Sodium*

## Why is this drug prescribed?

Fosamax is prescribed for the treatment of osteoporosis, the brittle-bone disease, in postmenopausal women and for Paget's disease, a painful weakening of the bones.

## Most important fact about this drug

For Fosamax to be effective, you must take the tablets without food or other medications, exactly as directed.

## How should you use this medication?

Fosamax is effective only when each tablet is taken with a full glass of water first thing in the morning, at least 30 minutes before the first food, beverage, or other medication. If you can wait longer before eating or drinking, the medication will be absorbed better. Do not lie down for at least 30 minutes after taking Fosamax.

You should take calcium and vitamin D supplements if you don't get enough in your diet. Avoid smoking and alcohol. Weight-bearing exercise can also strengthen bones.

■ *If you miss a dose...*
Take it as soon as you remember it. If it is almost time for the next dose, skip the one you missed and go back to your regular schedule.
■ *Storage instructions...*
Keep the container tightly closed and store at room temperature.

## What side effects may occur?

Side effects cannot be anticipated. If any develop or change in intensity, inform your doctor as soon as possible. Only your doctor can determine if it is safe for you to continue using Fosamax.

■ *More common side effects may include:*
Abdominal pain, constipation, diarrhea, indigestion, muscle and bone pain, nausea
■ *Less common side effects may include:*
Abdominal distention, acid backup, difficulty in swallowing, esophageal ulcers, gas, headache, vomiting
■ *Rare side effects may include:*
Changes in taste, inflammation of the stomach, rash, skin redness

### Why should this drug not be prescribed?
You should not take Fosamax if the calcium level in your blood is low. Avoid Fosamax if it causes an allergic reaction.

### Special warnings about this medication
Fosamax is not recommended for women on hormone replacement therapy, or for women with kidney problems.

Be sure to tell your doctor if you have trouble swallowing or have any digestive disease.

### Possible food and drug interactions when taking this medication
Combining aspirin with a Fosamax dose of more than 10 milligrams per day will increase the likelihood of stomach upset.

Calcium supplements such as Caltrate, antacids such as Riopan, and some other oral medications will interfere with the absorption of Fosamax, so wait at least 30 minutes after taking Fosamax before you take anything else.

### Special information if you are pregnant or breastfeeding
The effects of Fosamax during pregnancy and breastfeeding have not been adequately studied. If you are pregnant or plan to become pregnant, notify your doctor immediately. It is not known whether Fosamax appears in breast milk. The drug is not recommended for nursing mothers.

### Recommended dosage
POSTMENOPAUSAL OSTEOPOROSIS

The usual dose is 10 milligrams once a day. Treatment continues for years.

PAGET'S DISEASE

The usual dose is 40 milligrams once a day for 6 months.

### Overdosage
Any medication taken in excess can have serious consequences. If you suspect an overdose, seek medical attention immediately.

■ *Symptoms of Fosamax overdose may include:*
Heartburn, inflammation of the esophagus or stomach, ulcer, upset stomach

---

*Generic name:*

# Fosinopril

*See Monopril, page 335.*

---

*Brand name:*

# Fulvicin P/G

*See Gris-PEG, page 230.*

---

*Generic name:*

# Furosemide

*See Lasix, page 275.*

---

*Generic name:*

# Gabapentin

*See Neurontin, page 355.*

---

*Brand name:*

# Gantrisin

*Pronounced: GAN-tris-in*
*Generic name: Sulfisoxazole*

### Why is this drug prescribed?
Gantrisin is prescribed for the treatment of severe, repeated, or long-lasting urinary tract infections. These include pyelonephritis (bacterial kidney inflammation), pyelitis (inflammation of the part of the kidney that drains urine into the ureter), and cystitis (inflammation of the bladder).

This drug is also used to treat bacterial meningitis, and is prescribed as a preventive measure for people who have been exposed to meningitis.

Some middle ear infections are treated with Gantrisin in combination with penicillin or erythromycin.

Toxoplasmosis (parasitic disease transmitted by infected cats, their feces or litter boxes, and by undercooked meat) can be treated with Gantrisin in combination with pyrimethamine (Daraprim).

Malaria that does not respond to the drug chloroquine (Aralen) can be treated with Gantrisin in combination with other drug treatment.

Gantrisin is also used in the treatment of bacterial infections such as trachoma and inclusion inflammation conjunctivitis (eye infections), nocardiosis (bacterial disease affecting the lungs, skin, and brain), and chancroid (venereal disease causing enlargement and ulceration of lymph nodes in the groin).

## Most important fact about this drug

Notify your doctor at the first sign of a reaction such as skin rash, sore throat, fever, joint pain, cough, shortness of breath, or other breathing difficulties, abnormal skin paleness, reddish or purplish skin spots or yellowing of the skin or whites of the eyes.

Rare but severe reactions, sometimes fatal, have occurred with the use of sulfa drugs such as Gantrisin. These reactions include sudden and severe liver damage, agranulocytosis (a severe blood disorder), aplastic anemia (a lack of red and white blood cells because of a bone marrow disorder), and Stevens-Johnson syndrome (severe blistering).

Patients taking sulfa drugs such as Gantrisin should have frequent blood counts.

## How should you take this medication?

Take Gantrisin exactly as prescribed. It is important that you drink plenty of fluids while taking this medication in order to prevent crystals in the urine and the formation of stones.

Gantrisin Pediatric Suspension should be shaken well before each dose. To ensure an accurate dose, ask your pharmacist for a specially marked measuring spoon.

Gantrisin, like other antibacterials, works best when there is a constant amount in the blood and urine. To help keep a constant level, try not to miss any doses and take them at evenly spaced intervals, around the clock.

■ *If you miss a dose...*
Take it as soon as you remember. If it is almost time for your next dose, skip the one you missed and go back to your regular schedule. Never take 2 doses at the same time.

■ *Storage instructions...*
Keep this medication in the container it came in, tightly closed. Store it at room temperature, away from moist places and direct light.

## What side effects may occur?

Side effects cannot be anticipated. If any develop or change in intensity, inform your doctor as soon as possible. Only your doctor can determine if it is safe for you to continue taking Gantrisin.

■ *Side effects may include:*
Abdominal bleeding, abdominal pain, allergic reactions, anemia and other blood disorders, angioedema (swelling of face, lips, tongue and throat), anxiety, bluish discoloration of the skin, chills, colitis, convulsions, cough, dark, tarry stools, depression, diarrhea, disorientation, dizziness, drowsiness, enlarged salivary glands, enlarged thyroid, exhaustion, fainting, fatigue, fever, flushing, gas, hallucinations, headache, hearing loss, hepatitis, hives, inability to fall or stay asleep, inability to urinate, increased urination, inflammation of the mouth or tongue, itching, joint pain, kidney failure, lack of feeling or concern, lack of muscle coordination, lack or loss of appetite, low blood sugar, muscle pain, nausea, palpitations, presence of blood or crystals in urine, rapid heartbeat, reddish or purplish skin spots, retention of urine, ringing in the ears, sensitivity to light, serum sickness (fever, painful joints, enlarged lymph nodes, skin rash), severe skin welts or swelling, shortness of breath, skin eruptions, skin rash, swelling due to fluid retention, tingling or pins and needles, vertigo, vomiting, weakness, yellow eyes and skin

## Why should this drug not be prescribed?

If you are sensitive to or have ever had an allergic reaction to Gantrisin or other sulfa drugs, you should not take this medication. Make sure that your doctor is aware of any drug reactions that you have experienced.

Except in rare cases, doctors do not prescribe Gantrisin for infants less than 2 months of age. Also, you should not take Gantrisin if you are at the end of your pregnancy or if you are nursing a baby under 2 months.

### Special warnings about this medication

If you have impaired kidney or liver function, or if you have severe allergies or bronchial asthma make sure your doctor knows about it. Caution should be exercised when taking Gantrisin.

An analysis of your urine and kidney function should be performed by your doctor during treatment with Gantrisin, especially if you have a kidney problem.

If you develop diarrhea while taking Gantrisin notify your doctor.

### Possible food and drug interactions when taking this medication

If Gantrisin is taken with certain other drugs, the effects of either could be increased, decreased, or altered. It is especially important to check with your doctor before combining this drug with the following:

Blood-thinning drugs such as Coumadin
Methotrexate, an anticancer drug
Oral contraceptives
Oral diabetes drugs such as Micronase

### Special information if you are pregnant or breastfeeding

There are no adequate and well controlled studies in pregnant women. This medication should not be used during pregnancy unless your doctor has determined that the benefits outweigh the potential risks. Gantrisin appears in breast milk. If this medication is essential to your health, your doctor may advise you to discontinue breastfeeding until your treatment with this drug is finished.

### Recommended dosage

ADULTS

The recommended starting dose is 2 to 4 grams. Later, a regular dose of 4 to 8 grams per day, divided into 4 to 6 doses, is recommended.

CHILDREN

This medication should not be prescribed for infants under 2 months of age except in the treatment of congenital toxoplasmosis (a parasitic infection contracted by pregnant women and passed along to the fetus).

The usual dose for children 2 months of age or older is 150 milligrams per 2.2 pounds of body weight divided into 4 to 6 doses taken over 24 hours.

The usual starting dose is one-half of the regular dose, or 75 milligrams per 2.2 pounds of body weight divided into 4 to 6 doses taken over 24 hours. Doses should not exceed 6 grams over 24 hours.

Gantrisin tablets come in a half-gram (500 milligram) strength. Gantrisin pediatric suspension and syrup supply a half-gram (500 milligrams) in each teaspoonful.

### Overdosage

Any medication taken in excess can have serious consequences. If you suspect an overdose, seek emergency medical treatment immediately.

■ *Symptoms of an overdose of Gantrisin include:*
Blood or sediment in the urine, blue tinge to the skin, colic, dizziness, drowsiness, fever, headache, lack or loss of appetite, nausea, unconsciousness, vomiting, yellowing of skin and whites of eyes

*Brand name:*

# Garamycin Ophthalmic

*Pronounced: gar-uh-MY-sin*
*Generic name: Gentamicin sulfate*

### Why is this drug prescribed?

Garamycin Ophthalmic, an antibiotic, is applied to the eye for treatment of infections such as conjunctivitis (pinkeye) and other eye infections.

### Most important fact about this drug

To help clear up your infection completely, keep using Garamycin eyedrops or ointment for the full time of treatment, even if your symptoms have disappeared. Do not allow anyone else to use this medication, and do not save it for use on another infection.

### How should you use this medication?

Use this medication exactly as prescribed. To administer Garamycin, follow these steps:

Eyedrops
1. Wash your hands thoroughly.
2. Gently pull your lower eyelid down to form a pocket between your eye and the lid.
3. Brace the eyedrop bottle on your forehead or on the bridge of your nose.
4. Do not touch the applicator tip to your eye or any other surface.

5. Close your eyes gently and keep them closed for a minute or two.
6. Do not rinse the dropper.
7. If you are using a second type of eyedrop, wait 5 to 10 minutes before applying it.

Eye Ointment
1. Wash your hands thoroughly.
2. Pull your lower eyelid down away from the eye to form a pocket.
3. Squeeze a thin strip of ointment into the pouch.
4. Avoid touching the tip of the tube to your eye or any other surface.
5. Close your eyes for a couple of minutes.
6. Wipe the tip of the tube with tissue and immediately replace the cap tightly.

Your vision may be blurred for a few minutes following application of the ointment.

■ *If you miss a dose...*
Apply it as soon as you remember. If it is almost time for your next dose, skip the one you missed and go back to your regular schedule.
■ *Storage instructions...*
Store away from heat and light. Do not freeze.

### What side effects may occur?
Occasional eye irritation—with itching, redness and swelling—may occur with use of the eyedrops.

Occasional burning or stinging in the eye may occur with use of the ointment.

### Why should this drug not be prescribed?
If you are sensitive to or have ever had an allergic reaction to Garamycin or certain other antibiotics, such as Tobrex, you should not take this medication. Make sure your doctor is aware of any drug reactions you have experienced.

### Special warnings about this medication
Continued or prolonged use of this drug may result in a growth of bacteria or fungi that do not respond to this medication and can cause a second infection. Should this occur, notify your doctor.

Ophthalmic ointments may slow corneal healing.

### Possible food and drug interactions with this medication
No interactions have been reported.

### Special Information
### if you are pregnant or breastfeeding
There are no special recommendations for this medication. If you are pregnant or plan to become pregnant, ask your doctor for the best advice in your personal situation.

### Recommended dosage
ADULTS AND CHILDREN

*Garamycin Ophthalmic Solution*
Put 1 or 2 drops into the affected eye every 4 hours. For severe infections, your doctor may increase your dosage up to a maximum of 2 drops once every hour.

*Garamycin Ophthalmic Ointment*
Apply a thin strip—about one-third inch—of ointment to the affected eye 2 or 3 times a day.

### Overdosage
Although there is no information on overdose with Garamycin ophthalmic products, any medication taken in excess can have serious consequences. If you suspect an overdose, seek medical attention immediately.

*Brand name:*

# Gaviscon

*See Antacids, page 30.*

*Brand name:*

# Gelusil

*See Antacids, page 30.*

*Brand name:*

# Gemcor

*See Lopid, page 290.*

*Generic name:*

# Gemfibrozil

*See Lopid, page 290.*

*Brand name:*

# Genora

*See Oral Contraceptives, page 382.*

Generic name:

# Gentamicin

See Garamycin Ophthalmic, page 224.

Brand name:

# Genuine Bayer

See Aspirin, page 37.

Generic name:

# Glimepiride

See Amaryl, page 18.

Generic name:

# Glipizide

See Glucotrol, page 228.

Brand name:

# Glucophage

Pronounced: GLEW-co-faje
Generic name: Metformin hydrochloride

### Why is this drug prescribed?

Glucophage is an oral antidiabetic medication used to treat Type II (noninsulin-dependent) diabetes. Diabetes develops when the body proves unable to burn sugar and the unused sugar builds up in the bloodstream. Glucophage lowers the amount of sugar in your blood by decreasing sugar production and absorption and helping your body respond better to its own insulin, which promotes the burning of sugar. It does not, however, increase the body's production of insulin.

### Most important fact about this drug

Always remember that Glucophage is an aid to, not a substitute for, good diet and exercise. Failure to follow a sound diet and exercise plan can lead to serious complications such as dangerously high or low blood sugar levels. Remember, too, that Glucophage is not an oral form of insulin and cannot be used in place of insulin.

### How should you take this medication?

Do not take more or less of this medication than directed by your doctor. Glucophage should be taken with food to reduce the possibility of nausea or diarrhea, especially during the first few weeks of therapy.

■ *If you miss a dose...*
Take it as soon as you remember. If it is almost time for your next dose, skip the one you missed and go back to your regular schedule. Never take 2 doses at the same time.

■ *Storage instructions...*
Store it at room temperature.

### What side effects may occur?

Side effects cannot be anticipated. If any develop or change in intensity, tell your doctor as soon as possible. Only your doctor can determine if it is safe for you to continue taking Glucophage.

If side effects from Glucophage occur, they usually happen during the first few weeks of therapy. Most side effects are minor and will go away after you've taken Glucophage for a while.

■ *More common side effects may include:*
Abdominal bloating, diarrhea, gas, loss of appetite, metallic or unpleasant taste, nausea, vomiting

Glucophage, unlike other oral antidiabetics, does not usually cause hypoglycemia (low blood sugar). However, hypoglycemia remains a possibility, especially in older, weak, and undernourished people and those with kidney, liver, adrenal, or pituitary gland problems. The risk of hypoglycemia can be increased by missed meals, alcohol, other medications, fever, trauma, infection, surgery, or excessive exercise. To avoid hypoglycemia, you should closely follow the dietary and exercise plan suggested by your physician. If you feel hypoglycemia coming on, get some fast-acting sugar, such as a 4 to 6 ounce glass of fruit juice.

Glucophage can cause a serious side effect called lactic acidosis, a buildup of lactic acid in the blood. This problem is most likely to occur in people whose liver or kidneys are not working well. Although the condition is rare, it can be fatal. Lactic acidosis is a medical emergency that must be treated in a hospital.

■ *Symptoms of lactic acidosis may include:*
Feeling very weak, tired, or uncomfortable, feeling cold, dizzy, or light-headed, increasing sleepiness, muscle pain, slow or irregular heartbeat, trouble breathing, unexpected or unusual stomach discomfort

If you notice these symptoms, stop taking Glucophage and call your doctor right away.

### Why should this drug not be prescribed?

Avoid Glucophage if it has ever given you an allergic reaction.

Do not take Glucophage if you are suffering from acute or chronic metabolic acidosis, including diabetic ketoacidosis (a life-threatening medical emergency caused by insufficient insulin and marked by excessive thirst, nausea, fatigue, pain below the breastbone, and fruity breath).

You should not take Glucophage for 2 days before and after having an X-ray procedure with an injectable contrast agent (radioactive iodine). Also, if you are going to have surgery, except minor surgery, you should stop taking Glucophage. Once you have resumed normal food and fluid intake, your doctor will tell you when you can go back to therapy with Glucophage.

If you have kidney or liver disease or develop serious conditions such as a heart attack, severe infection, or a stroke, do not take Glucophage.

You should not take Glucophage if you are seriously dehydrated, having lost a large amount of fluid from severe vomiting, diarrhea, or high fever.

### Special warnings about this medication

Before you start therapy with Glucophage, and at least once a year thereafter, your doctor will do a complete assessment of your kidney function. If you develop kidney problems while on Glucophage, your doctor will discontinue this medication. If you are an older person, you will need to have your kidney function monitored more frequently, and your doctor may want to start you at a lower dosage.

If you are taking Glucophage, you should check your blood or urine periodically for abnormal sugar (glucose) levels. Your doctor will do annual blood checks to see if Glucophage is causing a vitamin $B_{12}$ deficiency or any other blood problem.

It's possible that drugs such as Glucophage may lead to more heart problems than diet treatment alone, or diet plus insulin. If you have a heart condition, you may want to discuss this with your doctor. The effectiveness of any oral antidiabetic, including Glucophage, may decrease with time. This may be due to either a diminished responsiveness to the medication or a worsening of the diabetes.

### Possible food and drug interactions when taking this medication

If Glucophage is taken with certain other drugs, the effects of either could be increased, decreased, or altered. It is especially important to check with your doctor before combining Glucophage with the following:

Amiloride (Moduretic)
Calcium channel blockers (heart medications) such as Calan, Isoptin, and Procardia
Cimetidine (Tagamet)
Decongestant, airway-opening drugs such as Sudafed and Ventolin
Digoxin (Lanoxin)
Estrogens such as Premarin
Furosemide (Lasix) and other diuretics
Isoniazid (Rifamate), a drug used for tuberculosis
Major tranquilizers such as Thorazine
Morphine
Niacin (Slo-Niacin, Nicobid)
Oral contraceptives
Phenytoin (Dilantin)
Procainamide (Procan SR)
Quinidine (Quinidex)
Quinine
Ranitidine (Zantac)
Steroids such as prednisone (Deltasone)
Thyroid hormones (Synthroid)
Trimethoprim (Bactrim, Trimpex)
Vancomycin (Vancocin HCl)

Do not drink too much alcohol, since excessive alcohol consumption can cause low blood sugar and alcohol enhances some effects of this drug.

### Special information if you are pregnant or breastfeeding

If you are pregnant or plan to become pregnant, tell your doctor immediately. Glucophage should not be taken during pregnancy. Since studies suggest the importance of maintaining normal blood sugar (glucose) levels during pregnancy, your doctor may prescribe insulin injections instead.

It is not known whether Glucophage appears in human breast milk. Therefore, women should discuss with their doctors whether to discontinue the medication or to stop breastfeeding. If the medication is discontinued and if diet alone does not control glucose levels, then your doctor may consider insulin injections.

### Recommended dosage

Your doctor will tailor your dosage to your individual needs.

ADULTS

The usual starting dose is one 500-milligram tablet twice a day, taken with morning and evening meals. Your doctor may increase your daily dose by 500 milligrams at weekly intervals, based on your response. Daily doses of greater than 2500 milligrams are not recommended. An alternative starting dose is one 850-milligram tablet a day, taken with the morning meal. Your doctor may increase this by 850 milligrams at 14-day intervals, to a maximum of 2550 milligrams a day.

The usual maintenance dose ranges from 1,500 to 2,550 milligrams daily.

OLDER ADULTS

Older people and those who are malnourished or in a weakened state are generally given lower doses of Glucophage because their kidneys may be weaker, making side effects more likely.

CHILDREN

The safety and effectiveness of Glucophage have not been established in children.

### Overdosage

An overdose of Glucophage can cause lactic acidosis. (See "What Side Effects May Occur?") If you suspect a Glucophage overdose, seek emergency treatment immediately.

*Brand name:*

# Glucotrol

*Pronounced: GLUE-kuh-troll*
*Generic name: Glipizide*
*Other brand name: Glucotrol XL*

### Why is this drug prescribed?

Glucotrol is an oral antidiabetic medication used to treat Type II (non-insulin-dependent) diabetes. In diabetics either the body does not make enough insulin or the insulin that is produced no longer works properly.

There are actually two forms of diabetes: Type I insulin-dependent and Type II non-insulin-dependent. Type I usually requires insulin injections for life, while Type II diabetes can usually be treated by dietary changes and/or oral antidiabetic medications such as Glucotrol. Apparently, Glucotrol controls diabetes by stimulating the pancreas to secrete more insulin. Occasionally, Type II diabetics must take insulin injections on a temporary basis, especially during stressful periods or times of illness.

### Most important fact about this drug

Always remember that Glucotrol is an aid to, not a substitute for, good diet and exercise. Failure to follow a sound diet and exercise plan can lead to serious complications, such as dangerously high or low blood sugar levels. Remember, too, that Glucotrol is *not* an oral form of insulin, and cannot be used in place of insulin.

### How should you take this medication?

In general, to achieve the best control over blood sugar levels, Glucotrol should be taken 30 minutes before a meal. However, the exact dosing schedule as well as the dosage amount must be determined by your physician.

Glucotrol XL should be taken with breakfast. Swallow the tablets whole; do not chew, crush, or divide them. Do not be alarmed if you notice something that looks like a tablet in your stool—it will be the empty shell that has been eliminated.

■ *If you miss a dose...*
Take it as soon as you remember. If it is almost time for your next dose, skip the one you missed and go back to your regular schedule. Never take 2 doses at the same time.
■ *Storage instructions...*
Glucotrol should be stored at room temperature and protected from moisture and humidity.

### What side effects may occur?

Side effects from Glucotrol are rare and seldom require discontinuation of the medication.

■ *More common side effects may include:*
Constipation, diarrhea, drowsiness, gas, hives, itching, low blood sugar, sensitivity to light, skin rash and eruptions, stomach pain
■ *Less common or rare side effects may include:*
Anemia and other blood disorders, yellow eyes and skin

Glucotrol and Glucotrol XL, like all oral antidiabetic drugs, can cause low blood sugar. This risk is increased by missed meals, alcohol, other medications, and/or excessive exercise. To avoid low blood sugar, you should closely follow the dietary and exercise regimen suggested by your physician.

■ *Symptoms of mild low blood sugar may include:*
Blurred vision, cold sweats, dizziness, fast heartbeat, fatigue, headache, hunger, light-headedness, nausea, nervousness

■ *Symptoms of more severe low blood sugar may include:*
Coma, disorientation, pale skin, seizures, shallow breathing

Ask your doctor what steps you should take if you experience mild hypoglycemia. If symptoms of severe low blood sugar occur, contact your doctor immediately. Severe hypoglycemia should be considered a medical emergency, and prompt medical attention is essential.

## Why should this drug not be prescribed?
You should not take Glucotrol if you have had an allergic reaction to it previously.

Glucotrol will be stopped if you are suffering from diabetic ketoacidosis (a life-threatening medical emergency caused by insufficient insulin and marked by excessive thirst, nausea, fatigue, pain below the breastbone, and a fruity breath).

## Special warnings about this medication
It's possible that drugs such as Glucotrol may lead to more heart problems than diet treatment alone, or diet plus insulin. If you have a heart condition, you may want to discuss this with your doctor.

If you are taking Glucotrol, you should check your blood and urine periodically for the presence of abnormal sugar (glucose) levels.

Even people with well-controlled diabetes may find that injury, infection, surgery, or fever results in a lack of control over their diabetes. In these cases, the physician may recommend that you stop taking Glucotrol temporarily and use insulin instead.

Glucotrol may not work well in patients with poor kidney or liver function.

In addition, the effectiveness of any oral antidiabetic, including Glucotrol, may decrease with time. This may occur because of either a diminished responsiveness to the medication or a worsening of the diabetes.

Be careful taking the extended-release form of the drug, Glucotrol XL, if you have any narrowing in your stomach or intestines. Also, if you have any stomach or intestinal disease, Glucotrol XL may not work as well.

## Possible food and drug interactions when taking this medication
It is essential that you closely follow your physician's dietary guidelines and that you inform your physician of any medication, either prescription or nonprescription, that you are taking. Specific medications that affect Glucotrol include:

Airway-opening drugs such as Sudafed
Antacids such as Mylanta
Aspirin
Chloramphenicol (Chloromycetin)
Cimetidine (Tagamet)
Clofibrate (Atromid-S)
Corticosteroids such as prednisone (Deltasone)
Diuretics such as HydroDIURIL
Estrogens such as Premarin
Fluconazole (Diflucan)
Gemfibrozil (Lopid)
Heart and blood pressure medications called beta
    blockers such as Tenormin and Lopressor
Heart medications called calcium channel blockers
    such as Cardizem and Procardia XL
Isoniazid (Nydrazid)
Itraconazole (Sporanox)
MAO inhibitors (antidepressant drugs such as
    Nardil)
Major tranquilizers such as Thorazine and Mellaril
Miconazole (Monistat)
Nicotinic acid (Nicobid)
Nonsteroidal anti-inflammatory drugs such as
    Motrin
Oral contraceptives
Phenytoin (Dilantin)
Probenecid (Benemid)
Rifampin (Rifadin)
Sulfa drugs such as Bactrim
Thyroid medications such as Synthroid
Warfarin (Coumadin)

Alcohol must be used carefully, since excessive alcohol consumption can cause low blood sugar.

## Special information if you are pregnant or breastfeeding
The effects of Glucotrol during pregnancy have not been adequately studied. Therefore, if you are pregnant, or planning to become pregnant, you should

take Glucotrol only on the advice of your physician. Since studies suggest the importance of maintaining normal blood sugar (glucose) levels during pregnancy, your physician may prescribe insulin during pregnancy. To minimize the risk of low blood sugar in newborn babies, Glucotrol, if taken during pregnancy, should be discontinued at least one month before the expected delivery date. Although it is not known if Glucotrol appears in breast milk, other oral antidiabetics do. Because of the potential for hypoglycemia in nursing infants, your doctor may advise you either to discontinue Glucotrol or to stop nursing. If Glucotrol is discontinued and if diet alone does not control glucose levels, your doctor may prescribe insulin.

### Recommended dosage

Dosage levels must be determined by each patient's needs.

ADULTS

*Glucotrol*
The usual recommended starting dose is 5 milligrams taken before breakfast. Depending upon blood glucose response, your doctor may increase the initial dose in increments of 2.5 to 5 milligrams. The maximum recommended daily dose is 40 milligrams; total daily dosages above 15 milligrams are usually divided into 2 equal doses that are taken before meals.

*Glucotrol XL*
The usual starting dose is 5 milligrams each day at breakfast. After 3 months, your doctor may increase the dose to 10 milligrams daily. The maximum recommended daily dose is 20 milligrams.

CHILDREN

The safety and effectiveness of this drug in children have not been established.

OLDER ADULTS

Older people or those with liver disease usually start Glucotrol therapy with 2.5 milligrams. They can start Glucotrol XL treatment with 5 milligrams.

### Overdosage

An overdose of Glucotrol can cause low blood sugar. (See side effects section for symptoms.) Eating sugar or a sugar-based product will often correct the condition. Otherwise, seek medical attention immediately.

---

*Generic name:*

# Glyburide

See Micronase, page 324.

---

*Brand name:*

# Glynase

See Micronase, page 324.

---

*Brand name:*

# Grisactin

See Gris-PEG, page 230.

---

*Generic name:*

# Griseofulvin

See Gris-PEG, page 230.

---

*Brand name:*

# Gris-PEG

*Pronounced: GRISS-peg*
*Generic name: Griseofulvin*
*Other brand names: Grisactin, Fulvicin P/G*

### Why is this drug prescribed?

Gris-PEG is prescribed for the treatment of the following ringworm infections:

Athlete's foot
Barber's itch (inflammation of the facial hair follicles)
Ringworm of the body
Ringworm of the groin and thigh
Ringworm of the nails
Ringworm of the scalp

Because Gris-PEG is effective for only certain types of fungal infections, before treatment your doctor may perform tests to identify the source of infection.

### Most important fact about this drug

To clear up your infection completely, continue taking Gris-PEG as prescribed until your doctor tells you to stop. Although some improvement may appear within a few days, you need to take Gris-PEG for an extended period.

## How should you take this medication?

To minimize stomach irritation and help your body absorb the drug, take Gris-PEG at meal times or with food or whole milk. If you are on a low fat diet, check with your doctor.

Observe good hygiene during treatment to help control infection and prevent reinfection.

■ *If you miss a dose...*
Take it as soon as you remember. If it is almost time for your next dose, skip the one you missed and go back to your regular schedule. Do not take 2 doses at once.

■ *Storage instructions...*
Store at room temperature in a tightly closed container. Protect from light. Keep the liquid from freezing.

## What side effects may occur?

Side effects cannot be anticipated. If any develop or change in intensity, inform your doctor as soon as possible. Only your doctor can determine if it is safe for you to continue taking Gris-PEG.

■ *More common side effects may include:*
Hives, skin rashes

■ *Less common side effects may include:*
Confusion, diarrhea, dizziness, fatigue, headache, impairment of performance of routine activities, inability to fall or stay asleep, nausea, oral thrush (mouth inflammation), upper abdominal pain, vomiting

■ *Rare side effects may include:*
Menstrual irregularities, swelling, itching, and shedding of areas of skin, tingling sensation in hands and feet

## Why should this drug not be prescribed?

If you are sensitive to or have ever had an allergic reaction to Gris-PEG or other drugs of this type, you should not take this medication. Make sure your doctor is aware of any drug reactions you have experienced.

Unless you are directed to do so by your doctor, do not take this medication if you have liver damage or porphyria (an inherited disorder of the liver or bone marrow).

Do not take Gris-PEG while pregnant.

## Special warnings about this medication

Gris-PEG is similar to penicillin. Although penicillin-sensitive people have used Gris-PEG without difficulty, notify your doctor if you are sensitive to or allergic to penicillin.

Because Gris-PEG can make you sensitive to light, avoid exposure to intense natural or artificial sunlight.

Notify your doctor if you develop lupus erythematosus (a form of rheumatism) or a lupus-like condition. Signs and symptoms of lupus include arthritis, red butterfly rash over the nose and cheeks, tiredness, weakness, sensitivity to sunlight, and skin eruptions.

If you are being treated with Gris-PEG for an extended period of time, your doctor should perform regular tests, including periodic monitoring of kidney function, liver function, and blood cell production.

Gris-PEG has not been proved safe and effective for the prevention of fungal infections.

Gris-PEG may decrease the effectiveness of birth-control pills. Use additional protection while you are taking Gris-PEG.

Men should wait at least 6 months after finishing therapy with griseofulvin before they father a child.

Women should avoid becoming pregnant while they are taking the drug.

## Possible food and drug interactions when taking this medication

Gris-PEG may intensify the effects of alcohol. If you drink alcohol while taking this medication, your heart may start beating faster and your skin may be flushed.

If Gris-PEG is taken with certain other drugs, the effects of either could be increased, decreased, or altered. It is especially important to check with your doctor before combining Gris-PEG with the following:

Blood-thinning drugs such as Coumadin
Barbiturates such as phenobarbital
Oral contraceptives

## Special information if you are pregnant or breastfeeding

Do not take Gris-PEG if you are pregnant. If you become pregnant while taking this drug, notify your doctor immediately. There is a potential hazard to the developing baby.

If you are breastfeeding, consult with your doctor before taking Gris-PEG.

## Recommended dosage

The usual treatment periods for various ringworm infections are:

Ringworm of the scalp—4 to 6 weeks
Ringworm of the body—2 to 4 weeks
Athlete's foot—4 to 8 weeks

The usual treatment period, depending on the rate of growth, for ringworm of the fingernails is at least 4 months and for ringworm of the toenails at least 6 months.

### ADULTS

*Ringworm of the Body, Groin and Thigh, Scalp*
The usual dosage is 375 milligrams a day taken as a single dose or divided into smaller doses, as determined by your doctor.

*Athlete's Foot, Ringworm of the Nails*
The usual dosage is 750 milligrams a day divided into smaller doses, as determined by your doctor.

### CHILDREN

A single daily dose is effective in children with ringworm of the scalp.

The usual dosage is 3.3 milligrams per pound of body weight per day. This means that children weighing 35 to 60 pounds will take 125 to 187.5 milligrams a day, and children weighing more than 60 pounds will take 187.5 to 375 milligrams a day.

No dosage has been established for children 2 years of age and under.

## Overdosage

Any medication taken in excess can have dangerous consequences. If you suspect an overdose of Gris-PEG, seek emergency medical treatment immediately.

*Generic name:*

# Guaifenesin with Codeine

*See Tussi-Organidin NR, page 569.*

*Generic name:*

# Guaifenesin with Phenylpropanolamine

*See Entex LA, page 194.*

*Generic name:*

# Guanabenz

*See Wytensin, page 594.*

*Generic name:*

# Guanfacine

*See Tenex, page 528.*

*Brand name:*

# Gyne-Lotrimin

*Pronounced: GUY-nuh-LOW-trim-in*
*Generic name: Clotrimazole*
*Other brand names: Lotrimin, Mycelex, Mycelex-7*

## Why is this drug prescribed?

Clotrimazole, the active ingredient in these medications, is used to treat fungal infections. In preparations for the skin, it is effective against ringworm, athlete's foot, and jock itch. In vaginal creams and tablets, it is used against vaginal yeast infections. In lozenge form, it is prescribed to treat oral yeast infections and to prevent them in people with weak immune systems.

## Most important fact about this drug

Keep using this medicine for the full time of treatment, even if the infection seems to have disappeared. If you stop too soon, the infection could return. You should continue using the vaginal forms of this medicine even during your menstrual period.

## How should you take this medication?

Keep all forms of this medicine away from your eyes.

Before applying the skin preparations, be sure to wash your hands. Massage the medication gently into the affected area and the surrounding skin.

If you are taking Mycelex troches, place the lozenge in your mouth and let it dissolve slowly for 15 to 30 minutes. Do not chew the lozenge or swallow it whole.

If you are using a vaginal cream or tablet, use the following administration technique:

1. Load the applicator to the fill line with cream, or unwrap a tablet, wet it with warm water, and place it in the applicator as shown in the instructions you receive with the product.

2. Lie on your back with your knees drawn up.
3. Gently insert the applicator high into the vagina and push the plunger.
4. Withdraw the applicator and discard it if disposable, or wash with soap and water.

To keep the vaginal medication from getting on your clothing, wear a sanitary napkin. Do not use a tampon because it will absorb the medicine. Wear underwear or pantyhose with a cotton crotch—avoid synthetic fabrics such as nylon or rayon. Do not douche unless your doctor tells you to do so.

■ *If you miss a dose...*
  Make up for it as soon as you remember. If it is almost time for the next dose, skip the one you missed and go back to your regular schedule.
■ *Storage instructions...*
  Store at room temperature, away from heat, light, and moisture.

### What side effects may occur?
Side effects cannot be anticipated. If any develop or change in intensity, inform your doctor as soon as possible. Only your doctor can determine if it is safe for you to continue using this medication.

■ *Side effects may include:*
  Blistering, burning, hives, irritated skin, itching, peeling, reddened skin, stinging, swelling due to fluid retention
■ *Side effects of clotrimazole vaginal preparations may include:*
  Abdominal/stomach cramps/pain, burning/irritation of penis of sexual partner, headache, pain during sexual intercourse, skin rash, hives, vaginal burning, vaginal irritation, vaginal itching, vaginal soreness during sexual intercourse

An unpleasant mouth sensation has been reported by some people taking Mycelex.

### Why should this drug not be prescribed?
You should not be using this medication if you have had an allergic reaction to any of its ingredients.

### Special warnings about this medication
Contact your doctor if you experience increased skin irritations (such as redness, itching, burning, blistering, swelling, or oozing).

  Check with your doctor before using this medication on a child.

In general, if your symptoms have not improved within 2 to 4 weeks of treatment, notify your doctor.

  Clotrimazole vaginal preparations should not be used if you have abdominal pain, fever, or a foul-smelling vaginal discharge. Contact your doctor immediately.

  While using the vaginal preparations, either avoid sexual intercourse or make sure your partner uses a condom. This will prevent reinfection. Oils used in some vaginal preparations can weaken latex condoms or diaphragms. To find out whether you can use your medication with latex products, check with your pharmacist.

### Possible food and drug interactions when taking this medication
None have been reported.

### Special information if you are pregnant or breastfeeding
The use of clotrimazole during the first trimester of pregnancy has not been adequately studied. It should be used during the first trimester only if clearly needed. Do not use clotrimazole at any time during pregnancy without the advice and supervision of your doctor.

  It is not known whether clotrimazole appears in breast milk. Nursing mothers should use this medication cautiously and only when clearly needed.

### Recommended dosage
LOTRIMIN

*Adults and Children*
Wash your hands before and after you use Lotrimin. Apply in the morning and evening. Use enough Lotrimin to massage into the affected area.

  Symptoms usually improve during the first week of treatment with Lotrimin.

GYNE-LOTRIMIN CREAM

*Adults*
Fill the applicator with the cream and insert 1 applicatorful into the vagina every day, preferably at bedtime. Repeat this procedure for 7 consecutive days.

MYCELEX TROCHE

*Adults*
The recommended dosage is 1 troche slowly dissolved in the mouth 5 times daily for 14 consecutive days. For prevention, the recommended dose is 1 troche 3 times daily.

## Overdosage

Although any medication used in excess can have serious consequences, an overdose of clotrimazole is unlikely. If you suspect an overdose, however, seek medical help immediately.

Brand name:

# Habitrol

See Nicotine Patches, page 359.

Brand name:

# Halcion

Pronounced: HAL-see-on
Generic name: Triazolam

### Why is this drug prescribed?

Halcion is used for short-term treatment of insomnia. It is a member of the benzodiazepine class of drugs, many of which are used as tranquilizers.

### Most important fact about this drug

Sleep problems are usually temporary, requiring treatment for only a short time, usually 1 or 2 days and no more than 1 to 2 weeks. Insomnia that lasts longer than this may be a sign of another medical problem. If you find you need this medicine for more than 7 to 10 days, be sure to check with your doctor.

### How should you take this medication?

Take this medication exactly as directed; never take more than your doctor has prescribed.

As with all prescription medications, never share Halcion with anyone else.

To help avoid upset stomach, Halcion can be taken with food.

■ *If you miss a dose...*
  Take Halcion only as needed.
■ *Storage instructions...*
  Keep this medication in the container it came in, tightly closed, and out of reach of children. Store it at room temperature.

### What side effects may occur?

Side effects cannot be anticipated. If any develop or change in intensity, inform your doctor as soon as possible. Only your doctor can determine if it is safe for you to continue taking Halcion.

■ *More common side effects may include:*
  Coordination problems, dizziness, drowsiness, headache, light-headedness, nausea/vomiting, nervousness
■ *Less common or rare side effects may include:*
  Aggressiveness, agitation, behavior problems, burning tongue, changes in sexual drive, chest pain, confusion, congestion, constipation, cramps/pain, delusions, depression, diarrhea, disorientation, dreaming abnormalities, drowsiness, dry mouth, exaggerated sense of well-being, excitement, fainting, falling, fatigue, hallucinations, impaired urination, inappropriate behavior, incontinence, inflammation of the tongue and mouth, irritability, itching, loss of appetite, loss of sense of reality, memory impairment, memory loss (e.g. traveler's amnesia), menstrual irregularities, morning "hangover" effects, muscle spasms in the shoulders or neck, nightmares, rapid heart rate, restlessness, ringing in the ears, skin inflammation, sleep disturbances including insomnia, sleepwalking, slurred or difficult speech, stiff awkward movements, taste changes, tingling or pins and needles, tiredness, visual disturbances, weakness, yellowing of the skin and whites of the eyes

### Why should this drug not be prescribed?

You should not take this drug if you are pregnant or if you have had an allergic reaction to it or to other benzodiazepine drugs such as Valium.

### Special warnings about this medication

When Halcion is used every night for more than a few weeks, it loses its effectiveness to help you sleep. This is known as tolerance. Also, it can cause dependence, especially when it is used regularly for longer than a few weeks or at high doses.

Abrupt discontinuation of Halcion should be avoided, since it has been associated with withdrawal symptoms (convulsions, cramps, tremor, vomiting, sweating, feeling ill, perceptual problems, and insomnia). A gradual dosage tapering schedule is usually recommended for patients taking more than the lowest dose of Halcion for longer than a few weeks. The usual treatment period is 7 to 10 days.

If you develop unusual and disturbing thoughts or behavior during treatment with Halcion, you should discuss them with your doctor immediately.

"Traveler's amnesia" has been reported by patients who took Halcion to induce sleep while traveling. To avoid this condition, do not take Halcion on an overnight airplane flight of less than 7 to 8 hours.

You may suffer increased anxiety during the daytime while taking Halcion.

When you first start taking Halcion, until you know whether the medication will have any "carry over" effect the next day, use extreme care while doing anything that requires complete alertness such as driving a car or operating machinery.

After discontinuing the drug, you may experience a "rebound insomnia" for the first 2 nights—that is, insomnia may be worse than before you took the sleeping pill.

You should be aware that anterograde amnesia (forgetting events after an injury) has been associated with benzodiazepine drugs such as Halcion.

You should be cautious about using this drug if you have liver or kidney problems, lung problems, or a tendency to temporarily stop breathing while you are asleep.

### Possible food and drug interactions when taking this medication

Avoid alcoholic beverages.

If Halcion is taken with certain other drugs, the effects of either could be increased, decreased, or altered. It is especially important to check with your doctor before combining Halcion with the following:

Antidepressant medications, including "tricyclic" drugs such as Elavil and MAO inhibitors such as Nardil and Parnate
Antihistamines such as Benadryl and Tavist
Barbiturates such as phenobarbital and Seconal
Cimetidine (Tagamet)
Erythromycin (E.E.S., PCE, E-Mycin, others)
Isoniazid (Nydrazid)
Narcotic painkillers such as Demerol
Major tranquilizers such as Mellaril and Thorazine
Other tranquilizers such as BuSpar, Valium, and Xanax
Oral contraceptives
Seizure medications such as Dilantin and Tegretol

### Special information if you are pregnant or breastfeeding

Since benzodiazepines have been associated with damage to the developing baby, you should not take Halcion if you are pregnant, think you may be pregnant, or are planning to become pregnant; or if you are breastfeeding.

### Recommended dosage

#### ADULTS

The usual dose is 0.25 milligram before bedtime. The dose should never be more than 0.5 milligram.

#### CHILDREN

Safety and effectiveness for children under the age of 18 have not been established.

#### OLDER ADULTS

To decrease the possibility of oversedation, dizziness, or impaired coordination, the usual starting dose is 0.125 milligram. This may be increased to 0.25 milligram if necessary.

### Overdosage

Any medication taken in excess can have serious consequences. Severe overdosage of Halcion can be fatal. If you suspect an overdose, seek medical help immediately.

■ *Symptoms of Halcion overdose may include:*
Apnea (temporary cessation of breathing), coma, confusion, excessive sleepiness, problems in coordination, seizures, shallow or difficult breathing, slurred speech

*Brand name:*

# Haldol

*Pronounced: HAL-dawl*
*Generic name: Haloperidol*

### Why is this drug prescribed?

Haldol is used to reduce the symptoms of mental disorders such as schizophrenia. It is also prescribed to control tics (uncontrolled muscle contractions of face, arms, or shoulders) and the unintended utterances that mark Gilles de la Tourette's syndrome. In addition, it is used in short-term treatment of children with severe behavior problems, including hyperactivity and combativeness.

Some doctors also prescribe Haldol to relieve severe nausea and vomiting caused by cancer drugs, to treat drug problems such as LSD flashback and PCP intoxication, and to control symptoms of hemiballismus, a condition that causes involuntary writhing of one side of the body.

### Most important fact about this drug

Haldol may cause tardive dyskinesia—a condition characterized by involuntary muscle spasms and twitches in the face and body. This condition can be permanent, and appears to be most common among the elderly, especially women. Ask your doctor for information about this possible risk.

### How should you take this medication?

Haldol may be taken with food or after eating. If taking Haldol in a liquid concentrate form, you will need to dilute it with milk or water.

You should not take Haldol with coffee, tea, or other caffeinated beverages, or with alcohol.

Haldol causes dry mouth. Sucking on a hard candy or ice chips may help alleviate the problem.

■ *If you miss a dose...*
Take it as soon as you remember. Take the rest of the doses for that day at equally spaced intervals. Do not take 2 doses at once.
■ *Storage instructions...*
Store away from heat, light, and moisture in a tightly closed container. Do not freeze the liquid.

### What side effects may occur?

Side effects cannot be anticipated. If any side effects develop or change in intensity, inform your doctor as soon as possible. Only your doctor can determine if it is safe for you to continue taking Haldol.

■ *Side effects may include:*
Abnormal secretion of milk, acne-like skin reactions, agitation, anemia, anxiety, blurred vision, breast pain, breast development in males, cataracts, catatonic (unresponsive) state, chewing movements, confusion, constipation, coughing, deeper breathing, dehydration, depression, diarrhea, dizziness, drowsiness, dry mouth, epileptic seizures, exaggerated feeling of well-being, exaggerated reflexes, excessive perspiration, excessive salivation, hair loss, hallucinations, headache, heat stroke, high fever, high or low blood pressure, high or low blood sugar, impotence, inability to urinate, increased sex drive, indigestion, involuntary movements, irregular menstrual periods, irregular pulse, lack of muscular coordination, liver problems, loss of appetite, muscle spasms, nausea, Parkinson-like symptoms, persistent abnormal erections, physical rigidity and stupor, protruding tongue, puckering of mouth, puffing of checks, rapid heartbeat, restlessness, rigid arms, feet, head, and muscles, rotation of eyeballs, sensitivity to light, skin rash, skin eruptions, sleeplessness, sluggishness, swelling of breasts, twitching in the body, neck, shoulders, and face, vertigo, visual problems, vomiting, wheezing or asthma-like symptoms, yellowing of skin and whites of eyes

### Why should this drug not be prescribed?

You should not take Haldol if you have Parkinson's disease or are sensitive to or allergic to the drug.

### Special warnings about this medication

You should use Haldol cautiously if you have ever had breast cancer, a severe heart or circulatory disorder, chest pain, the eye condition known as glaucoma, seizures, or any drug allergies.

Temporary muscle spasms and twitches may occur if you suddenly stop taking Haldol. Follow your doctor's instructions closely when discontinuing the drug.

This drug may impair your ability to drive a car or operate potentially dangerous machinery. Do not participate in any activities that require full alertness if you are unsure of your reaction to Haldol.

Haldol may make your skin more sensitive to sunlight. When spending time in the sun, use a sunscreen or wear protective clothing.

Avoid exposure to extreme heat or cold. Haldol interferes with the body's temperature-regulating mechanism, so you could become overheated or suffer severe chills.

### Possible food and drug interactions when taking this medication

Extreme drowsiness and other potentially serious effects can result if Haldol is combined with alcohol, narcotics, painkillers, sleeping medications, or other drugs that slow down the central nervous system.

If Haldol is taken with certain other drugs, the effects of either could be increased, decreased, or altered. It is especially important to check with your doctor before combining Haldol with the following:

Antiseizure drugs such as Dilantin or Tegretol
Antispasmodic drugs such as Bentyl and Cogentin

Blood-thinning medications such as Coumadin

Certain antidepressants, including Elavil, Tofranil, and Prozac

Epinephrine (EpiPen)

Lithium (Lithonate)

Methyldopa (Aldomet)

Propranolol (Inderal)

Rifampin (Rifadin)

## Special information if you are pregnant or breastfeeding

The effects of Haldol during pregnancy have not been adequately studied. Pregnant women should use Haldol only if clearly needed. If you are pregnant or plan to become pregnant, inform your doctor immediately. Haldol should not be used by women who are breastfeeding an infant.

## Recommended dosage

ADULTS

*Moderate Symptoms*

The usual dosage is 1 to 6 milligrams daily. This amount should be divided into 2 or 3 smaller doses.

*Severe Symptoms*

The usual dosage is 6 to 15 milligrams daily, divided into 2 or 3 smaller doses.

CHILDREN

Children younger than 3 years old should not take Haldol.

For children between the ages of 3 and 12, weighing approximately 33 to 88 pounds, doses should start at 0.5 milligram per day. Your doctor will increase the dose if needed.

*For Psychotic Disorders*

The daily dose may range from 0.05 milligram to 0.15 milligram for every 2.2 pounds of body weight.

*For Non-Psychotic Behavior Disorders and Tourette's Syndrome*

The daily dose may range from 0.05 milligram to 0.075 milligram for every 2.2 pounds of body weight.

OLDER ADULTS

In general, older people take dosages of Haldol in the lower ranges. Older adults (especially older women) may be more susceptible to tardive dyskinesia—a possibly irreversible condition marked by involuntary muscle spasms and twitches in the face and body. Consult your doctor for information about these potential risks.

Doses may range from 1 to 6 milligrams daily.

## Overdosage

Any medication taken in excess can have serious consequences. If you suspect an overdose, seek medical help immediately.

■ *Symptoms of Haldol overdose may include:*
Catatonic (unresponsive) state, coma, decreased breathing, low blood pressure, rigid muscles, sedation, tremor, weakness

*Brand name:*

# Halfprin

*See Aspirin, page 37.*

*Generic name:*

# Haloperidol

*See Haldol, page 235.*

*Brand name:*

# Hismanal

*Pronounced: HISS-man-al*
*Generic name: Astemizole*

## Why is this drug prescribed?

Hismanal is an antihistamine prescribed to relieve hay fever and to treat chronic hives. Hismanal is for long-term use; it will not provide immediate relief.

## Most important fact about this drug

Never take more than the prescribed dose of Hismanal in an attempt to speed its action. Higher doses have been known to cause dangerously irregular heartbeats.

## How should you take this medication?

Hismanal should be taken on an empty stomach—for example, 1 hour before you eat or 2 hours after eating. Taking the drug with food may make it less effective.

■ *If you miss a dose...*
Take it as soon as you remember. If it is almost time for your next dose, skip the one you

missed and go back to your regular schedule. Never take 2 doses at the same time.

■ *Storage instructions...*
Store at room temperature. Protect from moisture.

## What side effects may occur?

Side effects cannot be anticipated. If any develop or change in intensity, inform your doctor as soon as possible. Only your doctor can determine if it is safe for you to continue taking Hismanal.

■ *More common side effects may include:*
Drowsiness, dry mouth, fatigue, headache, increase in appetite, weight gain
■ *Less common side effects may include:*
Asthma-like symptoms, burning, prickling, or tingling, depression, diarrhea, dizziness, fluid retention, hepatitis, inflammation of the eyelids, itching, joint pain, muscle pain, nausea, nervousness, nosebleed, palpitations, sensitivity to light, skin rash, sore throat, stomach and intestinal pain
■ *Rare side effects may include:*
Low blood pressure

## Why should this drug not be prescribed?

Avoid Hismanal if you have a known allergy to it.

## Special warnings about this medication

Rare—but serious—heart-related side effects have been reported when Hismanal is used with erythromycin (PCE, E-Mycin), ketoconazole (Nizoral), or itraconazole (Sporanox). If you are taking these medicines, do not take Hismanal. The same reaction can be caused by combining Hismanal with a large dose of quinine. However, the amount of quinine in tonic water is too small to cause the problem under ordinary circumstances.

If you are being treated for a lower respiratory tract disease such as asthma or for liver or kidney disease, consult with your doctor before taking Hismanal.

## Possible food and drug interactions when taking this medication

Taking this drug with food can decrease its effectiveness.

If Hismanal is taken with certain other drugs the effects of either may be increased, decreased, or altered. It is especially important to check with your doctor before combining Hismanal with the following:

Alcohol
Antibiotics such as Flagyl
Antifungal drugs such as Diflucan, Nizoral, and Sporanox
Drugs that affect heart rhythms such as Vascor, Elavil, and Thorazine
"Macrolide" antibiotics such as Zithromax, Biaxin, E-Mycin, PCE, and Tao
Quinine

See "Special warnings about this medication" for more information.

## Special information if you are pregnant or breastfeeding

The effects of Hismanal during pregnancy have not been adequately studied. Therefore, this medication should be prescribed only when the benefits of therapy outweigh any potential risk to the fetus. It is not known whether Hismanal appears in breast milk. If this medication is essential to your health, your doctor may advise you to stop nursing your baby until your treatment with this drug is finished.

## Recommended dosage

### ADULTS

The usual dose for adults and children 12 years and over is 10 milligrams (1 tablet) once daily.

### CHILDREN

Safety and effectiveness in children under 12 have not been established.

## Overdosage

Hismanal is generally safe; however, large amounts may cause serious symptoms. If you suspect an overdose, get medical help immediately.

■ *Symptoms of Hismanal overdose may include:*
Cardiac arrest, fainting, irregular heartbeat, seizures

*Brand name:*

# Humulin

*See Insulin, page 258.*

*Brand name:*

# Hydergine

*Pronounced: HY-der-jeen*
*Generic name: Ergoloid mesylates*

## Why is this drug prescribed?

Hydergine helps relieve symptoms of declining mental capacity, thought to be related to aging or dementia, seen in some people over age 60. The symptoms include reduced understanding and motivation, and a decline in self-care and interpersonal skills.

### Most important fact about this drug

It may take several weeks or more for Hydergine to produce noticeable results. In fact, your doctor may need up to 6 months to determine whether the drug is right for you. Keep taking your regular doses even if you feel no effect.

### How should you take this medication?

Take Hydergine exactly as prescribed.

If you are taking sublingual tablets, allow them to dissolve completely under the tongue. Do not crush or chew them.

■ *If you miss a dose...*
Skip the dose you missed and go back to your regular schedule. Do not take 2 doses at once. If you miss 2 or more doses in a row, consult your doctor.

■ *Storage instructions...*
Store away from heat, light, and moisture. Do not freeze the oral solution.

### What side effects may occur?

Side effects cannot be anticipated. If any develop or change in intensity, notify your doctor as soon as possible. Only your doctor can determine whether it is safe to continue taking Hydergine.

■ *Side effects may include:*
Irritation below the tongue (with sublingual tablets), stomach upset, temporary nausea

### Why should this drug not be prescribed?

Do not use Hydergine if you have ever had an allergic reaction to or are sensitive to the drug, or if you have a mental disorder.

### Special warnings about this medication

Since the symptoms treated with Hydergine are of unknown origin and may change or evolve into a specific disease, your doctor will make a careful diagnosis before prescribing Hydergine and then watch closely for any changes in your condition.

### Possible food and drug interactions when taking this medication

No interactions have been reported.

### Special information if you are pregnant or breastfeeding

Hydergine is not intended for use by women of childbearing age.

### Recommended dosage

ADULTS

The usual dose of Hydergine is 1 milligram, 3 times a day.

### Overdosage

Any medication taken in excess can have serious consequences. If you suspect an overdose of Hydergine, seek medical attention immediately.

---

*Brand name:*

# Hydrocet

*See Vicodin, page 587.*

---

*Generic name:*

# Hydrochlorothiazide

*See HydroDIURIL, page 240.*

---

*Generic name:*

# Hydrochlorothiazide with Triamterene

*See Dyazide, page 181.*

---

*Generic name:*

# Hydrocodone with Acetaminophen

*See Vicodin, page 587.*

---

*Generic name:*

# Hydrocodone with Chlorpheniramine

*See Tussionex, page 568.*

*Generic name:*

# Hydrocortisone

*See Anusol-HC, page 33.*

*Brand name:*

# HydroDIURIL

*Pronounced: High-dro-DYE-your-il*
*Generic name: Hydrochlorothiazide*
*Other brand name: Esidrix*

### Why is this drug prescribed?

HydroDIURIL is used in the treatment of high blood pressure and other conditions that require the elimination of excess fluid (water) from the body. These conditions include congestive heart failure, cirrhosis of the liver, corticosteroid and estrogen therapy, and kidney disorders. When used for high blood pressure, HydroDIURIL can be used alone or with other high blood pressure medications. HydroDIURIL contains a form of thiazide, a diuretic that prompts your body to produce and eliminate more urine, which helps lower blood pressure.

### Most important fact about this drug

If you have high blood pressure, you must take HydroDIURIL regularly for it to be effective. Since blood pressure declines gradually, it may be several weeks before you get the full benefit of Hydro-DIURIL; and you must continue taking it even if you are feeling well. HydroDIURIL does not cure high blood pressure; it merely keeps it under control.

### How should you take this medication?

Take HydroDIURIL exactly as prescribed by your doctor.

■ *If you miss a dose...*
  If you forget a dose, take it as soon as you remember. If it is almost time for your next dose, skip the one you missed and go back to your regular schedule. Never take two doses at the same time.
■ *Storage instructions...*
  Keep container tightly closed. Protect from light, moisture, and freezing cold. Store at room temperature.

### What side effects may occur?

Side effects cannot be anticipated. If any develop or change in intensity, inform your doctor as soon as possible. Only your doctor can determine if it is safe for you to continue taking HydroDIURIL.

■ *Side effects may include:*
  Abdominal cramping, diarrhea, dizziness upon standing up, headache, loss of appetite, low blood pressure, low potassium (leading to symptoms such as dry mouth, excessive thirst, weak or irregular heartbeat, muscle pain or cramps), stomach irritation, stomach upset, weakness
■ *Less common or rare side effects may include:*
  Anemia, blood disorders, changes in blood sugar, constipation, difficulty breathing, dizziness, fever, fluid in the lung, hair loss, high levels of sugar in the urine, hives, hypersensitivity reactions, impotence, inflammation of the lung, inflammation of the pancreas, inflammation of the salivary glands, kidney failure, muscle spasms, nausea, rash, reddish or purplish spots on the skin, restlessness, sensitivity to light, skin disorders including Stevens-Johnson syndrome (blisters in the mouth and eyes), skin peeling, tingling or pins and needles, vertigo, vision changes, vomiting, yellow eyes and skin

### Why should this drug not be prescribed?

If you are unable to urinate, you should not take this medication.

If you are sensitive to or have ever had an allergic reaction to HydroDIURIL or similar drugs, or if you are sensitive to sulfa or other sulfonamide-derived drugs, you should not take this medication.

### Special warnings about this medication

Diuretics can cause your body to lose too much potassium. Signs of an excessively low potassium level include muscle weakness and rapid or irregular heartbeat. To boost your potassium level, your doctor may recommend eating potassium-rich foods or taking a potassium supplement.

If you are taking HydroDIURIL, your kidney function should be given a complete assessment, and should continue to be monitored.

If you have liver disease, diabetes, gout, or lupus erythematosus (a form of rheumatism), Hydro-DIURIL should be used with caution.

If you have bronchial asthma or a history of allergies, you may be at greater risk for an allergic reaction to this medication.

Dehydration, excessive sweating, severe diarrhea or vomiting could deplete your body's fluids and cause your blood pressure to become too low. Be careful when exercising and in hot weather.

### Possible food and drug interactions when taking this medication

HydroDIURIL may increase the effects of alcohol. Do not drink alcohol while taking this medication.

If HydroDIURIL is taken with certain other drugs, the effects of either could be increased, decreased, or altered. It is especially important to check with your doctor before combining Hydro-DIURIL with the following:

Barbiturates such as phenobarbital
Cholestyramine (Questran)
Colestipol (Colestid)
Corticosteroids such as prednisone and ACTH
Digoxin (Lanoxin)
Drugs to treat diabetes such as insulin or Micronase
Lithium (Lithonate)
Narcotics such as Percocet
Nonsteroidal anti-inflammatory drugs such as Naprosyn
Norepinephrine (Levophed)
Other high blood pressure medications such as Aldomet
Skeletal muscle relaxants, such as tubocurarine

### Special information if you are pregnant or breastfeeding

The effects of HydroDIURIL during pregnancy have not been adequately studied. If you are pregnant or plan to become pregnant, inform your doctor immediately. HydroDIURIL appears in breast milk and could affect a nursing infant. If this medication is essential to your health, your doctor may advise you to discontinue breastfeeding until your treatment is finished.

### Recommended dosage

Dosage should be adjusted to each individual's needs. The smallest dose that is effective should be used.

### ADULTS

#### Water Retention
The usual dose is 25 milligrams to 100 milligrams per day. Your doctor may tell you to take the drug in a single dose or to divide the total amount into more than one dose. Your doctor may put you on a day on, day off schedule or some other alternate day schedule to suit your needs.

#### High Blood Pressure
The usual dose is 25 milligrams as a single dose. Your doctor may increase the dose to 50 milligrams, as a single dose or divided into 2 doses. Dosages should be adjusted when used with other high blood pressure medications.

### CHILDREN

Dosages for children should be adjusted according to weight, generally 0.5 to 1 milligram per pound of body weight in 1 or 2 doses per day. Infants under 2 years should not receive more than 37.5 milligrams per day, and children aged 2 to 12 should not get more than 100 milligrams a day. Infants under 6 months may need 1.5 milligrams per pound per day in 2 doses.

#### Under 2 years
Based on age and body weight, the daily dosage is 12.5 milligrams to 37.5 milligrams per day.

#### 2 to 12 years
The daily dosage, based on body weight, is 37.5 milligrams to 100 milligrams.

HydroDIURIL tablets come in strengths of 25, 50 and 100 milligrams.

### Overdosage

Any medication taken in excess can cause symptoms of overdose. If you suspect an overdose, seek medical attention immediately.

■ *Symptoms of HydroDIURIL overdose may include:*
   Dry mouth, excessive thirst, muscle pain or cramps, nausea and vomiting, weak or irregular heartbeat, weakness and dizziness

*Generic name:*

# Hydromorphone

*See Dilaudid, page 163.*

*Generic name:*

# Hydroxychloroquine

*See Plaquenil, page 420.*

*Generic name:*

# Hydroxyzine

See Atarax, page 38.

*Brand name:*

# Hygroton

Pronounced: HIGH-grow-ton
Generic name: Chlorthalidone
Other brand name: Thalitone

### Why is this drug prescribed?

Hygroton is a diuretic (water pill) used to treat high blood pressure and fluid retention associated with congestive heart failure, cirrhosis of the liver (a disease of the liver caused by damage to its cells), corticosteroid and estrogen therapy, and kidney disease. When used for high blood pressure, Hygroton may be used alone or in combination with other high blood pressure medications. Diuretics help your body produce and eliminate more urine, which helps lower blood pressure.

### Most important fact about this drug

If you have high blood pressure, you must take Hygroton regularly for it to be effective. Since blood pressure declines gradually, it may be several weeks before you get the full benefit of Hygroton; and you must continue taking it even if you are feeling well. Hygroton does not cure high blood pressure; it merely keeps it under control.

### How should you take this medication?

Diuretics such as Hygroton increase urination; therefore Hygroton should be taken in the morning.

Do not interchange Hygroton or generic chlorthalidone with Thalitone without consulting your doctor or pharmacist.

Hygroton may be taken with food. Take it exactly as prescribed.

■ *If you miss a dose...*
Take it as soon as you remember. If it is almost time for the next dose, skip the one you missed and go back to your regular schedule. Do not take 2 doses at the same time.

■ *Storage instructions...*
Store at room temperature.

### What side effects may occur?

Side effects cannot be anticipated. If any side effects develop or change in intensity, tell your doctor immediately. Only your doctor can determine whether it is safe to continue taking Hygroton.

■ *Side effects may include:*
Allergic reaction, anemia, changes in blood sugar, change in potassium levels (causing such symptoms as dry mouth, excessive thirst, weak or irregular heartbeat, and muscle pain or cramps), constipation, cramping, diarrhea, dizziness, dizziness upon standing up, flaky skin, headache, hives, impotence, inflammation of the pancreas, itching, loss of appetite, low blood pressure, muscle spasms, nausea, rash, restlessness, sensitivity to light, stomach irritation, tingling or pins and needles, vision changes, vomiting, weakness, yellow eyes and skin

### Why should this drug not be prescribed?

If you are unable to urinate or if you have ever had an allergic reaction to or are sensitive to chlorthalidone or other sulfa drugs, do not take Hygroton.

### Special warnings about this medication

Diuretics can cause your body to lose too much potassium. Signs of an excessively low potassium level include muscle weakness and rapid or irregular heartbeat. To boost your potassium level, your doctor may recommend eating potassium-rich foods or taking a potassium supplement.

Tell your doctor if you have ever had an allergic reaction to other diuretics or if you have asthma, kidney or liver disease, gout, or lupus.

If you have a history of bronchial asthma, you are more likely to have an allergic reaction to Hygroton.

Be careful in hot weather not to become dehydrated. Contact your doctor if you experience excessive thirst, tiredness, restlessness, muscle pains or cramps, nausea, vomiting, or increased heart rate or pulse.

This medication may aggravate lupus erythematosus, a disease of the connective tissue.

Avoid prolonged exposure to sunlight.

### Possible food and drug interactions when taking this medication

Drinking alcohol may increase the chance of dizziness. Do not drink alcohol while taking this medication.

If Hygroton is taken with certain other drugs, the effects of either could be increased, decreased, or altered. It is especially important to check with your doctor before combining Hygroton with the following:

Appetite-control medicines such as Tenuate
Cholestyramine (Questran)
Colestipol (Colestid)
Decongestants (medicines for colds, cough, hay fever, or sinus)
Digitalis (Lanoxin)
Insulin
Lithium (Lithonate)
Oral diabetes drugs such as Micronase
Other high blood pressure medications such as Catapres and Aldomet
Steroids such as prednisone

### Special information
### if you are pregnant or breastfeeding

Information is not available about the safety of Hygroton during pregnancy. If you are pregnant or plan to become pregnant, inform your doctor immediately. Hygroton may appear in breast milk and could affect a nursing infant. If Hygroton is essential to your health, your doctor may advise you to stop breastfeeding until your treatment is finished.

### Recommended dosage

Your doctor will tailor your individual dose to the lowest possible amount that delivers a satisfactory response.

Once desired control of blood pressure or fluid retention has been achieved, your doctor may adjust your dose downward.

#### HIGH BLOOD PRESSURE

*Hygroton*
The usual initial dosage is a single dose of 25 milligrams. Your doctor may increase the dose to 100 milligrams once daily.

*Thalitone*
The usual initial dose is a single dose of 15 milligrams. Your doctor may increase the dose to 45 to 50 milligrams once daily.

#### FLUID RETENTION

*Hygroton*
The usual recommended initial dose is 50 to 100 milligrams daily or 100 milligrams every other day. Some people may require up to 150 to 200 milligrams at these intervals.

*Thalitone*
The usual initial dose is 30 to 60 milligrams daily or 60 milligrams on alternate days. Some people may require up to 90 to 120 milligrams at these intervals.

### Overdosage

Any medication taken in excess can have serious consequences. If you suspect an overdose, seek medical treatment immediately.

■ *Symptoms of Hygroton overdose may include:*
Confusion, dizziness, nausea, weakness

*Generic name:*

# Hyoscyamine

*See Levsin, page 278.*

*Brand name:*

# Hytone

*See Anusol-HC, page 33.*

*Brand name:*

# Hytrin

*Pronounced: HIGH-trin*
*Generic name: Terazosin hydrochloride*

### Why is this drug prescribed?

Hytrin is prescribed to reduce high blood pressure. It may be used alone or in combination with other blood pressure lowering drugs, such as Hydro-DIURIL (a diuretic) or Inderal, a beta blocker.

Hytrin is also prescribed to relieve the symptoms of benign prostatic hyperplasia or BPH. BPH is an enlargement of the prostate gland that surrounds the urinary canal. It leads to the following symptoms:

■ a weak or interrupted stream when urinating
■ a feeling that you cannot empty your bladder completely
■ a feeling of delay when you start to urinate
■ a need to urinate often, especially at night
■ a feeling that you must urinate right away

Hytrin relaxes the tightness of a certain type of muscle in the prostate and at the opening of the bladder. This can reduce the severity of the symptoms.

## Most important fact about this drug

If you have high blood pressure, you must take Hytrin regularly for it to be effective. Since blood pressure declines gradually, it may be several weeks before you get the full benefit of Hytrin; and you must continue taking it even if you are feeling well. Hytrin does not cure high blood pressure; it merely keeps it under control.

## How should you take this medication?

You may take Hytrin with or without food. Take your first dose at bedtime. Do not take more than the 1 milligram your doctor has prescribed.

■ *If you miss a dose...*
Take it as soon as you remember. If it is almost time for the next dose, skip the one you missed and go back to your regular schedule. Do not take 2 doses at the same time.

■ *Storage instructions...*
Store at room temperature in a cool, dry place. Protect from light.

## What side effects may occur?

Side effects cannot be anticipated. If any develop or change in intensity, inform your doctor as soon as possible. Only your doctor can determine if it is safe for you to continue taking Hytrin.

■ *More common side effects may include:*
Difficult or labored breathing, dizziness, headache, heart palpitations, light-headedness upon standing, nausea, pain in the arms and legs, sleepiness, stuffy nose, swollen wrists and ankles, weakness

If these symptoms persist, tell your doctor. Your dosage of Hytrin may be higher than needed.

■ *Less common or rare side effects may include:*
Anxiety, back pain, blurred vision, bronchitis, conjunctivitis (inflamed eyes), constipation, decreased sex drive, depression, diarrhea, dimmed vision, dry mouth, facial swelling, fainting, fever, flu or cold symptoms (cough, sore throat, runny nose), fluid retention, frequent urination, gas, gout, impotence, inability to hold urine, increased heart rate, indigestion, inflamed sinuses, insomnia, irregular heartbeat, itching, joint pain and inflammation, low blood pressure, muscle aches, nasal inflammation, nervousness, nosebleed, numbness or tingling, pain in the abdomen, chest, neck, or shoulder, rash, ringing

in the ears, severe allergic reaction, sweating, urinary tract infection, vertigo, vision changes, vomiting, weight gain

## Why should this drug not be prescribed?

Do not take Hytrin if you are sensitive to it or have ever had an allergic reaction to it.

## Special warnings about this medication

When your blood pressure falls in response to Hytrin, you may faint. Other less severe reactions include dizziness, heart palpitations, light-headedness, and drowsiness. You are also likely to feel dizzy or faint whenever you rise from a sitting or lying position; this should disappear as your body becomes accustomed to Hytrin. If your occupation is such that these symptoms might cause serious problems, make sure your doctor knows this from the start; he or she will increase your Hytrin dosage very cautiously.

Regardless of your occupation, avoid driving, climbing, and other hazardous tasks at the following times:

■ For 12 hours after your first dose of Hytrin
■ With each new dosage increase
■ When you re-start Hytrin after any treatment interruption

If you are taking Hytrin for benign prostatic hyperplasia, remember that although Hytrin helps relieve the symptoms of BPH, it does NOT change the size of the prostate, which may continue to grow. You may still need surgery in the future. In addition, it *is* possible to have BPH and prostate cancer at the same time.

## Possible food and drug interactions when taking this medication

If Hytrin is taken with certain other drugs, the effects of either could be increased, decreased, or altered. It is especially important to check with your doctor before combining Hytrin with the following:

Nonsteroidal anti-inflammatory painkillers such as Motrin and Naprosyn
Other blood pressure medications, such as Dyazide, Vasotec, Calan, and Verelan

## Special information if you are pregnant or breastfeeding

The effects of Hytrin during pregnancy have not been adequately studied. If you are pregnant or plan to become pregnant, notify your doctor immediately. Hytrin is not recommended during pregnancy unless the benefit outweighs the potential risk to the unborn baby. It is not known whether Hytrin appears in breast milk. Because many drugs do appear in breast milk, your doctor may advise you to stop breastfeeding until your treatment with this drug is finished.

## Recommended dosage

### ADULTS

*High blood pressure*
The usual initial dose is 1 milligram at bedtime. Your doctor may slowly increase the dose until your blood pressure has been lowered sufficiently. The usual recommended dosage range is 1 milligram to 5 milligrams taken once a day; however, some people may benefit from doses as high as 20 milligrams per day.

*Benign prostatic hyperplasia*
The starting dose is 1 milligram at bedtime. Your doctor will gradually increase the dose to 10 milligrams, taken once a day, usually for at least 4 to 6 weeks. A few men have needed a dose of 20 milligrams a day.

If you stop taking Hytrin for several days or longer, your doctor will re-start your treatment with 1 milligram at bedtime.

### CHILDREN

Safety and effectiveness of Hytrin in children have not been established.

## Overdosage

If you take too much Hytrin, dizziness, light-headedness, and fainting may occur within 90 minutes. A large overdose may lead to shock. If you suspect an overdose of Hytrin, seek medical attention immediately.

*Brand name:*

# Hyzaar

*Pronounced: HI-zuhr*
*Generic names: Losartan Potassium and Hydrochlorothiazide*

## Why is this drug prescribed?

Hyzaar is a combination medication used in the treatment of high blood pressure. One component, losartan, belongs to a new class of blood pressure medications that work by preventing the hormone angiotensin-II from constricting the blood vessels, thus allowing blood to flow more freely and keeping the blood pressure down. The other component, hydrochlorothiazide, is a diuretic that increases the output of urine, removing excess fluid from the body and thus lowering blood pressure.

## Most important fact about this drug

You must take Hyzaar regularly for it to be effective. Since blood pressure declines gradually, it may be several weeks before you get the full benefit of Hyzaar, and you must continue taking it even if you are feeling well. Hyzaar does not cure high blood pressure; it merely keeps it under control.

## How should you take this medication?

Hyzaar may be taken with or without food. Take Hyzaar exactly as directed. Try to take it at the same time each day so that it is easier to remember.

■ *If you miss a dose...*
Take the forgotten dose as soon as you remember. If it is almost time for your next dose, skip the one you missed and go back to your regular schedule.
■ *Storage instructions...*
Keep in a tightly closed container at room temperature. Protect from light.

## What side effects may occur?

Side effects cannot be anticipated. If any develop or change in intensity, inform your doctor as soon as possible. Only your doctor can determine if it is safe for you to continue taking Hyzaar.

■ *More common side effects include:*
Dizziness, upper respiratory infection
■ *Less common side effects include:*
Abdominal pain, back pain, cough, fluid retention and swelling, heart palpitations, sinus inflammation, skin rash

## Why should this drug not be prescribed?

If you have ever had an allergic reaction to losartan, hydrochlorothiazide, or sulfonamide-derived drugs, you should not take this medication. If you are unable to urinate, do not take Hyzaar.

## Special warnings about this medication

If you are taking Hyzaar and have kidney disease, your doctor will watch your kidney function carefully.

Hyzaar can cause low blood pressure, especially if you are also taking another diuretic. You may feel light-headed or faint, especially during the first few days of therapy. If these symptoms occur, contact your doctor. Your dosage may need to be adjusted or discontinued. If you actually faint, stop taking the medication until you have talked to your doctor.

If you have liver or kidney disease, diabetes, gout, or lupus erythematosus, Hyzaar should be used with caution. This drug may bring out hidden diabetes. If you are already taking insulin or oral diabetes drugs, your medication may have to be adjusted. If you have bronchial asthma or a history of allergies, you may be at greater risk for an allergic reaction to this medication.

Excessive sweating, severe diarrhea or vomiting could deplete your body fluids and cause your blood pressure to drop too low. Be careful when exercising and in hot weather. Call your doctor if your mouth becomes dry, you feel weak or tired or sluggish, you are unusually thirsty, you feel restless or confused, you ache all over, your heart starts beating faster, or you are nauseated.

### Possible food and drug interactions when taking this medication

Hyzaar may increase the effects of alcohol. Avoid alcohol while taking this medication.

If Hyzaar is taken with certain other drugs, the effects of either could be increased, decreased, or altered. It is especially important to check with your doctor before taking Hyzaar with the following:

Barbiturates such as phenobarbital and Seconal
Cholestyramine (Questran)
Colestipol (Colestid)
Corticosteroids (Prednisone)
Insulin
Ketoconazole (Nizoral)
Lithium (Eskalith, Lithobid)
Narcotic pain-killers such as Demerol, Tylenol with Codeine, and Percocet
Nonsteroidal anti-inflammatory drugs (NSAIDs) such as Aleve, Anaprox, and Motrin
Other blood pressure-lowering drugs such as Procardia XL and Tenormin
Oral diabetes drugs such as Diabinese, DiaBeta, and Glucotrol
Potassium supplements such as Slow-K

Salt substitutes containing potassium
Sulfaphenazole
Troleandomycin (Tao)

### Special Information
### if you are pregnant or breastfeeding

When used in the second or third trimester of pregnancy, Hyzaar can cause injury or even death to the unborn child. Stop taking Hyzaar as soon as you know you are pregnant. If you are pregnant or plan to become pregnant, tell your doctor immediately. Hyzaar appears in breast milk and can affect the nursing infant. If this medication is essential to your health, your doctor may advise you to stop breastfeeding while you are taking Hyzaar.

### Recommended dosage

ADULTS

The usual starting dose of Hyzaar is 1 tablet once daily (losartan 50 milligrams/hydrochlorothiazide 12.5 milligrams).

If your blood pressure does not respond to this dose, after about 3 weeks the dose may be increased to 2 tablets once daily. Taking more than 2 tablets daily is not recommended.

CHILDREN

The safety and effectiveness of Hyzaar in children have not been studied.

### Overdosage

Any medication taken in excess can have serious consequences. Information concerning Hyzaar overdosage is limited. However, extremely low blood pressure and abnormally rapid or slow heartbeat may be signs of an overdose. Other signs may include dryness and thirst, overall weakness and tiredness, restlessness and confusion, muscle pains, nausea, and vomiting.

If you suspect an overdose, seek medical attention immediately.

*Generic name:*

# Ibuprofen

*See Motrin, page 337.*

*Brand name:*

# Iletin

*See Insulin, page 258.*

Brand name:

# Ilosone

See Erythromycin, Oral, page 196.

Brand name:

# Imdur

Pronounced: IM-duhr
Generic name: Isosorbide mononitrate
Other brand names: Ismo, Monoket

## Why is this drug prescribed?

Imdur is prescribed to prevent angina pectoris (crushing chest pain that results when partially clogged arteries restrict the flow of needed oxygen-rich blood to the heart). This medication does not relieve angina attacks already underway.

## Most important fact about this drug

Imdur may cause severe low blood pressure (possibly marked by dizziness or fainting), especially when you are standing or if you sit up quickly. People taking blood pressure medication or those who have low blood pressure should use Imdur with caution.

## How should you take this medication?

To maintain this drug's protective effect, it is important that you take it exactly as prescribed.

Take Imdur once a day, when you get up in the morning. It may be taken with or without food. Imdur tablets should not be crushed or chewed. Swallow them with half a glass of liquid.

Do not switch to another brand of isosorbide mononitrate without consulting your doctor or pharmacist.

■ If you miss a dose...
Take it as soon as you remember. If it is almost time for your next dose, skip the one you missed and go back to your regular schedule. Do not take 2 doses at the same time.
■ Storage instructions...
Store at room temperature.

## What side effects may occur?

Side effects cannot be anticipated. If any develop or change in intensity, tell your doctor as soon as possible. Only your doctor can determine if it is safe for you to continue taking Imdur.

Headache is the most common side effect; usually, aspirin or acetaminophen will relieve the pain. The headaches associated with Imdur usually subside within a short time after treatment with the drug begins. Check with your doctor if your headaches persist or become more intense. Another common side effect is dizziness.

■ Less common or rare side effects may include:
Abdominal pain, abnormal hair texture, abnormal heart sounds, abnormal or terrifying dreams, abnormal vision, acne, anemia, anxiety, back pain, bacterial infection, black stools, breast pain, bronchitis, chest pain, confusion, constipation, coughing, decreased sex drive, depression, diarrhea, difficult or labored breathing, difficulty concentrating, diminished sense of touch, drooping eyelid, dry mouth, earache, excessive amount of urine, fatigue, fever, fluid retention and swelling, flu-like symptoms, flushing, frozen shoulder, gas, general feeling of illness, heart attack, heart failure, heart murmur, hemorrhoids, high blood pressure, hot flashes, impotence, inability to sleep, increased mucus from the lungs, increased sweating, indigestion, inflamed eyes, inflammation of the stomach, inflammation of the tongue, inflammation of the vagina, intolerance of light, irregular heartbeat, itching, joint pain, kidney stones, leg ulcer, loose stools, low blood pressure, migraine, muscle and/or bone pain, muscle weakness, nasal or sinus inflammation, nausea, nervousness, palpitations (throbbing or fluttering heartbeat), paralysis, perforated eardrum, pneumonia, purple or red spots on the skin, rapid heartbeat, rash, ringing in the ears, severe pain in calf muscles during walking, sleepiness, slow heartbeat, sore throat, stomach ulcer with or without bleeding, stuffy nose, tingling or pins and needles, tremor, twisted neck, urinary tract infection, varicose veins, vertigo, viral infection, vomiting, weakness, wheezing, worsening of angina pectoris, yeast infection

## Why should this drug not be prescribed?

You should not take Imdur if you have had a previous allergic reaction to it or to other heart medications containing nitrates or nitrites. Your doctor will probably not prescribe Imdur if you have had a recent heart attack or congestive heart failure. If the doctor decides that this medication is essential, your heart function and blood pressure will need to be closely monitored to avoid potential side effects.

### Special warnings about this medication

Do not abruptly stop taking this medication. Follow your doctor's plan for a gradual withdrawal.

Since Imdur can cause dizziness, you should be careful while driving, operating machinery, or performing other tasks that demand concentration.

Nitrate-type medications such as Imdur may aggravate angina caused by certain heart conditions.

Do not try to avoid a headache by changing your dose. If your headache stops, it may mean the drug has lost its effectiveness.

Be sure to tell your doctor about any medical conditions you have before starting Imdur therapy.

### Possible food and drug interactions
### when taking this medication

If Imdur is taken with certain other drugs, the effects of either could be increased, decreased, or altered. Extreme low blood pressure with dizziness and fainting upon standing up may occur if Imdur is taken with calcium-blocking blood pressure medications such as Calan, Cardizem, and Procardia.

Alcohol may interact with Imdur and cause a swift decrease in blood pressure, possibly resulting in light-headedness.

### Special information
### if you are pregnant or breastfeeding

The effects of Imdur during pregnancy have not been adequately studied. If you are pregnant or plan to become pregnant, tell your doctor immediately. Imdur should be used during pregnancy only if it is clearly needed.

It is not known whether Imdur appears in breast milk. If the drug is essential to your health, your doctor may advise you to stop nursing until your treatment is finished.

### Recommended dosage

ADULTS

The usual starting dose is 30 milligrams (taken as one-half of a 60-milligram tablet) or 60 milligrams once a day.

After several days, your doctor may increase the dose to 120 milligrams (two 60-milligram tablets) once daily.

Your doctor may further adjust the dosage according to your response to the medication.

CHILDREN

Safety and effectiveness of Imdur in children have not been established.

### Overdosage

Any medication taken in excess can have serious consequences. Severe overdosage of Imdur can be fatal. If you suspect an overdose, seek medical help immediately.

■ *Symptoms of Imdur overdose may include:*
Air hunger, bloody diarrhea, coma, confusion, difficulty breathing, fainting, fever, nausea, palpitations, paralysis, pressure in the head, profuse sweating, seizures, skin either cold and clammy or flushed, slow heartbeat, throbbing headache, vertigo, visual disturbances, vomiting

*Generic name:*

# Imipramine

*See Tofranil, page 549.*

*Brand name:*

# Imitrex

*Pronounced: IM-i-trex*
*Generic name: Sumatriptan succinate*

### Why is this drug prescribed?

Imitrex is prescribed for the treatment of a migraine attack with or without the presence of an aura (visual disturbances, usually sensations of halos or flickering lights, which precede an attack). This medication will not prevent or reduce the number of attacks you may experience.

### Most important fact about this drug

Imitrex should be used only to treat an acute, classic migraine attack. It should not be used for other types of headache, including cluster headache, or certain unusual types of migraine.

### How should you take this medication?

Imitrex Injection is administered just below the skin with an autoinjector (self-injection device). Your doctor should carefully instruct you on how to use the autoinjector and how to dispose of the empty syringes. You should carefully read the instruction pamphlet that comes with the medication.

Imitrex Tablets are swallowed whole, with liquid.

Imitrex should be taken as soon as your migraine symptoms appear, but may be used at any time during an attack.

A second injection may be given if your migraine symptoms return; however, never take more than 2 injections within 24 hours, and be sure to wait 1 hour between doses.

If you have had no relief 2 hours after taking Imitrex Tablets, you may take a second dose of up to 100 milligrams, if your doctor advises it. If the headache returns, you may take additional doses at intervals of at least 2 hours. You should not take more than 300 milligrams in one day. If your headache returns after you have had an Imitrex Injection, you may take single Imitrex Tablets, at intervals of at least 2 hours, up to a maximum of 200 milligrams in a day.

■ *If you miss a dose...*
Imitrex is *not* for regular use. Take it only during an attack.

■ *Storage instructions...*
Store Imitrex away from heat and light, at room temperature, in the case provided. If your medication has expired (the expiration date is printed on the treatment pack), throw it away as instructed, but keep the autoinjector. If your doctor decides to stop your treatment, do not keep any leftover medicine unless your doctor tells you to. Throw away your medicine as instructed.

## What side effects may occur?
Side effects cannot be anticipated. If any develop or change in intensity, inform your doctor as soon as possible. Only your doctor can determine if it is safe for you to continue taking Imitrex.

■ *More common side effects may include:*
Burning sensation, dizziness or vertigo, feeling of heaviness, feeling of tightness, flushing, mouth and tongue discomfort, muscle weakness, neck pain and stiffness, numbness, pressure sensation, redness at the site of injection, sore throat, tingling, warm/hot sensation

■ *Less common or rare side effects may include:*
Abdominal discomfort, agitation, allergic reactions (severe), anxiety, changes in heart rhythm, cold sensation, difficult or painful urination, difficulty swallowing, drowsiness/calmness, eye irritation, fatigue, feeling strange, general feeling of illness, headache, hives, itching, jaw discomfort, muscle cramps, muscle pain or tenderness, pressure in chest, rapid and throbbing heartbeat, rash, rise in blood pressure (temporary), shortness of breath, sinus or nasal discomfort, sweating, tight feeling in head, tightness in chest, vision changes

## Why should this drug not be prescribed?
If you are sensitive to or have had an allergic reaction to sumatriptan you should not use this drug again. Make sure your doctor is aware of any drug reactions you have experienced.

Imitrex should not be used if you have certain types of heart disease, including angina (crushing chest pain) or a history of heart attack, if you suffer from irregular heartbeat, shortness of breath, or uncontrolled blood pressure, or within 24 hours of taking a medication containing ergotamine (often used in other migraine medications) or drugs such as D.H.E. 45 Injection and Sansert.

You should not use Imitrex with antidepressant drugs known as MAO inhibitors, such as Nardil and Parnate, or within 2 weeks of discontinuing treatment with an MAO inhibitor.

## Special warnings about this medication
Your doctor may administer the first dose of Imitrex in the office. Although extremely rare, serious heart problems have occurred in people with heart disease when receiving this medication, and you should be carefully observed after the initial dose to make sure this medication is safe for you to use. Tell your doctor if you have high blood pressure, high cholesterol, or diabetes, if you smoke, if there is heart disease in your family, or if you have gone through menopause.

Do not use Imitrex Injection intravenously. This can cause a serious heart irregularity.

This medication should not be used for other types of migraine headache. If the first dose does not relieve your symptoms, your doctor will re-evaluate you; you may not have a migraine.

If your headache does not feel like any you have been experiencing, do not take Imitrex.

Use Imitrex cautiously if you have liver or kidney disease. Also, if you have any trouble with your eyes, tell your doctor.

Imitrex has not been tested in children or adults over age 65.

Although very rare, severe and even fatal allergic reactions have occurred in people taking Imitrex. Such reactions are more likely in people who have several allergies.

In rare cases, people have suffered seizures after taking Imitrex.

### Possible food and drug interactions while taking this medication

If Imitrex is taken with certain other drugs, the effects of either may be increased, decreased, or altered. Do not combine Imitrex with the following:

Antidepressants classified as MAO inhibitors, including Nardil and Parnate
Ergot-containing drugs such as Cafergot and Ergostat

### Special information if you are pregnant or breastfeeding

The effects of Imitrex during pregnancy have not been adequately studied. If you are pregnant or plan to become pregnant, inform your doctor immediately. Imitrex may appear in breast milk and could affect a nursing infant. If this medication is essential to your health, your doctor may advise you to discontinue breastfeeding until your treatment with Imitrex is finished.

### Recommended dosage

ADULTS

The maximum single recommended dose of Imitrex Injection is 6 milligrams injected under the skin.

The maximum recommended dose that may be given within 24 hours is two 6 milligram injections taken at least 1 hour apart.

The usual dose of Imitrex Tablets is one 25-milligram tablet taken with water or other liquid. The most you should take at one time is 100 milligrams, and the most you should take in 1 day is 300 milligrams. Doses should be spaced at least 2 hours apart.

If you have liver disease, you should not take more than 50 milligrams of Imitrex Tablets at one time.

### Overdosage

Any medication taken in excess can have serious consequences. If you suspect an overdose, seek medical attention immediately.

■ *Symptoms of Imitrex overdose may include:*
Bluish tinge to the skin, convulsions, dilated pupils, inactivity, lack of coordination, paralysis, redness in the arms and legs, skin changes at the site of injection, slow breathing, sluggishness, tremor

*Brand name:*

# Imodium

*Pronounced: i-MOH-dee-um*
*Generic name: Loperamide hydrochloride*

### Why is this drug prescribed?

Imodium is prescribed for the control and relief of symptoms of diarrhea not known to be caused by a specific germ, and for diarrhea associated with long-term inflammatory bowel disease. This drug is also prescribed for reducing the volume of discharge from an ileostomy (a surgical opening of the small intestine onto the abdominal wall for purposes of elimination).

Some doctors also prescribe Imodium, along with antibiotics such as Septra or Bactrim, to treat traveler's diarrhea.

### Most important fact about this drug

If your diarrhea does not stop after a couple of days, if you have blood in your stools, or a fever develops, notify your doctor immediately.

### How should you take this medication?

Do not take more than the prescribed dose of this medication.

Imodium may cause dryness of the mouth. Sucking on a hard candy or chewing gum can help relieve the problem.

■ *If you miss a dose...*
If you are taking Imodium on a regular schedule for chronic diarrhea and miss a dose, take it as soon as you remember then take the remaining doses for that day at evenly spaced intervals. However, if you are not having diarrhea, skip the missed dose completely.
■ *Storage instructions...*
Imodium should be stored at room temperature.

### What side effects may occur?

Side effects reported from the use of Imodium are difficult to distinguish from symptoms associated with diarrhea. Those reported, however, were more commonly observed during the treatment of long-lasting diarrhea.

■ *Side effects may include:*
Abdominal distention, abdominal pain or discomfort, allergic reactions, including skin rash, constipation, dizziness, drowsiness, dry mouth, nausea and vomiting, tiredness

## Why should this drug not be prescribed?
If you are sensitive to or have ever had an allergic reaction to Imodium, you should not take this medication. Make sure that your doctor is aware of any drug reactions that you have experienced.

Unless you are directed to do so by your doctor, do not take Imodium if constipation must be avoided.

## Special warnings about this medication
Imodium may cause drowsiness and/or dizziness. You should exercise extra caution while driving or performing tasks requiring mental alertness.

Imodium is not good for all types of diarrhea. It is not prescribed for acute dysentery (an inflammation of the intestines characterized by abdominal pain, watery—sometimes bloody—stools, and fever, caused by bacteria, viruses, or parasites).

Dehydration can be a problem when you have diarrhea. It is important that you drink plenty of fluids while taking Imodium.

Use special caution when giving Imodium to a young child. Response to the drug can be unpredictable.

If you have a liver problem, your doctor should closely watch for signs of central nervous system reactions, such as drowsiness or convulsions.

If you have colitis and develop abdominal distention, constipation or an intestinal blockage, notify your doctor immediately. The use of Imodium should be discontinued.

## Possible food and drug interactions when taking this medication
There are no reported food or drug interactions.

## Special information if you are pregnant or breastfeeding
The effects of Imodium during pregnancy have not been adequately studied. If you are pregnant or plan to become pregnant, notify your doctor. It is not known whether Imodium appears in breast milk. If this medication is essential to your health, your doctor may advise you to discontinue breastfeeding until your treatment is finished.

## Recommended dosage
ADULTS

*Severe Diarrhea*
The recommended starting dosage is 2 capsules (4 milligrams) followed by 1 capsule (2 milligrams) after each unformed stool. Daily dosage should not exceed 8 capsules (16 milligrams). Improvement should be observed within 48 hours.

*Long-Lasting or Frequently Recurring Diarrhea*
The recommended starting dosage is 2 capsules (4 milligrams) followed by 1 capsule (2 milligrams) after each unformed stool until diarrhea is controlled, after which the dosage of Imodium should be reduced by your doctor to meet your individual needs. When the ideal daily dosage has been established, this amount may then be given as a single dose or in divided doses. The average maintenance dosage is 2 to 4 capsules per day, not to exceed 8 capsules. If improvement is not observed after treatment with 8 capsules (16 milligrams) per day for at least 10 days, notify your doctor.

CHILDREN

Imodium is not recommended in children under 2 years of age.

*Severe Diarrhea*
In children 2 to 5 years of age or 44 pounds or less, the nonprescription liquid medication (Imodium A-D) should be used. For children between the ages of 6 and 12, either Imodium capsules (2 milligrams per capsule) or Imodium A-D Liquid (1 milligram per teaspoonful) may be used.

For children 2 to 12 years of age, the following schedule for capsules or liquid will usually fulfill starting dosage requirements:

2 to 5 years (28-44 pounds):
1 milligram (1 teaspoonful of Imodium A-D liquid) taken 3 times a day (3 milligrams daily)

6 to 8 years (45-66 pounds):
2 milligrams taken 2 times a day (4 milligrams daily)

8 to 12 years (67 pounds and over):
2 milligrams taken 3 times a day (6 milligrams daily)

After the first day of treatment, additional Imodium doses (1 milligram per 22 pounds of body weight) should be given only after a loose stool. The total daily dosage should not exceed the recommended dosages for the first day.

*Long-Lasting or Frequently Recurring Diarrhea*
A dosage has not been established for children with long-lasting or frequently recurring diarrhea.

### Overdosage
Any medication taken in excess can have serious consequences. If you suspect an Imodium overdose, seek medical attention immediately.

■ *Symptoms of an Imodium overdose may include:*
Constipation, drowsiness, lethargy, and depression, nausea

*Generic name:*

# Indapamide
*See Lozol, page 301.*

*Brand name:*

# Inderal
*Pronounced: IN-der-al*
*Generic name: Propranolol hydrochloride*
*Other brand name: Inderal LA*

### Why is this drug prescribed?
Inderal, a type of medication known as a beta blocker, is used in the treatment of high blood pressure, angina pectoris (chest pain, usually caused by lack of oxygen to the heart due to clogged arteries), changes in heart rhythm, prevention of migraine headache, hereditary tremors, hypertrophic subaortic stenosis (a condition related to exertional angina), and tumors of the adrenal gland. It is also used to reduce the risk of death from recurring heart attack.

When used for the treatment of high blood pressure, it is effective alone or combined with other high blood pressure medications, particularly thiazide-type diuretics. Beta blockers decrease the force and rate of heart contractions, reducing the heart's demand for oxygen and lowering blood pressure.

### Most important fact about this drug
If you have high blood pressure, you must take Inderal regularly for it to be effective. Since blood pressure declines gradually, it may be several weeks before you get the full benefit of Inderal; and you must continue taking it even if you are feeling well. Inderal does not cure high blood pressure; it merely keeps it under control.

### How should you take this medication?
Inderal works best when taken before meals. Take it exactly as prescribed, even if your symptoms have disappeared.

Try not to miss any doses. If this medication is not taken regularly, your condition may worsen.

■ *If you miss a dose...*
Take it as soon as you remember. If it is within 8 hours of your next scheduled dose, skip the one you missed and go back to your regular schedule. Never take 2 doses at the same time.
■ *Storage instructions...*
Store at room temperature in a tightly closed, light-resistant container. Protect from freezing or excessive heat.

### What side effects may occur?
Side effects cannot be anticipated. If any develop or change in intensity, inform your doctor as soon as possible. Only your doctor can determine if it is safe for you to continue taking Inderal.

■ *Side effects may include:*
Abdominal cramps, colitis, congestive heart failure, constipation, decreased sexual ability, depression, diarrhea, difficulty breathing, disorientation, dry eyes, fever with sore throat, hair loss, hallucinations, headache, light-headedness, low blood pressure, lupus erythematosus (a disease of the connective tissue), nausea, rash, reddish or purplish spots on the skin, short-term memory loss, slow heartbeat, tingling, prickling in hands, tiredness, trouble sleeping, upset stomach, visual changes, vivid dreams, vomiting, weakness, worsening of certain heartbeat irregularities

### Why should this drug not be prescribed?
If you have inadequate blood supply to the circulatory system (cardiogenic shock), certain types of irregular heartbeat, a slow heartbeat, bronchial asthma, or severe congestive heart failure, you should not take this medication.

## Special warnings about this medication

If you have a history of congestive heart failure, your doctor will prescribe Inderal cautiously.

Inderal should not be stopped suddenly. This can cause increased chest pain and heart attack. Dosage should be gradually reduced.

If you suffer from asthma or other bronchial conditions, coronary artery disease, or kidney or liver disease, this medication should be used with caution.

Ask your doctor if you should check your pulse while taking Inderal. This medication can cause your heartbeat to become too slow.

This medication may mask the symptoms of low blood sugar or alter blood sugar levels. If you are diabetic, discuss this with your doctor.

Notify your doctor or dentist that you are taking Inderal if you have a medical emergency, and before you have surgery or dental treatment.

## Possible food and drug interactions when taking this medication

If Inderal is taken with certain other drugs, the effects of either could be increased, decreased, or altered. It is especially important to check with your doctor before combining Inderal with the following:

Alcohol
Aluminum hydroxide gel (Amphojel)
Antipyrine (Auralgan)
Calcium-blocking blood pressure drugs such as
    Cardizem, Procardia, and Calan
Certain high blood pressure medications such as
    Diupres and Ser-Ap-Es
Chlorpromazine (Thorazine)
Cimetidine (Tagamet)
Epinephrine (EpiPen)
Haloperidol (Haldol)
Insulin
Lidocaine (Xylocaine)
Nonsteroidal anti-inflammatory drugs such as
    Motrin and Naprosyn
Oral diabetes drugs such as Micronase
Phenobarbitone
Phenytoin (Dilantin)
Rifampin (Rifadin)
Theophylline (Theo-Dur and others)
Thyroid medications such as Synthroid

## Special information if you are pregnant or breastfeeding

The effects of Inderal during pregnancy have not been adequately studied. If you are pregnant or plan to become pregnant, inform your doctor immediately. Inderal appears in breast milk and could affect a nursing infant. If this medication is essential to your health, your doctor may advise you to discontinue breastfeeding until your treatment with this medication is finished.

## Recommended dosage

ADULTS

All dosages of Inderal, for any problem, must be tailored to the individual. Your doctor will determine when and how often you should take this drug. Remember to take it exactly as directed.

*Hypertension*
The usual starting dose is 40 milligrams 2 times a day. This dose may be in combination with a diuretic. Dosages are gradually increased to between 120 milligrams and 240 milligrams per day for maintenance. In some cases, a dose of 640 milligrams per day may be needed. Depending on the individual, maximum effect of this drug may not be reached for a few days or even several weeks. Some people may do better taking this medication 3 times a day.

*Angina Pectoris*
The usual daily dosage is 80 milligrams to 320 milligrams, divided into 2, 3, or 4 smaller doses. When your treatment is being discontinued, your doctor will reduce the dosage gradually over a period of several weeks.

*Irregular Heartbeat*
The usual dose is 10 milligrams to 30 milligrams 3 or 4 times a day, before meals and at bedtime.

*Heart Attack*
The usual daily dosage is 180 milligrams to 240 milligrams divided into smaller doses. The usual maximum dose is 240 milligrams, although your doctor may increase the dose when treating heart attack with angina or high blood pressure.

*Migraine*
The usual starting dosage is 80 milligrams per day divided into smaller doses. Dosages can be increased gradually to between 160 milligrams and 240 milligrams per day. If this dose does not relieve your symptoms in 4 to 6 weeks, your doctor will slowly take you off the drug.

*Tremors*
The usual starting dose is 40 milligrams, 2 times per day. Symptoms will usually be relieved with a

dose of 120 milligrams per day; however, on occasion, dosages of 240 milligrams to 320 milligrams per day may be necessary.

### Hypertrophic Subaortic Stenosis
The usual dose is 20 milligrams to 40 milligrams, 3 to 4 times a day, before meals and at bedtime.

### Before Adrenal Gland Surgery
The usual dose is 60 milligrams a day divided into smaller doses for 3 days before surgery in combination with an alpha-blocker drug.

Inderal may also be taken by people with inoperable tumors in doses of 30 milligrams a day, divided into smaller doses.

### CHILDREN
Inderal will be carefully individualized for use in children and is used only for high blood pressure. Doses in children are calculated by body weight, and range from 2 milligrams to 4 milligrams per 2.2 pounds daily, divided into 2 equal doses. The maximum dose is 16 milligrams per 2.2 pounds per day.

If treatment is stopped, this drug must be gradually reduced over a 7- to 14-day period.

Inderal is also available in a sustained-release formulation, called Inderal LA, for once-a-day dosing.

### Overdosage
No specific information on Inderal overdosage is available; however, overdose symptoms with other beta blockers include:

Extremely slow heartbeat, irregular heartbeat, low blood pressure, severe congestive heart failure, seizures, wheezing

Any medication taken in excess can have serious consequences. If you suspect an overdose, seek medical attention immediately.

*Brand name:*

# Inderide

*Pronounced: IN-deh-ride*
*Generic ingredients: Inderal (Propranolol
  hydrochloride), Hydrochlorothiazide*
*Other brand name: Inderide LA*

### Why is this drug prescribed?
Inderide is used in the treatment of high blood pressure. It combines a beta blocker (Inderal) with a thi-azide diuretic (hydrochlorothiazide). Beta blockers decrease the force and rate of heart contractions, thus lowering blood pressure. Diuretics help your body produce and eliminate more urine, which also helps lower blood pressure.

### Most important fact about this drug
You must take Inderide regularly for it to be effective. Since blood pressure declines gradually, it may be several weeks before you get the full benefit of Inderide; and you must continue taking it even if you are feeling well. Inderide does not cure high blood pressure; it merely keeps it under control.

### How should you take this medication?
Take Inderide exactly as prescribed, even if your symptoms have disappeared.

Try not to miss any doses. If this medication is not taken regularly, your condition may worsen.

■ *If you miss a dose...*
Take it as soon as you remember. If the next dose is within 8 hours, skip the one you missed and go back to your regular schedule. Do not take 2 doses at the same time.
■ *Storage instructions...*
Store at room temperature in a tightly closed container, protected from moisture, freezing, and excessive heat.

### What side effects may occur?
Side effects cannot be anticipated. If any develop or change in intensity, inform your doctor as soon as possible. Only your doctor can determine if it is safe for you to continue taking Inderide.

■ *Side effects may include:*
Allergic reactions (including fever, rash, aching and sore throat), anemia, blood disorders, blurred vision, constipation, congestive heart failure, cramps, decreased mental clarity, depression, diarrhea, difficulty breathing, difficulty sleeping, disorientation, dizziness, dizziness when standing, dry eyes, emotional changeability, exhaustion, fatigue, hair loss, hallucinations, headache, high blood sugar, hives, increased skin sensitivity to sunlight, inflammation of the large intestine or the pancreas, inflammation of the salivary glands, light-headedness, loss of appetite, low blood pressure, lupus erythematosus (a connec-

tive tissue disease), male impotence, muscle spasms, nausea, restlessness, short-term memory loss, slow heartbeat, stomach irritation, sugar in the urine, tingling or pins and needles, upset stomach, vertigo, visual disturbances, vivid dreams, vomiting, weakness, wheezing, yellow eyes and skin

## Why should this drug not be prescribed?

If you have inadequate blood supply to the circulatory system (cardiogenic shock), certain types of irregular heartbeat, slow heartbeat, bronchial asthma, or congestive heart failure, you should not take this medication.

Do not take Inderide if you are unable to urinate or if you are sensitive to or have ever had an allergic reaction to any of its ingredients or to sulfa drugs.

## Special warnings about this medication

Inderide should not be stopped suddenly. This can cause chest pain and even heart attack. Dosage should be gradually reduced.

Diuretics can cause your body to lose too much potassium. Signs of an excessively low potassium level include muscle weakness and rapid or irregular heartbeat. To boost your potassium level, your doctor may recommend eating potassium-rich foods or taking a potassium supplement.

If you suffer from asthma, seasonal allergies or other bronchial conditions, or kidney or liver disease, your doctor will prescribe this medication with caution.

This medication may mask the symptoms of low blood sugar or alter blood sugar levels. If you are diabetic, discuss this with your doctor.

If you have a history of allergies or bronchial asthma, you are more likely to have an allergic reaction to Inderide.

Inderide may interfere with the screening test for glaucoma (excessive pressure in the eyes) and pressure within the eyes may increase when the medication is stopped.

Notify your doctor or dentist that you are taking Inderide if you have a medical emergency, and before you have surgery or dental treatment.

## Possible food and drug interactions
## when taking this medication

If Inderide is taken with certain other drugs, the effects of either could be increased, decreased, or altered. It is especially important to check with your doctor before combining Inderide with the following:

ACTH (adrenocorticotropic hormone)
Alcohol
Aluminum hydroxide gel (Amphojel)
Antipyrine (Auralgan)
Calcium-blocking blood pressure drugs such as
    Calan, Cardizem, and Procardia XL
Certain blood pressure medications such as Diupres
    and Ser-Ap-Es
Chlorpromazine (Thorazine)
Cimetidine (Tagamet)
Corticosteroids such as prednisone
Digitalis (Lanoxin)
Epinephrine (EpiPen)
Haloperidol (Haldol)
Insulin
Lidocaine (Xylocaine)
Nonsteroidal anti-inflammatory drugs such as
    Motrin
Norepinephrine (Levophed)
Oral diabetes drugs such as Micronase
Phenobarbitone
Phenytoin (Dilantin)
Rifampin (Rifadin)
Theophylline (Theo-Dur)
Thyroid medications such as Synthroid

## Special information
## if you are pregnant or breastfeeding

The effects of Inderide during pregnancy have not been adequately studied. If you are pregnant or plan to become pregnant, inform your doctor immediately. Inderide appears in breast milk and could affect a nursing infant. If Inderide is essential to your health, your doctor may advise you to discontinue breastfeeding until your treatment is finished.

## Recommended dosage

ADULTS

Your doctor will tailor your dosage according to your response to Inderide's main ingredients.

The usual dose is one Inderide tablet, 2 times per day.

Your doctor may use this medication in combination with other high blood pressure drugs to achieve the desired effect.

This drug is also available in a sustained-release formulation, called Inderide LA, for once-a-day dosing.

CHILDREN

The safety and effectiveness of this drug in children have not been established.

OLDER ADULTS

Your doctor will adjust your dosage with extra caution.

### Overdosage

Any medication taken in excess can have severe consequences. If you suspect an overdose, seek medical attention immediately.

■ *Symptoms of Inderide overdose may include:*
Coma, extremely slow heartbeat, heart failure, increased urination, irritation and overactivity of the stomach and intestines, low blood pressure, sluggishness, stupor, wheezing

*Generic name:*

# Indinavir

*See Crixivan, page 121.*

*Brand name:*

# Indocin

*Pronounced: IN-doh-sin*
*Generic name: Indomethacin*

### Why is this drug prescribed?

Indocin, a nonsteroidal anti-inflammatory drug, is used to relieve the inflammation, swelling, stiffness and joint pain associated with moderate or severe rheumatoid arthritis and osteoarthritis (the most common form of arthritis), and ankylosing spondylitis (arthritis of the spine). It is also used to treat bursitis, tendinitis (acute painful shoulder), acute gouty arthritis, and other kinds of pain.

### Most important fact about this drug

You should have frequent checkups with your doctor if you take Indocin regularly. Ulcers or internal bleeding can occur without warning.

### How should you take this medication?

Indocin should be taken with food or an antacid, and with a full glass of water. Never take on an empty stomach.

Take this medication exactly as prescribed by your doctor.

If you are using Indocin for arthritis, it should be taken regularly.

If you are taking the liquid form of this medicine, shake the bottle well before each use.

Indocin SR capsules should be swallowed whole, not crushed or broken.

Do not lie down for about 20 to 30 minutes after taking Indocin. This helps prevent irritation that could lead to trouble in swallowing.

If you are using the suppository form of this medicine:

1. If the suppository is too soft to insert, hold it under cool water or chill it before removing the wrapper
2. Remove the foil wrapper and moisten your rectal area with cool tap water.
3. Lie down your side and use your finger to push the suppository well up into the rectum. Hold your buttocks together for a few seconds.
4. Indocin suppositories should be kept inside the rectum for at least one hour so that all of the medicine can be absorbed by your body.

■ *If you miss a dose...*
Take the forgotten dose as soon as you remember. If it is time for your next dose, skip the one you missed and return to your regular schedule. Never take a double dose.
■ *Storage instructions...*
The liquid and suppository forms of Indocin may be stored at room temperature. Keep both forms from extreme heat, and protect the liquid from freezing.

### What side effects may occur?

Side effects cannot be anticipated. If any develop or change in intensity inform your doctor as soon as possible. Only your doctor can determine if it is safe for you to continue taking Indocin.

■ *More common side effects may include:*
Abdominal pain, constipation, depression, diarrhea, dizziness, fatigue, headache, heartburn, indigestion, nausea, ringing in the ears, sleepiness or excessive drowsiness, stomach pain, stomach upset, vertigo, vomiting
■ *Less common or rare side effects may include:*
Anemia, anxiety, asthma, behavior disturbances, bloating, blurred vision, breast changes, changes in heart rate, chest pain, coma, congestive heart failure, convulsions, decrease in white blood

cells, fever, fluid in lungs, fluid retention, flushing, gas, hair loss, hepatitis, high or low blood pressure, hives, itching, increase in blood sugar, insomnia, kidney failure, labored breathing, light-headedness, loss of appetite, mental confusion, muscle weakness, nosebleed, peptic ulcer, problems in hearing, rash, rectal bleeding, Stevens-Johnson syndrome (skin peeling), stomach or intestinal bleeding, sweating, twitching, unusual redness of skin, vaginal bleeding, weight gain, worsening of epilepsy, yellow eyes and skin

### Why should this drug not be prescribed?

If you are sensitive to or have ever had an allergic reaction to Indocin, aspirin, or similar drugs, or if you have had asthma attacks caused by aspirin or other drugs of this type, you should not take this medication. Make sure that your doctor is aware of any drug reactions that you have experienced.

Do not use Indocin suppositories if you have a history of rectal inflammation or recent rectal bleeding.

### Special warnings about this medication

Indocin prolongs bleeding time. If you are taking blood-thinning medication, this drug should be taken with caution.

Your doctor should prescribe the lowest possible effective dose. The incidence of side effects increases as dosage increases.

Peptic ulcers and bleeding can occur without warning.

This drug should be used with caution if you have kidney or liver disease, and it can cause liver inflammation in some people.

Do not take aspirin or any other anti-inflammatory medications while taking Indocin, unless your doctor tells you to do so.

If you have heart disease or high blood pressure, this drug can increase water retention.

This drug can mask the symptoms of an existing infection.

Indocin may cause you to become drowsy or less alert; therefore, driving or operating dangerous machinery or participating in any hazardous activity that requires full mental alertness is not recommended.

### Possible food and drug interactions when taking this medication

If Indocin is taken with certain other drugs, the effects of either could be increased, decreased or altered. It is especially important to check with your doctor before combining Indocin with the following:

Aspirin
Beta-adrenergic blockers such as Tenormin, Inderal
Blood-thinning medicines such as Coumadin
Captopril (Capoten)
Cyclosporine (Sandimmune)
Diflunisal (Dolobid)
Digoxin (Lanoxin)
Lithium (Eskalith)
Loop diuretics (Lasix)
Potassium-sparing diuretics such as Aldactone
Probenecid (Benemid, ColBENEMID)
The anticancer drug methotrexate
Thiazide-type diuretics such as Diuril
Triamterene (Dyazide)

### Special information if you are pregnant or breastfeeding

The effects of Indocin during pregnancy have not been adequately studied. If you are pregnant or plan to become pregnant inform your doctor immediately. Indocin appears in breast milk and could affect a nursing infant. If this medication is essential to your health, your doctor may advise you to discontinue breastfeeding until your treatment with this medication is finished.

### Recommended dosage

ADULTS

This medication is available in liquid, capsule, and suppository form. The following dosages are for the capsule form. If you prefer the liquid form ask your doctor to make the proper substitution. Do not try to convert the medication or dosage yourself.

*Moderate to Severe Rheumatoid Arthritis, Osteoarthritis, Ankylosing Spondylitis*
The usual dose is 25 milligrams 2 or 3 times a day, increasing to a total daily dose of 150 to 200 milligrams. Your doctor should monitor you carefully for side effects when you are taking this drug.

Your doctor may prescribe a single daily 75-milligram capsule of Indocin SR in place of regular Indocin.

*Bursitis or Tendinitis*
The usual dose is 75 to 150 milligrams daily divided into 3 to 4 small doses for 1 to 2 weeks, until symptoms disappear.

*Acute Gouty Arthritis*

The usual dose is 50 milligrams 3 times a day until pain is reduced to a tolerable level (usually 3 to 5 days). Your doctor will advise you when to stop taking this drug for this condition. Keep him informed of its effects on your symptoms.

### CHILDREN

The safety and effectiveness of Indocin have not been established in children under 14 years of age. However, your doctor may decide that the benefits of this medication may outweigh the potential risks.

### OLDER ADULTS

Your doctor will adjust the dosage as needed.

### Overdosage

Any medication taken in excess can cause symptoms of overdose. If you suspect an overdose seek medical attention immediately.

■ *The symptoms of Indocin overdose may include:*
Convulsions, disorientation, dizziness, intense headache, lethargy, mental confusion, nausea, vomiting, numbness, tingling or pins and needles

*Generic name:*

# Indomethacin

*See Indocin, page 256.*

*Brand name:*

# Insulatard

*See Insulin, page 258.*

*Generic name:*

# Insulin

*Pronounced: IN-suh-lin*
*Available formulations:*
*Insulin, Human:*
    Humulin
*Insulin, Human Isophane Suspension:*
    Humulin N
*Insulin, Human NPH:*
    Insulatard NPH Human
    Novolin N

*Insulin, Human Regular:*
    Novolin R
    Humulin BR & R
    Velosulin Human
*Insulin, Human Regular and Human NPH mixture:*
    Humulin 70/30
    Mixtard Human 70/30
    Novolin 70/30
*Insulin, Human, Zinc Suspension:*
    Humulin L & U
    Novolin L
*Insulin, NPH:*
    NPH Iletin I (also II, Beef; II, Pork)
    Insulatard NPH
    NPH Insulin
*Insulin Regular and NPH mixture:*
    Mixtard 70/30
*Insulin, Zinc Crystals:*
    NPH Iletin I
*Insulin, Regular:*
    Iletin I Regular (also II, Beef; II, Pork)
    Regular Insulin
    Velosulin
*Insulin, Zinc Suspension:*
    Iletin I, Lente
    Protamine, Zinc and Iletin
    Iletin I, Semilente
    Iletin I
    Lente Insulin
    Ultralente Insulin

### Why is this drug prescribed?

Insulin is prescribed for diabetes mellitus when this condition does not improve with oral medications or by modifying your diet. Insulin is a hormone produced by the pancreas, a large gland that lies near the stomach. This hormone is necessary for the body's correct use of food, especially sugar. Insulin apparently works by helping sugar penetrate the cell wall, where it is then utilized by the cell. In people with diabetes, the body either does not make enough insulin, or the insulin that is produced cannot be used properly.

There are actually two forms of diabetes: Type I insulin-dependent and Type II non-insulin-dependent. Type I usually requires insulin injection for life, while Type II diabetes can usually be treated by dietary changes and/or oral antidiabetic medications such as Diabinese and Glucotrol. Occasionally, Type II diabetics must take insulin injections on a temporary basis, especially during stressful periods or times of illness.

The various insulin brands above differ in several ways: in the source (animal, human, or genetically engineered), in the time requirements for the insulin to take effect, and in the length of time the insulin remains working.

Regular insulin is manufactured from beef and pork pancreas, begins working within 30 to 60 minutes, and lasts for 6 to 8 hours. Variations of insulin have been developed to satisfy the needs of individual patients. For example, zinc suspension insulin is an intermediate-acting insulin that starts working within 1 to 1¹/₂ hours and lasts approximately 24 hours. Insulin combined with zinc and protamine is a longer-acting insulin that takes effect within 4 to 6 hours and lasts up to 36 hours. The time and course of action may vary considerably in different individuals or at different times in the same individual.

Animal-based insulin is a very safe product. However, some components may cause an allergic reaction (see "What side effects may occur?"). Therefore, genetically engineered human insulin has been developed to lessen the chance of an allergic reaction. It is structurally identical to the insulin produced by your body's pancreas. However, some human insulin may be produced in a semi-synthetic process that begins with animal-based ingredients, which may cause an allergic reaction.

## Most important fact about this drug

Regardless of the type of insulin your doctor has prescribed, you should follow carefully the dietary and exercise guidelines he or she has recommended. Failure to follow these guidelines or to take your insulin as prescribed may result in serious and potentially life-threatening complications such as hypoglycemia (lowered blood sugar levels).

## How should you take this medication?

Take your insulin exactly as prescribed, being careful to follow your doctor's dietary and exercise recommendations.

■ *If you miss a dose...*
Your doctor should tell you what to do if you miss an insulin injection or meal.

■ *Storage instructions...*
Store insulin in a refrigerator (but not in the freezer) or in another cool, dark place. Do not expose insulin to heat or direct sunlight.

Some brands of prefilled syringes can be kept at room temperature for a week or a month. Check your product's label. Never use insulin after the expiration date which is printed on the label and carton.

## What side effects may occur?

While side effects from insulin use are rare, allergic reactions or low blood sugar (sometimes called "an insulin reaction") may pose significant health risks. Your doctor should be notified if any of the following occur:

■ *Mild allergic reactions:*
Swelling, itching or redness at the injection site (usually disappears within a few days or weeks)
■ *More serious allergic reactions:*
Fast pulse, low blood pressure, perspiration, rash over the entire body, shortness of breath, shallow breathing, or wheezing

Other side effects are virtually eliminated when the correct dose of insulin is matched with the proper diet and level of physical activity. Low blood sugar may develop in poorly controlled or unstable diabetes. Consuming sugar or a sugar-containing product will usually correct the condition, which can be brought about by taking too much insulin, missing or delaying meals, exercising or working more than usual, an infection or illness, a change in the body's need for insulin, drug interactions, or consuming alcohol.

■ *Symptoms of low blood sugar include:*
Abnormal behavior, anxiety, blurred vision, cold sweat, confusion, depressed mood, dizziness, drowsiness, fatigue, headache, hunger, inability to concentrate, light-headedness, nausea, nervousness, personality changes, rapid heartbeat, restlessness, sleep disturbances, slurred speech, sweating, tingling in the hands, feet, lips, or tongue, tremor, unsteady movement

Contact your physician if these symptoms persist.

■ *Symptoms of more severe low blood sugar include:*
Coma, disorientation

Remember, too, the symptoms associated with an under-supply of insulin, which can be brought on by taking too little of it, overeating, or fever and infection.

■ *Symptoms of insufficient insulin include:*
Drowsiness, flushing, fruity breath, heavy breathing, loss of appetite, rapid pulse, thirst

If you are ill, you should check your urine for ketones (acetone), and notify your doctor if the test is positive. This condition can be life-threatening.

**Why should this drug not be prescribed?**
Insulin should be used only to correct diabetic conditions.

**Special warnings about this medication**
Wear personal identification that states clearly that you are diabetic. Carry a sugar-containing product such as hard candy to offset any symptoms of low blood sugar.

Do not change the type of insulin or even the model and brand of syringe or needle you use without your physician's instruction. Failure to use the proper syringe may lead to improper dosage levels of insulin.

If you become ill from any cause, especially with nausea and vomiting or fever, your insulin requirements may change. It is important to eat as normally as possible. If you have trouble eating, drink fruit juices, soda, or clear soups, or eat small amounts of bland foods. Test your urine and/or blood sugar and tell your doctor at once. If you have severe and prolonged vomiting, seek emergency medical care.

If you are taking insulin, you should check your glucose levels with home blood and urine testing devices. If your blood tests consistently show above-normal sugar levels or your urine tests consistently show the presence of sugar, your diabetes is not properly controlled, and you should tell your doctor.

To avoid infection or contamination, use disposable needles and syringes or sterilize your reusable syringe and needle carefully.

Always keep handy an extra supply of insulin as well as a spare syringe and needle.

**Possible food and drug interactions
when taking this medication**
Follow your physician's dietary guidelines as closely as you can and inform your physician of

any medication, either prescription or non-prescription, that you are taking. Specific medications, depending on the amount present, that affect insulin levels or its effectiveness include:

Anabolic steroids such as Anadrol-50
Appetite suppressants such as Tenuate
Aspirin
Beta-blocking blood pressure medicines such as
    Tenormin and Lopressor
Diuretics such as Lasix and Dyazide
Epinephrine (EpiPen)
Estrogens such as Premarin
MAO inhibitors (antidepressant drugs such as Nardil
    and Parnate)
Phenytoin (Dilantin)
Steroid medications such as prednisone
Thyroid medications such as Synthroid

Use alcohol carefully, since excessive alcohol consumption can cause low blood sugar. Don't drink unless your doctor has approved it.

**Special information
if you are pregnant or breastfeeding**
Insulin is considered safe for pregnant women, but pregnancy may make managing your diabetes more difficult.

Properly controlled diabetes is essential for the health of the mother and the developing baby; therefore, it is extremely important that pregnant women follow closely their physician's dietary and exercise guidelines and prescribing instructions.

Since insulin does not pass into breast milk, it is safe for nursing mothers.

**Recommended dosage**
Your doctor will specify which insulin to use, how much, when, and how often to inject it. Your dosage may be affected by changes in food, activity, illness, medication, pregnancy, exercise, travel, or your work schedule. Proper control of your diabetes requires close and constant cooperation with your doctor. Failure to use your insulin as prescribed may result in serious and potentially fatal complications.

Some insulins should be clear, and some have a cloudy precipitate. Find out what your insulin should look like and check it carefully before using.

**Overdosage**
An overdose of insulin can cause low blood sugar (hypoglycemia). Symptoms include:

Depressed mood, dizziness, drowsiness, fatigue, headache, hunger, inability to concentrate, irritability, nausea, nervousness, personality changes, rapid heartbeat, restlessness, sleep disturbances, slurred speech, sweating, tingling, tremor, unsteady movements

■ *Symptoms of more severe low blood sugar include:*
Coma, disorientation, pale skin, seizures

Your doctor should be contacted immediately if these symptoms of severe low blood sugar occur.

Eating sugar or a sugar-based product will often correct the condition. If you suspect an overdose, seek medical attention immediately.

*Brand name:*

# Intal

*Pronounced: IN-tahl*
*Generic name: Cromolyn sodium*
*Other brand name: Nasalcrom*

## Why is this drug prescribed?
Intal contains the antiasthmatic/antiallergic medication cromolyn sodium.

Different forms of the drug are used to manage bronchial asthma, to prevent asthma attacks, and to prevent and treat seasonal and chronic allergies.

The drug works by preventing certain cells in the body from releasing substances that can cause allergic reactions or prompt too much bronchial activity. It also helps prevent bronchial constriction caused by exercise, aspirin, cold air, and certain environmental pollutants such as sulfur dioxide.

## Most important fact about this drug
Intal does not help an acute asthma attack. When taken to prevent severe bronchial asthma, it can be 4 weeks before you feel its maximum benefit, though some people get relief sooner. Do not discontinue the inhalation capsules or nasal solution abruptly without the advice of your doctor.

## How should you take this medication?
Intal capsules should not be swallowed. They are for inhalation using the Spinhaler turbo-inhaler. The contents of 1 capsule are usually inhaled 4 times daily at regular intervals. Wash the Spinhaler in warm water at least once a week; dry thoroughly. Replace the Spinhaler every 6 months.

Intal nebulizer solution should be inhaled using a power-operated nebulizer equipped with an appropriate face mask or mouthpiece. Hand-operated nebulizers are not suitable. It is important that the solution be inhaled at regular intervals, usually 4 times per day.

Intal aerosol spray can be used either for chronic asthma or to prevent an asthma attack. For chronic asthma, it must be inhaled at regular intervals, as directed by your doctor, usually 2 sprays inhaled 4 times daily. To prevent an asthma attack caused by exercise, cold air, or other irritants, the usual dose of 2 inhalation sprays should be taken between 10 and 60 minutes before exercising or exposure to cold or pollutants.

Nasalcrom nasal solution should be used with a metered nasal spray device, which should be replaced every 6 months. Blow your nose to clear your nasal passages before administering the spray. The nasal solution is used for nasal congestion due to seasonal or chronic allergies. For seasonal allergies, treatment is more effective if begun before the start of the allergy season. Treatment should then continue throughout the season. For year-round allergies, treatment may be required for up to 4 weeks before results are seen. Your doctor may find it necessary to add other allergy medications, such as antihistamines or decongestants, during initial treatment.

■ *If you miss a dose...*
Take it as soon as you remember. Then take the rest of that day's doses at equally spaced intervals. Do not take 2 doses at once.
■ *Storage instructions...*
Store at room temperature, away from light and heat. Keep the ampules in their foil pouch until you are ready to use them.

## What side effects may occur?
Side effects cannot be anticipated. If any develop or change in intensity, inform your doctor as soon as possible. Only your doctor can determine if it is safe for you to continue taking Intal.

■ *More common side effects may include:*
Cough, nasal congestion or irritation, nausea, sneezing, throat irritation, wheezing
■ *Less common or rare side effects may include:*
Angioedema (swelling of face around lips, tongue, and throat, swollen arms and legs), bad

taste in mouth, burning in chest, difficulty swallowing, dizziness, ear problems, headache, hives, joint swelling and pain, nosebleed, painful urination or frequent urination, postnasal drip, rash, severe allergic reaction, swollen glands, swollen throat, teary eyes, tightness in throat

## Why should this drug not be prescribed?

If you are sensitive to or have ever had an allergic reaction to cromolyn sodium or lactose, you should not take this medication. Make sure your doctor is aware of any drug reactions you have experienced.

## Special warnings about this medication

Asthma symptoms may recur if the recommended dosage of Intal is reduced or discontinued. Intal has no role in the treatment of an acute asthmatic attack once it has begun. Obtain medical help immediately if you experience a severe attack.

If you have liver or kidney problems, your doctor may have to reduce the dosage or even take you off the drug altogether.

When using the capsules, you may accidentally inhale some powder, which can irritate your throat or make you cough. Try rinsing your mouth or taking a drink of water immediately before and/or after using the Spinhaler.

If your heartbeat is ever irregular or if you have any other kind of heart trouble, be sure your doctor knows about it before you use Intal aerosol spray.

Intal aerosol spray may not help you if your attack has been brought on by exercise.

## Possible food and drug interactions when taking this medication

If you are taking other prescription or nonprescription drugs, discuss this with your doctor to determine if these drugs would interact with Intal.

## Special information if you are pregnant or breastfeeding

The effects of Intal during pregnancy have not been adequately studied. If you are pregnant or plan to become pregnant, inform your doctor immediately. It is not known whether Intal appears in breast milk. As with all medication, a nursing woman should use this drug only after careful consultation with her doctor.

## Recommended dosage

INTAL CAPSULES FOR INHALATION
INTAL NEBULIZER SOLUTION

*Adults and Children 2 years Old and Over*
For management of bronchial asthma, the usual dosage is 20 milligrams (1 capsule or ampule) inhaled 4 times daily at regular intervals, using the Spinhaler turbo-inhaler or power-operated nebulizer. If you have chronic asthma, this drug's effectiveness depends on your taking it regularly, as directed, and only after an attack has been controlled and you can inhale adequately.

For the prevention of an acute attack following exercise or exposure to cold, dry air or environmental irritants, the usual dose is 1 capsule or ampule inhaled shortly before exposure to the irritant. You may repeat the inhalation as needed for continued protection during prolonged exposure.

INTAL INHALER AEROSOL SPRAY

*Adults and Children 5 Years Old and Over*
For the management of bronchial asthma, the usual starting dose is 2 metered sprays taken at regular intervals, 4 times daily. This is the maximum dose that should be taken, and lower dosages may be effective in children. This drug should be used only after an asthma attack has been controlled and you can inhale adequately.

For the prevention of an acute asthma attack following exercise, exposure to cold air or environmental agents, the usual dose is inhalation of 2 metered sprays shortly (10 to 15 minutes but not more than 60 minutes) before exposure to the irritant.

NASALCROM NASAL SOLUTION

*Adults and Children 6 Years Old and Over*
For the prevention and treatment of allergies caused by exposure to certain irritants, the usual dosage is 1 spray in each nostril 3 to 4 times per day at regular intervals, using the metered spray device. Your doctor may have you use the spray 6 times a day if you need it.

## Overdosage

Any medication taken in excess can have serious consequences. If you suspect an overdose, seek medical attention immediately.

■ *Symptoms of Intal overdose may include:*
Difficulty breathing, heart failure, low blood pressure, slow heartbeat

*Brand name:*

# Invirase

*Pronounced: IN-vir-ace*
*Generic name: Saquinavir mesylate*

## Why is this drug prescribed?

Invirase is used in the treatment of advanced human immunodeficiency virus (HIV) infection. HIV causes the immune system to break down so that it can no longer fight off other infections. This virus leads to the fatal disease known as acquired immune deficiency syndrome (AIDS).

Invirase belongs to a new class of HIV drugs called protease inhibitors, which work by interfering with an important step in the virus's reproductive cycle. Invirase is used in combination with other HIV drugs called nucleoside analogues (Retrovir or Hivid). The combination produces an increase in the immune system's vital CD4 cells (white blood cells) and reduces the amount of virus in the bloodstream.

## Most important fact about this drug

Invirase will not cure an HIV infection. You will continue to face the possibility of complications, including opportunistic infections (rare infections that develop only when the immune system falters, such as certain types of pneumonia, tuberculosis, and fungal infections). Therefore, it is important that you remain under the care of a doctor and keep all your follow-up appointments.

## How should you take this medication?

Take this medication exactly as prescribed by your doctor. Do not share this medication with anyone and do not exceed your recommended dosage. Take Invirase within 2 hours after a full meal. This allows the drug to be properly absorbed by your body. Your doctor will perform laboratory tests before you start therapy with Invirase and at regular intervals during your therapy to see how you are reacting to the medication.

■ *If you miss a dose...*
Take it as soon as possible. If it is almost time for your next dose, skip the one you missed and go back to your regular schedule. Never take a double dose.

■ *Storage instructions...*
Store Invirase at room temperature in a tightly closed bottle.

## What side effects may occur?

Side effects cannot be anticipated. If any develop or change in intensity, tell your doctor as soon as possible. Only your doctor can determine if it is safe for you to continue taking Invirase.

■ *Possible side effects may include:*
Abdominal discomfort and pain, appetite disturbance, diarrhea, dizziness, headache, indigestion, mouth sores, muscle and bone pain, nausea, numbness in the arms and legs, tingling or "pins and needles" sensation, weakness

## Why should this drug not be prescribed?

If you suffer an allergic reaction to Invirase or any of its components, you must stop taking the drug.

## Special warnings about this medication

Invirase has been studied for only a limited period of time and only in patients with advanced HIV infections. Its long-term effects are still unknown.

This medication does not reduce the risk of transmission of HIV to others through sexual contact or blood contamination. Therefore, you should continue to avoid practices that could give HIV to others.

## Possible food and drug interactions when taking this medication

If Invirase is taken with certain other drugs. the effects of either could be increased, decreased, or altered. It is especially important to check with your doctor before combining Invirase with the following:

Astemizole (Hismanal)
Calcium channel blockers (blood pressure medications such as Calan, Verelan,
Cardizem, and Procardia)
Carbamazepine (Tegretol)
Clindamycin (Cleocin)
Dapsone (a drug used to treat leprosy)
Dexamethasone (Decadron)
Phenobarbital (Donnatal)
Phenytoin (Dilantin)
Quinidine (Quinidex)
Rifabutin (Mycobutin)
Rifampin (Rifadin)
Terfenadine (Seldane)
Triazolam (Halcion)

Be sure to tell your doctor and pharmacist about all the medications (both prescription and over-the-counter) that you are presently taking. Alert them, too, whenever you *stop* taking a medication.

### Special information
### if you are pregnant or breastfeeding
The effects of Invirase during pregnancy have not been adequately studied. If you are pregnant or plan to become pregnant, tell your doctor immediately. Do not breastfeed. HIV appears in breast milk and can be passed to a nursing infant.

### Recommended dosage
ADULTS

The recommended dosage is 600 milligrams (three 200-milligram capsules), taken 3 times a day within 2 hours after a full meal. Daily doses lower than 600 milligrams 3 times a day are not recommended, since they will not have the same antiviral activity. You should also take Retrovir or Hivid as directed.

CHILDREN

The safety and effectiveness of Invirase in children younger than 16 years of age have not been established.

### Overdosage
There have been no reports of Invirase poisoning. However, any medication taken in excess can have serious consequences. If you suspect an overdose, seek emergency medical treatment immediately.

---

*Brand name:*
# Ionamin

See Fastin, page 204.

---

*Generic name:*
# Ipratropium

See Atrovent, page 41.

---

*Brand name:*
# Ismo

See Imdur, page 247.

---

*Brand name:*
# Isollyl

See Fiorinal, page 210.

---

*Generic name:*
# Isometheptene, Dichloralphenazone, and Acetaminophen

See Midrin, page 326.

---

*Brand name:*
# Isoptin

See Calan, page 70.

---

*Brand name:*
# Isopto Carpine

See Pilocar, page 419.

---

*Brand name:*
# Isordil

*Pronounced: ICE-or-dill*
*Generic name: Isosorbide dinitrate*
*Other brand name: Sorbitrate*

### Why is this drug prescribed?
Isordil is prescribed to relieve or prevent angina pectoris (suffocating chest pain). Angina pectoris occurs when the arteries and veins become constricted and sufficient oxygen does not reach the heart. Isordil dilates the blood vessels by relaxing the muscles in their walls. Oxygen flow improves as the vessels relax, and chest pain subsides.

In swallowed capsules or tablets, Isordil helps to increase the amount of exercise you can do before chest pain begins.

In chewable or sublingual (held under the tongue) tablets, Isordil can help relieve chest pain that has already started or prevent pain expected from a strenuous activity such as walking up a hill or climbing stairs.

### Most important fact about this drug
Isordil may cause severe low blood pressure (possibly marked by dizziness or fainting), especially when you stand or sit up quickly. People taking diuretic medication or those who have low blood pressure should use Isordil with caution.

## How should you take this medication?

Swallowed capsules or tablets should be taken on an empty stomach. While regular tablets may be crushed for easier use, sustained- or prolonged-release products should not be chewed, crushed or altered.

Chewable tablets should be chewed thoroughly and held in the mouth for a couple of minutes. Do not eat, drink, smoke, or use chewing tobacco while a sublingual tablet is dissolving.

This drug's effectiveness is closely linked to the dose, so follow your doctor's instructions carefully.

■ *If you miss a dose...*
  If you are taking this drug regularly, take the forgotten dose as soon as you remember. If your next dose is within 2 hours—or 6 hours for controlled-release tablets and capsules—skip the one you missed and go back to your regular schedule. Do not take 2 doses at once.
■ *Storage information...*
  Store at room temperature in a tightly closed container, away from light.

## What side effects may occur?

Side effects cannot be anticipated. If any develop or change in intensity, inform your doctor as soon as possible. Only your doctor can determine if it is safe for you to continue taking Isordil.

Headache is the most common side effect; usually, standard headache treatments with over-the-counter pain products will relieve the pain. The headaches associated with Isordil usually subside within 2 weeks after treatment with the drug begins. Do not change your dose to avoid the headache. At a dose that eliminates headaches, the drug may not be as effective against angina.

■ *Other common side effects may include:*
  Dizziness, light-headedness, low blood pressure, weakness
■ *Less common or rare side effects may include:*
  Collapse, fainting, flushed skin, high blood pressure, nausea, pallor, perspiration, rash, restlessness, skin inflammation and flaking, vomiting

## Why should this drug not be prescribed?

You should not take Isordil if you have had a previous allergic reaction to it or to other nitrates or nitrites.

## Special warnings about this medication

You should use Isordil with caution if you have anemia, the eye condition called glaucoma, a previous head injury or heart attack, heart disease, low blood pressure, or thyroid disease.

If you stop using Isordil, you should follow your doctor's plan for a gradual withdrawal schedule. Abruptly stopping this medication could result in additional chest pain.

Some people may develop a tolerance to Isordil, which causes its effects to be reduced over time. Tell your doctor if you think Isordil is starting to lose its effectiveness.

## Possible food and drug interactions when taking this medication

If Isordil is taken with certain other drugs, the effects of either could be increased, decreased, or altered.

Extreme low blood pressure (marked by dizziness, fainting, and numbness) may occur if you take Isordil with certain other high blood pressure drugs such as Cardizem and Procardia.

Alcohol may interact with Isordil and produce a swift decrease in blood pressure, possibly causing dizziness and fainting.

## Special information if you are pregnant or breastfeeding

The effects of Isordil in pregnancy have not been adequately studied. Isordil should be used only when the benefits of therapy clearly outweigh the potential risks to the developing baby. If you are pregnant or plan to become pregnant, inform your doctor immediately. It is not known if Isordil appears in breast milk; therefore, nursing mothers should use Isordil with caution.

## Recommended dosage

Because you can develop a tolerance to this drug, your doctor may schedule a daily period of time when you do not take any drug.

ADULTS

The usual sublingual starting dose for the treatment of angina pectoris is 2.5 milligrams to 5 milligrams. Your doctor will increase this initial dose gradually until the pain subsides or side effects prove bothersome.

The usual sublingual starting dose for the prevention of an impending attack of angina pectoris is usually 5 or 10 milligrams every 2 to 3 hours.

To prevent chronic stable angina pectoris, the usual starting dose for swallowed, immediately released Isordil is 5 to 20 milligrams. Your doctor may increase this initial dose to 10 to 40 milligrams every 6 hours.

To prevent chronic stable angina pectoris with controlled-release Isordil, the usual initial dose is 40 milligrams. Your doctor may increase this dose from 40 to 80 milligrams given every 8 to 12 hours.

CHILDREN

The safety and effectiveness of Isordil have not been established for children.

### Overdosage

Any medication taken in excess can have serious consequences. Severe overdosage of Isordil can be fatal. If you suspect an overdose, seek medical help immediately.

■ *Symptoms of Isordil overdose may include:*
Bloody diarrhea, coma, confusion, convulsions, fainting, fever, flushed and perspiring skin (later cold and blue), nausea, palpitations paralysis, rapid decrease in blood pressure, rapid, then difficult and slow breathing, slow pulse, throbbing headache, vertigo, visual disturbances, vomiting

*Generic name:*

# Isosorbide dinitrate

*See Isordil, page 264.*

*Generic name:*

# Isosorbide mononitrate

*See Imdur, page 247.*

*Generic name:*

# Isotretinoin

*See Accutane, page 2.*

*Generic name:*

# Isradipine

*See DynaCirc, page 182.*

*Generic name:*

# Itraconazole

*See Sporanox, page 507.*

*Brand name:*

# Kaon-CL

*See Micro-K, page 323.*

*Brand name:*

# K-Dur

*See Micro-K, page 323.*

*Brand name:*

# Keflex

*Pronounced: KEF-lecks*
*Generic name: Cephalexin hydrochloride*
*Other brand name: Keftab*

### Why is this drug prescribed?

Keflex and Keftab are cephalosporin antibiotics. They are prescribed for bacterial infections of the respiratory tract including middle ear infection, bone, skin, and the reproductive and urinary systems. Because they are effective for only certain types of bacterial infections, before beginning treatment your doctor may perform tests to identify the organisms causing the infection.

Keflex is available in capsules and an oral suspension form for use in children. Keftab, available only in tablet form, is prescribed exclusively for adults.

### Most important fact about this drug

If you are allergic to either penicillin or cephalosporin antibiotics in any form, consult your doctor *before taking Keflex*. There is a possibility that you are allergic to both types of medication and if a reaction occurs, it could be extremely severe. If you take the drug and feel signs of a reaction, seek medical attention immediately.

### How should you take this medication?

Keflex may be taken with or without meals. However, if the drug upsets your stomach, you may want to take it after you have eaten.

Take Keflex at even intervals around the clock as prescribed by your doctor.

If you are taking the liquid form of Keflex, use the specially marked spoon to measure each dose accurately.

To obtain maximum benefit, it is important that you finish taking all of this medication, even if you are feeling better.

■ *If you miss a dose...*

Take it as soon as you remember. If it is almost time for the next dose, and you take 2 doses a day, take the one you missed and the next dose 5 to 6 hours later. If you take 3 or more doses a day, take the one you missed and the next dose 2 to 4 hours later, or double the next dose. Then go back to your regular schedule.

■ *Storage instructions...*

Store capsules and tablets at room temperature. Store the liquid suspension in a refrigerator; discard any unused medication after 14 days.

### What side effects may occur?

Side effects cannot be anticipated. If any develop or change in intensity, inform your doctor as soon as possible. Only your doctor can determine if it is safe for you to continue taking Keflex.

■ *More common side effects may include:*

Diarrhea

■ *Less common or rare side effects may include:*

Abdominal pain, agitation, colitis (inflammation of the large intestine), confusion, dizziness, fatigue, fever, genital and rectal itching, hallucinations, headache, hepatitis, hives, indigestion, inflammation of joints, inflammation of the stomach, joint pain, nausea, rash, seizures, severe allergic reaction, skin peeling, skin redness, swelling due to fluid retention, vaginal discharge, vaginal inflammation, vomiting, yellowing of skin and whites of eyes

### Why should this drug not be prescribed?

If you are sensitive to or have ever had an allergic reaction to the cephalosporin group of antibiotics, you should not use this medication. Make sure your doctor is aware of any drug reactions you have experienced.

### Special warnings about this medication

If you have a history of stomach or intestinal disease, especially colitis, check with your doctor before taking Keflex.

If you have ever had an allergic reaction, particularly to drugs, be sure to tell your doctor.

If diarrhea occurs while taking cephalexin, check with your doctor before taking a remedy. Certain diarrhea medications (for instance, Lomotil) may increase your diarrhea or make it last longer.

Prolonged use of Keflex may result in an overgrowth of bacteria that do not respond to the medication, causing a secondary infection. Your doctor will monitor your use of this drug on a regular basis.

If you have a kidney disorder, check with your doctor before taking Keflex. You may need a reduced dose.

If you are diabetic, it is important to note that Keflex may cause false results in tests for urine sugar. Notify your doctor that you are taking this medication before being tested. Do not change your diet or dosage of diabetes medication without first consulting with your doctor.

If your symptoms do not improve within a few days, or if they get worse, notify your doctor immediately.

Do not give this medication to other people or use it for other infections before checking with your doctor.

### Possible food and drug interactions when taking this medication

If Keflex is taken with certain other drugs, the effects of either could be increased, decreased, or altered. It is especially important to check with your doctor before combining Keflex with the following:

Certain diarrhea medications such as Lomotil
Oral contraceptives

### Special information if you are pregnant or breastfeeding

The effects of Keflex during pregnancy have not been adequately studied. If you are pregnant or plan to become pregnant, notify your doctor immediately. Keflex appears in breast milk and could affect a nursing infant. If this medication is essential to your health, your doctor may advise you to discontinue breastfeeding until your treatment is finished.

## Recommended dosage

ADULTS

*Throat, Skin, and Urinary Tract Infections*
The usual adult dosage is 500 milligrams taken every 12 hours. Cystitis (bladder infection) therapy should be continued for 7 to 14 days.

*Other Infections*
The usual recommended dosage is 250 milligrams taken every 6 hours. For more severe infections, larger doses may be needed, as determined by your doctor.

CHILDREN

*Keflex*
The usual dose is 25 to 50 milligrams for each 2.2 pounds of body weight per day, divided into smaller doses.

For strep throat in children over 1 year of age and for skin infections, the dose may be divided into 2 doses taken every 12 hours. For strep infections, the medication should be taken for at least 10 days. Your doctor may double the dose if your child has a severe infection.

For middle ear infection, the dose is 75 to 100 milligrams per 2.2 pounds per day, divided into 4 doses.

*Keftab*
Safety and effectiveness have not been established in children.

## Overdosage

Any medication taken in excess can have serious consequences.

If you suspect an overdose, seek emergency medical treatment immediately.

■ *Symptoms of Keflex overdose may include:*
Blood in the urine, diarrhea, nausea, upper abdominal pain, vomiting

*Brand name:*

# Keftab

See Keflex, page 266.

*Generic name:*

# Ketoconazole

See Nizoral, page 364.

*Generic name:*

# Ketoprofen

See Orudis, page 388.

*Generic name:*

# Ketorolac

See Toradol, page 556.

*Brand name:*

# Klonopin

Pronounced: KLON-uh-pin
Generic name: Clonazepam

## Why is this drug prescribed?

Klonopin is used alone or along with other medications to treat convulsive disorders such as epilepsy. It belongs to a class of drugs known as benzodiazepines.

## Most important fact about this drug

Klonopin works best when there is a constant amount in the bloodstream. To keep blood levels as constant as possible, take your doses at regularly spaced intervals and try not to miss any.

## How should you take this medication?

Klonopin should be taken exactly as prescribed by your doctor.

■ *If you miss a dose...*
If it is within an hour after the missed time, take the dose as soon as you remember. If you do not remember until later, skip the dose and go back to your regular schedule. Never take 2 doses at the same time.

■ *Storage instructions...*
Store away from heat, light, and moisture.

## What side effects may occur?

Side effects cannot be anticipated. If any develop or change in intensity, inform your doctor as soon as possible. Only your doctor can determine if it is safe for you to continue taking Klonopin.

■ *More common side effects may include:*
Behavior problems, drowsiness, lack of muscular coordination

■ *Less common or rare side effects may include:*
Abnormal eye movements, anemia, bed wetting, chest congestion, coated tongue, coma, confu-

sion, constipation, dehydration, depression, diarrhea, double vision, dry mouth, excess hair, fever, fluttery or throbbing heartbeat, "glassy-eyed" appearance, hair loss, hallucinations, headache, inability to fall or stay asleep, inability to urinate, increased sex drive, involuntary rapid movement of the eyeballs, loss of or increased appetite, loss of voice, memory loss, muscle and bone pain, muscle weakness, nausea, nighttime urination, painful or difficult urination, partial paralysis, runny nose, shortness of breath, skin rash, slowed breathing, slurred speech, sore gums, speech difficulties, stomach inflammation, swelling of ankles and face, tremor, uncontrolled body movement or twitching, vertigo, weight loss or gain

■ *Side effects due to rapid decrease or abrupt withdrawal from Klonopin may include:*
Abdominal and muscle cramps, behavior disorders, convulsions, depressed feeling, hallucinations, restlessness, sleeping difficulties, tremors

### Why should this drug not be prescribed?

If you are sensitive to or have ever had an allergic reaction to Klonopin or similar drugs, such as Librium and Valium, you should not take this medication. Make sure your doctor is aware of any reactions you have experienced.

You should not take this medication if you have severe liver disease or the eye condition known as acute narrow angle glaucoma.

### Special warnings about this medication

Klonopin may cause you to become drowsy or less alert; therefore, you should not drive or operate dangerous machinery or participate in any hazardous activity that requires full mental alertness until you know how this drug affects you.

If you have several types of seizures, this drug may increase the possibility of grand mal seizures (epilepsy). Inform your doctor if this occurs. Your doctor may wish to prescribe an additional anticonvulsant drug or increase your dose.

Klonopin can be habit-forming and can lose its effectiveness as you build up a tolerance to it. You may experience withdrawal symptoms—such as convulsions, hallucinations, tremor, and abdominal and muscle cramps—if you stop using this drug abruptly. Discontinue or change your dose only in consultation with your doctor.

### Possible food and drug interactions when taking this medication

Klonopin slows the nervous system and its effects may be intensified by alcohol. Do not drink while taking this medication.

If Klonopin is taken with certain other drugs, the effects of either could be increased, decreased, or altered. It is especially important to check with your doctor before combining Klonopin with the following:

Antianxiety drugs such as Valium
Antidepressant drugs such as Elavil, Nardil, Parnate, and Tofranil
Barbiturates such as phenobarbital
Major tranquilizers such as Haldol, Navane, and Thorazine
Narcotic pain relievers such as Demerol and Percocet
Other anticonvulsants such as Dilantin, Depakene, and Depakote
Sedatives such as Halcion

### Special information if you are pregnant or breastfeeding

The effects of Klonopin during pregnancy have not been adequately studied. If you are pregnant or plan to become pregnant, inform your doctor immediately. Klonopin appears in breast milk and could affect a nursing infant. If this medication is essential to your health, you should not breastfeed until your treatment with this medication is finished.

### Recommended dosage

ADULTS

The starting dose should be no more than 1.5 milligrams per day, divided into 3 doses. Your doctor may increase your daily dosage by 0.5 to 1 milligram every 3 days until your seizures are controlled or the side effects become too bothersome. The most you should take in 1 day is 20 milligrams.

CHILDREN

The starting dose for infants and children up to 10 years old or up to 66 pounds should be 0.01 to 0.03 milligram—no more than 0.05 milligram—per 2.2 pounds of body weight daily. The daily dosage should be given in 2 or 3 smaller doses. Your doctor may increase the dose by 0.25 to 0.5 milligram every 3 days until seizures are controlled or side effects become too bad. If the dose cannot be divided into 3 equal doses, the largest dose should be given at bedtime. The maximum maintenance dose is 0.1 to 0.2 milligram per 2.2 pounds daily.

### Overdosage
Any medication taken in excess can have serious consequences. If you suspect an overdose, seek medical attention immediately.

■ *The symptoms of Klonopin overdose may include:*
Coma, confusion, sleepiness, slowed reaction time

*Brand name:*

# Klor-Con

*See Micro-K, page 323.*

*Brand name:*

# Kwell

*Pronounced: QUELL*
*Generic name: Lindane*

### Why is this drug prescribed?
Kwell cream and lotion are used to treat scabies, a contagious skin disease caused by an almost invisible organism known as the "itch mite." Kwell shampoo is used to treat people with head lice and pubic (crab) lice and their eggs.

### Most important fact about this drug
Use Kwell only as directed by your doctor. Using too much or applying it more often than directed can result in seizures or even death, particularly in the young. Read the "Instructions to Patients" information sheet accompanying the Kwell package before using. If you have any questions, call your doctor.

### How should you use this medication?
CREAM AND LOTION

Shake the lotion well before using. Apply cream or lotion in a thin layer to dry skin, starting from the neck and working down, including the soles of your feet (unless otherwise directed by your doctor), and rub in thoroughly. Trim your nails and apply the medication under the nails with a toothbrush, then throw the toothbrush away. If you take a warm bath or shower before using Kwell, dry your skin thoroughly and let it cool completely before applying

the medication. Leave the cream or lotion on for no less than 8 and no more than 12 hours (usually overnight), then take a shower or bath to wash it off thoroughly. Apply only once, and use only enough to cover the body in a thin layer.

SHAMPOO

Before applying Kwell shampoo, wash your hair with regular shampoo, without conditioners, then rinse it and dry it completely. Shake the shampoo well, then apply directly to dry hair, without adding water. Work thoroughly into your hair and leave it on for 4 minutes. After 4 minutes, add a little water until you have a good lather. Immediately rinse all the lather away. Do not let the lather touch any other part of the body any more than necessary. Towel-dry your hair. Remove nits (eggs) with a nit comb or tweezers. If you are using Kwell on another person, try to keep it off your skin as much as possible. If you are using Kwell on more than one person, wear rubber gloves (this applies especially to pregnant women and nursing mothers).

■ *If you miss a dose...*
Use Kwell only once per infection. Multiple applications are dangerous.
■ *Storage instructions...*
Store away from heat and direct light. Keep out of the reach of children.

### What side effects may occur?
Side effects are extremely rare, but can be serious. If any develop, contact your doctor as soon as possible.

■ *Side effects may include:*
Convulsions, dizziness, seizures, skin eruptions, skin rash

### Why should this drug not be prescribed?
If you are sensitive to or have ever had an allergic reaction to Kwell or any of its ingredients, do not use it again. Do not use Kwell on premature infants, their skin is more sensitive and more drug could be absorbed into the body. Do not use Kwell if you have any kind of seizure disorder; and do not use the cream or lotion for Norwegian scabies (an extremely contagious skin disease with a thin, flaky, rash).

### Special warnings about this medication
Be careful to avoid contact with your eyes. If any Kwell does get in your eyes, immediately flush

them with cold water; if they become irritated or you have an allergic reaction, call your doctor.

Do not swallow Kwell. If you accidentally swallow any, call your doctor or your local poison control center immediately. Do not allow your child to apply Kwell without close adult supervision.

Be sure to cover an infant's hands and feet during treatment with Kwell cream or lotion to prevent the child from sucking or licking the medication.

Do not use Kwell on open wounds such as cuts or sores unless directed by your doctor. After one application of Kwell cream or lotion, your itching may continue for several weeks. The itching is quite normal and does not require a reapplication of Kwell. You will not usually need a second treatment with Kwell shampoo, but if you find living lice in your hair 7 days after treatment, call your doctor. You may need retreatment.

Wash all recently worn clothing, underwear and pajamas, used sheets, pillow cases, and towels in very hot water or have them dry cleaned.

Use Kwell cream or lotion cautiously on young children and the elderly because their skin may absorb more of the medication. To avoid reinfection, make sure that any sexual partners are treated at the same time that you are. Kwell cannot be used to prevent scabies or lice, since no effects remain after it has been washed off.

### Possible food and drug interactions when taking this medication

Oils may cause more Kwell to be absorbed through the skin into the body, possibly causing serious side effects. Therefore, do not use oils, creams, or ointments at the same time you are using Kwell cream or lotion and do not use oil treatments or oil-based hair dressings or conditioners immediately before and after you apply Kwell shampoo.

### Special information if you are pregnant or breastfeeding

If you are pregnant, follow your doctor's directions carefully. Do not use more Kwell than your doctor recommends, and do not use it more than twice during your pregnancy.

If you are breastfeeding, be sure to check with your doctor before using Kwell. Small amounts pass into breast milk, so even though Kwell has not been found to cause problems in nursing infants, your doctor may have you give up breastfeeding for 4 days after using Kwell.

### Recommended dosage
CREAM AND LOTION

*Adults and children aged 6 and over*
Use 1 to 2 ounces. Apply only once; and do not leave on for more than 12 hours.

*Children under age 6*
Use 1 ounce (half of a 2-ounce container). Apply only once.

SHAMPOO

Use 1 ounce (1/2 bottle) for short hair, 1 1/2 ounces (3/4 bottle) for medium-length hair, and 2 ounces (1 bottle) for long hair. Do not use more than 2 ounces.

### Overdosage
Any medication used in excess can have serious consequences. If you suspect an overdose, seek medical attention immediately.

■ *Symptoms of Kwell overdose may include:*
  Convulsions, dizziness

*Generic name:*
# Labetalol

*See Normodyne, page 368.*

*Generic name:*
# Lactulose

*See Chronulac Syrup, page 91.*

*Brand name:*
# Lamictal

*Pronounced: LAM-ic-tal*
*Generic name: Lamotrigine*

### Why is this drug prescribed?
Lamictal is prescribed to control partial seizures in people with epilepsy. It is used in combination with other antiepileptic medications such as Tegretol and Depakene.

### Most important fact about this drug
You may develop a rash during the first 4 to 6 weeks of Lamictal therapy, particularly if you are also taking Depakene. If this happens, notify your doctor immediately. The rash could become severe and even dangerous.

## How should you take this medication?

Take Lamictal exactly as prescribed by your doctor. Do not stop taking this medication without first discussing it with your doctor. An abrupt halt could increase your seizures. Your doctor can schedule a gradual reduction in dosage.

■ *If you miss a dose...*
Take it as soon as you remember. If it is almost time for your next dose, skip the one you missed and go back to your regular schedule. Do not take 2 doses at once.

■ *Storage instructions...*
Store in a tightly closed container at room temperature. Keep dry and protect from light.

## What side effects may occur?

Side effects cannot be anticipated. If any develop or change in intensity, tell your doctor as soon as possible. Only your doctor can determine if it is safe for you to continue taking Lamictal.

■ *More common side effects may include:*
Blurred vision, dizziness, double vision, headache, nausea, rash, sleepiness, uncoordinated movements, vomiting

■ *Less common side effects may include:*
Abdominal pain, accidental injury, anxiety, constipation, depression, diarrhea, fever, "flu-like" symptoms, increased cough, inflammation of vagina, irritability, painful menstruation, sore throat, tremor

■ *Rare side effects may include:*
Absence of menstrual periods, chills, confusion, dry mouth, ear pain, emotional changes, heart palpitations, hot flashes, joint disorders, memory decrease, mind racing, muscle weakness, muscle spasm, poor concentration, ringing in ears, sleep disorder, speech disorder

## Why should this drug not be prescribed?

If you are sensitive to or have ever had an allergic reaction to Lamictal, you should not take this medication. Make sure your doctor is aware of any drug reactions you have experienced.

## Special warnings about this medication

Lamictal may cause some people to become drowsy, dizzy, or less alert. Do not drive or operate dangerous machinery or participate in any activity that requires full mental alertness until you are certain the drug does not have this kind of effect on you. Remember to be alert for development of any type of rash, especially during the first 4 to 6 weeks of treatment.

Be sure to tell your doctor about any medical problems you have before starting therapy with Lamictal. If you have kidney or liver disease, or heart problems, Lamictal should be used with caution.

Lamictal may cause vision problems. If any develop, notify your doctor immediately. Also be sure to call your doctor if you find you have less control over your seizures.

## Possible food and drug interactions when taking this medication

Lamictal is not used alone; it is combined with other medications used to treat epilepsy, including the following:

Carbamazepine (Tegretol)
Phenobarbital (Donnatal, Quadrinal, others)
Phenytoin (Dilantin)
Primidone (Mysoline)
Valproic acid (Depakene)

Be sure to check with your doctor before combining any other drugs with your seizure medications. Lamictal, in particular, may inhibit the action of sulfa drugs such as Bactrim, Proloprim, and Septra.

## Special information if you are pregnant or breastfeeding

The effects of Lamictal during pregnancy have not been adequately studied. If you are pregnant or plan to become pregnant, tell your doctor immediately. Lamictal should be used during pregnancy only if clearly needed. Lamictal appears in breast milk. Because the effects of Lamictal on an infant exposed to this medication are unknown, breastfeeding is not recommended.

## Recommended dosage

ADULTS

*Lamictal combined with Tegretol, Dilantin, Phenobarbital, and Mysoline:*
One 50-milligram dose per day for 2 weeks, then two 50-milligram doses per day, for 2 weeks. After that, your doctor will have you take a total of 300 milligrams to 500 milligrams a day, divided into 2 doses.

*Lamictal combined with Depakene and any of the above medications:*
One 25-milligram dose every other day for 2 weeks, then 25 milligrams once a day for 2 weeks. After that, the doctor will prescribe a total of 100 milligrams to 150 milligrams a day, divided into 2 doses. You should not take more than 25 milligrams every other day because of the increased risk of rash with this combination of drugs.

CHILDREN

Safety and effectiveness of Lamictal in children below the age of 16 have not been studied.

### Overdosage

Any medication taken in excess can have serious consequences. If you suspect an overdose, seek medical treatment immediately. There has been little experience with Lamictal overdose. However, the following symptoms might be seen.

■ *Symptoms of Lamictal overdose may include:*
  Coma, dizziness, headache, sleepiness

*Generic name:*

# Lamotrigine

See Lamictal, page 271.

*Brand name:*

# Lanoxin

*Pronounced: la-NOCKS-in*
*Generic name: Digoxin*

### Why is this drug prescribed?

Lanoxin is used in the treatment of congestive heart failure, irregular heartbeat, and other heart problems. It improves the strength and efficiency of your heart, which leads to better circulation of blood and reduction of the uncomfortable swelling that is common in people with congestive heart failure. Lanoxin is in a class of drugs known as cardiac glycosides.

### Most important fact about this drug

You should not stop taking Lanoxin without first consulting your doctor. A sudden absence of the drug could cause a serious change in your heart function. You will probably have to take Lanoxin for a long time—possibly for the rest of your life.

### How should you take this medication?

Lanoxin usually is taken once daily. To help you remember your dose, try to take it at the same time every day, for instance when brushing your teeth in the morning or going to bed at night.

If you are taking the liquid form of Lanoxin, use the specially marked droppers that comes with it.

It's best to take this medicine on an empty stomach. However, if this upsets your stomach, you can take Lanoxin with food.

Avoid taking this medicine with high-bran/high-fiber foods, such as certain breakfast cereals.

Do not change from one brand of this drugs to another without first consulting your doctor or pharmacist.

Your doctor may ask you to check your pulse rate while taking Lanoxin. Slowing or quickening of your pulse could mean you are developing side effects to your prescribed dose. The amount of Lanoxin needed to help most people is very close to the amount that could cause serious problems from overdose, so monitoring your pulse can be very important.

■ *If you miss a dose...*
  If you remember within 12 hours, take it immediately. If you remember later, skip the dose you missed and go back to your regular schedule. Never take 2 doses at the same time. If you miss doses 2 or more days in a row, consult your doctor.
■ *Storage instructions...*
  Store this medication at room temperature in the container it came in, tightly closed, and away from moist places and direct light. Keep out of reach of children. Digitalis is a major cause of accidental poisoning in the young.

### What side effects may occur?

Side effects cannot be anticipated. If any develop or change in intensity, inform your doctor as soon as possible. Only your doctor can determine if it is safe for you to continue taking Lanoxin.

■ *Side effects may include:*
  Apathy, blurred vision, breast development in males, change in heartbeat, diarrhea, dizziness, headache, loss of appetite, lower stomach pain, nausea, psychosis, rash, vomiting, weakness, yellow vision

## Why should this drug not be prescribed?

If you are sensitive to or have ever had an allergic reaction to Lanoxin or other digitalis preparations, you should not take this medication. Make sure your doctor is aware of any drug reactions you have experienced.

Lanoxin should not be taken by people with the heart irregularity known as ventricular fibrillation.

Lanoxin should not be used, alone or with other drugs, for weight reduction. It can cause irregular heartbeat and other dangerous, even fatal, reactions.

## Special warnings about this medication

Tell the doctor that you are taking Lanoxin if you have a medical emergency and before you have surgery or dental treatment.

Even if you have no symptoms, do not change your dose or discontinue the use of Lanoxin before consulting with your doctor.

## Possible food and drug interactions when taking this medication

In general, you should avoid nonprescription medicines, such as antacids; laxatives; cough, cold, and allergy remedies; and diet aids, except on professional advice.

If Lanoxin is taken with certain other drugs, the effects of either can be increased, decreased, or altered. It is especially important to check with your doctor before combining Lanoxin with the following:

Airway-opening drugs such as Proventil and
    Ventolin
Alprazolam (Xanax)
Amiloride (Midamor)
Amiodarone (Cordarone)
Antacids such as Maalox and Mylanta
Antiarrhythmic drugs such as Quinidex
Antibiotics such as neomycin and tetracycline
Beta-blocking blood pressure drugs such as
    Tenormin and Inderal
Calcium (injectable form)
Calcium-blocking blood pressure drugs such as
    Calan SR, Cardizem, and Procardia
Certain anticancer drugs such as Neosar
Cholestyramine (Questran)
Colestipol (Colestid)
Cyclosporine (Sandimmune)
Diphenoxylate (Lomotil)
Disopyramide (Norpace)

Diuretics such as Lasix
Indomethacin (Indocin)
Itraconazole (Sporanox)
Kaolin-pectin
Metoclopramide (Reglan)
Propafenone (Rythmol)
Propantheline (Pro-Banthine)
Rifampin (Rifadin)
Steroids such as Decadron and Deltasone
Succinylcholine (Anectine)
Sucralfate (Carafate)
Sulfasalazine (Azulfidine)
Thyroid hormones such as Synthroid

## Special information
## if you are pregnant or breastfeeding

The effects of Lanoxin during pregnancy have not been adequately studied. If you are pregnant or plan to become pregnant, inform your doctor immediately. Lanoxin appears in breast milk and could affect a nursing infant. If this medication is essential to your health, your doctor may advise you to discontinue breastfeeding.

## Recommended dosage

Your doctor will determine your dosage based on several factors: (1) the disease being treated; (2) your body weight; (3) your kidney function; (4) your age; and (5) other diseases you have or drugs you are taking.

### ADULTS

If you are receiving Lanoxin for the first time, you may be rapidly "digitalized" (a larger first dose may be taken, followed by smaller maintenance doses), or gradually "digitalized" (maintenance doses only), depending on your doctor's recommendation. A typical maintenance dose might be a 0.125 milligram or 0.25 milligram tablet once daily, but individual requirements vary widely. The exact dose will be determined by your doctor, based on your needs.

### CHILDREN

Infants and young children usually have their daily dose divided into smaller doses; children over age 10 need adult dosages in proportion to body weight as determined by your doctor.

## Overdosage

Suspected overdoses of Lanoxin must be treated immediately; you should contact your doctor or emergency room without delay.

■ *Symptoms of Lanoxin overdose include:*
Abdominal pain, diarrhea, irregular heartbeat, loss of appetite, nausea, very slow pulse, vomiting

In infants and children, irregular heartbeat is the most common sign of overdose.

*Generic name:*

# Lansoprazole

See Prevacid, page 433.

*Brand name:*

# Lasix

Pronounced: LAY-six
Generic name: Furosemide

### Why is this drug prescribed?

Lasix is used in the treatment of high blood pressure and other conditions that require the elimination of excess fluid (water) from the body. These conditions include congestive heart failure, cirrhosis of the liver, and kidney disease. When used to treat high blood pressure, Lasix is effective alone or in combination with other high blood pressure medications. Diuretics help your body produce and eliminate more urine, which helps lower blood pressure. Lasix is classified as a "loop diuretic" because of its point of action in the kidneys.

Lasix is also used with other drugs in people with fluid accumulation in the lungs.

### Most important fact about this drug

Lasix acts quickly, usually within 1 hour when taken orally and within 5 minutes if you are given the drug intravenously. However, since blood pressure declines gradually, it may be several weeks before you get the full benefit of Lasix; and you must continue taking it even if you are feeling well. Lasix does not cure high blood pressure; it merely keeps it under control.

### How should you take this medication?

Take this medication exactly as prescribed by your doctor.

■ *If you miss a dose...*
Take the forgotten dose as soon as you remember. If it is almost time for your next dose, skip the one you missed and go back to your regular schedule. Never take two doses at the same time.

■ *Storage instructions...*
Keep this medication in the container it came in, tightly closed, and away from direct light. Store at room temperature. Discard an open bottle of oral solution after 60 days.

### What side effects may occur?

Side effects cannot be anticipated. If any develop or change in intensity, inform your doctor as soon as possible. Only your doctor can determine if it is safe for you to continue taking Lasix.

■ *Side effects may include:*
Anemia, blood disorders, blurred vision, constipation, cramping, diarrhea, dizziness, dizziness upon standing, fever, headache, hearing loss, high blood sugar, hives, itching, loss of appetite, low potassium (leading to symptoms like dry mouth, excessive thirst, weak or irregular heartbeat, muscle pain or cramps), muscle spasms, nausea, rash, reddish or purplish spots on the skin, restlessness, ringing in the ears, sensitivity to light, skin eruptions, skin inflammation and flaking, stomach or mouth irritation, tingling or pins and needles, vertigo, vision changes, vomiting, weakness, yellow eyes and skin

### Why should this drug not be prescribed?

If you are sensitive to or have ever had an allergic reaction to Lasix or diuretics, or if you are unable to urinate, you should not take this medication.

### Special warnings about this medication

Lasix can cause your body to lose too much potassium. Signs of an excessively low potassium level include muscle weakness and rapid or irregular heartbeat. To improve your potassium level, your doctor may prescribe a potassium supplement or recommend potassium-rich foods, such as bananas, raisins, and orange juice.

Make sure the doctor knows if you have kidney disease, liver disease, diabetes, gout, or the connective tissue disease, lupus erythematosus. Lasix should be used with caution.

If you are allergic to sulfa drugs, you may also be allergic to Lasix.

If you have high blood pressure, avoid over-the-counter medications that may increase blood pressure, including cold remedies and appetite suppressants.

Your skin may be more sensitive to the effects of sunlight.

## Possible food and drug interactions when taking this medication

If Lasix is taken with certain other drugs, the effects of either could be increased, decreased, or altered. It is especially important to consult with your doctor before taking Lasix with any of the following:

Aminoglycoside antibiotics such as Garamycin
Aspirin and other salicylates
Ethacrynic acid (Edecrin)
Indomethacin (Indocin)
Lithium (Lithonate)
Norepinephrine (Levophed)
Other high blood pressure medications such as Hytrin and Cardura
Sucralfate (Carafate)

## Special information if you are pregnant or breastfeeding

The effects of Lasix during pregnancy have not been adequately studied. If you are pregnant or plan to become pregnant, inform your doctor immediately. Lasix appears in breast milk and could affect a nursing infant. If this medication is essential to your health, your doctor may advise you to discontinue breastfeeding until your treatment is finished.

## Recommended dosage

Your doctor will adjust the dosages of this medication, which is a strong diuretic, to meet your specific needs. It is available in both oral and injectable form. The injectable form is used only in emergency situations or in cases where patients cannot take oral medication. Dosages shown here are for oral tablets or solution only.

### ADULTS

#### Fluid Retention

You will probably be started at a single dose of 20 to 80 milligrams. If needed, the same dose can be repeated 6 to 8 hours later, or the dose may be increased. Your doctor may raise the dosage by 20 milligrams or 40 milligrams with each successive administration— each 6 to 8 hours after the previous dose—until the desired effect is achieved. This dosage is then taken once or twice daily thereafter. Your doctor should monitor you carefully using laboratory tests. The maximum daily dose is 600 milligrams.

#### High Blood Pressure

The usual starting dose is 80 milligrams per day divided into 2 doses. Your doctor will adjust the dosages and may add other high blood pressure medications if Lasix is not enough.

### CHILDREN

The usual initial dose is 2 milligrams per 2.2 pounds of body weight given in a single oral dose. The doctor may increase subsequent doses by 1 to 2 milligrams per 2.2 pounds. Doses are spaced 6 to 8 hours apart. A child's dosage will be adjusted to the lowest needed to achieve maximum effect, and should not exceed 6 milligrams per 2.2 pounds.

### ELDERLY

The doctor will determine the dosage based on the particular needs of the individual.

## Overdosage

Any medication taken in excess can have serious consequences. An overdose of Lasix can cause symptoms of severe dehydration. If you suspect an overdose, seek medical attention immediately.

■ *Symptoms of Lasix overdose may include:*
Dry mouth, excessive thirst, low blood pressure, muscle pain or cramps, nausea and vomiting, weak or irregular heartbeat, weak & shyness or drowsiness

*Brand name:*

# Lescol

*Pronounced: LESS-cahl*
*Generic name: Fluvastatin sodium*

## Why is this drug prescribed?

Lescol is a cholesterol-lowering drug. Your doctor may prescribe Lescol if you have been unable to reduce your blood cholesterol level sufficiently with a low-fat, low-cholesterol diet alone.

## Most important fact about this drug

Lescol is usually prescribed only if diet, exercise, and weight-loss fail to bring your cholesterol levels under control. It's important to remember that Lescol is a supplement—not a substitute—for those other measures. To get the full benefit of the medication, you need to stick to the diet and exercise program prescribed by your doctor. All these efforts to keep your cholesterol levels normal are important because together they may lower your risk of heart disease.

### How should you take this medication?
Take Lescol at bedtime; you may take it with or without food.

■ *If you miss a dose...*
If you miss a dose of this medication, take it as soon as you remember. However, if it is almost time for your next dose, skip the one you missed and go back to your regular schedule. Do not take 2 doses at the same time.

■ *Storage instructions...*
Store at room temperature. Protect from direct light and excessive heat. Keep out of reach of children.

### What side effects may occur?
Side effects cannot be anticipated. If any develop or change in intensity, tell your doctor as soon as possible. Only your doctor can determine if it is safe for you to continue taking Lescol.

■ *More common side effects may include:*
Abdominal pain, accidental injury, back pain, diarrhea, fatigue, flu-like symptoms, headache, indigestion, joint disease, muscle pain, nasal inflammation, nausea, sore throat, upper respiratory infection

■ *Less common side effects may include:*
Allergy, bronchitis, constipation, coughing, dizziness, dental problems, gas, inflamed sinuses, insomnia, rash

### Why should this drug not be prescribed?
Do not take Lescol while pregnant or nursing. Also avoid Lescol if you are experiencing liver problems, or if you have ever been found to be excessively sensitive to it.

### Special warnings about this medication
Because Lescol may damage the liver, your doctor may order a blood test to check your liver enzyme levels before you start taking this medication. Blood tests will probably be done at 6 and 12 weeks after you start Lescol therapy and periodically after that. If your liver enzymes rise too high, your doctor may tell you to stop taking Lescol. Your doctor will monitor you especially closely if you have ever had liver disease or if you are, or have ever been, a heavy drinker.

Since Lescol may cause damage to muscle tissue, be sure to tell your doctor of any unexplained muscle pain, tenderness, or weakness right away, especially if you also have a fever or feel sick. Your doctor may want to do a blood test to check for signs of muscle damage. If your blood test shows signs of muscle damage, your doctor may suggest discontinuing this medication.

If your risk of muscle and/or kidney damage suddenly increases because of major surgery or injury, or conditions such as low blood pressure, severe infection, or seizures, your doctor may tell you to stop taking Lescol for a while.

Be sure to tell your doctor about any medical conditions you may have before starting therapy with Lescol.

### Possible food and drug interactions when taking this medication
If you take Lescol with certain drugs, the effects of either could be increased, decreased, or altered. It is especially important to check with your doctor before combining Lescol with the following:

Cholestyramine (Questran)
Cimetidine (Tagamet)
Clofibrate (Atromid-S)
Cyclosporine (Sandimmune, Neoral)
Digoxin (Lanoxin, Lanoxicaps)
Erythromycin (E-Mycin, E.E.S.)
Gemfibrozil (Lopid)
Ketoconazole (Nizoral)
Omeprazole (Prilosec)
Ranitidine (Zantac)
Rifampin (Rifadin)
Spironolactone (Aldactone, Aldactazide)

### Special information if you are pregnant or breastfeeding
You must not become pregnant while taking Lescol. This medication lowers cholesterol, and cholesterol is needed for a baby to develop properly. Because of the possible risk of birth defects, your doctor will prescribe Lescol only if you are highly unlikely to get pregnant while taking this medication. If you do become pregnant while taking Lescol, stop taking the drug and notify your doctor right away.

Lescol does appear in breast milk. Therefore, Lescol could cause severe side effects in a nursing baby. Do not take Lescol while breastfeeding your baby.

### Recommended dosage

Your doctor will put you on a cholesterol-lowering diet before starting treatment with Lescol. You should continue on this diet while you are taking Lescol.

ADULTS

The usual starting dose is 20 milligrams per day, taken as a single dose at bedtime. The usual range after that is 20 to 40 milligrams per day as a single dose in the evening. After 4 weeks of therapy with Lescol, your doctor will check your cholesterol level and adjust your dosage if necessary.

*Combined Drug Therapy*

If you are taking Lescol with another cholesterol medication such as Questran, make sure you take the other drug at least 2 hours before your dose of Lescol.

CHILDREN

The safety and effectiveness of Lescol in children under 18 years old have not been established. Do not give Lescol to children under 18 years of age.

### Overdosage

Although no specific information about Lescol overdose is available, any medication taken in excess can have serious consequences. If you suspect an overdose of Lescol, seek medical attention immediately.

*Brand name:*

# Levbid

See Levsin, page 278.

*Brand name:*

# Levlen

See Oral Contraceptives, page 382.

*Generic name:*

# Levobunolol

See Betagan, page 59.

*Brand name:*

# Levothroid

See Synthroid, page 516.

*Generic name:*

# Levothyroxine

See Synthroid, page 516.

*Brand name:*

# Levoxyl

See Synthroid, page 516.

*Brand name:*

# Levsinex

See Levsin, page 278.

*Brand name:*

# Levsin

Pronounced: LEV-sin
Generic name: Hyoscyamine sulfate
Other brand names: Anaspaz, Levbid, Levsinex

### Why is this drug prescribed?

Levsin is an antispasmodic medication given to help treat various stomach, intestinal, and urinary tract disorders that involve cramps, colic, or other painful muscle contractions. Because Levsin has a drying effect, it may also be used to dry a runny nose or to dry excess secretions before anesthesia is administered.

For inflammation of the pancreas, Levsin may be used to help control excess secretions and reduce pain. Levsin may also be taken in Parkinson's disease to help reduce muscle rigidity and tremors and to help control drooling and excess sweating.

Doctors also give Levsin as part of the preparation for certain diagnostic x-rays (for example, of the stomach, intestines, or kidneys).

Levsin comes in several forms, including regular tablets, tablets to be dissolved under the tongue, sustained-release capsules (Levsinex Timecaps) and tablets (Levbid), liquid, drops, and an injectable solution.

### Most important fact about this drug

Levsin may make you sweat less, causing your body temperature to increase and putting you at the risk of heatstroke. Try to stay inside as much as possible on hot days, and avoid warm places such as very hot baths and saunas.

## How should you take this medication?

If you take Levsin for a stomach disorder, you may also need to take antacid medication. However, antacids make Levsin more difficult for the body to absorb. To minimize this problem, take Levsin before meals and the antacid after meals.

Take Levsin exactly as prescribed. Although the sublingual tablets (Levsin/SL) are designed to be dissolved under the tongue, they may also be chewed or swallowed. The regular tablets may also be dissolved under the tongue or swallowed.

Levsin can cause dry mouth. For temporary relief, suck on a hard candy or chew gum.

■ *If you miss a dose...*
Take it as soon as you remember. If it is almost time for your next dose, skip the one you missed and go back to your regular schedule. Do not take 2 doses at once.

■ *Storage instructions...*
Store at room temperature.

## What side effects may occur?

Side effects cannot be anticipated. If any side effects develop or change in intensity, tell your doctor immediately. Only your doctor can determine whether it is safe for you to continue taking Levsin.

■ *Side effects may include:*
Allergic reactions, bloating, blurred vision, confusion, constipation, decreased sweating, dilated pupils, dizziness, drowsiness, dry mouth, excitement, headache, hives, impotence, inability to urinate, insomnia, itching, heart palpitations, lack of coordination, loss of sense of taste, nausea, nervousness, rapid heartbeat, skin reactions, speech problems, vomiting, weakness

## Why should this drug not be prescribed?

Do not take Levsin if you have ever had an allergic reaction to it or similar drugs such as scopolamine. Also, you should not be given Levsin if you have any of the following:

Bowel or digestive tract obstruction or paralysis
Glaucoma (excessive pressure in the eyes)
Myasthenia gravis (a disorder in which muscles become weak and tire easily)
Ulcerative colitis (severe bowel inflammation)
Urinary obstruction

Levsin is not appropriate if you have diarrhea, especially if you have a surgical opening to the bowels (an ileostomy or colostomy).

## Special warnings about this medication

Be careful using Levsin if you have an overactive thyroid gland, heart disease, congestive heart failure, irregular heartbeats, high blood pressure, or kidney disease.

Because Levsin may make you dizzy or drowsy, or blur your vision, do not drive, operate other machinery, or do any other hazardous work while taking this medication.

While you are taking Levsin, you may experience confusion, disorientation, short-term memory loss, hallucinations, difficulty speaking, lack of coordination, coma, an exaggerated sense of well-being, decreased anxiety, fatigue, sleeplessness and agitation. These symptoms should disappear 12 to 48 hours after you stop taking the drug.

## Possible food and drug interactions when taking this medication

If Levsin is taken with certain other drugs, the effects of either drug could be increased, decreased, or altered. It is especially important to check with your doctor before combining Levsin with the following:

Amantadine (Symmetrel)
Antacids
Antidepressant drugs such as Elavil, Nardil, Parnate, and Tofranil
Antihistamines such as Benadryl
Major tranquilizers such as Thorazine and Haldol
Other antispasmodic drugs such as Bentyl
Potassium supplements such as Slow-K

## Special information if you are pregnant or breastfeeding

If you are pregnant or plan to become pregnant, inform your doctor immediately. Although it is not known whether Levsin can cause birth defects, pregnant women should avoid all drugs except those necessary to health.

Levsin appears in breast milk. Your doctor may ask you to forgo breastfeeding when taking this drug.

## Recommended dosage

LEVSIN/SL AND LEVSIN TABLETS

The tablets may be swallowed or placed under the tongue. Levsin/SL tablets may also be chewed.

*Adults and Children 12 Years of Age and Older*
The usual dose is 1 to 2 tablets every four hours or
as needed. Do not take more than 12 tablets in 24
hours.

*Children 2 to Under 12 Years of Age*
The usual dose is one-half to 1 tablet every four
hours or as needed. Do not give a child more than 6
tablets in 24 hours.

LEVSIN ELIXIR

*Adults and Children 12 Years of Age and Older*
The recommended dosage is 1 to 2 teaspoonfuls
every four hours or as needed, but no more than 12
teaspoonfuls in 24 hours.

*Children 2 to 12 Years of Age*
Dosage is by body weight. Doses may be given
every 4 hours or as needed. Do not give a child
more than 6 teaspoonfuls in 24 hours.

| Weight | Dose |
|---|---|
| 22 pounds | 1/4 teaspoon |
| 44 pounds | 1/2 teaspoon |
| 88 pounds | 3/4 teaspoon |
| 110 pounds | 1 teaspoon |

LEVSIN DROPS

*Adults and Children 12 Years of Age and Older*
The recommended dosage is 1 to 2 milliliters every
4 hours or as needed, but no more than 12 milliliters in 24 hours.

*Children 2 to 12 Years of Age*
The usual dosage is one-quarter to 1 milliliter every
4 hours or as needed. Do not give a child more than
6 milliliters in 24 hours.

*Children under 2 Years of Age*
Your doctor will determine the dosage based on
body weight. The doses may be repeated every 4
hours or as needed.

| Weight | Usual Dose | Do Not Exceed in 24 Hours |
|---|---|---|
| 7.5 pounds | 4 drops | 24 drops |
| 11 pounds | 5 drops | 30 drops |
| 15 pounds | 6 drops | 36 drops |
| 22 pounds | 8 drops | 48 drops |

LEVSINEX TIMECAPS

*Adults and Children 12 Years of Age and Older*
The recommended dosage is 1 to 2 capsules every
12 hours. Your doctor may adjust the dosage to 1
capsule every 8 hours if needed. Do not take more
than 4 capsules in 24 hours.

LEVBID EXTENDED-RELEASE TABLETS

*Adults and Children 12 Years of Age and Older*
The dosage is 1 to 2 tablets every 12 hours. The
tablets are scored so that you can break them in half
if your doctor wants you to. You should not take
more than 4 tablets in 24 hours.

**Overdosage**
Any medication taken in excess can have serious
consequences. If you suspect an overdose, seek
medical attention immediately.

■ *Symptoms of Levsin overdose may include:*
Blurred vision, dilated pupils, dizziness, dry
mouth, excitement, headache, hot dry skin,
nausea, swallowing difficulty, vomiting

*Brand name:*

# Librax

*Pronounced: LIB-racks*
*Generic ingredients: Chlordiazepoxide*
*hydrochloride, Clidinium bromide*
*Other brand name: Clindex*

**Why is this drug prescribed?**
Librax is used, in combination with other therapy,
for the treatment of peptic ulcer, irritable bowel
syndrome (spastic colon), and acute enterocolitis
(inflammation of the colon and small intestine).
Librax is a combination of a benzodiazepine
(chlordiazepoxide) and an antispasmodic medication (clidinium).

**Most important fact about this drug**
Because of its sedative effects, you should not
operate heavy machinery, drive, or engage in other
hazardous tasks that require you to be mentally
alert while you are taking Librax.

**How should you take this medication?**
Take Librax as directed by your doctor. Other
therapy may be prescribed to be used at the
same time.

Librax can make your mouth dry. For temporary relief, suck a hard candy or chew gum.

Take Librax before meals and at bedtime.

■ *If you miss a dose...*

Take it as soon as you remember. If it is almost time for your next dose, skip the one you missed and go back to your regular schedule. Do not take 2 doses at once.

■ *Storage instructions...*

Store away from heat, light, and moisture.

## What side effects may occur?

Side effects cannot be anticipated. If any develop or change in intensity, inform your doctor as soon as possible. Only your doctor can determine if it is safe for you to continue taking Librax.

■ *Side effects may include:*

Blurred vision, changes in sex drive, confusion, constipation, drowsiness, dry mouth, fainting, lack of coordination, liver problems, minor menstrual irregularities, nausea, skin eruptions, swelling due to fluid retention, urinary difficulties, yellowing of skin and eyes

## Why should this drug not be prescribed?

You should not take this drug if you have glaucoma (elevated pressure in the eye), prostatic hypertrophy (enlarged prostate), or a bladder obstruction. If you are sensitive to or have ever had an allergic reaction to Librax or any of its ingredients, you should not take this medication. Make sure your doctor is aware of any drug reactions you have experienced.

## Special warnings about this medication

Librax can be habit-forming and has been associated with drug dependence and addiction. Be very careful taking this medication if you have ever had problems with alcohol or drug abuse. Never take more than the prescribed amount.

In addition, you should not stop taking Librax suddenly, because of the risk of withdrawal symptoms (convulsions, cramps, tremors, vomiting, sweating, feeling depressed, and insomnia). If you have been taking Librax over a long period of time, your doctor will have you taper off gradually.

The elderly are more likely to develop side effects such as confusion, excessive drowsiness, and uncoordinated movements when taking Librax. The doctor will probably prescribe a low dose.

Long-term treatment with Librax may call for periodic blood and liver function tests.

## Possible food and drug interactions when taking this medication

If Librax is taken with certain other drugs, the effects of either can be increased, decreased, or altered. It is especially important to check with your doctor before combining Librax with the following:

Antidepressant drugs known as MAO inhibitors, such as Nardil and Parnate
Blood-thinning drugs such as Coumadin
Certain diarrhea medications such as Donnagel and Kaopectate
Ketoconazole (Nizoral)
Major tranquilizers such as Stelazine and Thorazine
Potassium supplements such as Micro-K

In addition, you may experience excessive drowsiness and other potentially dangerous side effects if you combine Librax with alcohol or other drugs, such as Benadryl and Valium, that make you drowsy.

## Special information if you are pregnant or breastfeeding

Several studies have found an increased risk of birth defects if Librax is taken during the first 3 months of pregnancy. Therefore, Librax is rarely recommended for use by pregnant women. If you are pregnant, plan to become pregnant, or are breastfeeding, inform your doctor immediately.

## Recommended dosage

ADULTS

The usual dose is 1 or 2 capsules, 3 or 4 times a day before meals and at bedtime.

OLDER ADULTS

Your doctor will have you take the lowest dose that is effective.

## Overdosage

Any medication taken in excess can have serious consequences. A severe overdose of Librax can be fatal. If you suspect an overdose, seek medical help immediately.

■ *Symptoms of Librax overdose may include:*

Blurred vision, coma, confusion, constipation, excessive sleepiness, excessively dry mouth, slow reflexes, urinary difficulties

*Brand name:*

# Libritabs

*See Librium, page 282.*

*Brand name:*

# Librium

*Pronounced: LIB-ree-um*
*Generic name: Chlordiazepoxide*
*Other brand name: Libritabs*

### Why is this drug prescribed?

Librium is used in the treatment of anxiety disorders. It is also prescribed for short-term relief of the symptoms of anxiety, symptoms of withdrawal in acute alcoholism, and anxiety and apprehension before surgery. It belongs to a class of drugs known as benzodiazepines.

### Most important fact about this drug

Librium is habit-forming and you can become dependent on it. You could experience withdrawal symptoms if you stopped taking it abruptly (See "What side effects may occur?"). Discontinue or change your dose only on advice of your doctor.

### How should you take this medication?

Take this medication exactly as prescribed.

■ *If you miss a dose...*
Take it as soon as you remember if it is within an hour or so of your scheduled time. If you do not remember until later, skip the dose you missed and go back to your regular schedule. Do not take 2 doses at once.
■ *Storage instructions...*
Store away from heat, light, and moisture.

### What side effects may occur?

Side effects cannot be anticipated. If any develop or change in intensity, inform your doctor as soon as possible. Only your doctor can determine if it is safe for you to continue taking Librium.

■ *Side effects may include:*
Confusion, constipation, drowsiness, fainting, increased or decreased sex drive, liver problems, lack of muscle coordination, minor menstrual irregularities, nausea, skin rash or eruptions, swelling due to fluid retention, yellow eyes and skin

■ *Side effects due to rapid decrease or abrupt withdrawal from Librium include:*
Abdominal and muscle cramps, convulsions, exaggerated feeling of depression, sleeplessness, sweating, tremors, vomiting

### Why should this drug not be prescribed?

If you are sensitive to or have ever had an allergic reaction to Librium or similar tranquilizers, you should not take this medication.

Anxiety or tension related to everyday stress usually does not require treatment with Librium. Discuss your symptoms thoroughly with your doctor.

### Special warnings about this medication

Librium may cause you to become drowsy or less alert; therefore, you should not drive or operate dangerous machinery or participate in any hazardous activity that requires full mental alertness until you know how you react to this drug.

If you are severely depressed or have suffered from severe depression, consult with your doctor before taking this medication.

This drug may cause children to become less alert.

If you have a hyperactive, aggressive child taking Librium, inform your doctor if you notice contrary reactions such as excitement, stimulation, or acute rage.

Consult with your doctor before taking Librium if you are being treated for porphyria (a rare metabolic disorder) or kidney or liver disease.

### Possible food and drug interactions when taking this medication

Librium is a central nervous system depressant and may intensify the effects of alcohol or have an additive effect. Do not drink alcohol while taking this medication.

If Librium is taken with certain other drugs, the effects of either can be increased, decreased, or altered. It is especially important to check with your doctor before combining Librium with the following:

Antacids such as Maalox and Mylanta
Antidepressant drugs known as MAO inhibitors,
    including Nardil and Parnate
Barbiturates such as phenobarbital
Blood-thinning drugs such as Coumadin
Cimetidine (Tagamet)

Disulfiram (Antabuse)

Levodopa (Larodopa)

Major tranquilizers such as Stelazine and Thorazine

Narcotic pain relievers such as Demerol and Percocet

Oral contraceptives

## Special information
## if you are pregnant or breastfeeding

Do not take Librium if you are pregnant or planning to become pregnant. There may be an increased risk of birth defects. This drug may appear in breast milk and could affect a nursing infant. If the medication is essential to your health, your doctor may advise you to discontinue breastfeeding until your treatment with the drug is finished.

## Recommended dosage

ADULTS

*Mild or Moderate Anxiety*

The usual dose is 5 or 10 milligrams, 3 or 4 times a day.

*Severe Anxiety*

The usual dose is 20 to 25 milligrams, 3 or 4 times a day.

*Apprehension and Anxiety before Surgery*

On days preceding surgery, the usual dose is 5 to 10 milligrams, 3 or 4 times a day.

*Withdrawal Symptoms of Acute Alcoholism*

The usual starting oral dose is 50 to 100 milligrams; the doctor will repeat this dose, up to a maximum of 300 milligrams per day, until agitation is controlled. The dose will then be reduced as much as possible.

CHILDREN

The usual dose for children 6 years of age and older is 5 milligrams, 2 to 4 times per day. Some children may need to take 10 milligrams, 2 or 3 times per day. The drug is not recommended for children under 6.

OLDER ADULTS

Your doctor will limit the dose to the smallest effective amount in order to avoid oversedation or lack of coordination. The usual dose is 5 milligrams, 2 to 4 times per day.

## Overdosage

Any medication taken in excess can cause symptoms of overdose. If you suspect an overdose, seek medical attention immediately.

■ *The symptoms of Librium overdose may include:*
Coma, confusion, sleepiness, slow reflexes

*Brand name:*

# Lidex

*Pronounced: LYE-decks*
*Generic name: Fluocinonide*
*Other brand name: Dermacin*

## Why is this drug prescribed?

Lidex is a steroid medication that relieves the itching and inflammation of a wide variety of skin problems, including redness and swelling.

## Most important fact about this drug

When you use Lidex, you inevitably absorb some of the medication through your skin and into the bloodstream. Too much absorption can lead to unwanted side effects elsewhere in the body. To keep this problem to a minimum, avoid using large amounts of Lidex over large areas, and do not cover it with airtight dressings such as plastic wrap or adhesive bandages unless specifically told to by your doctor.

## How should you use this medication?

Lidex is for use only on the skin. Be careful to keep it out of your eyes. If the medication gets in your eyes and causes irritation, immediately flush your eyes with a large amount of water.

Apply Lidex as directed by your doctor. Do not use more of the medication than suggested by your doctor.

■ *If you miss a dose...*
Apply it as soon as you remember. If it is almost time for the next dose, skip the one you missed and go back to your regular schedule.

■ *Storage instructions...*
Store at room temperature. Avoid excessive heat.

## What side effects may occur?

Side effects cannot be anticipated. If any develop or change in intensity, inform your doctor immediately. Only your doctor can determine if it is safe for you to continue using Lidex.

■ *Side effects may include:*
Acne-like eruptions, burning, dryness, excessive hair growth, infection of the skin, irritation, itching, lack of skin color, prickly heat, skin inflammation, skin loss or softening, stretch marks

### Why should this drug not be prescribed?

You should not be using Lidex if you are allergic to any of its components.

### Special warnings about this medication

Do not use Lidex more often or for a longer time than your doctor ordered. If enough of the drug is absorbed through the skin, it may produce unusual side effects, including increased sugar in your blood and urine and a group of symptoms called Cushing's syndrome, characterized by a moon-shaped face, emotional disturbances, high blood pressure, weight gain, and growth of body hair in women.

Some factors that may increase absorption include:

Using bandages over the area where the medication is applied;

Using the medication over a large area of skin or on broken skin; or

Using the medication for an extended period of time.

Children may absorb a proportionally greater amount of steroid drugs and may be more sensitive to the effects of these drugs. Avoid covering a treated area with waterproof diapers or plastic pants. They can increase absorption of Lidex.

*Effects experienced by children may include:*
  Bulges on the head
  Delayed weight gain
  Headache
  Slow growth

Lidex should be discontinued if irritation develops, and another treatment should be used.

Extended treatment time with any steroid product may cause skin to waste away. This may also occur with short-term use on the face, armpits, and skin creases.

### Possible food and drug interactions when taking this medication

No interactions have been reported with Lidex.

### Special information if you are pregnant or breastfeeding

Pregnant women should not use steroids on the skin in large amounts or for long periods of time. During pregnancy, these medications should be used only if the possible gains outweigh the possible risks to the baby.

Steroids do appear in breast milk. Women who breastfeed an infant should use them cautiously.

### Recommended dosage

ADULTS

Lidex is applied to the affected areas in a thin film 2 to 4 times a day. If hair covers the infected area, part the hair so that the medication can be applied directly.

CHILDREN

Children should be given the smallest effective dose.

### Overdosage

Lidex can be absorbed in amounts large enough to have temporary effects on the adrenal, hypothalamic, and pituitary glands.

■ *Some effects of steroid drugs may include:*
  Abnormal sugar levels in urine, excessive blood sugar levels, symptoms of Cushing's syndrome

■ *Symptoms of Cushing's syndrome may include:*
  Easily bruised skin, increased blood pressure, mood swings, water retention, weak muscles, weight gain

If you suspect a Lidex overdose, seek medical help immediately.

*Generic name:*

# Lindane

*See Kwell, page 270.*

*Generic name:*

# Lisinopril

*See Zestril, page 604.*

*Generic name:*

# Lisinopril with Hydrochlorothiazide

*See Zestoretic, page 602.*

*Generic name:*

# Lithium

*See Lithonate, page 285.*

*Brand name:*

# Lithobid

See Lithonate, page 285.


*Brand name:*

# Lithonate

Pronounced: LITH-oh-nate
Generic name: Lithium carbonate
Other brand names: Cibalith-S (lithium citrate),
  Eskalith, Lithobid, Lithotabs

## Why is this drug prescribed?

Lithonate is used to treat the manic episodes of manic-depressive illness, a condition in which a person's mood swings from depression to excessive excitement. A manic episode may involve some or all of the following symptoms:

Aggressiveness
Elation
Fast, urgent talking
Frenetic physical activity
Grandiose, unrealistic ideas
Hostility
Little need for sleep
Poor judgment

Once the mania subsides, Lithonate treatment may be continued over the long term, at a somewhat lower dosage, to prevent or reduce the intensity of future manic episodes.

Some doctors also prescribe lithium for premenstrual tension, eating disorders such as bulimia, certain movement disorders, and sexual addictions.

## Most important fact about this drug

If the Lithonate dosage is too low, you will derive no benefit; if it is too high, you could suffer lithium poisoning. You and your doctor will need to work together to find the correct dosage. Initially, this means frequent blood tests to find out how much of the drug is actually circulating in your bloodstream. As long as you take Lithonate, you will need to watch for side effects. Signs of lithium poisoning include vomiting, unsteady walking, diarrhea, drowsiness, tremor, and weakness. Stop taking the drug and call your doctor if you have any of these symptoms.

## How should you take this medication?

To avoid stomach upset, take Lithonate immediately after meals or with food or milk.

Do not change from one brand of lithium to another without consulting your doctor or pharmacist. Take the drug exactly as prescribed.

While taking Lithonate, you should drink 10 to 12 glasses of water or fluid a day. To minimize the risk of harmful side effects, eat a balanced diet that includes some salt and lots of liquids. If you have been sweating a great deal or have had diarrhea, make sure you get extra liquids and salt.

If you develop an infection with a fever, you may need to cut back on your Lithonate dosage or even quit taking it temporarily. While you are ill, keep in close touch with your doctor.

Long-acting forms of lithium, such as Eskalith CR or Lithobid, should be swallowed whole. Do not chew, crush, or break.

If you are taking a syrup form of lithium, such as Cibalith-S, dilute it with fruit juice or another flavored beverage. You may obtain a specially marked measuring spoon from your pharmacist to ensure an accurate dose.

■ *If you miss a dose...*
  Ask your doctor what to do; requirements vary for each individual. Do not take 2 doses at once.
■ *Storage instructions...*
  Store at room temperature.

## What side effects may occur?

The possibility of side effects varies with the level of lithium in your bloodstream. If you experience unfamiliar symptoms of any kind, inform your doctor as soon as possible.

■ *Side effects that may occur when you start taking lithium include:*
  Discomfort, frequent urination, hand tremor, mild thirst, nausea
■ *Side effects that may occur at a high dosage include:*
  Diarrhea, drowsiness, lack of coordination, muscular weakness, vomiting

## Why should this drug not be prescribed?

Although your doctor will be cautious under certain conditions, lithium may be prescribed for anyone.

## Special warnings about this medication

Lithonate may affect your judgment or coordination. Do not drive, climb, or perform hazardous tasks until you find out how this drug affects you.

Your doctor will prescribe Lithonate with extra caution if you have a heart or kidney problem, brain or spinal cord disease, or a weak, run-down, or dehydrated condition.

Also make sure your doctor is aware of any medical problems you may have, including diabetes, epilepsy, thyroid problems, Parkinson's disease, and difficulty urinating.

You should be careful in hot weather to avoid activities that cause you to sweat heavily. Also avoid drinking large amounts of coffee, tea, or cola, which can cause dehydration through increased urination. Do not make a major change in your eating habits or go on a weight loss diet without consulting your doctor. The loss of water and salt from your body could lead to lithium poisoning.

### Possible food and drug interactions when taking this medication

If Lithonate is taken with certain other drugs, the effects of either could be increased, decreased, or altered. It is especially important to check with your doctor before combining Lithonate with the following:

ACE-inhibitor blood pressure drugs such as Capoten or Vasotec
Acetazolamide (Diamox)
Amphetamines such as Dexedrine
Anti-inflammatory drugs such as Indocin and Feldene
Bicarbonate of soda
Caffeine (No-Doz)
Calcium-blocking blood pressure drugs such as Calan and Cardizem
Carbamazepine (Tegretol)
Diuretics such as Lasix or HydroDIURIL
Fluoxetine (Prozac)
Iodine-containing preparations such as potassium iodide (Quadrinal)
Major tranquilizers such as Haldol and Thorazine
Methyldopa (Aldomet)
Metronidazole (Flagyl)
Sodium bicarbonate
Tetracyclines such as Achromycin V and Sumycin
Theophylline (Theo-Dur, Quibron, others)

### Special information if you are pregnant or breastfeeding

The use of Lithonate during pregnancy is usually not recommended because of the possibility that it might cause birth defects. If you are pregnant or plan to become pregnant, inform your doctor immediately.

Lithonate is excreted in breast milk and is considered potentially harmful to a nursing infant. If this medication is essential to your health, your doctor may advise you to discontinue breastfeeding while you are taking it.

### Recommended dosage

ADULTS

*Acute Episodes*
The usual dosage is a total of 1,800 milligrams per day. Immediate-release forms are taken in 3 doses per day; long-acting forms are taken twice a day. The usual dose of syrup is 2 teaspoons, taken 3 times a day.

Your doctor will individualize your dosage according to the levels of the drug in your blood. Your blood levels will be checked at least twice a week when the drug is first prescribed and on a regular basis thereafter.

*Long-term Control*
Dosage will vary from one individual to another, but a total of 900 milligrams to 1,200 milligrams per day is typical. Immediate-release forms are taken in 3 or 4 doses per day; long-acting forms are taken two or three times a day. The usual dose of syrup is 1 teaspoon 3 or 4 times a day.

Blood levels in most cases should be checked every 2 months.

CHILDREN

Safety and effectiveness of Lithonate in children under 12 years of age have not been established.

OLDER ADULTS

Older people often need less Lithonate and may show signs of overdose at a dosage younger people can handle well.

### Overdosage

Any medication taken in excess can have serious consequences. If you suspect symptoms of an overdose of Lithonate, seek medical attention immediately.

The harmful levels are close to those that will treat your condition. Watch for early signs of overdose, such as diarrhea, drowsiness, lack of coordination, vomiting, and weakness. If you develop any of these signs, stop taking the drug and call your doctor.

*Brand name:*

# Lithotabs

See Lithonate, page 285.

*Brand name:*

# Lodine

*Pronounced: LOW-deen*
*Generic name: Etodolac*

## Why is this drug prescribed?

Lodine, a nonsteroidal anti-inflammatory drug, is used to relieve the inflammation, swelling, stiffness, and joint pain associated with acute and long-term treatment of osteoarthritis (the most common form of arthritis).

## Most important fact about this drug

You should have frequent checkups with your doctor if you take Lodine regularly. Ulcers or internal bleeding can occur without warning.

## How should you take this medication?

Your doctor may ask you to take Lodine with food or an antacid, and with a full glass of water. Never take it on an empty stomach.

Take this medication exactly as prescribed by your doctor.

If you are using Lodine for arthritis, it should be taken regularly.

■ *If you miss a dose...*
Take the forgotten dose as soon as you remember. If it is almost time for the next dose, skip the one you missed and go back to your regular schedule. Never try to "catch up" by doubling the dose.

■ *Storage instructions...*
Store at room temperature. Protect capsules from moisture.

## What side effects may occur?

Side effects cannot be anticipated. If any develop or change in intensity, inform your doctor as soon as possible. Only your doctor can determine if it is safe for you to continue taking Lodine.

■ *More common side effects may include:*
Abdominal pain, black stools, blurred vision, chills, constipation, depression, diarrhea, dizziness, fever, gas, increased frequency of urination, indigestion, itching, nausea, nervousness, rash, ringing in ears, painful or difficult urination, vomiting, weakness

■ *Less common or rare side effects may include:*
Abdominal bleeding, abnormal intolerance of light, anemia, asthma, blood disorders, congestive heart failure, dry mouth, fainting, flushing, hepatitis, high blood pressure, high blood sugar in some diabetics, hives, inability to sleep, inflamed blood vessels, inflammation of mouth, kidney problems, including kidney failure, loss of appetite, peptic ulcer, rapid heartbeat, rash, severe allergic reactions, skin disorders including increased pigmentation, sleepiness, Stevens-Johnson syndrome (peeling skin), sweating, swelling (fluid retention), thirst, visual disturbances, yellowed skin and eyes

## Why should this drug not be prescribed?

If you are sensitive to or have ever had an allergic reaction to Lodine, aspirin, or similar drugs, or if you have had asthma attacks caused by aspirin or other drugs of this type, you should not take this medication. Make sure that your doctor is aware of any drug reactions that you have experienced.

## Special warnings about this medication

Peptic ulcers and bleeding can occur without warning.

This drug should be used with caution if you have kidney or liver disease; and it can cause liver inflammation in some people.

Do not take aspirin or any other anti-inflammatory medications while taking Lodine, unless your doctor tells you to do so.

If you are taking Lodine over an extended period of time, your doctor should check your blood for anemia.

This drug can increase water retention. Use with caution if you have heart disease or high blood pressure.

## Possible food and drug interactions when taking this medication

If Lodine is taken with certain other drugs, the effects of either could be increased, decreased, or altered. It is especially important to check with your doctor before combining Lodine with the following:

Aspirin
Cyclosporine (Sandimmune, Neoral)

Diuretics such as HydroDIURIL
Digoxin (Lanoxin)
Lithium (Lithobid, others)
Methotrexate
Phenylbutazone (Butazolidin)
The blood-thinning drug warfarin (Coumadin)

### Special information
### if you are pregnant or breastfeeding

The effects of Lodine during pregnancy have not been adequately studied. If you are pregnant or plan to become pregnant, inform your doctor immediately. Lodine may appear in breast milk and could affect a nursing infant. If this medication is essential to your health, your doctor may advise you to discontinue breastfeeding until your treatment with this medication is finished.

### Recommended dosage

ADULTS

*General Pain Relief*

Take 200 to 400 milligrams every 6 to 8 hours as needed. Do not take more than 1,200 milligrams a day. For individuals weighing less than 132 pounds, the maximum dose is 20 milligrams per 2.2 pounds.

*Osteoarthritis*

Starting dose is a total of 800 to 1,200 milligrams per day divided into smaller doses, followed by 600 to 1,200 milligrams per day in divided doses (i.e., 400 milligrams 2 or 3 times a day; 300 milligrams 2, 3 or 4 times a day). For those weighing less than 132 pounds the maximum dose is 20 milligrams per 2.2 pounds.

The lowest dose that proves beneficial should be used.

CHILDREN

The safety and effectiveness of Lodine have not been established in children.

### Overdosage

Any medication taken in excess can cause symptoms of overdose. If you suspect an overdose, seek medical attention immediately.

■ *Symptoms of Lodine overdose may include:*
Drowsiness, lethargy, nausea, stomach pain, vomiting

*Brand name:*

# Loestrin

*See Oral Contraceptives, page 382.*

*Generic name:*

# Lomefloxacin

*See Maxaquin, page 307.*

*Brand name:*

# Lomotil

*Pronounced: loe-MOE-till*
*Generic ingredients: Diphenoxylate hydrochloride,*
*    Atropine sulfate*

### Why is this drug prescribed?

Lomotil is used, along with other drugs, in the treatment of diarrhea.

### Most important fact about this drug

Lomotil is not a harmless drug, so never exceed your recommended dosage. An overdose could be fatal.

### How should you take this medication?

Lomotil can be habit-forming. Take it exactly as prescribed.

Be sure to drink plenty of liquids to replace lost body fluids. Eat bland foods, such as cooked cereals, breads and crackers.

Lomotil may cause dry mouth. Suck on a hard candy or chew gum to relieve this problem.

■ *If you miss a dose...*
Take it as soon as you remember. If it is almost time for your next dose, skip the one you missed and go back to your regular schedule. Do not take 2 doses at once.
■ *Storage instructions...*
Store away from heat, light, and moisture. Keep the liquid from freezing.

### What side effects may occur?

Side effects cannot be anticipated. If any develop or change in intensity, inform your doctor as soon as possible. Only your doctor can determine if it is safe for you to continue taking Lomotil.

■ *Side effects may include:*
Abdominal discomfort, confusion, depression, difficulty urinating, dizziness, dry mouth and

skin, exaggerated feeling of elation, fever, flushing, general feeling of not being well, headache, hives, intestinal blockage, itching, lack or loss of appetite, nausea, numbness of arms and legs, rapid heartbeat, restlessness, sedation/drowsiness, severe allergic reaction, sluggishness, swelling due to fluid retention, swollen gums, vomiting

## Why should this drug not be prescribed?

If you are sensitive to or have ever had an allergic reaction to the ingredients of Lomotil, diphenoxylate or atropine, you should not take this medication. Make sure your doctor is aware of any drug reactions you have experienced.

Unless you are directed to do so by your doctor, do not take Lomotil if you have obstructive jaundice (a disease in which bile made in the liver does not reach the intestines because of a bile duct obstruction such as gallstones). Do not take Lomotil if you have diarrhea associated with pseudomembranous enterocolitis (inflammation of the intestines) or an infection with enterotoxin-producing bacteria (an enterotoxin is a poisonous substance that affects the stomach and intestines).

## Special warnings about this medication

Certain antibiotics such as Ceclor, Cleocin, PCE and Achromycin V may cause diarrhea. Lomotil can make this type of diarrhea worse and longer-lasting. Check with your doctor before using Lomotil while taking an antibiotic.

Lomotil may cause drowsiness or dizziness. Therefore, you should not drive a car, operate dangerous machinery, or participate in any hazardous activity that requires full mental alertness until you know how this drug affects you.

Lomotil slows activity of the digestive system; this can result in a buildup of fluid in the intestine, which may worsen the dehydration and imbalance in normal body salts that usually occur with diarrhea.

If you have severe ulcerative colitis (an inflammation of the intestines), your doctor will want to monitor your condition while you are taking this drug. If your abdomen becomes distended, or enlarged, notify your doctor.

Use Lomotil with extreme caution if you have kidney and liver disease or if your liver is not functioning normally.

Lomotil should be used with caution in children, since side effects may occur even with recommended doses, especially in children with Down's syndrome (congenital mental retardation).

Since addiction to diphenoxylate hydrochloride is possible at high doses, you should never exceed the recommended dosage.

## Possible food and drug interactions when taking this medication

Lomotil may intensify the effects of alcohol. It's better not to drink alcohol while taking this medication.

If Lomotil is taken with certain other drugs, the effects of either could be increased, decreased, or altered. It is especially important to check with your doctor before combining Lomotil with the following:

Barbiturates (anticonvulsants and sedatives such as phenobarbital)
MAO inhibitors (antidepressants such as Nardil and Parnate)
Tranquilizers (such as Valium and Xanax)

## Special information if you are pregnant or breastfeeding

The effects of Lomotil during pregnancy have not been adequately studied. If you are pregnant or plan to become pregnant, notify your doctor immediately. Lomotil appears in breast milk and could affect a nursing infant. If this medication is essential to your health, your doctor may advise you to discontinue breastfeeding until your treatment is finished.

## Recommended dosage

ADULTS

The recommended starting dosage is 2 tablets 4 times a day or 2 regular teaspoonfuls (10 milliliters) of liquid 4 times per day.

Once your diarrhea is under control, your doctor may reduce the dosage; you may need as little as 5 milligrams (2 tablets or 10 milliliters of liquid) per day.

You should see improvement within 48 hours. If your diarrhea persists after you have taken 20 milligrams a day for 10 days, the drug is not likely to work for you.

CHILDREN

Lomotil is not recommended in children under 2 years of age.

Your doctor will take into account your child's nutritional status and degree of dehydration before prescribing this drug.

In children under 13 years of age, use only Lomotil liquid and administer with the plastic dropper. The recommended starting dosage is 0.3 to 0.4 milligram per 2.2 pounds of body weight per day, divided into 4 equal doses. The following table provides approximate starting dosage recommendations for children:

2 years (24-31 pounds):
   1.5-3.0 milligrams, 4 times daily
3 years (26-35 pounds):
   2.0-3.0 milligrams, 4 times daily
4 years (31-44 pounds):
   2.0-4.0 milligrams, 4 times daily
5 years (35-51 pounds):
   2.5-4.5 milligrams, 4 times daily
6-8 years (38-71 pounds):
   2.5-5.0 milligrams, 4 times daily
9-12 years (51-121 pounds):
   3.5-5.0 milligrams, 4 times daily

Your doctor may reduce the dosage as soon as symptoms are controlled. A maintenance dosage may be as low as one-quarter of the starting dose. If your child does not show improvement within 48 hours, Lomotil is unlikely to work.

### Overdosage
An overdose of Lomotil can be dangerous and even fatal. If you suspect an overdose, seek medical attention immediately.

■ *Symptoms of Lomotil overdose may include:*
   Coma, dry skin and mucous membranes, enlarged pupils of the eyes, extremely high body temperature, flushing, involuntary eyeball movement, lower than normal muscle tone, pinpoint pupils, rapid heartbeat, restlessness, sluggishness, suppressed breathing

Suppressed breathing may be seen as late as 30 hours after an overdose.

*Brand name:*
# Lo/Ovral

*See Oral Contraceptives, page 382.*

*Generic name:*
# Loperamide

*See Imodium, page 250.*

*Brand name:*
# Lopid

*Pronounced: LOH-pid*
*Generic name: Gemfibrozil*
*Other brand name: Gemcor*

### Why is this drug prescribed?
Lopid is prescribed, along with a special diet, for treatment of people with very high levels of serum triglycerides (a fatty substance in the blood) who are at risk of developing pancreatitis (inflammation of the pancreas) and who do not respond adequately to a strict diet.

This drug can also be used to reduce the risk of coronary heart disease in people who have failed to respond to weight loss, diet, exercise, and other triglyceride- or cholesterol-lowering drugs.

### Most important fact about this drug
Lopid is usually prescribed only if diet, exercise, and weight-loss fail to bring your cholesterol levels under control. It's important to remember that Lopid is a supplement—not a substitute—for these other measures. To get the full benefit of the medication, you need to stick to the diet and exercise program prescribed by your doctor. All these efforts to keep your cholesterol levels normal are important because together they may lower your risk of heart disease.

### How should you take this medication?
Take this medication 30 minutes before the morning and evening meal, exactly as prescribed.

■ *If you miss a dose...*
   Take it as soon as you remember. If it is almost time for the next dose, skip the one you missed and go back to your regular schedule. Do not take 2 doses at the same time.
■ *Storage instructions...*
   Store at room temperature.

### What side effects may occur?
Side effects cannot be anticipated. If any develop or change in intensity, inform your doctor as soon as possible. Only your doctor can determine if it is safe for you to continue taking Lopid.

■ *More common side effects may include:*
Abdominal pain, acute appendicitis, constipation, diarrhea, eczema, fatigue, headache, indigestion, nausea/vomiting, rash, vertigo

■ *Less common or rare side effects may include:*
Anemia, blood disorders, blurred vision, confusion, convulsions, decreased male fertility, decreased sex drive, depression, dizziness, fainting, hives, impotence, inflammation of the colon, irregular heartbeat, itching, joint pain, laryngeal swelling, muscle disease, muscle pain, muscle weakness, painful extremities, sleepiness, tingling sensation, weight loss, yellow eyes and skin

## Why should this drug not be prescribed?

There is a slight possibility that Lopid may cause malignancy, gallbladder disease, abdominal pain leading to appendectomy, or other serious, possibly fatal, abdominal disorders. This drug should not be used by those who have only mildly elevated cholesterol levels, since the benefits do not outweigh the risk of these severe side effects.

If you are sensitive to or have ever had an allergic reaction to Lopid or similar drugs such as Atromid-S, you should not take this medication. Make sure your doctor is aware of any drug reactions you have experienced.

Unless you are directed to do so by your doctor, do not take this medication if you are being treated for severe kidney or liver disorders or gallbladder disease.

## Special warnings about this medication

Excess body weight and excess alcohol intake may be important risk factors leading to unusually high levels of fats in the body. Your doctor will probably want you to lose weight and stop drinking before he or she tries to treat you with Lopid.

Your doctor will probably do periodic blood level tests during the first 12 months of therapy with Lopid because of blood diseases associated with the use of this medication.

Liver disorders have occurred with the use of this drug. Therefore, your doctor will probably test your liver function periodically.

If you are being treated for any disease that contributes to increased blood cholesterol, such as an overactive thyroid, diabetes, nephrotic syndrome (kidney and blood vessel disorder), dysproteinemia (excess of protein in the blood), or obstructive liver disease, consult with your doctor before taking Lopid.

Lopid should begin to reduce cholesterol levels during the first 3 months of therapy. If your cholesterol is not lowered sufficiently, this medication should be discontinued. Therefore, it is important that your doctor check your progress regularly.

The use of this medication may cause gallstones leading to possible gallbladder surgery. If you develop gallstones, your doctor will have you stop taking the drug.

The use of this drug may be associated with myositis, a muscle disease. If you have muscle pain, tenderness, or weakness, consult with your doctor. If myositis is suspected, your doctor will stop treating you with this drug.

## Possible food and drug interactions when taking this medication

If Lopid is taken with certain other drugs, the effects of either could be increased, decreased, or altered. It is especially important to check with your doctor before combining Lopid with the following:

Blood-thinning drugs such as Coumadin
Fluvastatin (Lescol)
Lovastatin (Mevacor)
Pravastatin (Pravachol)
Simvastatin (Zocor)

## Special information if you are pregnant or breastfeeding

The effects of Lopid during pregnancy have not been adequately studied. If you are pregnant or plan to become pregnant, inform your doctor immediately. Because this medication causes tumors in animals, it may have an effect on nursing infants. If Lopid is essential to your health, your doctor may advise you to discontinue breastfeeding until your treatment with Lopid is finished.

## Recommended dosage

ADULTS

The recommended dose is 1,200 milligrams divided into 2 doses, given 30 minutes before the morning and evening meals.

CHILDREN

Safety and effectiveness of Lopid have not been established for use in children.

OLDER ADULTS

This drug should be used with caution by older adults.

### Overdosage

There have been no reported cases of overdose with Lopid. However, should you suspect a Lopid overdose, seek medical attention immediately.

Brand name:

# Lopressor

Pronounced: low-PRESS-or
Generic name: Metoprolol tartrate

### Why is this drug prescribed?

Lopressor, a type of medication known as a beta blocker, is used in the treatment of high blood pressure, angina pectoris (chest pain, usually caused by lack of oxygen to the heart due to clogged arteries), and heart attack. When prescribed for high blood pressure, it is effective when used alone or in combination with other high blood pressure medications. Beta blockers decrease the force and rate of heart contractions, thereby reducing the demand for oxygen and lowering blood pressure.

Occasionally doctors prescribe Lopressor for the treatment of aggressive behavior, prevention of migraine headache, and relief of temporary anxiety.

### Most important fact about this drug

If you have high blood pressure, you must take Lopressor regularly for it to be effective. Since blood pressure declines gradually, it may be several weeks before you get the full benefit of Lopressor; and you must continue taking it even if you are feeling well. Lopressor does not cure high blood pressure; it merely keeps it under control.

### How should you take this medication?

Lopressor should be taken with food or immediately after you have eaten.

Take Lopressor exactly as prescribed, even if your symptoms have disappeared.

Try not to miss any doses. If this medication is not taken regularly, your condition may worsen.

■ *If you miss a dose...*
If it is within 4 hours of your next dose, skip the one you missed and go back to your regular schedule. Never take 2 doses at the same time.

■ *Storage instructions...*
Store at room temperature in a tightly closed container, away from light. Protect from moisture.

### What side effects may occur?

Side effects cannot be anticipated. If any develop or change in intensity, inform your doctor as soon as possible. Only your doctor can determine if it is safe for you to continue taking Lopressor.

■ *More common side effects may include:*
Depression, diarrhea, dizziness, itching, rash, shortness of breath, slow heartbeat, tiredness
■ *Less common or rare side effects may include:*
Blurred vision, cold hands and feet, confusion, congestive heart failure, constipation, difficult or labored breathing, dry eyes, dry mouth, gas, hair loss, headache, heart attack, heartburn, low blood pressure, muscle pain, nausea, nightmares, rapid heartbeat, ringing in the ears, short-term memory loss, stomach pain, swelling due to fluid retention, trouble sleeping, wheezing, worsening of heart irregularities

### Why should this drug not be prescribed?

If you have a slow heartbeat, certain heart irregularities, low blood pressure, inadequate output from the heart, or heart failure, you should not take this medication.

### Special warnings about this medication

If you have a history of congestive heart failure, Lopressor should be used with caution.

Do not stop Lopressor abruptly. This can cause increased chest pain and heart attack. Dosage should be gradually reduced.

If you suffer from asthma, seasonal allergies or other bronchial conditions, or liver disease, this medication should be used with caution.

Ask your doctor if you should check your pulse while taking Lopressor. This medication can cause your heartbeat to become too slow.

This medication may mask some symptoms of low blood sugar in diabetics or alter blood sugar levels. If you are diabetic, discuss this with your doctor.

Lopressor may cause you to become drowsy or less alert; therefore, driving or operating dangerous machinery or participating in any hazardous activity that requires full mental alertness is not recommended until you know how you respond to this medication.

Notify your doctor or dentist that you are taking Lopressor if you have a medical emergency, or before you have surgery or dental treatment.

Notify your doctor if you have any difficulty in breathing.

## Possible food and drug interactions when taking this medication

If Lopressor is taken with certain other drugs, the effects of either could be increased, decreased, or altered. It is especially important to check with your doctor before combining Lopressor with certain high blood pressure drugs such as reserpine (Ser-Ap-Es).

*Other medications that might interact with Lopressor include:*
   Albuterol (Proventil, Ventolin)
   Amiodarone (Cordarone)
   Barbiturates such as phenobarbital
   Calcium channel blockers such as Calan and Cardizem
   Cimetidine (Tagamet)
   Ciprofloxacin (Cipro)
   Clonidine (Catapres)
   Epinephrine (EpiPen)
   Hydralazine (Apresoline)
   Insulin
   Nonsteroidal anti-inflammatory drugs such as Motrin and Indocin
   Oral diabetes drugs such as Glucotrol and Micronase
   Prazosin (Minipress)
   Quinidine (Quinaglute)
   Ranitidine (Zantac)
   Rifampin (Rifadin)

## Special information if you are pregnant or breastfeeding

The effects of Lopressor during pregnancy have not been adequately studied. If you are pregnant or plan to become pregnant, inform your doctor immediately. Lopressor appears in breast milk and could affect a nursing infant. If this medication is essential to your health, your doctor may advise you to discontinue breastfeeding until your treatment with this medication is finished.

## Recommended dosage

ADULTS

Dosages of Lopressor should be individualized by your doctor. It should be taken with or immediately following meals.

*Hypertension*

The usual starting dosage is a total of 100 milligrams a day taken in 1 or 2 doses, whether taken alone or with a diuretic. Your doctor may gradually increase the dosage up to 400 milligrams a day. Generally, the effectiveness of each dosage increase will be seen within a week.

*Angina Pectoris*

The usual starting dosage is a total of 100 milligrams a day taken in 2 doses. Your doctor may gradually increase the dosage up to 400 milligrams a day.

Generally, the effectiveness of each dosage increase will be seen within a week. If treatment is to be discontinued, your doctor will withdraw the drug gradually over a period of 1 to 2 weeks.

*Heart Attack*

Lopressor can be used for treatment of heart attack both in the hospital during the early phases and after the individual's condition has stabilized. Your doctor will determine the dosage according to your needs.

CHILDREN

The safety and effectiveness of Lopressor have not been established in children.

## Overdosage

Any medication taken in excess can cause symptoms of overdose. If you suspect an overdose, seek medical attention immediately.

■ *The symptoms of Lopressor overdose may include:* Asthma-like symptoms, heart failure, low blood pressure, slow heartbeat

*Brand name:*

# Loprox

*Pronounced: LOW-prox*
*Generic name: Ciclopirox olamine*

## Why is this drug prescribed?

Loprox is prescribed for the treatment of the following fungal skin infections:

Athlete's foot
Fungal infection of the groin (jock itch)
Fungal infection of non-hairy parts of the skin

Candidiasis (yeastlike fungal infection of the skin, nails, mouth, vagina, and lungs)

Tinea versicolor—infection of the skin that is characterized by brown or tan patches on the trunk.

Loprox is available in cream and lotion forms.

### Most important fact about this drug
Loprox is for external treatment of skin infections. Do not use Loprox in the eyes.

### How should you use this medication?
Use this medication for the full treatment time even if your symptoms have improved. Notify your doctor if there is no improvement after 4 weeks.

Shake Loprox lotion vigorously before each use.

■ *If you miss a dose...*
Apply the forgotten dose as soon as you remember. If it is almost time for your next dose, skip the one you missed and go back to your regular schedule.

■ *Storage instructions...*
Store at room temperature.

### What side effects may occur?
Loprox rarely causes side effects. If any develop or change in intensity, inform your doctor as soon as possible. Only your doctor can determine if it is safe for you to continue using Loprox.

■ *Rare side effects may include:*
Burning, itching, worsening of infection symptoms

### Why should this drug not be prescribed?
If you are sensitive to or have ever had an allergic reaction to ciclopirox olamine or any other ingredient in Loprox, you should not take this medication. Make sure your doctor is aware of any drug reactions you have experienced.

### Special warnings about this medication
If the affected area of skin shows signs of increased irritation (redness, itching, burning, blistering, swelling, oozing), notify your doctor.

Avoid the use of airtight dressings or bandages.

### Special information
### if you are pregnant or breastfeeding
The effects of Loprox during pregnancy have not been adequately studied. If you are pregnant or plan to become pregnant, inform your doctor immediately. It is not known whether this drug appears in

breast milk. If this medication is essential to your health, your doctor may advise you to discontinue breastfeeding your baby until your treatment is finished.

### Recommended dosage
ADULTS

Gently massage Loprox into the affected and surrounding skin areas 2 times a day, in the morning and evening. For most infections, improvement usually occurs within the first week of treatment. People with tinea versicolor usually show signs of improvement after 2 weeks of treatment.

CHILDREN

Safety and effectiveness have not been established in children under 10 years of age.

### Overdosage
Any medication taken in excess can have serious consequences. If you suspect an overdose, seek medical treatment immediately.

---

*Brand name:*

# Lopurin

*See Zyloprim, page 613.*

---

*Brand name:*

# Lorabid

*Pronounced: LOR-a-bid*
*Generic name: Loracarbef*

### Why is this drug prescribed?
Lorabid is used to treat mild-to-moderate bacterial infections of the lungs, ears, throat, sinuses, skin, urinary tract, and kidneys.

### Most important fact about this drug
If you have ever had an allergic reaction to Lorabid, penicillin, cephalosporins, or any other drug, be sure your doctor is aware of it before you take Lorabid. You may experience a severe reaction if you are sensitive to penicillin-type medications.

### How should you take this medication?
Take Lorabid at least 1 hour before or 2 hours after eating. It is best to take your medication at evenly spaced intervals, day and night.

Do not stop taking your medication even if you begin to feel better after a few days. If you stop taking your medicine too soon, your symptoms may return. If you have a "strep" infection, you should take your medication for at least 10 days.

■ *If you miss a dose...*
Take it as soon as possible. This will help keep a constant amount of medicine in your system. If it is almost time for your next dose, skip the one you missed and go back to your regular schedule. Do not take 2 doses at once.

■ *Storage instructions...*
Lorabid can be stored at room temperature. The liquid form can be kept in the refrigerator, but not in the freezer. Discard any unused portion.

## What side effects may occur?

Side effects cannot be anticipated. If any develop or change in intensity, tell your doctor as soon as possible. Only your doctor can determine if it is safe for you to continue taking Lorabid.

■ *More common side effects in children may include:*
Diarrhea, inflamed, runny nose, vomiting
■ *Less common or rare side effects in children may include:*
Headache, loss of appetite, rash, sleepiness
■ *More common side effects in adults may include:*
Diarrhea, headache
■ *Less common side effects in adults may include:*
Abdominal pain, nausea, rhinitis, skin rashes, vaginitis (inflammation of the vaginal tissues), vomiting, yeast infection
■ *Rare side effects may include:*
Blood disorders, dizziness, hives, insomnia, itching, loss of appetite, nervousness, red bumps on skin, sleepiness, vasodilation (widening of the blood vessels)
■ *Side effects for other drugs of this class may include:*
Allergic reactions (sometimes severe), anemia, blood disorders, hemorrhage, kidney problems, serum sickness (fever, skin rash, joint pain, swollen lymph nodes), skin peeling

## Why should this drug not be prescribed?

If you are allergic to penicillin, cephalosporins, or other medications, you should not take Lorabid. Make sure you tell your doctor about any drug reactions you have experienced.

## Special warnings about this medication

As with many antibiotics, Lorabid can cause colitis—an inflammation of the bowel. This condition can range from mild to life-threatening. If you develop diarrhea while taking Lorabid, notify your doctor, and do not take any diarrhea medication without your doctor's approval.

Prolonged use of Lorabid may result in development of bacteria that do not respond to the medication, leading to a second infection. Because of this danger, you should not use any left-over Lorabid for later infections, even if they have similar symptoms. Take Lorabid only when your doctor prescribes it for you.

If you have known or suspected kidney problems, your doctor will perform blood tests to check your urine and kidney function before and during Lorabid therapy.

## Possible food and drug interactions when taking this medication

If Lorabid is taken with certain other drugs, the effects of either could be increased, decreased, or altered. It is especially important to check with your doctor before combining Lorabid with the following:

Diuretics such as Lasix and Bumex
Probenecid (the gout medication Benemid)

## Special information if you are pregnant or breastfeeding

The effects of Lorabid during pregnancy have not been adequately studied. If you are pregnant or plan to become pregnant, tell your doctor immediately. Lorabid should be used during pregnancy only if clearly needed. It is not known whether Lorabid appears in human breast milk. Your doctor will determine whether it is safe for you to take Lorabid while breastfeeding.

## Recommended dosage

ADULTS (13 YEARS AND OLDER)

*Bronchitis*
The usual dose is 200 to 400 milligrams every 12 hours for 7 days.

*Pneumonia*
The usual dose is 400 milligrams every 12 hours for 14 days.

*Sinusitis*
The usual dose is 400 milligrams every 12 hours for 10 days.

*Skin and Soft Tissue Infections*
The usual dose is 200 milligrams every 12 hours for 7 days.

*Streptococcal Pharyngitis ("strep throat") and Tonsillitis*
The usual dose is 200 milligrams every 12 hours for 10 days. For strep throat, take Lorabid for at least 10 days.

*Bladder Infections*
The usual dose is 200 milligrams every 24 hours for 7 days.

*Kidney Infections*
The usual dose is 400 milligrams every 12 hours for 14 days.

If you have impaired kidney function, your doctor will adjust the dosage according to your needs.

CHILDREN (6 MONTHS TO 12 YEARS OF AGE)

*Otitis Media*
This infection of the middle ear should be treated with the suspension. Do not use the pulvules.

The dose is based on body weight. The usual dose is 30 milligrams of liquid per 2.2 pounds of body weight per day in divided doses (half the dose every 12 hours), for 10 days.

*Streptococcal Pharyngitis (strep throat) and Tonsillitis*
The dose is based on body weight. The usual dose is 15 milligrams per 2.2 pounds of body weight per day in divided doses (half the dose every 12 hours), for at least 10 days.

*Impetigo (Skin Infection)*
The dose is based on body weight. The usual dose is 15 milligrams of liquid per 2.2 pounds of body weight per day in divided doses (half the dose every 12 hours), for 7 days.

**Overdosage**
Any medication taken in excess can have serious consequences. If you suspect an overdose, seek medical attention immediately.

■ *Symptoms of Lorabid overdose may include:*
Diarrhea, nausea, stomach upset, vomiting

*Generic name:*

# Loracarbef

*See Lorabid, page 294.*

*Generic name:*

# Loratadine

*See Claritin, page 94.*

*Generic name:*

# Loratadine with Pseudoephedrine

*See Claritin-D, page 95.*

*Generic name:*

# Lorazepam

*See Ativan, page 40.*

*Brand name:*

# Lorcet

*See Vicodin, page 587.*

*Brand name:*

# Lortab

*See Vicodin, page 587.*

*Generic name:*

# Losartan

*See Cozaar, page 120.*

*Generic name:*

# Losartan with Hydrochlorothiazide

*See Hyzaar, page 245.*

*Brand name:*

# Lotensin

*Pronounced: Lo-TEN-sin*
*Generic name: Benazepril hydrochloride*

**Why is this drug prescribed?**
Lotensin is used in the treatment of high blood pressure. It is effective when used alone or in com-

bination with thiazide diuretics. Lotensin is in a family of drugs called ACE (angiotensin-converting enzyme) inhibitors. It works by preventing a chemical in your blood called angiotensin I from converting into a more potent form that increases salt and water retention in your body. Lotensin also enhances blood flow throughout your blood vessels.

## Most important fact about this drug

You must take Lotensin regularly for it to be effective. Since blood pressure declines gradually, it may be several weeks before you get the full benefit of Lotensin; and you must continue taking it even if you are feeling well. Lotensin does not cure high blood pressure; it merely keeps it under control.

## How should you take this medication?

Lotensin can be taken with or without food. Do not use salt substitutes containing potassium.

Take Lotensin exactly as prescribed. Suddenly stopping Lotensin could cause your blood pressure to increase.

■ *If you miss a dose...*
Take the forgotten dose as soon as you remember. If it is almost time for the next dose, skip the one you missed and go back to your regular schedule. Never try to "catch up" by doubling the dose.

■ *Storage instructions...*
Store at room temperature in a tightly closed container. Protect from light.

## What side effects may occur?

Side effects cannot be anticipated. If any develop or change in intensity, inform your doctor as soon as possible. Only your doctor can determine if it is safe for you to continue taking Lotensin.

■ *More common side effects may include:*
Cough, dizziness, fatigue, headache, high potassium levels (dry mouth, excessive thirst, weak or irregular heartbeat, muscle pain or cramps), nausea

If you develop swelling of your face, around the lips, tongue, or throat; swelling of arms and legs; sore throat, fever, and chills; or difficulty swallowing, you should contact your doctor immediately. You may need emergency treatment.

■ *Less common or rare side effects may include:*
Allergic reactions, anxiety, arthritis, asthma, bronchitis, chest pain, constipation, dark tarry stool containing blood, decreased sex drive, difficulty sleeping, dizziness when standing, fainting, fluid retention, flushing, impotence, infection, inflammation of the skin, inflammation of the stomach or pancreas, itching, joint pain, low blood pressure, muscle pain, nervousness, pounding heartbeat, rash, sensitivity to light, shortness of breath, sinus inflammation, sweating, swelling of arms, legs, face, tingling or pins and needles, urinary infections, vomiting, weakness

## Why should this drug not be prescribed?

If you are sensitive to or have ever had an allergic reaction to Lotensin or other angiotensin-converting enzyme (ACE) inhibitors, do not take this medication.

## Special warnings about this medication

Your kidney function should be assessed when you start taking Lotensin and then monitored for the first few weeks. If you are on kidney dialysis, your doctor may need to use a different medication.

Lotensin can cause low blood pressure, especially if you are also taking a diuretic. You may feel light-headed or faint, especially during the first few days of therapy. If these symptoms occur, contact your doctor. Your dosage may need to be adjusted or discontinued.

If you have congestive heart failure, this drug should be used with caution.

Do not use potassium supplements or salt substitutes containing potassium without talking to your doctor first.

If you develop a sore throat or fever, you should contact your doctor immediately. It could indicate a more serious illness.

Excessive sweating, dehydration, severe diarrhea, or vomiting could make you lose too much water, causing your blood pressure to become too low.

## Possible food and drug interactions when taking this medication

If Lotensin is taken with certain other drugs, the effects of either could be increased, decreased, or altered. It is especially important to check with your doctor before combining Lotensin with the following:

Diuretics such as Lasix and HydroDIURIL
Lithium (Lithonate)
Potassium supplements such as Slow-K
Potassium-sparing diuretics such as Moduretic and
   Dyazide

## Special information
## if you are pregnant or breastfeeding

Lotensin can cause injury or death to developing and newborn babies, especially if taken during the second and third trimesters of pregnancy. If you are pregnant or plan to become pregnant and are taking Lotensin, contact your doctor immediately to discuss the potential hazard to your unborn child. Minimal amounts of Lotensin appear in breast milk. If this medication is essential to your health, your doctor may advise you to discontinue breastfeeding until your treatment with this medication is finished.

## Recommended dosage
### ADULTS

For people not taking a diuretic drug, the usual starting dose is 10 milligrams, once a day. Regular total dosages range from 20 to 40 milligrams per day taken in either a single dose or divided into 2 equal doses. The maximum dose is 80 milligrams per day. Your doctor will closely monitor the effect of this drug and adjust it according to your individual needs.

For people already taking a diuretic, the diuretic should be stopped, if possible, 2 to 3 days before taking Lotensin. This reduces the possibility of fainting or light-headedness. If blood pressure cannot be controlled by Lotensin alone, then diuretic use should begin again. If the diuretic cannot be discontinued, the starting dosage of Lotensin should be 5 milligrams.

For people with reduced kidney function, the dosages should be individualized according to the amount of reduced function. The usual starting dose in these instances is 5 milligrams per day, adjusted upwards to a maximum of 40 milligrams per day. If you are on kidney dialysis, your doctor may need to use a different medication.

### CHILDREN

The safety and effectiveness of Lotensin have not been established in children.

## Overdosage

Although there is no specific information available, a sudden drop in blood pressure would most likely be the primary symptom of Lotensin overdose. If you suspect a Lotensin overdose, seek medical attention immediately.

*Brand name:*

# Lotrel

*Pronounced: LOW-trel*
*Generic names: Amlodipine and Benazepril*
   *Hydrochloride*

## Why is this drug prescribed?

Lotrel is used in the treatment of high blood pressure. It is a combination medicine that is used when treatment with a single drug has not been successful or has caused side effects.

One component, amlodipine, is a calcium channel blocker. It eases the workload of the heart by slowing down the passage of nerve impulses and hence the contractions of the heart muscle. This improves blood flow through the heart and throughout the body and reduces blood pressure. The other component, benazepril, is an angiotensin-converting enzyme (ACE) inhibitor. It works by preventing the transformation of a hormone called angiotensin I into a more potent substance that increases salt and water retention in your body.

## Most important fact about this drug

You must take Lotrel regularly for it to be effective. Since blood pressure declines gradually, it may take 1 to 2 weeks for the full effect of Lotrel to be seen. Even if you are feeling well, you must continue to take the medication. Lotrel does not cure high blood pressure; it merely keeps it under control.

## How should you take this medication?

Take Lotrel exactly as prescribed by your doctor. Try to take your medication at the same time each day, such as before or after breakfast, so that it is easier to remember.

■ *If you miss a dose...*
   Take it as soon as you remember. However, if it is almost time for your next dose, skip the one you missed and go back to your regular schedule. Do not take 2 doses at once.

■ *Storage instructions...*
   Store at room temperature. Store away from moisture and light; avoid excessive heat.

## What side effects may occur?

Side effects cannot be anticipated. If any develop or change in intensity, tell your doctor as soon as possible. Only your doctor can determine if it is safe for you to continue taking Lotrel.

■ *More common side effects may include:*
   cough

If you develop swelling of your face, around the lips, tongue, or throat; swelling of arms and legs; or difficulty swallowing, you should contact your doctor immediately. You may need emergency treatment.

■ *Less common side effects may include:*
   Abdominal pain, anxiety, back pain, bloating and gas, constipation, cramps, decreased sex drive, diarrhea, dizziness, dry mouth, excessive urination, fluid retention and swelling, flushing, headache, hot flashes, impotence, insomnia, muscle and bone pain, muscle cramps, nausea, nervousness, rash, skin disorders, sore throat, tremor, weakness and fatigue
■ *Rare side effects may include:*
   Anemia, heart attack, pancreatitis (inflammation of the pancreas) worsening of angina pectoris (crushing chest pain)

### Why should this drug not be prescribed?

If you are sensitive to or have ever had an allergic reaction to amlodipine, benazepril, or any angiotensin-converting enzyme (ACE) inhibitors, do not take this medication.

### Special warnings about this medication

Your kidney function should be assessed when you start taking Lotrel, then monitored for the first few weeks.

   Lotrel can cause low blood pressure, especially if you are taking high doses of diuretics. You may feel light-headed or faint, especially during the first few days of therapy. If these symptoms occur, contact your doctor. Your dosage may need to be adjusted or discontinued.

   If you have congestive heart failure, use this drug with caution. If you have kidney disease or severe liver disease, diabetes, lupus erythematosus, or scleroderma (a rare disease affecting the blood vessels or connective tissue), use Lotrel with caution.

   Excessive sweating, severe diarrhea, or vomiting could make you lose too much water, causing a severe drop in blood pressure. If you notice a yellow coloring to your skin or the whites of your eyes, stop taking the drug and notify your doctor immediately. You could be developing liver problems.

If you develop a persistent, dry cough, tell your doctor. It may be due to the medication and, if so, will disappear if you stop taking Lotrel. In a medical emergency and before you have surgery, notify your doctor or dentist that you are taking Lotrel.

### Possible food and drug interactions when taking this medication

If Lotrel is taken with certain other drugs, the effects of either could be increased, decreased, or altered. It is especially important to check with your doctor before combining Lotrel with the following:

Diuretics such as Diuril, Lasix, Hydrodiuril
Lithium (Eskalith, Lithobid)
Potassium supplements (Slow-K)
Potassium-sparing diuretics (Aldactazide,
   Moduretic, Maxzide)

### Special information if you are pregnant or breastfeeding

Lotrel can cause injury or death to developing and newborn babies, especially if taken during the second and third trimesters of pregnancy. If you are pregnant and are taking Lotrel, contact your doctor immediately to discuss the potential hazard to your unborn child. Minimal amounts of benazepril appear in breast milk. If this medication is essential to your health, your doctor may advise you to discontinue breastfeeding while you are taking Lotrel.

### Recommended dosage

ADULTS

Your doctor will closely monitor the effects of this drug and adjust the dosage according to your blood pressure response. For small, older, frail, or liver-impaired individuals, the usual starting dose is a capsule containing 2.5 milligrams amlodipine and 10 milligrams benazepril.

CHILDREN

Safety and effectiveness in children have not been established.

### Overdosage

Any medication taken in excess can have serious consequences. Although there is no specific information available, a sudden drop in blood pressure and rapid heartbeat would be the primary symptoms of a Lotrel overdose. If you suspect an overdose, seek medical attention immediately.

*Brand name:*

# Lotrimin

*See Gyne-Lotrimin, page 232.*

*Brand name:*

# Lotrisone

*Pronounced: LOE-trih-sone*
*Generic ingredients: Clotrimazole, Betamethasone*
*dipropionate*

### Why is this drug prescribed?

Lotrisone, a combination of a steroid (betamethasone) and an antifungal drug (clotrimazole), is used to treat skin infections caused by fungus, such as athlete's foot, jock itch, and ringworm of the body.

Betamethasone treats symptoms (such as itching, redness, swelling, and inflammation) that result from fungus infections, while clotrimazole treats the cause of the infection by inhibiting the growth of certain yeast and fungus organisms.

### Most important fact about this drug

When you use Lotrisone, you inevitably absorb some of the medication through your skin and into the bloodstream. Too much absorption can lead to unwanted side effects elsewhere in the body. To keep this problem to a minimum, avoid using large amounts of Lotrisone over wide areas, and do not cover it with airtight dressings such as plastic wrap or adhesive bandage unless specifically told to by your doctor.

### How should you use this medication?

Wash your hands before and after applying Lotrisone. Gently massage it into the affected area and surrounding skin twice a day, in the morning and evening. Do not get it in your eyes.

Use Lotrisone for the full time prescribed, even if your condition has improved.

Lotrisone should be applied sparingly to the groin area, and it should not be used for longer than 2 weeks. Wear loose-fitting clothing.

■ *If you miss a dose...*
Apply it as soon as you remember. If it is almost time for your next dose, skip the one you missed and go back to your regular schedule.
■ *Storage instructions...*
Store at room temperature.

### What side effects may occur?

Side effects cannot be anticipated. If any develop or change in intensity, inform your doctor as soon as possible. Only your doctor can determine if it is safe for you to continue using Lotrisone.

■ *More common side effects may include:*
Blistering, hives, infection, irritated skin, itching, peeling, reddened skin, skin eruptions and rash, stinging, swelling due to fluid retention, tingling sensation
■ *Less common side effects may include:*
Acne, burning, dryness, excessive hair growth, inflamed hair follicles, inflamed skin, irritated skin around mouth, loss of skin color, softening of the skin, streaks in the skin

### Why should this drug not be prescribed?

You should not use Lotrisone if you are sensitive to clotrimazole or betamethasone or any of its other ingredients, or to similar steroid and antifungal medications.

### Special warnings about this medication

Steroid drugs (such as betamethasone) can affect the functioning of the adrenal, hypothalamic, and pituitary glands and temporarily produce sugar in the urine, excessive blood sugar levels, and a disorder called Cushing's syndrome. Symptoms of Cushing's syndrome include easily bruised skin, increased blood pressure, low potassium levels, low sex hormone levels, mood swings, water retention, weak muscles, and weight gain.

Do not take Lotrisone internally and be sure to keep it away from your eyes.

If you are using Lotrisone to treat jock itch (tinea cruris) or a fungal infection of the skin, called tinea corporis, and there has been no improvement after 1 week, notify your doctor.

If you are using Lotrisone to treat athlete's foot (tinea pedis), notify your doctor if there is no improvement after 2 weeks of treatment.

Do not use Lotrisone for any condition other than the one for which it was prescribed, and do not use it for longer than 4 weeks.

Lotrisone is not for use on diaper rash.

### Possible food and drug interactions when taking this medication

No interactions have been reported.

## Special information
## if you are pregnant or breastfeeding

Pregnant women should not use steroid drugs in large amounts or for prolonged periods of time. The effects of Lotrisone during pregnancy have not been adequately studied. The medication should be used during pregnancy only if the potential benefits justify the potential risk to the developing baby. It is not known whether Lotrisone appears in breast milk. Nursing mothers should use Lotrisone with caution and only when clearly needed.

## Recommended dosage

ADULTS AND CHILDREN OVER 12 YEARS OLD

*"Jock Itch" (Tinea Cruris) or Fungal Skin Infections (Tinea Corporis)*

Gently massage Lotrisone into the affected and surrounding skin areas twice a day, in the morning and the evening, for 2 weeks. Lotrisone should be applied sparingly to the groin area. Notify your doctor if there has been no improvement after 1 week of treatment.

*Athlete's Foot (Tinea Pedis)*

Gently massage Lotrisone into the affected and surrounding skin areas twice a day, in the morning and the evening, for 4 weeks. Notify your doctor if there has been no improvement after 2 weeks of treatment.

CHILDREN

The safety and effectiveness of Lotrisone have not been established for children under 12 years of age. Children may absorb proportionally larger amounts of topical Lotrisone and be more sensitive to its effects than are adults.

## Overdosage

Any medication used in excess can have serious consequences. A serious overdose of Lotrisone, which is applied to the skin, is unlikely. However, seek medical help immediately if you suspect an overdose.

*Generic name:*

# Lovastatin

See Mevacor, page 318.

*Brand name:*

# Lozol

*Pronounced: LOW-zoll*
*Generic name: Indapamide*

## Why is this drug prescribed?

Lozol is used in the treatment of high blood pressure, either alone or in combination with other high blood pressure medications. Lozol is also used to relieve salt and fluid retention. During pregnancy, your doctor may prescribe Lozol to relieve fluid retention caused by a specific condition or when fluid retention causes extreme discomfort that is not relieved by rest.

## Most important fact about this drug

If you have high blood pressure, you must take Lozol regularly for it to be effective. Since blood pressure declines gradually, it may be several weeks before you get the full benefit of Lozol; and you must continue taking it even if you are feeling well. Lozol does not cure high blood pressure; it merely keeps it under control.

## How should you take this medication?

Take Lozol exactly as prescribed by your doctor. Suddenly stopping Lozol could cause your condition to worsen.

Lozol is best taken in the morning.

■ *If you miss a dose...*
Take the forgotten dose as soon as you remember. If it is almost time for your next dose, skip the one you missed and go back to your regular schedule. Never take two doses at the same time.

■ *Storage instructions...*
Store Lozol at room temperature. Protect from excessive heat. Keep the container tightly closed.

## What side effects may occur?

Side effects cannot be anticipated. If any side effects develop or change in intensity, tell your doctor immediately. Only your doctor can determine whether it is safe to continue taking Lozol. Most side effects are mild and temporary.

■ *More common side effects may include:*
Agitation, anxiety, back pain, dizziness, headache, infection, irritability, muscle cramps or spasms, nasal inflammation, nervousness, numbness in hands and feet, pain, tension, weakness, fatigue, loss of energy or tiredness

■ *Less common or rare side effects may include:*
Abdominal pain or cramps, blurred vision, chest pain, conjunctivitis, constipation, cough, depression, diarrhea, dizziness when standing up too quickly, drowsiness, dry mouth, excessive urination at night, fluid retention, flu-like symptoms, flushing, fluttering heartbeat, frequent urination, hives, impotence or reduced sex drive, indigestion, insomnia, irregular heartbeat, itching, lightheadedness, loss of appetite, nausea, nervousness, premature heart contractions, production of large amounts of pale urine, rash, runny nose, sore throat, stomach irritation, tingling in hands and feet, vertigo, vomiting, weakness, weak or irregular heartbeat, weight loss

### Why should this drug not be prescribed?
Avoid using Lozol if you are unable to urinate or if you have ever had an allergic reaction or are sensitive to indapamide or other sulfa-containing drugs.

### Special warnings about this medication
Diuretics such as Lozol can cause the body to lose too much salt and potassium, especially among elderly women. Signs of an excessively low potassium level include muscle weakness and rapid or irregular heartbeat. To boost your potassium level, your doctor may recommend eating potassium-rich foods or taking a potassium supplement.

The risk of potassium loss increases when larger doses are used, if you have cirrhosis, or if you are also using corticosteroids or ACTH. Your doctor should check your blood regularly, especially if you have an irregular heartbeat or are taking heart medications.

Lozol should be used with care if you have gout or high uric acid levels, liver disease, diabetes, or lupus erythematosus, a disease of the connective tissue.

This medication should be used with caution if you have severe kidney disease. Your kidney function should be given a complete assessment and should continue to be monitored.

In general, diuretics should not be taken if you are taking lithium, as they increase the risk of lithium poisoning.

### Possible food and drug interactions when taking this medication
If Lozol is taken with certain other drugs, the effects of either could be increased, decreased, or altered. It is especially important to check with your doctor before combining Lozol with the following:

Lithium (Eskalith)
Norepinephrine (a drug used to treat cardiac arrest and to maintain blood pressure)
Other high blood pressure medications such as Aldomet and Tenormin

### Special information
### if you are pregnant or breastfeeding
If you are pregnant or plan to become pregnant, tell your doctor immediately. No information is available about the safety of Lozol during pregnancy.

Lozol may appear in breast milk and could affect a nursing infant. If Lozol is essential to your health, your doctor may advise you to stop breast-feeding until your treatment is finished.

### Recommended dosage
ADULTS

*High Blood Pressure*
The usual starting dose is 1.25 milligrams as a single daily dose taken in the morning. If Lozol does not seem to be working for you, your doctor may gradually increase your dosage up to 5 milligrams taken once a day.

*Fluid Buildup in Congestive Heart Failure*
The usual starting dose is 2.5 milligrams as a single daily dose taken in the morning. Your doctor may increase your dosage to 5 milligrams taken once daily.

### Overdosage
Any medication taken in excess can have serious consequences. If you suspect an overdose, seek medical treatment immediately.

■ *Symptoms of Lozol overdose may include:*
Electrolyte imbalance (potassium or salt depletion due to too much fluid loss), nausea, stomach disorders, vomiting, weakness

*Brand name:*

# Luride

*Pronounced: LUHR-ide*
*Generic name: Sodium fluoride*

### Why is this drug prescribed?
Luride is prescribed to strengthen children's teeth against decay during the period when the teeth are still developing.

Studies have shown that children who live where the drinking water contains a certain level of fluoride have fewer cavities than others. Fluoride helps prevent cavities in three ways: by increasing the teeth's resistance to dissolving on contact with acid, by strengthening teeth, and by slowing down the growth of mouth bacteria.

Luride may be given to children who live where the water fluoride level is 0.6 parts per million or less.

### Most important fact about this drug

Before Luride is prescribed, it is important for the doctor to know the fluoride content of the water your child drinks every day. Your water company, or a private laboratory, can tell you the level of fluoride in your water.

### How should you take this medication?

Give your child Luride exactly as prescribed by your doctor. It is preferable to give the tablet at bedtime after the child's teeth have been brushed. The youngster may chew and swallow the tablet or simply suck on it until it dissolves. The liquid form of this medicine is to be taken by mouth. It may be dropped directly into the mouth or mixed with water or fruit juice. Always store Luride drops in the original plastic dropper bottle.

■ *If you miss a dose...*
Take it as soon as you remember. If it is almost time for your next dose, skip the one you missed and go back to your regular schedule. Do not take 2 doses at once.

■ *Storage instructions...*
Store away from heat, light, and moisture. Keep the liquid from freezing.

### What side effects may occur?

Side effects cannot be anticipated. If any develop, tell your doctor immediately. Only your doctor can determine whether it is safe for your child to continue taking Luride.

In rare cases, Luride may cause an allergic rash or some other unexpected effect.

### Why should this drug not be prescribed?

Your child should not take Luride if he or she is sensitive to it or has had an allergic reaction to Sodium Fluoride in the past.

Your child should not take the 1-milligram strength of Luride if the drinking water in your area contains 0.3 parts per million of fluoride or more. He or she should not take the other forms of Luride if the water contains 0.6 parts per million of fluoride or more.

### Special warnings about this medication

Do not give full-strength tablets (1 milligram) to children under the age of 6.

### Possible food and drug interactions when taking this medication

Avoid giving your child Luride with dairy products. The calcium in dairy products may interact with the fluoride to create calcium fluoride, which the body cannot absorb well.

### Recommended dosage

Since this drug is used to supplement water with low fluoride content, consult your physician to determine the proper amount based on the local water content. Also check with your doctor if you move to a new area, change to bottled water, or begin using a water-filtering device. Dosages are determined by both age and the fluoride content of the water.

INFANTS AND CHILDREN

The following daily dosages are recommended for areas where the drinking water contains fluoride at less than 0.3 parts per million:

*Children 6 Months to 3 Years of Age*
1 quarter-strength (0.25 milligram) tablet or ½ dropperful of liquid

*3 to 6 Years of Age*
1 half-strength (0.5 milligram) tablet or 1 dropperful of liquid

*6 to 16 Years of Age*
1 full-strength (1 milligram) tablet or 2 droppersful of liquid

For areas where the fluoride content of drinking water is between 0.3 and 0.6 parts per million, the recommended daily dosage of the tablets is one-half the above dosages. Dosage of the liquid should be reduced to ½ dropperful for children ages 3 to 6 and 1 dropperful for children over 6.

### Overdosage

Any medication taken in excess can have serious consequences. Taking too much fluoride for a long period of time may cause discoloration of the teeth. Notify your doctor or dentist if you notice white, brown, or black spots on the teeth.

Brand name:

# Luvox

Pronounced: LOO-voks
Generic name: Fluvoxamine maleate

### Why is this drug prescribed?

Luvox is prescribed for obsessive compulsive behavior. Obsessive behavior may include continual, unwanted thoughts that prevent functioning properly in everyday living. Compulsive behavior is typified by ritualistic actions such as repetitious washing, repeating certain phrases, completing steps in a process over and over, counting and recounting, checking and rechecking to make sure that something has not been forgotten, excessive neatness, and hoarding of useless items.

### Most important fact about this drug

Before starting therapy with Luvox, it is very important to tell your doctor what medications you are taking, either prescription or over-the-counter, since combining Luvox with certain drugs may cause serious or even life-threatening effects. You should never take Luvox with the antihistamines Seldane and Hismanal. You should also avoid taking Luvox within 14 days of taking an antidepressant drug known as an MAO inhibitor, including Nardil and Parnate.

### How should you take this medication?

Take this medication only as directed by your doctor.

Luvox may be taken with or without food.

■ *If you miss a dose...*
If you are taking 1 dose a day, skip the missed dose and go back to your regular schedule. If you are taking 2 doses a day, take the missed dose as soon as possible, then go back to your regular schedule. Never take 2 doses at the same time.

■ *Storage instructions...*
Store at room temperature and protect from humidity.

### What side effects may occur?

Side effects cannot be anticipated. If any develop or change in intensity, tell your doctor immediately.

Only your doctor can determine if it is safe for you to continue taking Luvox.

■ *More common side effects may include:*
Abnormal ejaculation, abnormal tooth decay and toothache, anxiety, blurred vision, constipation, decreased appetite, diarrhea, dizziness, dry mouth, feeling "hot or flushed", "flu-like" symptoms, frequent urination, gas and bloating, headache, heart palpitations, inability to fall asleep, indigestion, nausea, nervousness, sleepiness, sweating, taste alteration, tremor, unusual tiredness or weakness, upper respiratory infection, vomiting

■ *Less common side effects may include:*
Abnormal muscle tone, agitation, chills, decreased sex drive, depression, difficult or labored breathing, difficulty swallowing, extreme excitability, impotence, inability to urinate, lack of orgasm, yawning

### Why should this drug not be prescribed?

If you are sensitive to or have ever had an allergic reaction to Luvox or similar drugs, such as Prozac and Zoloft, do not take this medication. Make sure your doctor is aware of any drug reactions you have experienced.

Never combine Luvox with Seldane or Hismanal, or take it within 14 days of taking an MAO inhibitor such as Nardil or Parnate. (See "Most important fact about this drug.")

### Special warnings about this medication

You should discuss all your medical problems with your doctor before starting therapy with Luvox, as certain physical conditions or diseases may affect your reaction to Luvox.

If you suffer from seizures, use this medication cautiously. If you experience a seizure while taking Luvox, stop taking the drug and call your doctor immediately.

If you have or have ever had suicidal thoughts, be sure to tell your doctor, as your dosage may need to be adjusted.

If you have a history of mania (excessively energetic, out-of-control behavior), use this medication cautiously.

If you have liver disease, your doctor will adjust the dosage.

Luvox may cause you to become drowsy or less alert and may affect your judgment. Therefore, avoid driving, operating dangerous machinery, or participating in any hazardous activity that requires full mental alertness until you know your reaction to this medication.

If you develop a rash or hives, or any other allergic-type reaction, notify your physician immediately.

## Possible food and drug interactions when taking this medication

Do not drink alcohol while taking this medication. If you smoke, be sure to tell your doctor before starting Luvox therapy, as your dosage may need adjustment.

If Luvox is taken with certain other drugs, the effects of either could be increased, decreased, or altered. It is especially important to check with your doctor before combining Luvox with the following:

Anticoagulant drugs such as Coumadin
Antidepressant medications such as Anafranil, Elavil, and Tofranil, as well as the MAO inhibitors Nardil and Parnate
Blood pressure medications known as beta blockers, including Inderal and Lopressor
Carbamazepine (Tegretol)
Clozapine (Clozaril)
Diazepam (Valium)
Diltiazem (Cardizem)
Lithium (Lithonate)
Methadone (Dolophine)
Phenytoin (Dilantin)
Theophylline (Theo-Dur)
Tranquilizers and sedatives such as Halcion, Valium, Versed, and Xanax
Tryptophan

## Special information if you are pregnant or breastfeeding

The effects of Luvox in pregnancy have not been adequately studied. If you are pregnant or plan to become pregnant, consult your doctor immediately. Luvox passes into breast milk and may cause serious reactions in a nursing baby. If this medication is essential your health, your doctor may advise you to discontinue breastfeeding until your treatment with Luvox is finished.

## Recommended dosage

ADULTS

The usual starting dose is one 50-milligram tablet taken at bedtime.

Your doctor may increase your dose, depending upon your response. The maximum daily dose is 300 milligrams. If you take more than 100 milligrams a day, your doctor will divide the total amount into 2 doses; if the doses are not equal, you should take the larger dose at bedtime.

CHILDREN

The safety and effectiveness of Luvox have not been established in children under age 18.

## Overdosage

Any medication taken in excess can have serious consequences. If you suspect an overdose, seek medical attention immediately.

■ *Symptoms of Luvox overdose may include:*
Breathing difficulties, changes in pulse rate, coma, convulsions, diarrhea, dizziness, drowsiness, low blood pressure, liver problems, vomiting

*Brand name:*

# Maalox

*See Antacids, page 30.*

*Brand name:*

# Macrobid

*See Macrodantin, page 305.*

*Brand name:*

# Macrodantin

*Pronounced: Mack-row-DAN-tin*
*Generic name: Nitrofurantoin*
*Other brand name: Macrobid*

## Why is this drug prescribed?

Nitrofurantoin, an antibacterial drug, is prescribed for the treatment of urinary tract infections caused by certain strains of bacteria.

## Most important fact about this drug

Breathing disorders have occurred in people taking nitrofurantoin. The drug can cause inflammation of the lungs characterized by coughing, difficulty breathing, and wheezing. Pulmonary fibrosis (an abnormal increase in fibrous tissue of the lungs) can develop gradually without symptoms and can cause death. An allergic reaction to this drug is also possible and may occur without warning. Symptoms include a feeling of ill health and a persistent cough. However, these reactions occur rarely and generally in those receiving nitrofurantoin therapy for 6 months or longer.

Sudden and severe lung reactions are characterized by fever, chills, cough, chest pain, and difficulty breathing. These acute reactions usually occur within the first week of treatment and subside when therapy with nitrofurantoin is stopped.

Your doctor should monitor your condition closely, especially if you are receiving long-term treatment with this medication.

### How should you take this medication?
To improve absorption of the drug, nitrofurantoin should be taken with food.

Follow your doctor's instructions carefully. Take the full amount prescribed, even if you are feeling better.

This medication works better if your urine is acidic. Ask your doctor whether you should be taking special measures to assure its acidity.

Nitrofurantoin may turn the urine brown.

■ *If you miss a dose...*
Take the forgotten dose as soon as you remember, then space out the rest of the day's doses at equal intervals.
■ *Storage instructions...*
Store at room temperature. Protect from light and keep the container tightly closed.

### What side effects may occur?
Side effects cannot be anticipated. If any develop or change in intensity, inform your doctor as soon as possible. Only your doctor can determine if it is safe for you to continue taking nitrofurantoin.

■ *More common side effects may include:*
Lack or loss of appetite, nausea, vomiting
■ *Less common or rare side effects may include:*
Abdominal pain/discomfort, blue skin, chills, confusion, cough, chest pain, depression, diarrhea, difficulty breathing, dizziness, drowsiness, exaggerated sense of well-being, eye disorder, fever, hair loss, headache, hepatitis, hives, inflammation of the nerves causing symptoms of numbness, tingling, pain, or muscle weakness, intestinal inflammation, involuntary eye movement, irregular heartbeat, itching, itchy red skin

patches, joint pain, muscle pain, peeling skin, psychotic reactions, rash, severe allergic reactions, skin inflammation with flaking, skin swelling or welts, vertigo, yellowing of the skin and whites of the eyes, weakness

### Why should this drug not be prescribed?
If you are sensitive to or have ever had an allergic reaction to nitrofurantoin or other drugs of this type, such as Furoxone, you should not take this medication. Make sure that your doctor is aware of any drug reactions that you have experienced.

Unless you are directed to do so by your doctor, do not take this medication if your kidneys are not functioning properly, if they are unable to produce urine, or if they produce only a small amount.

Nitrofurantoin should not be taken at term of pregnancy or during labor and delivery; it should not be given to infants under 1 month of age.

### Special warnings about this medication
Tell your doctor if you have any unusual symptoms while you are taking this drug.

Fatalities have been reported from hepatitis (liver disease) during treatment with nitrofurantoin. Long-lasting, active hepatitis can occur without symptoms; therefore, if you are receiving long-term treatment with this drug, your doctor should check you periodically for changes in liver function.

Fatalities from peripheral neuropathy—disease of the nerves—have been reported in people taking nitrofurantoin.

If you have a kidney disorder, anemia, diabetes mellitus, a debilitating disease, or a vitamin B deficiency, caution should be exercised when taking this medication. These conditions make peripheral neuropathy more likely. Consult your doctor.

If you experience diarrhea, tell your doctor. It may be a sign of serious intestinal inflammation.

Hemolytic anemia (below-normal hemoglobin content in the blood caused by the destruction of red blood cells) has occurred in people taking nitrofurantoin.

Continued or prolonged use of this drug may result in growth of bacteria that do not respond to it. This can cause a secondary infection, so it is important that your doctor monitor your condition on a regular basis.

## Possible food and drug interactions when taking this medication

If nitrofurantoin is taken with certain other drugs, the effects of either could be increased, decreased, or altered. It is especially important to check with your doctor before combining nitrofurantoin with the following:

Magnesium trisilicate (Gaviscon Antacid Tablets)
Uricosuric drugs (medications that increase the amount of the uric acid eliminated in the urine), such as the antigout drugs Benemid and Anturane

## Special information if you are pregnant or breastfeeding

The safety of nitrofurantoin during pregnancy and breastfeeding has not been established. Nitrofurantoin does appear in human breast milk. If you are pregnant or breastfeeding or you plan to become pregnant or breastfeed, inform your doctor immediately.

## Recommended dosage

Treatment with nitrofurantoin should be continued for 1 week or for at least 3 days after obtaining a urine specimen free of infection. If your infection has not cleared up, your doctor should re-evaluate your case.

ADULTS

The recommended dosage of Macrodantin is 50 to 100 milligrams taken 4 times a day. For long-term treatment, your doctor may reduce your dosage to 50 to 100 milligrams taken at bedtime.

The recommended dosage of Macrobid is one 100 milligram capsule every 12 hours for 7 days.

CHILDREN

This medication should not be prescribed for children under 1 month of age.

The recommended daily dosage of Macrodantin for infants and children over 1 month of age is 5 to 7 milligrams per 2.2 pounds of body weight, divided into 4 doses over 24 hours.

For the long-term treatment of children, the doctor may prescribe daily doses as low as 1 milligram per 2.2 pounds of body weight taken in 1 or 2 doses per day.

The dosage of Macrobid for children over 12 years of age is one 100 milligram capsule every 12 hours for 7 days. Safety and effectiveness have not been established for children under 12.

## Overdosage

An overdose of nitrofurantoin has not resulted in any specific symptoms other than vomiting. If vomiting does not occur soon after an excessive dose, it should be induced.

If you suspect an overdose, seek emergency medical treatment immediately.

*Brand name:*

# Materna

*See Stuartnatal Plus, page 511.*

*Brand name:*

# Maxaquin

*Pronounced: MAX-ah-kwin*
*Generic name: Lomefloxacin hydrochloride*

## Why is this drug prescribed?

Maxaquin is a quinolone antibiotic used to treat lower respiratory infections, including chronic bronchitis, and urinary tract infections, including cystitis (inflammation of the inner lining of the bladder). Maxaquin is also given before bladder surgery to prevent the infections that sometimes follow this operation.

## Most important fact about this drug

During and following treatment, Maxaquin causes sensitivity reactions in people exposed to sunlight or sunlamps. The reactions can occur despite use of sunscreens and sunblocks, and can be prompted by shaded or diffused light or exposure through glass. Avoid even indirect sunlight while taking Maxaquin and for several days following therapy.

## How should you take this medication?

It is important to finish your prescription of Maxaquin completely. If you stop taking your medication too soon, your symptoms may return.

Maxaquin may be taken with or without food. Take it with a full 8-ounce glass of water; and be sure to drink plenty of fluids while on this medication.

You can reduce the risk of a reaction to sunlight by taking Maxaquin in the evening.

■ *If you miss a dose...*
Take it as soon as you remember. If it is almost time for your next dose, skip the one you missed

and go back to your regular schedule. Do not take 2 doses at the same time.

■ *Storage instructions...*
Store at room temperature.

## What side effects may occur?

Side effects cannot be anticipated. If any develop or change in intensity, tell your doctor as soon as possible. Only your doctor can determine if it is safe for you to continue taking Maxaquin.

■ *More common side effects may include:*
Headache, nausea
■ *Less common side effects may include:*
Diarrhea, dizziness, sensitivity to light
■ *Rare side effects may include:*
Abdominal pain, abnormal or terrifying dreams, abnormal vision, agitation, allergic reaction, altered taste, angina pectoris (crushing chest pain), anxiety, back pain, bleeding between menstrual periods, bleeding in the stomach and intestines, blood clots in the lungs, blood in the urine, blue skin color, chest pain, chills, coma, confusion, conjunctivitis (pinkeye), constipation, convulsions, cough, decreased heat tolerance, depression, difficult or labored breathing, difficulty swallowing, dry mouth, earache, eye pain, facial swelling, fainting, fatigue, fluid retention and swelling, flu-like symptoms, flushing, gas, general feeling of illness, gout, harsh, high-pitched sound during breathing, heart attack, heart failure, high blood pressure, hives, inability to sleep, increased appetite, increased mucus from the lungs, increased sweating, indigestion, inflammation in the male genital area, inflammation of the stomach and intestines, inflammation of the vagina, irregular heartbeat, itching, joint pain, lack of urine, leg cramps, loss of appetite, loss of sense of identity, low blood pressure, low blood sugar, lung infection or other problems, muscle pain, nervousness, nosebleed, overactivity, pain in the genital-rectal area, problems with urination, purple or red spots on the skin, rapid heartbeat, rash, ringing in the ears, skin disorders, skin eruptions or peeling, sleepiness, slow heartbeat, thirst, tingling or a "pins and needles" feeling, tongue discoloration, tremor, vaginal yeast infection, vertigo, vomiting, weakness, wheezing, white or yellow vaginal discharge

## Why should this drug not be prescribed?

If you are sensitive to or have ever had an allergic reaction to Maxaquin or other quinolone antibiotics such as Cipro and Floxin, you should not take this medication. Make sure your doctor is aware of any drug reactions you have experienced.

## Special warnings about this medication

Use Maxaquin cautiously if you have disorders such as epilepsy, severe hardening of the arteries in the brain, and other conditions that can lead to seizures. Maxaquin may cause convulsions.

In rare cases, people taking antibiotics similar to Maxaquin have experienced severe, even fatal reactions, sometimes after only one dose. These reactions may include confusion, convulsions, difficulty breathing, hallucinations, hives, itching, light-headedness, loss of consciousness, rash, restlessness, swelling in the face or throat, tingling, and tremors. If you develop any of these symptoms, stop taking Maxaquin immediately and seek medical help.

If other antibiotics have given you diarrhea, or it develops while you are taking Maxaquin, be sure to tell your doctor. Maxaquin may cause inflammation of the bowel, ranging from mild to life-threatening.

Maxaquin may cause dizziness or light-headedness and may impair your ability to drive a car or operate potentially dangerous machinery. Do not participate in any activities that require full alertness until you know how Maxaquin affects you.

## Possible food and drug interactions when taking this medication

If Maxaquin is taken with certain other drugs, the effects of either could be increased, decreased, or altered. It is especially important to check with your doctor before combining Maxaquin with the following:

Antacids containing magnesium or aluminum, such as Maalox or Gaviscon
Caffeine (including coffee, tea, and some soft drinks)
Cimetidine (Tagamet)
Cyclosporine (Sandimmune and Neoral)
Probenecid (Benemid)
Sucralfate (Carafate)
Theophylline (Theo-Dur)
Warfarin (Coumadin)
Vitamins or products containing iron or zinc

## Special information
## if you are pregnant or breastfeeding

The effects of Maxaquin in pregnancy have not been adequately studied. If you are pregnant or plan to become pregnant, notify your doctor immediately. It is not known if Maxaquin appears in breast milk. Because many drugs do make their way into breast milk, your doctor may have you stop nursing while you are taking Maxaquin.

## Recommended dosage

ADULTS

*Chronic Bronchitis*

The usual dosage is 400 milligrams once a day for 10 days.

*Cystitis*

The usual dosage is 400 milligrams once a day for 10 days.

*Complicated Urinary Tract Infections*

The dosage is 400 milligrams once a day for 14 days.

*People With Impaired Renal Function or Cirrhosis*

Your doctor will adjust the dosage according to your needs.

*People on Dialysis*

The recommended dosage for people on dialysis is 400 milligrams, followed by daily maintenance doses of 200 milligrams (one half tablet) once a day for the duration of treatment.

CHILDREN

Safety and efficacy have not been established for children under the age of 18.

## Overdosage

There is no information on overdosage with Maxaquin. However, any medication taken in excess can have serious consequences. If you suspect an overdose, seek medical help immediately.

*Brand name:*

# Maxzide

*Pronounced: MAX-ide*
*Generic ingredients: Triamterene,*
  *Hydrochlorothiazide*

## Why is this drug prescribed?

Maxzide is a diuretic combination used in the treatment of high blood pressure or other conditions that require the elimination of excess fluid (water) from the body. When used for high blood pressure, Maxzide can be used alone or with other high blood pressure medications. Diuretics help your body produce and eliminate more urine, which helps lower blood pressure. Triamterene, one of the ingredients, helps to minimize potassium loss, which can be caused by the other component, hydrochlorothiazide.

## Most important fact about this drug

If you have high blood pressure, you must take Maxzide regularly for it to be effective. Since blood pressure declines gradually, it may be several weeks before you get the full benefit of Maxzide; and you must continue taking it even if you are feeling well. Maxzide does not cure high blood pressure; it merely keeps it under control.

## How should you take this medication?

Take Maxzide exactly as prescribed. Stopping Maxzide suddenly could cause your condition to worsen.

■ *If you miss a dose...*
  Take it as soon as you remember. If it is almost time for the next dose, skip the one you missed and go back to your regular schedule. Do not take 2 doses at the same time.
■ *Storage instructions...*
  Store at room temperature in a tightly closed container away from light.

## What side effects may occur?

Side effects cannot be anticipated. If any develop or change in intensity, inform your doctor as soon as possible. Only your doctor can determine if it is safe for you to continue taking Maxzide.

■ *Side effects may include:*
  Abdominal cramps, anemia, anxiety, change in potassium levels (causing such symptoms as dry mouth, excessive thirst, weak or irregular heartbeat, muscle pain or cramps), change in taste, chest pain, constipation, decreased sexual performance, depression, diarrhea, difficulty breathing, difficulty sleeping, discolored urine, dizziness, dizziness on standing up, drowsiness, dry mouth, fatigue, fever, headache, hives, hypersensitivity reaction, inflammation of the pancreas, inflammation of the salivary glands, kidney stones, loss of appetite, muscle cramps, muscle weakness,

nausea, rapid heartbeat, rash, reddish or purplish spots on the skin, restlessness, sensitivity to light, shortness of breath, stomach irritation, tingling or pins and needles, vertigo, vision changes, vomiting, yellow eyes and skin

### Why should this drug not be prescribed?

If you are unable to urinate or have any serious kidney disease, if you have high potassium levels in your blood, or if you are taking other drugs that prevent loss of potassium, you should not take this medication.

If you are sensitive to or have ever had an allergic reaction to triamterene, hydrochlorothiazide, or similar drugs, or if you are sensitive to other sulfa drugs, you should not take this medication. Make sure your doctor is aware of any drug reactions you may have experienced.

### Special warnings about this medication

This medication should be used only if your doctor has determined that the precise amount of each ingredient in Maxzide meets your specific needs. It cannot be exchanged with Dyazide, a combination of the same ingredients in different amounts.

If you are taking Maxzide and have kidney disease, your doctor will do a complete assessment of your kidney function and will continue to monitor it.

If you are taking an ACE-inhibitor type of blood pressure medication such as Vasotec, Maxzide should be used with extreme caution.

If you have liver disease, diabetes, gout, or the connective tissue disease, lupus erythematosus, make sure your doctor knows about it. Maxzide should be prescribed with caution.

If you have bronchial asthma or a history of allergies, you may be at greater risk for an allergic reaction to this medication.

Dehydration, excessive sweating, severe diarrhea, or vomiting could deplete your fluids and cause your blood pressure to become too low. Be careful when exercising and in hot weather.

Avoid potassium-containing salt substitutes, potassium supplements, and potassium-enriched diets.

Notify your doctor or dentist that you are taking Maxzide if you have a medical emergency, and before you have surgery.

### Possible food and drug interactions when taking this medication

Maxzide may increase the effects of alcohol. Avoid alcohol while taking this medication.

If Maxzide is taken with certain other drugs, the effects of either could be increased, decreased, or altered. It is especially important to check with your doctor before taking Maxzide with the following:

ACE inhibitors such as Vasotec
Amantadine (Symmetrel)
Barbiturates such as phenobarbital
Beta-blocking blood pressure medications such as Inderal
Cholestyramine (Questran)
Fluconazole (Diflucan)
Indomethacin (Indocin)
Lithium (Lithonate)
Narcotics such as Percocet
Norepinephrine (Levophed)
Oral diabetes drugs such as Micronase
Other diuretics that minimize loss of potassium, such as Midamor
Other high blood pressure medications (Aldomet)
Potassium-containing salt substitutes
Tubocurarine

### Special information if you are pregnant or breastfeeding

The effects of Maxzide during pregnancy have not been adequately studied. If you are pregnant or plan to become pregnant, inform your doctor immediately. Maxzide appears in breast milk and could affect a nursing infant. If this medication is essential to your health, your doctor may advise you to discontinue breastfeeding until your treatment with this medication is finished.

### Recommended dosage

ADULTS

It is important that potassium levels be carefully monitored when you are taking either strength of this medication. Your doctor will adjust your dosage based on your individual condition.

The usual dose of Maxzide-25 MG is 1 or 2 tablets a day in a single dose.

The usual dose of Maxzide is 1 tablet daily.

CHILDREN

The safety and effectiveness of Maxzide have not been established in children.

### Overdosage

Any medication taken in excess can have serious consequences. If you suspect an overdose, seek medical attention immediately.

No specific information is available on Maxzide. However, an overdose of triamterene can cause dehydration, nausea, vomiting, and weakness. An overdose of hydrochlorothiazide can cause dehydration, sluggishness—possibly leading to coma—and stomach and intestinal irritation.

*Generic name:*

# Meclizine

*See Antivert, page 32.*

*Brand name:*

# Medrol

*Pronounced: MED-rohl*
*Generic name: Methylprednisolone*

### Why is this drug prescribed?

Medrol, a corticosteroid drug, is used to reduce inflammation and improve symptoms in a variety of disorders, including rheumatic arthritis, acute gouty arthritis, and severe cases of asthma. Medrol may be given to people to treat primary or secondary adrenal cortex insufficiency (inability of the adrenal gland to produce sufficient hormone). It is also given to help treat the following disorders:

Severe allergic conditions (including drug-induced allergic states)
Blood disorders (leukemia and various anemias)
Certain cancers (along with other drugs)
Skin diseases (including severe psoriasis)
Connective tissue diseases such as systemic lupus erythematosus
Digestive tract diseases such as ulcerative colitis
High serum levels of calcium associated with cancer
Fluid retention due to nephrotic syndrome (a condition in which damage to the kidney causes loss of protein in urine)
Various eye diseases
Lung diseases such as tuberculosis
Worsening of multiple sclerosis

### Most important fact about this drug

Medrol lowers your resistance to infections and can make them harder to treat. Medrol may also mask some of the signs of an infection, making it difficult for your doctor to diagnose the actual problem.

### How should you take this medication?

Take Medrol exactly as prescribed. It can be taken every day or every other day, depending on the condition being treated.

Do not abruptly stop taking Medrol without checking with your doctor. If you have been using Medrol for a long time, the dose should be reduced gradually.

Medrol may cause stomach upset. Take Medrol with meals or snacks.

■ *If you miss a dose...*
If you take your dose once a day, take it as soon as you remember. Then go back to your regular schedule. If you don't remember until the next day, skip the one you missed. Do not take 2 doses at once.

If you take it several times a day, take it as soon as you remember. Then go back to your regular schedule. If you don't remember until your next dose, double the dose you take.

If you take your dose every other day, and you remember it the same morning, take it as soon as you remember and go back to your regular schedule. If you don't remember until the afternoon, do not take it until the following morning, then skip a day and go back to your regular schedule.

■ *Storage instructions...*
Store at room temperature.

### What side effects may occur?

Side effects cannot be anticipated. If any develop or change in intensity, tell your doctor immediately. Only your doctor can determine whether it is safe for you to continue taking Medrol.

■ *Side effects may include:*
Abdominal swelling, allergic reactions, bone fractures, bruising, congestive heart failure, cataracts, convulsions, Cushingoid symptoms (moon face, weight gain, high blood pressure, emotional disturbances, growth of facial hair in women), face redness, fluid and salt retention, headache, high blood pressure, increased eye pressure, increased sweating, increase in amounts of insulin or hypoglycemic medications needed, inflammation of the pancreas, irregular menstruation, muscle wasting and weakness, osteoporosis, poor healing of wounds, protruding eyes,

stomach ulcer, suppression of growth in children, symptoms of diabetes, thin, fragile skin, tiny red or purplish spots on the skin, vertigo

### Why should this drug not be prescribed?
Medrol should not be used if you have a fungal infection or if you are sensitive to or allergic to steroids (corticosteroids).

### Special warnings about this medication
The 24-milligram Medrol tablet contains FD&C Yellow No. 5 (tartrazine), which has caused allergic reactions (including asthma) in some people. Although this is rare, it is more common in people who are sensitive to aspirin.

Medrol can alter the way your body responds to unusual stress. If you are injured, need surgery, or develop an acute illness, inform your doctor. Your dosage may need to be increased.

You should avoid immunization shots with live or live, attenuated vaccines while taking high doses of Medrol, because Medrol can suppress the im-mune system. Immunization with killed or inactivated vaccines is safe, but may have diminished effect.

Long-term use of Medrol may cause cataracts, glaucoma (increased eye pressure), and eye infections.

Large doses of Medrol may cause high blood pressure, salt and water retention, and potassium and calcium loss. It may be necessary to restrict your salt intake and take a potassium supplement.

Medrol may reactivate dormant cases of tuberculosis. If you have inactive tuberculosis and must take Medrol for an extended period of time, your doctor will prescribe anti-TB medication as well.

Medrol should be used cautiously if you have an underactive thyroid, liver cirrhosis, or herpes simplex (virus) infection of the eye.

This medication may aggravate existing emotional problems or cause new ones. You may experience euphoria (an exaggerated sense of well-being) and difficulty sleeping, mood swings, or mental problems. If you have any changes in mood, contact your doctor.

People taking corticosteroids, such as Medrol, have developed Kaposi's sarcoma, a form of cancer.

Medrol should also be taken with caution if you have any of the following conditions:

Diverticulitis or other inflammatory conditions of the intestine
High blood pressure
Certain kidney diseases
Active or dormant peptic ulcer
Myasthenia gravis (a muscle weakness disorder)
Osteoporosis (brittle bones)
Ulcerative colitis with impending danger of infection

Long-term use of Medrol can slow the growth and development of infants and children.

Use aspirin cautiously with Medrol if you have a blood-clotting disorder.

Avoid exposure to chickenpox and measles.

### Possible food and drug interactions when taking this medication
If Medrol is taken with certain other drugs, the effects of either drug could be increased, decreased, or altered. It is especially important to check with your doctor before combining Medrol with the following:

Aspirin
Barbiturates such as phenobarbital
Carbamazepine (Tegretol)
Cyclosporine (Sandimmune, Neoral)
Diuretics such as Lasix and HydroDIURIL
Estrogen medications such as Premarin
Insulin
Ketoconazole (Nizoral)
Nonsteroidal anti-inflammatory medications such as Indocin
Oral anticoagulants (blood thinners) such as Coumadin
Oral diabetes drugs such as Glucotrol
Phenytoin (Dilantin)
Rifampin (Rifadin)
Troleandomycin (Tao)

### Special information if you are pregnant or breastfeeding
If you are pregnant or plan to become pregnant, tell your doctor immediately. There is no information about the safety of Medrol during pregnancy. Babies born to mothers who have taken doses of Medrol (corticosteroids) during pregnancy should be carefully watched for adrenal problems. Medrol may appear in breast milk and could affect a nursing infant. If Medrol is essential to your health, your doctor may advise you to stop breastfeeding until your treatment with Medrol is finished.

## Recommended dosage

The starting dose of Medrol tablets may vary from 4 milligrams to 48 milligrams per day, depending on the specific problem being treated.

Once the doctor is satisfied with your response, he or she will gradually lower the dosage to the smallest effective amount.

For a worsening of multiple sclerosis, the dosage is 160 milligrams a day for one week, then 64 milligrams every other day for a month.

## Overdosage

Any medication taken in excess can have serious consequences. If you suspect an overdose of Medrol, seek medical treatment immediately.

*Generic name:*

# Medroxyprogesterone

*See Provera, page 448.*

*Generic name:*

# Mefenamic acid

*See Ponstel, page 425.*

*Brand name:*

# Mellaril

*Pronounced: MEL-ah-rill*
*Generic name: Thioridazine hydrochloride*

## Why is this drug prescribed?

Mellaril is used to reduce the symptoms of psychotic disorders such as schizophrenia, and to treat depression and anxiety in adults. Mellaril is also used in the treatment of agitation, fears, sleep disturbances, tension, depression, and anxiety in elderly people, and for certain behavior problems in children.

## Most important fact about this drug

Mellaril may cause tardive dyskinesia—a condition marked by involuntary muscle spasms and twitches in the face and body. This condition may be permanent, and appears to be most common among the elderly, especially women. Ask your doctor for information about this possible risk.

## How should you take this medication?

If you are taking Mellaril in a liquid concentrate form, you can dilute it with a liquid such as distilled water, soft tap water, or juice just before taking it.

Do not change from one brand of thioridazine to another without consulting your doctor.

■ *If you miss a dose...*
If you take 1 dose a day and remember later in the day, take the dose immediately. If you don't remember until the next day, skip the dose and go back to your regular schedule.

If you take more than 1 dose a day and remember the forgotten dose within an hour or so after its scheduled time, take it immediately. If you don't remember until later, skip the dose and go back to your regular schedule.

Never try to "catch up" by doubling a dose.

■ *Storage instructions...*
Store at room temperature, tightly closed, in the container the medication came in.

## What side effects may occur?

Side effects cannot be anticipated. If any develop or change in intensity, inform your doctor as soon as possible. Only your doctor can determine if it is safe for you to continue taking Mellaril.

■ *Side effects may include:*
Abnormal and excessive secretion of milk, agitation, anemia, asthma, blurred vision, body spasm, breast development in males, changed mental state, changes in sex drive, chewing movements, confusion (especially at night), constipation, diarrhea, discolored eyes, drowsiness, dry mouth, excitement, eyeball rotation, fever, fluid accumulation and swelling, headache, inability to hold urine, inability to urinate, inhibition of ejaculation, intestinal blockage, involuntary movements, irregular blood pressure, pulse, and heartbeat, irregular or missed menstrual periods, jaw spasm, loss of appetite, loss of muscle movement, mouth puckering, muscle rigidity, nasal congestion, nausea, overactivity, painful muscle spasm, paleness, pinpoint pupils, protruding tongue, psychotic reactions, puffing of cheeks, rapid heartbeat, redness of the skin, restlessness, rigid and masklike face, sensitivity to light, skin pigmentation and rash, sluggishness, stiff, twisted

neck, strange dreams, sweating, swelling in the throat, swelling or filling of breasts, swollen glands, tremors, vomiting, weight gain, yellowing of the skin and whites of eyes

## Why should this drug not be prescribed?

Never combine this drug with excessive amounts of central nervous system depressants such as alcohol, barbiturates, or narcotics. Do not take Mellaril if you have heart disease accompanied by severe high or low blood pressure.

## Special warnings about this medication

This drug may impair your ability to drive a car or operate potentially dangerous machinery. Do not participate in any activities that require full alertness until you are certain the drug will not interfere.

If you have ever had breast cancer, make sure your doctor is aware of it.

Mellaril may cause false positive results in tests for pregnancy.

## Possible food and drug interactions when taking this medication

If Mellaril is taken with certain other drugs, the effects of either could be increased, decreased, or altered. It is especially important to check with your doctor before combining Mellaril with the following:

Epinephrine (EpiPen)
Phosphorus insecticides
Pindolol (Visken)
Propranolol (Inderal)

Extreme drowsiness and other potentially serious effects can result if Mellaril is combined with alcohol or other central nervous system depressants such as narcotics, painkillers, and sleeping medications.

## Special information if you are pregnant or breastfeeding

Pregnant women should use Mellaril only if clearly needed. If you are pregnant or plan to become pregnant, inform your doctor immediately.

## Recommended dosage

Your doctor will tailor your dose to your needs, using the smallest effective amount.

### ADULTS

*Psychotic Disorders*

The starting dose ranges from 150 to 300 milligrams a day, divided into 3 equal doses. Your doctor may increase your dosage to as much as 800 milligrams a day, taken in 2 to 4 small doses. Once your symptoms improve, your doctor will decrease the dosage to the lowest effective amount.

*Depression and Anxiety*

The initial dose is 75 milligrams a day, divided into 3 doses per day. Dosage may range from 20 to 200 milligrams a day, divided into 2 to 4 doses.

### CHILDREN

*Behavior Problems*

Mellaril should not be given to children younger than 2 years old. For children 2 to 12 years old, doses are determined by body weight. Total daily doses range from 0.5 milligram to 3 milligrams for every 2.2 pounds of body weight.

The usual beginning dose for children with moderate disorders is from 20 to 30 milligrams a day, divided into 2 or 3 doses.

### OLDER ADULTS

In general, older people take dosages of Mellaril in the lower range. Older people (especially older women) may be more susceptible to tardive dyskinesia—a possibly irreversible condition marked by involuntary muscle spasms and twitches in the face and body. Consult your doctor for information about these potential risks.

*Depression, Anxiety and Sleep Disturbances*

The starting dose is 75 milligrams a day, divided into 3 doses per day. The dosage may range from 20 to 200 milligrams a day, divided into 2 to 4 doses.

## Overdosage

Any medication taken in excess can have serious consequences. An overdose of Mellaril can be fatal. If you suspect an overdose, seek medical help immediately.

■ *Symptoms of Mellaril overdose may include:*
Agitation, blurred vision, coma, confusion, constipation, difficulty breathing, dilated or constricted pupils, diminished flow of urine, dry mouth, dry skin, excessively high or low body temperature, extremely low blood pressure, fluid in the lungs, heart abnormalities, inability to urinate, intestinal blockage, nasal congestion, restlessness, sedation, seizures, shock

Generic name:

# Meperidine

See Demerol, page 145.

Generic name:

# Meprobamate

See Miltown, page 327.

Generic name:

# Mesalamine

See Rowasa, page 480.

Brand name:

# Metaprel

See Alupent, page 16.

Generic name:

# Metaproterenol

See Alupent, page 16.

Generic name:

# Metformin

See Glucophage, page 226.

Generic name:

# Methazolamide

See Neptazane, page 354.

Generic name:

# Methenamine

See Urised, page 577.

Brand name:

# Methergine

Pronounced: METH-er-jin
Generic name: Methylergonovine maleate

## Why is this drug prescribed?

Methergine, a blood-vessel constrictor, is given to prevent or control excessive bleeding following childbirth. It works by causing the uterine muscles to contract, thereby reducing the mother's blood loss.

Methergine comes in tablet and injectable forms.

## Most important fact about this drug

Some blood-vessel disorders and certain infections make the use of Methergine dangerous. Make sure your doctor is aware of any medical conditions you may have.

## How should you take this medication?

Take Methergine tablets exactly as prescribed.

■ *If you miss a dose...*
Do not take the missed dose at all and do not double the next one. Instead, go back to your regular schedule.
■ *Storage instructions...*
Store at room temperature in a tightly closed container, away from light.

## What side effects may occur?

Side effects cannot be anticipated. If any develop or change in intensity, inform your doctor as soon as possible. Only your doctor can determine if it is safe for you to continue taking Methergine.

The most common side effect is high blood pressure, which may cause a headache or even a seizure. In some people, however, Methergine may cause low blood pressure.

■ *Less common or rare side effects may include:*
Bad taste, blood clots, blood in urine, chest pains (temporary), diarrhea, difficult or labored breathing, dizziness, edema, hallucinations, heart attack, leg cramps, nasal congestion, nausea, palpitations (throbbing heartbeat), ringing in the ears, sweating, vomiting

## Why should this drug not be prescribed?

You should not take Methergine if you are allergic to it, if you are pregnant, or if you have high blood pressure or toxemia (poisons circulating in the blood).

## Special warnings about this medication

It may be dangerous to take Methergine if you have an infection, certain blood vessel disorders, or a liver or kidney problem. Inform your doctor if you think you have any such condition.

Your doctor will use intravenous Methergine only when necessary, because of the possibility of a sudden rise in blood pressure or a stroke.

## Possible food and drug interactions when taking this medication

If Methergine is taken with certain other drugs, the effects of either may be increased, decreased, or altered. It is especially important to check with your doctor before combining Methergine with the following:

Other blood-vessel constrictors such as EpiPen
Other ergot-derived medications such as Ergotrate

## Special information if you are pregnant or breastfeeding

Methergine should not be taken during pregnancy. Methergine appears in breast milk. Although no specific information is available about possible effects of Methergine on a nursing baby, the general rule is that a mother who is breastfeeding should not take any drug unless it is clearly needed.

## Recommended dosage

The usual dose is 1 tablet (0.2 milligram) 3 or 4 times daily after childbirth for a maximum of 1 week.

## Overdosage

Any medication taken in excess can have serious consequences. If you suspect symptoms of a Methergine overdose, seek medical attention immediately.

■ *Symptoms of Methergine overdose may include:*
   Abdominal pain, coma, convulsions, elevated blood pressure, hypothermia (drop in body temperature), lowered blood pressure, nausea, numbness, slowed breathing, tingling of the arms and legs, vomiting

*Generic name:*

# Methocarbamol

*See Robaxin, page 476.*

*Generic name:*

# Methotrexate

*Pronounced: meth-oh-TREX-ate*
*Brand name: Rheumatrex*

## Why is this drug prescribed?

Methotrexate is an anticancer drug used in the treatment of lymphoma (cancer of the lymph nodes) and certain forms of leukemia. It is also given to treat some forms of cancers of the uterus, breast, lung, head, neck, and ovary. Methotrexate is also given to treat rheumatoid arthritis when other treatments have proved ineffective, and is sometimes used to treat very severe and disabling psoriasis (a skin disease characterized by thickened patches of red, inflamed skin often covered by silver scales).

## Most important fact about this drug

Be certain to remember that in the treatment of psoriasis and rheumatoid arthritis, methotrexate is taken once a *week*, not once a day. Accidentally taking the recommended weekly dosage on a daily basis can lead to fatal overdosage. Be sure to read the patient instructions that come with the package.

## How should you take this medication?

Take methotrexate exactly as prescribed, and promptly report to your doctor any new symptoms that may develop.

Methotrexate is given at a higher dosage for cancer than for psoriasis or rheumatoid arthritis. After high-dose methotrexate treatment, a drug called leucovorin may be given to limit the toxic effects.

■ *If you miss a dose...*
   Skip it and go back to your regular schedule. Do not take 2 doses at once.
■ *Storage instructions...*
   Store at room temperature, away from light.

## What side effects may occur?

Side effects cannot be anticipated. If any develop or change in intensity, inform your doctor as soon as possible. Only your doctor can determine whether it is safe for you to continue taking methotrexate.

■ *More common side effects may include:*
   Abdominal pain and upset, chills and fever, decreased resistance to infection, dizziness, fatigue, general feeling of illness, mouth ulcers, nausea

■ *Less common side effects may include:*

Abortion, acne, anemia, birth defects, black or tarry stool, blurred vision, boils, bruises, changes in skin coloration, convulsions, diarrhea, drowsiness, fatigue, hair loss, headaches, hives, inability to speak, infection of hair follicles, infertility, inflammation of the gums or mouth, intestinal inflammation, kidney failure, loss of appetite, lung disease, menstrual problems, partial or complete paralysis, rash or itching, red patches on skin, sensitivity to light, sore throat, stomach and intestinal ulcers and bleeding, stomach pain, vaginal discharge, vomiting, vomiting blood

■ *Rare side effects may include:*

Diabetes, impotence, infection, joint pain, loss of sexual desire, muscular pain, osteoporosis, ringing in the ears, severe allergic reaction, shortness of breath, sleepiness, sudden death, sweating

If you are taking methotrexate for psoriasis, you may also experience hair loss and/or sun sensitivity, and your patches of psoriasis may give a burning sensation.

Methotrexate can sometimes cause serious lung damage that makes it necessary to limit the treatment. If you experience a dry cough, fever, or breathing difficulties while taking methotrexate, be sure to tell your doctor right away.

During and immediately after treatment with methotrexate, fertility may be impaired. Men may have an abnormally low sperm count; women may have menstrual irregularities.

### Why should this drug not be prescribed?

Do not take this medication if you are sensitive to it or it has given you an allergic reaction.

Do not take this medication if you are pregnant.

Methotrexate treatment is not suitable for you if you suffer from psoriasis or rheumatoid arthritis and also have one of the following conditions:

Abnormal blood cell count
Alcoholic liver disease or other chronic liver disease
Alcoholism
Anemia
Immune-system deficiency

### Special warnings about this medication

Before you start taking methotrexate, your doctor will do a chest X-ray plus blood tests to determine your blood cell counts, liver enzyme levels, and the efficiency of your kidney function. While you are taking methotrexate, the blood tests will be repeated at regular intervals; if you develop a cough or chest pain, the chest X-ray will be repeated.

Older or physically debilitated people are particularly vulnerable to toxic effects from methotrexate.

Your doctor will prescribe methotrexate with great caution if you have any of the following:

Active infection
Liver disease
Peptic ulcer
Ulcerative colitis

### Possible food and drug interactions when taking this medication

If you are being given methotrexate for the treatment of cancer or psoriasis, you should not take aspirin or other nonsteroidal painkillers such as Advil or Naprosyn; this combination could increase the toxic effects of methotrexate. If you are taking methotrexate for rheumatoid arthritis, you may be able to continue taking aspirin or a nonsteroidal painkiller, but your doctor should monitor you carefully.

Other drugs that may increase the toxic effects of methotrexate include:

Cisplatin (Platinol)
Phenylbutazone
Phenytoin (Dilantin)
Probenecid (Benemid)
Sulfa drugs such as Bactrim and Gantrisin

Sulfa drugs may increase methotrexate's toxic effect on the bone marrow, where new blood cells are made.

Certain antibiotics, including tetracycline (Achromycin) and chloramphenicol (Chloromycetin) may reduce the effectiveness of methotrexate. This is also true of vitamin preparations that contain folic acid.

### Special information if you are pregnant or breastfeeding

A woman should not start methotrexate therapy until the doctor is sure she is not pregnant. Because methotrexate causes birth defects and miscarriages, it must not be taken during pregnancy by women with psoriasis or rheumatoid arthritis. It should be taken by women being treated for cancer only if the potential benefit outweighs the risk to the developing baby. In fact, a couple should avoid pregnancy if either the man or the woman is taking methotrexate. After the end of methotrexate treatment, a man should wait at least 3 months, and a woman should wait for the completion of at least one menstrual cycle, before attempting to conceive a child.

Methotrexate should not be taken by a woman who is breastfeeding; it does pass into breast milk and may harm a nursing baby.

### Recommended dosage

Treatment with methotrexate is highly individualized. Your doctor will carefully tailor your dosage of methotrexate in order to avoid serious side effects and possible under- or overdosing.

### Overdosage

Taken in excess, methotrexate can cause serious and even fatal damage to the liver, kidneys, bone marrow, lungs, or other parts of the body. Symptoms of overdosage may include lung or breathing problems, mouth ulcers, or diarrhea. Initially, however, serious damage caused by methotrexate may be apparent only in the results of blood tests. For this reason, careful, regular monitoring by your doctor is necessary. If for any reason you suspect symptoms of an overdose of metho-trexate, seek medical attention immediately.

Generic name:

# Methyldopa

See Aldomet, page 12.

Generic name:

# Methylergonovine

See Methergine, page 315.

Generic name:

# Methylphenidate

See Ritalin, page 474.

Generic name:

# Methylprednisolone

See Medrol, page 311.

Generic name:

# Metoclopramide

See Reglan, page 458.

Generic name:

# Metolazone

See Zaroxolyn, page 599.

Generic name:

# Metoprolol

See Lopressor, page 292.

Generic name:

# Metronidazole

See Flagyl, page 214.

Brand name:

# Mevacor

Pronounced: MEV-uh-core
Generic name: Lovastatin

### Why is this drug prescribed?

Mevacor is used, along with diet, to lower cholesterol levels in the blood of people with primary hypercholesterolemia (too much cholesterol), a condition caused by a lack of the low-density lipoprotein (LDL) receptors that remove cholesterol from the bloodstream. However, Mevacor is usually prescribed only when a low-fat, low-cholesterol diet does not lower cholesterol levels enough. Mevacor is also used to slow down hardening of arteries in people with coronary heart disease.

### Most important fact about this drug

Mevacor is usually prescribed only if diet, exercise, and weight-loss fail to bring your cholesterol levels under control. It's important to remember that Mevacor is a supplement—not a substitute—for these other measures. To get the full benefit of the medication, you need to stick to the diet and exercise program prescribed by your doctor. All these efforts to keep your cholesterol levels normal are important because together they may lower your risk of heart disease.

## How should you take this medication?

Take Mevacor exactly as prescribed by your doctor. Mevacor should be taken with meals.

■ *If you miss a dose...*

Take it as soon as you remember. If it is almost time for your next dose, skip the one you missed and go back to your regular schedule. Never take 2 doses at the same time.

■ *Storage instructions...*

Protect Mevacor from light. Store at room temperature. Keep container tightly closed.

## What side effects may occur?

Mevacor is generally well tolerated. Any side effects that have occurred have usually been mild and short-lived. If any side effects develop or change in intensity, inform your doctor as soon as possible. Only your doctor can determine if it is safe for you to continue taking Mevacor.

■ *Side effects may include:*

Abdominal pain/cramps, altered sense of taste, blurred vision, constipation, diarrhea, dizziness, gas, headache, heartburn, indigestion, itching, muscle cramps, muscle pain, nausea, rash, weakness

## Why should this drug not be prescribed?

If you are sensitive to or have ever had an allergic reaction to Mevacor or similar anticholesterol drugs, you should not take this medication. Make sure that your doctor is aware of any drug reactions that you have experienced.

Unless you are directed to do so by your doctor, do not take this medication if you are being treated for liver disease.

Do not take this drug if you are pregnant or nursing.

## Special warnings about this medication

If you are being treated for any disease that contributes to increased blood cholesterol, such as hypothyroidism, diabetes, nephrotic syndrome (kidney and blood vessel disorder), dysproteinemia (an excess of protein in the blood), or liver disease, your doctor will closely monitor your reaction to Mevacor.

It is recommended that liver function tests be performed by your doctor before treatment with Mevacor begins, at 6 and 12 weeks after your treatment has started or your dosage has been raised, and periodically (about 6-month intervals) thereafter.

This drug should be used with caution if you consume substantial quantities of alcohol or have a past history of liver disease.

## Possible food and drug interactions when taking this medication

If Mevacor is taken with certain other drugs, the effects of either could be increased, decreased, or altered. It is especially important to check with your doctor before combining Mevacor with the following:

Blood-thinning drugs such as Coumadin
Cyclosporine (Sandimmune, Neoral) and other immunosuppressive drugs (medications that lower the body's defense reaction to a foreign or invading substance)
Erythromycin (E.E.S., PCE, others)
Gemfibrozil (Lopid)
Itraconazole (Sporanox)
Nicotinic acid or niacin (Nicobid)

If you are taking Mevacor in combination with nicotinic acid, Lopid, or immunosuppressive drugs such as cyclosporine, alert your doctor immediately if you experience muscle pain, tenderness, or weakness, especially with fever or general bodily discomfort. This could be the first sign of impending kidney damage.

If you are taking cyclosporine and need to take Sporanox as well, the doctor will temporarily take you off Mevacor.

## Special information if you are pregnant or breastfeeding

You should take Mevacor only if pregnancy is highly unlikely. If you become pregnant while taking this drug, discontinue using it and notify your physician immediately. There may be a potential hazard to the developing baby. This medication may appear in breast milk and may have an effect on nursing infants. If this medication is essential to your health, you should discontinue breastfeeding until your treatment with this medication is finished.

## Recommended dosage

ADULTS

The recommended starting dose is 20 milligrams once a day, taken with the evening meal. The maximum recommended dose is 80 milligrams per day, taken as a single dose or divided into smaller doses, as determined by your doctor. Adjustments to any dose, as determined by your doctor, should be made at intervals of 4 weeks or more.

If you are taking immunosuppressive drugs in combination with Mevacor, your dose of Mevacor should begin with 10 milligrams and should not exceed 20 milligrams per day.

Cholesterol levels should be monitored periodically by your doctor, who may decide to reduce the dose if your cholesterol level falls below the targeted range.

If you have reduced kidney function, your doctor will be cautious about increasing your dosage.

CHILDREN

The safety and effectiveness of this drug have not been established in children.

### Overdosage

There have been no reported cases of overdose with Mevacor. However, if you suspect an overdose, seek medical attention immediately.

---

*Generic name:*

# Mexiletine

*See Mexitil, page 320.*

---

*Brand name:*

# Mexitil

*Pronounced: MEX-ih-till*
*Generic name: Mexiletine hydrochloride*

### Why is this drug prescribed?

Mexitil is used to treat severe irregular heartbeat (arrhythmia). Irregular heart rhythms are generally divided into two main types: heartbeats that are faster than normal (tachycardia) and heartbeats that are slower than normal (bradycardia). Arrhythmias are often caused by drugs or disease but can occur in otherwise healthy people with no history of heart disease or other illness.

### Most important fact about this drug

While you are taking Mexitil, your doctor should carefully monitor your heartbeat to make sure the drug is working properly.

### How should you take this medication?

Take Mexitil with food or an antacid. Take it exactly as prescribed.

■ *If you miss a dose...*
If you remember within 4 hours, take it immediately. If more than 4 hours have passed, skip the missed dose and return to your regular schedule. Never take 2 doses at the same time.
■ *Storage instructions...*
Store at room temperature.

### What side effects may occur?

Side effects cannot be anticipated. If any develop or change in intensity, inform your doctor as soon as possible. Only your doctor can determine if it is safe for you to continue taking Mexitil.

■ *More common side effects may include:*
Blurred vision, changes in sleep habits, chest pain, constipation, depression, diarrhea, difficult or labored breathing, dizziness, headache, heartburn, light-headedness, nausea, nervousness, numbness, poor coordination, rash, swelling due to fluid retention, throbbing heartbeat, tingling or pins and needles, tremors, upset stomach, vision changes, vomiting
■ *Less common or rare side effects may include:*
Abdominal pain/cramps, angina (crushing chest pain), appetite changes, behavior changes, bleeding from the stomach, confusion, congestive heart failure, decreased sex drive, depression, difficulty swallowing, difficulty urinating, dry mouth, dry skin, excessive perspiration, fainting, fatigue, fever, hallucinations, hair loss, hepatitis, hiccups, high blood pressure, hot flashes, impotence, joint pain, loss of consciousness, low blood pressure, peptic ulcer, ringing in the ears, seizures, short-term memory loss, skin inflammation and flaking, skin peeling, slow heartbeat, sore throat, speech difficulties, taste changes, vague feeling of bodily discomfort, weakness, worsening of irregular heartbeat

### Why should this drug not be prescribed?

This drug should not be used if you have heart failure, a heartbeat irregularity called heart block that has not been corrected by a pacemaker, structural heart disease, or if you have recently had a heart attack.

## Special warnings about this medication

If you have heart block and a pacemaker Mexitil may be prescribed, but you should be continuously monitored while taking it.

Mexitil can aggravate low blood pressure and severe congestive heart failure so will be prescribed cautiously for people with these conditions.

You should be monitored carefully if you have liver disease or abnormal liver function as a result of congestive heart failure.

Diets that change the pH (acid/alkaline content) of your urine can alter the excretion of Mexitil from your body. Talk to your doctor or pharmacist about proper diet.

*Blood disorders have occurred with Mexitil use. Make sure your doctor performs periodic blood tests while you are using this medication.*

If you have a seizure disorder, use Mexitil with caution.

## Possible food and drug interactions when taking this medication

If Mexitil is taken with certain other drugs, the effects of either may be increased, decreased, or altered. It is especially important that you consult with your doctor before taking any of the following:

Antacids such as Maalox
Caffeine products such as No-Doz
Cimetidine (Tagamet)
Other antiarrhythmic drugs such as Norpace and
    Quinidex
Phenobarbital
Phenytoin (Dilantin)
Rifampin (Rifadin)
Theophylline products such as Theo-Dur

## Special information if you are pregnant or breastfeeding

The effects of Mexitil during pregnancy have not been adequately studied. If you are pregnant or plan to become pregnant, inform your doctor immediately. Mexitil appears in breast milk and could affect a nursing infant. If this medication is essential to your health, your doctor may advise you to discontinue breastfeeding until your treatment is finished.

## Recommended dosage

Treatment is usually begun in the hospital.

ADULTS

The dosage of Mexitil will be adjusted to your individual needs on the basis of your response to the drug.

The usual starting dose is 200 milligrams every 8 hours when quick control of an irregular heartbeat is not necessary. Your doctor may adjust the dose by 50 or 100 milligrams up or down every 2 to 3 days.

Most people will do well on 200 to 300 milligrams taken every 8 hours with food or antacids. If you do not, your doctor may raise your dose to 400 milligrams every 8 hours. You should not take more than 1,200 milligrams in a day.

When fast relief is needed, your doctor may start you on 400 milligrams of Mexitil, followed by 200 milligrams in 8 hours. You should see the effects of this drug within 30 minutes to 2 hours.

In general, people with reduced kidney function are prescribed the usual doses of Mexitil, but those with severe liver disease may require lower doses and will be monitored closely.

Some people who handle this drug well may be transferred to a 12-hour dosage schedule that will make it easier and more convenient to take Mexitil. If you do well on a Mexitil dose of 300 milligrams or less every 8 hours, your doctor may decide to divide the daily total into 2 doses taken every 12 hours.

CHILDREN

The safety and efficacy of this drug have not been established in children.

OLDER ADULTS

Dosages will be adjusted according to the individual's needs.

## Overdosage

Any medication taken in excess can have serious consequences. There have been deaths from Mexitil overdose. If you suspect an overdose, seek medical attention immediately.

■ *The symptoms of Mexitil overdose may include:*
    Low blood pressure, nausea, seizures, slow heartbeat, tingling or pins and needles

*Brand name:*

# Miacalcin

*Pronounced: my-ah-CAL-sin*
*Generic name: Calcitonin-salmon*
*Other brand name: Calcimar*

## Why is this drug prescribed?

Miacalcin is a synthetic form of calcitonin, a naturally occurring hormone produced by the thyroid gland. Miacalcin reduces the rate of calcium loss from bones. Since less calcium passes from the bones to the blood, Miacalcin also helps control blood calcium levels. Miacalcin Nasal Spray is used to treat postmenopausal osteoporosis (bone loss occurring after menopause) in women who cannot or will not take estrogen. Calcimar is also used to treat Paget's disease (abnormal bone growth leading to deformities) and hypercalcemia (abnormally high calcium blood levels).

### Most important fact about this drug

Although no allergic reactions have been reported with Miacalcin Nasal Spray, the injectable form of the drug, Calcimar, has been reported to cause serious allergic reactions (such as shock, difficulty breathing, wheezing, and swelling of the throat or tongue) in a few people. The possibility exists for such a reaction with the nasal spray. Your doctor may give you a skin test to see if you are allergic to calcitonin-salmon.

### How should you take this medication?

Spray Miacalcin into one nostril one day, the other the next.

Follow the manufacturer's instructions for activating the pump before the first dose.

Keep your head upright. Put the nozzle into your nostril and depress the pump toward the bottle.

Be sure your diet provides enough calcium and vitamin D. Foods that are good sources of calcium include dairy products (such as milk and cheese) and fish. Good sources of vitamin D include fish (such as salmon, sardines, and tuna), liver, and dairy products. Sunlight is an indirect source of vitamin D.

■ *If you miss a dose...*
Take it as soon as you remember. Never take 2 doses at once.

■ *Storage instructions...*
Store the unopened medication in the refrigerator. Protect from freezing. Once the pump has been activated, you can keep the bottle at room temperature until you have finished the medication (2 weeks).

### What side effects may occur?

Side effects cannot be anticipated. If any develop or change in intensity, inform your doctor as soon as possible. Only your doctor can determine if it is safe for you to continue using Miacalcin Nasal Spray.

■ *More common side effects may include:*
Back pain, headache, joint pain, nasal inflammation, nasal symptoms (crusts, dryness, redness, sores, irritation, itching, thick feeling, soreness, paleness, infection, narrowing of passages, runny or blocked nose, small wounds, bleeding wound, uncomfortable feeling), nosebleed

■ *Less common side effects may include:*
Flushing, nausea, possible allergic reaction, respiratory tract irritation

### Why should this drug not be prescribed?

You should not be using Miacalcin if you are allergic to calcitonin-salmon.

### Special warnings about this medication

Your doctor will examine your nose before you use Miacalcin Nasal Spray and periodically while you are using it.

If your nose becomes very irritated, notify your doctor.

Miacalcin may cause small wounds or ulcers in your nose.

### Possible food and drug interactions when taking this medication

There are no interactions listed for this drug. However, people with Paget's disease who have taken a diphosphonate such as Didronel may find that Miacalcin Nasal Spray is not working as well as it should.

### Special information if you are pregnant or breastfeeding

The effects of calcitonin-salmon in pregnancy have not been adequately studied, but use of Miacalcin Nasal Spray if you are pregnant is not recommended.

It is not known whether Miacalcin appears in breast milk. Women are usually advised not to use Miacalcin while breastfeeding an infant.

### Recommended dosage

The usual dose is 200 I.U. a day, sprayed into the nose. Alternate nostrils. Ask your doctor about taking supplemental Vitamin D and calcium.

Miacalcin Nasal Spray should not be used by children.

### Overdosage

Any medication taken in excess can have serious consequences. If you suspect an overdose, seek medical help immediately.

■ *Symptoms of Miacalcin overdose may include:*
Spasms

*Generic name:*

# Miconazole

*See Monistat, page 334.*

*Brand name:*

# Micro-K

*Pronounced: MY-kroe kay*
*Generic name: Potassium chloride*
*Other brand names: Klor-Con, K-Dur, Kaon-CL,*
*Slow-K, Ten-K*

### Why is this drug prescribed?

Micro-K is used to treat or prevent low potassium levels in people who may face potassium loss caused by digitalis (Lanoxin) and non-potassium-sparing diuretics (such as Diuril and Dyazide) and certain diseases.

Potassium plays an essential role in the proper functioning of a wide range of systems in the body, including the kidneys, muscles, and nerves. As a result, a potassium deficiency may have a wide range of effects, including dry mouth, thirst, reduced urination, weakness, fatigue, drowsiness, low blood pressure, restlessness, muscle cramps, abnormal heart rate, nausea, and vomiting.

Micro-K, Klor-Con, K-Dur, Kaon-CL, Slow-K and Ten-K are slow-release potassium formulations.

### Most important fact about this drug

There have been reports of intestinal and gastric ulcers and bleeding associated with use of slow-release potassium chloride medications. Micro-K should be used only by people who cannot take potassium chloride in liquid or effervescent forms.

Do not change from one brand of potassium chloride to another without consulting your doctor or pharmacist.

### How should you take this medication?

Take Micro-K with meals and with water or some other liquid.

Tell your doctor if you have difficulty swallowing Micro-K. You may sprinkle the contents of the capsule onto a spoonful of soft food. Capsules should not be crushed, chewed, or sucked.

■ *If you miss a dose...*
If it is within 2 hours of the scheduled time, take it as soon as you remember. If you do not remember until later, skip the dose you missed and go back to your regular schedule. Do not take 2 doses at once.

■ *Storage instructions...*
Store at room temperature in a tightly closed container.

### What side effects may occur?

Side effects cannot be anticipated. If any develop or change in intensity, inform your doctor as soon as possible. Only your doctor can determine if it is safe for you to continue taking Micro-K.

■ *Side effects may include:*
Abdominal pain or discomfort, diarrhea, nausea, stomach and intestinal ulcers and bleeding, blockage, or perforation, vomiting

### Why should this drug not be prescribed?

You should not be using Micro-K in a solid form if you are taking any drug or have any condition that could stop or slow Micro-K as it goes through the gastrointestinal tract.

If you have high potassium levels, you should not use Micro-K.

### Special warnings about this medication

Before taking Micro-K, tell your doctor if you have ever had acute dehydration, heat cramps, adrenal insufficiency, diabetes, heart disease, kidney disease, liver disease, ulcers, or severe burns.

Tell your doctor immediately if you notice that your stools are black or tarry.

### Possible food and drug interactions when taking this medication

If Micro-K is taken with certain other drugs, the effects of either could be increased, decreased, or altered. It is important to check with your doctor before combining Micro-K with the following:

Antispasmodic drugs such as Bentyl
Blood pressure medications classified as ACE
 inhibitors, such as Vasotec and Capoten
Digitalis (Lanoxin)
Potassium-sparing diuretics such as Midamor and
 Aldactone

Also tell your doctor if you use salt substitutes.

### Special information if you are pregnant or breastfeeding

Micro-K is generally considered safe for pregnant women or women who breastfeed their babies.

## Recommended dosage

Dosages must be adjusted for each individual. Safety and effectiveness in children have not been established. The following are typical dosages for Micro-K and other leading slow-release potassium supplements.

### TO TREAT LOW POTASSIUM LEVELS

*Micro-K, Klor-Con 8, Slow-K*
The usual dosage is 5 to 12 tablets or capsules per day.

*Micro-K 10, Klor-Con 10, K-Dur 10, Kaon-CL 10, Ten-K*
The usual dose is 4 to 10 tablets or capsules per day.

*K-DUR 20*
The usual dose is 2 to 5 tablets per day.

### TO PREVENT LOW POTASSIUM LEVELS

*Micro-K, Klor-Con 8, Slow-K, K-Dur 10, Kaon-CL 10, Ten-K*
The usual dosage is 2 or 3 tablets or capsules per day.

*Micro-K 10, Klor-Con 10*
The usual dose is 2 tablets or capsules per day.

If you are taking more than 2 tablets or capsules per day, your total daily dose will be divided into smaller doses.

## Overdosage

Any medication taken in excess can have serious consequences. Overdoses of these supplements can result in potentially fatal levels of potassium. Overdose symptoms may not be noticeable in their early stages. Therefore, if you have any reason to suspect an overdose, seek medical help immediately.

■ *Symptoms of potassium overdose may include:*
Blood in stools, cardiac arrest, irregular heartbeat, muscle paralysis, muscle weakness

*Brand name:*

# Micronase

*Pronounced: MIKE-roh-naze*
*Generic name: Glyburide*
*Other brand names: DiaBeta, Glynase*

## Why is this drug prescribed?

Micronase is an oral antidiabetic medication used to treat Type II (non-insulin-dependent) diabetes. Diabetes occurs either when the body does not make enough insulin or when the insulin that is produced no longer works properly. Insulin works by helping sugar get inside the cell, where it is then used for energy.

There are two forms of diabetes: Type I (insulin-dependent) and Type II (non-insulin-dependent). Type I diabetes usually requires insulin injections for life, while Type II diabetes can usually be treated by dietary changes, exercise, and/or oral antidiabetic medications such as Micronase. This medication controls diabetes by stimulating the pancreas to secrete more insulin and by helping insulin to work better. Type II diabetics may need insulin injections, sometimes only temporarily during stressful periods such as illness, or if an oral antidiabetic medication fails to control blood sugars, on a long-term basis.

## Most important fact about this drug

Always remember that Micronase is an aid to, not a substitute for, good diet and exercise. Failure to follow a sound diet and exercise plan can lead to serious complications, such as dangerously high or low blood sugar levels. Remember, too, that Micronase is *not* an oral form of insulin, and cannot be used in place of insulin.

## How should you take this medication?

In general, Micronase should be taken with breakfast or the first main meal of the day.

■ *If you miss a dose...*
Take it as soon as you remember. If it is almost time for your next dose, skip the one you missed and go back to your regular schedule. Never take 2 doses at the same time.
■ *Storage instructions...*
Keep this medication in the container it came in, tightly closed. Store it at room temperature.

## What side effects may occur?

Side effects cannot be anticipated. If any develop or change in intensity, inform your doctor as soon as possible. Only your doctor can determine if it is safe for you to continue taking Micronase.

Many side effects from Micronase are rare and seldom require discontinuation of the medication.

■ *More common side effects may include:*
Bloating, heartburn, nausea
■ *Less common or rare side effects may include:*
Anemia and other blood disorders, blurred vision, changes in taste, headache, hives, itching,

joint pain, liver problems, muscle pain, reddening of the skin, skin eruptions, skin rash, yellowing of the skin

Micronase, like all oral antidiabetics, may cause hypoglycemia (low blood sugar) especially in elderly, weak, and undernourished people, and those with kidney, liver, adrenal, or pituitary gland problems. The risk of hypoglycemia can be increased by missed meals, alcohol, other medications, fever, trauma, infection, surgery, or excessive exercise. To avoid hypoglycemia, you should closely follow the dietary and exercise plan suggested by your physician.

■ *Symptoms of mild hypoglycemia may include:*
Cold sweat, drowsiness, fast heartbeat, headache, nausea, nervousness
■ *Symptoms of more severe hypoglycemia may include:*
Coma, pale skin, seizures, shallow breathing

Eating sugar or a sugar-based product will often correct mild hypoglycemia.

Severe hypoglycemia should be considered a medical emergency, and prompt medical attention is essential.

### Why should this drug not be prescribed?
You should not take Micronase if you have had an allergic reaction to it or to similar drugs such as Glucotrol or Diabinese.

Micronase should not be taken if you are suffering from diabetic ketoacidosis (a life-threatening medical emergency caused by insufficient insulin and marked by excessive thirst, nausea, fatigue, pain below the breastbone, and fruity breath).

### Special warnings about this medication
It's possible that drugs such as Micronase may lead to more heart problems than diet treatment alone, or diet plus insulin. If you have a heart condition, you may want to discuss this with your doctor.

If you are taking Micronase, you should check your blood or urine periodically for abnormal sugar (glucose) levels.

It is important that you closely follow the diet and exercise plan recommended by your doctor.

The effectiveness of any oral antidiabetic, including Micronase, may decrease with time. This may occur either because of a diminished responsiveness to the medication or a worsening of the diabetes.

### Possible food and drug interactions when taking this medication
If Micronase is taken with certain other drugs, the effects of either could be increased, decreased, or altered. It is especially important to check with your doctor before combining Micronase with the following:

Airway-opening drugs such as Proventil and Ventolin
Anabolic steroids such as testosterone and Danazol
Antacids such as Mylanta
Aspirin
Beta blockers such as Inderal and Tenormin
Blood thinners such as Coumadin
Calcium channel blockers such as Cardizem and Procardia
Certain antibiotics such as Cipro
Chloramphenicol (Chloromycetin)
Cimetidine (Tagamet)
Clofibrate (Atromid-S)
Estrogens such as Premarin
Fluconazole (Diflucan)
Furosemide (Lasix)
Gemfibrozil (Lopid)
Isoniazid (a drug used for tuberculosis)
Itraconazole (Sporanox)
Major tranquilizers such as Stelazine and Mellaril
MAO inhibitors (antidepressants such as Nardil and Parnate)
Niacin (Nicolar, Nicobid)
Nonsteroidal anti-inflammatory drugs such as Advil, Motrin, Naprosyn, and Voltaren
Oral contraceptives
Phenytoin (Dilantin)
Probenecid (Benemid, ColBENEMID)
Steroids such as prednisone
Sulfa drugs such as Gantrisin
Thiazide diuretics such as Diuril and HydroDIURIL
Thyroid medications such as Synthroid

Be careful about drinking alcohol, since excessive alcohol consumption can cause low blood sugar.

### Special information if you are pregnant or breastfeeding
The effects of Micronase during pregnancy have not been adequately studied in humans. This drug should be used during pregnancy only if the benefit outweighs the potential risk to the unborn baby. Since studies suggest the importance of maintaining

normal blood sugar (glucose) levels during pregnancy, your physician may prescribe insulin injections during pregnancy.

While it is not known if Micronase appears in breast milk, other oral diabetes medications do. Therefore, women should discuss with their doctors whether to discontinue the medication or to stop breastfeeding. If the medication is discontinued, and if diet alone does not control glucose levels, then your doctor may consider insulin injections.

### Recommended dosage

Your doctor will tailor your dosage to your individual needs.

### ADULTS

Usually the doctor will prescribe an initial daily dose of 2.5 to 5 milligrams. Maintenance therapy usually ranges from 1.25 to 20 milligrams daily. Daily doses greater than 20 milligrams are not recommended. In most cases, Micronase is taken once a day; however, people taking more than 10 milligrams a day may respond better to twice-a-day dosing.

### CHILDREN

The safety and effectiveness of Micronase have not been established in children.

### OLDER ADULTS

Older, malnourished or debilitated individuals, or those with impaired kidney and liver function, usually receive lower initial and maintenance doses to minimize the risk of low blood sugar (hypoglycemia).

### Overdosage

An overdose of Micronase can cause low blood sugar (hypoglycemia).

■ *Symptoms of severe hypoglycemia include:*
Coma, pale skin, seizure, shallow breathing

If you suspect a Micronase overdose, seek medical attention immediately.

*Brand name:*

# Micronor

*See Oral Contraceptives, page 382.*

*Brand name:*

# Midrin

*Pronounced: MID-rin*
*Generic ingredients: Isometheptene mucate,*
*   Dichloralphenazone, Acetaminophen*

### Why is this drug prescribed?

Midrin is prescribed for the treatment of tension headaches. It is also used to treat vascular headaches such as migraine.

### Most important fact about this drug

Midrin can be used only after the headache starts. It does not prevent headaches.

### How should you take this medication?

You should start taking Midrin at the first sign of a migraine attack.

Do not take more than the maximum dose of Midrin.

Take this medication exactly as prescribed by your doctor.

■ *If you miss a dose...*
Take this medication only as needed.
■ *Storage instructions...*
Store at room temperature in a dry place.

### What side effects may occur?

Side effects cannot be anticipated. If any develop or change in intensity, tell your doctor immediately. Only your doctor can determine whether it is safe for you to continue taking Midrin.

■ *Side effects may include:*
Short periods of dizziness, skin rash

### Why should this drug not be prescribed?

Unless directed to do so by your doctor, do not take Midrin if you have the eye condition called glaucoma or severe kidney disease, high blood pressure, a physical defect of the heart, or liver disease, or if you are currently taking antidepressant drugs known as MAO inhibitors, including Nardil and Parnate.

### Special warnings about this medication

Take Midrin cautiously if you have high blood pressure or any abnormal condition of the blood vessels outside of the heart, or have recently had a cardiovascular attack such as a heart attack or stroke.

## Possible food and drug interactions when taking this medication

Avoid alcoholic beverages.

If Midrin is taken with certain other drugs, the effects of either drug could be increased, decreased, or altered. It is especially important to check with your doctor before combining Midrin with the following:

Acetaminophen-containing pain relievers such as Tylenol

Antidepressants classified as MAO inhibitors, including

Nardil and Parnate

Antihistamines such as Benadryl

Central nervous system depressants such as Halcion, Valium and Xanax

## Special information if you are pregnant or breastfeeding

If you are pregnant, plan to become pregnant, or are breastfeeding your baby, check with your doctor before taking Midrin.

## Recommended dosage

ADULTS

*Relief of Migraine Headache*

The usual dosage is 2 capsules at once, followed by 1 capsule every hour until the headache is relieved; do not take more than 5 capsules within a 12-hour period.

*Relief of Tension Headache*

The usual dosage is 1 or 2 capsules every 4 hours up to a maximum of 8 capsules a day.

## Overdosage

Any medication taken in excess can have serious consequences. If you suspect a Midrin overdose, seek emergency medical treatment immediately.

*Brand name:*

# Miltown

*Pronounced: MILL-town*
*Generic name: Meprobamate*
*Other brand name: Equanil*

## Why is this drug prescribed?

Miltown is a tranquilizer used in the treatment of anxiety disorders and for short-term relief of the symptoms of anxiety.

## Most important fact about this drug

Miltown can be habit forming. You can develop tolerance and dependence, and you may experience withdrawal symptoms if you stop using this drug abruptly. Discontinue this drug or change your dose only on your doctor's advice.

## How should you take this medication?

Take Miltown exactly as prescribed.

■ *If you miss a dose...*
Take it as soon as you remember if it is within an hour of your scheduled time. If you do not remember until later, skip the dose you missed and go back to your regular schedule. Never take 2 doses at the same time.

■ *Storage instructions...*
Store at room temperature in a tightly closed container.

## What side effects may occur?

Side effects cannot be anticipated. If any develop or change in intensity, inform your doctor as soon as possible. Only your doctor can determine if it is safe for you to continue taking Miltown.

■ *More common side effects may include:*
Allergic reactions, blood disorders, bruises, diarrhea, dizziness, drowsiness, exaggerated feeling of well-being, fainting, fast throbbing heartbeat, fever, headache, inappropriate excitement, itchy rash, loss of muscle coordination, nausea, rapid or irregular heartbeat, skin eruptions, slurred speech, small, purplish spots on the skin, sudden severe drop in blood pressure, swelling due to fluid retention, tingling sensation or numbness, vertigo, vision problems, vomiting, weakness

■ *Less common or rare side effects may include:*
Breathing difficulty, chills, high fever, inflammation of mouth, inflammation of the rectum, little or no urine, redness and swelling of skin, severe allergic reaction, skin inflammation and flaking, Stevens-Johnson syndrome (peeling skin)

■ *Side effects due to rapid decrease in dose or abrupt withdrawal from Miltown:*
Anxiety, confusion, convulsions, hallucinations, inability to fall or stay asleep, loss of appetite, loss of coordination, muscle twitching, tremors, vomiting

Withdrawal symptoms usually become apparent within 12 to 48 hours after discontinuation of this medication and should disappear in another 12 to 48 hours.

### Why should this drug not be prescribed?

If you are sensitive to or have ever had an allergic reaction to Miltown or related drugs such as carisoprodol (Soma), you should not take this medication.

You should not take Miltown if you have acute intermittent porphyria, an inherited disease of the body's metabolism. It can make your symptoms worse.

Anxiety or tension related to everyday stress usually does not require treatment with Miltown. Discuss your symptoms thoroughly with your doctor.

### Special warnings about this medication

If you develop a skin rash, sore throat, fever, or shortness of breath, contact your doctor immediately. You may be having an allergic reaction to the drug.

Miltown may cause you to become drowsy or less alert; therefore, you should not drive or operate dangerous machinery, or participate in any hazardous activity that requires full mental alertness until you know how this drug affects you.

Long-term use of this drug should be evaluated by your doctor periodically for its usefulness.

If you have liver or kidney disorders, make sure your doctor is aware of these conditions before you begin using this medication.

If you have epilepsy, use of this drug may bring on seizures. Consult your doctor before taking it.

### Possible food and drug interactions when taking this medication

Miltown may intensify the effects of alcohol. Do not drink alcohol while taking this medication.

If Miltown is taken with certain other drugs, the effects of either could be increased, decreased, or altered. It is especially important to check with your doctor before combining Miltown with mood-altering drugs and central nervous system depressants such as the following:

Antidepressant drugs such as Elavil, Nardil, and Tofranil
Barbiturates such as Seconal and phenobarbital
Major tranquilizers such as Thorazine and Mellaril
Narcotics such as Percocet or Demerol
Tranquilizers such as Halcion, Restoril, and Valium

### Special information if you are pregnant or breastfeeding

Do not take Miltown if you are pregnant or planning to become pregnant. There is an increased risk of birth defects. Miltown appears in breast milk and could affect a nursing infant. If this medication is essential to your health, your doctor may advise you to discontinue breastfeeding until your treatment is finished.

### Recommended dosage

ADULTS

*Miltown 200 and 400*
The usual dosage is 1,200 milligrams to 1,600 milligrams per day divided into 3 or 4 doses. You should not take more than 2,400 milligrams a day.

*Miltown 600*
The usual dose is one 600-milligram tablet, 2 times a day. Do not take more than 2,400 milligrams a day.

CHILDREN

*Miltown 200 and 400*
The usual dose for children 6 to 12 years of age is 200 to 600 milligrams per day divided into 2 or 3 doses.

Miltown 200 and 400 are not recommended for use in children under age 6. Miltown 600 is not recommended for use in children.

OLDER ADULTS

Your doctor will limit your dose to the smallest effective amount to avoid oversedation.

### Overdosage

Any medication taken in excess can cause symptoms of overdose. If you suspect an overdose, seek emergency medical attention immediately.

■ *The symptoms of Miltown overdose may include:* Coma, drowsiness, loss of muscle control, severely impaired breathing, shock, sluggishness and unresponsiveness

*Brand name:*

# Minipress

*Pronounced: MIN-ee-press*
*Generic name: Prazosin hydrochloride*

### Why is this drug prescribed?

Minipress is used to treat high blood pressure. It is effective used alone or with other high blood pressure medications such as diuretics or beta-blocking medications (drugs that ease heart contractions) such as Tenormin.

Minipress is also prescribed for the treatment of benign prostatic hyperplasia (BPH), an abnormal enlargement of the prostate gland.

### Most important fact about this drug

If you have high blood pressure, you must take Minipress regularly for it to be effective. Since blood pressure declines gradually, it may be several weeks before you get the full benefit of Minipress; and you must continue taking it even if you are feeling well. Minipress does not cure high blood pressure; it merely keeps it under control.

### How should you take this medication?

Minipress can be taken with or without food.

This medication should be taken exactly as prescribed by your doctor even if your symptoms have disappeared. Try not to miss any doses. If this medication is not taken regularly, your blood pressure will increase.

■ *If you miss a dose...*
  Take it as soon as you remember. If it is almost time for your next dose, skip the one you missed and go back to your regular schedule. Never take 2 doses at the same time.
■ *Storage instructions...*
  Protect from heat, light, and moisture.

### What side effects may occur?

Side effects cannot be anticipated. If any develop or change in intensity, inform your doctor as soon as possible. Only your doctor can determine if it is safe for you to continue taking Minipress.

■ *More common side effects may include:*
  Dizziness, drowsiness, headache, lack of energy, nausea, palpitations (pounding heartbeat), weakness
■ *Less common side effects may include:*
  Blurred vision, constipation, depression, diarrhea, dizziness on standing up, dry mouth, fainting, fluid retention, frequent urination, nasal congestion, nervousness, nosebleeds, rash, red eyes, shortness of breath, vertigo, vomiting
■ *Rare side effects may include:*
  Abdominal discomfort/pain, excessive perspiration, fever, hair loss, hallucinations, impotence, inability to hold urine, inflammation of the pancreas, itching, itchy purple spots on wrists, forearms, and thighs, joint pain, persistent, painful erection, rapid heartbeat, ringing in ears, tingling or pins and needles

### Why should this drug not be prescribed?

There are no known reasons to avoid this drug.

### Special warnings about this medication

Minipress can cause low blood pressure, especially when you first start taking the medication. This can cause you to become faint, dizzy, or light-headed, particularly on standing up. You should avoid driving or any hazardous tasks where injury could occur for 24 hours after taking the first dose or after your dose has been increased. Dizziness, fainting, or light-headedness may also occur in hot weather, when exercising, or when standing for long periods of time. Ask your doctor what precautions you should take.

### Possible food and drug interactions when taking this medication

Minipress can intensify the effects of alcohol. Be careful of the amount you drink.

If Minipress is taken with certain other drugs, the effects of either could be increased, decreased, or altered. It is especially important that you check with your doctor before combining Minipress with the following:

Beta blockers such as Inderal
Dextroamphetamine (Dexedrine)
Diuretics such as Dyazide
Ibuprofen (Motrin, Advil, others)
Other high blood pressure medications
Verapamil (Calan, Verelan)

### Special information if you are pregnant or breastfeeding

The effects of Minipress during pregnancy have not been adequately studied. If you are pregnant or plan to become pregnant, notify your doctor immediately. Minipress appears in breast milk and can affect a nursing infant. If this medication is essential to your health, your doctor may advise you to discontinue breastfeeding until your treatment is finished.

### Recommended dosage

ADULTS

Dosages of this drug should be adjusted by your doctor according to your response.

The usual starting dose is 1 milligram, 2 or 3 times per day.

To determine your regular dose, your doctor may slowly increase this medication to as much as

20 milligrams per day, divided into smaller doses. The commonly prescribed daily dose is 6 milligrams to 15 milligrams per day, divided into smaller doses. Although doses higher than 20 milligrams per day have not been found to be effective, there are some people who may benefit from a daily dose of 40 milligrams, divided into smaller doses.

If Minipress is used with a diuretic or other high blood pressure drug, the dose can be reduced to 1 to 2 milligrams, 3 times a day.

CHILDREN

Safety and effectiveness of this drug have not been established in children.

### Overdosage

Any medication taken in excess can have serious consequences. If you suspect a Minipress overdose, seek medical treatment immediately.

■ *The symptoms of Minipress overdose may include:*
Extreme drowsiness, low blood pressure

*Brand name:*

# Minocin

*Pronounced: MIN-o-sin*
*Generic name: Minocycline hydrochloride*
*Other brand name: Dynacin*

### Why is this drug prescribed?

Minocin is a form of the antibiotic tetracycline.

It is given to help treat many different kinds of infection, including:

Acne
Amebic dysentery
Anthrax (a rare skin infection)
Cholera
Gonorrhea (when penicillin cannot be given)
Plague
Respiratory infections such as pneumonia
Rocky Mountain spotted fever
Syphilis (when penicillin cannot be given)
Urinary tract infections caused by certain microbes

### Most important fact about this drug

To help clear up your infection completely, keep taking Minocin for the full time of treatment, even if you begin to feel better after a few days. Minocin, like other antibiotics, works best when

there is a constant amount in the body. To help keep the level constant, take the doses at evenly spaced times around the clock.

### How should you take this medication?

You may take Minocin with or without food. Take Minocin exactly as directed. Your doctor will prescribe it for a specific number of days according to the condition you are being treated for; keep taking the medication until you have used it all up.

To reduce the risk of throat irritation, take the capsule form of Minocin with plenty of fluids.

You should avoid use of antacids that contain aluminum, calcium, or magnesium, such as Maalox and Mylanta, and iron preparations such as Feosol. If you must take these medicines, take them 2 to 3 hours before or after taking Minocin.

■ *If you miss a dose...*
Take it as soon as you remember, then space out evenly any remaining doses for that day. Never take 2 doses at the same time.
■ *Storage instructions...*
Store capsules and liquid at room temperature. Keep capsules away from moist places and direct light. Do not freeze the liquid.

### What side effects may occur?

Side effects cannot be anticipated. If any develop or change in intensity, inform your doctor as soon as possible. Only your doctor can determine if it is safe for you to continue taking Minocin.

■ *Side effects may include:*
Aching, inflamed joints, anal or genital sores with fungus infection, anaphylaxis (life-threatening allergic reaction), anemia, appetite loss, blurry vision, bulging of soft spots in infants' heads, decreased hearing, diarrhea, difficulty swallowing, discoloration of children's teeth, fever, fluid retention, headache, hepatitis, hives, inflammation of the penis, inflammation of the intestines, inflammation of the tongue, joint pain, kidney or liver failure, nausea, rash, sensitivity to light, skin coloration, skin eruptions, skin inflammation and peeling, throat irritation, thyroid gland problems, vomiting

### Why should this drug not be prescribed?

Do not take Minocin if you have ever had an allergic reaction to it or to any other tetracycline antibiotic.

Although Minocin may be given to kill meningococcal (spinal) bacteria in people who are carriers, it should not be given to treat actual meningococcal meningitis (inflammation in the spinal canal).

Minocin is not a first-choice drug for treating any staphylococcal ("staph") infection.

### Special warnings about this medication

If you have a kidney problem, a normal dose of Minocin may amount to an overdose for you. It is likely that you will need a lower-than-average dosage; if you need to take Minocin for an extended period of time, your doctor may order frequent blood tests to make sure you are not getting too much of the drug.

Because Minocin may make you dizzy or lightheaded or cause a whirling feeling, do not drive, climb, or perform hazardous tasks until you know how the medication affects you.

Minocin should not be given to children 8 years old or younger, since it may cause discoloration of the teeth. Occasionally, Minocin has also caused tooth discoloration in adults.

Like other tetracycline antibiotics, Minocin may cause a sensitivity to light, and you may sunburn very easily. Be careful in sun and under sunlamps. If your skin turns red and hot, stop taking Minocin immediately.

While taking Minocin you may be especially susceptible to infections, including fungus infections such as vaginal yeast infection. If you do get an infection, check with your doctor immediately.

If you get a headache and blurry vision while taking Minocin, or if an infant receiving Minocin develops bulging of the "soft spots" (fontanels) on the head, this could mean that the drug is causing a buildup of fluid within the skull. It is important to stop taking Minocin and see a doctor immediately.

Minocin liquid contains a sulfite that can cause severe allergic reactions in susceptible people.

### Possible food and drug interactions when taking this medication

If Minocin is taken with certain other drugs, the effects of either could be increased, decreased, or altered. It is especially important to check with your doctor before combining Minocin with the following:

Antacids containing aluminum, calcium, or magnesium, such as Mylanta
Blood thinners such as Coumadin
Iron-containing preparations such as Feosol
Oral contraceptives
Penicillin (Pen-Vee K)

### Special information if you are pregnant or breastfeeding

If you are pregnant or plan to become pregnant, inform your doctor immediately. If you take Minocin during the second half of pregnancy, it may cause permanent yellow, gray, or brown discoloration of your baby's teeth.

There is reason to believe that taking Minocin during pregnancy could also harm the baby in other ways. Therefore, Minocin should be taken during pregnancy only if an antibiotic is clearly needed and only if a non-tetracycline antibiotic cannot be used instead. Because Minocin appears in breast milk and could harm the baby, it should not be taken by a woman who is breastfeeding. If this drug is essential to your health, your doctor may advise you to discontinue breastfeeding until treatment is finished.

### Recommended dosage

Minocin differs from the other tetracyclines in the usual dosage and number of times it is taken per day.

You may experience more side effects if you take more than the recommended dosage.

ADULTS

The usual dosage of Minocin is 200 milligrams to start with, followed by 100 milligrams every 12 hours. If your doctor wants you to take more frequent doses, he or she may prescribe two or four 50-milligram capsules initially, and then one 50-milligram capsule 4 times daily.

The dosage and the length of time you take the drug can vary according to your condition and the specific infection.

CHILDREN ABOVE 8 YEARS OF AGE

The usual dosage of Minocin is 4 milligrams per 2.2 pounds of body weight to start, followed by 2 milligrams per 2.2 pounds every 12 hours.

### Overdosage

Although no specific information is available, any medication taken in excess can have serious consequences. If you suspect symptoms of an overdose of Minocin, seek medical attention immediately.

*Generic name:*

# Minocycline

*See Minocin, page 330.*

*Generic name:*

# Minoxidil

*See Rogaine, page 478.*

*Generic name:*

# Misoprostol

*See Cytotec, page 127.*

*Brand name:*

# Modicon

*See Oral Contraceptives, page 382.*

*Brand name:*

# Moduretic

*Pronounced: mod-your-ET-ik*
*Generic ingredients: Amiloride,*
*Hydrochlorothiazide*

## Why is this drug prescribed?

Moduretic is a diuretic combination used in the treatment of high blood pressure and congestive heart failure, conditions which require the elimination of excess fluid (water) from the body. When used for high blood pressure, Moduretic can be used alone or with other high blood pressure medications. Diuretics help your body produce and eliminate more urine, which helps lower blood pressure. Amiloride, one of the ingredients, helps minimize the potassium loss that can be caused by the other component, hydrochlorothiazide.

## Most important fact about this drug

If you have high blood pressure, you must take Moduretic regularly for it to be effective. Since blood pressure declines gradually, it may be several weeks before you get the full benefit of Moduretic; and you must continue taking it even if you are feeling well. Moduretic does not cure high blood pressure; it merely keeps it under control.

## How should you take this medication?

Take this medication with food.

Take Moduretic exactly as prescribed by your doctor. Stopping Moduretic suddenly could cause your condition to worsen.

■ *If you miss a dose...*
Take the forgotten dose as soon as you remember. If it is almost time for your next does, skip the one you missed and go back to your regular schedule. Never take a double dose.

■ *Storage instructions...*
Store at room temperature. Keep this medication in the container it came in, tightly closed, and protected from moisture, light, and freezing.

## What side effects may occur?

Side effects cannot be anticipated. If any develop or change in intensity, inform your doctor as soon as possible. Only your doctor can determine if it is safe for you to continue taking Moduretic.

■ *More common side effects may include:*
Diarrhea, dizziness, elevated potassium levels, fatigue, headache, irregular heartbeat, itching, leg pain, loss of appetite, nausea, rash, shortness of breath, stomach and intestinal pain, weakness

■ *Less common or rare side effects may include:*
Anemia, appetite changes, back pain, bad taste, breast development in males, changes in liver function, changes in potassium levels leading to symptoms such as dry mouth, excessive thirst, weak or irregular heartbeat, muscle pain or cramps, chest pain, constipation, cough, decreased sex drive, dehydration, depression, dermatitis, dizziness on standing up, dry mouth, excessive perspiration, excessive urination at night, fainting, fever, fluid in lungs, flushing, frequent urination, fullness in abdomen, gas, gout, hair loss, heartburn, hiccups, hives, impotence, incontinence, indigestion, insomnia, itching, joint pain, mental confusion, muscle cramps, nasal congestion, neck and shoulder ache, nervousness, numbness, painful or difficult urination, rapid heartbeat, ringing in ears, sensitivity to light, sleepiness, Stevens-Johnson Syndrome (severe blisters), stomach and intestinal bleeding, stupor, sugar in blood or urine, thirst, tingling or pins and needles, tremors, vague feeling of bodily discomfort, vertigo, vision changes, vomiting, yellow eyes and skin

## Why should this drug not be prescribed?

If you are unable to urinate or have serious kidney disease, or if you have high potassium levels in your blood, you should not take this medication.

If you are sensitive to or have ever had an allergic reaction to amiloride, hydrochlorothiazide or similar drugs, or if you are sensitive to other sulfonamide-derived drugs, you should not take this medication. Make sure your doctor is aware of any drug reactions you may have experienced.

## Special warnings about this medication

Potassium supplements, potassium-containing salt substitutes, and other diuretics (such as Dyazide) that minimize loss of potassium should not be used while you are taking moduretic unless your doctor specifically says otherwise. You should also limit your consumption of potassium-rich foods such as bananas, prunes, raisins, orange juice, and whole and skim milk. Ask your doctor for advice on how much of these foods to consume.

If you are taking Moduretic, a complete assessment of your kidney function should be done; kidney function should continue to be monitored.

If you are taking an ACE-inhibitor type of blood pressure medication such as Vasotec, this drug should be used with extreme caution.

If you have liver disease, diabetes, gout, or collagen vascular disease (lupus erythematosus), Moduretic should be used with caution.

If you have bronchial asthma or a history of allergies, you may be at risk for an allergic reaction to this medication.

Dehydration, excessive sweating, severe diarrhea or vomiting could deplete your fluids and cause your blood pressure to become too low. Be careful when exercising and in hot weather.

Notify your doctor or dentist that you are taking Moduretic if you have a medical emergency or before you have surgery.

## Possible food and drug interactions when taking this medication

Moduretic may increase the effects of alcohol. Avoid alcohol while taking this medication.

If Moduretic is taken with certain other drugs, the effects of either could be increased, decreased, or altered. It is especially important to check with your doctor before combining Moduretic with the following:

ACE inhibitors such as Vasotec
Barbiturates such as phenobarbital
Cholestyramine (Questran)
Colestipol (Colestid)
Corticosteroids such as prednisone
Insulin
Lithium (Lithonate)
Muscle relaxants such as tubocurarine
Narcotics such as Percocet
Nonsteroidal anti-inflammatory drugs such as
    Naprosyn
Norepinephrine (Levophed)
Oral drugs for treating diabetes such as Micronase,
    DiaBeta
Other high blood pressure medications

## Special information
## if you are pregnant or breastfeeding

The effects of Moduretic during pregnancy have not been adequately studied. If you are pregnant or plan to become pregnant, inform your doctor immediately. Moduretic appears in breast milk and could affect a nursing infant. If this medication is essential to your health, your doctor may advise you to discontinue breastfeeding until your treatment is finished.

## Recommended dosage

Your doctor will tailor the dosage to meet your individual requirements, taking into consideration other medical conditions you may have and other medications you may be taking.

### ADULTS

The usual starting dose is 1 tablet per day, which may be increased to 2 tablets per day taken at the same time or separately.

### CHILDREN

The safety and effectiveness of Moduretic have not been established in children.

## Overdosage

Any medication taken in excess can cause symptoms of overdose. If you suspect an overdose, seek medical attention immediately.

No specific information on symptoms of Moduretic overdose is available, but dehydration might be expected.

Generic name:

# Moexipril

*See Univasc, page 576.*

Generic name:

# Mometasone

*See Elocon, page 191.*

Brand name:

# Monistat

Pronounced: MON-ih-stat
Generic name: Miconazole nitrate

### Why is this drug prescribed?

Monistat is available in several formulations, including Monistat 3 vaginal suppositories, Monistat 7 vaginal cream and suppositories, and Monistat-Derm skin cream. Monistat's active ingredient, Miconazole, fights fungal infections.

Monistat 3 and Monistat 7 are used for vaginal yeast infections. Monistat-Derm is used for skin infections such as athlete's foot, ringworm, jock itch, yeast infection on the skin (cutaneous candidiasis), and tinea versicolor (a common skin condition that produces patches of white, tan, or brown finely flaking skin over the neck and trunk).

### Most important fact about this drug

Keep using this medicine regularly for the full time of the treatment, even if the infection seems to have disappeared. If you stop too soon, the infections could return. You should continue using the vaginal forms of the medicine even during your menstrual period.

### How should you use this medication?

Use this medication exactly as prescribed.

Keep all forms of this medicine away from your eyes.

Before applying Monistat-Derm to your skin, be sure to wash your hands. Massage the medication gently into the affected area and the surrounding skin.

If you are using the vaginal cream or suppository, follow these steps:

1. Load the applicator to the fill line with cream, or unwrap a tablet, wet it with warm water, and place it in the applicator as shown in the instructions you received with the product.
2. Lie on your back with your knees drawn up.
3. Gently insert the application high into the vagina and push the plunger.
4. Withdraw the applicator and discard it if disposable, or wash with soap and water.

To keep the vaginal medication from getting on your clothing, wear a sanitary napkin. Do not use tampons because they will absorb the medicine. Wear cotton underwear—avoid synthetic fabrics such as rayon or nylon. Do not douche unless your doctor tells you to do so.

Dry the genital area thoroughly after a shower, bath, or swim. Change out of a wet bathing suit or damp workout clothes as soon as possible. Yeast is less likely to flourish in a dry environment.

Do not scratch if you can help it. Scratching can cause more irritation and can spread the infection.

■ *If you miss a dose...*
Make up for it as soon as you remember. However, if it is almost time for your next dose, skip the one you missed and go back to your regular schedule.

■ *Storage instructions...*
Store at room temperature.

### What side effects may occur?

Side effects cannot be anticipated. If any develop or change in intensity, inform your doctor. Only your doctor can determine whether it is safe for you to continue taking Monistat.

■ *Side effects may include:*
Burning sensation, cramping, headaches, hives, irritation, rash, vulval or vaginal itching

### Why should this drug not be prescribed?

If you have ever had an allergic reaction to or are sensitive to miconazole nitrate, you should not use this medication. Make sure your doctor is aware of any drug reactions you have experienced.

### Special warnings about this medication

If symptoms persist, or if an irritation or allergic reaction develops while you are using Monistat, notify your doctor.

The hydrogenated vegetable oil base of Monistat 3 may interact with the latex in vaginal diaphragms, so concurrent use of these two products is not recommended.

Your doctor may recommend Monistat 7 Vaginal Cream if you are using a diaphragm. However, you should be aware that the mineral oil in the vaginal cream can weaken the latex in condoms and diaphragms, making them less reliable for prevention of pregnancy or sexually transmitted disease.

If you are using Monistat 3 or Monistat 7 suppositories, you should either avoid sexual intercourse or make sure your partner uses a condom.

Do not give Monistat 7 to girls less than 12 years of age. Also avoid using Monistat 7 if you have any of the following symptoms:

Fever above 100°F orally
Foul-smelling vaginal discharge
Pain in the lower abdomen, back, or either shoulder

If these symptoms develop while you are using Monistat 7, stop treatment and contact your doctor right away. You may have a more serious infection.

If the infection fails to improve or worsens within 3 days, or you do not obtain complete relief within 7 days, or symptoms return within two months, you may have something other than a yeast infection.

### Possible food and drug interactions when taking this medication

No interactions have been reported.

### Special information if you are pregnant or breastfeeding

Unless you are directed to do so by your doctor, do not use Monistat during the first trimester (three months) of pregnancy because it is absorbed in small amounts from the vagina. It is not known whether miconazole appears in breast milk. If Monistat is essential to your health, your doctor may advise you to discontinue breastfeeding until your treatment with this medication is finished.

### Recommended dosage

MONISTAT-7 VAGINAL CREAM

The usual daily dose is 1 applicatorful inserted into the vagina at bedtime for 7 consecutive days.

MONISTAT-7 VAGINAL SUPPOSITORIES

The usual daily dose is 1 suppository inserted into the vagina at bedtime for 7 consecutive days.

MONISTAT-DERM

For jock itch, ringworm, athlete's foot, or yeast infection of the skin, apply a thin layer of Monistat-Derm over the affected area morning and night. For tinea versicolor, apply a thin layer over the affected area once daily.

### Overdosage

Overdose of Monistat has not been reported. However any medication used in excess can have serious consequences. If you suspect an overdose, seek medical attention immediately.

*Brand name:*

# Monoket

*See Imdur, page 247.*

*Brand name:*

# Monopril

*Pronounced: MON-oh-prill*
*Generic name: Fosinopril sodium*

### Why is this drug prescribed?

Monopril is a high blood pressure medication known as an ACE inhibitor. It is effective when used alone or in combination with other medications for the treatment of high blood pressure. Monopril is also prescribed for heart failure.

Monopril works by preventing the conversion of a chemical in your blood called angiotensin I into a more potent substance that increases salt and water retention in your body. Monopril also enhances blood flow in your circulatory system.

### Most important fact about this drug

You must take Monopril regularly for it to be effective. Since blood pressure declines gradually, it may be several weeks before you get the full benefit of Monopril; and you must continue taking it even if you are feeling well. Monopril does not cure high blood pressure; it merely keeps it under control.

### How should you take this medication?

Monopril is best taken one hour before meals; but it can be taken with food if it upsets your stomach.

Take this medication exactly as prescribed by your doctor.

■ *If you miss a dose...*

Suddenly stopping Monopril could cause your blood pressure to increase. If you forget to take a dose, take it as soon as you remember. If it is almost time for your next dose, skip the one you missed and go back to your regular schedule. Never take 2 doses at the same time.

■ *Storage instructions...*
Store Monopril at room temperature in a tightly closed container to protect the medication from moisture.

## What side effects may occur?

Side effects cannot be anticipated. If any develop or change in intensity, inform your doctor as soon as possible. Only your doctor can determine if it is safe for you to continue taking Monopril.

WHEN TAKEN FOR HIGH BLOOD PRESSURE

■ *More common side effects may include:*
Cough, dizziness, nausea, vomiting

■ *Less common or rare side effects may include:*
Abdominal pain, anaphylaxis (severe allergic reaction), changes in appetite and weight, changes in sexual performance, confusion, constipation, decreased sex drive, diarrhea, drowsiness, dry mouth, excessive sweating, eye irritation, fatigue, gas, headache, heartburn, itching, kidney failure, liver failure, muscle cramps, rash, ringing in ears, skin sensitivity to sunlight, sleep disturbances, tremors, vertigo, vision disturbances, weakness, yellow eyes and skin

WHEN TAKEN FOR HEART FAILURE

■ *More common side effects may include:*
Cough, dizziness, low blood pressure, muscle and bone pain

■ *Less common or rare side effects may include:*
Abnormal breathing, arm or leg weakness, behavior change, bronchitis, chest pain, constipation, decreased appetite, depression, diarrhea, distended abdomen, dry mouth, excessive sweating, fainting, fever, flu, fluid retention/swelling, gas, gout, heart rhythm disturbances, high blood pressure, itching, kidney pain, lightheadedness on standing up, muscle ache, nasal inflammation, nausea, numbness, pain, pins and needles, rapid or slow heartbeat, sensation of cold, sexual problems, shock, sinus problems, speaking abnormality, stoppage of breathing/heart, stroke, swelling in legs or arms, taste disturbance, tremor, upper respiratory infection, urinary problems, vertigo, vision problems, vomiting, weakness, weight gain

## Why should this drug not be prescribed?

If you are sensitive to or have ever had an allergic reaction to Monopril or other ACE inhibitors such as Capoten, you should not take this medication. Make sure that your doctor is aware of any drug reactions that you have experienced.

## Special warnings about this medication

If you develop a sore throat or fever, you should contact your doctor immediately for medical attention. It could indicate a more serious illness.

If you develop swelling of your face, lips, tongue or throat, or arms and legs, or have difficulty swallowing, you should contact your doctor immediately. You may need emergency treatment.

Make sure your doctor knows about any kidney or liver problems you may have. If you notice your skin or the whites of your eyes turning yellow, stop taking Monopril and contact your doctor immediately.

Your kidney function should be monitored while you are taking Monopril for either high blood pressure or heart failure. If you have heart failure and your kidneys are not functioning properly, you may develop low blood pressure. Also, certain blood tests may be needed if you have a disease of the connective tissue.

If you are taking high doses of diuretic and Monopril, you may develop excessively low blood pressure.

You may experience light-headedness while taking Monopril, especially during the first few days of therapy. If this occurs, notify your doctor. If you actually faint, discontinue the use of this medication and notify your doctor immediately.

Do not use potassium-containing salt substitutes without consulting your doctor.

If you have heart failure, this drug should be started under close medical supervision. Your doctor should continue to monitor your progress for the first 2 weeks of treatment and whenever your dosage is increased.

Excessive sweating, dehydration, severe diarrhea, or vomiting could lead to excessive loss of water and cause your blood pressure to drop dangerously. Take precautions to avoid excessive water loss while exercising.

This drug should be used with caution if you are on dialysis. There have been reports of extreme allergic reactions during dialysis in people taking

ACE inhibitors such as Monopril. There have also been reports of severe allergic reactions in people given bee or wasp venom to protect against stings.

### Possible food and drug interactions when taking this medication

If Monopril is taken with certain other drugs, the effects of either could be increased, decreased, or altered. It is especially important to check with your doctor before combining Monopril with the following:

Antacids such as Mylanta and Maalox
Lithium (Eskalith, Lithonate)
Potassium preparations such as K+10 and K-Lyte
Potassium-sparing diuretics such as Moduretic and
 Aldactone
Thiazide diuretics such as Esidrix and Diuril

### Special information if you are pregnant or breastfeeding

ACE inhibitors such as Monopril have been shown to cause injury and even death in the developing baby when used in pregnancy during the second or third trimesters. If you are pregnant your doctor should discontinue the use of this medication as soon as possible. If you plan to become pregnant and are taking Monopril, contact your doctor immediately to discuss the potential hazard to your unborn child. Monopril appears in breast milk and could affect a nursing infant. If this medication is essential to your health, your doctor may advise you to discontinue breastfeeding until your treatment with this medication is finished.

### Recommended dosage

ADULTS

*High Blood Pressure*
The usual initial dose is 10 milligrams, taken once a day, either alone or when added to a diuretic. Dosage, after blood pressure is adjusted, should be 20 to 40 milligrams a day in a single dose. For some patients, the doctor may divide the daily total into several smaller doses.

Diuretic use should, if possible, be stopped before using Monopril. If not, your physician may give an initial dose of 10 milligrams under his supervision before any further medication is prescribed.

*Heart Failure*
The usual starting dose is 10 milligrams once a day, with diuretics and possibly digitalis. Your doctor

will gradually increase the dose to one that works for you—usually between 20 milligrams daily and the maximum dose of 40 milligrams per day. If your kidneys are impaired you will probably start with a dose of 5 milligrams.

CHILDREN

The safety and effectiveness of Monopril have not been established in children.

### Overdosage

Any medication taken in excess can have serious consequences. If you suspect an overdose, seek medical attention immediately.

The primary effect of a Monopril overdose is likely to be a sudden drop in blood pressure.

*Generic name:*

# Morphine

*See MS Contin, page 339.*

*Brand name:*

# Motrin

*Generic name: Ibuprofen*
*Other brand names: Advil, Rufen*

### Why is this drug prescribed?

Motrin is a nonsteroidal anti-inflammatory drug available in both prescription and nonprescription forms. Prescription Motrin is used in adults for relief of the symptoms of rheumatoid arthritis and osteoarthritis, treatment of menstrual pain, and relief of mild to moderate pain. In children aged 6 months and older it can be given to reduce fever and relieve mild to moderate pain. It is also used to relieve the symptoms of juvenile arthritis.

Motrin IB tablets, caplets, and gelcaps; Children's Motrin Suspension; and Advil tablets and caplets are available without a prescription. Check the packages for uses, dosage, and other information on these products.

### Most important fact about this drug

You should have frequent checkups with your doctor if you take Motrin regularly. Ulcers or internal bleeding can occur without warning.

## How should you take this medication?

Your doctor may ask you to take Motrin with food or an antacid to avoid stomach upset. The suspension can be given with meals or milk if it upsets the stomach.

A drink of water or other fluid after taking a chewable tablet can help your body absorb the drug.

If you are using Motrin for arthritis, you should take it regularly, exactly as prescribed.

■ *If you miss a dose...*
Take it as soon as you remember. If it is almost time for your next dose, skip the one you missed and go back to your regular schedule. Never take 2 doses at the same time.
■ *Storage information...*
Store at room temperature.

## What side effects may occur?

Side effects cannot be anticipated. If any develop or change in intensity, inform your doctor as soon as possible. Only your doctor can determine if it is safe for you to continue taking Motrin.

■ *More common side effects may include:*
Abdominal cramps or pain, abdominal discomfort, bloating and gas, constipation, diarrhea, dizziness, fluid retention and swelling, headache, heartburn, indigestion, itching, loss of appetite, nausea, nervousness, rash, ringing in ears, stomach pain, vomiting
■ *Less common or rare side effects may include:*
Abdominal bleeding, anemia, black stool, blood in urine, blurred vision, changes in heartbeat, chills, confusion, congestive heart failure, depression, dry eyes and mouth, emotional volatility, fever, hair loss, hearing loss, hepatitis, high or low blood pressure, hives, inability to sleep, inflammation of nose, inflammation of the pancreas or stomach, kidney or liver failure, severe allergic reactions, shortness of breath, skin eruptions or peeling, sleepiness, stomach or upper intestinal ulcer, ulcer of gums, vision loss, vomiting blood, wheezing, yellow eyes and skin

## Why should this drug not be prescribed?

If you are sensitive to or have ever had an allergic reaction to ibuprofen, aspirin, or similar drugs, such as Aleve and Naprosyn, or if you have had asthma attacks caused by aspirin or other drugs of this type, or if you have angioedema, a condition whose symptoms are skin eruptions, you should not take this medication.

Make sure that your doctor is aware of any drug reactions that you have experienced.

## Special warnings about this medication

Peptic ulcers and bleeding can occur without warning. Tell your doctor if you have bleeding or any other problems.

This drug should be used with caution if you have kidney or liver disease, or are severely dehydrated; it can cause liver or kidney inflammation or other problems in some people.

Do not take aspirin or any other anti-inflammatory medications while taking Motrin unless your doctor tells you to do so.

If you have a severe allergic reaction, seek medical help immediately.

Motrin may cause vision problems. If you experience any changes in your vision, inform your doctor.

Motrin may prolong bleeding time. If you are taking blood-thinning medication, this drug should be taken with caution.

This drug can cause water retention. It should be used with caution if you have high blood pressure or poor heart function.

Avoid the use of alcohol while taking this medication.

Motrin may mask the usual signs of infection or other diseases. Use with care in the presence of an existing infection.

If you have diabetes, remember that the suspension contains 1.5 grams of sucrose and 8 calories per teaspoonful.

Motrin chewable tablets contain phenylalanine. If you have a hereditary disease called phenylketonuria, you should be aware of this.

## Possible food and drug interactions when taking this medication

If Motrin is taken with certain other drugs, the effects of either could be increased, decreased, or altered. It is especially important to check with your doctor before combining Motrin with the following:

Aspirin
Blood pressure medications known as ACE
inhibitors, including Vasotec and Capoten
Blood-thinning drugs such as Coumadin
Diuretics such as Lasix and HydroDIURIL
Lithium (Lithonate)
Methotrexate (Rheumatrex)

## Special information
## if you are pregnant or breastfeeding

The effects of ibuprofen during pregnancy have not been adequately studied. If you are pregnant or plan to become pregnant, inform your doctor immediately. Ibuprofen may appear in breast milk and could affect a nursing infant. If this medication is essential to your health, your doctor may advise you to discontinue breastfeeding until your treatment with this medication is finished.

## Recommended dosage

### ADULTS

*Rheumatoid Arthritis and Osteoarthritis*

The usual dosage is 1,200 to 3,200 milligrams per day divided into 3 or 4 doses. Your doctor will tailor the dose to your individual needs. Symptoms should be reduced within 2 weeks. Daily dosage should not be greater than 3,200 milligrams.

*Mild to Moderate Pain*

The usual dose is 400 milligrams every 4 to 6 hours as necessary.

*Menstrual Pain*

The usual dose is 400 milligrams every 4 hours as necessary. Begin treatment when symptoms first appear.

### CHILDREN 6 MONTHS TO 12 YEARS OF AGE

*Fever reduction*

The recommended dose is 5 milligrams per 2.2 pounds of body weight if temperature is less than 102.5°F or 10 milligrams per 2.2 pounds of body weight if temperature is 102.5°F or greater. The fever should go down for 6 to 8 hours. Do not give the child more than 40 milligrams per 2.2 pounds of body weight in one day.

*Mild to Moderate Pain*

The usual dose is 10 milligrams per 2.2 pounds of body weight every 6 to 8 hours. Do not give the child more than 4 such doses per day.

*Juvenile Arthritis*

The usual dose is 30 to 40 milligrams daily per 2.2 pounds of body weight, divided into 3 or 4 doses. Some children may need only 20 milligrams daily per 2.2 pounds.

## Overdosage

Any medication taken in excess can have serious consequences. An overdose of Motrin can be fatal. If you suspect an overdose, seek medical attention immediately.

■ *Symptoms of Motrin overdose may include:*
Abdominal pain, breathing difficulties, coma, drowsiness, headache, irregular heartbeat, kidney failure, low blood pressure, nausea, ringing in the ears, seizures, sluggishness, vomiting

*Brand name:*

# MS Contin

*Pronounced: em-ess KON-tin*
*Generic name: Morphine sulfate*

## Why is this drug prescribed?

MS Contin, a controlled-release tablet containing morphine, is used to relieve moderate to severe pain. While regular morphine is usually given every four hours, MS Contin is typically given every 12 hours—only twice a day. MS Contin is intended for people who need a morphine painkiller for more than just a few days.

## Most important fact about this drug

Like other narcotics, MS Contin is potentially addictive. If you take MS Contin for some time and then stop abruptly, you could experience withdrawal symptoms. For this reason, do not make dosage changes on your own; always consult your doctor.

## How should you take this medication?

Take MS Contin exactly as prescribed by your doctor—typically one tablet every 12 hours. Swallow the tablets whole. If you crush or chew the tablets, a dangerously large amount of morphine could enter your bloodstream all at once.

Do not increase the dose or take the drug more frequently than prescribed. It will take a little time for the drug to begin working.

Do not drink alcoholic beverages while using MS Contin.

■ *If you miss a dose...*
Take the forgotten dose as soon as you remember. If it is almost time for your next dose, skip the one you missed and go back to your regular schedule. Do not take 2 doses at once.

■ *Storage instructions...*
Store at room temperature in a tightly closed container, away from light.

## What side effects may occur?

Side effects cannot be anticipated. If any develop or change in intensity, tell your doctor immediately.

Only your doctor can determine whether it is safe for you to continue taking MS Contin.

As with other narcotics, the most hazardous potential side effect of MS Contin is respiratory depression (dangerously slow breathing). If you are older or in a weakened condition, you are particularly vulnerable to respiratory depression; you may be at special risk at any age if you have a lung or breathing problem.

■ *More common side effects may include:*
Constipation, depressed or irritable mood, dizziness, exaggerated sense of well-being, lightheadedness, nausea, sedation, sweating, vomiting

You may be able to lessen some of these side effects by lying down.

■ *Less common side effects may include:*
Agitation, appetite loss, apprehension, blurred vision, chills, constipation, cramps, depression, diarrhea, difficult urination, disorientation, double vision, dreams, dry mouth, facial flushing, fainting, faintness, floating feeling, hallucinations, headache, high blood pressure, hives, inability to urinate, insomnia, involuntary movement of the eyeball, itching, low blood pressure, mood changes, nervousness, "pinpoint" pupils, rapid heartbeat, rash, rigid muscles, seizure, sexual drive or performance problems, slow heartbeat, sweating, swelling due to fluid retention, taste alterations, throbbing heartbeat, tingling or pins and needles, tremor, uncoordinated muscle movements, vision disturbances, weakness

If you stop taking MS Contin after a long period of use, you will probably experience some degree of narcotic withdrawal syndrome. During the first 24 hours, you may have: dilated pupils, goose bumps, restlessness, restless sleep, runny nose, sweating, tearing, or yawning.

Over the next 72 hours, the following may be added:

Abdominal and leg pains, abdominal and muscle cramps, anxiety, diarrhea, hot and cold flashes, inability to fall or stay asleep, increase in body temperature, blood pressure and breathing and heart rate, kicking movements, loss of appetite, nasal discharge, nausea, severe backache, sneezing, twitching and spasm of muscles, vomiting, weakness

Even without treatment, your withdrawal symptoms will probably disappear within a week or two. However, you could experience a second phase of withdrawal, involving aching muscles, irritability, and insomnia, which might last for 2 to 6 months.

## Why should this drug not be prescribed?

Do not take MS Contin if you have ever had an allergic reaction to morphine or are sensitive to it, or if you have bronchial asthma.

If your breathing is abnormally slow, you should not be given MS Contin unless there is resuscitation equipment nearby.

MS Contin should not be prescribed if you are suffering an intestinal blockage.

## Special warnings about this medication

MS Contin should not be given to anyone who might have a brain injury, or the beginnings of an abdominal problem requiring surgery; the drug could mask the symptoms, making correct diagnosis difficult or impossible.

Caution is advised in giving MS Contin to people facing biliary tract surgery, since the drug could make their condition worse. Your doctor will also prescribe MS Contin with extreme caution if you have any of the following conditions:

Alcoholism
Coma
Curvature of the spine
Delirium tremens (severe alcohol withdrawal)
Drug-related psychosis
Enlarged prostate or constricted urinary canal
Kidney disorder
Liver disorder
Low adrenalin levels
Low thyroid levels
Lung disorder
Swallowing difficulty

If taken by an epileptic person, MS Contin could increase the likelihood of a seizure.

Since MS Contin can impair judgment and coordination, do not drive, climb, or operate hazardous equipment while taking this drug.

MS Contin can lower blood pressure; you may feel dizzy or light-headed, especially when you just stand up.

## Possible food and drug interactions when taking this medication

If MS Contin is taken with certain other drugs, the effects of either could be increased, decreased, or altered. It is especially important to check with your doctor before combining MS Contin with the following:

Alcohol
Certain analgesics such as Talwin, Nubain, Stadol, and Buprenex
Major tranquilizers such as Thorazine and Phenergan
Muscle relaxants such as Flexeril and Valium
Sedatives such as Dalmane and Halcion
Tranquilizers such as Librium and Xanax

## Special information if you are pregnant or breastfeeding

If you are pregnant or plan to become pregnant, inform your doctor immediately. Although there is no evidence so far that a pregnant woman's short-term use of MS Contin can harm her unborn baby, this drug should be taken during pregnancy only if the benefit to the mother outweighs a possible risk to the child.

MS Contin is not recommended for use as a painkiller during childbirth. If a woman takes this drug shortly before giving birth, her baby may have trouble breathing. Babies born to mothers who use morphine chronically may suffer from drug withdrawal symptoms.

Since some of the morphine from MS Contin appears in breast milk, do not take this medication while breastfeeding. If you do nurse while using MS Contin, your baby could experience withdrawal symptoms once you stop taking this medication.

## Recommended dosage

ADULTS

MS Contin tablets are swallowed whole, and are not to be broken, chewed, or crushed.

Because MS Contin is so potent, your doctor will determine which dosage form will work best and how often you should take the drug, based on your individual needs.

## Overdosage

Any medication taken in excess can have serious consequences. An overdose of MS Contin can be fatal. If you suspect an overdose, seek medical attention immediately.

■ *Symptoms of MS Contin overdose may include:*
Cold, clammy skin, flaccid muscles, lowered blood pressure, "pinpoint" pupils, sleepiness leading to stupor and coma, slowed breathing, slow pulse rate

*Category:*
# Multivitamins

*Brand names: Centrum, Theragran, Vi-Daylin*

## Why is this supplement prescribed?

Multivitamins are nutritional supplements for people whose diet may be deficient in certain vitamins and minerals. You may need a supplement if you are on a special diet, or don't eat the right foods. A supplement may also be necessary if you are a strict vegetarian, take medications that prevent the body from using certain nutrients, or have an illness that affects your appetite. In addition, special formulas are available for use during pregnancy.

Vitamin/mineral supplements come in a wide range of formulations. Three of the most widely used are Centrum, Theragran, and Vi-Daylin. Each of these brands offers a variety of formulas tailored to the needs of different groups.

*Centrum* is a multivitamin/multimineral supplement that includes all antioxidants, the vitamins that strengthen the body's natural defenses against cell damage. *Centrum Silver* contains higher strengths of the vitamins that people 50 years of age or older need the most. *Centrum, Jr.*, formulations are geared to children's needs.

*Theragran* is a multivitamin supplement. *Theragran-M* adds minerals to the formulation. *Theragran Stress Formula* contains higher strengths of the B vitamins that may be needed for people under stress, plus extra vitamin C.

*Vi-Daylin* is a multivitamin supplement; *Vi-Daylin + Iron* is a multivitamin plus iron, which may be needed by women who have heavy menstrual periods. Some Vi-Daylin formulations also contain fluoride. *Vi-Daylin drops* are given to infants and young children.

## Most important fact about this supplement

Do not use supplements as a replacement for a diet rich in essential vitamins and minerals. Food contains many important ingredients not available in supplements.

## How should you take this supplement?

Follow the dosing instructions on the bottle, or use as directed by your doctor.

Do not take more than suggested.

■ *If you miss a dose...*
If you forget to take your multivitamin for a day, don't be concerned. Resume your regular schedule the following day.

■ *Storage instructions...*
Keep out of the reach of children. Store at room temperature, and keep tightly closed.

## Why should this supplement not be used?

If you have any serious chronic medical conditions check with your doctor before starting on a multivitamin supplement. You may have special requirements.

If your multivitamin supplement contains fluoride, check with your doctor. You should not use it if your drinking water contains more than 0.7 parts per million of fluoride.

## Special warnings about this supplement

Do not take more of a multivitamin supplement than suggested on the packaging, or directed by your doctor. Very high doses of some vitamins and minerals can be harmful or even dangerous.

## Possible food and drug interactions when taking this supplement

When taken as suggested on the packaging, there are no known supplement interactions.

## Special information if you are pregnant or breastfeeding

Ask your doctor whether you should take a multivitamin supplement while you are pregnant or breastfeeding. Taking too much of any supplement may be harmful to you or your unborn child.

## Recommended dosage

ADULTS

The usual dose is 1 tablet, teaspoonful, or tablespoonful daily according to package instructions, or as directed by your doctor.

CHILDREN

The usual dose of children's formulations is 1 tablet, teaspoonful, or dropperful daily or as directed by your doctor. Younger children may require only half this dose. Check the instructions on the package.

## Overdosage

Megadoses of some vitamins and minerals can be harmful when taken for extended periods. If you have unexplained symptoms and suspect an overdose, check with your doctor.

*Generic name:*

# Mupirocin

*See Bactroban, page 52.*

*Brand name:*

# Mycelex

*See Gyne-Lotrimin, page 232.*

*Brand name:*

# Mycolog-II

*Pronounced: MY-koe-log too*
*Generic ingredients: Nystatin, Triamcinolone acetonide*
*Other brand names: Myco-Triacet II, Mytrex*

## Why is this drug prescribed?

Mycolog-II Cream and Ointment are prescribed for the treatment of candidiasis (a yeast-like fungal infection) of the skin. The combination of an antifungal (nystatin) and a steroid (triamcinolone acetonide) provides greater benefit than nystatin alone during the first few days of treatment. Nystatin kills the fungus or prevents its growth; triamcinolone helps relieve the redness, swelling, itching, and other discomfort that can accompany a skin infection.

## Most important fact about this drug

Absorption of this drug through the skin can affect the whole body instead of just the surface of the skin being treated. Although unusual, it is possible that you could experience symptoms of steroid excess such as weight gain, reddening and rounding of the face and neck, growth of excess body and facial hair, high blood pressure, emotional disturbances, increased blood sugar, and urinary excretion of glucose (marked by an increase in frequency of urination).

Use of this medication over large surface areas, for prolonged periods, or with airtight dressings or bandages, could cause these problems. Your doctor will watch your condition and periodically check for symptoms.

### How should you use this medication?
Use this medicine for the full course of treatment, even if your symptoms are gone. Apply a thin layer to the affected area and gently rub it in. Do not bandage or wrap the area being treated, unless your doctor tells you to. Keep the area cool and dry.

Use this medication exactly as prescribed by your doctor. Do not use it more often or for a longer time. It is for external use only. Avoid contact with the eyes.

■ *If you miss a dose...*
Apply it as soon as you remember. If it is almost time for your next dose, skip the one you missed and go back to your regular schedule.

■ *Storage instructions...*
Store away from heat and light. Do not freeze.

### What side effects may occur?
Side effects cannot be anticipated. If any develop or change in intensity, inform your doctor as soon as possible. Only your doctor can determine if it is safe for you to continue taking Mycolog-II.

■ *Side effects may include:*
Blistering, burning, dryness, eruptions resembling acne, excessive discoloring of the skin, excessive growth of hair (especially on the face), hair loss (especially on the scalp), inflammation around the mouth, inflammation of hair follicles, irritation, itching, peeling, prickly heat, reddish purple lines on skin, secondary infection, severe inflammation of the skin, softening of the skin, stretch marks, stretching or thinning of the skin

### Why should this drug not be prescribed?
If you are sensitive to or have ever had an allergic reaction to nystatin, triamcinolone acetonide, or other antifungals or steroids, you should not take this medication. Make sure your doctor is aware of any drug reactions you have experienced.

### Special warnings about this medication
Do not use this drug for any disorder other than the one for which it was prescribed.

Remember to avoid wrapping or bandaging the affected area. The use of tight-fitting diapers or plastic pants is not recommended for a child being treated in the diaper area with Mycolog-II. These garments may act in the same way as airtight dressings or bandages.

If an irritation or allergic reaction develops while using Mycolog-II, notify your doctor.

If used in the groin area, apply Mycolog-II sparingly and wear loose-fitting clothing.

If your condition does not show improvement after 2 to 3 weeks, or if it gets worse, consult your doctor.

### Possible food and drug interactions when taking this medication
No interactions have been reported.

### Special information if you are pregnant or breastfeeding
The effects of Mycolog-II in pregnancy have not been adequately studied. If you are pregnant or plan to become pregnant, inform your doctor before using Mycolog-II.

It is not known whether this medication appears in breast milk. If this drug is essential to your health, your doctor may advise you to discontinue breastfeeding until your treatment with this medication is finished.

### Recommended dosage
ADULTS

*Mycolog-II Cream*
Mycolog-II Cream is usually applied to the affected areas 2 times a day, in the morning and evening, by gently and thoroughly massaging the preparation into the skin. Your doctor will have you stop using the cream if your symptoms persist after 25 days of treatment.

*Mycolog-II Ointment*
A thin film of Mycolog-II Ointment is usually applied to the affected areas 2 times a day, in the morning and the evening. Your doctor will have you stop using the ointment if your symptoms persist after 25 days of treatment.

CHILDREN

Your doctor will limit use of Mycolog-II for children to the least amount that is effective. Long-term treatment may interfere with the growth and development of children.

### Overdosage
An acute overdosage is unlikely with the use of Mycolog-II; however, long-term or prolonged use can produce reactions throughout the body. See "Most important fact about this drug."

*Brand name:*

# Myco-Triacet II

See Mycolog-II, page 342.

*Brand name:*

# Mykrox

See Zaroxolyn, page 599.

*Brand name:*

# Mylanta

See Antacids, page 30.

*Brand name:*

# Mysoline

Pronounced: MY-soh-leen
Generic name: Primidone

## Why is this drug prescribed?

Mysoline is used to treat epileptic and other seizures. It can be used alone or with other anticonvulsant drugs. It is chemically similar to barbiturates.

## Most important fact about this drug

Mysoline should not be stopped suddenly; this could cause you to have seizures. If you no longer need the medication, your doctor will reduce the dosage gradually.

## How should you take this medication?

Take Mysoline exactly as prescribed. Do not change from one manufacturer's product to another without consulting your doctor.

If using Mysoline Suspension, shake well before using.

■ *If you miss a dose...*
Take it as soon as you remember. If it is within an hour of your next dose, skip the one you missed and go back to your regular schedule. Never take 2 doses at the same time.

■ *Storage instructions...*
Store at room temperature in a tightly closed container, away from light.

## What side effects may occur?

Side effects cannot be anticipated. If any develop or change in intensity, inform your doctor as soon as possible. Only your doctor can determine if it is safe for you to continue taking Mysoline.

■ *More common side effects may include:*
Lack of muscle coordination, vertigo or severe dizziness

■ *Less common side effects may include:*
Double vision, drowsiness, emotional disturbances, excessive irritability, fatigue, impotence, loss of appetite, nausea, skin eruptions that resemble measles, uncontrolled movement of the eyeballs, vomiting

## Why should this drug not be prescribed?

You should not take Mysoline if you have porphyria (an inherited metabolic disorder) or if you are allergic to phenobarbital.

## Special warnings about this medication

Remember that you must not stop taking Mysoline suddenly.

It can take several weeks for the full effectiveness of Mysoline to be seen.

Since Mysoline is generally given for long periods of time, your doctor will check your blood count every 6 months.

## Possible food and drug interactions when taking this medication

If Mysoline is taken with certain other drugs, the effects of either could be increased, decreased, or altered. It is especially important to check with your doctor before combining Mysoline with the following:

Antidepressants called MAO inhibitors, such as Parnate and Nardil
Blood-thinning drugs such as Coumadin
Doxycycline (Doryx, Vibramycin)
Estrogen-containing oral contraceptives such as Ortho-Novum and Triphasil
Griseofulvin (Fulvicin-U/F, Grifulvin V)
Steroid drugs such as Decadron

Avoid alcoholic beverages while you are taking Mysoline.

## Special information if you are pregnant or breastfeeding

Although the effects of Mysoline in pregnancy and nursing infants are not known, recent studies show an increase in birth defects in infants born to epileptic women taking anticonvulsant medications (particularly Dilantin and phenobarbital). Although most pregnant women taking anticonvulsant medication give birth to normal, healthy babies, this possibility may also exist with Mysoline. If you are pregnant or plan to become pregnant, inform your doctor immediately. Mysoline appears in breast milk and can affect a nursing infant, causing excessive sleepiness and drowsiness. If this medication is essential to your health, your doctor may advise you to stop breastfeeding.

### Recommended dosage

ADULTS

For people 8 years of age and older who have not been treated before, the doctor will start Mysoline as follows, using either 50-milligram or scored 250-milligram Mysoline tablets:

Days 1 to 3: 100 to 125 milligrams at bedtime
Days 4 to 6: 100 to 125 milligrams 2 times a day
Days 7 to 9: 100 to 125 milligrams 3 times a day
Day 10 to maintenance: 250 milligrams 3 times
    a day

For most adults and children 8 years of age and over, the usual maintenance dosage is 250 milligrams 3 or 4 times a day. If you need more, your doctor may increase the dose to five or six 250-milligram tablets. You should not take more than 500 milligrams 4 times a day (2000 milligrams or 2 grams).

In patients already receiving other anticonvulsants, the usual starting dose of Mysoline is 100 to 125 milligrams at bedtime; your doctor will gradually increase this dose to a maintenance level as the other drug is gradually decreased. Your doctor will either find a working level for the combination or withdraw the other medication completely. When Mysoline is to be used as a single drug, it will take at least 2 weeks to make the transition from two drugs to one.

CHILDREN UNDER AGE 8

Days 1 to 3: 50 milligrams at bedtime
Days 4 to 6: 50 milligrams 2 times a day
Days 7 to 9: 100 milligrams 2 times a day
Day 10 to maintenance: 125 milligrams 3 times a
    day to 250 milligrams 3 times day

The usual maintenance dosage is 125 to 250 milligrams 3 times daily or 10 to 25 milligrams per 2.2 pounds of body weight per day, divided into smaller doses.

### Overdosage

Any medication taken in excess can have serious consequences. If you suspect a Mysoline overdose, seek medical attention immediately.

*Brand name:*

# Mytrex

*See Mycolog-II, page 342.*

*Generic name:*

# Nabumetone

*See Relafen, page 460.*

*Generic name:*

# Nadolol

*See Corgard, page 113.*

*Generic name:*

# Nadolol with Bendroflumethiazide

*See Corzide, page 116.*

*Generic name:*

# Naltrexone

*See ReVia, page 466.*

*Generic name:*

# Naphazoline with Pheniramine

*See Naphcon-A, page 346.*

*Brand name:*

# Naphcon-A

*Pronounced: NAFF-kon ay*
*Generic ingredients: Naphazoline hydrochloride,*
  *Pheniramine maleate*
*Other brand name: Opcon-A*

### Why is this drug prescribed?

Naphcon-A, an eyedrop containing both a decongestant and an antihistamine, is used to relieve itchy, red eyes caused by ragweed, pollen, and animal hair.

### Most important fact about this drug

If this medication causes changes in your vision, be careful when driving or performing other tasks that could be hazardous.

### How should you use this medication?

Remove contact lenses before administering this medication. Do not use the solution if it becomes cloudy or changes color.

  To administer the eyedrops, follow these steps:

1. Wash your hands thoroughly.
2. Gently pull your lower eyelid down to form a pocket between your eye and the lid.
3. Hold the eyedrop bottle on your forehead or the bridge of your nose.
4. Do not touch the applicator tip to your eye or any other surface.
5. Tilt your head back and squeeze the medication into your eye.
6. Close your eyes gently and keep them closed for a minute or two.
7. Do not rinse the dropper.

■ *If you miss a dose...*
  Use this medication only as needed.
■ *Storage instructions...*
  Store at room temperature in a tightly closed bottle. Protect from light.

### What side effects may occur?

Naphcon is unlikely to cause side effects. However, overuse can cause reddening of the eyes.

### Why should this drug not be prescribed?

Do not take Naphcon-A if you have ever had an allergic reaction to it or are sensitive to any of its ingredients.

Do not use Naphcon-A if you have heart disease, high blood pressure, or trouble urinating because of enlargement of the prostate gland.

Do not use this medication if you have glaucoma.

### Special warnings about this medication

Contact your doctor before giving Naphcon-A to infants or children under 6 years of age. Swallowing this medication can cause stupor or coma and a serious drop in body temperature in an infant or child.

If your eyes hurt or continue to be red or irritated, if you experience changes in vision, if your eyes get worse, or if the itching and redness last more than 72 hours, stop using Naphcon-A and call your doctor.

### Recommended dosage

ADULTS

Place 1 or 2 drops in the affected eyes, up to 4 times a day.

### Overdosage

Overdose from accidental oral use can have serious consequences, especially in young children. If you suspect an overdose, seek medical attention immediately.

---

*Brand name:*

# Naprosyn

*Pronounced: NA-proh-sinn*
*Generic name: Naproxen*
*Other brand name: EC-Naprosyn*

### Why is this drug prescribed?

Naprosyn, a nonsteroidal anti-inflammatory drug, is used to relieve the inflammation, swelling, stiffness, and joint pain associated with rheumatoid arthritis, osteoarthritis (the most common form of arthritis), juvenile arthritis, ankylosing spondylitis (spinal arthritis), tendinitis, bursitis, and acute gout; it is also used to relieve menstrual cramps and other types of mild to moderate pain.

### Most important fact about this drug

You should have frequent checkups with your doctor if you take Naprosyn regularly. Ulcers or internal bleeding can occur without warning.

## How should you take this medication?

Naprosyn may be taken with food or an antacid, and with a full glass of water to avoid stomach upset. Avoid taking it on an empty stomach.

If you are using Naprosyn for arthritis, it should be taken regularly; take it exactly as prescribed.

Do not break, crush, or chew an EC-Naprosyn tablet.

■ *If you miss a dose...*

And you take the drug on a regular schedule, take the dose as soon as you remember. If it is almost time for your next dose, skip the one you missed and go back to your regular schedule. Do not take 2 doses at once.

■ *Storage instructions...*

Store at room temperature in a well-closed container. Protect from light and extreme heat.

## What side effects may occur?

Side effects cannot be anticipated. If any develop or change in intensity, inform your doctor as soon as possible. Only your doctor can determine if it is safe for you to continue taking Naprosyn.

■ *More common side effects may include:*

Abdominal pain, bruising, constipation, difficult or labored breathing, dizziness, drowsiness, headache, heartburn, indigestion, itching, nausea, ringing in ears, skin eruptions, swelling due to fluid retention

■ *Less common or rare side effects may include:*

Abdominal bleeding, black stools, blood in the urine, changes in liver function, chills and fever, colitis, congestive heart failure, depression, diarrhea, dream abnormalities, general feeling of illness, hair loss, hearing disturbances or loss, inability to concentrate, inability to sleep, inflammation of the lungs, inflammation of the mouth, kidney disease or failure, light-headedness, menstrual disorders, muscle pain and weakness, peptic ulcer, red or purple spots on the skin, severe allergic reaction, skin inflammation due to sensitivity to light, skin rashes and hives, sweating, thirst, throbbing heartbeat, vertigo, visual disturbances, vomiting, vomiting of blood, yellow skin and eyes

## Why should this drug not be prescribed?

If you are sensitive to or have ever had an allergic reaction to Naprosyn, EC-Naprosyn, Anaprox, Anaprox DS, or Aleve, you should not take this drug. Also, if aspirin or other nonsteroidal anti-inflammatory drugs have ever given you asthma or nasal inflammation or tumors, you should not take this medication. Make sure your doctor is aware of any drug reactions you have experienced.

## Special warnings about this medication

Remember that peptic ulcers and bleeding can occur without warning. Call your doctor immediately if you suspect a problem.

Use this drug with caution if you have kidney or liver disease; it can cause liver or kidney problems in some people.

Naprosyn may prolong bleeding time. If you are taking blood-thinning medication, your doctor will prescribe Naprosyn with caution.

By reducing fever and inflammation, Naprosyn may hide an underlying condition.

This medication may cause vision problems. If you experience any changes in your vision, inform your doctor.

This drug can increase water retention. It will be prescribed with caution if you have heart disease or high blood pressure. Naprosyn suspension contains a significant amount of sodium. If you are on a low-sodium diet, discuss this with your doctor.

Naprosyn may cause you to become drowsy or less alert; therefore, avoid driving, operating dangerous machinery, or participating in any hazardous activity that requires full mental alertness until you are sure of the drug's effect on you.

## Possible food and drug interactions when taking this medication

If Naprosyn is taken with certain other drugs, the effects of either could be increased, decreased, or altered. It is especially important to check with your doctor before combining Naprosyn with the following:

ACE inhibitors such as Capoten
Aspirin
Beta blockers such as Tenormin
Blood-thinning drugs such as Coumadin
Furosemide (Lasix)
Lithium (Lithonate)
Methotrexate
Naproxen sodium (Aleve, Anaprox)
Oral diabetes drugs such as Diabinese and
Micronase

Phenytoin (Dilantin)
Probenecid (Benemid)
Sulfa drugs such as Bactrim and Septra

EC-Naprosyn should not be used with antacids, $H_2$ blockers such as Tagamet, or sucralfate (Carafate).

### Special information
### if you are pregnant or breastfeeding

The effects of Naprosyn during pregnancy have not been adequately studied. If you are pregnant or plan to become pregnant, inform your doctor immediately. Naprosyn appears in breast milk and could affect a nursing infant. If this medication is essential to your health, your doctor may advise you to discontinue breastfeeding until your treatment with this medication is finished.

### Recommended dosage

Naprosyn is available in tablet and liquid form. When taking the liquid, use a teaspoon or the measuring cup, marked in one-half teaspoon and 2.5 milliliter increments, that comes with Naprosyn suspension.

#### ADULTS

*Rheumatoid Arthritis, Osteoarthritis, and Ankylosing Spondylitis*

The usual dose of Naprosyn is 250 milligrams (10 milliliters or 2 teaspoons of suspension), 375 milligrams (15 milliliters or 3 teaspoons), or 500 milligrams (20 milliliters or 4 teaspoons) 2 times a day (morning and evening). EC-Naprosyn is taken in doses of 375 or 500 milligrams twice a day. Your dose may be adjusted by your doctor over your period of treatment. Improvement of symptoms should be seen in 2 to 4 weeks.

*Acute Gout*

Starting dose of Naprosyn is 750 milligrams (30 milliliters or 6 teaspoons), followed by 250 milligrams (10 milliliters or 2 teaspoons) every 8 hours until the symptoms are relieved. EC-Naprosyn should not be used to treat gout.

*Mild to Moderate Pain, Menstrual Cramps, Acute Tendinitis and Bursitis*

Starting dose is 500 milligrams (20 milliliters or 4 teaspoons of suspension), followed by 250 milligrams (10 milliliters or 2 teaspoons) every 6 to 8 hours as needed. The most you should take in a day is 1,250 milligrams (50 milliliters or 10 teaspoons). Do not take EC-Naprosyn for these problems.

#### CHILDREN

*Juvenile Arthritis*

The usual daily dose is 10 milligrams per 2.2 pounds of body weight, divided into 2 doses. Follow your doctor's directions carefully when giving a child this medicine.

The safety and effectiveness of Naprosyn have not been established in children under 2 years of age.

#### OLDER ADULTS

Your doctor will probably have you take a reduced dose.

### Overdosage

Any medication taken in excess can have serious consequences. If you suspect an overdose, seek medical attention immediately.

■ *Symptoms of Naprosyn overdose may include:*
Drowsiness, heartburn, indigestion, nausea, vomiting

---

*Generic name:*

# Naproxen

*See Naprosyn, page 346.*

---

*Generic name:*

# Naproxen sodium

*See Anaprox, page 26.*

---

*Brand name:*

# Nardil

*Pronounced: NAHR-dill*
*Generic name: Phenelzine sulfate*

### Why is this drug prescribed?

Nardil is a monoamine oxidase (MAO) inhibitor used to treat depression as well as anxiety or phobias mixed with depression. MAO is an enzyme responsible for breaking down certain neurotransmitters (chemical messengers) in the brain. By inhibiting MAO, Nardil helps restore more normal mood states. Unfortunately, MAO inhibitors such as Nardil also block MAO activity throughout the body, an action that can have serious, even fatal, side effects—especially if MAO inhibitors are combined with other foods or drugs containing a substance called tyramine.

### Most important fact about this drug

Avoid the following foods, beverages, and medications while taking Nardil and for 2 weeks thereafter:

Beer (including alcohol-free or reduced-alcohol beer)
Caffeine (in excessive amounts)
Cheese (except for cottage cheese and cream cheese)
Chocolate (in excessive amounts)
Dry sausage (including Genoa salami, hard salami, pepperoni, and Lebanon bologna)
Fava bean pods
Liver
Meat extract
Pickled herring
Pickled, fermented, aged, or smoked meat, fish, or dairy products
Sauerkraut
Spoiled or improperly stored meat, fish, or dairy products
Wine (including alcohol-free or reduced-alcohol wine)
Yeast extract (including large amounts of brewer's yeast)
Yogurt

*Medications to avoid:*
   Amphetamines
   Appetite suppressants such as Tenuate
   Antidepressants and related medications such as Prozac, Elavil, Triavil, Tegretol, and Flexeril
   Asthma inhalants such as Proventil and Ventolin
   Cold and cough preparations including those with dextromethorphan, such as Robitussin DM
   Hay fever medications such as Contac and Dristan
   L-tryptophan-containing products
   Nasal decongestants in tablet, drop, or spray form such as Sudafed
   Sinus medications such as Sinutab

Taking Nardil with any of the above foods, beverages, or medications can cause serious, potentially fatal, high blood pressure. Therefore, when taking Nardil you should immediately report the occurrence of a headache, heart palpitations, or any other unusual symptom. In addition, make certain that you inform any other physician or dentist you see that you are currently taking Nardil or have taken Nardil within the last 2 weeks.

### How should you take this medication?

Nardil may be taken with or without food. Take it exactly as prescribed. It can take up to 4 weeks for the drug to begin working.

   Use of Nardil may complicate other medical treatment. Always carry a card that says you take Nardil, or wear a Medic Alert bracelet.

■ *If you miss a dose...*
   Take it as soon as you remember. If it is within 2 hours of your next dose, skip the one you missed and go back to your regular schedule. Do not take 2 doses at once.
■ *Storage instructions...*
   Store at room temperature.

### What side effects may occur?

Side effects cannot be anticipated. If any develop or change in intensity, inform your doctor as soon as possible. Only your doctor can determine if it is safe for you to continue taking Nardil.

■ *More common side effects may include:*
   Constipation, disorders of the stomach and intestines, dizziness, drowsiness, dry mouth, excessive sleeping, fatigue, headache, insomnia, low blood pressure (especially when rising quickly from lying down or sitting up), muscle spasms, sexual difficulties, strong reflexes, swelling due to fluid retention, tremors, twitching, weakness, weight gain
■ *Less common or rare side effects may include:*
   Anxiety, blurred vision, coma, convulsions, delirium, exaggerated feeling of well-being, fever, glaucoma, inability to urinate, involuntary eyeball movements, jitteriness, lack of coordination, liver damage, mania, muscular rigidity, onset of the mental disorder schizophrenia, rapid breathing, rapid heart rate, repetitive use of words and phrases, skin rash, sweating, swelling in the throat, tingling sensation, yellowed skin and whites of eyes

### Why should this drug not be prescribed?

You should not take this drug if you have pheochromocytoma (a tumor of the adrenal gland), congestive heart failure, or a history of liver disease, or if you have had an allergic reaction to it.

You should not take Nardil if you are taking medications that may increase blood pressure (such as amphetamines, cocaine, allergy and cold medications, or Ritalin), other MAO inhibitors, L-dopa, methyldopa (Aldomet), phenylalanine, L-tryptophan, L-tyrosine, fluoxetine (Prozac), buspirone (BuSpar), bupropion (Wellbutrin), guanethidine (Ismelin), meperidine (Demerol), dextromethorphan, or central nervous system depressants such as alcohol and narcotics; or if you must consume the foods, beverages, or medications listed above in the "Most important fact about this drug" section.

### Special warnings about this medication

You must follow the food and drug limitations established by your physician; failure to do so may lead to potentially fatal side effects. While taking Nardil, you should promptly report the occurrence of a headache or any other unusual symptoms.

If you are diabetic, your doctor will prescribe Nardil with caution, since it is not clear how MAO inhibitors affect blood sugar levels.

If you are taking Nardil, talk to your doctor before you decide to have elective surgery.

If you stop taking Nardil abruptly, you may have withdrawal symptoms. They may include nightmares, agitation, strange behavior, and convulsions.

### Possible food and drug interactions
### when taking this medication

If Nardil is taken with certain other drugs, the effects of either could be increased, decreased, or altered. It is important that you closely follow your doctor's dietary and medication limitations when taking Nardil. Consult the "Most important fact about this drug" and "Why should this drug not be prescribed?" sections for lists of the foods, beverages, and medications that should be avoided while taking Nardil.

In addition, you should use blood pressure medications (including diuretics and beta blockers) with caution when taking Nardil, since excessively low blood pressure may result. Symptoms of low blood pressure include dizziness when rising from a lying or sitting position, fainting, and tingling in the hands or feet.

### Special information
### if you are pregnant or breastfeeding

The effects of Nardil during pregnancy have not been adequately studied. Nardil should be used during pregnancy only if the benefits of therapy clearly outweigh the potential risks to the fetus. If you are pregnant or plan to become pregnant, inform your doctor immediately. Nursing mothers should use Nardil only after consulting their physician, since it is not known whether Nardil appears in human milk.

### Recommended dosage

ADULTS

The usual starting dose is 15 milligrams (1 tablet) 3 times a day. Your doctor may increase the dosage to 90 milligrams per day.

It may be 4 weeks before the drug starts to work.

Once you have had good results, your doctor may gradually reduce the dose, possibly to as low as 15 milligrams daily or every 2 days.

CHILDREN

Nardil is not recommended, since safety and efficacy for children under the age of 16 have not been determined.

### Overdosage

Any medication taken in excess can have serious consequences. An overdose of Nardil can be fatal. If you suspect an overdose, seek medical help immediately.

■ *Symptoms of overdose may include:*
Agitation, backward arching of the head, neck, and back, cool, clammy skin, coma, convulsions, difficult breathing, dizziness, drowsiness, faintness, hallucinations, high blood pressure, high fever, hyperactivity, irritability, jaw muscle spasms, low blood pressure, pain in the heart area, rapid and irregular pulse, rigidity, severe headache, sweating

*Brand name:*

# Nasacort

*See Azmacort, page 46.*

*Brand name:*

# Nasalcrom

*See Intal, page 261.*

Brand name:

# Nasalide

*See AeroBid, page 7.*

Brand name:

# Natalins Rx

*See Stuartnatal Plus, page 511.*

Brand name:

# Navane

Pronounced: NA-vain
Generic name: Thiothixene

### Why is this drug prescribed?

Navane is used to treat psychotic disorders (a severe sense of distorted reality). Researchers theorize that antipsychotic medications such as Navane work by lowering levels of dopamine, a neurotransmitter (or chemical messenger) in the brain. Excessive levels of dopamine are believed to be related to psychotic behavior.

### Most important fact about this drug

Navane may cause tardive dyskinesia—a condition marked by involuntary muscle spasms and twitches in the face and body. This condition can be permanent and appears to be most common among the elderly, especially women. Ask your doctor for information about this possible risk.

### How should you take this medication?

Navane may be taken in liquid or capsule form. In liquid form, a dropper is supplied.

■ *If you miss a dose...*
Take it as soon as you remember. If it is within 2 hours of your next dose, skip the one you missed and go back to your regular schedule. Do not take 2 doses at once.

■ *Storage instructions...*
Store at room temperature away from heat, light, and moisture. Keep the liquid form from freezing.

### What side effects may occur?

Side effects cannot be anticipated. If any develop or change in intensity, inform your doctor as soon as possible. Only your doctor can determine if it is safe for you to continue taking Navane.

■ *Side effects may include:*
Abnormal muscle rigidity, abnormal secretion of milk, abnormalities in movements and posture, agitation, anemia, blurred vision, breast development in males, chewing movements, constipation, diarrhea, dizziness, drowsiness, dry mouth, excessive thirst, eyeball rotation or state of fixed gaze, fainting, fatigue, fluid accumulation and swelling, headache, high fever, high or low blood sugar, hives, impotence, insomnia, intestinal blockage, involuntary movements of the arms and legs, irregular menstrual periods, itching, light-headedness, loss or increase of appetite, low blood pressure, narrow or dilated pupils of the eye, nasal congestion, nausea, painful muscle spasm, protruding tongue, puckering of mouth, puffing of cheeks, rapid heartbeat, rash, restlessness, salivation, sedation, seizures, sensitivity to light, severe allergic reaction, skin inflammation and peeling, strong reflexes, sweating, swelling of breasts, tremors, twitching in the body, neck, shoulders, and face, visual problems, vomiting, weakness, weight increase, worsening of psychotic symptoms

### Why should this drug not be prescribed?

Do not give Navane to comatose individuals. Do not take Navane if you are known to be hypersensitive to it. Also, you should not be using Navane if the activity of your central nervous system is slowed down for any reason—for example, by a sleeping medication, if you have had circulatory system collapse, or if you have an abnormal bone marrow or blood condition.

### Special warnings about this medication

Navane may hide symptoms of brain tumor and intestinal obstruction. Your doctor will prescribe Navane cautiously if you have or have ever had a brain tumor, breast cancer, convulsive disorders, the eye condition called glaucoma, intestinal blockage, or heart disease; or if you are exposed to extreme heat or are recovering from alcohol addiction.

This drug may impair your ability to drive a car or operate potentially dangerous machinery. Do not participate in any activities that require full alertness if you are unsure of your ability.

### Possible food and drug interactions when taking this medication

If Navane is taken with certain other drugs, the effects of either could be increased, decreased, or altered. It is especially important to check with your doctor before combining Navane with the following:

Antihistamines such as Benadryl
Barbiturates such as phenobarbital
Drugs that contain atropine, such as Donnatal

Extreme drowsiness and other potentially serious effects can result if Navane is combined with alcohol or other central nervous system depressants such as painkillers, narcotics, or sleeping medications.

### Special information
### if you are pregnant or breastfeeding
If you are pregnant or plan to become pregnant, inform your doctor immediately; pregnant women should use Navane only if clearly needed. Consult your doctor if you are breastfeeding; he or she may have you stop while you are taking Navane.

### Recommended dosage
Dosages of Navane are tailored to the individual. Usually treatment begins with a small dose, which is increased if needed.

ADULTS

*For Milder Conditions*
The usual starting dosage is a daily total of 6 milligrams, divided into doses of 2 milligrams and taken 3 times a day. Your doctor may increase the dose to a total of 15 milligrams a day.

*For More Severe Conditions*
The usual starting dosage is a daily total of 10 milligrams, taken in 2 doses of 5 milligrams each. Your doctor may increase this dose to a total of 60 milligrams a day.

Taking more than 60 milligrams a day rarely increases the benefits of Navane.

Some people are able to take Navane once a day. Check with your doctor to see whether you can follow this schedule.

CHILDREN

Navane is not recommended for children younger than 12 years old.

OLDER ADULTS

In general, older adults are prescribed dosages of Navane in the lower ranges. Because older adults may develop low blood pressure while taking Navane, their doctors will monitor them closely.

Older adults (especially women) may be more susceptible to such side effects as involuntary muscle spasms and twitches in the face and body. Check with your doctor for more information about these potential risks.

### Overdosage
Any medication taken in excess can have serious consequences. If you suspect an overdose, seek medical help immediately.

■ *Symptoms of Navane overdose may include:*
Central nervous system depression, coma, difficulty swallowing, dizziness, drowsiness, head tilted to the side, low blood pressure, muscle twitching, rigid muscles, salivation, tremors, walking disturbances, weakness

---

*Generic name:*

# Nedocromil

*See Tilade, page 545.*

---

*Generic name:*

# Nefazodone

*See Serzone, page 497.*

---

*Brand name:*

# Neodecadron Ophthalmic Ointment and Solution

*Pronounced: Nee-oh-DECK-uh-drohn*
*Generic ingredients: Dexamethasone sodium phosphate, Neomycin sulfate*

### Why is this drug prescribed?
Neodecadron is a steroid and antibiotic combination that is used to treat inflammatory eye conditions in which there is also a bacterial infection or the possibility of a bacterial infection. Dexamethasone (the steroid) decreases inflammation. Neomycin, the antibiotic, kills some of the more common bacteria.

### Most important fact about this drug
The prolonged use of Neodecadron may increase the possibility of developing additional eye infections. It could also cause vision problems or even

result in glaucoma and cataracts. If you take this medication for 10 days or longer, your doctor will routinely check your eye pressure.

## How should you use this medication?
*Neodecadron Ophthalmic Solution*
1. Wash your hands thoroughly before use.
2. Tilt your head backward or lie down and gaze upward.
3. Gently pull the lower eyelid away from the eye to form a pouch.
4. Drop the medicine in the pouch and gently close your eyes. Try not to blink.
5. Keep your eye closed for a couple of minutes. Do not rub the eye.
6. Do not touch the applicator tip or dropper to any surface (including the eye).

*Neodecadron Ophthalmic Ointment*
1. Wash your hands thoroughly before use.
2. Hold the ointment tube in your hand for a few minutes to warm the ointment and make it flow more smoothly.
3. Tilt your head backward or lie down and gaze upward.
4. Gently pull the lower eyelid away from the eye to form a pouch.
5. Squeeze the tube gently, and with a sweeping motion along the inside of the lower lid, apply 0.25 to 0.5 inch of ointment.
6. Close your eyes for a couple of minutes and roll them in all directions.

■ *If you miss a dose...*
Take the forgotten dose as soon as you remember. If it is almost time for the next dose, skip the one you missed and go back to your regular schedule. Never try to "catch up" by doubling the dose.

■ *Storage instructions...*
Store at room temperature. Protect solution from light.

## What side effects may occur?
Side effects cannot be anticipated. If any develop or change in intensity, notify your doctor as soon as possible. Only your doctor can determine whether it is safe to continue using Neodecadron.

■ *Side effects may include:*
Allergic skin reactions, cataracts, delay in healing of wounds, development of additional eye infections, increased eye pressure with possible glaucoma and optic nerve damage

## Why should this drug not be prescribed?
Neodecadron should be avoided if you have an inflammation of the cornea (the transparent surface of the eye); chickenpox; or other bacterial, fungal, or viral eye infections. Do not use Neodecadron if you have ever had an allergic reaction or are sensitive to any of its ingredients.

Neodecadron solution contains a sulfite that can cause an allergic reaction in susceptible people.

## Special warnings about this medication
Neodecadron is absorbed into your bloodstream when applied to your eye. Its steroid component can lower your resistance to infection and it can prolong or worsen the severity of many viral infections of the eye. Diseases such as measles and chickenpox can be serious and even fatal in adults. If you are using Neodecadron and are exposed to chickenpox or measles, notify your doctor immediately.

Using Neodecadron for a long time may result in increased pressure in the eye, including glaucoma, as well as vision changes and cataracts. Long-term use also increases the chances of developing an additional eye infection. If you use Neodecadron for 10 days or longer, your doctor should check your eye pressure regularly.

If you have high pressure in your eyes, your doctor will watch you closely and check your pressure frequently.

Eye medications can become contaminated if they are not used properly, causing dangerous infections. Do not let the tip of the container touch anything. If your eyes continue to be red, irritated, swollen, or painful, or if they get worse, notify your doctor immediately.

A preservative in Neodecadron solution can be absorbed by soft contact lenses. If you wear contacts, wait at least 15 minutes after using the solution before you insert your lenses.

If you develop a skin rash or any other allergic reaction, stop using the medication and contact your doctor.

If you have had cataract surgery, Neodecadron may delay healing.

Neodecadron may cause temporary blurring of vision or stinging.

This prescription should not be renewed unless your doctor has re-examined your eyes.

If your signs and symptoms have not improved after two days, your doctor will reconsider your treatment.

### Possible food and drug interactions when taking this medication
No interactions have been reported.

### Special information if you are pregnant or breastfeeding
Neodecadron has not been adequately studied during pregnancy. If you are pregnant or plan to become pregnant, inform your doctor immediately. Steroids can appear in breast milk. Your doctor may advise you not to breastfeed while you are using Neodecadron.

### Recommended dosage
The length of treatment varies with the type of condition being treated. Treatment can take a few days or several weeks.

NEODECADRON OPHTHALMIC OINTMENT

Apply a thin coating of Neodecadron Ophthalmic Ointment 3 or 4 times a day. When the condition gets better, daily applications should be reduced to 2 and later to 1 if a maintenance dose is required to control the symptoms.

NEODECADRON OPHTHALMIC SOLUTION

The recommended initial dose is to place 1 or 2 drops into the conjunctival sac every hour during the day and every 2 hours during the night. When your condition improves, the doctor will lower the dose to 1 drop every 4 hours, and then to 1 drop 3 or 4 times a day.

### Overdosage
Any medication taken in excess can have serious consequences. If you suspect a Neodecadron overdose, seek medical treatment immediately.

*Brand name:*

# Neoral

*See Sandimmune, page 486.*

*Brand name:*

# Neptazane

*Pronounced: NEP-tuh-zayne*
*Generic name: Methazolamide*

### Why is this drug prescribed?
Neptazane, anhydrase is used to treat the eye condition called chronic open-angle glaucoma. This type of glaucoma is caused by a gradual blockage of the outflow of fluid in the front compartment of the eye over a period of years, causing a slow rise in pressure. It rarely occurs before the age of 40. Neptazane is also used in the type called acute angle-closure glaucoma when pressure within the eye must be lowered before surgery.

### Most important fact about this drug
This medication is related to sulfa drugs and can cause allergic reactions, including fever, rash, redness and peeling of the skin, hives, difficulty breathing, serious skin and blood disorders, and even death. Make sure your doctor is aware of any drug reactions you have experienced. He or she should monitor your blood while you are taking this drug. Call your doctor immediately if you experience any allergic symptoms.

### How should you take this medication?
Take Neptazane exactly as prescribed. Your doctor may have you use it with other eye medications.

■ *If you miss a dose...*
Take it as soon as you remember. If it is almost time for your next dose, skip the one you missed and go back to your regular schedule. Do not take 2 doses at once.
■ *Storage instructions...*
Store at room temperature.

### What side effects may occur?
Side effects cannot be anticipated. If any occur or change in intensity, inform your doctor as soon as possible. Only your doctor can determine if it is safe for you to continue taking Neptazane. Most reactions to Neptazane have been mild and disappear when the medication is stopped or the dosage is adjusted.

■ *More common side effects may include:*
Confusion, depression, diarrhea, dizziness, drowsiness, excessive urination, fatigue, fever, general feeling of not being well, headache,

hearing problems, loss of appetite, nausea and vomiting, rash, ringing in the ears, severe allergic reaction, taste changes, temporary nearsightedness, tingling in fingers, toes, hands, or feet

■ *Rare side effects may include:*
Black, tarry stools, blood in the urine, convulsions, hives, increased sensitivity to light, kidney stones, paralysis

### Why should this drug not be prescribed?

Neptazane is not for use against all types of glaucoma—only the ones mentioned in "Why is this drug prescribed?" Also, you should not use Neptazane if you have kidney or liver disease, adrenal gland disorders, or low sodium or potassium levels.

### Special warnings about this medication

Neptazane can aggravate acidosis, a condition in which the blood is too acidic.

If you have emphysema or a lung blockage, this drug will be prescribed cautiously.

### Possible food and drug interactions when taking this medication

If Neptazane is taken with certain other drugs, the effects of either could be increased, decreased, or altered.

Neptazane and high-dose aspirin taken at the same time can cause loss of appetite, rapid breathing, lethargy, coma, and even death.

Use of Neptazane with steroids may lower your potassium level.

### Special information if you are pregnant or breastfeeding

The effects of Neptazane in pregnancy have not been adequately studied. Neptazane should be used by a pregnant woman only if the potential benefit outweighs the potential risk to the developing baby. If you are pregnant or plan to become pregnant, inform your doctor immediately. Neptazane may appear in breast milk and could affect a nursing infant. If this medication is essential to your health, your doctor may advise you to stop breastfeeding until your treatment with Neptazane is finished.

### Recommended dosage

ADULTS

The usual dosage is 50 milligrams to 100 milligrams taken 2 to 3 times a day.

### Overdosage

Any drug taken in excess can have serious consequences. If you suspect an overdose of Neptazane, seek medical attention immediately.

*Brand name:*

# Neurontin

*Pronounced: NUHR-on-tin*
*Generic name: Gabapentin*

### Why is this drug prescribed?

Neurontin, an epilepsy medication, is used with other medications to treat certain types of difficult to manage seizures, including elementary partial seizures (brief and no loss of consciousness) and complex partial seizures (consciousness impaired), with and without secondary generalization (grand mal epilepsy with loss of consciousness).

### Most important fact about this drug

Take Neurontin exactly as directed by your doctor. To effectively control your seizures, it is important that you take Neurontin 3 times a day, approximately every 8 hours. You should not go longer than 12 hours without a dose of medication.

### How should you take this medication?

Do not increase or decrease dosage of this medication without your doctor's approval; and do not suddenly stop taking it, as this may cause an increase in the frequency of your seizures. If you are taking an antacid such as Maalox, take Neurontin at least 2 hours after the antacid.

You may take Neurontin with or without food.

■ *If you miss a dose...*
Try not to allow more than 12 hours to pass between doses. Do not double doses.
■ *Storage instructions...*
Store at room temperature.

### What side effects may occur?

Side effects cannot be anticipated. If any develop or change in intensity, inform your doctor as soon as possible. Because Neurontin is used with other anti-seizure drugs, it may not be possible to determine whether a side effect is due to Neurontin alone. Only your doctor can determine if it is safe for you to continue taking Neurontin.

■ *More common side effects may include:*
Blurred, dimmed, or double vision, dizziness, drowsiness, fatigue, involuntary eye movement, itchy, runny nose, lack of muscular coordination, nausea, tremor, vomiting

■ *Less common or rare side effects may include:*
Abnormal coordination, abnormal dreams, abnormal thinking, agitation, allergy, altered reflexes, anemia, angina pectoris (crushing chest pain), anxiety, apathy, arthritis, back pain, behavioral or psychological problems, bladder problems, bleeding gums, bloody stools, bruising, cataracts, chill, conjunctivitis (pinkeye), constipation, cough, cysts, decreased sensitivity to touch, depression, difficult or labored breathing, dry eyes, dry mouth or throat, dry or scaly skin, ear problems, exaggerated feeling of well-being, excessive body hair, eye pain or disorder, fainting, feeling "high", "fever" blisters on lips and mouth, fluid retention, fracture, gas, general feeling of illness, hair loss, hallucination, heart murmur, heartburn, hemorrhoids, high blood pressure, hostility, hyperactivity, increased appetite, increased salivation, increased sweating, indigestion, inflammation of the mouth, gums, or tongue, inflammation of the stomach and intestinal lining, irregular heartbeat, itching, joint pain, stiffness, or swelling, liver enlargement, loss of appetite, loss of bowel control, loss of memory, low blood pressure, menstrual problems, migraines, mouth sores, muscle pain or weakness, nervousness, nosebleeds, paralysis, pneumonia, sexual problems, shortness of breath, skin disorders, sore throat, speech difficulties, stupor, swelling of the face, taste loss, tendinitis, thirst, tingling or pins and needles, twitching, vaginal hemorrhage, vertigo, weight increase or decrease

## Why should this drug not be prescribed?

You should not take Neurontin if you have ever had an allergic reaction to it.

## Special warnings about this medication

Neurontin causes some people to become drowsy and less alert. Do not drive or operate dangerous machinery or participate in any hazardous activity that requires full mental alertness until you are certain Neurontin does not have this effect on you.

Be sure to tell your doctor if you have any kidney problems or are on hemodialysis, as your doctor will need to adjust your dosage of Neurontin.

Tell your doctor about any medications you are taking, including over-the-counter drugs.

## Possible food and drug interactions when taking this medication

If Neurontin is taken with certain other drugs, the effects of either can be increased, decreased, or altered. It is especially important to check with your doctor before combining Neurontin with the following:

Antacids such as Maalox

## Special information if you are pregnant or breastfeeding

The effects of Neurontin on pregnant women have not been adequately studied, although birth defects have occurred in babies whose mothers took an antiepileptic drug while they were pregnant. It should be used during pregnancy only if clearly needed. If you are pregnant or plan to become pregnant, tell your doctor immediately. This medication may appear in breast milk and could affect a nursing infant. Check with your doctor if you plan to breastfeed your baby.

## Recommended dosage

ADULTS AND CHILDREN 12 YEARS AND OVER

Your doctor will probably start your therapy with one 300-milligram dose at bedtime on the first day, two 300-milligram doses the second day, and three 300-milligram doses the third day. After that, the usual daily dosage ranges from 900 to 1,800 milligrams divided into 3 doses, using 300-milligram or 400-milligram capsules.

If Neurontin is discontinued or another drug added to therapy, your doctor will do this gradually, over a 1-week period.

## Overdosage

Any medication taken in excess can have serious consequences. If you suspect an overdose, seek medical treatment immediately.

■ *Symptoms of Neurontin overdose may include:*
Diarrhea, double vision, drowsiness, lethargy, slurred speech

*Generic name:*

# Nicardipine

See Cardene, page 78.

*Brand name:*

# Nicoderm

See Nicotine Patches, page 359.

*Brand name:*

# Nicorette

*Pronounced: Nik-ho-RET*
*Generic name: Nicotine polacrilex*

## Why is this drug prescribed?

Nicorette and Nicorette DS (double strength) chewing gums are used as a temporary aid by cigarette smokers who want to stop. Used as directed, Nicorette reduces withdrawal symptoms such as nicotine craving. The gum is available without a prescription.

Nicorette is most effective when used in a medically supervised behavior modification program offering education, counseling, and psychological support.

## Most important fact about this drug

Nicorette contains nicotine—an addicting and toxic substance. Nicorette is a powerful, potentially addicting medication that must be used according to your doctor's instructions.

## How should you take this medication?

The following are general, medically approved guidelines for taking Nicorette. Consult the Nicorette package for further information.

1) You must give up smoking completely and immediately when you start using Nicorette.
2) When you want to smoke, put 1 piece of Nicorette in your mouth.
3) Chew Nicorette very slowly; chewing Nicorette too fast may release the nicotine in the product too quickly, causing the same effects as inhaling for the first time or smoking too fast (lightheadedness, nausea, vomiting, throat and mouth soreness, hiccups, and upset stomach).

4) Stop chewing when you get a peppery taste or feel a slight tingling in your mouth. This usually happens after about 15 chews.
5) "Park" the gum by placing it between your cheek and gums.
6) Start slowly chewing again when the peppery taste or tingling feeling is almost gone (about 1 minute). Stop chewing when the peppery taste or tingling returns.
7) "Park" the gum again in a different part of the mouth.
8) Repeat this procedure until most of the nicotine is gone from the gum (about 30 minutes).
9) Do not use more than 30 pieces of Nicorette or 20 pieces of Nicorette DS a day.
10) As your urge to smoke fades, gradually use fewer pieces of Nicorette. This may be possible in 2 to 3 months.
11) Stop using Nicorette when you are satisfied with 1 or 2 pieces a day, unless your doctor tells you otherwise. If you have trouble reducing your use of Nicorette, contact your doctor. Do not use Nicorette for more than 6 months.
12) Carry Nicorette with you at all times in case you feel the urge to smoke again.

The effects of Nicorette may be reduced by many foods or drinks such as coffee, juices, wine or soft drinks. Do not eat or drink 15 minutes before or while chewing Nicorette.

■ *If you miss a dose...*
With Nicorette, the goal is to take as few doses as possible. Don't make up a missed dose, and never double the dose.

■ *Storage instructions...*
Keep Nicorette below 86 degrees. (Remember, the inside of a parked car can get much hotter than this.) Protect the chewing pieces from light.

## What side effects may occur?

Side effects cannot be anticipated. If any develop or change in intensity, inform your doctor as soon as possible. Only your doctor can determine if it is safe for you to continue taking this medication.

■ *More common side effects may include:*
Bleeding gums, excessive saliva in mouth, hiccups, indigestion, inflammation of the mouth, injury to teeth or cheeks, nausea, stomach and intestinal discomfort, throat soreness, tingling or pins and needles

■ *Less common or rare side effects may include:*
Diarrhea, dry mouth, inflammation of the gums, tongue, throat, mouth sores, muscle pain, rash, sweating, tongue sores

### Why should this drug not be prescribed?
Do not smoke, chew tobacco, or use snuff powder while using Nicorette. Never use Nicorette and nicotine patches at the same time.

### Special warnings about this medication
Using Nicorette on a long-term basis is not recommended because nicotine, if consumed for a long enough time, can be harmful and addicting.

You must chew Nicorette slowly to avoid side effects and addiction.

If you develop an allergic reaction such as hives or rash, stop using Nicorette and contact your doctor.

Check with your doctor before using Nicorette if you have heart disease or an irregular heartbeat, or have recently had a heart attack. Check first, too, if you have uncontrolled high blood pressure, a stomach ulcer, or diabetes, and if you are taking prescription drugs for asthma or depression.

Nicorette may stick to dentures; if this becomes a problem, stop chewing Nicorette and tell your doctor.

### Possible food and drug interactions when taking this medication
If Nicorette is taken with certain other drugs, the effects of either could be increased, decreased, or altered. It is especially important to check with your doctor before combining Nicorette with the following:

Acetaminophen (Tylenol)
Caffeine
Furosemide (Lasix)
Glutethimide
Imipramine (Tofranil)
Insulin
Isoproterenol (Isuprel)
Labetalol (Normodyne)
Oxazepam (Serax)
Pentazocine (Talwin)
Phenacetin, the pain and fever reducer
Phenylephrine (Entex)
Prazosin (Minipress)
Propoxyphene (Darvon)
Propranolol (Inderal)
Theophylline (Theo-Dur)

### Special information if you are pregnant or breastfeeding
If you are pregnant or nursing your baby, you should not use Nicorette. If you become pregnant while using Nicorette, contact your doctor immediately.

Nicotine, either from smoking or from chewing Nicorette, does appear in breast milk and can affect the baby.

### Recommended dosage
ADULTS

Follow package instructions carefully. Chew 1 piece of Nicorette every 1 to 2 hours. Most adults require 9 to 12 pieces of Nicorette a day during the first month of treatment. Do not use more than 30 pieces of Nicorette or 20 pieces of Nicorette DS per day. After 2 to 3 months, follow your doctor's plan for gradual withdrawal of Nicorette.

Gradual withdrawal of Nicorette is recommended to avoid the return of symptoms that may lead you to start smoking again. Suggested procedures are as follows:

1. Decrease the total number of pieces of Nicorette used per day by 1 or more pieces every 4-7 days.
2. Decrease the chewing time with each piece of Nicorette from the normal 30 minutes to 10 to 15 minutes. Then gradually decrease the total number of pieces used per day. You can also chew each piece longer than 30 minutes and cut down the number of pieces you chew a day.
3. Substitute 1 or more pieces of sugarless gum for an equal number of pieces of Nicorette. Increase the number of pieces of sugarless gum substituted for Nicorette every 4 to 7 days.

CHILDREN

Safety and effectiveness for children and adolescents who smoke have not been established. Adolescents under 18 years of age should check with their doctor before using Nicorette. If a child swallows a piece of Nicorette accidentally, contact your doctor or local poison control center immediately.

OLDER ADULTS

Use Nicorette cautiously.

### Overdosage
Any medication taken in excess can have serious consequences. Overdose may occur if you chew

many pieces of Nicorette at one time or in rapid succession, or if you smoke while you are using Nicorette. Accidentally swallowing a piece of Nicorette will probably not cause side effects, but if you have any reason to suspect an overdose, seek medical help immediately.

- *Symptoms of Nicorette overdose are similar to symptoms of acute nicotine poisoning and may include:*
  Abdominal pain, blurred vision, cold sweat, diarrhea, difficulty breathing, disturbed hearing, dizziness, exhaustion, fainting, headache, low blood pressure, mental confusion, nausea, paleness, rapid and irregular pulse, salivation, tremor, upset stomach, vomiting, weakness

A large overdose can result in prostration and respiratory failure.

*Category:*
# Nicotine Patches

*Brand names: Habitrol, Nicoderm, Nicotrol, ProStep*

### Why is this drug prescribed?
Nicotine patches, which are available under several brand names, are designed to help you quit smoking by reducing your craving for tobacco. Each adhesive patch contains a specific amount of nicotine embedded in a pad or gel.

Nicotine, the habit-forming ingredient in tobacco, is a stimulant and a mood lifter. When you give up smoking, lack of nicotine makes you crave cigarettes and may also cause anger, anxiety, concentration problems, irritability, frustration, or restlessness.

When you wear a nicotine patch, a specific amount of nicotine steadily travels out of the patch, through your skin, and into your bloodstream, keeping a constant low level of nicotine in your body. Although the resulting level of nicotine is less than you would get from smoking, it may be enough to keep you from craving cigarettes or experiencing other withdrawal symptoms.

Habitrol patches are round and come in three strengths: 21, 14, or 7 milligrams of nicotine per patch. You wear a Habitrol patch 24 hours a day.

Nicoderm patches are rectangular and come in three strengths: 21, 14, or 7 milligrams of nicotine per patch. You wear a Nicoderm patch 24 hours a day.

Nicotrol patches are rectangular and come in three strengths: 15, 10, or 5 milligrams of nicotine per patch. You put on a Nicotrol patch in the morning, wear it all day, and remove it at bedtime. You do not use it when you sleep.

ProStep patches are round and come in two strengths: 22 or 11 milligrams of nicotine per patch. You wear a Prostep patch 24 hours a day.

### Most important fact about this drug
Nicotine patch therapy should be part of an overall stop-smoking program that also includes behavior modification, counseling, and support. The goal of the therapy should be complete cessation of smoking, not just "cutting down."

### How should you use this medication?
Use nicotine patches exactly as prescribed. The general procedure is as follows:

- Take a fresh patch out of its packaging and remove the protective liner from the adhesive. Save the wrapper for later disposal of the used patch.
- Stick the patch onto your outer upper arm or any clean, non-hairy part of your trunk.
- Press the patch firmly onto your skin for about 10 seconds, making sure that the edges are sticking well.
- Wash your hands. Any nicotine sticking to your hands could get into your eyes or nose, causing irritation.
- After 16 or 24 hours (depending on the brand), remove that patch and apply a fresh patch to a different spot on your body. To reduce the chances of irritation, do not return to a previously used spot for at least a week.
- Fold the used patch in half, place it back in its own wrapper, and throw it in a trash container that cannot be reached by children or pets.

Water will not harm the nicotine patch. You may keep wearing your patch while bathing, showering, swimming, or using a hot tub.

If your patch does fall off, dispose of it carefully and apply a new patch.

As a memory aid, pick a specific time of day and always apply a fresh patch at that time. You may change the schedule if you need to. Just remember not to wear any single patch for more than the recommended time (16 or 24 hours), since after that time the patch will begin to lose strength and may begin to irritate your skin.

Do not change brands without consulting your doctor.

If you are unable to stop smoking by your fourth week of wearing nicotine patches, it is likely that patch treatment will not work for you. At this point, your doctor may stop prescribing the patches for you.

■ *If you miss a dose...*
Apply the patch as soon as you remember. Never use 2 patches at once.
■ *Storage instructions...*
Do not remove a patch from its wrapping until you are ready to use it. Store your supply of patches at temperatures no higher than 86 degrees Fahrenheit; remember that in warm weather the inside of a car can get much hotter than this.

## What side effects may occur?

Side effects cannot be anticipated. If any develop or change in intensity, inform your doctor as soon as possible. Only your doctor can determine if it is safe for you to continue using nicotine patches.

■ *Most common side effects may include:*
Itching and burning at the application site, rash, redness of the skin
■ *Less common side effects may include:*
Abnormal dreaming, allergic reactions, back pain, chest pain, constipation, cough, diarrhea, dizziness, drowsiness, dry mouth, headache, high blood pressure, impaired concentration, indigestion, inflammation of sinuses, menstrual irregularities, nausea, nervousness, numbness, pain, pins and needles sensation, sleeplessness, sore throat, stomach pain, sweating, taste changes, tingling, vomiting, weakness

## Why should this drug not be prescribed?

Do not take this medication if you are sensitive to or have ever had an allergic reaction to nicotine. Be cautious if you have ever had a bad reaction to a different brand of nicotine patch or to adhesive tape or other adhesive material.

## Special warnings about this medication

Do not smoke any form of tobacco while wearing a patch; doing so could give you an overdose of nicotine. Be aware that for several hours after you remove a patch, nicotine from the patch is still in your skin and passing into your bloodstream.

The use of nicotine patches may aggravate certain medical conditions. Before you use any brand of nicotine patch, make sure your doctor knows if you have, or have ever had, any of the following conditions:

Allergies to drugs, adhesive tape, or bandages
Chest pain from a heart condition (angina)
Diabetes requiring insulin injections
Heart attack
High blood pressure (severe)
Irregular heartbeat (heart arrhythmia)
Kidney disease
Liver disease
Overactive thyroid
Skin disease
Stomach ulcer

Nicotine, from any source, can be toxic and addictive. Thoroughly discuss with your doctor the benefits and risks of nicotine replacement therapy.

Because a used nicotine patch still contains enough nicotine to poison a child or a pet, you must dispose of used patches with special care. Wrap each patch in the opened pouch or aluminum foil in which it came and throw it in a trash receptacle that is out of the reach of youngsters and animals.

## Possible food and drug interactions when taking this medication

If nicotine patches are used with certain other drugs, the effects of either could be increased, decreased, or altered. It is especially important to check with your doctor before combining nicotine patches with the following:

Acetaminophen-containing drugs such as Tylenol
Caffeine-containing drugs such as No Doz
Certain airway-opening drugs such as Isuprel, Dristan, and Neo-Synephrine
Certain blood pressure medicines such as Minipress, Trandate, and Normodyne
Cimetidine (Tagamet)
Haloperidol (Haldol)
Imipramine (Tofranil)
Insulin

Lithium (Lithonate)
Oxazepam (Serax)
Pentazocine (Talwin)
Propranolol (Inderal)
Theophylline (Theo-Dur)

## Special information
## if you are pregnant or breastfeeding

If you are pregnant or plan to become pregnant, inform your doctor immediately. Ideally, a pregnant woman should not take nicotine in any form. Do your best to quit smoking with the aid of counseling and support and without drug therapy. If you are unable to quit, you and your doctor should discuss which is more likely to harm your unborn baby: continued smoking or use of nicotine patches to help you quit smoking. Because nicotine passes very readily into breast milk, ideally it should not be taken in any form during breastfeeding. If you are breastfeeding and are unable to quit smoking, discuss with your doctor the pros and cons of using nicotine patches.

Remember that if you smoke while wearing a patch, you are giving your body a "double dose" of nicotine; if you are pregnant or breastfeeding, your baby will get the "double dose", too.

## Recommended dosage

Nicotine patches come in two or three strengths, depending on the brand; larger patches contain higher doses of nicotine. The usual starting dose is 1 high-strength patch per day. If you weigh less than 100 pounds, however, or if you smoke less than half a pack of cigarettes a day or have heart disease, your doctor may start you on a lower-dose patch.

Your doctor will work closely with you to determine the best product and the most effective cessation program.

## Overdosage

Any medication used in excess, including nicotine patches, can have serious consequences. If you suspect symptoms of an overdose of nicotine, either from a patch or from smoking while wearing a patch, seek medical attention immediately.

■ *Symptoms of nicotine overdose may include:*
Abdominal pain, blurred vision, breathing abnormalities, cold sweat, confusion, diarrhea, dizziness, drooling, fainting, hearing difficulties, heart palpitations, low blood pressure, nausea, pallor, salivation, severe headaches, sweating, tremor, upset stomach, vision problems, vomiting, weakness

*Generic name:*

# Nicotine polacrilex

*See Nicorette, page 357.*

*Brand name:*

# Nicotrol

*See Nicotine Patches, page 359.*

*Generic name:*

# Nifedipine

*See Procardia, page 438.*

*Brand name:*

# Nitro-Bid

*See Nitroglycerin, page 361.*

*Brand name:*

# Nitro-Dur

*See Nitroglycerin, page 361.*

*Generic name:*

# Nitrofurantoin

*See Macrodantin, page 305.*

*Generic name:*

# Nitroglycerin

*Pronounced: NIGHT-row-GLISS-err-in*
*Brand names: Nitro-Bid, Nitro-Dur, Nitrolingual*
*Spray, Nitrostat Tablets, Transderm-Nitro*

## Why is this drug prescribed?

Nitroglycerin is prescribed to prevent and treat angina pectoris (suffocating chest pain). This condition occurs when the arteries and veins become constricted and are not able to carry sufficient oxygen to the heart. Nitroglycerin is thought to improve oxygen flow by relaxing the muscles of arteries and veins, thus allowing them to dilate.

Nitroglycerin is used in different forms. As a patch or ointment, nitroglycerin may be applied to the skin. The patch and the ointment are for *prevention* of chest pain.

Swallowing nitroglycerin in capsule or tablet form also helps to *prevent* chest pain from occurring.

In the form of sublingual (held under the tongue) or buccal (held in the cheek) tablets, or in oral spray (sprayed on or under the tongue), nitroglycerin helps relieve chest pain that has *already occurred*. The spray can also prevent anginal pain. The type of nitroglycerin you use will depend on your condition.

## Most important fact about this drug

Nitroglycerin may cause severe low blood pressure (possibly marked by dizziness or light-headedness), especially if you are in an upright position or have just gotten up from sitting or lying down. You may also find your heart rate slowing and your chest pain increasing. People taking diuretic medication, or who have low systolic blood pressure (less than 90 mm Hg) should use nitroglycerin with caution.

## How should you take this medication?

Since nitroglycerin is available in many forms, it is crucial for you to follow your doctor's directions for taking the type of nitroglycerin prescribed for you. Never interchange brands.

Ideally, you should take nitroglycerin while sitting down—especially if you feel dizzy or light-headed—so as to avoid a fall.

■ *If you miss a dose...*
If you are using a skin patch or ointment:

Apply it as soon as you remember. If it is almost time for your regular dose, skip the one you missed and go back to your regular schedule. Never apply 2 skin patches at the same time.

If you are taking oral tablets or capsules:

Take the forgotten dose as soon as you remember. However, if it is within 2 hours of your next dose, skip the one you missed and go back to your regular schedule. Never take 2 doses at the same time.

■ *Storage instructions...*
Keep this medication in the container it came in, tightly closed. Store it at room temperature. Do not refrigerate.

Avoid puncturing the spray container and keep it away from excess heat.

Do not open the container of sublingual tablets until you need a dose. Close the container tightly immediately after each use. Do not put other medications, a cotton plug, or anything else in the container. Keep the sublingual tablets handy at all times. Keep the patches in the protective pouches they come in until use.

## What side effects may occur?

Side effects cannot be anticipated. If any develop or change in intensity, inform your doctor as soon as possible. Only your doctor can determine if it is safe for you to continue taking nitroglycerin.

■ *More common side effects may include:*
Dizziness, flushed skin (neck and face), headache, light-headedness, worsened angina pain
■ *Less common or rare side effects may include:*
Diarrhea, fainting, heart pounding, low blood pressure, nausea, numbness, pallor, restlessness, severe allergic reactions, skin rashes and eruptions, sweating, vertigo, vomiting, weakness

## Why should this drug not be prescribed?

You should not be using nitroglycerin if you are allergic to it or to the adhesive in the patch, if you have a head injury, or if you have any condition caused by increased fluid pressure in your head. Nitroglycerin should not be taken if you have severe anemia or if you recently had a heart attack. The capsule form should not be used if you have closed-angle glaucoma (pressure in the eye) or suffer from postural hypotension (dizziness upon standing up).

## Special warnings about this medication

If your vision becomes blurry or your mouth becomes dry while taking nitroglycerin, it should be discontinued. Contact your doctor immediately if these symptoms develop.

You may develop acute headaches if you take nitroglycerin excessively. Also, some people may develop a tolerance to nitroglycerin, and it may become less beneficial over time, especially if used in excess.

Take no more than the smallest possible amount needed to relieve pain.

Daily headaches may be an indicator of the drug's activity. Do not change your dose to avoid the headache, because you may reduce the drug's effectiveness at the same time.

Before taking nitroglycerin, tell your doctor if you have had a recent heart attack, head injury, or stroke; or if you have anemia, glaucoma (pressure in the eye), or heart, kidney, liver, or thyroid disease.

If you use a patch, dispose of it carefully. There is enough drug left in a used patch to be harmful to children and pets.

Since nitroglycerin can cause dizziness, you should observe caution while driving, operating machinery, or performing other tasks that demand concentration.

The benefits of applying nitroglycerin to the skin of people experiencing heart attacks or congestive heart failure have not been established. If you are using the medication for these conditions, your doctor will monitor you to prevent low blood pressure and pounding heartbeat.

## Possible food and drug interactions when taking this medication

If nitroglycerin is taken with certain other drugs, the effects of either could be increased, decreased, or altered.

Taken with many high blood pressure drugs, nitroglycerin may cause extreme low blood pressure (dizziness, fainting, numbness). Take particular care with calcium channel blockers such as Calan and Procardia XL, with isosorbide dinitrate (Sorbitrate, Isordil, others), isosorbide mononitrate (Ismo, others), blood vessel dilators such as Loniten, and beta-blocker medications such as Tenormin.

Alcohol may interact with nitroglycerin and cause a swift decrease in blood pressure, possibly causing dizziness and fainting.

Also be alert for an interaction with dihydroergotamine (D.H.E.). Check with your doctor if you are uncertain about any combination.

## Special information if you are pregnant or breastfeeding

It has not been determined whether nitroglycerin might harm a fetus or a pregnant woman. As a result, nitroglycerin should be used only when the benefits of therapy clearly outweigh the potential risks to the fetus and woman. It is not known if nitroglycerin appears in breast milk; therefore, a nursing mother should use nitroglycerin only on advice of her doctor.

## Recommended dosage

The following section is intended to provide guidelines for taking nitroglycerin. Follow your doctor's instructions carefully for using nitroglycerin in the form prescribed for you.

### ADULTS

*Sublingual or Buccal Tablets*
At the first sign of chest pain, 1 tablet should be dissolved under the tongue or inside the cheek. You may repeat the dose every 5 minutes until the pain is relieved. If your pain continues after you have taken 3 tablets in a 15-minute period, notify your doctor or seek medical attention immediately.

You may take sublingual or buccal nitroglycerin from 5 to 10 minutes before starting activities that may cause chest pain.

*Patch Form*
A patch is applied to the skin for 12 to 14 hours. After this time, the patch is removed; it is not applied again for 10 to 12 hours (a "patch-off" period). Apply the patch as soon as you remove it from its protective pouch.

*Spray Form*
At the first sign of chest pain, spray 1 or 2 pre-measured doses onto or under the tongue. You should not use more than 3 doses within a 15-minute period. If your chest pain continues, you should contact your doctor or seek medical attention immediately.

The spray can be used 5 to 10 minutes before activity that might precipitate an attack.

*Ointment Form*
Your initial dose may be a daily total of 1 inch of ointment. Apply one-half inch on rising in the morning, and the remaining one-half inch 6 hours later. If needed, follow your doctor's instructions for increasing your dosage. Apply in a thin, uniform layer, regardless of the amount of your dosage. There should be a daily period where no ointment is applied. Usually, the "ointment-off" period will last from 10 to 12 hours.

Absorption varies with site of application—more is absorbed through the chest.

### Sustained-Release Capsules or Tablets
The smallest effective amount should be taken 2 or 3 times a day at 8- to 12-hour intervals.

### CHILDREN
The safety and effectiveness of nitroglycerin have not been established for children.

### OLDER ADULTS
In general, dosages less than the above adult dosages are recommended, since the elderly may be more susceptible to low blood pressure and headaches.

### Overdosage
Any medication taken in excess can have serious consequences. Severe overdosage of nitroglycerin may result in death. If you suspect an overdose, seek medical attention immediately.

■ *Symptoms of overdose may include:*
Bluish skin, clammy skin, colic, coma, confusion, diarrhea (may be bloody), difficult and/or slow breathing, dizziness, fainting, fever, flushed skin, headache (persistent, throbbing), increased pressure within the skull, irregular pulse, loss of appetite, nausea, palpitations (an abnormally rapid throbbing or fluttering of the heart), paralysis, rapid decrease in blood pressure, seizures, slow pulse/heartbeat, sweating, vertigo, visual disturbances, vomiting

*Brand name:*
# Nitrolingual Spray
*See Nitroglycerin, page 361.*

*Brand name:*
# Nitrostat Tablets
*See Nitroglycerin, page 361.*

*Generic name:*
# Nizatidine
*See Axid, page 45.*

*Brand name:*
# Nizoral
*Pronounced: NYE-zore-al*
*Generic name: Ketoconazole*

### Why is this drug prescribed?
Nizoral, a broad-spectrum antifungal drug available in tablet form, may be given to treat several fungal infections within the body, including oral thrush and candidiasis.

It may also be given to treat severe, hard-to-treat fungal skin infections that have not cleared up after treatment with creams or ointments, or the oral drug griseofulvin (Fulvicin, Grisactin).

### Most important fact about this drug
In some people, Nizoral may cause serious or even fatal damage to the liver. Before starting to take Nizoral, and at frequent intervals while you are taking it, you should have blood tests to evaluate your liver function. Tell your doctor immediately if you experience any signs or symptoms that could mean liver damage: these include unusual fatigue, loss of appetite, nausea or vomiting, jaundice, dark urine, or pale stools.

### How should you take this medication?
Take Nizoral exactly as prescribed.

You should keep taking the drug until tests show that your fungal infection has subsided. If you stop too soon, the infection might return.

You may want to take Nizoral Tablets with meals to avoid stomach upset.

Avoid alcohol and do not take with antacids. If antacids are necessary, you should wait 2 to 3 hours before taking them.

■ *If you miss a dose...*
Take the forgotten dose as soon as you remember. This will help to keep the proper amount of medicine in the body. However, if it is almost time for your next dose, skip the one you missed and go back to your regular schedule. Do not take double doses.
■ *Storage instructions...*
Nizoral should be stored at room temperature.

### What side effects may occur?
Side effects from Nizoral cannot be anticipated. If any develop or change in intensity, inform your doctor as soon as possible. Only your doctor can determine if it is safe for you to continue taking Nizoral.

■ *More common side effects may include:*
Nausea, vomiting
■ *Less common side effects may include:*
Abdominal pain, itching
■ *Rare side effects may include:*
  Breast swelling (in men), depression, diarrhea, dizziness, drowsiness, fever and chills, headache, hives, impotence, light-sensitivity, rash

## Why should this drug not be prescribed?

Do not take Nizoral if you are sensitive to it or have ever had an allergic reaction to it. Never take Nizoral together with Seldane, Hismanal, Halcion, or Propulsid. Rare, but sometimes fatal reactions have been reported when these drugs are combined.

## Special warnings about this medication

In rare cases, people have had anaphylaxis (a life-threatening allergic reaction) after taking their first dose of Nizoral.

Observe caution when driving or performing other tasks requiring alertness, due to potential side effects of headache, dizziness, and drowsiness.

## Possible food and drug interactions when taking this medication

If Nizoral is taken with certain other drugs, the effects of either could be increased, decreased, or altered. It is especially important to check with your doctor before combining Nizoral with the following:

Alcoholic beverages
Antacids such as Di-Gel, Maalox, Mylanta, and
   others
Anticoagulants such as Coumadin, Dicumarol, and
   others
Anti-ulcer medications such as Axid, Pepcid,
   Tagamet, and Zantac
Astemizole (Hismanal)
Cisapride (Propulsid)
Cyclosporine (Sandimmune, Neoral)
Digoxin (Lanoxin)
Drugs that relieve spasms, such as Donnatal
Isoniazid (Nydrazid)
Methylprednisolone (Medrol)
Midazolam (Versed)
Oral diabetes drugs such as Diabinese and
   Micronase,
Phenytoin (Dilantin)
Rifampin (Rifadin, Rifamate, and Rimactane)
Tacrolimus (Prograf)

Terfenadine (Seldane)
Theophyllines such as Theo 24, Slo-Phyllin, Theo-
   Dur, and others
Triazolam (Halcion)

## Special information if you are pregnant or breastfeeding

If you are pregnant or plan to become pregnant, inform your doctor immediately. Nizoral should be taken during pregnancy only if the benefit outweighs the possible harm to your unborn child.

Since Nizoral can probably make its way into breast milk, it should not be taken during breastfeeding. If you are a new mother, check with your doctor. You may need to stop breastfeeding while you are taking Nizoral.

## Recommended dosage

### ADULTS

The recommended starting dose of Nizoral is a single daily dose of 200 milligrams (1 tablet).

In very serious infections, or if the problem does not clear up within the expected time, the dose of Nizoral may be increased to 400 milligrams (2 tablets) once daily. Treatment lasts at least 1 to 2 weeks, and for some infections much longer.

### CHILDREN

In small numbers of children over 2 years of age, a single daily dose of 3.3 to 6.6 milligrams per 2.2 pounds of body weight has been used.

Nizoral has not been studied in children under 2 years of age.

## Overdosage

Although no specific information is available, any medication taken in excess can have serious consequences. If you suspect an overdose of Nizoral, seek medical attention immediately.

*Brand name:*

# Nolvadex

*Pronounced: NOLL-vah-decks*
*Generic name: Tamoxifen citrate*

## Why is this drug prescribed?

Nolvadex, an anticancer drug, may be given to treat breast cancer. It also has proved effective when cancer has spread to other parts of the body. Nolvadex is most effective in stopping the kind of breast cancer that thrives on estrogen.

## Most important fact about this drug

Women taking Nolvadex should have routine gynecological examinations and report any abnormal
vaginal bleeding, changes in menstrual periods,
change in vaginal discharge, or pelvic pain or pressure to the doctor immediately. Even after
Nolvadex therapy has stopped, any abnormal
vaginal bleeding should be reported at once.

## How should you take this medication?

Take Nolvadex exactly as prescribed. Do not stop
taking this medication without first consulting your
doctor. It may be necessary to continue taking the
drug for several years.

■ *If you miss a dose...*
Do not try to make it up. Go back to your regular
schedule with the next dose.
■ *Storage instructions...*
Nolvadex should be stored away from heat
and light.

## What side effects may occur?

Side effects from Nolvadex are usually mild and
rarely require the drug to be stopped. If any develop
or change in intensity, inform your doctor as soon
as possible. Only your doctor can determine if it is
safe for you to continue taking Nolvadex.

■ *More common side effects may include:*
Hot flashes, nausea, vomiting
■ *Less common side effects may include:*
Bone pain, diarrhea, menstrual irregularities, skin
rash, tumor pain, vaginal bleeding, vaginal discharge
■ *Rare side effects may include:*
Blood clots, depression, distaste for food, dizziness, hair thinning or partial loss, headache,
light-headedness, liver disorders, swelling of
arms or legs, vaginal itching or dryness, visual
problems

## Why should this drug not be prescribed?

Do not take Nolvadex if you are sensitive to it or
have ever had an allergic reaction to it.

## Special warnings about this medication

If you experience visual problems while taking
Nolvadex, notify your doctor immediately.

In a few women Nolvadex may raise the level of
cholesterol and other fats in the blood. Your doctor
may periodically do blood tests to check your cholesterol and triglyceride levels.

Nolvadex may produce an abnormally high level
of calcium in the blood. Symptoms include muscle
pain and weakness, loss of appetite, and, if severe,
kidney failure. If you experience any of these
symptoms, notify your doctor as soon as possible.

If tests show that your blood contains too few
white blood cells or platelets while you are taking
Nolvadex, your doctor should monitor you with
special care. These problems have sometimes been
found in women taking Nolvadex; whether the drug
caused the blood-cell abnormalities is uncertain.

## Possible food and drug interactions when taking this medication

If Nolvadex is taken with certain other drugs, the
effects of either could be increased, decreased, or
altered. It is especially important to check with
your doctor before combining Nolvadex with the
following:

Blood-thinning drugs such as Coumadin
Bromocriptine (Parlodel)
Cancer drugs such as Hydrea
Phenobarbital

## Special information if you are pregnant or breastfeeding

It is important to avoid pregnancy while taking
Nolvadex, because the drug could harm the unborn
child. Since Nolvadex is an anti-estrogen drug, you
will need to use a non-hormonal form of contraception, such as a condom and/or diaphragm, and not
birth control pills. If you accidentally become pregnant while taking Nolvadex, or within 2 months
after you have stopped taking it, discuss this with
your doctor immediately.

Because Nolvadex might cause serious harm to
a nursing infant, you should not breastfeed your
baby while taking this drug. If this medication is
essential to your health, your doctor may advise
you to discontinue breastfeeding until your treatment is finished.

## Recommended dosage

ADULTS

The recommended dosage is one or two 10-mil-
ligram tablets in the morning and evening. 20 milligram tablets are also available. The recommended
dosage is a single tablet once or twice a day.

## Overdosage

Any medication taken in excess can have serious consequences. If you suspect an overdose of Nolvadex, seek medical attention immediately.

■ *Symptoms of Nolvadex overdose may include:*
Dizziness, overactive reflexes, tremor, unsteady gait

*Brand name:*

# Nordette

*See Oral Contraceptives, page 382.*

*Brand name:*

# Norethin

*See Oral Contraceptives, page 382.*

*Generic name:*

# Norfloxacin

*See Noroxin, page 370.*

*Brand name:*

# Norgesic

*Pronounced: nor-JEE-zic*
*Generic ingredients: Orphenadrine citrate, Aspirin, Caffeine*
*Other brand name: Norgesic Forte*

## Why is this drug prescribed?

Norgesic is prescribed, along with rest, physical therapy, and other measures, for the relief of mild to moderate pain of severe muscle disorders.

## Most important fact about this drug

Norgesic may impair your ability to drive a car or operate dangerous machinery. Do not participate in potentially hazardous activities until you know how you react to this medication.

## How should you take this medication?

If aspirin upsets your stomach, you may take Norgesic with food. Take it exactly as prescribed.

■ *If you miss a dose...*
If it is within an hour of your scheduled time, take it as soon as you remember. If you do not remember until later, skip the dose you missed and go back to your regular schedule. Do not take 2 doses at once.

■ *Storage instructions...*
Store at room temperature.

## What side effects may occur?

Side effects cannot be anticipated. If any develop or change in intensity, inform your doctor as soon as possible. Only your doctor can determine if it is safe for you to continue taking Norgesic.

■ *Side effects may include:*
Blurred vision, confusion (in the elderly), constipation, difficulty in urinating, dilation of the pupils, dizziness, drowsiness, dry mouth, fainting, hallucinations, headache, hives, light-headedness, nausea, palpitations, rapid heart rate, skin diseases, stomach and intestinal bleeding, vomiting, weakness

## Why should this drug not be prescribed?

If you are sensitive to or have ever had an allergic reaction to the ingredients of Norgesic, orphenadrine, aspirin, caffeine, you should not take this medication. Make sure your doctor is aware of any drug reactions you have experienced.

You should not be taking Norgesic if you have the eye condition called glaucoma, a stomach or intestinal blockage, an enlarged prostate gland, a bladder obstruction, achalasia (failure of stomach or intestinal muscles to relax), or myasthenia gravis (muscle weakness and fatigue).

Because taking aspirin while you have chickenpox or flu may cause a rare but serious condition called Reye's syndrome, do not give Norgesic to anyone with these diseases. Call your doctor if fever or swelling develops.

## Special warnings about this medication

Because the safety of continuous, long-term therapy with Norgesic has not been established, your doctor should monitor your blood, urine, and liver function if you use this drug for a prolonged period of time.

Because Norgesic contains aspirin, you should be careful taking it if you have a peptic ulcer or problems with blood clotting.

## Possible food and drug interactions when taking this medication

If Norgesic is taken with certain other drugs, the effects of either could be increased, decreased, or altered. It is especially important to check with your doctor before combining Norgesic with propoxyphene (Darvon). The combination can cause confusion, anxiety, and tremors.

## Special information
## if you are pregnant or breastfeeding

The effects of Norgesic during pregnancy have not been adequately studied. If you are pregnant or plan to become pregnant, inform your doctor immediately. This drug may appear in breast milk and could affect a nursing infant. If this medication is essential to your health, your doctor may advise you to discontinue breastfeeding until your treatment is finished.

## Recommended dosage

### ADULTS

The usual dose of Norgesic is 1 to 2 tablets taken 3 or 4 times a day.

The usual dosage of Norgesic Forte, which is exactly twice the strength of Norgesic, is one-half to 1 tablet, taken 3 or 4 times per day.

### CHILDREN

The safety and effectiveness of Norgesic have not been established in children. It is not recommended for children under 12 years of age.

### OLDER ADULTS

Some older adults have experienced confusion when taking this drug. Your doctor may adjust the dosage accordingly.

## Overdosage

Any medication taken in excess can have serious consequences. If you suspect an overdose of Norgesic, seek emergency medical treatment immediately.

*Brand name:*

# Norinyl

*See Oral Contraceptives, page 382.*

*Brand name:*

# Normodyne

*Pronounced: NORM-oh-dine*
*Generic name: Labetalol hydrochloride*
*Other brand name: Trandate*

## Why is this drug prescribed?

Normodyne is used in the treatment of high blood pressure. It is effective when used alone or in combination with other high blood pressure medications, especially thiazide diuretics such as HydroDIURIL and "loop" diuretics such as Lasix.

## Most important fact about this drug

You must take Normodyne regularly for it to be effective. Since blood pressure declines gradually, it may be several weeks before you get the full benefit of Normodyne; and you must continue taking it even if you are feeling well. Normodyne does not cure high blood pressure; it merely keeps it under control.

## How should you take this medication?

Normodyne can be taken with or without food. The amount of Normodyne absorbed into your bloodstream is actually increased by food.

This medication should be taken exactly as prescribed by your doctor, even if your symptoms have disappeared.

Try not to miss any doses. If Normodyne is not taken regularly, your condition may worsen.

■ *If you miss a dose...*
Take it as soon as you remember. If it is almost time for your next dose, skip the one you missed and go back to your regular schedule. Never take 2 doses at the same time.

■ *Storage instructions...*
Store at room temperature.

## What side effects may occur?

Side effects cannot be anticipated. If any develop or change in intensity, inform your doctor as soon as possible. Only your doctor can determine if it is safe for you to continue taking Normodyne.

■ *More common side effects may include:*
Dizziness, fatigue, indigestion, nausea, stuffy nose

■ *Less common or rare side effects may include:*
Anaphylaxis (severe allergic reaction), angioedema (swelling of the face, lips, tongue and throat, difficulty swallowing), changes in taste,

depression, diarrhea, difficulty urinating, dizziness upon standing up (especially among the elderly), drowsiness, dry eyes, ejaculation failure, fainting, fluid retention, hair loss, headache, heart block (conduction disorder), hives, impotence, increased sweating, itching, low blood pressure, lupus erythematosus (fever, arthritis, skin eruptions), muscle cramps, rash, shortness of breath, slow heartbeat, tingling or pins and needles, tingling scalp, vertigo, vision changes, weakness, wheezing or asthma-like symptoms, vomiting, yellow eyes and skin

### Why should this drug not be prescribed?

You should not take Normodyne if you are currently suffering from bronchial asthma, congestive heart failure, heart block (a heart irregularity), inadequate blood supply to the circulatory system (cardiogenic shock), a severely slow heartbeat, or any other condition that causes severe and continued low blood pressure.

If you are sensitive to or have ever had an allergic reaction to Normodyne or any of its ingredients you should not take this medication.

### Special warnings about this medication

Normodyne has caused severe liver damage in some people. Although this is a rare occurrence, if you develop any symptoms of abnormal liver function—itching, dark urine, continuing loss of appetite, yellow eyes and skin, or unexplained "flu-like" symptoms—contact your doctor immediately.

If you have a history of congestive heart failure, or kidney or liver disease, Normodyne should be used with caution.

Normodyne should not be stopped suddenly. This can cause chest pain and heart attack. Dosage should be gradually reduced.

If you suffer from asthma, chronic bronchitis, emphysema, or other bronchial diseases, Normodyne should be used cautiously.

This medication may mask the symptoms of low blood sugar or alter blood sugar levels. If you are diabetic, discuss this with your doctor.

Notify your doctor or dentist that you are taking Normodyne if you have a medical emergency, and before you have surgery or dental treatment.

### Possible food and drug interactions when taking this medication

If Normodyne is taken with certain other drugs, the effects of either could be increased, decreased, or altered. It is especially important to check with your doctor before taking Normodyne with the following:

Airway opening drugs such as Proventil and Ventolin
Antidepressant medications such as Elavil
Cimetidine (Tagamet)
Diabetes drugs such as Micronase
Epinephrine (EpiPen)
Insulin
Nitroglycerin products such as Transderm-Nitro
Nonsteroidal anti-inflammatory drugs such as Advil and Motrin
Ritodrine (Yutopar)
Verapamil (Calan)

### Special information if you are pregnant or breastfeeding

The effects of Normodyne during pregnancy have not been adequately studied. If you are pregnant or plan to become pregnant, inform your doctor immediately. Normodyne appears in breast milk and could affect a nursing infant. If this medication is essential to your health, your doctor may advise you to discontinue breastfeeding until your treatment is finished.

### Recommended dosage

ADULTS

Your doctor will adjust the dosages to fit your needs. Your doctor may observe the drug's effect in his or her office over a 1- to 3-hour period after you begin taking it, and then check your pressure again at regular office visits (12 hours after a dose) to make sure that the medicine is effective.

The usual starting dose is 100 milligrams, 2 times per day, alone or with a diuretic drug. After 2 to 3 days of checking your blood pressure, your doctor may begin increasing your dose by 100 milligrams, 2 times per day, at intervals of 2 to 3 days.

The regular dose ranges from 200 to 400 milligrams, 2 times per day. Some people may require total daily dosage of as much as 1,200 to 2,400 milligrams, either alone or with a thiazide diuretic. In these cases, your doctor will observe the drug's effect and adjust your dose accordingly.

CHILDREN

The safety and effectiveness of this drug in children have not been established.

## OLDER ADULTS

The usual starting dose is the same as younger people's—100 milligrams twice a day. Your doctor may increase the dose, but usually to no more than 200 milligrams twice a day.

### Overdosage

Any medication taken in excess can have serious consequences. If you suspect an overdose, seek medical treatment immediately.

■ *Symptoms of Normodyne overdose may include:*
Dizziness when standing up
Severely low blood pressure
Severely slow heartbeat

*Brand name:*

# Noroxin

*Pronounced: Nor-OX-in*
*Generic name: Norfloxacin*

### Why is this drug prescribed?

Noroxin is an antibacterial used to treat infections of the urinary tract, including cystitis (inflammation of the inner lining of the bladder caused by a bacterial infection), prostatitis (inflammation of the prostate gland), and certain sexually transmitted diseases, such as gonorrhea.

### Most important fact about this drug

Noroxin is not given for the treatment of syphilis. When used in high doses for a short period of time to treat gonorrhea, it may actually mask or delay the symptoms of syphilis. Your doctor may perform certain tests for syphilis at the time of diagnosing gonorrhea, and after treatment with Noroxin.

### How should you take this medication?

Noroxin should be taken, with a glass of water, either 1 hour *before* or 2 hours *after* eating a meal. Do not take more than the dosage prescribed by your doctor.

It is important to drink plenty of fluids while taking Noroxin.

Take all the Noroxin your doctor prescribes. If you stop taking the medicine too soon, you may have a relapse.

■ *If you miss a dose...*
Be sure to take it as soon as possible. This will help to keep a constant amount of Noroxin in your body. However, if it is almost time for your next dose, skip the one you missed and go back to your regular schedule. Do not take two doses at the same time.

■ *Storage instructions...*
Store at room temperature. Keep container tightly closed. Store out of reach of children.

### What side effects may occur?

Side effects cannot be anticipated. If any develop or change in intensity, inform your doctor as soon as possible. Only your doctor can determine whether it is safe for you to continue taking Noroxin.

■ *More common side effects may include:*
Abdominal cramping, dizziness, headache, nausea, weakness
■ *Other side effects may include:*
Abdominal pain or swelling, allergies, anal itching, anal/rectal pain, anxiety, arthritis, back pain, bitter taste, blood abnormalities, blurred vision, bursitis, chest pain, chills, confusion, constipation, depression, diarrhea, difficult breathing, double vision, dry mouth, extreme sleepiness, fever, fluid retention and swelling, gas, heart attack, heartburn, heart palpitations, hives, indigestion, insomnia, intestinal inflammation, itching, joint pain, kidney failure (symptoms may include reduced amount of urine, drowsiness, nausea, vomiting, and coma), lack of coordination, loose stools, loss of appetite, menstrual disorders, mouth ulcer, muscle pain, peeling skin, rash, reddened skin, ringing in the ears, severe skin reaction to light, stomach pain, sweating, swelling of feet or hands, temporary hearing loss, tingling in fingers, vision problems, vomiting, yellow eyes and skin

### Why should this drug not be prescribed?

You should not be using Noroxin if you are sensitive to it or to other drugs of the same type, such as Cipro. See "Special Warnings" section.

### Special warnings about this medication

Noroxin is not recommended for:

Children (under the age of 18)
Nursing mothers
Pregnant women

People with disorders such as epilepsy, severe cerebral arteriosclerosis, and other conditions that might lead to seizures should use Noroxin cautiously. There have been reports of convulsions in some people taking Noroxin.

If you develop diarrhea, tell your doctor. It could be a symptom of a potentially serious intestinal inflammation.

Some people taking drugs chemically similar to Noroxin have experienced severe, sometimes fatal reactions, occasionally after only one dose.

*These reactions may include:*
Confusion, convulsions, difficulty breathing, hallucinations, heart collapse, hives, increased pressure in the head, itching, light-headedness, loss of consciousness, psychosis, rash, restlessness, shock, swelling in the face or throat, tingling, tremors.

If you experience any of these reactions you should immediately stop taking Noroxin and seek medical help.

Some people find needle-shaped crystals in their urine after taking Noroxin. Drink plenty of fluids while taking Noroxin. This will increase urine output and reduce crystallization.

Noroxin may cause dizziness or light-headedness and might impair your ability to drive a car or operate potentially dangerous machinery. Use caution when undertaking any activities that require full alertness if you are unsure of your ability.

You should avoid excessive exposure to direct sunlight while taking Noroxin. Stop taking Noroxin and contact your doctor immediately if you have a severe reaction to sunlight, such as a skin rash.

## Possible food and drug interactions when taking this medication

If Noroxin is taken with certain other drugs, the effects of either could be increased, decreased, or altered. It is especially important to check with your doctor before combining Noroxin with the following:

Antacids such as Maalox and Tums
Caffeine (including coffee, tea, and some soft drinks)
Calcium supplements
Cyclosporine (Sandimmune, Neoral)
Multivitamins and other products containing iron or zinc
Nitrofurantoin (Macrodantin, Macrobid)
Oral anticoagulants, such as warfarin (Coumadin)
Probenecid (Benemid)
Sucralfate (Carafate)
Theophylline (Theo-Dur)

## Special information if you are pregnant or breastfeeding

The effects of Noroxin during pregnancy have not been adequately studied. Inform your doctor if you are pregnant or planning a pregnancy.

Do not take Noroxin while breastfeeding. There is a possibility of harm to the infant.

## Recommended dosage

Take Noroxin with a full glass of water 1 hour before, or 2 hours after, eating a meal. Drink plenty of liquids while taking Noroxin.

*Uncomplicated Urinary Tract Infections*
The suggested dose is 800 milligrams per day; 400 milligrams should be taken twice a day for 3 to 10 days, depending upon the kind of bacteria causing the infection. People with impaired kidney function may take 400 milligrams once a day for 3 to 10 days.

*Complicated Urinary Tract Infections*
The suggested dose is 800 milligrams per day; 400 milligrams should be taken twice a day for 10 to 21 days.

*Prostatitis*
The usual daily dose is 800 milligrams, divided into 2 doses of 400 milligrams each, taken for 28 days.

*Sexually Transmitted Diseases (Gonorrhea)*
The usual recommended dose is one single dose of 800 milligrams for 1 day.

The total daily dosage of Noroxin should not be more than 800 milligrams.

## Overdosage

The symptoms of overdose with Noroxin are not known. However, any medication taken in excess can have serious consequences. If you suspect a Noroxin overdose, seek medical help immediately.

*Brand name:*

# Norpace

*Pronounced: NOR-pace*
*Generic name: Disopyramide phosphate*
*Other brand name: Norpace CR*

## Why is this drug prescribed?

Norpace is used to treat severe irregular heartbeat. It relaxes an overactive heart and improves the efficiency of the heart's pumping action.

## Most important fact about this drug

Do not stop taking Norpace without first consulting your doctor. Stopping suddenly can cause serious changes in heart function.

## How should you take this medication?

Be sure to take this medication exactly as prescribed.

Norpace may cause dry mouth. For temporary relief suck on a hard candy, chew gum, or melt ice chips in your mouth.

■ *If you miss a dose...*
Take it as soon as you remember, if the next dose is 4 or more hours away. If you do not remember until later, skip the dose you missed and go back to your regular schedule. Do not take 2 doses at once.

■ *Storage instructions...*
Store at room temperature.

## What side effects may occur?

Side effects cannot be anticipated. If any develop or change in intensity, inform your doctor as soon as possible. Only your doctor can determine if it is safe for you to continue taking Norpace.

■ *More common side effects may include:*
Abdominal pain, aches and pains, bloating and gas, blurred vision, constipation, dizziness, dry eyes, nose, and throat, dry mouth, fatigue, headache, inability to urinate, increased urinary frequency and urgency, muscle weakness, nausea, vague feeling of bodily discomfort

■ *Less common or rare side effects may include:*
Breast development in males, chest pain, congestive heart failure, depression, diarrhea, difficulty breathing, difficulty sleeping, fainting, fever, impotence, itching, low blood pressure, low blood sugar (hypoglycemia), nervousness, numbness or tingling, painful urination, rash, psychosis, shortness of breath, skin diseases, swelling due to fluid retention, vomiting, weight gain, yellow eyes and skin

## Why should this drug not be prescribed?

This drug should not be used if the output of your heart is inadequate (cardiogenic shock) or if you are sensitive to or have ever had an allergic reaction to Norpace.

Norpace can be used for only certain types of irregular heartbeat, and must not be used for others.

## Special warnings about this medication

If you have structural heart disease, inflammation of the heart muscle, or other heart disorders, use this medication with extreme caution.

Norpace may cause or worsen congestive heart failure and can cause severe low blood pressure. If you have a history of heart failure, your doctor will carefully monitor your heart function while you are taking this medication.

Norpace can cause low blood sugar (hypoglycemia), especially if you have congestive heart failure; poor nutrition; or kidney, liver, or other diseases; or if you are taking beta-blocking blood pressure drugs such as Tenormin or drinking alcohol.

Your doctor will prescribe Norpace along with other heart-regulating drugs, such as quinidine, procainamide, encainide, flecainide, propafenone, and propranolol, only if the irregular rhythm is considered life-threatening and other antiarrhythmic medication has not worked.

If you have the eye condition called glaucoma, myasthenia gravis, or difficulty urinating (particularly if you have a prostate condition), use this drug cautiously.

You will take lower dosages if you have liver or kidney disease.

Your doctor should check your potassium levels before starting you on Norpace. Low potassium levels may make this drug ineffective; high levels may increase its toxic effects.

## Possible food and drug interactions when taking this medication

Avoid alcoholic beverages while taking Norpace.

If Norpace is taken with certain other drugs, the effects of either could be increased, decreased, or altered. It is especially important to check with your doctor before combining Norpace with the following:

Other heart-regulating drugs such as quinidine
  (Quinidex), procainamide
(Procan SR), lidocaine (Xylocaine), propranolol
  (Inderal), Verapamil (Calan)
Phenytoin (Dilantin)

## Special information if you are pregnant or breastfeeding

The effects of Norpace during pregnancy have not been adequately studied. If you are pregnant or plan to become pregnant, inform your doctor immediately. Norpace appears in breast milk and may affect a nursing infant. If this medication is essential to your health, your doctor may advise you to discontinue breastfeeding until your treatment with this medication is finished.

### Recommended dosage

Treatment with Norpace should be started in the hospital.

ADULTS

Your doctor will adjust your dosage according to your own response to, and tolerance of, Norpace or Norpace CR.

The usual dosage range of Norpace and Norpace CR is 400 milligrams to 800 milligrams per day, divided into smaller doses.

The recommended dosage for most adults is 600 milligrams per day, divided into smaller doses (either 150 milligrams every 6 hours for immediate-release Norpace or 300 milligrams every 12 hours for Norpace CR).

For those who weigh less than 110 pounds, the recommended dosage is 400 milligrams per day, divided into smaller doses (either 100 milligrams every 6 hours for immediate-release Norpace or 200 milligrams every 12 hours for Norpace CR.

For people with severe heart disease, the starting dose will be 100 milligrams of immediate-release Norpace every 6 to 8 hours. Your doctor will adjust the dosage gradually and watch you closely for any signs of low blood pressure or heart failure.

For people with moderately reduced kidney or liver function, the dosage is 400 milligrams per day, divided into smaller doses (either 100 milligrams every 6 hours for immediate-release Norpace or 200 milligrams every 12 hours for Norpace CR).

For those who have severe kidney impairment, the dosage of immediate-release Norpace is 100 milligrams; the times will vary with the individual as determined by your doctor.

Norpace CR is not recommended for people with severe kidney disease.

CHILDREN

Dosage in children to age 18 is based on body weight. The total daily dosage should be divided into equal doses taken orally every 6 hours or at intervals that are best for the individual.

### Overdosage

Any medication taken in excess can have serious consequences. An overdose of Norpace can be fatal. If you suspect an overdose, seek medical treatment immediately.

■ *The symptoms of Norpace overdose may include:*
Cessation of breathing, irregular heartbeat, loss of consciousness, low blood pressure, slow heartbeat, worsening of congestive heart failure

*Brand name:*

# Norpramin

*Pronounced: NOR-pram-in*
*Generic name: Desipramine hydrochloride*

### Why is this drug prescribed?

Norpramin is used in the treatment of depression. It is one of a family of drugs called tricyclic antidepressants. Drugs in this class are thought to work by affecting the levels of the brain's natural chemical messengers (called neurotransmitters), and adjusting the brain's response to them.

Norpramin has also been used to treat bulimia and attention deficit disorders, and to help with cocaine withdrawal.

### Most important fact about this drug

Serious, sometimes fatal, reactions have been known to occur when drugs such as Norpramin are taken with another type of antidepressant called an MAO inhibitor. Drugs in this category include Nardil and Parnate. Do not take Norpramin within two weeks of taking one of these drugs. Make sure your doctor and pharmacist know of all the medications you are taking.

### How should you take this medication?

Norpramin should be taken exactly as prescribed.

Do not stop taking Norpramin if you feel no immediate effect. It can take up to 2 or 3 weeks for improvement to begin.

Norpramin can cause dry mouth. Sucking hard candy or chewing gum can help this problem.

■ *If you miss a dose...*
If you take several doses per day, take the forgotten dose as soon as you remember, then take any remaining doses for the day at evenly spaced intervals. If you take Norpramin once a day at

bedtime and don't remember until morning, skip the missed dose. Never try to "catch up" by doubling the dose.

■ *Storage instructions...*

Norpramin can be stored at room temperature. Protect it from excessive heat.

### What side effects may occur?

Side effects cannot be anticipated. If any develop or change in intensity, inform your doctor as soon as possible. Only your doctor can determine if it is safe for you to continue taking Norpramin.

■ *Side effects may include:*

Abdominal cramps, agitation, anxiety, black tongue, black, red, or blue spots on skin, blurred vision, breast development in males, breast enlargement in females, confusion, constipation, delusions, diarrhea, dilated pupils, disorientation, dizziness, drowsiness, dry mouth, excessive or spontaneous flow of milk, fatigue, fever, flushing, frequent urination or difficulty or delay in urinating, hallucinations, headache, heart attack, heartbeat irregularities, hepatitis, high or low blood pressure, high or low blood sugar, hives, impotence, increased or decreased sex drive, inflammation of the mouth, insomnia, intestinal blockage, lack of coordination, light-headedness (especially when rising from lying down), loss of appetite, loss of hair, mild elation, nausea, nightmares, odd taste in mouth, painful ejaculation, palpitations, purplish spots on the skin, rapid heartbeat, restlessness, ringing in the ears, seizures, sensitivity to light, skin itching and rash, sore throat, stomach pain, stroke, sweating, swelling due to fluid retention (especially in face or tongue), swelling of testicles, swollen glands, tingling, numbness and pins and needles in hands and feet, tremors, urinating at night, visual problems, vomiting, weakness, weight gain or loss, worsening of psychosis, yellowed skin and whites of eyes

### Why should this drug not be prescribed?

Norpramin should not be used if you are known to be hypersensitive to it, or if you have had a recent heart attack.

People who take antidepressant drugs known as MAO inhibitors (including Nardil and Parnate) should not take Norpramin.

### Special warnings about this medication

Before using Norpramin, tell your doctor if you have heart or thyroid disease, a seizure disorder, a history of being unable to urinate, or glaucoma.

Nausea, headache, and uneasiness can result if you suddenly stop taking Norpramin. Consult your doctor and follow instructions closely when discontinuing Norpramin.

This drug may impair your ability to drive a car or operate potentially dangerous machinery. Do not participate in any activities that require full alertness if you are unsure about your ability.

Norpramin may increase your skin's sensitivity to sunlight. Overexposure could cause rash, itching, redness, or sunburn. Avoid direct sunlight or wear protective clothing.

If you are planning to have elective surgery, make sure that your doctor is aware that you are taking Norpramin. It should be discontinued as soon as possible prior to surgery.

Tell your doctor if you develop a fever and sore throat while you are taking Norpramin. He may want to do some blood tests.

### Possible food and drug interactions when taking this medication

People who take antidepressant drugs known as MAO inhibitors (including Nardil and Parnate) should not take Norpramin.

If Norpramin is taken with certain other drugs, the effects of either could be increased, decreased, or altered. It is especially important to check with your doctor before combining Norpramin with the following:

Cimetidine (Tagamet)
Drugs that improve breathing, such as Proventil
Drugs that relax certain muscles, such as Bentyl
Fluoxetine (Prozac)
Guanethidine (Ismelin)
Sedatives/hypnotics (Halcion, Valium)
Thyroid medications (Synthroid)

Extreme drowsiness and other potentially serious effects can result if Norpramin is combined with alcohol or other depressants, including narcotic painkillers such as Percocet and Demerol, sleeping medications such as Halcion and Nembutal, and tranquilizers such as Valium and Xanax.

### Special information if you are pregnant or breastfeeding

Pregnant women or mothers who are nursing an infant should use Norpramin only when the potential benefits clearly outweigh the potential risks. If you are pregnant or planning to become pregnant, inform your doctor immediately.

### Recommended dosage

Your doctor will tailor the dose to your individual needs.

#### ADULTS

The usual dose ranges from 100 to 200 milligrams per day, taken in 1 dose or divided into smaller doses. If needed, dosages may gradually be increased to 300 milligrams a day. Dosages above 300 milligrams per day are not recommended.

#### CHILDREN

Norpramin is not recommended for children.

#### OLDER ADULTS AND ADOLESCENTS

The usual dose ranges from 25 to 100 milligrams per day. If needed, dosages may gradually be increased to 150 milligrams a day. Doses above 150 milligrams per day are not recommended.

### Overdosage

Any medication taken in excess can have serious consequences. An overdosage of Norpramin can be fatal. If you suspect an overdose, seek medical help immediately.

■ *Symptoms of overdose may include:*
Agitation, coma, confusion, delirium, difficult breathing, dilated pupils, extremely low blood pressure, fever, inability to urinate, irregular heart rate, kidney failure, restlessness, rigid muscles, seizures, shock, stupor, vomiting

Generic name:

# Nortriptyline

*See Pamelor, page 390.*

Brand name:

# Norvasc

*Pronounced: NOR-vask*
*Generic name: Amlodipine besylate*

### Why is this drug prescribed?

Norvasc is prescribed for angina, a condition characterized by episodes of crushing chest pain usually resulting from a lack of oxygen in the heart due to clogged arteries. Norvasc is also prescribed for high blood pressure. It is a type of medication called a calcium channel blocker. These drugs dilate blood vessels and slow the heart to reduce blood pressure and the pain of angina.

### Most important fact about this drug

If you have high blood pressure, you must take Norvasc regularly for it to be effective. Since blood pressure declines gradually, it may be several weeks before you get the full benefit of Norvasc; and you must continue taking it even if you are feeling well. Norvasc does not cure high blood pressure; it merely keeps it under control.

### How should you take this medication?

Norvasc may be taken with or without food. A once-a-day medication, Norvasc may be used alone or in combination with other drugs for high blood pressure or angina.

You should take this medication exactly as prescribed, even if your symptoms have disappeared.

■ *If you miss a dose...*
If you forget to take a dose, take it as soon as you remember. If it is almost time for your next dose, skip the one you missed and go back to your regular schedule. Never take 2 doses at the same time.
■ *Storage instructions...*
Store at room temperature in a tightly closed container, away from light.

### What side effects may occur?

Side effects cannot be anticipated. If any develop or change in intensity, tell your doctor as soon as possible. Only your doctor can determine if it is safe for you to continue taking Norvasc.

■ *More common side effects may include:*
Dizziness, fatigue, flushing, fluid retention and swelling, headache, palpitations (fluttery or throbbing heartbeat)
■ *Less common side effects may include:*
Abdominal pain, nausea, sleepiness
■ *Rare side effects may include:*
Abnormal dreams, agitation, altered sense of smell or taste, anxiety, apathy, back pain, chest pain, cold and clammy skin, conjunctivitis (pinkeye), constipation, coughing, depression, diarrhea, difficult or labored breathing, difficult

or painful urination, difficulty swallowing, dizziness or light-headedness when standing, double vision, dry mouth, dry skin, excessive urination, eye pain, fainting, frequent urination, gas, general feeling of illness, hair loss, heart failure, hives, hot flashes, inability to sleep, increased appetite, increased sweating, indigestion, irregular heartbeat, irregular pulse, itching, joint pain or problems, lack of coordination, lack of sensation, loose stools, loss of appetite, loss of memory, loss of sense of identity, low blood pressure, migraine, muscle cramps or pain, muscle weakness, nasal inflammation, nervousness, nosebleed, pain, purple or red spots on the skin, rapid heartbeat, rash, ringing in the ears, sexual problems, skin discoloration, skin inflammation, slow heartbeat, stomach inflammation, thirst, tingling or "pins and needles", tremor, twitching, urinating at night, urinating problems, vertigo, vision problems, vomiting, weakness, weight gain

### Why should this drug not be prescribed?
If you are sensitive to or have ever had an allergic reaction to Norvasc, do not take this medication.

### Special warnings about this medication
Check with your doctor before you stop taking Norvasc, as a slow reduction in the dose may be needed.

Your doctor will prescribe Norvasc with caution if you have certain heart conditions or liver disease. Make sure the doctor is aware of all your medical problems before you start therapy with Norvasc.

Although very rare, if you have severe heart disease, you may experience an increase in frequency and duration of angina attacks, or even have a heart attack, when you are starting on Norvasc or your dosage is increased.

Safety and effectiveness in children have not been established.

### Possible food and drug interactions
There are no known food or drug interactions with this medication.

### Special information
### if you are pregnant or breastfeeding
The effects of Norvasc during pregnancy have not been adequately studied. If you are pregnant or planning to become pregnant, tell your doctor immediately. Norvasc should be used during preg-

nancy only if clearly needed. Norvasc may appear in breast milk. If this medication is essential to your health, your doctor may tell you to discontinue breastfeeding your baby until your treatment with Norvasc is finished.

### Recommended dosage
HIGH BLOOD PRESSURE

*Adults*
The usual starting dose is 5 milligrams taken once a day. The most you should take in a day is 10 milligrams. If your doctor is adding Norvasc to other high blood pressure medications, the dose is 2.5 milligrams once daily. The lower 2.5-milligram starting dose also applies if you have liver disease.

*Older Adults*
You will be prescribed a lower starting dose of 2.5 milligrams.

ANGINA

*Adults*
The usual starting dose is 5 to 10 milligrams once daily. If you have liver disease, the lower 5-milligram dose will be used at the start.

*Older Adults*
The usual starting dose is 5 milligrams. Your doctor may adjust the dose based on your response to the drug.

### Overdosage
Experience with Norvasc is limited; but if you suspect an overdose of Norvasc, seek medical attention immediately. The most likely symptoms are a drop in blood pressure and a faster heartbeat.

*Brand name:*

# Norvir

*Pronounced: NOR-veer*
*Generic name: Ritonavir*

### Why is this drug prescribed?
Norvir is prescribed to slow the progress of HIV (human immunodeficiency virus) infection. HIV causes the immune system to break down so that it can no longer respond effectively to infection, leading to the fatal disease known as acquired immune deficiency syndrome (AIDS). Without treatment, HIV takes over certain human cells, especially white blood cells, and uses the inner

workings of the infected cell to make additional copies of itself. Norvir belongs to a new class of HIV drugs, called protease inhibitors, which work by interfering with an important step in this process. Although Norvir cannot get rid of HIV already present in the body, it can reduce the amount of virus available to infect other cells.

Norvir is used alone or in combination with other HIV drugs called nucleoside analogues (Retrovir, Hivid, and others). Because these two types of drugs act against HIV in different ways, your doctor may prescribe a combination of Norvir and Retrovir or Hivid.

### Most important fact about this drug

Do not take Norvir with the following medications. The combination could cause serious, even life-threatening, effects.

Amiodarone (Cordarone), astemizole (Hismanal), bepridil (Vascor), bupropion (Wellbutrin), cisapride (Propulsid), clozapine (Clozaril), encainide (Enkaid), flecainide (Tambocor), meperidine (Demerol), piroxicam (Feldene), propafenone (Rythmol), propoxyphene (Darvon), quinidine (Quinidex), rifabutin (Mycobutin), terfenadine (Seldane)

Norvir may also increase the effects of certain sedative and sleeping medications, leading to extreme sedation and difficulty breathing. Never combine Norvir with the following:

Alprazolam (Xanax), clorazepate (Tranxene), diazepam (Valium), estazolam (ProSom), flurazepam (Dalmane), midazolam (Versed), triazolam (Halcion), zolpidem (Ambien)

Be sure to tell your doctor and pharmacist what medications you are taking, both prescription and over-the-counter, and let them know when you *stop* taking any medication.

### How should you take this medication?

Take Norvir every day, exactly as prescribed by your doctor. Do not share this medication with anyone and do not take more than your recommended dosage.

Take Norvir with food, if possible, or the medication may not work properly.

If you are taking Norvir oral solution and want to improve the taste, you can mix the liquid with chocolate milk or a liquid nutritional product (Ensure or Advera) within 1 hour of taking the dose. Use a measuring cup or spoon to measure each dose of the oral solution accurately. A household teaspoon may not hold the correct amount of oral solution.

■ *If you miss a dose...*
Take it as soon as possible. If it is almost time for the next dose, skip the one you missed and go back to your regular schedule. Never double the dose.

■ *Storage instructions...*
Capsules should be refrigerated and protected from light. The oral solution is best kept in the refrigerator, although it does not require refrigeration if used within 30 days and stored below 77°F. Avoid exposure to extreme heat and keep the cap tightly closed. Keep the oral solution in its original container.

### What side effects may occur?

Side effects cannot be anticipated. If any develop or change in intensity, tell your doctor as soon as possible. Only your doctor can determine if it is safe for you to continue taking Norvir.

■ *Possible side effects may include:*
Abdominal pain, bodily weakness, constipation, diarrhea, disturbed thoughts, dizziness, drowsiness, fever, gas, general feeling of illness, headache, indigestion, insomnia, loss of appetite, muscle aches, nausea, numbness or tingling sensation around the face or mouth, "pins and needles" sensation in the arms and legs, rash, sore or irritated throat, sweating, taste alteration, vomiting

### Why should this drug not be prescribed?

If you have ever had an allergic reaction to Norvir or any of its ingredients, do not take the drug. Never combine Norvir with the drugs listed under "Most important fact about this drug."

### Special warnings about this medication

Norvir is very new and has been studied for only a limited period of time. Its long-term effects are still unknown.

Norvir is not a cure for AIDS or HIV infection. You may contine to experience symptoms and develop complications, including opportunistic infections (rare diseases that attack when the immune system falters, such as certain types of pneumonia, tuberculosis, and fungal infections).

Norvir does not reduce the danger of transmission of HIV to others through sexual contact or blood contamination. Therefore, you should continue to avoid practices that could give HIV to others. If you have liver disease, you should take this medication with caution.

### Possible food and drug interactions when taking this medication

Combining Norvir with certain drugs (see "Most important fact about this drug") may cause serious or life-threatening effects. Other drugs may cause less dangerous—but still worrisome—effects. It is especially important to check with your doctor before combining Norvir with the following:

Clarithromycin (Biaxin)
Desipramine (Norpramin)
Disulfiram (Antabuse)
Metronidazole (Flagyl)
Oral contraceptives
Saquinavir (Invirase)
Theophylline (Theo-Dur)

Less significant interactions may occur with many other drugs. Your wisest course is to check with your doctor before combining *any* drug with Norvir.

Tobacco use decreases the effects of Norvir. The effects of antacids taken with Norvir have not been studied.

### Special information if you are pregnant or breastfeeding

The effects of Norvir during pregnancy have not been adequately studied. If you are pregnant or plan to become pregnant, tell your doctor immediately. This drug may appear in breast milk and could affect a nursing infant. To avoid transmitting HIV to a newborn baby, HIV-positive women should not breastfeed.

### Recommended dosage

ADULTS AND ADOLESCENTS OVER 12 YEARS OF AGE

The recommended dose of Norvir is 600 milligrams twice a day with food.

Should you experience nausea when first starting on Norvir, your doctor may lower your starting dosage to 300 milligrams twice a day for 1 day, 400 milligrams twice a day for 2 days, 500 milligrams twice a day for 1 day, and then 600 milligrams twice a day thereafter.

If Norvir is to be used in combination with other HIV drugs, your doctor may suggest taking Norvir alone at first and adding the second drug later in the first 2 weeks of therapy. This approach may cause fewer stomach problems.

CHILDREN

The safety and effectiveness of Norvir in children below the age of 12 have not been established at this time.

### Overdosage

Information on acute overdose with Norvir is limited. However, any medication taken in excess can have serious consequences. If you suspect an overdose, seek emergency medical treatment immediately.

■ *Symptoms of Norvir overdose may include:*
Numbness, tingling, or a "pins and needles" sensation, particularly in the arms and legs

*Brand name:*

# Novolin

*See Insulin, page 258.*

*Generic name:*

# Nystatin with Triamcinolone

*See Mycolog-II, page 342.*

*Brand name:*

# Oby-Cap

*See Fastin, page 204.*

*Generic name:*

# Ofloxacin

*See Floxin, page 217.*

*Brand name:*

# Ogen

*Pronounced: OH-jen*
*Generic name: Estropipate*
*Other brand name: Ortho-Est*

## Why is this drug prescribed?

Ogen and Ortho-Est are estrogen replacement drugs. The tablets are used to reduce symptoms of menopause, including feelings of warmth in face, neck, and chest, and the sudden intense episodes of heat and sweating known as "hot flashes." They also may be prescribed for teenagers who fail to mature at the usual rate.

In addition, either the tablets or Ogen vaginal cream can be used for other conditions caused by lack of estrogen, such as dry, itchy external genitals and vaginal irritation.

Along with diet, calcium supplements, and exercise, Ogen tablets are also prescribed to prevent osteoporosis, a condition in which the bones become brittle and easily broken.

Some doctors also prescribe these drugs to treat breast cancer and cancer of the prostate.

## Most important fact about this drug

Because estrogens have been linked with increased risk of endometrial cancer (cancer in the lining of the uterus) in women who have had their menopause, it is essential to have regular check-ups and to report any unusual vaginal bleeding to your doctor immediately.

## How should you take this medication?

Be careful to follow the cycle of administration your doctor establishes for you. Take the medication exactly as prescribed.

When using Ogen Vaginal Cream, follow the instructions printed on the carton. It is for short-term use only. Remove the cap from the tube and make sure the plunger of the applicator is all the way into the barrel. Screw the nozzle of the applicator onto the tube and squeeze the cream into the applicator. The number on the plunger, which indicates the dose you should take, should be level with the top of the barrel. Unscrew the applicator and replace the cap on the tube. Insert the applicator into the vagina and push the plunger all the way down. Between uses, take the plunger out of the barrel and wash the applicator with warm, soapy water. Never use hot or boiling water.

■ *If you miss a dose...*
Take the forgotten dose as soon as you remember. If it is almost time for the next dose, skip the one you missed and go back to your regular schedule. Never try to "catch up" by doubling the dose.

■ *Storage instructions...*
Store at room temperature.

## What side effects may occur?

Side effects cannot be anticipated. If any develop or change in intensity, notify your doctor as soon as possible. Only your doctor can determine if it is safe for you to continue taking estrogen.

■ *Side effects may include:*
Abdominal cramps, bloating, breakthrough bleeding, breast enlargement, breast tenderness and secretions, change in amount of cervical secretion, changes in sex drive, changes in vaginal bleeding patterns, chorea (irregular, rapid, jerky movements, usually affecting the face and limbs), depression, dizziness, enlargement of benign tumors (fibroids), excessive hairiness, fluid retention, hair loss, headache, inability to use contact lenses, menstrual changes, migraine, nausea, reduced ability to tolerate carbohydrates, spotting, spotty darkening of the skin, especially around the face, skin eruptions (especially on the legs and arms) with bleeding, skin irritation, skin redness and scaling, vaginal yeast infection, vision problems, vomiting, weight gain or loss, yellow eyes and skin

## Why should this drug not be prescribed?

Estrogens should not be used if you know or suspect you have breast cancer or other cancers promoted by estrogen. Do not use estrogen if you are pregnant or think you may be pregnant. Also avoid estrogen if you have abnormal, undiagnosed genital bleeding, or if you have blood clots or a blood clotting disorder or a history of blood clotting disorders associated with previous estrogen use.

Ogen Vaginal Cream should not be used if you are sensitive to or have ever had an allergic reaction to any of its components.

## Special warnings about this medication

The risk of cancer of the uterus increases when estrogen is used for a long time or taken in large doses. There also may be increased risk of breast cancer in women who take estrogen for an extended period of time.

Women who take estrogen after menopause are more likely to develop gallbladder disease.

Ogen also increases the risk of blood clots. These blood clots can cause stroke, heart attack, or other serious disorders.

Your doctor will check your blood pressure regularly. It could go up or down.

While taking estrogen, get in touch with your doctor right away if you notice any of the following:

Abdominal pain, tenderness, or swelling
Abnormal bleeding from the vagina
Breast lumps
Coughing up blood
Pain in your chest or calves
Severe headache, dizziness, or faintness
Speech changes
Sudden shortness of breath
Vision changes
Vomiting
Weakness or numbness in an arm or leg
Yellowing of the skin

Ogen may cause fluid retention in some people. If you have asthma, epilepsy, migraine, or heart or kidney disease, use this medication with care.

Estrogen therapy may cause uterine bleeding or breast pain.

## Possible food and drug interactions when taking this medication

If Ogen is taken with certain other drugs, the effects of either could be increased, decreased, or altered. It is especially important to check with your doctor before combining Ogen with the following:

Barbiturates such as phenobarbital
Blood thinners such as Coumadin
Epilepsy drugs (Tegretol, Dilantin, others)
Insulin
Tricyclic antidepressants (Elavil, Tofranil, others)
Rifampin (Rifadin)

## Special information if you are pregnant or breastfeeding

Estrogens should not be used during pregnancy. If you are pregnant or plan to become pregnant, notify your doctor immediately. These drugs may appear in breast milk and could affect a nursing infant. If this medication is essential to your health, your doctor may advise you to discontinue breastfeeding until your treatment is finished.

## Recommended dosage

### HOT FLASHES AND NIGHT SWEATS

Ogen Tablets: The usual dose ranges from one .625 tablet to two 2.5 tablets per day. Tablets should be taken in cycles, according to your doctor's instructions.

Ortho-Est Tablets: The usual dose ranges from $\frac{1}{2}$ tablet to 4 tablets per day of Ortho-Est 1.25 or 1 to 8 tablets of Ortho-Est .625. Tablets should be taken in cycles, according to your doctor's instructions.

### VAGINAL INFLAMMATION AND DRYNESS

Ogen Tablets: The usual dose ranges from one .625 tablet to two 2.5 tablets per day. Tablets should be taken in cycles, according to your doctor's instructions.

Ortho-Est Tablets: The usual dose ranges from $\frac{1}{2}$ tablet to 4 tablets per day of Ortho-Est 1.25 or 1 to 8 tablets of Ortho-Est .625. Tablets should be taken in cycles, according to your doctor's instructions.

Ogen Vaginal Cream: The usual dose is 2 to 4 grams daily. Cream should be used in cycles, and only for limited periods of time.

### ESTROGEN HORMONE DEFICIENCY

Ogen Tablets: The usual dose ranges from one 1.25 tablet to three 2.5 tablets per day, taken for 3 weeks, followed by a rest period of 8 to 10 days.

Ortho-Est Tablets: The usual dose ranges from 1 to 6 tablets per day of Ortho-Est 1.25 or 2 to 12 tablets of Ortho-Est .625, given for 3 weeks, followed by a rest period of 8 to 10 days.

### OVARIAN FAILURE

Ogen Tablets: The usual dose ranges from one 1.25 tablet to three 2.5 tablets per day for 3 weeks, followed by a rest period of 8 to 10 days. Your doctor may increase or decrease your dosage according to your response.

Ortho-Est Tablets: The usual dose ranges from 1 to 6 tablets per day of Ortho-Est 1.25 or 2 to 12 tablets of Ortho-Est. .625 for 3 weeks, followed by a rest period of 8 to 10 days. Your doctor may increase or decrease your dosage according to your response.

### PREVENTION OF OSTEOPOROSIS

Ogen Tablets: The usual dose is one .625 tablet per day for 25 days of a 31-day monthly cycle.

## Overdosage

Any medication taken in excess can have serious consequences. If you suspect an overdose, seek emergency medical treatment immediately.

■ *Symptoms of Ogen overdose may include:*
  Nausea, vomiting, withdrawal bleeding

*Generic name:*

# Olsalazine

*See Dipentum, page 166.*

*Generic name:*

# Omeprazole

*See Prilosec, page 435.*

*Brand name:*

# Omnipen

*Pronounced: AHM-nee-pen*
*Generic name: Ampicillin*
*Other brands: Principen, Totacillin*

## Why is this drug prescribed?

Omnipen is a penicillin-like antibiotic prescribed for a wide variety of infections, including gonorrhea and other genital and urinary infections, respiratory infections, and gastrointestinal infections, as well as meningitis (inflamed membranes of the spinal cord or brain).

## Most important fact about this drug

If you are allergic to either penicillin or cephalosporin antibiotics in any form, consult your doctor *before taking Omnipen.* There is a possibility that you are allergic to both types of medication; and if a reaction occurs, it could be extremely severe. If you take the drug and develop a skin reaction, diarrhea, shortness of breath, wheezing, sore throat, or fever, seek medical attention immediately.

## How should you use this medication?

Take Omnipen capsules with a full glass of water, a half hour before or 2 hours after a meal.

Omnipen Oral Suspension should be shaken well before using.

Take Omnipen exactly as prescribed. It works best when there is a constant amount in the body.

Take your doses at evenly spaced times around the clock, and try not to miss a dose.

■ *If you miss a dose...*
  Take it as soon as you remember. If it is almost time for the next dose, and you take 2 doses a day, take the one you missed and the next dose 5 to 6 hours later. If you take 3 or more doses a day, take the one you missed and the next dose 2 to 4 hours later. Then go back to your regular schedule. Do not take 2 doses at once.

■ *Storage information...*
  Store Omnipen Capsules at room temperature in a tightly closed container.

  Keep Omnipen Oral Suspension in the refrigerator, in a tightly closed container. Discard the unused portion after 14 days.

## What side effects may occur?

Side effects cannot be anticipated. If any develop or change in intensity, inform your doctor as soon as possible. Only your doctor can determine whether it is safe for you to continue taking Omnipen.

■ *Side effects may include:*
  Colitis (inflammation of the bowel), diarrhea, fever, itching, nausea, rash or other skin problems, sore tongue or mouth, vomiting

## Why should this drug not be prescribed?

You should not take Omnipen if you are allergic to penicillin or cephalosporin antibiotics.

## Special warnings about this medication

If you have an allergic reaction, stop taking Omnipen and contact your doctor immediately.

After you have taken Omnipen for a long time, you may get a new infection (called a superinfection) due to an organism this medication cannot treat. Consult your doctor if your symptoms do not improve or seem to get worse.

Omnipen sometimes causes diarrhea. Some diarrhea medications can make the diarrhea worse. Check with your doctor before taking any diarrhea remedy.

Oral contraceptives may not work properly while you are taking Omnipen. For greater certainty, use other measures while taking Omnipen.

If you are diabetic, be aware that Omnipen may cause a *false positive* in certain urine glucose tests. You should talk to your doctor about the right tests to use while you are taking Omnipen.

For infections such as strep throat, it is important to take Omnipen for the entire amount of time your doctor has prescribed. Even if you feel better, you need to continue taking the medication.

### Possible food and drug interactions when taking this medication

If Omnipen is taken with certain other drugs the effects of either could be increased, decreased, or altered. It is especially important to check with your doctor before combining Omnipen with any of the following:

Allopurinol (Zyloprim)
Atenolol (Tenormin)
Chloroquine (Aralen)
Mefloquine (Lariam)
Oral contraceptives

### Special information if you are pregnant or breastfeeding

The effects of Omnipen during pregnancy have not been adequately studied. If you are pregnant or plan to become pregnant, inform your doctor immediately. Omnipen should be used during pregnancy only if the potential benefit justifies the potential risk to the developing baby.

Omnipen appears in breast milk and could affect a nursing infant. If this medication is essential to your health, your doctor may advise you to stop breastfeeding until your treatment with Omnipen is finished.

### Recommended dosage

Unless you are being treated for gonorrhea, your doctor will have you continue taking Omnipen for 2 to 3 days after your symptoms have disappeared. Dosages are for capsules and oral suspension.

ADULTS

*Infections of the Genital, Urinary, or Gastrointestinal Tracts*
The usual dose is 500 milligrams, taken every 6 hours.

*Gonorrhea*
The usual dose is 3.5 grams in a single oral dose along with 1 gram of probenecid

*Respiratory Tract Infections*
The usual dose is 250 milligrams, taken every 6 hours.

CHILDREN

Children weighing over 44 pounds should follow the adult dose schedule.

Children weighing 44 pounds or less should have their dosage determined by their weight.

*Infections of the Genital, Urinary, or Gastrointestinal Tracts*
The usual dose is 100 milligrams for each 2.2 pounds of body weight daily, divided into 4 doses for the capsules, and 3 to 4 doses for the suspension.

*Respiratory Tract Infections*
The usual dose is 50 milligrams for each 2.2 pounds of body weight daily, divided into 3 to 4 doses.

### Overdosage

Although no specific symptoms have been reported, any medication taken in excess can have serious consequences. If you suspect an overdose of Omnipen, seek medical attention immediately.

*Generic name:*

# Ondansetron

*See Zofran, page 609.*

*Brand name:*

# Opcon-A

*See Naphcon-A, page 346.*

*Category:*

# Oral Contraceptives

*Brand names: Brevicon, Demulen, Desogen, Genora, Levlen, Loestrin, Lo/Ovral, Micronor, Modicon, Nordette, Norethin, Norinyl, Ortho-Cept, Ortho-Cyclen, Ortho-Novum, Ortho Tri-Cyclen, Ovcon, Ovral, Triphasil*

### Why is this drug prescribed?

Oral contraceptives (also known as "The Pill") are highly effective means of preventing pregnancy. Oral contraceptives consist of synthetic forms of two hormones produced naturally in the body: either progestin alone or estrogen and progestin. Estrogen and progestin regulate a woman's menstrual cycle, and the fluctuating levels of these hormones play an essential role in fertility.

To reduce side effects, oral contraceptives are available in a wide range of estrogen and progestin concentrations. Progestin-only products (such as Micronor) are usually prescribed for women who should avoid estrogens; however, they may not be as effective as estrogen/progestin contraceptives.

### Most important fact about this drug

Cigarette smoking increases the risk of serious heart-related side effects (stroke, heart attack, blood clots, etc.) in women who use oral contraceptives. This risk increases with heavy smoking (15 or more cigarettes per day) and with age. There is an especially significant increase in heart disease risk in women over 35 years old who smoke and use oral contraceptives.

### How should you take this medication?

Oral contraceptives should be taken daily, no more than 24 hours apart, for the duration of the prescribed cycle of 21 or 28 days. Ideally, you should take your pill at the same time every day to reduce the chance of forgetting a dose.

■ *If you miss a dose...*

If you neglect to take only one estrogen/progestin pill, take it as soon as you remember, take the next pill at your regular time, and continue taking the rest of the medication cycle. The risk of pregnancy is small if you miss only one combination pill per cycle. If you miss more than one tablet, check your product's patient information for instructions.

Missing a single progestin-only tablet increases the chance of pregnancy. Consult your doctor immediately if you miss a single dose and use another method of birth control until your next period begins or pregnancy is ruled out.

■ *Storage instructions...*

To help keep track of your doses, use the original container. Store at room temperature.

### What side effects may occur?

Side effects cannot be anticipated. If any develop or change in intensity, inform your doctor as soon as possible. Only your doctor can determine if it is safe for you to continue taking an oral contraceptive.

■ *Side effects may include:*

Abdominal cramps, acne, appetite changes, bladder infection, bleeding in spots during a menstrual period, bloating, blood clots, breast tenderness or enlargement, cataracts, chest pain, contact lens discomfort, decreased flow of milk when given immediately after birth, depression, difficulty breathing, dizziness, fluid retention, gallbladder disease, growth of face, back, chest, or stomach hair, hair loss, headache, heart attack, high blood pressure, inflammation of the large intestine, kidney trouble, lack of menstrual periods, liver tumors, lumps in the breast, menstrual pattern changes, migraine, muscle, joint, or leg pain, nausea, nervousness, premenstrual syndrome (PMS), secretion of milk, sex drive changes, skin infection, skin rash or discoloration, stomach cramps, stroke, swelling, temporary infertility, unexplained bleeding in the vagina, vaginal discharge, vaginal infections (and/or burning and itching), visual disturbances, vomiting, weight gain or loss, yellow skin or whites of eyes

### Why should this drug not be prescribed?

You should not take oral contraceptives if you have had an allergic reaction to them or if you are pregnant (or think you might be).

If you have ever had breast cancer or cancer in the reproductive organs or liver tumors, you should not take oral contraceptives.

If you have or have ever had a stroke, heart disease, angina (severe chest pain), or blood clots, you should not take oral contraceptives. Women who have had pregnancy-related jaundice or jaundice stemming from previous use of oral contraceptives should not take them.

If you have undiagnosed and/or unexplained abnormal vaginal bleeding, do not take oral contraceptives.

### Special warnings about this medication

Oral contraceptives should be used with caution if you are over 40 years old; smoke tobacco; have liver, heart, gallbladder, kidney, or thyroid disease; have high blood pressure, high cholesterol, diabetes, epilepsy, asthma, or porphyria (a blood disorder); or are obese.

In addition, you should use oral contraceptives with caution if you have a family history of breast cancer or other cancers, or you have a personal history of depression, migraine or other headaches, irregular menstrual periods, or visual disturbances.

Since the blood's clotting ability may be affected by oral contraceptives, your doctor may take you off them prior to surgery. If bleeding lasts more than 8 days while you are on a progestin-only oral contraceptive, be sure to let your doctor know.

Oral contraceptives do not protect against HIV infection (AIDS) or any other sexually transmitted disease.

If you miss a menstrual period but have taken your pills regularly, contact your doctor but do not stop taking your pills. If you miss a period and have not taken your pills regularly, or if you miss two consecutive periods, you may be pregnant; stop taking your pills and check with your doctor immediately to see if you are pregnant. Use another form of birth control while you are not taking your pills.

### Possible food and drug interactions when taking this medication

If oral contraceptives are taken with certain other drugs, the effects of either could be increased, decreased, or altered. It is especially important to check with your doctor before combining oral contraceptives with the following:

Amitriptyline (Elavil, Endep)
Ampicillin (Principen, Totacillin)
Barbiturates (phenobarbital, Seconal)
Carbamazepine (Tegretol)
Chloramphenicol (Chloromycetin)
Clomipramine (Anafranil)
Diazepam (Valium)
Doxepin (Sinequan)
Glipizide (Glucotrol)
Griseofulvin (Fulvicin, Grisactin)
Imipramine (Tofranil)
Lorazepam (Ativan)
Metoprolol (Lopressor)
Oxazepam (Serax)
Penicillin (Veetids, Pen-Vee K)
Phenylbutazone (Butazolidin)
Phenytoin (Dilantin)
Prednisolone (Prelone, Pediapred)
Prednisone (Deltasone)
Primidone (Mysoline)
Propranolol (Inderal)
Rifampin (Rifadin, Rimactane)

Sulfonamides (Bactrim, Septra)
Tetracycline (Achromycin V, Sumycin)
Theophylline (Theo-Dur, Slo-bid)
Warfarin (Coumadin, Panwarfin)

In addition, oral contraceptives may affect tests for blood sugar levels and thyroid function and may cause an increase in blood cholesterol levels.

### Special information
### if you are pregnant or breastfeeding

If you are pregnant (or think you might be), you should not use oral contraceptives, since they are not safe during pregnancy. In addition, wait at least 4 weeks after delivery before starting an oral contraceptive.

In general, nursing mothers should not use oral contraceptives, since these drugs can appear in breast milk and may cause jaundice and enlarged breasts in nursing infants. Your doctor may advise you to use a different form of contraception while you are nursing your baby.

### Recommended dosage

If you have any questions about how you should take oral contraceptives, consult your doctor or the patient instructions that come in the drug package. The following is a partial list of instructions for taking oral contraceptives; it should not be used as a substitute for consultation with your doctor.

Some brands can be started on the first day of your menstrual cycle or on the first Sunday afterwards. Others must be started on the fifth day of the cycle or the first Sunday afterwards. The instructions below are for the first-Sunday schedule.

Oral contraceptives are supplied in 21-day and 28-day packages.

FOR A 21-DAY SCHEDULE

Oral contraceptives are taken every day for a 3-week period, followed by 1 week of no oral contraceptives; this cycle is repeated each month.

1) Starting on the first Sunday after the beginning of your menstrual period, take one tablet daily (at the same time each day) for the next 21 days. Note: If your period begins on Sunday, take the first tablet that day.
2) Wait 1 week before taking any tablets. Your menstrual period should occur during this time.
3) Following this 1-week waiting time, begin taking a daily tablet again for the next 21 days.

## FOR A 28-DAY SCHEDULE

Starting on the first Sunday after the beginning of your menstrual period, take one tablet daily (at the same time each day) for the next 28 days. Continue taking the oral contraceptives according to your physician's instructions. Note: If your period begins on Sunday, take the first tablet that day.

## FOR BOTH 21- AND 28-DAY REGIMENS

When following a regimen with a Sunday or Day 5 start, use an additional method of birth control for the first 7 days of the cycle.

Progestin-only tablets should be taken every day of the year.

### Overdosage

While any medication taken in excess can cause overdose, the risk associated with oral contraceptives is minimal. Even young children who have taken large amounts of oral contraceptives have not experienced serious adverse effects. However, if you suspect an overdose, seek medical help immediately.

■ *Symptoms of overdose may include:*
Nausea, withdrawal bleeding in females

*Brand name:*

# Orasone

*See Deltasone, page 142.*

*Brand name:*

# Orinase

*Pronounced: OR-in-aze*
*Generic name: Tolbutamide*

### Why is this drug prescribed?

Orinase is an oral antidiabetic medication used to treat Type II (non-insulin-dependent) diabetes. Diabetes occurs when the body does not make enough insulin, or when the insulin that is produced no longer works properly. Insulin works by helping sugar get inside the body's cells, where it is then used for energy.

There are two forms of diabetes: Type I (insulin-dependent) and Type II (non-insulin-dependent). Type I diabetes usually requires taking insulin injections for life, while Type II diabetes can usually be treated by dietary changes, exercise, and/or oral antidiabetic medications such as Orinase. Orinase controls diabetes by stimulating the pancreas to secrete more insulin and by helping insulin work better.

Occasionally, Type II diabetics must take insulin injections temporarily during stressful periods or times of illness. When diet, exercise, and an oral antidiabetic medication fail to reduce symptoms and/or blood sugar levels, a person with Type II diabetes may require long-term insulin injections.

### Most important fact about this drug

Always remember that Orinase is an aid to, not a substitute for, good diet and exercise. Failure to follow a sound diet and exercise plan can lead to serious complications, such as dangerously high or low blood sugar levels. Remember, too, that Orinase is *not* an oral form of insulin, and cannot be used in place of insulin.

### How should you take this medication?

In general, Orinase should be taken 30 minutes before a meal to achieve the best control over blood sugar levels. However, the exact dosing schedule, as well as the dosage amount, must be determined by your physician. Ask your doctor when it is best for you to take this medication.

To help prevent low blood sugar levels (hypoglycemia) you should:

Understand the symptoms of hypoglycemia.
Know how exercise affects your blood sugar levels.
Maintain an adequate diet.
Keep a product containing quick-acting sugar with you at all times.
Limit alcohol intake. If you drink alcohol, it may cause breathlessness and facial flushing.

■ *If you miss a dose...*
Take it as soon as you remember. If it is almost time for the next dose, skip the one you missed and go back to your regular schedule. Do not take 2 doses at the same time.
■ *Storage instructions...*
Store at room temperature.

### What side effects may occur?

Side effects cannot be anticipated. If any develop or change in intensity, inform your doctor as soon as possible. Only your doctor can determine if it is safe for you to continue taking Orinase.

Side effects from Orinase are rare and seldom require discontinuation of the medication.

■ *More common side effects may include:*
Bloating, heartburn, nausea
■ *Less common or rare side effects may include:*
Anemia and other blood disorders, blistering, changes in taste, headache, hepatic porphyria (a condition frequently characterized by sensitivity to light, stomach pain, and nerve damage, caused by excessive levels of a substance called porphyrin in the liver), hives, itching, redness of the skin, skin eruptions, skin rash

Orinase, like all oral antidiabetics, may cause hypoglycemia (low blood sugar). The risk of hypoglycemia can be increased by missed meals, alcohol, other medications, fever, trauma, infection, surgery, or excessive exercise. To avoid hypoglycemia, you should closely follow the dietary and exercise plan suggested by your physician.

■ *Symptoms of mild hypoglycemia may include:*
Cold sweat, drowsiness, fast heartbeat, headache, nausea, nervousness.
■ *Symptoms of more severe hypoglycemia may include:*
Coma, pale skin, seizures, shallow breathing.

Contact your doctor immediately if these symptoms of severe low blood sugar occur.

Ask your doctor what you should do if you experience mild hypoglycemia. Severe hypoglycemia should be considered a medical emergency, and prompt medical attention is essential.

### Why should this drug not be prescribed?
You should not take Orinase if you have had an allergic reaction to it.

Orinase should not be taken if you are suffering from diabetic ketoacidosis (a life-threatening medical emergency caused by insufficient insulin and marked by excessive thirst, nausea, fatigue, pain below the breastbone, and fruity breath).

In addition, Orinase should not be used as the sole therapy in treating Type I (insulin-dependent) diabetes.

### Special warnings about this medication
It's possible that drugs such as Orinase may lead to more heart problems than diet treatment alone, or diet plus insulin. If you have a heart condition, you may want to discuss this with your doctor.

If you are taking Orinase, you should check your blood or urine periodically for abnormal sugar (glucose) levels.

It is important that you closely follow the diet and exercise plan recommended by your doctor.

Even people with well-controlled diabetes may find that stress, illness, surgery, or fever results in a loss of control over their diabetes. In these cases, your physician may recommend that you temporarily stop taking Orinase and use injected insulin instead.

In addition, the effectiveness of any oral antidiabetic, including Orinase, may decrease with time. This may occur because of either a diminished responsiveness to the medication or a worsening of the diabetes.

Like other antidiabetic drugs, Orinase may produce severe low blood sugar if the dosage is wrong. While taking Orinase, you are particularly susceptible to episodes of low blood sugar if:

You suffer from a kidney or liver problem;
You have a lack of adrenal or pituitary hormone;
You are elderly, run-down, malnourished, hungry, exercising heavily, drinking alcohol, or using more than one glucose-lowering drug.

### Possible food and drug interactions when taking this medication
If Orinase is taken with certain other drugs, the effects of either could be increased, decreased, or altered. It is especially important to check with your doctor before combining Orinase with the following:

Adrenal corticosteroids such as prednisone (Deltasone) and cortisone (Cortone)
Airway-opening drugs such as Proventil and Ventolin
Anabolic steroids such as testosterone
Barbiturates such as Amytal, Seconal, and phenobarbital
Beta blockers such as Inderal and Tenormin
Blood-thinning drugs such as Coumadin
Calcium channel blockers such as Cardizem and Procardia
Chloramphenicol (Chloromycetin)
Cimetidine (Tagamet)
Clofibrate (Atromid-S)
Colestipol (Colestid)
Epinephrine (EpiPen)

Estrogens (Premarin)
Fluconazole (Diflucan)
Furosemide (Lasix)
Isoniazid (Laniazid, Rifamate)
Itraconazole (Sporanox)
Major tranquilizers such as Stelazine and Mellaril
MAO inhibitors such as Nardil and Parnate
Methyldopa (Aldomet)
Miconazole (Monistat)
Niacin (Nicobid, Nicolar)
Nonsteroidal anti-inflammatory agents such as
   Advil, aspirin, Motrin, Naprosyn, and Voltaren
Oral contraceptives
Phenytoin (Dilantin)
Probenecid (Benemid)
Rifampin (Rifadin)
Sulfa drugs such as Bactrim and Septra
Thiazide and other diuretics such as Diuril and
   HydroDIURIL
Thyroid medications such as Synthroid

Be cautious about drinking alcohol, since excessive alcohol can cause low blood sugar.

## Special information
## if you are pregnant or breastfeeding

The effects of Orinase during pregnancy have not been adequately established in humans. Since Orinase has caused birth defects in rats, it is not recommended for use by pregnant women. Therefore, if you are pregnant or planning to become pregnant, you should take Orinase only on the advice of your physician. Since studies suggest the importance of maintaining normal blood sugar (glucose) levels during pregnancy, your physician may prescribe injected insulin during your pregnancy. While it is not known if Orinase enters breast milk, other similar medications do. Therefore, you should discuss with your doctor whether to discontinue the medication or to stop breastfeeding. If the medication is discontinued, and if diet alone does not control glucose levels, your doctor will consider giving you insulin injections.

## Recommended dosage

Dosage levels are based on individual needs.

### ADULTS

Usually an initial daily dose of 1 to 2 grams is recommended. Maintenance therapy usually ranges from 0.25 to 3 grams daily. Daily doses greater than 3 grams are not recommended.

### CHILDREN

Safety and effectiveness have not been established in children.

### OLDER ADULTS

Older, malnourished, or debilitated people, or those with impaired kidney or liver function, are usually prescribed lower initial and maintenance doses to minimize the risk of low blood sugar (hypoglycemia).

## Overdosage

Any medication taken in excess can have serious consequences. An overdose of Orinase can cause low blood sugar (see "Special warnings about this medication"). Eating sugar or a sugar-based product will often correct mild hypoglycemia. If you suspect an overdose, seek medical attention immediately.

*Generic name:*

# Orphenadrine, Aspirin, and Caffeine

*See Norgesic, page 367.*

*Brand name:*

# Ortho-Cept

*See Oral Contraceptives, page 382.*

*Brand name:*

# Ortho-Cyclen

*See Oral Contraceptives, page 382.*

*Brand name:*

# Ortho-Est

*See Ogen, page 379.*

*Brand name:*

# Ortho-Novum

*See Oral Contraceptives, page 382.*

*Brand name:*

# Ortho Tri-Cyclen

*See Oral Contraceptives, page 382.*

*Brand name:*

# Orudis

*Pronounced: Oh-ROO-dis*
*Generic name: Ketoprofen*
*Other brand names: Orudis KT, Oruvail*

## Why is this drug prescribed?

Orudis, a nonsteroidal anti-inflammatory drug, is used to relieve the inflammation, swelling, stiffness, and joint pain associated with rheumatoid arthritis and osteoarthritis (the most common form of arthritis). It is also used to relieve mild to moderate pain, as well as menstrual pain. Oruvail, an extended-release form of the drug, is used to treat the signs and symptoms of rheumatoid arthritis and osteoarthritis over the long term, not severe attacks that come on suddenly.

## Most important fact about this drug

You should have frequent check-ups with your doctor if you take Orudis regularly. Ulcers or internal bleeding can occur without warning.

## How should you take this medication?

To minimize side effects, your doctor may recommend that you take Orudis with food, an antacid, or milk.

If you are using Orudis for arthritis, it should be taken regularly.

Orudis and Oruvail should not be taken together.

■ *If you miss a dose...*
If you take Orudis on a regular schedule, take the forgotten dose as soon as you remember. If it is almost time for your next dose, skip the one you missed and go back to your regular schedule. Do not take 2 doses at once.
■ *Storage instructions...*
Store at room temperature in a tightly closed container. Protect Oruvail capsules from direct light and excessive heat and humidity.

## What side effects may occur?

Side effects cannot be anticipated. If any develop or change in intensity, inform your doctor as soon as possible. Only your doctor can determine if it is safe for you to continue taking Orudis.

■ *More common side effects may include:*
Abdominal pain, changes in kidney function, constipation, diarrhea, dreams, fluid retention, gas, headache, inability to sleep, indigestion, nausea, nervousness
■ *Less common or rare side effects may include:*
Allergic reaction, amnesia, anemia, asthma, belching, blood in the urine, bloody or black stools, change in taste, chills, confusion, congestive heart failure, coughing up blood, conjunctivitis (pinkeye), depression, difficult or labored breathing, dizziness, dry mouth, eye pain, facial swelling due to fluid retention, general feeling of illness, hair loss, high blood pressure, hives, impaired hearing, impotence, increase in appetite, increased salivation, infection, inflammation of the mouth, irregular or excessive menstrual bleeding, itching, kidney failure, loosening of fingernails, loss of appetite, migraine, muscle pain, nasal inflammation, nosebleed, pain, peptic or intestinal ulcer, rapid heartbeat, rash, rectal bleeding, red or purple spots on the skin, ringing in the ears, sensitivity to light, skin discoloration, skin eruptions, skin inflammation and flaking, sleepiness, sore throat, stomach inflammation, sweating, swelling of the throat, thirst, throbbing heartbeat, tingling or pins and needles, vertigo, visual disturbances, vomiting, vomiting blood, weight gain or loss

## Why should this drug not be prescribed?

If you are sensitive to or have ever had an allergic reaction to Orudis, or if you have had asthma attacks, hives, or other allergic reactions caused by aspirin or other nonsteroidal anti-inflammatory drugs, you should not take this medication. Make sure your doctor is aware of any drug reactions you have experienced.

## Special warnings about this medication

Remember that stomach ulcers and bleeding can occur without warning.

This drug should be used with caution if you have kidney or liver disease.

If you are taking Orudis for an extended period of time, your doctor will check your blood for anemia.

This drug can increase water retention. Use with caution if you have heart disease or high blood pressure.

## Possible food and drug interactions when taking this medication

If Orudis is taken with certain other drugs, the effects of either could be increased, decreased, or altered. It is especially important to check with your doctor before combining Orudis with the following:

Aspirin
Blood thinners such as Coumadin
Diuretics such as hydrochlorothiazide
   (HydroDIURIL)
Lithium (Lithonate)
Methotrexate
Probenecid (the gout medication Benemid)

Orudis can prolong bleeding time. If you are taking blood-thinning medication, use this drug cautiously.

## Special information if you are pregnant or breastfeeding

The effects of Orudis during pregnancy have not been adequately studied. If you are pregnant or plan to become pregnant, inform your doctor immediately. Orudis may appear in breast milk and could affect a nursing infant. If this medication is essential to your health, your doctor may advise you to discontinue breastfeeding until your treatment with this medication is finished.

## Recommended dosage

ADULTS

*Rheumatoid Arthritis and Osteoarthritis*
The starting dose of Orudis is 75 milligrams 3 times a day or 50 milligrams 4 times a day; for Oruvail, 200 milligrams taken once a day. The most you should take in a day is 300 milligrams of Orudis or 200 milligrams of Oruvail. Some side effects, such as headache or upset stomach, increase in severity as the dose gets higher.

*Mild to Moderate Pain and Menstrual Pain*
The usual dose of Orudis is 25 to 50 milligrams every 6 to 8 hours as needed.

Smaller people, older people, and those with kidney or liver disease need smaller doses of Orudis. Doses above 75 milligrams have no additional effect.

CHILDREN

The safety and effectiveness of Orudis have not been established in children.

OLDER ADULTS

You may need a lower dosage.

## Overdosage

Any medication taken in excess can have serious consequences. If you suspect an overdose of Orudis, seek medical attention immediately.

- *Symptoms of Orudis overdose may include:*
  Breathing difficulty, coma, convulsions, drowsiness, high blood pressure, kidney failure, low blood pressure, nausea, sluggishness, stomach and intestinal bleeding, stomach pain, vomiting

*Brand name:*
# Oruvail

See Orudis, page 388.

*Brand name:*
# Ovcon

See Oral Contraceptives, page 382.

*Brand name:*
# Ovral

See Oral Contraceptives, page 382.

*Generic name:*
# Oxaprozin

See Daypro, page 133.

*Generic name:*
# Oxazepam

See Serax, page 496.

*Generic name:*
# Oxiconazole

See Oxistat, page 390.

*Brand name:*

# Oxistat

*Pronounced: OX-ee-stat*
*Generic name: Oxiconazole nitrate*

## Why is this drug prescribed?

Oxistat is used to treat fungal skin diseases commonly called ringworm (tinea). Oxistat is prescribed for athlete's foot (tinea pedis), jock itch (tinea cruris), and ringworm of the entire body (tinea corporis). It is available as a cream or lotion.

## Most important fact about this drug

Oxistat should not be used in, on, or near the eyes, or applied to the vagina.

## How should you use this medication?

Use Oxistat exactly as prescribed.

Wash and dry the area to be treated before applying Oxistat and then apply the cream or lotion so that it covers the entire affected area and the area right around it.

Be careful when applying to raw, blistered, or oozing skin.

■ *If you miss a dose...*
Apply the cream or lotion when you remember, then return to your regular schedule.
■ *Storage instructions...*
Store Oxistat at room temperature.

## What side effects may occur?

Side effects cannot be anticipated. If any develop or change in intensity, notify your doctor as soon as possible. Only your doctor can determine whether it is safe for you to continue using Oxistat.

■ *Side effects may include:*
Allergic skin inflammation, burning, cracks in the skin, eczema, irritation, itching, pain, rash, scaling, skin redness, skin softening, small, firm, raised skin eruptions similar to those of chickenpox, stinging, tingling

## Why should this drug not be prescribed?

Do not use Oxistat if you have ever had an allergic reaction or are sensitive to oxiconazole or any other ingredients in the cream.

## Special warnings about this medication

If you develop an irritation or sensitivity to the medication, notify your doctor.

## Possible food and drug interactions when taking this medication

No interactions have been reported.

## Special information if you are pregnant or breastfeeding

Oxistat has not been proved safe during pregnancy. If you are pregnant or plan to become pregnant, inform your doctor immediately.

Oxistat appears in breast milk and could affect a nursing infant. If Oxistat is essential to your health, your doctor may advise you to stop breastfeeding until your treatment is finished.

## Recommended dosage

ADULTS AND CHILDREN

Apply Oxistat Cream or Lotion to cover the affected area once or twice a day. Athlete's foot (tinea pedis) is treated for 1 month. Jock itch (tinea cruris) and ringworm of the body (tinea corporis) are treated for 2 weeks. If your does not improve, your doctor will re-evaluate the diagnosis.

## Overdosage

Overdose of Oxistat has not been reported. However, if you suspect an overdose, seek medical attention immediately.

---

*Generic name:*

# Oxybutynin

See Ditropan, page 170.

---

*Brand name:*

# Pamelor

*Pronounced: PAM-eh-lore*
*Generic name: Nortriptyline hydrochloride*
*Other brand name: Aventyl*

## Why is this drug prescribed?

Pamelor is prescribed for the relief of symptoms of depression. Pamelor is in the class of drugs known as tricyclic antidepressants.

Some doctors also prescribe Pamelor to treat chronic hives, premenstrual depression, attention deficit hyperactivity disorder in children, and bedwetting.

## Most important fact about this drug

Pamelor must be taken regularly to be effective and it may be several weeks before you begin to feel better. Do not skip doses, even if they seem to make no difference.

## How should you take this medication?

Take Pamelor exactly as prescribed. Pamelor may make your mouth dry. Sucking on hard candy, chewing gum, or melting ice chips in your mouth can provide relief.

■ *If you miss a dose...*

Take it as soon as you remember. If it is almost time for the next dose, skip the one you missed and go back to your regular schedule. If you take Pamelor once a day at bedtime and you miss a dose, do not take it in the morning, since disturbing side effects could occur. Never take 2 doses at once.

■ *Storage instructions...*

Keep Pamelor in the container it came in, tightly closed and away from light. Be sure to keep this drug out of reach of children; an overdose is particularly dangerous in the young. Store at room temperature.

## What side effects may occur?

Side effects cannot be anticipated. If any develop or change in intensity, inform your doctor as soon as possible. Only your doctor can determine if it is safe for you to continue taking Pamelor.

■ *Side effects may include:*

Abdominal cramps, agitation, anxiety, black tongue, blurred vision, breast development in males, breast enlargement, confusion, constipation, delusions, diarrhea, dilation of pupils, disorientation, dizziness, drowsiness, dry mouth, excessive or spontaneous flow of milk, excessive urination at night, fatigue, fever, fluid retention, flushing, frequent urination, hair loss, hallucinations, headache, heart attack, high or low blood pressure, high or low blood sugar, hives, impotence, inability to sleep, inability to urinate, increased or decreased sex drive, inflammation of the mouth, intestinal blockage, itching, loss of appetite, loss of coordination, nausea, nightmares, numbness, panic, perspiration, pins and needles in the arms and legs, rapid, fluttery, or irregular heartbeat, rash, reddish or purplish spots on skin, restlessness, ringing in the ears, seizures, sensitivity to light, stomach upset, strange taste, stroke, swelling of the testicles, swollen glands,

tingling, tremors, vision problems, vomiting, weakness, weight gain or loss, yellow eyes and skin

■ *Side effects due to rapid decrease or abrupt withdrawal from Pamelor after a long term of treatment include:*

Headache, nausea, vague feeling of bodily discomfort

These side effects do not indicate addiction to this drug.

## Why should this drug not be prescribed?

If you are sensitive to or have ever had an allergic reaction to Pamelor or similar drugs, you should not take this medication. Make sure your doctor is ware of any drug reactions you have experienced.

Do not take Pamelor if you are taking—or have taken one within the past 14 days—an antidepressant drug classified as an MAO inhibitor. Drugs in this category include Nardil and Parnate. Combining these drugs with Pamelor can cause fever and convulsions, and could even be fatal.

Unless you are directed to do so by your doctor, do not take this medication if you are recovering from a heart attack or are taking any other antidepressant drugs.

If you have been taking Prozac, you may have to wait at least 5 weeks before beginning therapy with Pamelor. A drug interaction could result.

## Special warnings about this medication

Pamelor may cause you to become drowsy or less alert; therefore, you should not drive or operate dangerous machinery or participate in any hazardous activity that requires full mental alertness until you know how this drug affects you.

Use Pamelor with caution if you have a history of seizures, difficulty urinating, diabetes, or chronic eye conditions such as glaucoma. Be careful, also, if you have heart disease, high blood pressure, an overactive thyroid, or are receiving thyroid medication. You should discuss all of your medical problems with your doctor before taking this medication.

If you are being treated for a severe mental disorder (schizophrenia or manic depression), tell your doctor before taking Pamelor.

Pamelor may make your skin more sensitive to sunlight. Try to stay out of the sun, wear protective clothing, and apply a sun block.

Before having surgery, dental treatment or any diagnostic procedure, tell your doctor that you are taking Pamelor. Certain drugs used during these procedures, such as anesthetics and muscle relaxants, may interact with Pamelor.

### Possible food and drug interactions when taking this medication

Combining Pamelor and MAO inhibitors can be fatal.

Pamelor may intensify the effects of alcohol. Do not drink alcohol while taking this medication.

If Pamelor is taken with certain other drugs, the effects of either can be increased, decreased, or altered. It is especially important to check with your doctor before combining Pamelor with the following:

Airway-opening drugs such as Ventolin and Proventil
Antidepressants such as Wellbutrin and Desyrel
Antidepressants that act on serotonin, such as
    Prozac, Paxil and Zoloft
Antispasmodic drugs such as Donnatal and Bentyl
Blood pressure medications such as Catapres and
    Esimil
Cimetidine (Tagamet)
Chlorpropamide (Diabinese)
Drugs for heart irregularities, such as Tambocor
    and Rythmol
Levodopa (Larodopa)
Major tranquilizers such as Thorazine and Mellaril
Quinidine (Quinidex)
Reserpine (Diupres)
Stimulants such as Dexedrine
Thyroid medication such as Synthroid
Warfarin (Coumadin)

### Special information if you are pregnant or breastfeeding

The effects of Pamelor during pregnancy have not been adequately studied. If you are pregnant or planning to become pregnant, inform your doctor immediately. Also consult your doctor before breastfeeding.

### Recommended dosage

This medication is available in tablet and liquid form. Only tablet dosages are listed. Consult your doctor if you cannot take the tablet form of this medication.

ADULTS

Your doctor will monitor your response to this medication carefully and will gradually increase or decrease the dose to suit your needs.

The usual starting dosage is 25 milligrams, 3 or 4 times per day.

Alternatively, your doctor may prescribe that the total daily dose be taken once a day.

Doses above 150 milligrams per day are not recommended.

Your doctor may want to perform a blood test to help in deciding the best dose you should receive.

CHILDREN

The safety and effectiveness of Pamelor have not been established for children and its use is not recommended. However, adolescents may be given 30 to 50 milligrams per day, either in a single dose or divided into smaller doses, as determined by your doctor.

OLDER ADULTS

The usual dose is 30 to 50 milligrams taken in a single dose or divided into smaller doses, as determined by your doctor.

### Overdosage

An overdose of this type of antidepressant can be fatal. If you suspect an overdose, seek medical help immediately.

■ *Symptoms of Pamelor overdose may include:*
    Agitation, coma, confusion, congestive heart failure, convulsions, decreased breathing, excessive reflexes, extremely high fever, rapid heartbeat, restlessness, rigid muscles, shock, stupor, vomiting

If you suspect a Pamelor overdose, seek medical attention immediately.

*Brand name:*

# Panadol

See Tylenol, page 571.

*Brand name:*

# Pancrease

*Pronounced: PAN-kree-ace*
*Generic name: Pancrelipase*
*Other brand names: Creon, Pancrease MT,*
    *Viokase, Ultrase*

### Why is this drug prescribed?

Pancrease is used to treat pancreatic enzyme deficiency. It is often prescribed for people with cystic fibrosis, chronic inflammation of the pancreas, or blockages of the pancreas or common bile duct caused by cancer. It is also taken by people who have had their pancreas removed or who have had gastrointestinal bypass surgery. Pancrease is taken to help with digestion of proteins, starches, and fats.

### Most important fact about this drug

Pancrease capsules should not be chewed or crushed.

### How should you take this medication?

Take this medication exactly as prescribed. If you are taking Pancrease for cystic fibrosis, your doctor may also prescribe a special diet for you. Be sure to follow the diet closely, as well as taking Pancrease.

Do not change brands or dosage forms of this medication without first checking with your doctor.

If swallowing the Pancrease capsule is difficult, open the capsule and shake the contents (microspheres) onto a small amount of soft food, such as applesauce or gelatin, that does not require chewing, then swallow immediately. Avoid mixing it with alkaline foods, such as ice cream or milk. They can reduce the medication's effect.

Pancrease should be taken with meals and snacks. Drink plenty of fluids while you are taking Pancrease.

■ *If you miss a dose...*
Resume taking the medication with your next meal or snack.
■ *Storage instructions...*
Store at room temperature in a tightly closed container away from moisture. Do not refrigerate.

### What side effects may occur?

Side effects cannot be anticipated. If any develop or change in intensity, inform your doctor as soon as possible. Only your doctor can determine if it is safe for you to continue taking Pancrease.

■ *More common side effects may include:*
Stomach and intestinal upset
■ *Less common or rare side effects may include:*
Allergic-type reactions

### Why should this drug not be prescribed?

Pancrease should not be used if you are sensitive to or have ever had an allergic reaction to pork protein, if you have a recently inflamed pancreas, or if you have a disease of the pancreas that gets worse.

### Special warnings about this medication

If you develop an allergic reaction to Pancrease, stop taking the medication and inform your doctor immediately. If you have cystic fibrosis and develop any signs of an intestinal blockage, call your doctor.

### Possible food and drug interactions when taking this medication

If Pancrease is taken with certain other drugs, the effects of either can be increased, decreased, or altered. It is especially important that you check with your doctor before combining Pancrease with the following:

Certain antacids such as Tums and Milk of Magnesia
Ulcer medications classified as $H_{+72}$ histamine antagonists, such as Pepcid and Zantac

### Special information if you are pregnant or breastfeeding

The effects of Pancrease during pregnancy have not been adequately studied. If you are pregnant or plan to become pregnant, inform your doctor immediately.

It is not known whether Pancrease appears in breast milk. Your doctor may advise you not to nurse while you are taking this drug.

### Recommended dosage

ADULTS

Doses range from 4,000 units to 20,000 units (more if necessary) with each meal and with snacks. The dosage will be adjusted based on your response. Any increase in dosage should be made slowly. People with cystic fibrosis may require less.

CHILDREN

Your doctor will determine the best dosage of Pancrease based on the child's individual needs.

### Overdosage

Although no specific information is available, any medication taken in excess can have serious consequences. If you suspect an overdose of Pancrease, seek medical treatment immediately.

*Generic name:*

# Pancrelipase

*See Pancrease, page 392.*

*Brand name:*

# Parafon Forte DSC

*Pronounced: PAIR-a-fahn FOR-tay DEE-ESS-SEE*
*Generic name: Chlorzoxazone*

## Why is this drug prescribed?

Parafon Forte DSC is prescribed, along with rest and physical therapy, for the relief of discomfort associated with severe, painful muscle spasms.

## Most important fact about this drug

Although rare, serious, sometimes fatal liver problems have been reported in people using Parafon Forte DSC. You should stop taking this medication and notify your doctor immediately if you develop any of the following signs of liver toxicity: fever, rash, loss of appetite, nausea, vomiting, fatigue, pain in the upper right part of your abdomen, dark urine, or yellow skin or eyes.

## How should you take this medication?

Take Parafon Forte DSC exactly as prescribed by your doctor. Do not increase the dose or take it more often than prescribed.

Parafon Forte DSC occasionally discolors urine orange or purple red.

■ *If you miss a dose...*
Take it as soon as you remember, if it is within an hour or so of the missed time. Otherwise, skip the dose and go back to your regular schedule. Do not take 2 doses a once.

■ *Storage instructions...*
Store at room temperature in a tightly closed container.

## What side effects may occur?

Parafon Forte DSC is generally well tolerated and rarely produces undesirable side effects. However, if any develop or change in intensity, inform your doctor as soon as possible. Only your doctor can determine if it is safe for you to continue taking Parafon Forte DSC.

■ *Uncommon and rare side effects may include:*
Bruises, dizziness, drowsiness, feeling of illness, fluid retention, light-headedness, overstimulation, red or purple spots on the skin, severe allergic reaction, skin rashes, stomach or intestinal disturbances or bleeding, urine discoloration

## Why should this drug not be prescribed?

If you have had any reaction to this drug, notify your doctor. Make sure he or she is aware of any drug reactions you have experienced.

## Special warnings about this medication

Be careful using this drug if you have allergies or have ever had an allergic reaction to a drug. If you have a sensitivity reaction such as hives, redness, or itching of skin while you are taking Parafon Forte DSC, notify your doctor immediately.

## Possible food and drug interactions when taking this medication

Parafon Forte DSC may intensify the effects of alcohol. Be cautious about drinking alcohol while taking this medication.

If Parafon Forte DSC is taken with certain other drugs, the effects of either could be increased, decreased, or altered. It is especially important to check with your doctor before combining Parafon Forte DSC with drugs that slow the action of the central nervous system, such as Percocet, Valium, and Xanax.

## Special information if you are pregnant or breastfeeding

The effects of Parafon Forte DSC during pregnancy have not been adequately studied. If you are pregnant or plan to become pregnant, inform your doctor immediately. This drug may appear in breast milk and could affect a nursing infant. If this medication is essential to your health, your doctor may advise you to discontinue breastfeeding until your treatment is finished.

## Recommended dosage

ADULTS

The usual dosage of Parafon Forte DSC is 1 caplet taken 3 or 4 times per day. If you do not respond to this dosage, your doctor may increase it to one and a half caplets (750 milligrams) taken 3 or 4 times per day.

## Overdosage

Any medication taken in excess can have serious consequences. If you suspect an overdose, seek medical treatment immediately.

■ *Symptoms of Parafon Forte DSC overdose may include:*
Diarrhea, dizziness, drowsiness, headache, light-headedness, nausea, vomiting

■ *Symptoms that may develop after a period of time include:*
Feeling of illness, loss of muscle strength, lowered blood pressure, sluggishness, troubled or rapid breathing

*Brand name:*

# Parlodel

*Pronounced: PAR-luh-del*
*Generic name: Bromocriptine mesylate*

### Why is this drug prescribed?

Parlodel inhibits the secretion of the hormone pro-lactin from the pituitary gland. It also mimics the action of dopamine, a chemical lacking in the brain of someone with Parkinson's disease. It is used to treat a variety of medical conditions, including:

■ Infertility in some women
■ Menstrual problems such as the abnormal stoppage or absence of flow, with or without excessive production of milk
■ Growth hormone overproduction leading to acromegaly, a condition characterized by an abnormally large skull, jaw, hands, and feet
■ Parkinson's disease
■ Pituitary gland tumors

Some doctors also prescribe Parlodel to treat cocaine addiction, the eye condition known as glaucoma, erection problems in certain men, restless leg syndrome, and a dangerous reaction to major tranquilizers called neuroleptic malignant syndrome.

### Most important fact about this drug

Notify your doctor immediately if you develop a severe headache that does not let up or continues to get worse. It could be a warning of the possibility of other dangerous reactions, including seizure, stroke, or heart attack.

### How should you take this medication?

Parlodel should be taken with food. Take the first dose while lying down. You may faint or become dizzy due to lower blood pressure, especially following the first dose.

You may not feel the full effect of this medication for a few weeks. Do not stop taking Parlodel without first checking with your doctor.

■ *If you miss a dose...*
Take it as soon as you remember if it is within 4 hours of the scheduled time. Otherwise, skip the dose you missed and go back to your regular schedule. Do not take 2 doses at once.
■ *Storage information...*
Store at room temperature in a tightly closed, light-resistant container. Protect from excessive heat.

### What side effects may occur?

The number and severity of side effects depend on many factors, including the condition being treated, dosage, and duration of treatment. Side effects cannot be anticipated. If any develop or change in intensity, inform your doctor as soon as possible. Only your doctor can determine if it is safe for you to continue taking Parlodel.

■ *More common side effects may include:*
Abdominal cramps or discomfort, confusion, constipation, depression, diarrhea, dizziness, drop in blood pressure, drowsiness, dry mouth, fainting, fatigue, hallucinations (particularly in Parkinson's patients), headache, inability to sleep, indigestion, light-headedness, loss of appetite, loss of coordination, nasal congestion, nausea, shortness of breath, uncontrolled body movement, vertigo, visual disturbance, vomiting, weakness
■ *Less common side effects may include:*
Abdominal bleeding, anxiety, difficulty swallowing, frequent urination, heart attack, inability to hold urine, inability to urinate, nightmares, nervousness, rash, seizures, splotchy skin, stroke, swelling in feet and ankles, twitching of eyelids

Some of the above side effects are also symptoms of Parkinson's disease.

■ *Rare side effects may include:*
Abnormal heart rhythm, blurred vision or temporary blindness, cold feet, fast or slow heartbeat, hair loss, heavy-headedness, increase in blood pressure, lower back pain, muscle cramps, muscle cramps in feet and legs, numbness, pale face, paranoia, prickling or tingling, reduced tolerance to cold, severe or continuous headache, shortness of breath, sluggishness, tingling of ears or fingers

## Why should this drug not be prescribed?

You should not be using Parlodel if you have high blood pressure that is not under control or if you are pregnant (unless your doctor finds it medically necessary). You should also not take Parlodel if you are allergic to it or to any other drugs considered to be ergot alkaloids, such as Bellergal-S and Cafergot.

## Special warnings about this medication

Your doctor will check your pituitary gland thoroughly before you are treated with Parlodel.

Since Parlodel can restore fertility and pregnancy can result, women who do not want to become pregnant should use a "barrier" method of contraception during treatment with this medication. Do not use the "Pill" or oral contraceptives, as they may prevent Parlodel from working properly.

Notify your doctor immediately if you become pregnant while you are being treated with Parlodel.

If you have kidney or liver disease, consult your doctor before taking Parlodel.

If you are being treated with Parlodel for endocrine problems related to a tumor and stop taking this medication, the tumor may grow back rapidly.

If you are being treated for Parkinson's disease, the use of Parlodel alone or Parlodel with levodopa may cause hallucinations, confusion, and low blood pressure. If this happens, notify your doctor immediately.

If you have an abnormal heartbeat rhythm caused by a previous heart attack, consult your doctor before taking Parlodel.

If you experience a persistent watery nasal discharge while taking Parlodel, notify your doctor.

This drug may impair your ability to drive a car or operate potentially dangerous machinery. Do not participate in any activities that require full alertness if you are unsure about your ability to do so.

Your first dose of Parlodel may cause dizziness. If so, check with your doctor.

## Possible food and drug interactions when taking this medication

Combining alcohol with Parlodel can cause blurred vision, chest pain, pounding heartbeat, throbbing headache, confusion, and other problems. Do not drink alcoholic beverages while taking this medication.

Certain drugs used for psychotic conditions, including Thorazine and Haldol, inhibit the action of Parlodel. It is important that you consult your doctor before taking these drugs while on Parlodel therapy.

*Other drugs that may interact with Parlodel include:*

Blood pressure-lowering drugs such as Aldomet and Catapres

Metoclopramide (Reglan)

Oral contraceptives

Other ergot derivatives such as Hydergine

## Special information if you are pregnant or breastfeeding

The use of Parlodel during pregnancy should be discussed thoroughly with your doctor. If Parlodel is essential to your treatment, your doctor will carefully monitor you throughout your pregnancy.

You should not take Parlodel while breastfeeding.

## Recommended dosage

ADULTS

Parlodel is available as 2.5-milligram tablets and 5-milligram capsules. Dosage information given is for 2.5-milligram tablets.

*Excess Prolactin Hormone*

If you are being treated for conditions associated with excess prolactin, such as menstrual problems, with or without excessive milk production, infertility, or pituitary gland tumors, the usual starting dose is one-half to 1 tablet daily. Your doctor may add a tablet every 3 to 7 days, until the treatment works. The usual longer term dose is 5 to 7.5 milligrams per day and ranges from 2.5 to 15 milligrams per day.

*Growth Hormone Overproduction*

Treatment for the overproduction of growth hormones is usually one-half to 1 tablet with food at bedtime for 3 days. Your doctor may add one-half to 1 tablet every 3 to 7 days. The usual treatment dose varies from 20 to 30 milligrams per day. The dose should not exceed 100 milligrams per day. Your doctor will do a monthly re-evaluation.

*Parkinson's Disease*

Parlodel taken in combination with levodopa may provide additional treatment benefits if you are currently taking high doses of levodopa, are beginning to develop a tolerance to levodopa, or are experiencing "end of dose failure" on levodopa therapy.

The usual starting dose of Parlodel is one-half tablet twice a day with meals. Your dose will be monitored by your doctor at 2-week intervals. If necessary, your doctor may increase the dose every 14 to 28 days by 1 tablet per day.

CHILDREN

The safety and effectiveness of Parlodel have not been established in children under 15 years of age.

## Overdosage

Any medication taken in excess can have serious consequences. If you suspect an overdose of Parlodel, contact your doctor immediately or seek other medical attention.

Generic name:

# Paroxetine

See Paxil, page 397.

Brand name:

# Paxil

Pronounced: PACKS-ill
Generic name: Paroxetine hydrochloride

## Why is this drug prescribed?

Paxil is prescribed for a serious, continuing depression that interferes with your ability to function. Symptoms of this type of depression often include changes in appetite and sleep patterns, a persistent low mood, loss of interest in people and activities, decreased sex drive, feelings of guilt or worthlessness, suicidal thoughts, difficulty concentrating, and slowed thinking.

## Most important fact about this drug

Your depression may seem to improve within 1 to 4 weeks after beginning treatment with Paxil. Even if you feel better, continue to take the medication as long as your doctor tells you to do so.

## How should you take this medication?

Take this medication exactly as prescribed by your doctor. Inform your doctor if you are taking or plan to take any prescription or over-the-counter drugs, since they may interact unfavorably with Paxil.

■ If you miss a dose...
Skip the forgotten dose and go back to your regular schedule with the next dose. Do not take a double dose to make up for the one you missed.
■ Storage instructions...
Paxil can be stored at room temperature.

## What side effects may occur?

Side effects cannot be anticipated. If any develop or change in intensity, inform your doctor as soon as possible. Only your doctor can determine whether it is safe for you to continue taking this medication.

Over a 4 to 6 week period, you may find some side effects less troublesome (nausea and dizziness, for example) than others (dry mouth, drowsiness, and weakness).

■ More common side effects may include:
Constipation, decreased appetite, diarrhea, dizziness, drowsiness, dry mouth, gas, male genital disorders, nausea, nervousness, sleeplessness, sweating, tremor, weakness
■ Less common side effects may include:
Agitation, altered taste sensation, anxiety, blurred vision, burning or tingling sensation, decreased sex drive, drugged feeling, increased appetite, muscle tenderness or weakness, pounding heartbeat, rash, tightness in throat, twitching, upset stomach, urinary disorders, vomiting, yawning

## Why should this drug not be prescribed?

Do not take Paxil if you are also taking an MAO inhibitor antidepressant or within 14 days after you discontinue treatment with this type of medication.

## Special warnings about this medication

Paxil should be used cautiously by people with a history of manic disorders.

If you have a history of seizures, make sure your doctor knows about it. Paxil should be used with caution in this situation. If you develop seizures once therapy has begun, the drug should be discontinued.

If you have a disease or condition that affects your metabolism or blood circulation, make sure your doctor is aware of it. Paxil should be used cautiously in this situation.

Paxil may impair your judgment, thinking, or motor skills. Do not drive, operate dangerous machinery, or participate in any hazardous activity that requires full mental alertness until you are sure the medication is not affecting you in this way.

## Possible food and drug interactions when taking this medication

Do not drink alcohol during your treatment with Paxil.

If Paxil is taken with certain other drugs, the effects of either could be increased, decreased, or altered. It is especially important to check with your doctor before combining Paxil with any of the following:

Antidepressants such as Elavil, Tofranil,
   Norpramin, Pamelor, Prozac, Nardil, and Parnate
Cimetidine (Tagamet)
Diazepam (Valium)
Digoxin (Lanoxin)
Flecainide (Tambocor)
Lithium (Lithonate)
Phenobarbital
Phenytoin (Dilantin)
Procyclidine (Kemadrin)
Propafenone (Rythmol)
Propranolol (Inderal, Inderide)
Quinidine (Quinaglute)
Thioridazine (Mellaril)
Tryptophan
Warfarin (Coumadin)

## Special information if you are pregnant or breastfeeding

The effects of Paxil during pregnancy have not been adequately studied. If you are pregnant or plan to become pregnant, inform your doctor immediately. Paxil appears in breast milk and could affect a nursing infant. If this medication is essential to your health, your doctor may advise you to discontinue breastfeeding until your treatment with Paxil is finished.

## Recommended dosage

### ADULTS

The usual starting dose is 20 milligrams a day, taken as a single dose, usually in the morning. Your physician may increase your dosage by 10 milligrams a day, up to a maximum of 50 milligrams a day.

### CHILDREN

The safety and effectiveness of this drug in children have not been established.

### OLDER ADULTS

The recommended initial dose for older adults or weak individuals or those with severe kidney or liver disease is 10 milligrams a day. Your doctor may increase the dosage if needed, but it should not exceed 40 milligrams a day.

## Overdosage

Any medication taken in excess can have serious consequences. If you suspect an overdose, seek medical attention immediately.

■ *The symptoms of Paxil overdose may include:* Drowsiness, enlarged pupils, nausea, rapid heartbeat, vomiting

Brand name:

# PCE

*See Erythromycin, Oral, page 196.*

Brand name:

# Pediapred

*Pronounced: PEE-dee-uh-pred*
*Generic name: Prednisolone sodium phosphate*

## Why is this drug prescribed?

Pediapred, a steroid drug, is used to reduce inflammation and improve symptoms in a variety of disorders, including rheumatic arthritis, acute gouty arthritis, and severe cases of asthma. It may be given to people to treat primary or secondary adrenal cortex insufficiency (lack of or insufficient adrenal cortical hormone in the body). It is also given to help treat the following disorders:

Blood disorders such as leukemia and various anemias
Certain cancers (along with other drugs)
Connective tissue diseases such as systemic lupus erythematosus
Digestive tract diseases such as ulcerative colitis
Eye diseases of various kinds
Fluid retention due to nephrotic syndrome (a condition in which damage to the kidney causes a loss of protein in the urine)
High serum levels of calcium associated with cancer
Lung diseases such as tuberculosis
Severe allergic conditions such as drug-induced allergic reactions
Skin diseases such as severe psoriasis

Studies have shown that high doses of Pediapred are effective in controlling severe symptoms of multiple sclerosis, although they do not affect the ultimate outcome or natural history of the disease.

### Most important fact about this drug

Pediapred decreases your resistance to infection; thus it is possible for you to get a new infection while taking this medication. Pediapred may also mask some of the signs and symptoms of new infection, which makes it difficult for a doctor to diagnose the actual problem.

### How should you take this medication?

Pediapred may cause stomach upset and should be taken with food. Take this medication exactly as prescribed.

■ *If you miss a dose...*

Take it as soon as you remember. If it is almost time for your next dose, skip the one you missed and go back to your regular schedule. Never take 2 doses at the same time.

■ *Storage instructions...*

Store Pediapred in a cool place, and keep the bottle tightly closed. This medication may be refrigerated.

### What side effects may occur?

Side effects cannot be anticipated. If any develop or change in intensity, inform your doctor as soon as possible. Only your doctor can determine if it is safe for you to continue taking Pediapred.

■ *Side effects may include:*

Abnormal loss of bony tissue causing fragile bones, abnormal redness of the face, backbone break that collapses the spinal column, bruising, cataracts, convulsions, dizziness, fluid retention (edema), fracture of long bones, glaucoma (increased eye pressure), headache, high blood pressure, increased sweating, loss of muscle mass, menstrual irregularities, mental capacity changes, muscle disease, muscle weakness, peptic ulcer (stomach ulcer with possible bleeding), protrusion of eyeball, salt retention, slow growth in children, slow wound healing, sugar diabetes, swelling of the abdomen, thinning of the skin, vertigo

### Why should this drug not be prescribed?

This drug should not be used for fungal infections of the body.

### Special warnings about this medication

You should not be vaccinated against smallpox while being treated with Pediapred. Avoid other immunizations as well, especially if you are taking Pediapred in high doses, because of the possible hazards of nervous system complications and a lack of natural immune response.

People who have never had measles or chickenpox should avoid exposure to these diseases. They can cause a serious or, in children, even fatal reaction.

If you are taking Pediapred and are subjected to unusual stress, notify your doctor. The drug reduces the function of your adrenal glands, and they may be unable to cope. Your doctor may therefore increase your dosage of this rapidly acting steroid before, during, and after the stressful situation.

Prolonged use of steroids may produce posterior subcapsular cataracts (a disorder under the envelope-like structure at the back of the eye that causes the lens to become less transparent) or the eye disease glaucoma, and may intensify additional eye infections due to fungi or viruses.

Average and high doses of this medication may cause an increase in blood pressure, salt and water retention, and an increased loss of potassium. Your doctor may have you decrease your salt intake and increase your potassium intake.

The effects of Pediapred may be intensified if you have an underactive thyroid or long-term liver disease.

If you have ocular herpes simplex (painful blisters of the eye), you should be careful using this drug because of the possibility of corneal perforation (puncture of the outer, transparent part of the eye).

The use of Pediapred may cause mood swings, feelings of elation, insomnia, personality changes, severe depression, or even severe mental disorders.

If you are being treated for a blood clotting factor deficiency, use aspirin with caution when taking Pediapred. Do not use this drug for any disorder other than that for which it was prescribed.

Your doctor will prescribe this medication very cautiously if you have ulcerative colitis (inflammation of the colon and rectum) where there is a possibility of a puncture, abscess, or other infection; diverticulitis (inflammation of a sac formed at weak points of the colon); recent intestinal anastomoses (a surgical connection between two separate parts of the colon); active or inactive peptic (stomach) ulcers; unsatisfactory kidney function; high blood pressure; osteoporosis (brittle bones that may fracture); and myasthenia gravis (a long-term disease characterized by abnormal fatigue and weakness of certain muscles).

Do not discontinue the use of Pediapred abruptly or without medical supervision.

If you should develop a fever or other signs of infection while taking Pediapred, notify your doctor immediately.

### Possible food and drug interactions when taking this medication

If Pediapred is taken with certain other drugs, the effects of either could be increased, decreased, or altered. It is especially important to check with your doctor before combining Pediapred with the following:

Amphotericin B
Aspirin
Barbiturates such as phenobarbital and
    Seconal
Carbamazepine (Tegretol)
Cyclosporine (Sandimmune and Neoral)
Diabetes drugs such as Glucotrol
Diuretics such as Lasix
Estrogens such as Premarin
Isoniazid (Nydrazid)
Ketoconazole (Nizoral)
Nonsteroidal anti-inflammatory drugs such
    as Motrin
Oral contraceptives
Phenytoin (Dilantin)
Rifampin (Rifadin)

### Special information if you are pregnant or breastfeeding

The effects of Pediapred during pregnancy have not been adequately studied. If you are pregnant or plan to become pregnant, inform your doctor immediately. This medication may appear in breast milk and could affect a nursing infant. If this drug is essential to your health, your doctor may advise you to discontinue breastfeeding until your treatment is finished.

### Recommended dosage

The starting dosage of Pediapred may vary from 5 milliliters to 60 milliliters, depending on the specific disease being treated.

Your doctor will adjust the dose until he or she is satisfied with the results. If your condition does not improve after a reasonable period of time, your doctor may switch you to another medication.

Once you have a favorable response, your doctor will determine your maintenance dosage by gradually decreasing the doses until you are taking the smallest amount that will keep an adequate response.

If you stop taking Pediapred after long-term therapy, your doctor will have you withdraw slowly, rather than abruptly.

For acute flare-ups of multiple sclerosis (MS), the usual dose is 200 milligrams per day of Pediapred for one week followed by 80 milligrams every other day or 4 to 8 milligrams of dexamethasone every other day for 1 month.

### Overdosage

Although no specific information is available, any medication taken in excess can have serious consequences. If you suspect an overdose of Pediapred seek medical treatment immediately.

*Brand name:*

# Pediazole

*Pronounced: PEE-dee-uh-zole*
*Generic ingredients: Erythromycin ethylsuccinate,*
    *Sulfisoxazole acetyl*

### Why is this drug prescribed?

Pediazole is prescribed for the treatment of severe middle ear infections in children.

### Most important fact about this drug

Sulfisoxazole is one of a group of drugs called sulfonamides, which prevent the growth of certain bacteria in the body. However, sulfonamides have been known to cause rare but sometimes fatal reactions such as Stevens-Johnson syndrome (a rare skin condition characterized by severe blisters and bleeding in the mucous membrane of the lips, mouth, nose, and eyes), sudden and severe liver damage, a severe blood disorder (agranulocytosis), and a lack of red and white blood cells because of a bone marrow disorder.

Notify your doctor at the first sign of a side effect such as skin rash, sore throat, fever, abnormal skin paleness, darkened urine, reddish or purplish skin spots, or yellowing of the skin or whites of the eyes.

## How should you take this medication?

Be sure to keep giving Pediazole for the full time prescribed, even if your child begins to feel better after the first few days. Keep to a regular schedule; the medication works best when there is a constant amount in the blood.

Pediazole can be given with or without food. However, you should not give this medication with or immediately after carbonated beverages, fruit juice, or tea. If the child develops an upset stomach, give the medicine with crackers or a light snack.

To prevent sediment in the urine and the formation of stones, make sure that the child drinks plenty of fluids during treatment with Pediazole.

This medication increases the skin's sensitivity to sunlight. Overexposure can cause a rash, itching, redness, or sunburn. Keep the child out of direct sunlight, or provide protective clothing.

Shake well before using.

■ *If you miss a dose...*
Give the forgotten dose as soon as you remember, then give the rest of the day's doses at evenly spaced intervals.

■ *Storage instructions...*
Store Pediazole in the refrigerator. Keep tightly closed. Do not allow it to freeze. Use within 14 days; discard unused portion.

## What side effects may occur?

Side effects cannot be anticipated. If any develop or change in intensity, inform your doctor as soon as possible. Only your doctor can determine if it is safe to continue giving Pediazole.

■ *More common side effects may include:*
Abdominal cramping and discomfort, diarrhea, lack or loss of appetite, nausea, vomiting

■ *Less common or rare side effects may include:*
Anxiety, blood disorders, blood or stone formation in the urine, bluish discoloration of skin, chills, colitis, convulsions, cough, dark, tarry stools, depression, difficulty in urinating or inability to urinate, disorientation, dizziness, drowsiness, exhaustion, fainting, fatigue, fluid retention, flushing, fever, gas, hallucinations, headache, hepatitis, hives, inability to fall or stay asleep (insomnia), increased urine, inflammation of the mouth, irregular heartbeat, itching, lack of muscle coordination, low blood sugar, palpitations, rapid heartbeat, redness and swelling of the tongue, ringing in the ears, scaling of dead skin due to inflammation, sensitivity to light, severe allergic reactions, severe skin welts or swelling, shortness of breath, skin eruptions, skin rash, Stevens-Johnson syndrome, stomach or intestinal bleeding, swelling around the eye, temporary hearing loss, tingling or pins and needles, vertigo, weakness, yellow eyes and skin

## Why should this drug not be prescribed?

If your child is sensitive to or has ever had an allergic reaction to erythromycin, sulfonamides, or drugs of this type, do not use this medication. Make sure that your doctor is aware of any drug reactions that your child has experienced.

Pediazole should not be used if you are taking Seldane or Hismanal.

This medication should not be prescribed for infants under 2 months of age.

Pediazole should not be taken by pregnant women at the end of their pregnancy or by mothers nursing infants under 2 months of age.

## Special warnings about this medication

If your child has impaired kidney or liver function or a history of severe allergies or bronchial asthma, caution should be exercised when giving Pediazole. Consult with your doctor.

Prolonged or repeated use of Pediazole may cause new infections. If your child develops a new infection (called a superinfection), talk to your doctor. A different antibiotic may be needed.

Your doctor may recommend frequent urine tests while your child is taking Pediazole.

## Possible food and drug interactions when taking this medication

If Pediazole is taken with certain other drugs, the effects of either could be increased, decreased, or altered. It is especially important to check with your doctor before combining Pediazole with the following:

Astemizole (Hismanal)
Blood thinners such as Warfarin (Coumadin)
Bromocriptine (Parlodel)
Carbamazepine (Tegretol)
Cyclosporine (Sandimmune)
Digoxin (Lanoxin)
Disopyramide (Norpace)
Ergotamine (Cafergot, Ergostat)
Lovastatin (Mevacor)

Methotrexate (Rheumatrex)
Oral antidiabetic drugs such as Micronase
Phenytoin (Dilantin)
Terfenadine (Seldane)
Theophylline (Theo-Dur)
Triazolam (Halcion)

### Special information
### if you are pregnant or breastfeeding

This drug is not prescribed for adults, and should never be taken at term of pregnancy or when breastfeeding.

### Recommended dosage

CHILDREN

The recommended dose for children 2 months of age or older is determined by weight. The total daily dose should be given in equally divided doses 3 or 4 times a day for 10 days.

*Four-times-a-day schedule*
Less than 18 pounds: Determined by doctor
18 pounds: ¹/₂ teaspoonful
35 pounds: 1 teaspoonful
53 pounds: 1¹/₂ teaspoonfuls
Over 70 pounds: 2 teaspoonfuls

*Three-times-a-day schedule*
Less than 13 pounds: Determined by doctor
13 pounds: ¹/₂ teaspoonful
26 pounds: 1 teaspoonful
40 pounds: 1¹/₂ teaspoonfuls
53 pounds: 2 teaspoonfuls
Over 66 pounds: 2¹/₂ teaspoonfuls

### Overdosage

Any medication taken in excess can have serious consequences. If you suspect an overdose, seek medical treatment immediately.

*Generic name:*

# Pemoline

*See Cylert, page 125.*

*Brand name:*

# Penetrex

*Pronounced: PEN-eh-trecks*
*Generic name: Enoxacin*

### Why is this drug prescribed?

Penetrex is used to treat urinary tract infections, including cystitis (inflammation of the inner lining of the bladder caused by bacterial infection), and certain sexually transmitted diseases such as gonorrhea. It is a quinolone antibiotic.

### Most important fact about this drug

Penetrex, like other antibiotics, works best when there is a constant amount in the blood and urine. To help keep the level constant try not to miss any doses, and take them at evenly spaced intervals around the clock.

### How should you take this medication?

Penetrex should be taken with a full glass of water, either 1 hour before or 2 hours after a meal. Do not take more than the prescribed dosage. Use up all the medicine. If you stop taking Penetrex too soon, your symptoms may return.

Be sure to drink plenty of fluids while taking Penetrex.

■ *If you miss a dose...*
Take it as soon as you remember. If it is almost time for your next dose, skip the one you missed and go back to your regular schedule. Do not take 2 doses at the same time.

■ *Storage instructions...*
Store at room temperature.

### What side effects may occur?

Side effects cannot be anticipated. If any develop or change in intensity, tell your doctor as soon as possible. Only your doctor can determine whether it is safe for you to continue taking this medication.

■ *More common side effects may include:*
Nausea, vomiting

■ *Less common or rare side effects may include:*
Abdominal pain, agitation, back pain, bloody stools, chest pain, chills, confusion, constipation, convulsions, cough, depression, diarrhea, difficulty or labored breathing, dizziness, dry mouth and throat, emotional changeability, excessive sweating, fainting, fatigue, fever, fluid retention and swelling, fungal infection, gas, general feeling of illness, hallucinations, headache, hives, inability to hold urine, indigestion, inflammation of the large intestine, inflammation of the mouth, inflammation of the stomach, inflammation of the vagina, inflamed eyes, joint pain, kidney failure, lack of coordination, loss of appetite, loss of feeling of identity, loss of memory, mental disorders, muscle pain, nosebleed, overactivity,

palpitations (throbbing or fluttering heartbeat), purple or red spots on the skin, rapid heartbeat, ringing in the ears, sensitivity to light, skin eruptions, skin peeling, sleepiness, tingling or pins and needles, tremor, twitching, vaginal yeast infection, vision disturbances, weakness

### Why should this drug not be prescribed?

You should not take Penetrex if you are sensitive to this medication or to other quinolone antibiotics such as Cipro and Floxin.

### Special warnings about this medication

Use Penetrex cautiously if you have disorders such as epilepsy, severe hardening of the arteries in the brain, and other conditions that might lead to seizures. Penetrex may cause convulsions.

In rare cases, other drugs in this class have caused severe, even fatal reactions, sometimes after a single dose. These reactions may include confusion, convulsions, difficulty breathing, hallucinations, hives, itching, light-headedness, loss of consciousness, rash, restlessness, swelling in the face or throat, tingling, and tremors. If you develop any of these symptoms, you should immediately stop taking Penetrex and seek medical help.

If you have experienced diarrhea when taking other antibacterial medications or develop it after you start taking Penetrex, be sure to tell your doctor. Penetrex may cause an inflammation of the bowel, ranging from mild to life-threatening.

Penetrex may cause dizziness or light-headedness and could impair your ability to drive a car or operate potentially dangerous machinery. Do not participate in any activities that require full alertness if you are unsure about the drug's effect on you.

You should avoid excessive exposure to direct sunlight while taking Penetrex. Stop taking Penetrex immediately if you have a severe reaction to sunlight, such as a skin rash.

### Possible food and drug interactions when taking this medication

If Penetrex is taken with certain other drugs, the effects of either could be increased, decreased, or altered. It is especially important to check with your doctor before combining Penetrex with the following:

Antacids containing calcium, magnesium, or aluminum, such as Maalox and Tums

Bismuth subsalicylate (Pepto-Bismol)
Caffeine (including certain drugs, coffee, tea, chocolate, and some soft drinks)
Cyclosporine (Sandimmune)
Digoxin (Lanoxin)
Ranitidine (Zantac)
Sucralfate (Carafate)
Theophylline (Theo-Dur)
Vitamins or products containing iron or zinc
Warfarin (Coumadin)

### Special information
### if you are pregnant or breastfeeding

The effects of Penetrex during pregnancy have not been adequately studied. If you are pregnant or plan to become pregnant, notify your doctor. Penetrex may appear in breast milk and may affect a nursing infant. Your doctor may have you stop nursing while you are taking this medication.

### Recommended dosage

ADULTS

*Uncomplicated Urinary Tract Infections*
The usual dose is 200 milligrams every 12 hours for 7 days.

*Other Urinary Tract Infections*
The usual dose is 400 milligrams every 12 hours for 14 days.

*Sexually Transmitted Disease (Gonorrhea)*
The usual dose is 400 milligrams taken in a single dose.

CHILDREN

Safety and efficacy of Penetrex have not been established for children under 18 years of age.

### Overdosage

There is no information on overdosage with Penetrex. However, any medication taken in excess can have serious consequences. If you suspect a Penetrex overdose, seek medical help immediately.

*Generic name:*

# Penicillin V Potassium

*Brand names: Beepen-VK, Pen-Vee K, V-cillin K, Veetids*

### Why is this drug prescribed?

Penicillin V potassium is used to treat infections, including:

Dental infection, infections in the heart, middle ear infections, rheumatic fever, scarlet fever, skin infections, upper and lower respiratory tract infections

Penicillin V works against only certain types of bacteria—it is ineffective against fungi, viruses, and parasites.

### Most important fact about this drug

If you are allergic to either penicillin or cephalosporin antibiotics in any form, consult your doctor before taking penicillin V. There is a possibility that you are allergic to both types of medication; and if a reaction occurs, it could be extremely severe. If you take the drug and feel signs of a reaction, seek medical attention immediately.

### How should you take this medication?

Penicillin V may be taken on a full or empty stomach, though it is better absorbed when the stomach is empty. Be sure to take it for the full time of treatment.

Doses of the oral solution of penicillin V should be measured with a calibrated measuring spoon. Shake the solution well before using.

■ *If you miss a dose...*
Take it as soon as you remember. If it is almost time for the next dose, and you take 2 doses a day, take the one you missed and the next dose 5 to 6 hours later. If you take 3 or more doses a day, take the one you missed and the next dose 2 to 4 hours later, or double the next dose. Then go back to your regular schedule.

■ *Storage instructions...*
Store in a tightly closed container. The reconstituted oral solution must be refrigerated; discard any unused solution after 14 days.

Tablets and powder for oral solution may be stored at room temperature.

### What side effects may occur?

Side effects cannot be anticipated. If any develop or change in intensity, inform your doctor as soon as possible. Only your doctor can determine if it is safe for you to continue taking this medication.

■ *Side effects may include:*
Anemia, black, hairy tongue, diarrhea, fever, hives, nausea, skin eruptions, stomach upset or pain, swelling in throat, vomiting

### Why should this drug not be prescribed?

You should not be using penicillin V if you have had an allergic reaction to penicillin or cephalosporin antibiotics.

### Special warnings about this medication

If any allergic reactions occur, stop taking penicillin V and contact your doctor immediately.

If new infections (called superinfections) occur, consult your doctor.

If you have ever had allergic reactions such as rashes, hives, or hay fever, consult with your doctor before taking penicillin V.

Before taking penicillin V, tell your doctor if you have ever had asthma, colitis (inflammatory bowel disease), diabetes, or kidney or liver disease.

For infections such as strep throat, it is important to take penicillin V for the entire amount of time your doctor has prescribed. Even if you feel better, you need to continue taking this medication. If you stop taking this medication before your treatment time is complete, your infection may recur.

### Possible food and drug interactions when taking this medication

If penicillin V is taken with certain other drugs, the effects of either could be increased, decreased, or altered. It is especially important to check with your doctor before combining penicillin V with the following:

Chloramphenicol (Chloromycetin)
Oral contraceptives
Tetracyclines such as Achromycin V and Sumycin

### Special information if you are pregnant or breastfeeding

The effects of penicillin V in pregnancy have not been adequately studied. If you are pregnant or planning to become pregnant, inform your doctor immediately. Penicillin V should be used during pregnancy only if your doctor determines that the potential benefit justifies the potential risk to the fetus. Since penicillin V appears in breast milk, you should consult with your doctor if you plan to breastfeed your baby. If this medication is essential to your health, your doctor may advise you to discontinue breastfeeding until your treatment is finished.

## Recommended dosage

ADULTS AND CHILDREN 12 YEARS OLD
AND OVER

Continue taking penicillin V for the full time of treatment, even if you begin to feel better after a few days. Failure to take a full course of therapy may prevent complete elimination of the infection. It is best to take the doses at evenly spaced times, around the clock.

*For mild to moderately severe strep infections of the upper respiratory tract and skin, and scarlet fever*
The usual dosage is 125 to 250 milligrams every 6 to 8 hours for 10 days.

*For mild to moderately severe pneumococcal infections of the respiratory tract, including middle ear infections*
The usual dosage is 250 milligrams to 500 milligrams every 6 hours until you have been without a fever for at least 2 days.

*For mild staph infections of skin*
The usual dosage is 250 milligrams to 500 milligrams every 6 to 8 hours.

*For mild to moderately severe gum infections known as Vincent's gingivitis*
The usual dosage is 250 milligrams to 500 milligrams every 6 to 8 hours.

*To prevent recurring rheumatic fever and/or chorea (infective disorder of the nervous system)*
The usual dosage is 125 milligrams to 250 milligrams 2 times a day on a continuing basis.

*Prevention of bacterial endocarditis (inflammation of the heart membrane) in people with heart disease who are undergoing dental or surgical procedures*
For oral therapy, the usual dose is 2 grams of penicillin V $\frac{1}{2}$ to 1 hour before the procedure, then 1 gram 6 hours later.

## Overdosage

Any medication taken in excess can have serious consequences. If you suspect an overdose, seek medical attention immediately.

■ *Symptoms of penicillin V overdose may include:*
Diarrhea, nausea, vomiting

*Brand name:*

# Pentasa

*See Rowasa, page 480.*

*Generic name:*

# Pentazocine with Aspirin

*See Talwin Compound, page 520.*

*Generic name:*

# Pentoxifylline

*See Trental, page 559.*

*Brand name:*

# Pen-Vee K

*See Penicillin V Potassium, page 403.*

*Brand name:*

# Pepcid

*Pronounced: PEP-sid*
*Generic name: Famotidine*
*Other brand name: Pepcid AC*

### Why is this drug prescribed?

Pepcid is prescribed for the short-term treatment of active duodenal ulcer (in the upper intestine) for 4 to 8 weeks and for active, benign gastric ulcer (in the stomach) for 6 to 8 weeks. It is prescribed for maintenance therapy, at reduced dosage, after a duodenal ulcer has healed. It is also used for short-term treatment of GERD, a condition in which the acid contents of the stomach flow back into the esophagus, and for resulting inflammation of the esophagus. And it is prescribed for certain diseases that cause the stomach to produce excessive quantities of acid, such as Zollinger-Ellison syndrome. Pepcid belongs to a class of drugs known as histamine $H_2$ blockers.

An over-the-counter formulation, Pepcid AC, is used to relieve and prevent heartburn, acid indigestion, and sour stomach.

### Most important fact about this drug

To cure your ulcer, you need to take Pepcid for the full time of treatment your doctor prescribes. Keep taking the drug even if you begin to feel better.

## How should you take this medication?

It may take several days for Pepcid to begin relieving stomach pain. You can use antacids for the pain, but should avoid taking them within 1 hour of a dose of Pepcid.

If you are taking Pepcid suspension, shake it vigorously for 5 to 10 seconds before use.

Take Pepcid AC with water. To prevent symptoms take it 1 hour before a meal you expect will cause trouble.

■ *If you miss a dose...*

Take it as soon as you remember. If it is almost time for your next dose, skip the one you missed and go back to your regular schedule. Do not take 2 doses at once.

■ *Storage instructions...*

Store at room temperature in a dry place. Protect the suspension from freezing, and discard any unused portion after 30 days.

## What side effects may occur?

Side effects cannot be anticipated. If any develop or change in intensity, inform your doctor as soon as possible. Only your doctor can determine if it is safe for you to continue taking Pepcid.

The most common side effect is headache.

■ *Less common or rare side effects may include:*

Abdominal discomfort, acne, agitation, altered taste, anxiety, breast development in males, changes in behavior, confusion, constipation, decreased sex drive, depression, diarrhea, difficulty sleeping, dizziness, dry mouth, dry skin, facial swelling due to fluid retention, fatigue, fever, flushing, grand mal seizures, hair loss, hallucinations, hives, impotence, irregular heartbeat, itching, loss of appetite, muscle, bone, or joint pain, nausea, pounding heartbeat, prickling, tingling, or pins and needles, rash, ringing in ears, severe allergic reaction, sleepiness, vomiting, weakness, wheezing, yellow eyes and skin

## Why should this drug not be prescribed?

If you are sensitive to or have ever had an allergic reaction to Pepcid, you should not take this medication. Make sure your doctor is aware of any drug reactions you have experienced.

## Special warnings about this medication

If you have stomach cancer, Pepcid may relieve the symptoms without curing the disease. Your doctor will be careful to rule out this possibility.

Use Pepcid with caution if you have severe kidney disease.

Although heartburn and acid indigestion are common, see your doctor if you have trouble swallowing or abdominal pain that does not let up.

Do not take 2 tablets of Pepcid AC a day continuously for more than 2 weeks unless your doctor tells you to.

You can help avoid heartburn and acid indigestion by:

Not lying down soon after eating
Keeping your weight down
Stopping smoking, or at least cutting down
Avoiding or limiting caffeine, chocolate, fatty
    foods, and alcohol
Not eating just before bedtime

## Possible food and drug interactions when taking this medication

If Pepcid is taken with certain other drugs, the effects of either can be increased, decreased, or altered. It is especially important that you check with your doctor before combining Pepcid with the following:

Itraconazole (Sporanox)
Ketoconazole (Nizoral)

## Special information if you are pregnant or breastfeeding

The effects of Pepcid during pregnancy have not been adequately studied. If you are pregnant or plan to become pregnant, inform your doctor immediately. Pepcid may appear in breast milk and could affect a nursing infant. If this medication is essential to your health, your doctor may advise you to discontinue breastfeeding until your treatment with this medication is finished.

## Recommended dosage

PEPCID

The safety and effectiveness of Pepcid have not been established in children.

### For Duodenal Ulcer

The usual starting dose is 40 milligrams or 5 milliliters (1 teaspoonful) once a day at bedtime. Results should be seen within 4 weeks, and this medication should not be used at full dosage longer than 6 to 8 weeks. Your doctor may have you take 20 milligrams or 2.5 milliliters (1/2 teaspoonful) twice a day. The normal maintenance dose after your ulcer has healed is 20 milligrams or 2.5 milliliters (1/2 teaspoonful) once a day at bedtime.

*Benign Gastric Ulcer*
The usual dose is 40 milligrams or 5 milliliters (1 teaspoonful) once a day at bedtime.

*Gastroesophageal Reflux Disease (GERD)*
The usual dose is 20 milligrams or 2.5 milliliters (1/2 teaspoonful) twice a day for up to 6 weeks. For inflammation of the esophagus due to GERD, the dose is 20 or 40 milligrams or 2.5 to 5 milliliters twice a day for up to 12 weeks.

*Excess Acid Conditions (such as Zollinger-Ellison Syndrome)*
The usual starting dose is 20 milligrams every 6 hours, although some people need a higher dose.

If your kidneys are not functioning properly, your doctor will adjust the dosage.

PEPCID AC

Pepcid AC should not be given to children under age 12. Take no more than 2 tablets per day.

*Relief*
Swallow 1 tablet with water.

*Prevention*
Take 1 tablet 1 hour before a meal that could cause symptoms.

## Overdosage

Any medication taken in excess can have serious consequences. If you suspect an overdose, seek medical attention immediately.

*Brand name:*

# Percocet

*Pronounced: PERK-o-set*
*Generic ingredients: Acetaminophen, Oxycodone hydrochloride*
*Other brand names: Roxicet, Tylox*

## Why is this drug prescribed?

Percocet, a narcotic analgesic, is used to treat moderate to moderately severe pain. It contains two drugs—acetaminophen and oxycodone. Acetaminophen is used to reduce both pain and fever. Oxycodone, a narcotic analgesic, is used for its calming effect and for pain.

## Most important fact about this drug

Percocet contains a narcotic and, even if taken only in prescribed amounts, can cause physical and psychological dependence when taken for a long time.

## How should you take this medication?

Percocet may be taken with meals or with milk.

■ *If you miss a dose...*
If you take Percocet on a regular schedule, take it as soon as you remember. If it is almost time for the next dose, skip the one you missed and go back to your regular schedule. Never take 2 doses at once.

■ *Storage instructions...*
Store at room temperature.

## What side effects may occur?

Side effects cannot be anticipated. If any develop or change in intensity, inform your doctor as soon as possible. Only your doctor can determine if it is safe for you to continue taking Percocet.

■ *More common side effects may include:*
Dizziness, light-headedness, nausea, sedation, vomiting

You may be able to alleviate some of these side effects by lying down.

■ *Less common or rare side effects may include:*
Constipation, depressed feeling, exaggerated feeling of well-being, itchy skin, skin rash, slowed breathing (at higher doses)

## Why should this drug not be prescribed?

You should not use Percocet if you are sensitive to either acetaminophen or oxycodone.

## Special warnings about this medication

You should take Percocet cautiously and according to your doctor's instructions, as you would take any medication containing a narcotic. If you have ever had a problem with alcohol addiction, make sure your doctor is aware of it.

If you have experienced a head injury, consult your doctor before taking Percocet. The effects of Percocet may be stronger for people with head injuries, and using it may delay recovery.

If you have stomach problems, such as an ulcer, check with your doctor before taking Percocet. Percocet may hide the symptoms of stomach problems, making them difficult to diagnose and treat.

If you have ever had liver, kidney, thyroid gland, or Addison's disease (a disease of the adrenal glands), difficulty urinating, or an enlarged prostate, consult your doctor before taking Percocet.

Elderly people or those in a weakened condition should take Percocet cautiously.

This drug may impair your ability to drive a car or operate potentially dangerous machinery. Do not participate in any activities that require full alertness if you are unsure about the drug's effect on you.

### Possible food and drug interactions when taking this medication

Alcohol may increase the sedative effects of Percocet. You should not take Percocet with alcohol.

If Percocet is taken with certain other drugs, the effects of either could be increased, decreased, or altered. It is especially important to check with your doctor before combining Percocet with the following:

Antidepressants such as Elavil, Nardil, Pamelor, and Parnate
Antispasmodic drugs such as Cogentin, Bentyl, and Donnatal
Major tranquilizers such as Thorazine and Mellaril
Other narcotic painkillers such as Darvon and Demerol
Sedatives such as phenobarbital and Seconal
Tranquilizers such as Xanax and Valium

### Special information if you are pregnant or breastfeeding

It is not known whether Percocet can injure a developing baby or affect a woman's reproductive capacity. Using any medication that contains a narcotic during pregnancy may cause physical addiction for your newborn baby. If you are pregnant or plan to become pregnant, inform your doctor immediately. As with other narcotic painkillers, taking Percocet shortly before delivery (especially at higher dosages) may cause some degree of impaired breathing in the mother and newborn. It is not known whether Percocet appears in breast milk, possibly harming a nursing infant. If you are breastfeeding use Percocet only under a doctor's directions.

### Recommended dosage

ADULTS

The usual dose is 1 tablet every 6 hours as needed.

CHILDREN

The safety and effectiveness of Percocet have not been established in children.

### Overdosage

A severe overdose of Percocet can be fatal. If you suspect an overdose, seek medical help immediately.

■ *Symptoms of Percocet overdose may include:*
Bluish skin, eyes or skin with yellow tone, cold and clammy skin, decreased or irregular breathing (ceasing in severe overdose), extreme sleepiness progressing to stupor or coma, heart attack, low blood pressure, muscle weakness, nausea, slow heartbeat, sweating, vague bodily discomfort, vomiting

*Brand name:*

# Periactin

*Pronounced: pair-ee-AK-tin*
*Generic name: Cyproheptadine hydrochloride*

### Why is this drug prescribed?

Periactin is an antihistamine given to help relieve cold- and allergy-related symptoms such as hay fever, nasal inflammation, stuffy nose, red and inflamed eyes, hives, and swelling. Periactin may also be given after epinephrine to help treat anaphylaxis, a life-threatening allergic reaction.

Some doctors prescribe Periactin to treat cluster headache and to stimulate appetite in underweight people.

### Most important fact about this drug

Like other antihistamines, Periactin may make you feel sleepy and sluggish. However, some people, particularly children, may have the opposite reaction and become excited.

### How should you take this medication?

Take Periactin exactly as prescribed by your doctor.

■ *If you miss a dose...*
Take it as soon as you remember. If it is almost time for your next dose, skip the one you missed and go back to your regular schedule. Do not take 2 doses at once.
■ *Storage instructions...*
Store at room temperature in a tightly closed container.

## What side effects may occur?

Side effects cannot be anticipated. If any develop or change in intensity, tell your doctor immediately. Only your doctor can determine whether it is safe for you to continue taking Periactin.

■ *Side effects may include:*

Anaphylaxis (life-threatening allergic reaction), anemia, appetite loss, chest congestion or tightness, chills, confusion, constipation, convulsions, diarrhea, difficulty urinating, dizziness, dry mouth, nose, or throat, earlier-than-expected menstrual period, exaggerated feeling of well-being, excessive perspiration, excitement, faintness, fatigue, fluttery or throbbing heartbeat, frequent urination, hallucinations, headache, hives, hysteria, inability to urinate, increased appetite and weight gain, insomnia, irritability, lack of coordination, light sensitivity, low blood pressure, nausea, nervousness, rapid heartbeat, rash and swelling, restlessness, ringing in the ears, sleepiness, stomach pain, stuffy nose, tingling or pins and needles, tremor, vertigo, vision problems (double vision, blurred vision), vomiting, weight gain, wheezing, yellow eyes and skin

Older people, in particular, are likely to become dizzy or drowsy, or develop low blood pressure in response to Periactin.

## Why should this drug not be prescribed?

Do not take Periactin if you are sensitive to it, or have ever had an allergic reaction to it or to a similar antihistamine.

Do not take Periactin if you are taking an antidepressant drug known as an MAO inhibitor. Drugs in this category include Nardil and Parnate.

Do not take Periactin if you have the eye condition called angle-closure glaucoma, a peptic ulcer, an enlarged prostate, obstruction of the neck of the bladder, or obstruction of the outlet of the stomach.

Newborn or premature infants should not be given this drug, nor should it be used by women who are breastfeeding an infant.

The elderly and those in a weakened condition should not take this drug.

## Special warnings about this medication

Like other antihistamines, Periactin may make you drowsy or impair your coordination. Be very careful about driving, climbing, or operating machinery, or doing hazardous tasks until you know how you react to this medication.

Be cautious about taking Periactin if you have bronchial asthma, the eye condition called glaucoma, an overactive thyroid gland, high blood pressure, heart disease, or circulatory problems.

## Possible food and drug interactions when taking this medication

Avoid alcoholic beverages while taking Periactin.

If Periactin is taken with certain other drugs, the effects of either could be increased, decreased, or altered. It is especially important to check with your doctor before combining Periactin with the following:

Antidepressant drugs classified as MAO inhibitors, including Nardil and Parnate
Sedatives such as Nembutal and Seconal
Tranquilizers such as Librium and Valium

## Special information if you are pregnant or breastfeeding

Because of possible harm to the unborn baby, Periactin should not be used during pregnancy unless it is clearly needed. Periactin should not be taken by a woman who is breastfeeding. If you have just given birth, you will need to choose between breastfeeding and taking Periactin.

## Recommended dosage

### ADULTS

The usual initial dose is 4 milligrams (1 tablet or 2 teaspoonfuls) 3 times daily. Dosage may range from 4 to 20 milligrams a day, but most people will take between 12 and 16 milligrams. Some may need as much as 32 milligrams a day.

### CHILDREN

*Ages 2 to 6 Years*
The usual dose is 2 milligrams (one-half tablet or 1 teaspoon) 2 or 3 times a day; your doctor may adjust the dose if necessary. A child this age should not take more than 12 milligrams a day.

*Ages 7 to 14 Years*
The usual dose is 4 milligrams (1 tablet or 2 teaspoons) 2 or 3 times a day; your doctor may adjust the dose if needed. A child this age should not take more than 16 milligrams a day.

## Overdosage

Any drug taken in excess may have serious consequences. An overdose of Periactin can be fatal. If you suspect an overdose, seek medical attention immediately.

■ *Symptoms of Periactin overdose may include:*
Dilated pupils, dry mouth, extreme excitement and agitation, fever, flushing, stomach or bowel distress, stupor or coma

Overdosage in children may produce hallucinations and convulsions.

*Brand name:*

# Peridex

Pronounced: PAIR-i-decks
Generic name: Chlorhexidine gluconate

### Why is this drug prescribed?
Peridex is an oral rinse used to treat gingivitis, a condition in which the gums become red and swollen. Peridex is also used to control gum bleeding caused by gingivitis.

### Most important fact about this drug
Peridex may stain front-tooth fillings, especially those with a rough surface. These stains have no adverse effect on the gums, and usually can be removed by a professional cleaning.

### How should you take this medication?
You should get a thorough dental cleaning and examination before beginning treatment with Peridex.

After brushing, thoroughly rinsing, and flossing your teeth, rinse with Peridex by swishing one-half fluid ounce (marked in the cap) around in your mouth for 30 seconds, then spit it out. Do not dilute Peridex and do not eat or drink for several hours after using this medication.

■ *If you miss a dose...*
Resume your regular schedule the next time you brush.
■ *Storage instructions...*
Protect from freezing.

### What side effects may occur?
Side effects cannot be anticipated. If any develop or change in intensity, inform your doctor as soon as possible. Only your doctor can determine if it is safe for you to continue using Peridex.

■ *More common side effects may include:*
Change in taste, increase in plaque, staining of teeth, mouth, tooth fillings, dentures, or other appliances in the mouth

■ *Less common or rare side effects may include:*
Irritation of the mouth, scaling of the lining of the mouth

### Why should this drug not be prescribed?
Unless you are directed to do so by your doctor, do not use Peridex if you have shown a sensitivity to or are allergic to Peridex.

### Special warnings about this medication
If you have both gingivitis and periodontitis (disease of the tissue that supports and attaches the teeth), remember that Peridex is used only for gingivitis. Periodontitis may require additional treatment by your doctor or dentist.

The use of Peridex may leave a bitter after-taste. Rinsing your mouth with or drinking water after using Peridex may increase the bitterness.

In addition to staining, Peridex can also cause an excess of tartar build-up on your teeth. It is recommended that you have your teeth cleaned at least every 6 months.

Foods may taste different to you for several hours after rinsing with Peridex. In most cases, this effect becomes less noticeable after continued use. Taste should return to normal when treatment with Peridex is finished.

### Possible food and drug interactions when taking this medication
No interactions with other drugs have been reported.

### Special information if you are pregnant or breastfeeding
The effects of Peridex during pregnancy have not been adequately studied. If you are pregnant or plan to become pregnant, inform your doctor immediately. It is not known whether this medication appears in breast milk. If it is essential for you to use Peridex, your doctor may advise you to stop breastfeeding until your treatment is finished.

### Recommended dosage
ADULTS

The usual dose of undiluted Peridex is one-half fluid ounce. Rinse for 30 seconds twice a day, morning and evening, after brushing. Peridex should be spit out after rinsing and never swallowed.

CHILDREN

The effectiveness and safety of Peridex have not been established in children under 18 years of age.

## Overdosage

If you suspect that a child of 22 pounds or less has swallowed 4 or more ounces of Peridex, seek medical attention immediately.

Also seek immediate medical attention if any child shows signs of alcohol intoxication such as slurred speech, staggering, or sleepiness, and you suspect he or she has swallowed Peridex.

If a small child swallows 1 or 2 ounces of Peridex, he or she may have an upset stomach and nausea.

*Brand name:*

# Persantine

*Pronounced: per-SAN-teen*
*Generic name: Dipyridamole*

## Why is this drug prescribed?

Persantine helps reduce the formation of blood clots in people who have had heart valve surgery. It is used in combination with blood thinners such as Coumadin.

Some doctors also prescribe Persantine in combination with other drugs, such as aspirin, to reduce the damage from a heart attack and prevent a recurrence, to treat angina, and to prevent complications during heart bypass surgery.

## Most important fact about this drug

Persantine is sometimes used with aspirin to provide better protection against the formation of blood clots. However, the risk of bleeding may also be increased. To reduce this risk, take *only* the amount of aspirin prescribed by the *same* doctor who directed you to take Persantine. If you need a medication for pain or a fever, do not take extra aspirin without first consulting your doctor.

## How should you take this medication?

Persantine must be taken exactly as your doctor prescribes, at regularly scheduled times.

It is best to take Persantine on an empty stomach, with a full glass of water. However, if this upsets your stomach, you can take the drug with food or milk.

Do not change from one brand of dipyridamole to another without consulting your doctor or phar-

macist. Products manufactured by different companies may not be equally effective.

■ *If you miss a dose...*
Take it as soon as you remember. If it is within 4 hours of your next scheduled dose, skip the dose you missed and go back to your regular schedule. Never take 2 doses at the same time.

■ *Storage instructions...*
Store at room temperature. Protect from excessive heat.

## What side effects may occur?

Side effects cannot be anticipated. If any develop or change in intensity, inform your doctor as soon as possible. Only your doctor can determine if it is safe for you to continue taking Persantine.

■ *More common side effects may include:*
Abdominal distress, dizziness
■ *Less common or rare side effects may include:*
Angina pectoris (crushing chest pain), diarrhea, feeling flushed, headache, itching, liver problems, skin rash, vomiting

## Why should this drug not be prescribed?

There is no known reason to avoid this drug.

## Special warnings about this medication

Use this medication carefully if you have low blood pressure.

Tell the doctor that you are taking Persantine if you have a medical emergency, and before you have surgery or dental treatment.

## Possible food and drug interactions when taking this medication

If Persantine is taken with certain other drugs, the effects of either could be increased, decreased, or altered. It is especially important to check with your doctor before combining Persantine with the following:

Aspirin
Blood thinners such as Coumadin
Indomethacin (Indocin)
Ticlopidine (Ticlid)
Valproic acid (Depakene)

## Special information if you are pregnant or breastfeeding

The effects of Persantine during pregnancy have not been adequately studied. If you are pregnant or plan to become pregnant, inform your doctor immediately. This drug appears in breast milk and may affect a nursing infant. If this medication is essential to your health, your doctor may advise you to discontinue breastfeeding until your treatment with this medication is finished.

### Recommended dosage

ADULTS

The usual recommended dose is 75 milligrams to 100 milligrams, 4 times a day.

CHILDREN

The safety and effectiveness of this medication have not been established in children under 12 years of age.

### Overdosage

Low blood pressure is the most common symptom of overdose and usually lasts for a short period of time. If this occurs, contact your doctor or emergency room immediately.

---

*Brand name:*

# Phenaphen with Codeine

*See Tylenol with Codeine, page 572.*

---

*Generic name:*

# Phenazopyridine

*See Pyridium, page 453.*

---

*Generic name:*

# Phenelzine

*See Nardil, page 348.*

---

*Brand name:*

# Phenergan

*Pronounced: FEN-er-gan*
*Generic name: Promethazine hydrochloride*

### Why is this drug prescribed?

Phenergan is an antihistamine that relieves nasal stuffiness and inflammation and red, inflamed eyes caused by hay fever and other allergies. It is also used to treat itching, swelling, and redness from hives and other rashes; allergic reactions to blood transfusions; and, with other medications, anaphylactic shock (severe allergic reaction).

Phenergan is also used as a sedative and sleep aid for both children and adults, and is prescribed to prevent and control nausea and vomiting before and after surgery and to prevent and treat motion sickness. It is also used, with other medications, for pain after surgery.

Antihistamines work by decreasing the effects of histamine, a chemical the body releases in response to certain irritants. Histamine narrows air passages in the lungs and contributes to inflammation. Antihistamines reduce itching and swelling and dry up secretions from the nose, eyes, and throat.

### Most important fact about this drug

Phenergan may cause considerable drowsiness. You should not drive or operate dangerous machinery or participate in any hazardous activity that requires full mental alertness until you know how you react to Phenergan. Children should be carefully supervised while they are bike-riding, roller-skating, or playing until the drug's effect on them is established.

### How should you take this medication?

Take Phenergan exactly as prescribed.

■ *If you miss a dose...*
   If you are taking Phenergan on a regular schedule, take the forgotten dose as soon as you remember. If it is almost time for your next dose, skip the one you missed and go back to your regular schedule. Never take 2 doses at once.
■ *Storage instructions...*
   Tablets should be stored at room temperature, away from light. Suppositories should be stored in the refrigerator, in a tightly closed container.

### What side effects may occur?

Side effects cannot be anticipated. If any develop or change in intensity, inform your doctor as soon as possible. Only your doctor can determine if it is safe for you to continue taking Phenergan.

■ *More common side effects may include:*
   Blurred vision, dizziness, dry mouth, increased/decreased blood pressure, nausea, rash, sedation (extreme calm), sleepiness, vomiting
■ *Rare side effects may include:*
   Abnormal eye movements, blood disorders, confusion, disorientation, protruding tongue, sensitivity to light, stiff neck

## Why should this drug not be prescribed?

Phenergan should not be used to treat asthma or other breathing difficulties or if you are sensitive to or have ever had an allergic reaction to it or to related medications, such as Thorazine, Mellaril, Stelazine, or Prolixin.

## Special warnings about this medication

If you are taking other medications that cause sedation, your doctor may reduce the dosage of these medications or eliminate them while you are using Phenergan.

If you have a seizure disorder, Phenergan may cause your seizures to occur more often.

Avoid this medication if you have sleep apnea (periods during sleep when breathing stops).

Use Phenergan cautiously if you have heart disease, high blood pressure or circulatory problems, liver problems, the eye condition called narrow-angle glaucoma, peptic ulcer or other abdominal obstructions, or urinary bladder obstruction due to an enlarged prostate.

Phenergan may affect the results of pregnancy tests and can raise your blood sugar.

Some people have developed jaundice (yellow eyes and skin) while on this medication.

Tell your doctor if you have any uncontrolled movements or seem to be unusually sensitive to sunlight.

Remember that Phenergan can cause drowsiness.

## Possible food and drug interactions when taking this medication

Phenergan may increase the effects of alcohol. Do not drink alcohol, or at least substantially reduce the amount you drink, while taking this medication.

If Phenergan is taken with certain other drugs, the effects of either could be increased, decreased, or altered. It is especially important to check with your doctor before combining Phenergan with the following:

Certain antidepressant drugs, including Elavil and Tofranil
Narcotic pain relievers such as Demerol and Dilaudid
Sedatives such as Halcion, Dalmane, and Seconal
Tranquilizers such as Xanax and Valium

## Special information if you are pregnant or breastfeeding

The effects of Phenergan during pregnancy have not been adequately studied. If you are pregnant or plan to become pregnant, inform your doctor immediately. Phenergan may appear in breast milk and may affect a nursing infant. If this medication is essential to your health, your doctor may advise you to discontinue breastfeeding until your treatment is finished.

## Recommended dosage

Phenergan is available in tablet, syrup, and suppository form. Phenergan tablets and suppositories are not recommended for children under 2 years of age.

ALLERGY

*Adults*
The average oral dose is 25 milligrams taken before bed; however, your doctor may have you take 12.5 milligrams before meals and before bed.

*Children*
The usual dose is a single 25-milligram dose at bedtime, or 6.25 to 12.5 milligrams 3 times daily.

MOTION SICKNESS

*Adults*
The average adult dose is 25 milligrams taken twice daily. The first dose should be taken one-half to 1 hour before you plan to travel, and the second dose 8 to 12 hours later, if necessary. On travel days after that, the recommended dose is 25 milligrams when you get up and again before the evening meal.

*Children*
The usual dose of Phenergan tablets, syrup, or rectal suppositories is 12.5 to 25 milligrams taken twice a day.

NAUSEA AND VOMITING

The average dose of Phenergan for nausea and vomiting in children or adults is 25 milligrams. When oral medication cannot be tolerated, use the rectal suppository. Your doctor may have you take 12.5 to 25 milligrams every 4 to 6 hours, if necessary.

For nausea and vomiting in children, the dose is usually calculated at 0.5 milligram per pound of body weight and will also be based on the age of the child and the severity of the condition being treated.

INSOMNIA

*Adults*

The usual dose is 25 to 50 milligrams for nighttime sedation.

*Children*

The usual dose is 12.5 to 25 milligrams by tablets or rectal suppository at bedtime.

## Overdosage

Any medication taken in excess can have serious consequences. If you suspect an overdose, seek medical treatment immediately.

■ *Symptoms of Phenergan overdose may include:*
Difficulty breathing, dry mouth, fixed, dilated pupils, flushing, loss of consciousness, slowdown in brain activity, slowed heartbeat, stomach and intestinal problems, very low blood pressure

Children may become overstimulated and have nightmares; rarely, they may have convulsions. The elderly may also become overstimulated.

*Brand name:*

# Phenergan with Codeine

*Pronounced: FEN-er-gan*
*Generic ingredients: Promethazine hydrochloride,*
*Codeine phosphate*

## Why is this drug prescribed?

Phenergan with Codeine is used to relieve coughs and other symptoms of allergies and the common cold. Promethazine, an antihistamine, helps reduce itching and swelling and dries up secretions from the nose, eyes, and throat. It also has sedative effects and helps control nausea and vomiting. Codeine, a narcotic analgesic, helps relieve pain and stops coughing.

## Most important fact about this drug

Phenergan with Codeine may cause considerable drowsiness. You should not drive or operate dangerous machinery or participate in any hazardous activity that requires full mental alertness until you know how you react to this medication. Children should be carefully supervised while they are bike-riding, roller-skating, or playing until the drug's effect on them is established.

## How should you take this medication?

Take this medication exactly as prescribed.

■ *If you miss a dose...*
If you take Phenergan with Codeine on a regular schedule, take the forgotten dose as soon as you remember. If it is almost time for your next dose, skip the one you missed and go back to your regular schedule. Never take 2 doses at once.

■ *Storage instructions...*
Store at room temperature, away from light.

## What side effects may occur?

Side effects cannot be anticipated. If any develop or change in intensity, inform your doctor as soon as possible. Only your doctor can determine if it is safe for you to continue taking Phenergan with Codeine.

■ *Side effects may include:*
Blurred vision, constipation, convulsions, decreased amount of urine, depressed feeling, difficulty breathing, disorientation, dizziness, dizziness on standing, dry mouth, exaggerated sense of well-being, fainting, faintness, fast, fluttery heartbeat, feeling of anxiety, restlessness, flushing, headache, hives, inability to urinate, increased/decreased blood pressure, itching, light-headedness, nausea, passing hallucinations, rapid heartbeat, rash, sedation (extreme calm), sleepiness, slow heartbeat, sweating, swelling due to fluid retention (including the throat), vision changes, vomiting, weakness, yellowed skin or whites of eyes

■ *Side effects seen rarely include:*
Abnormal eye movements, blood disorders, confusion, skin sensitivity to light, protruding tongue, stiff neck

## Why should this drug not be prescribed?

Phenergan with Codeine should not be used if you have asthma or other breathing difficulties or if you are sensitive to or have ever had an allergic reaction to codeine, promethazine, or related medications, such as Thorazine, Mellaril, Stelazine, or Prolixin.

## Special warnings about this medication

It is possible to develop psychological and physical dependence on codeine. Although the likelihood of this is quite low with oral codeine, be cautious if you have a history of drug abuse or dependence.

Never take more cough syrup than has been prescribed. If your cough does not seem better within 5 days, check back with your doctor.

Codeine can cause or worsen constipation.

Phenergan with Codeine should be used with extreme caution in young children.

Use this medication very carefully if you have a head injury, the eye condition called narrow-angle glaucoma, peptic ulcer or other abdominal obstruction, urinary bladder obstruction due to an enlarged prostate, heart disease, high blood pressure or circulatory problems, liver or kidney disease, fever, seizures, an underactive thyroid gland, intestinal inflammation, or Addison's disease (a disorder of the adrenal glands). Be cautious, too, if you have had recent stomach/intestinal or urinary tract surgery. The very young, the elderly, and people in a weakened condition may have problems taking Phenergan with Codeine.

This medication may make you dizzy when you first stand up. Getting up slowly can help prevent this problem.

If you are taking other medications with sedative effects, your doctor may reduce their dosage or eliminate them altogether while you are using Phenergan with Codeine.

If you have a seizure disorder, this medication may cause your seizures to occur more often.

Avoid using Phenergan with Codeine if you have sleep apnea (periods during sleep when breathing stops).

Phenergan with Codeine may affect the results of pregnancy tests; and it can raise your blood sugar.

Tell your doctor if you have any involuntary muscle movements or seem to be unusually sensitive to sunlight.

### Possible food and drug interactions when taking this medication

Phenergan with Codeine may increase the effects of alcohol. Do not drink alcohol, or at least substantially reduce the amount you drink, while taking this medication.

If Phenergan with Codeine is taken with certain other drugs, the effects of either could be increased, decreased, or altered. It is especially important to check with your doctor before combining Phenergan with Codeine with the following:

All antidepressant drugs, including Marplan, Nardil, Elavil and Prozac
Narcotic pain relievers such as Demerol and Dilaudid
Sedatives such as Seconal, Halcion and Dalmane
Tranquilizers such as Xanax and Valium

### Special information if you are pregnant or breastfeeding

The effects of Phenergan with Codeine during pregnancy have not been adequately studied. If you are pregnant or plan to become pregnant, inform your doctor immediately. Phenergan with Codeine may appear in breast milk and may affect a nursing infant. If this medication is essential to your health, your doctor may advise you to discontinue breastfeeding until your treatment is finished.

### Recommended dosage

#### ADULTS

The usual dosage is 1 teaspoon (5 milliliters) every 4 to 6 hours, not to exceed 6 teaspoons, or 30 milliliters, in 24 hours.

#### CHILDREN 6 YEARS TO UNDER 12 YEARS

The usual dose is one-half to 1 teaspoon (2.5 to 5 milliliters) every 4 to 6 hours, not to exceed 6 teaspoons, or 30 milliliters, in 24 hours.

#### CHILDREN UNDER 6 YEARS

The usual dose is one-quarter to one-half teaspoon (1.25 to 2.5 milliliters) every 4 to 6 hours. The total daily dose should not exceed 9 milliliters for children weighing 40 pounds, 8 milliliters for 35 pounds, 7 milliliters for 30 pounds, and 6 milliliters for 25 pounds.

Phenergan with Codeine is not recommended for children under 2 years of age.

### Overdosage

Any medication taken in excess can have serious consequences. An overdose of codeine can be fatal. If you suspect an overdose, seek medical treatment immediately.

■ Symptoms of an overdose of Phenergan with Codeine may include:
Bluish skin, cold, clammy skin, coma, convulsions, difficulty breathing, dilated pupils, dry mouth, extreme sleepiness, flushing, low blood pressure, muscle softness, nightmares, overexcitability, slow heartbeat, small pupils, stomach and intestinal problems, stupor, unconsciousness

Generic name:

# Phenobarbital, Hyoscyamine, Atropine, and Scopolamine

See Donnatal, page 174.

*Generic name:*

# Phenobarbital

*Pronounced: fee-noe-BAR-bi-tal*

### Why is this drug prescribed?
Phenobarbital, a barbiturate, is used as a sleep aid and in the treatment of certain types of epilepsy, including generalized or grand mal seizures and partial seizures.

### Most important fact about this drug
Phenobarbital can be habit-forming. You may become tolerant (needing more and more of the drug to achieve the same effect) and physically and psychologically dependent with continued use. Never increase the amount of phenobarbital you take without checking with your doctor.

### How should you take this medication?
Take this medication exactly as prescribed.

If you are taking phenobarbital for seizures, do not discontinue it abruptly.

■ *If you miss a dose...*
Take it as soon as you remember. If it is almost time for your next dose, skip the one you missed and go back to your regular schedule. Never take 2 doses at once.
■ *Storage instructions...*
Store at room temperature in a tightly closed container.

### What side effects may occur?
Side effects cannot be anticipated. If any develop or change in intensity, notify your doctor as soon as possible. Only your doctor can determine whether it is safe for you to continue taking phenobarbital.

■ *Side effects may include:*
Abnormal thinking, aggravation of existing emotional disturbances and phobias, agitation, anemia, angioedema (swelling of face around lips, tongue, and throat, swollen arms and legs, difficulty breathing), allergic reactions (localized swelling, especially of the eyelids, cheeks, or lips, skin redness and inflammation), anxiety, confusion, constipation, decreased breathing, delirium, difficulty sleeping, dizziness, drowsiness, excitement, fainting, fever, hallucinations, headache, increased physical activity and muscle movement, irritability and hyperactivity in children, lack of muscle coordination, low blood pressure, muscle, nerve, or joint pain, especially in people with insomnia, nausea, nervousness, nightmares, psychiatric disturbances, rash, residual drowsiness, restlessness, excitement, and delirium when taken for pain, shallow breathing, sleepiness, slow heartbeat, slowdown of the nervous system, sluggishness, softening of bones, temporary cessation of breathing, vertigo, vomiting

### Why should this drug not be prescribed?
Phenobarbital should not be used if you suffer from porphyria (an inherited metabolic disorder), liver disease, or a lung disease that causes blockages or breathing difficulties, or if you have ever had an allergic reaction to or are sensitive to phenobarbital or other barbiturates.

### Special warnings about this medication
Remember that phenobarbital may be habit-forming. Make sure you take the medication exactly as prescribed.

Phenobarbital should be used with extreme caution, or not at all, by people who are depressed, or have a history of drug abuse.

Be sure to tell your doctor if you are in pain, or if you have constant pain, before you take phenobarbital.

Phenobarbital may cause excitement, depression, or confusion in elderly or weakened individuals, and excitement in children.

If you have been diagnosed with liver disease or your adrenal glands are not functioning properly, make sure the doctor knows about it. Phenobarbital should be prescribed with caution.

Barbiturates such as phenobarbital may cause you to become tired or less alert. Be careful driving, operating machinery, or doing any activity that requires full mental alertness until you know how you react to this medication.

### Possible food and drug interactions when taking this medication
Phenobarbital may increase the effects of alcohol. Avoid alcoholic beverages while taking phenobarbital.

If phenobarbital is taken with certain other drugs, the effects of either could be increased, decreased, or altered. It is especially important to check with your doctor before combining phenobarbital with the following:

Antidepressant drugs known as MAO inhibitors,
  including Nardil and Parnate
Antihistamines such as Benadryl
Blood-thinning medications such as Coumadin
Doxycycline (Doryx, Vibramycin)
Griseofulvin (Fulvicin-P/G, Grifulvin V)
Narcotic pain relievers such as Percocet
Oral contraceptives
Other epilepsy drugs such as Dilantin, Depakene,
  and Depakote
Other sedatives such as Nembutal and Seconal
Steroids such as Medrol and Deltasone
Tranquilizers such as Xanax and Valium

## Special information
## if you are pregnant or breastfeeding

Barbiturates such as phenobarbital may cause
damage to the developing baby during pregnancy.
Withdrawal symptoms may occur in an infant
whose mother took barbiturates during the last
3 months of pregnancy. If you are pregnant or
plan to become pregnant, inform your doctor
immediately.

Phenobarbital appears in breast milk and could
affect a nursing infant. If phenobarbital is essential
to your health, your doctor may advise you to stop
breastfeeding until your treatment is finished.

## Recommended dosage

### ADULTS

*Sedation*
The usual initial dose of phenobarbital is a single
dose of 30 to 120 milligrams. Your doctor may
repeat this dose at intervals, depending on how you
respond to this medication.

You should not take more than 400 milligrams
during a 24-hour period.

*Daytime Sedation*
The usual dose is 30 to 120 milligrams a day,
divided into 2 to 3 doses.

*To Induce Sleep*
The usual dose is 100 to 200 milligrams.

*Anticonvulsant Use*
Phenobarbital dosage must be individualized on the
basis of specific laboratory tests. Your doctor will
determine the exact dose best for you. The usual
dose is 60 to 200 milligrams daily.

### CHILDREN

*Anticonvulsant Use*
The phenobarbital dosage must be individualized
on the basis of specific laboratory tests. Your
doctor will determine the exact dose best for your
child.

The usual dose is 3 to 6 milligrams per 2.2
pounds of body weight per day.

### OLDER ADULTS

If you are old or debilitated, your dose may be
lower than the regular adult dose. People who have
liver or kidney disease may also require a lower
dose of phenobarbital.

## Overdosage

Barbiturate overdose can be fatal. If you
suspect an overdose, seek medical treatment
immediately.

■ *Symptoms of phenobarbital overdose may
  include:*
  Congestive heart failure, diminished breathing,
  extremely low body temperature, fluid in lungs,
  involuntary eyeball movements, irregular heartbeat, kidney failure, lack of muscle coordination,
  low blood pressure, poor reflexes, skin reddening
  or bloody blisters, slowdown of the central
  nervous system

*Generic name:*

# Phentermine

*See Fastin, page 204.*

*Generic name:*

# Phenylephrine,
# Chlorpheniramine, and
# Pyrilamine

*See Rynatan, page 484.*

*Generic name:*

# Phenytoin

*See Dilantin, page 161.*

*Brand name:*

# Phospholine Iodide

*Pronounced: FOS-foh-lin I-o-dide*
*Generic name: Echothiophate iodide*

## Why is this drug prescribed?

Phospholine Iodide is used to treat chronic open-angle glaucoma, a partial loss of vision or blindness resulting from a gradual increase in pressure of fluid in the eye. Because the vision loss occurs slowly, people often do not experience any symptoms and do not realize that their vision has declined. By the time the loss is noticed, it may be irreversible. Phospholine Iodide helps by reducing fluid pressure in the eye.

Phospholine Iodide is also used to treat secondary glaucoma (such as glaucoma following surgery to remove cataracts), for subacute or chronic angle-closure glaucoma after iridectomy (surgical removal of a portion of the iris) or when someone cannot have surgery or refuses it. The drug is also prescribed for children with accommodative esotropia ("cross-eye").

## Most important fact about this drug

Avoid exposure to certain pesticides or insecticides such as Sevin and Trolene. They can boost the side effects of Phospholine Iodide. If you work with these chemicals, wear a mask over your nose and mouth, wash and change your clothing frequently, and wash your hands often.

## How should you use this medication?

To use Phospholine Iodide:

1. To minimize drainage of Phospholine Iodide into your nose, your doctor may instruct you to apply pressure with the middle finger to the inside corner of the eye for 1 to 2 minutes after placing the drops in your eyes.
2. Wipe off any excess Phospholine Iodide around the eye with a tissue.
3. Wash off any Phospholine Iodide that may get onto your hands.

■ *If you miss a dose...*
If you use 1 dose every other day: Apply the dose you missed as soon as you remember, if it is still the scheduled day. If you do not remember until the next day, apply it as soon as you remember, then skip a day and start your schedule again.

If you use 1 dose a day: Apply the dose you missed as soon as you remember. If you do not remember until the next day, skip the dose you missed and go back to your regular schedule.

If you use 2 doses a day: Apply the dose you missed as soon as you remember. If it is almost time for your next dose, skip the one you missed and go back to your regular schedule.

Never apply 2 doses at once.

■ *Storage instructions...*
You may keep the eye drops at room temperature for up to 4 weeks.

## What side effects may occur?

Side effects cannot be anticipated. If any develop or change in intensity, tell your doctor immediately. Only your doctor can determine whether it is safe to continue taking Phospholine Iodide.

■ *Side effects may include:*
Ache above the eyes, blurred vision, burning, clouded eye lens, cyst formation, decreased pupil size, decreased visual sharpness, excess tears, eye pain, heart irregularities, increased eye pressure, inflamed iris, lid muscle twitching, nearsightedness, red eyes, stinging

## Why should this drug not be prescribed?

You should not use Phospholine Iodide if you have an inflammation in the eye.

Most people with angle-closure glaucoma (a condition in which there is a sudden increase in pressure of fluid in the eye) should not use Phospholine Iodide.

If you have ever had an allergic reaction to or are sensitive to Phospholine Iodide or any of its ingredients, you should not use this medication.

## Special warnings about this medication

Drugs such as Phospholine Iodide should be used cautiously (if at all) if you have or have ever had:

Bronchial asthma
Detached retina
Epilepsy
Extreme low blood pressure
Parkinson's disease
Peptic ulcer
Recent heart attack
Slow heartbeat
Stomach or intestinal problems

If you notice any problems with your heart, notify your doctor immediately.

Stop taking the drug and notify your doctor immediately if you experience any of the following: breathing difficulties, diarrhea, inability to hold urine, muscle weakness, profuse sweating, or salivation.

If you will be using Phospholine Iodide for a long time, your doctor should schedule regular examinations to make sure that Phospholine Iodide is not causing unwanted effects.

Phospholine Iodide may cause vision problems. Be careful when driving at night or performing tasks in dim or poor light.

### Possible food and drug interactions when taking this medication

If Phospholine Iodide is taken with certain other drugs, the effects of either could be increased, decreased, or altered. It is especially important to check with your doctor before combining Phospholine Iodide with drugs such as Enlon, Mestinon, or Tensilon, used to treat myasthenia gravis, a condition of muscle weakness that usually affects muscles in the eyes, face, limbs, and throat.

### Special information if you are pregnant or breastfeeding

If you are pregnant or plan to become pregnant, inform your doctor immediately. No information is available about the safety of Phospholine Iodide during pregnancy.

Phospholine Iodide should not be used by women who are breastfeeding.

### Recommended dosage

ADULTS

*For Glaucoma*

A dose of 0.03 percent should be used 2 times a day, in the morning and at bedtime. Your doctor may increase the dose if necessary. Your doctor may have you take 1 dose a day or 1 dose every other day, instead.

CHILDREN

*For Accommodative Esotropia*

Place 1 drop of 0.125 percent solution in both eyes at bedtime for 2 or 3 weeks to diagnose the condition.

Your doctor may then change the schedule to 0.125 percent every other day or reduce the dose to 0.06 percent every day.

The maximum dose usually recommended is 0.125 percent solution once daily.

If the eye drops are slowly withdrawn after a year or two of treatment, and the eye problem returns, your doctor may want you to consider surgery.

### Overdosage

Any medication used in excess can have serious consequences. If you suspect an overdose of Phospholine Iodide, seek medical help immediately.

*Brand name:*

# Pilocar

*Pronounced: PYE-low-car*
*Generic name: Pilocarpine hydrochloride*
*Other brand names: Isopto Carpine, Pilopine HS Gel*

### Why is this drug prescribed?

Pilocar causes constriction of the pupils (miosis) and reduces pressure within the eye. It is used to treat the increased pressure of open-angle glaucoma and to lower eye pressure before surgery for acute angle-closure glaucoma. It can be used alone or in combination with other medications. Glaucoma, one of the leading causes of blindness in the United States, is characterized by increased pressure in the eye that can damage the optic nerve and cause loss of vision.

### Most important fact about this drug

There is no cure for glaucoma. Pilocar and similar drugs can keep ocular pressure under control, but only as long as you take them. You will probably need to continue treatment for life; and you must be sure to take the medication regularly.

### How should you use this medication?

Follow these steps to administer Pilocar:

1. Wash your hands thoroughly.
2. Gently pull your lower eyelid down to form a pocket next to your eye.
3. Brace the eyedrop bottle on the bridge of your nose or your forehead.
4. Tilt your head back and squeeze the medication into your eye.
5. Close your eyes gently. Keep them closed for 1 to 2 minutes.
6. Do not rinse the dropper.
7. Wait for 5 to 10 minutes before using a second eye medication.

To avoid contaminating the dropper and solution, do not touch the eyelids or surrounding areas with the tip of the dropper.

Do not use if the solution is discolored.

■ *If you miss a dose...*
Apply it as soon as you remember. If it is almost time for your next dose, skip the one you missed and go back to your regular schedule. Do not take 2 doses at once.

■ *Storage instructions...*
Store away from heat and light. Do not freeze.

Keep the bottle tightly closed when it is not being used.

### What side effects may occur?
Side effects cannot be anticipated. If any develop or change in intensity, inform your doctor as soon as possible. Only your doctor can determine if it is safe for you to continue using Pilocar.

■ *More common side effects may include:*
Cloudy vision, detached retina, headache over your eye, nearsightedness, reduced vision in poor light, spasms of the eyelids, tearing eyes

■ *Rare side effects may include:*
Breathing difficulty, diarrhea, excessive salivation, fluid in lungs, high blood pressure, nausea, rapid heartbeat, sweating, vomiting

### Why should this drug not be prescribed?
Pilocar should not be used if you are sensitive to or have ever had an allergic reaction to any of the components of this solution. Your doctor will not prescribe it for you if you have an eye condition in which your pupils should not be constricted.

### Special warnings about this medication
Pilocar may make it difficult for you to see in the dark. Be careful driving at night, or doing any hazardous activity in dim light.

### Possible food and drug interactions when using this medication
No interactions have been reported.

### Special information if you are pregnant or breastfeeding
The effects of Pilocar during pregnancy have not been adequately studied. If you are pregnant or plan to become pregnant, inform your doctor immediately. Pilocar may appear in breast milk and could affect a nursing infant. If this medication is essen-

tial to your health, your doctor may advise you to stop breastfeeding until your treatment with Pilocar is finished.

### Recommended dosage
ADULTS

The usual starting dose is 1 or 2 drops up to 6 times a day, depending on the severity of the glaucoma and your response. During a severe attack, your doctor will tell you to put drops into the unaffected eye as well.

### Overdosage
Any medication taken in excess can have serious consequences. If you suspect an overdose seek medical attention immediately.

---

*Generic name:*

# Pilocarpine

See Pilocar, page 419.

---

*Brand name:*

# Pilopine HS Gel

See Pilocar, page 419.

---

*Generic name:*

# Pindolol

See Visken, page 588.

---

*Generic name:*

# Piroxicam

See Feldene, page 207.

---

*Brand name:*

# Plaquenil

*Pronounced: PLAK-en-ill*
*Generic name: Hydroxychloroquine sulfate*

### Why is this drug prescribed?
Plaquenil is prescribed for the prevention and treatment of certain forms of malaria.

Plaquenil is also used to treat the symptoms of rheumatoid arthritis such as swelling, inflammation, stiffness, and joint pain. It is also prescribed for lupus erythematosus, a chronic inflammation of the connective tissue.

### Most important fact about this drug

Children are especially sensitive to Plaquenil. Relatively small doses of this medication have caused fatalities. Keep this drug in a child-proof container and out of the reach of children.

### How should you take this medication?

Take Plaquenil exactly as prescribed for the full course of therapy.

If you have been prescribed Plaquenil for rheumatoid arthritis, it will take several weeks for beneficial effects to appear. Take each dose with a meal or a glass of milk.

■ *If you miss a dose...*

And you take 1 dose every 7 days, take it as soon as you remember, then go back to your regular schedule.

If you take 1 dose a day and you miss your dose, take it as soon as you remember. If you do not remember until the next day, skip the one you missed and go back to your regular schedule.

If you take more than one dose a day, take it as soon as you remember if it is within an hour or so of the missed time. If you do not remember until later on, skip the missed dose and go back to your regular schedule. Do not take 2 doses at once.

■ *Storage information...*

Store away from heat, light, and moisture.

### What side effects may occur?

Side effects cannot be anticipated. If any develop or change in intensity, inform your doctor as soon as possible. Only your doctor can determine if it is safe for you to continue taking Plaquenil.

■ *Side effects of treatment for an acute malarial attack may include:*

Abdominal cramps, diarrhea, dizziness, lack or loss of appetite, mild headache, nausea, vomiting

■ *Side effects of treatment for lupus erythematosus and rheumatoid arthritis may include:*

Abdominal cramps, abnormal eye pigmentation, anemia, bleaching of hair, blind spots, blood disorders, blurred vision, convulsions, decreased vision, diarrhea, difficulty focusing the eyes, dizziness, emotional changes, excessive coloring

of the skin, eye muscle paralysis, "foggy vision," halos around lights, headache, hearing loss, hives, involuntary eyeball movement, irritability, itching, lack of muscle coordination, light flashes and streaks, light intolerance, loss of hair, loss or lack of appetite, muscle weakness, nausea, nervousness, nightmares, psoriasis (dry, scaly, red skin patches), reading difficulties, ringing in the ears, skin eruptions, skin inflammation and scaling, skin rash, vertigo, vomiting, weariness, weight loss

### Why should this drug not be prescribed?

If you are sensitive to or have ever had an allergic reaction to Plaquenil or similar drugs such as Aralen and Chloroquine, you should not take this medication. Make sure your doctor is aware of any drug reactions you have experienced.

Plaquenil should not be prescribed if you have suffered partial or complete loss of vision in small areas while taking this medication or similar drugs. Notify your doctor of any past or present visual changes you have experienced.

This drug should not be used for long-term therapy in children.

### Special warnings about this medication

Unless you are directed to do so by your doctor, do not take this medication if you have psoriasis (a recurrent skin disorder characterized by patches of red, dry, scaly skin) or porphyria (an inherited metabolic disorder affecting the liver or bone marrow). The use of Plaquenil may cause a severe attack of psoriasis and may increase the severity of porphyria.

Disorders of the retina causing impairment or loss of vision may be related to the length of time and the dose of Plaquenil given for lupus and rheumatoid arthritis. Problems have occurred several months to several years after beginning daily therapy. When you are on prolonged therapy your doctor will perform eye examinations at the beginning of treatment and every 3 months after that. Visual disturbances may progress, even after you have stopped taking this drug. If you have any problem with your vision or your eyes, notify your doctor immediately.

All people on long-term therapy with this drug should have a physical examination periodically, including testing of knee and ankle reflexes, to detect any evidence of muscular weakness.

Consult your doctor if you experience ringing in the ears, or other hearing problems.

If you are being treated for rheumatoid arthritis and have shown no improvement (such as reduced joint swelling or increased mobility) within 6 months, your doctor may decide to discontinue this drug.

Plaquenil should be used with caution by alcoholics and those who have liver disease or kidney problems.

Your doctor should conduct periodic blood cell counts if you are on prolonged therapy with this medication. If any severe blood disorder develops that is not attributed to the disease you are being treated for, your doctor may discontinue use of this drug.

Consult your doctor if you are taking a drug that has a tendency to produce dermatitis (inflammation of the skin), because you may have some skin reactions while taking Plaquenil.

### Possible food and drug interactions when taking this medication

If Plaquenil is taken with certain other drugs, the effects of either could be increased, decreased, or altered. It is especially important to check with your doctor before combining Plaquenil with the following:

Any medication that may cause liver damage
Aurothioglucose (Solganal)
Cimetidine (Tagamet)
Digoxin (Lanoxin)

### Special information if you are pregnant or breastfeeding

Use of this drug during pregnancy should be avoided except in the suppression or treatment of malaria when, in the judgment of your doctor, the benefit outweighs the possible hazard. This drug may appear in breast milk and could affect a nursing infant. If this medication is essential to your health, your doctor may advise you to discontinue breastfeeding until your treatment is finished.

### Recommended dosage

ADULTS

*Restraint or Prevention of Malaria*

The usual dose is 400 milligrams taken once every 7 days on exactly the same day of each week. If circumstances permit, preventive therapy should begin 2 weeks prior to exposure. If this is not possible,

your doctor will have you take a starting dose of 800 milligrams, which may be divided into 2 doses taken 6 hours apart. You should continue this suppressive therapy for 8 weeks after leaving the area where malaria occurs.

*Acute Attack of Malaria*

The usual starting dose is 800 milligrams, to be followed by 400 milligrams in 6 to 8 hours and 400 milligrams on each of 2 consecutive days.

Alternatively, your doctor may prescribe a single dose of 800 milligrams.

*Lupus Erythematosus*

The usual starting dose for adults is 400 milligrams once or twice daily. You will continue to take this dose for several weeks or months, depending on your response. For longer-term maintenance therapy, your doctor may reduce the dose to 200 to 400 milligrams per day.

*Rheumatoid Arthritis*

The usual starting dose for adults is 400 to 600 milligrams a day taken with a meal or a glass of milk. If your condition improves, usually within 4 to 12 weeks, your doctor will reduce the dose to a maintenance level of 200 to 400 milligrams daily.

CHILDREN

For the treatment of malaria, your doctor will calculate the dosage on the basis of your child's weight.

This drug has not been proved safe for treatment of juvenile arthritis.

### Overdosage

Any medication taken in excess can have serious consequences. If you suspect an overdose, seek emergency medical treatment immediately.

■ *Symptoms of an overdose of Plaquenil may occur within 30 minutes. They include:*
Convulsions, drowsiness, headache, heart problems and failure, inability to breathe, visual problems

Brand name:

# Plendil

Pronounced: PLEN-dill
Generic name: Felodipine

### Why is this drug prescribed?

Plendil is prescribed for the treatment of high blood pressure. It is effective alone or in combination with other high blood pressure medications. A type of medication called a calcium channel blocker, Plendil eases the workload of the heart by slowing down its muscle contractions and the passage of nerve impulses through it. This improves blood flow through the heart and throughout the body, reduces blood pressure, and helps prevent angina pain (chest pain, often accompanied by a feeling of choking, usually caused by lack of oxygen in the heart due to clogged arteries).

### Most important fact about this drug

If you have high blood pressure, you must take Plendil regularly for it to be effective. Since blood pressure declines gradually, it may be several weeks before you get the full benefit of Plendil; you must continue taking it even if you are feeling well. Plendil does not cure high blood pressure; it merely keeps it under control.

### How should you take this medication?

Plendil can be taken with or without food. The tablets should be swallowed whole, not crushed or chewed.

Try not to miss any doses. If Plendil is not taken regularly, your blood pressure may increase.

■ *If you miss a dose...*
Take the forgotten dose as soon as you remember. If it is almost time for the next dose, skip the one you missed and go back to your regular schedule. Never try to "catch up" by doubling the dose.

■ *Storage instructions...*
Store at room temperature. Protect from light.

### What side effects may occur?

Side effects cannot be anticipated. If any develop or change in intensity, inform your doctor as soon as possible. Only your doctor can determine if it is safe for you to continue taking Plendil.

■ *More common side effects may include:*
Flushing, headache, swelling of the legs and feet

■ *Less common or rare side effects may include:*
Anemia, angina pectoris (chest pain), ankle pain, anxiety disorders, arm pain, arthritis, back pain, blurred vision, bronchitis, bruising, constipation, cough, diarrhea, dizziness, decreased sex drive, depression, difficulty sleeping, dry mouth, enlarged gums, excessive nighttime urination, excessive perspiration, facial swelling, fainting,

fatigue, flu, foot pain, frequent urination, gas, muscle pain, heart attack, hip pain, hives, impotence, inflammation of the nose, irregular heartbeat, irritability, itching, joint pain, knee pain, leg pain, low blood pressure, nausea, neck pain, nervousness, nosebleeds, painful or difficult urination, rapid heartbeat, rash, respiratory infections, ringing in the ears, shortness of breath, shoulder pain, sinus inflammation, sleepiness, sneezing, sore throat, stomach and intestinal pain, tingling sensation, tremor, urgent urination, vomiting, warm sensation, weakness

### Why should this drug not be prescribed?

If you are sensitive to or have ever had an allergic reaction to Plendil or other calcium channel blockers, such as Calan and Procardia, you should not take this medication. Make sure your doctor is aware of any drug reactions you have experienced.

### Special warnings about this medication

Plendil can cause your blood pressure to become too low. If you feel light-headed or faint, or if you feel your heart racing or you experience chest pain, contact your doctor immediately.

If you have congestive heart failure, Plendil should be used with caution, especially if you are also taking one of the "beta-blocker" family of drugs, such as Inderal or Tenormin.

Your legs and feet may swell when you start taking Plendil, usually within the first 2 to 3 weeks of treatment.

If you have liver disease or are over age 65, your doctor should monitor your blood pressure carefully while adjusting your dosage of Plendil.

Your gums may become swollen and sore while you are taking Plendil. Good dental hygiene will help control this problem.

### Possible food and drug interactions when taking this medication

If Plendil is taken with certain other drugs, the effects of either could be increased, decreased, or altered. It is especially important to check with your doctor before combining Plendil with the following:

Beta-blocking blood pressure medicines such as
  Lopressor, Inderal, and Tenormin
Cimetidine (Tagamet)
Digoxin (Lanoxin)
Epilepsy medications such as Tegretol and Dilantin

Erythromycin (PCE, ERYC, others)
Phenobarbital
Theophylline (Theo-Dur)

Taking Plendil with double-concentrated grapefruit juice can more than double the effect of the drug.

### Special information
### if you are pregnant or breastfeeding

Although the effects of Plendil during pregnancy have not been adequately studied in humans, birth defects have occurred in animal studies. If you are pregnant or plan to become pregnant, inform your doctor immediately. Plendil may appear in breast milk and may affect a nursing infant. If this medication is essential to your health, your doctor may advise you to discontinue breastfeeding until your treatment is finished.

### Recommended dosage

ADULTS

Your doctor will adjust the dosage according to your response to the drug.

The usual starting dose is 5 milligrams once a day; your doctor will adjust the dose at intervals of not less than 2 weeks.

The usual dosage range is 2.5 to 10 milligrams once daily.

CHILDREN

The safety and effectiveness of Plendil in children have not been established.

OLDER ADULTS

If you are over 65 years of age, your doctor will monitor your blood pressure closely during dosage adjustment. In general, you should not take more than 10 milligrams a day.

### Overdosage

Any medication taken in excess can have serious consequences. If you suspect an overdose, seek medical treatment immediately.

■ *Symptoms of Plendil overdose may include:*
Severely low blood pressure, slow heartbeat

*Generic name:*

# Polymyxin B, Neomycin, and Hydrocortisone

*See Cortisporin Ophthalmic Suspension, page 115.*

*Brand name:*

# Poly-Vi-Flor

*Pronounced: pol-ee-VIE-floor*
*Generic ingredients: Vitamins, Fluoride*

### Why is this drug prescribed?

Poly-Vi-Flor is a multivitamin and fluoride supplement with 10 essential vitamins plus the mineral fluoride. It is prescribed for children aged 2 and older to provide fluoride where the drinking water contains less than the amount recommended by the American Dental Association to build strong teeth and prevent cavities. Poly-Vi-Flor supplies significant amounts of other vitamins to avoid deficiencies. The American Academy of Pediatrics recommends that children up to age 16 take a fluoride supplement if they live in areas where the drinking water contains less than the recommended amount of fluoride.

### Most important fact about this drug

Do not give your child more than the recommended dose. Too much fluoride can cause discoloration and pitting of teeth.

### How should you take this medication?

Do not give your child more than your doctor prescribes.

Poly-Vi-Flor should be chewed or crushed before swallowing.

■ *If you miss a dose...*
Take it as soon as you remember. If it is almost time for the next dose, skip the one you missed and go back to your regular schedule. Do not take 2 doses at once.

■ *Storage instructions...*
Store away from heat, light, and moisture.

### What side effects may occur?

Rarely, an allergic rash has occurred.

### Why should this drug not be prescribed?

Children should not take Poly-Vi-Flor if they are getting significant amounts of fluoride from other medications or sources.

### Special warnings about this medication

Do not give your child more than the recommended dosage. Your child's teeth should be checked periodically for discoloration or pitting. Notify your doctor if white, brown, or black spots appear on your child's teeth.

The fluoride level of your drinking water should be determined before Poly-Vi-Flor is prescribed.

Let your doctor know if you change drinking water or filtering systems.

Fluoride does not replace proper dental habits, such as brushing, flossing, and having dental checkups.

### Recommended dosage
The usual dose is 1 tablet every day as prescribed by the doctor.

### Overdosage
Although overdose is unlikely, any medication taken in excess can have serious consequences. If you suspect an overdose, seek medical treatment immediately.

*Brand name:*

# Ponstel

*Pronounced: PON-stel*
*Generic name: Mefenamic acid*

### Why is this drug prescribed?
Ponstel, a nonsteroidal anti-inflammatory drug, is used for the relief of moderate pain (when treatment will not last for more than 7 days) and for the treatment of menstrual pain.

### Most important fact about this drug
You should have frequent checkups with your doctor if you take Ponstel regularly. Ulcers or internal bleeding can occur without warning.

### How should you take this medication?
Take Ponstel with food if possible. If it upsets your stomach, be sure to take it with food or an antacid or with a full glass of milk.

Take Ponstel exactly as prescribed by your doctor.

■ *If you miss a dose...*
If you take Ponstel on a regular schedule, take the forgotten dose as soon as you remember. If it is almost time for your next dose, skip the one you missed and go back to your regular schedule. Do not take 2 doses at once.

■ *Storage instructions...*
Store away from heat, light, and moisture.

### What side effects may occur?
Side effects cannot be anticipated. If any develop or change in intensity, inform your doctor as soon as possible. Only your doctor can determine if it is safe for you to continue taking Ponstel.

■ *More common side effects may include:*
Abdominal pain, diarrhea, nausea, stomach and intestinal upset, vomiting

■ *Less common or rare side effects may include:*
Anemia, blurred vision, blood in the urine, changes in liver function, constipation, difficult or painful urination, dizziness, drowsiness, ear pain, eye irritation, facial swelling due to fluid retention, fluttery or throbbing heartbeat, gas, headache, heartburn, hives, inability to sleep, increased need for insulin in a diabetic, kidney failure, labored breathing, loss of appetite, loss of color vision, nervousness, rash, red or purple spots on the skin, sweating, ulcers and internal bleeding

### Why should this drug not be prescribed?
Do not take Ponstel if you are sensitive to or have ever had an allergic reaction to it. You should not take it, either, if you have had asthma attacks, hay fever, or hives caused by aspirin or other nonsteroidal anti-inflammatory drugs, such as Motrin and Nuprin. Make sure your doctor is aware of any drug reactions you have experienced.

Do not take Ponstel if you have ulcerations or frequently recurring inflammation of your stomach or intestines.

Avoid this drug if you have serious kidney disease.

### Special warnings about this medication
If you develop a rash, diarrhea, or other stomach problems, stop taking this medication and contact your doctor.

Ponstel should be used with caution if you have kidney disease, heart failure, or liver disease; it can cause liver inflammation in some people.

This drug may prolong bleeding time. If you are taking blood-thinning medication, take Ponstel with caution.

### Possible food and drug interactions when taking this medication
If Ponstel is taken with certain other drugs, the effects of either can be increased, decreased, or altered. It is especially important to check with your doctor before combining Ponstel with the following:

Aspirin
Blood-thinning medications such as Coumadin
Diuretics such as Lasix and HydroDIURIL
Lithium (Lithonate)
Methotrexate

### Special information
### if you are pregnant or breastfeeding

The effects of Ponstel during pregnancy have not
been adequately studied. If you are pregnant or plan
to become pregnant, inform your doctor immediately. You should not use Ponstel in late pregnancy
because nonsteroidal anti-inflammatory drugs
affect the heart and blood vessels of the developing
baby. Ponstel may appear in breast milk and could
affect a nursing infant. If this medication is essential to your health, your doctor may advise you to
discontinue breastfeeding until your treatment is
finished.

### Recommended dosage

ADULTS AND CHILDREN OVER 14

*Moderate Pain*

The usual starting dose is 500 milligrams, followed
by 250 milligrams every 6 hours, if needed, for
1 week.

*Menstrual Pain*

The usual starting dose, once symptoms appear, is
500 milligrams, followed by 250 milligrams every
6 hours for 2 to 3 days.

CHILDREN

The safety and effectiveness of Ponstel have not
been established in children under 14.

### Overdosage

Although there is no information available on overdosage with Ponstel, any medication taken in
excess can have serious consequences. If you
suspect an overdose of Ponstel, seek medical attention immediately.

*Generic name:*

# Potassium chloride

*See Micro-K, page 323.*

*Brand name:*

# Pravachol

*Pronounced: PRAV-a-coll*
*Generic name: Pravastatin sodium*

### Why is this drug prescribed?

Pravachol is a cholesterol-lowering drug. Your
doctor may prescribe it along with a cholesterol-
lowering diet if your blood cholesterol level is dangerously high, and if you have not been able to
lower it by diet alone.

The drug works by helping to clear harmful low-
density lipoprotein (LDL) cholesterol out of the
blood and by limiting the body's ability to form
new LDL cholesterol.

### Most important fact about this drug

Pravachol is usually prescribed only if diet, exercise, and weight-loss fail to bring your cholesterol
levels under control. It's important to remember
that Pravachol is a supplement—not a substitute—
for those other measures. To get the full benefit of
the medication, you need to stick to the diet and
exercise program prescribed by your doctor. All
these efforts to keep your cholesterol levels normal
are important because together they may lower
your risk of heart disease.

### How should you take this medication?

For an even greater cholesterol-lowering effect,
your doctor may prescribe Pravachol along with
a different kind of lipid-lowering drug such as
Questran or Colestid. However, you must not
take Pravachol at the same time of day as the
other cholesterol-lowering drug. Take Pravachol
at least 1 hour before or 4 hours after taking the
other drug.

Pravachol should be taken once daily at
bedtime. You may take it with or without food.

Your doctor will probably do blood tests for
cholesterol levels every 4 weeks to determine the
effectiveness of the dose.

■ *If you miss a dose...*
Take the forgotten dose as soon as you remember. If it is almost time for your next dose, skip
the one you missed and go back to your regular
schedule. Do not take a double dose.
■ *Storage instructions...*
Store at room temperature, in a tightly closed
container, away from moisture and light.

## What side effects may occur?

Side effects from Pravachol cannot be anticipated. If any develop or change in intensity, inform your doctor as soon as possible. Only your doctor can determine if it is safe for you to continue taking Pravachol.

■ *Side effects may include:*

Abdominal pain, chest pain, cold, constipation, cough, diarrhea, dizziness, fatigue, flu, gas, headache, heartburn, inflammation of nasal passages, muscle aching or weakness, nausea, rash, urinary problems, vomiting

## Why should this drug not be prescribed?

Do not take Pravachol if you are sensitive or have ever had an allergic reaction to it.

Do not take Pravachol if you have liver disease.

## Special warnings about this medication

Pravachol should not be used to try to lower high cholesterol that stems from a medical condition such as alcoholism, poorly controlled diabetes, an underactive thyroid gland, or a kidney or liver problem.

Because Pravachol may cause damage to the liver, your doctor will do blood tests regularly. Your doctor should monitor you especially closely if you have ever had liver disease or if you are or have ever been a heavy drinker.

Since Pravachol may cause damage to muscle tissue, promptly report to your doctor any unexplained muscle pain, tenderness, or weakness, especially if you also have a fever or you just generally do not feel well.

## Possible food and drug interactions when taking this medication

If Pravachol is taken with certain other drugs, the effects of either could be increased, decreased, or altered. It is especially important to check with your doctor before combining Pravachol with the following:

Cholestyramine (Questran)
Cimetidine (Tagamet)
Colestipol (Colestid)
Erythromycin (E.E.S., Erythrocin, others)
Gemfibrozil (Lopid)

Immunosuppressive drugs such as Sandimmune and Neoral
Niacin (Nicobid, Nicolar)
Warfarin (Coumadin)

## Special information if you are pregnant or breastfeeding

You must not become pregnant while taking Pravachol. Because this drug lowers cholesterol, and cholesterol is necessary for the proper development of an unborn baby, there is some suspicion that Pravachol might cause birth defects. Your doctor will prescribe Pravachol only if you are highly unlikely to become pregnant while taking the drug. If you do become pregnant while taking Pravachol, inform your doctor immediately.

Because Pravachol appears in breast milk, and because its cholesterol-lowering effects might prove harmful to a nursing baby, you should not take Pravachol while you are breastfeeding.

## Recommended dosage

ADULTS

The usual starting dose is 10 to 20 milligrams once a day at bedtime.

For ongoing therapy, the recommended dose is 10 to 40 milligrams, once a day at bedtime.

OLDER ADULTS

The usual starting dose is 10 milligrams a day at bedtime; for ongoing therapy, the dose is 20 milligrams per day or less.

## Overdosage

Although no specific information is available, any medication taken in excess can have serious consequences. If you suspect an overdose of Pravachol, seek medical attention immediately.

*Generic name:*

# Pravastatin

*See Pravachol, page 426.*

*Generic name:*

# Prazosin

*See Minipress, page 328.*

*Brand name:*

# Precose

*Pronounced: PREE-cohs*
*Generic name: Acarbose*

### Why is this drug prescribed?

Precose is an oral medication used to treat Type II (noninsulin-dependent) diabetes when high blood sugar levels cannot be controlled by diet alone. Precose works by slowing the body's digestion of carbohydrates so that blood sugar levels won't surge upward after a meal. Precose may be taken alone or in combination with certain other diabetes medications such as Diabinase and Micronase.

### Most important fact about this drug

Always remember that Precose is an aid to, not a substitute for, good diet and exercise. Failure to follow the diet and exercise plan recommended by your doctor can lead to serious complications such as dangerously high or low blood sugar levels. If you are overweight, losing pounds and exercising are critically important in controlling your diabetes. Remember, too, that Precose is not an oral form of insulin and cannot be used in place of insulin.

### How should you take this medication?

Do not take more or less of this medication than directed by your doctor. Precose is usually taken 3 times a day with the first bite of each main meal.

■ *If you miss a dose...*
Take it as soon as you remember. If it is almost time for your next dose, skip the one you missed and go back to your regular schedule. Never take 2 doses at the same time. Taking Precose with your 3 main meals will help you to remember your medication schedule.
■ *Storage instructions...*
Keep the container tightly closed. Protect from temperatures above 77°F. Store away from moisture.

### What side effects may occur?

Side effects cannot be anticipated. If any develop or change in intensity, tell your doctor as soon as possible. Only your doctor can determine if it is safe for you to continue taking Precose.

If side effects do occur, they usually appear during the first few weeks of therapy and generally become less intense and less frequent over time. They are rarely severe.

■ *More common side effects may include:*
Abdominal pain, diarrhea, gas

### Why should this drug not be prescribed?

Do not take Precose when suffering diabetic ketoacidosis (a life-threatening medical emergency caused by insufficient insulin and marked by mental confusion, excessive thirst, nausea, vomiting, headache, fatigue, and a sweet fruity smell to the breath).

You should not take Precose if you have cirrhosis (chronic degenerative liver disease). Also avoid Precose therapy if you have inflammatory bowel disease, ulcers in the colon, any intestinal obstruction or chronic intestinal disease associated with digestion, or any condition that could become worse as a result of gas in the intestine.

### Special warnings about this medication

Every 3 months during your first year of treatment, your doctor will give you a blood test to check your liver and see how it is reacting to Precose. While you are taking Precose, you should check your blood and urine periodically for the presence of abnormal sugar (glucose) levels.

Even people with well-controlled diabetes may find that stress such as injury, infection, surgery, or fever results in a loss of control over their blood sugar. If this happens to you, your doctor may recommend that Precose be discontinued temporarily and injected insulin used instead.

When taken alone, Precose does not cause hypoglycemia (low blood sugar), but when you take it in combination with other medications such as Diabinese or Glucotrol, or with insulin, your blood sugar may fall too low. If you have any questions about combining Precose with other medications, be sure to discuss them with your doctor.

If you are taking Precose along with other diabetes medications, be sure to have some source of glucose, such as Glutose tablets, available in case you experience any symptoms of mild or moderate low blood sugar. (Table sugar won't work because Precose inhibits its absorption.)

■ *Symptoms of mild hypoglycemia may include:*
Cold sweat, fast heartbeat, fatigue, headache, nausea, and nervousness.
■ *Symptoms of more severe hypoglycemia may include:*
Coma, pale skin, and shallow breathing.

Severe hypoglycemia is an emergency. Contact your doctor immediately if the symptoms occur.

### Possible food and drug interactions when taking this medication

When you take Precose with certain other drugs, the effects of either could be increased, decreased, or altered. It is especially important to check with your doctor before taking Precose with the following:

Airway-opening drugs such as Sudafed and
　　Proventil
Calcium channel blockers such as Cardizem and
　　Procardia
Charcoal tablets
Digestive enzyme preparations such as Creon 20
　　and Donnazyme
Diuretics such as HydroDIURIL, Enduron,
　　Moduretic
Estrogens such as Premarin
Isoniazid (Rifamate)
Major tranquilizers such as Compazine and Mellaril
Nicotinic acid (Nicobid, Nicolar)
Oral contraceptives
Phenytoin (Dilantin)
Steroid medications such as Deltasone and Prelone
Thyroid medications such as Synthroid and
　　Thyrolar

### Special information
### if you are pregnant or breastfeeding

The effects of Precose during pregnancy have not been adequately studied. If you are pregnant or plan to become pregnant, tell your doctor immediately. Since studies suggest the importance of maintaining normal blood sugar levels during pregnancy, your doctor may prescribe injected insulin. It is not known whether Precose appears in breast milk. Because many drugs do appear in breast milk, you should not take Precose while breastfeeding.

### Recommended dosage

ADULTS

The recommended starting dose of Precose is 25 milligrams (half of a 50-milligram tablet) 3 times a day, taken with the first bite of each main meal. Your doctor will adjust your dosage at 4- to 8-week intervals, based on blood tests and your individual response to Precose. The doctor may increase the medication to 50 milligrams 3 times a day or, if needed, 100 milligrams 3 times a day. You should not take more than 100 milligrams 3 times a day or, if you weigh less than 132 pounds, 50 milligrams 3 times a day.

If you are also taking another oral antidiabetic medication and you show signs of low blood sugar, your doctor will adjust the dosage of both medications.

CHILDREN

Safety and effectiveness of Precose in children have not been established.

### Overdosage

An overdose in Precose alone will not cause hypoglycemia. An overdose may cause a temporary increase in gas, diarrhea, and abdominal discomfort, which will disappear quickly.

*Brand name:*

# Pred Forte

*Pronounced: PRED FORT*
*Generic name: Prednisolone acetate*

### Why is this drug prescribed?

Pred Forte contains a steroid medication that eases redness, irritation, and swelling due to inflammation of the eye.

### Most important fact about this drug

Do not use Pred Forte more often or for a longer period than you doctor orders. Overuse can increase the risk of side effects and can lead to eye damage. If your eye problems return, do not use any leftover Pred Forte without first consulting your doctor.

### How should you use this medication?

Keep using Pred Forte for the full time prescribed.

To avoid spreading infection, do not let anyone else use your prescription.

Pred Forte may increase the chance of infection from contact lenses. Your doctor may advise you to stop wearing your contacts while using this medication.

Follow these steps to administer Pred Forte:

1. Wash your hands thoroughly.
2. Vigorously shake the dropper bottle.
3. Gently pull your lower eyelid down to form a pocket next to your eye.
4. Do not touch the applicator tip to any surface including your eye.

5. Brace the bottle against the bridge of your nose or your forehead.
6. Tilt your head back and squeeze the medication into your eye.
7. Close your eyes gently. Keep them closed for 1 to 2 minutes.
8. Do not rinse the dropper.
9. Wait for 5 to 10 minutes before using a second eye medication.

■ *If you miss a dose...*
Apply it as soon as you remember. If it is almost time for your next dose, skip the one you missed and go back to your regular schedule.

■ *Storage instructions...*
Store away from heat and direct light. Protect from freezing.

## What side effects may occur?

Side effects cannot be anticipated. If any develop or change in intensity, inform your doctor as soon as possible. Only your doctor can determine if it is safe for you to continue taking Pred Forte.

■ *Side effects may include:*
Cataract formation, increased pressure inside the eyeball, perforation of the eyeball, secondary infection with fungi or viruses

Since any one of these developments could affect your vision temporarily or permanently, it is important to keep in close contact with your doctor while using Pred Forte eyedrops, and to use the drops only as directed.

Occasionally, long-term use of Pred Forte eyedrops may cause bodywide side effects due to an overload of steroid hormone. Such side effects may include a "moon-faced" appearance, obese trunk, humped upper back, wasted limbs, and purple stretch marks on the skin. These effects are likely to disappear once the medication is withdrawn. If bodywide side effects occur, you will need to stop using the eye drops gradually rather than all at once.

## Why should this drug not be prescribed?

Do not use Pred Forte if you have an untreated, pus-forming eye infection.

You should not take Pred Forte if you have herpes or other viral diseases of the eye, tuberculosis of the eye, or a fungal disease of the eye.

Do not use Pred Forte if you are allergic to prednisolone or any other ingredients.

## Special warnings about this medication

You must stay in close touch with your doctor while using this medication, for the following reasons:

If you use Pred Forte eyedrops extensively and/or for an extended period of time, you may be at increased risk for cataracts.

If you use Pred Forte eyedrops for a condition that causes thinning of the cornea, you are at increased risk for perforation of the eyeball.

If you have a persistent ulceration of the cornea of your eye while using Pred Forte eyedrops, the problem may be a secondary fungus infection which Pred Forte cannot cure. An eye doctor should evaluate this possibility.

While you are using Pred Forte eyedrops, an eye doctor should check your intraocular pressure (pressure inside the eyeball) frequently, since steroids may increase this pressure. If increased pressure is allowed to continue, it may cause loss of vision.

Pred Forte contains sodium bisulfite, which can cause allergic-type reactions, including severe or even life-threatening asthmatic episodes. Sulfite sensitivity is seen more frequently in asthmatic than in non-asthmatic people.

## Possible food and drug interactions when using this medication

Prednisolone acetate, the active ingredient in Pred Forte eyedrops, is also available in tablet and injectable forms for the treatment of other disorders. If these other forms of prednisolone acetate are taken with certain other drugs, the effects of either could be increased, decreased, or altered. Therefore, it's wise to check with your doctor before combining Pred Forte eyedrops with other medications.

## Special information if you are pregnant or breastfeeding

If you are pregnant or plan to become pregnant, inform your doctor immediately. Pred Forte eyedrops should be used during pregnancy only if the potential benefit outweighs the potential risk to the developing baby.

It is not known whether the hormone in Pred Forte eyedrops appears in breast milk. If it does, the small quantity involved would be unlikely to harm a breastfeeding baby. Nevertheless, caution is advised when using Pred Forte eyedrops while breastfeeding.

### Recommended dosage

ADULTS

Put 1 to 2 drops under the eyelid 2 to 4 times daily. During the first 24 to 48 hours, your doctor may want you to use more frequent doses.

### Overdosage

A one-time accidental overdose of Pred Forte eyedrops ordinarily will not cause acute problems. Over time, however, overdosage may have serious consequences (see "What side effects may occur?"). If you suspect symptoms of a chronic overdose with Pred Forte eyedrops, seek medical attention immediately.

If you accidentally swallow Pred Forte eyedrops, drink fluids to dilute the medication. Call your local poison center or your doctor for assistance.

Generic name:

# Prednisolone acetate

See Pred Forte, page 429.

Generic name:

# Prednisolone sodium phosphate

See Pediapred, page 398.

Generic name:

# Prednisone

See Deltasone, page 142.

Brand name:

# Premarin

Pronounced: PREM-uh-rin
Generic name: Conjugated estrogens
Other brand names: Premphase, Prempro

### Why is this drug prescribed?

Premarin is an estrogen replacement drug. The tablets are used to reduce symptoms of menopause, including feelings of warmth in face, neck, and chest, and the sudden intense episodes of heat and sweating known as "hot flashes." They also may be prescribed for teenagers who fail to mature at the usual rate, and to relieve the symptoms of certain types of cancer, including some forms of breast and prostate cancer.

In addition, either the tablets or Premarin vaginal cream can be used for other conditions caused by lack of estrogen, such as dry, itchy external genitals and vaginal irritation.

Along with diet, calcium supplements, and exercise, Premarin tablets are also prescribed to prevent osteoporosis, a condition in which the bones become brittle and easily broken.

Premphase and Prempro both combine a daily Premarin tablet with tablets of medroxyprogesterone acetate (Cycrin). The addition of progesterone to estrogen-replacement therapy has been shown to reduce the risk of uterine cancer.

### Most important fact about this drug

Because estrogens have been linked with increased risk of endometrial cancer (cancer in the lining of the uterus), it is essential to have regular checkups and to report any unusual vaginal bleeding to your doctor immediately.

### How should you take this medication?

Take Premarin exactly as prescribed. Do not share it with anyone else.

If you are taking calcium supplements as a part of the treatment to help prevent brittle bones, check with your doctor about how much to take.

You should take a few moments to read the patient package insert provided with your prescription.

If you are using Premarin vaginal cream, apply it as follows:

1. Remove cap from tube.
2. Screw nozzle end of applicator onto tube.
3. Gently squeeze tube from the bottom to force sufficient cream into the barrel to provide the prescribed dose. Use the marked stopping points on the applicator as a guide.
4. Unscrew applicator from tube.
5. Lie on back with knees drawn up. Gently insert applicator deeply into the vagina and press plunger downward to its original position.

To cleanse the applicator, pull the plunger to remove it from the barrel, then wash with mild soap and warm water. Do not boil or use hot water.

■ *If you miss a dose...*

Take the forgotten dose as soon as you remember. If it is almost time for the next dose, skip the one you missed and go back to your regular schedule. Never try to "catch up" by doubling the dose.

■ *Storage instructions...*

Store at room temperature.

## What side effects may occur?

Side effects cannot be anticipated. If any develop or change in intensity, inform your doctor immediately. Only your doctor can determine whether it is safe to continue taking Premarin.

■ *Side effects may include:*

Abdominal cramps, abnormal vaginal bleeding, bloating, breast swelling and tenderness, depression, dizziness, enlargement of benign tumors in the uterus, fluid retention, gallbladder disease, hair loss from the scalp, increased body hair, inflammation of the pancreas, intolerance to contact lenses, migraine headache, nausea, vomiting, sex-drive changes, skin darkening, especially on the face, skin rash or redness, swelling of wrists and ankles, vaginal yeast infection, vomiting, weight gain or loss, yellow eyes and skin

■ *Other possible side effects of Premphase and Prempro:*

Appetite changes, backache, blood clots, changes in blood pressure, excessive flow of breast milk, eye disorders, fatigue, fever, headache, nervousness, sleep disturbances, twitching

## Why should this drug not be prescribed?

Do not take Premarin if you have ever had a bad reaction to it, or have undiagnosed abnormal vaginal bleeding.

Except in certain special circumstances, you should not be given Premarin if you have breast cancer or any other "estrogen-dependent" cancer.

Do not take Premarin if you have had any heart or circulation problem including a tendency for abnormal blood clotting.

## Special warnings about this medication

The risk of cancer of the uterus increases when estrogen is used for a long time or taken in large doses.

There may be an increased risk of breast cancer in women who take estrogen for a long time. If you have a family history of breast cancer or have ever had an abnormal mammogram, you need to have more frequent breast examinations.

Women who take Premarin after menopause are more likely to develop gallbladder disease.

Premarin also increases the risk of blood clots. These blood clots can cause stroke, heart attack, or other serious disorders.

While taking Premarin, get in touch with your doctor right away if you notice any of the following:

Abdominal pain, tenderness, or swelling
Abnormal bleeding from the vagina
Breast lumps
Coughing up blood
Pain in your chest or calves
Severe headache, dizziness, or faintness
Sudden shortness of breath
Vision changes
Yellowing of the skin

## Possible food and drug interactions when taking this medication

If Premarin is taken with certain other drugs, the effects of either could be increased, decreased, or altered. It is especially important to check with your doctor before combining Premarin with the following:

Barbiturates such as phenobarbital
Blood thinners such as Coumadin
Drugs used for epilepsy, such as Dilantin
Major tranquilizers such as Thorazine
Oral diabetes drugs such as Micronase
Rifampin (Rifadin)
Steroid medications such as Deltasone
Thyroid preparations such as Synthroid
Tricyclic antidepressants such as Elavil and
   Tofranil
Vitamin C

## Special information
## if you are pregnant or breastfeeding

If you are pregnant or plan to become pregnant, notify your doctor immediately. Premarin should not be taken during pregnancy because of the possibility of harm to the unborn child. Premarin cannot prevent a miscarriage. Estrogens can decrease the quantity and quality of breast milk, and progestins appear in breast milk. Your doctor may advise you not to breastfeed while you are taking this drug.

## Recommended dosage

Your doctor will start therapy with this medication at a low dose. He or she will want to check you periodically at 3- to 6-month intervals to determine the need for continued therapy.

### PREMARIN TABLETS

*Hot Flashes Associated with Menopause*
The usual dosage is 0.3 to 1.25 milligrams daily. If you are still having periods, the doctor will start the Premarin on the fifth day of your cycle, have you take it for 3 weeks, then give you 1 week off.

*Tissue Degeneration in the Vagina*
The usual dosage is 0.3 to 1.25 milligrams or more daily. The drug is taken cyclically (3 weeks on and 1 week off).

*Low Estrogen Levels Due to Reduced Ovary Function*
The usual dosage is 2.5 to 7.5 milligrams daily, taken in several small doses, for 20 days, followed by a 10-day rest period. If you do not have your period by the end of this time, the same dosage schedule is repeated.

If you start to bleed before the end of the 10-day period your doctor will start you on another 20-day cycle, with an oral progestin added during the last 5 days. If you start to bleed before the second cycle is over, stop taking the medication and tell your doctor.

*Ovary Removal or Ovarian Failure*
The usual dosage is 1.25 milligrams daily, cyclically (3 weeks on and 1 week off). Your doctor will adjust the dosage according to the severity of your symptoms and your response to treatment.

*Osteoporosis (Loss of Bone Mass)*
The usual dosage is 0.625 milligram daily, taken cyclically (3 weeks on and 1 week off).

*Advanced Androgen-Dependent Cancer of the Prostate, for Relief of Symptoms Only*
The usual dosage is 1.25 to 2.5 milligrams 3 times daily.

*Breast Cancer (for Relief of Symptoms Only) in Appropriately Selected Women and Men with Metastatic Disease*
The suggested dosage is 10 milligrams 3 times daily for a period of at least 3 months. Tell your doctor if you have any unusual bleeding.

### PREMARIN VAGINAL CREAM

Given cyclically for short-term use only.

*Degeneration of Genital Tissue or Severe Itching in the Genital Area*
The recommended dosage is $1/2$ to 2 grams daily, inserted into the vagina, depending on the severity of the condition. You will use the cream for 3 weeks, then stop for 1 week. Tell your doctor if you notice any unusual bleeding.

### PREMPHASE TABLETS

Take 1 maroon Premarin tablet every day for 28 days; on the 15th day, begin taking 1 light-purple Cycrin tablet along with the Premarin.

### PREMPRO TABLETS

Take 1 maroon Premarin tablet and 1 white Cycrin tablet together each day.

## Overdosage

Any medication taken in excess can have serious consequences. If you suspect an overdose of Premarin, seek medical attention immediately.

■ *Symptoms of Premphase/Prempro overdose may include:*
Nausea, vomiting, withdrawal bleeding

*Brand name:*

# Premphase

*See Premarin, page 431.*

*Brand name:*

# Prempro

*See Premarin, page 431.*

*Generic name:*

# Prenatal vitamins and minerals

*See Stuartnatal Plus, page 511.*

*Brand name:*

# Prevacid

*Pronounced: PREH-va-sid*
*Generic name: Lansoprazole*

## Why is this drug prescribed?

Prevacid blocks the production of stomach acid. It is prescribed for the short-term treatment (up to 4 weeks) of active duodenal ulcer, and is used for up to 8 weeks in the treatment of erosive esophagitis (a severe inflammation of the passage to the stomach). It is also used as long-term therapy for certain diseases marked by excessive acid production, such as Zollinger-Ellison syndrome.

### Most important fact about this drug

To relieve your symptoms and to heal your ulcer, you need to take Prevacid for the full time of treatment your doctor prescribes. Keep taking the drug even if you begin to feel better, and be sure to keep your appointments with your doctor.

### How should you take this medication?

Prevacid should be taken before meals. Do not open, chew, or crush the Prevacid capsule; it must be swallowed whole. If you are taking antacids for pain, you may continue to do so. You also may continue to take sucralfate (Carafate), but take your dose of Prevacid at least 30 minutes prior to the Carafate.

■ *If you miss a dose...*
Take it as soon as you remember. If it is almost time for your next dose, skip the one you missed and go back to your regular schedule. Do not take 2 doses at once.
■ *Storage instructions...*
Store at room temperature in a tightly closed container. Keep away from moisture.

### What side effects may occur?

Side effects cannot be anticipated. If any develop or change in intensity, tell your doctor as soon as possible. Only your doctor can determine if it is safe for you to continue taking Prevacid.

■ *More common side effects may include:*
Diarrhea
■ *Less common side effects may include:*
Abdominal pain, nausea
■ *Rare side effects may include:*
Abnormal thinking, acne, aggravation of hostility, agitation, anemia, anxiety, apathy, arthritis, asthma, bad breath, belching, black or discolored stools, blood in the urine, breast development in males, breast enlargement, breast tenderness, bronchitis, chest pain (including severe pain), colitis, confusion, constipation, cough, coughing up blood, deafness, decreased sex drive, depression, diabetes, difficult or labored breathing, difficulty swallowing, dizziness, dry mouth, ear

infection, eye pain, fainting, fever, fluid retention, "flu-like" symptoms, flushing, gallstones, gas, general feeling of illness, gout, hair loss, hallucinations, heart attack, hiccups, high blood pressure, high or low blood sugar, hives, impotence, increased appetite, increased salivation, indigestion, infection, inflammation of the esophagus or mouth, inflammation of the stomach lining, itching, kidney problems, kidney stones, loss of appetite, low blood pressure, memory loss, menstrual problems, muscle, bone, or joint pain, nervousness, nosebleeds, paralysis, pneumonia, prickling, tingling, or pins and needles, rash, rectal hemorrhage, rectal and bladder spasms, ringing in ears, shock, sore throat, stomach and intestinal hemorrhage, stroke, taste alteration, thirst, throbbing heartbeat, thyroid problems, visual disturbances, vomiting blood, weakness, weight gain or loss, wheezing, yeast infection

### Why should this drug not be prescribed?

Avoid Prevacid if you have ever had an allergic reaction to it.

### Special warnings about this medication

Do not take Prevacid any longer than your doctor has prescribed; this medication should not be used for long-term therapy of duodenal ulcer or erosive esophagitis.

If you have liver disease, be sure your doctor knows about it. Prevacid should be used cautiously.

If you do not begin to feel better on Prevacid therapy, or if your symptoms become worse, be sure to call your doctor.

Prevacid has no effect on stomach cancer. It could be present even if Prevacid relieves your symptoms.

### Possible food and drug interactions when taking this medication

If Prevacid is taken with certain other drugs, the effects of either could be increased, decreased, or altered. It is especially important to check with your doctor before combining Prevacid with the following:

Ampicillin
Digoxin (Lanoxin)
Iron salts (Ferro-Sequels, Ferro-Sulfate)
Ketoconazole (Nizoral)
Sucralfate (Carafate)
Theophylline (Theo-Dur)

## Special information
## if you are pregnant or breastfeeding

The effects of Prevacid in pregnant women have not been adequately studied. If you are pregnant or plan to become pregnant, tell your doctor. It is not known whether Prevacid appears in human breast milk. If this medication is essential to your health, your doctor may have you stop breastfeeding your baby while you are taking it.

## Recommended dosage:

ADULTS

*For treatment of duodenal ulcer*
The usual dose is 15 milligrams daily, before eating, for 4 weeks.

*For treatment of erosive esophagitis*
The usual dose is 30 milligrams daily, before eating, for up to 8 weeks. Depending on your response to the medication your doctor may suggest another 8-week treatment regimen.

*Other excess acid conditions (such as Zollinger-Ellison syndrome)*
The usual starting dose is 60 milligrams once daily. This dose can be adjusted upward by your doctor, depending on your response. Dosages totalling more than 120 milligrams a day should be divided into smaller doses. If you have severe liver disease, your doctor will tailor your dosage to fit your needs.

CHILDREN

The safety and effectiveness of Prevacid have not been established in children.

## Overdosage

Overdoses of Prevacid are not known to cause any problems. Nevertheless, no medication should be taken in excess. If you suspect an overdose, seek medical attention immediately.

*Brand name:*

# Prilosec

*Pronounced: PRILL-oh-sek*
*Generic name: Omeprazole*

## Why is this drug prescribed?

Prilosec is prescribed for the short-term treatment (4 to 8 weeks) of active duodenal ulcer, gastroesophageal reflux disease (backflow of acid stomach contents), and erosive esophagitis (inflammation of the esophagus). It is also used to maintain healing of erosive esophagitis and for the long-term treatment of conditions in which too much stomach acid is secreted such as Zollinger-Ellison syndrome, multiple endocrine adenomas (benign tumors), and systemic mastocytosis (cancerous cells).

## Most important fact about this drug

Prilosec's healing effect can mask the signs of stomach cancer. Your doctor should be careful to rule out this possibility.

## How should you take this medication?

Prilosec works best when taken before meals. It can be taken with an antacid.

The capsule should be swallowed whole. It should not be opened, chewed, or crushed.

Avoid excessive amounts of caffeine while taking this drug.

It may take several days for Prilosec to begin relieving stomach pain. Be sure to continue taking the drug exactly as prescribed even if it seems to have no effect.

■ *If you miss a dose...*
Take it as soon as you remember. If it is almost time for your next dose, skip the one you missed and go back to your regular schedule. Do not take 2 doses at once.
■ *Storage information...*
Store at room temperature in a tightly closed container, away from light and moisture.

## What side effects may occur?

Side effects cannot be anticipated. If any develop or change in intensity, inform your doctor as soon as possible. Only your doctor can determine if it is safe for you to continue taking Prilosec.

■ *More common side effects may include:*
Abdominal pain, diarrhea, headache, nausea, vomiting
■ *Less common or rare side effects may include:*
Abdominal swelling, abnormal dreams, aggression, anemia, anxiety, apathy, back pain, breast development in males, blood in urine, changes in liver function, chest pain, confusion, constipation, cough, depression, difficulty sleeping, discolored feces, dizziness, dry mouth, dry skin, fatigue, fever, fluid retention and swelling, fluttery heartbeat, frequent urination, gas, general

feeling of illness, hair loss, hallucinations, hepatitis, high blood pressure, hives, irritable colon, itching, joint and leg pain, loss of appetite, low blood sugar, muscle cramps and pain, nervousness, nosebleeds, pain, pain in testicles, rapid heartbeat, rash, ringing in ears, skin inflammation, sleepiness, slow heartbeat, stomach tumors, taste distortion, tingling or pins and needles, throat pain, tremors, upper respiratory infection, urinary tract infection, vertigo, weakness, weight gain, yellow eyes and skin

## Why should this drug not be prescribed?

If you are sensitive to or have ever had an allergic reaction to Prilosec or any of its ingredients, you should not take this medication. Make sure your doctor is aware of any drug reactions you have experienced.

## Special warnings about this medication

Long-term use of this drug can cause severe stomach inflammation.

## Possible food and drug interactions when taking this medication

If Prilosec is taken with certain other drugs, the effects of either could be increased, decreased, or altered. It is especially important to check with your doctor before combining Prilosec with the following:

Ampicillin-containing drugs such as Unasyn
Cyclosporine (Sandimmune, Neoral)
Diazepam (Valium)
Disulfiram (Antabuse)
Iron
Ketoconazole (Nizoral)
Phenytoin (Dilantin)
Warfarin (Coumadin)

## Special information if you are pregnant or breastfeeding

The effects of Prilosec during pregnancy have not been adequately studied. If you are pregnant or plan to become pregnant, inform your doctor immediately. Prilosec may appear in breast milk and could affect a nursing infant. If this medication is essential to your health, your doctor may advise you to discontinue breastfeeding until your treatment with this medication is finished.

## Recommended dosage

### ADULTS

*Short-term Treatment of Active Duodenal Ulcer*
The usual dose is 20 milligrams once a day. Most people heal within 4 weeks.

*Erosive Esophagitis or Poorly Responsive Gastroesophageal Reflux Disease (GERD)*
The usual dose is 20 milligrams daily for 4 to 8 weeks. The dose may be continued to maintain healing.

*Pathological Hypersecretory Conditions*
The usual starting dose is 60 milligrams once a day. If you take more than 80 milligrams a day, your doctor will divide the total into smaller doses. The dosing will be based on your needs.

### CHILDREN

The safety and effectiveness of Prilosec in children have not been established.

## Overdosage

No specific symptoms of Prilosec overdose are known, but any medication taken in excess can have serious consequences. If you suspect an overdose of Prilosec, seek medical attention immediately.

*Generic name:*

# Primidone

*See Mysoline, page 344.*

*Brand name:*

# Principen

*See Omnipen, page 381.*

*Brand name:*

# Prinivil

*See Zestril, page 604.*

*Brand name:*

# Prinzide

*See Zestoretic, page 602.*

*Generic name:*

# Procainamide

*See Procan SR, page 437.*

*Brand name:*

# Procan SR

*Pronounced: PROH-can*
*Generic name: Procainamide hydrochloride*
*Other brand name: Pronestyl-SR*

### Why is this drug prescribed?

Procan SR is used to treat severe irregular heartbeats (arrhythmias). Arrhythmias are generally divided into two main types: heartbeats that are faster than normal (tachycardia), and heartbeats that are slower than normal (bradycardia). Irregular heartbeats are often caused by drugs or disease but can occur in otherwise healthy people with no history of heart disease or other illness.

### Most important fact about this drug

Procan SR can cause serious blood disorders, especially during the first 3 months of treatment. Be sure to notify your doctor if you notice any of the following: joint or muscle pain, dark urine, yellowing of skin or eyes, muscular weakness, chest or abdominal pain, appetite loss, diarrhea, hallucinations, dizziness, depression, wheezing, cough, easy bruising or bleeding, tremors, palpitations, rash, soreness or ulcers in the mouth, sore throat, fever, and chills.

### How should you take this medication?

Take only your prescribed doses of Procan SR; never take more.

Procan SR should be swallowed whole. Do not break or chew the tablet. You may see the tablet matrix of Procan SR in your stool, since it does not disintegrate following release of procainamide.

Try not to miss any doses. Skipping doses, changing the intervals between doses, or "making up" missed doses by doubling up later may cause your condition to worsen and could be dangerous.

■ *If you miss a dose...*
Take it as soon as you remember if it is within 4 hours of your scheduled time. If you do not remember until later, skip the dose you missed and go back to your regular schedule. Never take 2 doses at the same time.

■ *Storage instructions...*
Store away from heat, light, and moisture.

### What side effects may occur?

Side effects cannot be anticipated. If any develop or change in intensity, inform your doctor as soon as possible. Only your doctor can determine if it is safe for you to continue taking Procan SR.

■ *More common side effects may include:*
Abdominal pain, bitter taste, diarrhea, loss of appetite, nausea, symptoms similar to those of lupus erythematosus, an inflammatory disease of the connective tissue (joint pain or inflammation, abdominal or chest pain, fever, chills, muscle pain, skin lesions), vomiting

■ *Less common side effects may include:*
Depression, dizziness, fluid retention, flushing, giddiness, hallucinations, hives, itching, rash, weakness

■ *Rare side effects may include:*
Anemia, changes in blood counts, low blood pressure

### Why should this drug not be prescribed?

Procan SR should not be taken if you have the heart irregularity known as complete heart block or incomplete heart block without a pacemaker, or if you have ever had an allergic reaction to procaine or similar local anesthetics.

Your doctor will not prescribe this drug if you have been diagnosed with the connective-tissue disease lupus erythematosus or the heartbeat irregularity known as torsade de pointes.

### Special warnings about this medication

To check for the serious blood disorders that can develop during Procan SR therapy, your doctor will do a complete blood count weekly for the first 12 weeks and will continue to monitor your blood count carefully after that.

If you develop a fever, chills, sore throat or mouth, bruising or bleeding, infections, chest or abdominal pain, loss of appetite, weakness, muscle or joint pain, skin rash, nausea, fluttery heartbeat, vomiting, diarrhea, hallucinations, dizziness, depression, wheezing, yellow eyes and skin, or dark urine, contact your doctor immediately. It could indicate a serious illness.

Use Procan SR cautiously if you have ever had congestive heart failure or other types of heart disease.

Your doctor will prescribe Procan SR along with other antiarrhythmic drugs, such as quinidine or disopyramide, only if they have been tried and have not worked when used alone.

If you have ever had kidney disease, liver disease, or myasthenia gravis (a disease that causes muscle weakness, especially in the face and neck), your doctor will watch you carefully while you are taking Procan SR.

Make sure your doctor is aware of any drug reactions you have experienced, especially to procaine, other local anesthetics, or aspirin.

### Possible food and drug interactions when taking this medication

If Procan SR is taken with certain other drugs, the effects of either could be increased, decreased, or altered. It is especially important to check with your doctor before combining Procan SR with the following:

Antiarrhythmic drugs such as quinidine (Quinidex), propranolol (Inderal), and mexiletine (Mexitil)
Drugs that ease muscle spasms, such as Cogentin and Artane
Lidocaine
Neuromuscular blocking agents such as Anectine

### Special information if you are pregnant or breastfeeding

The effects of Procan SR during pregnancy have not been adequately studied. If you are pregnant or plan to become pregnant, inform your doctor immediately. Procan SR appears in breast milk and may affect a nursing infant. If this medication is essential to your health, your doctor may advise you to discontinue breastfeeding until your treatment is finished.

### Recommended dosage

ADULTS

Dosages and intervals between doses will be adjusted for you, based on your doctor's assessment of the degree of underlying heart disease, your age, and the way your kidneys are functioning.

Younger people with normal kidney function will start with a total daily oral dose of up to 50 milligrams per 2.2 pounds of body weight, divided into smaller doses and taken every 6 hours.

Older people, especially those over 50 years of age, or those with reduced kidney, liver, or heart function will get lower doses or wait a longer time between doses; this may decrease the probability of side effects that are related to the size of the dose.

CHILDREN

The safety and effectiveness of this drug have not been established in children.

### Overdosage

Any medication taken in excess can have serious consequences. If you suspect an overdose, seek medical treatment immediately.

■ *Symptoms of Procan SR overdose may include:*
   Changes in heart function and heartbeat

Brand name:

# Procardia

*Pronounced: pro-CAR-dee-uh*
*Generic name: Nifedipine*
*Other brand names: Procardia XL, Adalat, Adalat CC*

### Why is this drug prescribed?

Procardia and Procardia XL are used to treat angina (chest pain caused by lack of oxygen to the heart due to clogged arteries or spasm of the arteries). Procardia XL is also used to treat high blood pressure. Procardia and Procardia XL are calcium channel blockers. They ease the workload of the heart by relaxing the muscles in the walls of the arteries, allowing them to dilate. This improves blood flow through the heart and throughout the body, reduces blood pressure, and helps prevent angina. Procardia XL is taken once a day and provides a steady rate of medication over a 24-hour period.

### Most important fact about this drug

If you have high blood pressure, you must take Procardia XL regularly for it to be effective. Since blood pressure declines gradually, it may be several weeks before you get the full benefit of Procardia XL; and you must continue taking it even if you are feeling well. Procardia XL does not cure high blood pressure; it merely keeps it under control.

### How should you take this medication?

Procardia and Procardia XL should be taken exactly as prescribed by your doctor, even if your symptoms have disappeared.

Procardia XL tablets are specially designed to release the medication into your bloodstream slowly. As a result, something that looks like a tablet may occasionally appear in your stool. This is normal and simply means that the medication has been released, and the shell that contained the medication has been eliminated from your body.

Procardia and Procardia XL tablets should be swallowed whole. Do not break, crush, or chew.

Procardia and Procardia XL can be taken with or without food.

Do not substitute another brand of nifedipine for Procardia or Procardia XL unless your doctor directs.

Procardia XL should be taken once a day. You can take it in the morning or evening, but should hold to the same time each day.

■ *If you miss a dose...*
Take the forgotten dose as soon as you remember. If it is almost time for your next dose, skip the one you missed. Never take 2 doses at the same time.

■ *Storage instructions...*
Procardia and Procardia XL can be stored at room temperature. Protect from moisture, light, humidity, and excessive heat.

### What side effects may occur?
Side effects cannot be anticipated. If any develop or change in intensity, inform your doctor as soon as possible. Only your doctor can determine whether it is safe for you to continue taking Procardia or Procardia XL.

■ *More common side effects may include:*
Constipation, cough, dizziness, fatigue, flushing, giddiness, headache, heartburn, heat sensation, light-headedness, mood changes, muscle cramps, nasal congestion, nausea, sore throat, swelling of arms, legs, hands, and feet, tremors, wheezing

■ *Less common side effects may include:*
Abdominal pain, blurred vision, chest congestion, chills, cramps, diarrhea, difficult or labored breathing, difficulty in balance, difficulty sleeping, drowsiness, dry cough, dry mouth, excessive sweating, fever, fluttering heartbeat, gas, general chest pain, hives, impotence, indigestion, itching, jitteriness, joint pain, leg cramps, muscle and bone inflammation, nervousness, pain, production of large amounts of pale urine, rash, sexual difficulties, shakiness, shortness of breath, skin inflammation, sleep disturbances, sleepiness, stiff joints, tingling or pins and needles, weakness

■ *Rare side effects may include:*
Abnormal or terrifying dreams, anemia, anxiety, arthritis, back pain, belching, blood in the urine, breast pain, breathing disorders, dark stools containing blood, decreased sex drive, depression, distorted taste, dulled sense of touch, excessive urination at night, facial swelling, fainting, fever, gout, gum overgrowth, hair loss, hepatitis, hives, hot flashes, increased angina, increased sweating, inflammation of the sinuses, irregular heartbeat, migraine, muscle incoordination, muscle pain, muscle tension, nosebleeds, painful or difficult urination, paranoia, rapid heartbeat, reddish or purplish spots under the skin, ringing in the ears, swelling around the eyes, tearing eyes, temporary blindness, upper respiratory tract infection, vague feeling of illness, vertigo, vision changes, vomiting, weight gain

### Why should this drug not be prescribed?
Procardia should not be used if you have ever had an allergic reaction to it or are sensitive to it or other calcium channel blockers (Adalat, Calan, others). Make sure your doctor is aware of any drug reactions you have experienced.

### Special warnings about this medication
Procardia and Procardia XL may cause your blood pressure to become too low, which may make you feel light-headed or faint. This is more likely to happen when you start taking the medication and when the amount you take is increased. It is also more likely to occur if you are also taking a beta-blocker heart medication such as Tenormin or Inderal. Your doctor should check your blood pressure when you start taking Procardia or Procardia XL and continue monitoring it while your dosage is being adjusted.

There is a remote possibility of experiencing increased angina when you start taking Procardia or Procardia XL, or when your dosage is increased. If this happens, contact your doctor immediately.

You may have angina pain if you suddenly stop taking beta blockers when beginning Procardia therapy. Your doctor will taper you off the other drug.

If you have tight aortic stenosis (a narrowing of the aortic valve that obstructs blood flow from the heart to the body) and have been taking a beta blocker, your doctor will monitor you carefully while you are taking Procardia or Procardia XL.

If you develop swelling of the arms, hands, legs, and feet, your doctor can prescribe a diuretic (water pill) to relieve the problem.

Procardia XL should be used cautiously if you have any stomach or intestinal narrowing.

Notify your doctor or dentist that you are taking Procardia if you have a medical emergency, and before you have surgery or dental treatment.

### Possible food and drug interactions when taking this medication

If Procardia or Procardia XL is taken with certain other drugs, the effects of either could be increased, decreased, or altered. It is especially important to check with your doctor before combining Procardia or Procardia XL with the following:

Cimetidine (Tagamet)
Digoxin (Lanoxin)

Taking Procardia with double-concentrated grapefruit juice can dramatically increase the effect of the drug.

### Special information if you are pregnant or breastfeeding

The effects of Procardia and Procardia XL during pregnancy have not been adequately studied, although new animal research points to possible birth defects in humans. If you are pregnant or plan to become pregnant, inform your doctor immediately. It is not known whether Procardia or Procardia XL appears in breast milk and can affect a nursing infant. If this medication is essential to your health, your doctor may advise you to discontinue breastfeeding until your treatment is finished.

### Recommended dosage

ADULTS

The usual starting dose of Procardia is one 10-milligram capsule, 3 times a day. The usual range is 10 to 20 milligrams 3 times a day. Some people may need 20 to 30 milligrams, 3 or 4 times a day. Usually you will not take more than 120 milligrams in a day and should take no more than 180 milligrams.

The starting dose of Procardia XL is usually a 30- or 60-milligram tablet, taken once daily. Your doctor may increase the dose over 1 to 2 weeks if not satisfied with the way the drug is working. Doses above 120 milligrams per day are not recommended.

Although no serious side effects have been reported when Procardia XL is stopped, your doctor will probably have you lower the dose gradually under close supervision.

### Overdosage

Any medication taken in excess can have serious consequences. If you suspect an overdose, seek medical treatment immediately.

■ *Symptoms of Procardia overdose may include:*
Dizziness, drowsiness, nausea, slurred speech, weakness

---

*Generic name:*

# Prochlorperazine

*See Compazine, page 111.*

---

*Brand name:*

# ProctoCream-HC

*See Anusol-HC, page 33.*

---

*Generic name:*

# Promethazine

*See Phenergan, page 412.*

---

*Generic name:*

# Promethazine with Codeine

*See Phenergan with Codeine, page 414.*

---

*Brand name:*

# Pronestyl-SR

*See Procan SR, page 437.*

---

*Generic name:*

# Propafenone

*See Rythmol, page 485.*

*Brand name:*

# Propine

*Pronounced: PROH-peen*
*Generic name: Dipivefrin hydrochloride*

## Why is this drug prescribed?

Propine is used to treat chronic open-angle glaucoma, the most common form of the disease. In glaucoma, the fluid inside the eyeball is under abnormally high pressure, a condition which can cause vision problems or even blindness.

Propine belongs to a class of medication called "prodrugs," drugs that generally are not active by themselves, but are converted in the body to an active form. This makes for better absorption, stability, and comfort and reduces side effects.

## Most important fact about this drug

There is no cure for glaucoma. Propine and similar drugs can keep ocular pressure under control, but only as long as you take them. You will probably need to continue treatment for life; and you must be sure to take the medication regularly.

## How should you use this medication?

Use this medication exactly as prescribed. If you use too much, or use it too often, Propine may cause side effects.

Wash your hands before and after you use the eyedrops. Once the drops are in your eye, keep your eye closed for 1 to 2 minutes, applying pressure to the inside corner of your eye, so the medicine can be properly absorbed.

To keep the medication free of contamination, do not touch the applicator tip to your eye or any other surface.

A number appears on the cap of the dropper bottle to tell you what dose you are taking. When you are ready to take the first dose, make sure the number 1 appears in the window. After each dose, replace the cap and rotate it to the next number. Turn until you hear a click.

■ *If you miss a dose...*
Apply it as soon as you remember. If it is almost time for your next dose, skip the one you missed and go back to your regular schedule. Never apply more than 1 dose at a time.

■ *Storage instructions...*
Keep Propine in the plastic dropper bottle it came in.

## What side effects may occur?

Side effects cannot be anticipated. If any develop or change in intensity, inform your doctor as soon as possible. Only your doctor can determine if it is safe for you to continue taking Propine.

■ *More common side effects may include:*
Burning and stinging, red eye
■ *Less common or rare side effects may include:*
Allergic reactions, change in heart rhythm, conjunctivitis, extreme dilation of pupils, increased heart rate or blood pressure, increased sensitivity to light

## Why should this drug not be prescribed?

If you are sensitive to or have ever had an allergic reaction to Propine or any of its ingredients, you should not use this medication. Make sure your doctor is aware of any drug reactions you have experienced.

Unless you are directed to do so by your doctor, do not use this medication if you have narrow-angle glaucoma.

## Special warnings about this medication

Propine may cause vision problems, including blurry vision, for a short time after the eyedrops are applied. If this occurs, make sure you do not drive, use machinery, or participate in any hazardous activity that requires clear vision.

## Possible food and drug interactions when taking this medication

No significant interactions have been reported.

## Special information if you are pregnant or breastfeeding

The effects of Propine during pregnancy have not been adequately studied. If you are pregnant or plan to become pregnant, inform your doctor immediately. Propine may appear in breast milk and could affect a nursing infant. If this medication is essential to your health, your doctor may advise you to discontinue breastfeeding your baby until your treatment is finished.

## Recommended dosage

ADULTS

The usual dose is 1 drop in the eye(s) every 12 hours. It usually takes about 30 minutes for Propine to start working. You should feel the maximum effects of the drug within 1 hour.

CHILDREN

The safety and effectiveness of Propine have not been established in children.

## Overdosage

Any medication taken in excess can have serious consequences. If you suspect an overdose of Propine, seek medical attention immediately.

---

*Generic name:*

# Propoxyphene

*See Darvocet-N, page 131.*

---

*Generic name:*

# Propranolol

*See Inderal, page 252.*

---

*Generic name:*

# Propranolol with Hydrochlorothiazide

*See Inderide, page 254.*

---

*Brand name:*

# Propulsid

*Pronounced: pro-PUHL-sid*
*Generic name: Cisapride*

## Why is this drug prescribed?

Propulsid is prescribed to treat nighttime heartburn caused by gastroesophageal reflux disease, a condition in which the valve between the esophagus and the stomach opens or leaks, allowing stomach acid to back up and cause burning or "heartburn."

## Most important fact about this drug

There have been rare reports of dangerous heartbeat irregularities developing when Propulsid is combined with certain drugs. If you are taking any other medications, be sure to check "Why should this drug not be prescribed?" below.

## How should you take this medication?

Take your medication 15 minutes before meals and at bedtime. Take Propulsid exactly as prescribed, even if your symptoms disappear.

■ *If you miss a dose...*
Take the forgotten dose as soon as you remember. If it is almost time for your next dose, skip the one you missed and go back to your regular schedule. Do not take 2 doses at once.

■ *Storage instructions...*
Store at room temperature. Protect from moisture.

## What side effects may occur?

Side effects cannot be anticipated. If any develop or change in intensity, tell your doctor as soon as possible. Only your doctor can determine if it is safe for you to continue taking Propulsid.

■ *More common side effects may include:*
Abdominal pain, bloating/gas, constipation, diarrhea, headache, inflamed nasal passages and sinuses, nausea, pain, upper respiratory and viral infections

■ *Less common side effects may include:*
Abnormal vision, anxiety, back pain, chest pain, coughing, depression, dehydration, dizziness, fever, fatigue, frequent urination, indigestion, insomnia, itching, inflammation of the vagina, joint pain, muscle pain, nervousness, rash, sore throat, urinary tract infection, vomiting

## Why should this drug not be prescribed?

You should not use Propulsid if you have bleeding, blockage, or leakage in the stomach or intestines. Do not use this drug if you are taking Nizoral, Sporanox, Monistat IV, Tao, Biaxin, erythromycin, or Diflucan. Also avoid Propulsid if you are sensitive to or have ever had an allergic reaction to it.

## Special warnings about this medication

Propulsid is used only for nighttime heartburn. It has not been shown to be effective for daytime heartburn.

Because irregular heartbeats have occurred in a few people taking Propulsid, be sure to tell your doctor if you have had any heart trouble.

Propulsid by itself rarely causes drowsiness. However, it may increase the effects of alcoholic beverages and tranquilizers.

## Possible food and drug interactions when taking this medication

If Propulsid is taken with certain other drugs, the effects of either could be increased, decreased, or altered. It is especially important to check with your doctor before combining Propulsid with the following:

Antispasmodic drugs such as Bentyl and Cogentin
Cimetidine (Tagamet)
Clarithromycin (Biaxin)
Erythromycin (E-Mycin, Eryc)
Fluconazole (Diflucan)
Itraconazole (Sporanox)
Ketoconazole (Nizoral)
Miconazole (Monistat IV)
Ranitidine (Zantac)
Tranquilizers such as Librium, Valium, and Xanax
Troleandomycin (TAO)
Warfarin (Coumadin)

Remember that Propulsid may increase the effects of alcohol. If you are taking blood thinners (warfarin), your doctor will give you a blood test 1 week after you start on Propulsid and after your therapy is completed. Your blood-thinning medication may need to be adjusted.

## Special information
## if you are pregnant or breastfeeding

The effects of Propulsid during pregnancy have not been adequately studied. If you are pregnant or plan to become pregnant, tell your doctor immediately. The drug appears in breast milk and could affect a nursing infant. If this medication is essential to your health, your doctor may advise you to discontinue breastfeeding until your treatment is finished.

## Recommended dosage

ADULTS

The usual starting dose is 10 milligrams of Propulsid 4 times daily, taken at least 15 minutes before meals and at bedtime.

Your doctor may need to adjust your dosage to 20 milligrams 4 times daily, depending on how well the drug works for you.

CHILDREN

The safety and effectiveness of Propulsid in children have not been established.

## Overdosage

Any medication taken in excess can have serious consequences. If you suspect an overdose, seek medical attention immediately.

■ *Symptoms of Propulsid overdose may include:*
  Frequent urination or bowel movements, gas, gurgling and rumbling in the stomach, retching

*Brand name:*

# Proscar

*Pronounced: PRAHS-car*
*Generic name: Finasteride*

## Why is this drug prescribed?

Proscar is prescribed to help shrink an enlarged prostate.

The prostate, a chestnut-shaped gland present in males, produces secretions that form part of the semen. This gland completely encloses the upper part of the urethra, the tube through which urine flows out of the bladder. Many men over age 50 suffer from a benign (noncancerous) enlargement of the prostate. The enlarged gland squeezes the urethra, obstructing the normal flow of urine. Resulting problems may include difficulty in starting urination, weak flow of urine, and the need to urinate urgently or frequently. Sometimes surgical removal of the prostate is necessary.

By shrinking the enlarged prostate, Proscar may alleviate the various associated urinary problems, making surgery unnecessary.

Some doctors are also prescribing Proscar for baldness and as a preventive measure against prostate cancer.

## Most important fact about this drug

Different men have different responses to Proscar:

■ You may experience early relief from your urinary problems.
■ You may need to take the drug for 6 months or even a year before noticing any improvement.
■ Or you may find that, even after a year of treatment, Proscar simply has not helped you.

## How should you take this medication?

You may take Proscar either with a meal or between meals.

■ *If you miss a dose...*
  Take it as soon as you remember. If it is almost time for your next dose, skip the one you missed and go back to your regular schedule. Never take 2 doses at the same time.
■ *Storage instructions...*
  Store at room temperature in a tightly closed container. Protect from light.

## What side effects may occur?

Side effects cannot be anticipated. If any develop or change in intensity, inform your doctor as soon as

possible. Only your doctor can determine if it is safe for you to continue taking Proscar.

■ *Side effects may include:*
Decreased amount of semen per ejaculation, decreased sex drive, impotence

### Why should this drug not be prescribed?
Proscar should never be taken by a woman or a child.

Do not take Proscar if you are sensitive to it or have ever had an allergic reaction to it.

### Special warnings about this medication
Even if Proscar does relieve your urinary symptoms, periodic checkups are necessary to test for possible development of cancer of the prostate. Proscar is not an effective treatment for prostate cancer.

Benign enlargement of the prostate is not the only condition that can cause male urinary inefficiency and discomfort. Other possibilities include infection, obstruction, cancer of the prostate, and bladder disorders. Before prescribing Proscar, your doctor will want to do various tests to determine the cause of your urinary problems.

If accidentally absorbed by a pregnant woman who is carrying a male fetus, Proscar may cause abnormal development of the unborn baby's genital organs. Thus, a woman who is pregnant or who may become pregnant should never even touch a crushed Proscar tablet. If she is going to have intercourse with a man who is taking Proscar, she should insist that he wear a condom to protect her from his semen, which may contain small amounts of the medication.

It is important to read the patient information that comes in the Proscar package every time you renew your prescription so that you are aware of the latest information on the drug.

### Possible food and drug interactions when taking this medication
No significant drug interactions have been reported.

### Special information if you are pregnant or breastfeeding
As noted above, if a pregnant woman who is carrying a male fetus absorbs Proscar accidentally, the drug may cause defective development of the baby's genital organs. Any woman of childbearing age should be careful never to touch a crushed

Proscar tablet. If her sexual partner is taking Proscar, he should always wear a condom when they have intercourse to avoid any possible transfer of the drug to her body via his semen.

### Recommended dosage
ADULTS

The recommended dosage, for men only, is one 5-milligram tablet per day.

### Overdosage
Although no specific information is available, any medication taken in excess can have serious consequences. If you suspect an overdose of Proscar, seek medical attention immediately.

*Brand name:*

# ProSom

*Pronounced: PROE-som*
*Generic name: Estazolam*

### Why is this drug prescribed?
ProSom, a sleeping pill, is given for the short-term treatment of insomnia. Insomnia may involve difficulty falling asleep, frequent awakenings during the night, or too-early morning awakening.

### Most important fact about this drug
As a chemical cousin of Valium and similar tranquilizers, ProSom is potentially addictive; thus, you should plan on taking this drug only as a temporary sleeping aid. Even after relatively short-term use of ProSom, you may experience some withdrawal symptoms when you stop taking the medication.

### How should you take this medication?
Take ProSom exactly as prescribed by your doctor. A typical schedule is 1 tablet every night at bedtime. For small, physically run-down, or older people, one-half a tablet may be a safer starting dose.

Avoid drinking alcoholic beverages while taking ProSom.

If you have ever had seizures, do not abruptly stop taking ProSom, even if you are taking anti-seizure medication. Instead, taper off from ProSom under your doctor's supervision.

Even if you have never had seizures, it is better to taper off from ProSom than to stop taking the medication abruptly. Experience suggests that tapering off can help prevent drug withdrawal symptoms.

Typically, the only withdrawal symptoms caused by ProSom are mild and temporary insomnia or irritability. Occasionally, however, withdrawal can involve considerable discomfort or even danger, with symptoms such as abdominal and muscle cramps, convulsions, sweating, tremors, and vomiting.

■ *If you miss a dose...*
Take at bedtime only as needed. It is not necessary to make up a missed dose.

■ *Storage instructions...*
Store at room temperature.

### What side effects may occur?
Side effects cannot be anticipated. If any develop or change in intensity, inform your doctor as soon as possible. Only your doctor can determine whether it is safe for you to continue taking ProSom.

■ *More common side effects may include:*
Abnormal coordination, cold symptoms, decreased movement or activity, dizziness, general feeling of illness, hangover, headache, leg and foot pain, nausea, nervousness, sleepiness, weakness

■ *Less common or rare side effects may include:*
Abdominal pain, abnormal dreaming, abnormal thinking, abnormal vision, acne, agitation, allergic reaction, altered taste, anxiety, apathy, arm and hand pain, arthritis, asthma, back pain, black stools, body pain, chest pain, chills, confusion, constant, involuntary eye movement, constipation, cough, decreased appetite, decreased hearing, decreased reflexes, depression, difficult/labored breathing, double vision, dry mouth, dry skin, ear pain, emotional changeability, fainting, fever, flushing, frequent urination, gas, hallucinations, hostility, inability to hold urine, inability to urinate, increased appetite, indigestion, inflamed sinuses, itching, lack of coordination, little or no urine flow, loss of memory, menstrual cramps, muscle stiffness, nasal inflammation, neck pain, nighttime urination, nosebleed, numbness or tingling around the mouth, purple or reddish spots on the skin, rapid, heavy breathing, rash, ringing in the ears, seizure, sleep problems, sore throat, stupor, swollen breast, thirst, throbbing or fluttering heartbeat, tingling or "pins and needles", tremor, twitch, urgent need to urinate, vaginal discharge/itching, vomiting, weight gain or loss

### Why should this drug not be prescribed?
Do not take ProSom if you are sensitive or allergic to it, or if you have ever had an adverse reaction to another Valium-type medication.

Do not take ProSom if you are pregnant or planning to become pregnant. Drugs in this class may cause damage to the unborn child.

### Special warnings about this medication
Since ProSom may cloud your thinking, impair your judgment, or interfere with your normal physical coordination, do not drive, climb, or perform hazardous tasks until you know your reaction to this medication. It is important to remember that the tablet you took in the evening may continue to affect you well into the following day.

If you are older or physically run-down, or if you have liver or kidney damage or breathing problems, you will be particularly vulnerable to side effects from ProSom, and you should use this medication with special caution.

### Possible food and drug interactions when taking this medication
Do not drink alcohol while you are taking ProSom; this combination could make you comatose or dangerously slow your breathing.

For the same reason, do not combine ProSom with any other medication that might calm or slow the functioning of your central nervous system. Among such drugs are:

Antiseizure drugs such as Dilantin, Tegretol, and Depakene
Antihistamines such as Benadryl and Chlor-Trimeton
Major tranquilizers such as Haldol and Mellaril
Barbiturates such as phenobarbital
MAO inhibitor antidepressants such as Nardil and Parnate
Narcotics such as Percodan and Tylox
Tranquilizers such as Valium and Xanax

If you smoke, you will tend to process and eliminate ProSom fairly quickly compared with a non-smoker.

### Special information if you are pregnant or breastfeeding
If you are pregnant, you must not take ProSom; it could cause birth defects in your child.

When a pregnant woman takes ProSom or a similar medication shortly before giving birth, her baby is likely to have poor muscle tone (flaccidity) and/or experience drug withdrawal symptoms.

Because ProSom is thought to pass into breast milk, you should not take this medication while breastfeeding.

### Recommended dosage

ADULTS

The recommended initial dose is 1 milligram at bedtime; however, some patients may need a 2-milligram dose.

CHILDREN

There is no information on the safety and effectiveness of ProSom in patients under age 18.

OLDER ADULTS

The recommended usual dosage for older adults is 1 milligram. However, some patients may require only 0.5 milligram.

### Overdosage

Any medication taken in excess can have serious consequences. If you suspect an overdose, seek medical attention immediately.

■ *Symptoms of a ProSom overdose may include:*
Confusion, depressed breathing, drowsiness and eventually coma, lack of coordination, slurred speech

Brand name:

# ProStep

*See Nicotine Patches, page 359.*

Brand name:

# Protostat

*See Flagyl, page 214.*

Brand name:

# Proventil

*Pronounced: Proh-VEN-till*
*Generic name: Albuterol sulfate*
*Other brand names: Ventolin, Volmax Extended-*
  *Release Tablets*

### Why is this drug prescribed?

Drugs containing albuterol are prescribed for the prevention and relief of bronchial spasms. This especially applies to the treatment of asthma. This medication is also used for the prevention of bronchial spasm due to exercise.

### Most important fact about this drug

Do not take albuterol more frequently than your doctor recommends. Increasing the number of doses can be dangerous and may actually make symptoms of asthma worse.

If the dose your doctor recommends does not provide relief of your symptoms, or if your symptoms become worse, consult with your doctor immediately.

### How should you take this medication?

If you are using a metered-dose inhaler, follow the instructions carefully. If you are taking extended-release tablets, swallow them whole with some liquid—never chew or crush them.

■ *If you miss a dose...*
Take the forgotten dose as soon as you remember; then take any remaining doses for that day at equally spaced intervals. Never take a double dose.

■ *Storage instructions...*
This medication can be kept in the refrigerator or at room temperature.

### What side effects may occur?

Side effects cannot be anticipated. If any develop or change in intensity, inform your doctor as soon as possible. Only your doctor can determine if it is safe for you to continue taking albuterol.

■ *More common side effects may include:*
Aggression, agitation, cough, diarrhea, dizziness, excitement, general bodily discomfort, headache, heartburn, increased appetite, increased blood pressure, increased difficulty breathing, indigestion, irritability, labored breathing, light-headedness, muscle cramps, nausea, nervousness, nightmares, nosebleed, overactivity, palpitations, rapid heartbeat, rash, ringing in the ears, shakiness, sleeplessness, stomachache, stuffy nose, throat irritation, tooth discoloration, tremors, vomiting, wheezing

■ *Less common side effects may include:*
Chest pain (sometimes crushing) or discomfort, difficulty urinating, drowsiness, dry mouth and throat, flushing, high blood pressure, muscle spasm, restlessness, sweating, unusual taste, vertigo, weakness

■ *Rare side effects following the use of inhaled albuterol include:*

Hoarseness, increased breathing or wheezing, skin rash or hives, unusual and unexpected swelling of mouth and throat

## Why should this drug not be prescribed?

If you are sensitive to or have ever had an allergic reaction to albuterol or other bronchodilators, you should not take this medication. Make sure that your doctor is aware of any drug reactions that you have experienced.

## Special warnings about this medication

When taking albuterol inhalation aerosol, you should not use other inhaled medications before checking with your doctor.

Consult with your doctor before using this medication if you have a cardiovascular or convulsive disorder, high blood pressure, abnormal heartbeat, overactive thyroid gland, or diabetes.

You may have an immediate, serious allergic reaction to the first dose of albuterol. There have also been rare reports of skin reddening and peeling in children taking albuterol syrup.

Do not exceed your doctor's recommended dose of albuterol. Do not change brands without first consulting your doctor or pharmacist.

## Possible food and drug interactions when taking this medication

Albuterol inhalation aerosol should not be used with other aerosol bronchodilators.

If albuterol is taken with certain other drugs, the effects of either could be increased, decreased, or altered. It is especially important to check with your doctor before combining albuterol with the following:

Antidepressants such as Elavil and Nardil
Beta blockers (heart and blood pressure drugs such as Inderal, Tenormin, and Sectral)
Digoxin (Lanoxin)
Drugs similar to albuterol, such as Alupent, Brethaire, Isuprel, and epinephrine
Drugs that lower potassium levels (water pills such as HydroDIURIL)

## Special information if you are pregnant or breastfeeding

The effects of albuterol during pregnancy have not been adequately studied. If you are pregnant or plan to become pregnant, inform your doctor immediately. It is not known whether albuterol appears in breast milk. If this drug is essential to your health, your doctor may advise you to stop nursing your baby until your treatment is finished.

## Recommended dosage

ADULTS

*Inhalation Aerosol*

Patient instructions are available with both products.

If you are being treated for a sudden or severe bronchial spasm or the prevention of asthma symptoms, the usual dosage of albuterol inhalation aerosol for adults and children aged 4 and over (Ventolin) or 12 and over (Proventil) is 2 inhalations repeated every 4 to 6 hours. More frequent use is not recommended. In some individuals, 1 inhalation every 4 hours may be sufficient.

The recommended dose of Proventil Inhalation Aerosol for prevention of recurring symptoms is 2 inhalations, 4 times a day.

For exercise-induced bronchial spasm, the usual dosage for adults and children 12 years and older is 2 inhalations, 15 minutes prior to exercise.

*Tablets*

The usual starting dose for adults and children 12 years of age and older is 2 or 4 milligrams 3 to 4 times a day.

*Syrup*

The usual starting dose for adults and children over 14 years of age is 1 or 2 teaspoonfuls 3 or 4 times a day.

*Ventolin Rotacaps for Inhalation*

The usual dosage for adults and children 4 years and older is the contents of one 200-microgram capsule inhaled every 4 to 6 hours using a Rotahaler inhalation device. Some people may require two 200-microgram capsules every 4 to 6 hours.

*Inhalation Solution*

The usual dosage for adults and children 12 years of age and older is 2.5 milligrams administered 3 to 4 times daily by nebulization. To administer 2.5 milligrams, dilute 0.5 milliliter of the 0.5 percent solution for inhalation with 2.5 milliliters of sterile normal saline solution.

*Ventolin Nebules Inhalation Solution*
The usual dosage for adults and children 12 years and older is 2.5 milligrams of Ventolin taken 3 to 4 times a day by nebulization.

*Proventil Repetabs and Volmax Extended-Release Tablets*
The usual recommended dosage for adults and children 12 years of age and older is 8 milligrams every 12 hours. In some people, 4 milligrams every 12 hours may be sufficient. If the desired effect is not achieved with the standard dosage, your doctor may increase doses to a maximum of 32 milligrams per day, divided into two 16-milligram doses spaced 12 hours apart. Those taking Ventolin Tablets or Ventolin Syrup can switch to Volmax Extended-Release Tablets. One Volmax tablet every 12 hours is equivalent to one 2-milligram Ventolin Tablet every 6 hours.

CHILDREN

*Inhalation Aerosol*
Safety and effectiveness in children below the age of 12 (Proventil, Volmax) and below the age of 4 (Ventolin) have not been established. For dosage in children above these ages, see adult section.

*Tablets*
The usual starting dose for children 6 to 12 years of age is 2 milligrams 3 or 4 times a day. The dose can be increased with caution but should not exceed 24 milligrams per day.

*Syrup*
The usual starting dose for children 6 to 14 years of age is 1 teaspoonful 3 to 4 times a day. For children 2 to 6 years of age, the starting dose is 0.1 milligram per 2.2 pounds of body weight, to a maximum of 4 milligrams, 3 times a day.

OLDER ADULTS

*Oral Dosage*
The usual starting dose of tablets or syrup is 2 milligrams 3 or 4 times a day.

### Overdosage

■ *Symptoms of albuterol overdose may include:*
   High blood pressure, low potassium level, radiating chest pain, rapid heartbeat, seizures

Exaggerated side effects may also be a sign of an overdose. If you suspect an overdose, seek medical attention immediately.

*Brand name:*

# Provera

*Pronounced: pro-VAIR-uh*
*Generic name: Medroxyprogesterone acetate*
*Other brand name: Cycrin*

### Why is this drug prescribed?

Provera is derived from the female hormone progesterone. You may be given Provera if your menstrual periods have stopped or a female hormone imbalance is causing your uterus to bleed abnormally.

Other forms of medroxyprogesterone, such as Depo-Provera, are used as a contraceptive injection and prescribed in the treatment of endometrial cancer.

Some doctors prescribe Provera to treat endometriosis, menopausal symptoms, premenstrual tension, sexual aggressive behavior in men, and sleep apnea (temporary failure to breath while sleeping).

### Most important fact about this drug

You should never take Provera during the first 4 months of pregnancy. During this formative period, even a few days of treatment with Provera might put your unborn baby at increased risk for birth defects. If you take Provera and later discover that you were pregnant when you took it, discuss this with your doctor right away.

### How should you take this medication?

Provera may be taken with or between meals.

Do not change from one brand to another without consulting your doctor or pharmacist.

Your doctor will probably have you take Provera for 5 to 10 days and then stop; you should have your period within 3 to 7 days after the last dose.

If you are being treated for lack of regular menstrual periods, your doctor may have you start taking Provera at any time. If you are being treated for abnormal uterine bleeding due to a female-hormone imbalance, your doctor will probably have you start taking Provera on day 16 or 21 of your menstrual cycle (i.e., 16 or 21 days after the start of your last period). You should have your period within 3 to 7 days after the last dose.

■ *If you miss a dose...*
   Take it as soon as you remember. If it is almost time for your next dose, skip the one you missed

and go back to your regular schedule. Never take 2 doses at the same time.

■ *Storage instructions...*
Store at room temperature.

## What side effects may occur?

Side effects cannot be anticipated. If any develop or change in intensity, inform your doctor as soon as possible. Only your doctor can determine if it is safe for you to continue taking Provera.

■ *Side effects may include:*
Acne, anaphylaxis (life-threatening allergic reaction), blood clot in a vein, lungs, or brain, breakthrough bleeding (between menstrual periods), breast tenderness or sudden or excessive flow of milk, cervical erosion or changes in secretions, depression, excessive growth of hair, fever, fluid retention, hair loss, headache, hives, insomnia, itching, lack of menstruation, menstrual flow changes, spotting, nausea, rash, skin discoloration, sleepiness, weight gain or loss, yellowed eyes and skin

## Why should this drug not be prescribed?

Do not take Provera if you are sensitive to it or have ever had an allergic reaction to it.

If you suspect you may have become pregnant, do not take Provera as a test for pregnancy. Doctors once prescribed Provera for this purpose, but no longer do so for 2 reasons:

■ Quicker, safer pregnancy tests are now available.
■ If you are in fact pregnant, Provera might injure the baby.

Do not take Provera during your first 4 months of pregnancy. In the past, Provera was sometimes given to try to prevent miscarriage. However, doctors now believe that this treatment is not only ineffective but also potentially harmful to the baby.

Do not take Provera if you have:

■ Cancer of the breast or genital organs
■ Liver disease or a liver condition
■ A dead fetus still in the uterus
■ Undiagnosed bleeding from the vagina

Do not take Provera if you have, or have ever developed, blood clots.

## Special warnings about this medication

Before you start to take Provera, your doctor will give you a complete physical exam, including examination of your breasts and pelvic organs. You should also have a cervical smear (Pap test).

Provera may cause some degree of fluid retention. If you have a medical condition that could be made worse by fluid retention—such as epilepsy, migraine, asthma, or a heart or kidney problem—make sure your doctor knows about it.

Provera may mask the onset of menopause. In other words, while taking Provera you may continue to experience regular menstrual bleeding even if your menopause has started.

Provera may make you depressed, especially if you have suffered from depression in the past. If you become seriously depressed, tell your doctor; you should probably stop taking Provera.

If you are diabetic, Provera could make your diabetes worse; your doctor will want to watch you closely while you are taking this drug.

There is some concern that Provera, like birth control pills, may increase your risk for a blood clot in a vein. If you experience any symptoms that might suggest the onset of such a condition—pain with swelling, warmth, and redness in a leg vein, coughing or shortness of breath, vision problems, migraine, or weakness or numbness in an arm or leg—see your doctor immediately.

Tell your doctor right away if you lose some or all of your vision or you start seeing double. You may have to stop taking the medication.

## Possible food and drug interactions when taking this medication

If Provera is taken with certain other drugs, the effects of either may be increased, decreased, or altered. It is especially important to check with your doctor before combining Provera with aminoglutethimide (Cytadren).

## Special information if you are pregnant or breastfeeding

You should not take Provera during pregnancy. If you are pregnant or plan to become pregnant, inform your doctor immediately.

Provera appears in breast milk. If you are a new mother, you may need to choose between taking Provera and breastfeeding your baby.

## Recommended dosage

ADULTS

*To Restore Menstrual Periods*
Provera Tablets are taken in dosages of 5 to 10 milligrams daily for 5 to 10 days. Make sure you

discuss what effect this will have on your menstrual cycle with your doctor. You should have bleeding 3 to 7 days after you stop taking Provera.

### ABNORMAL UTERINE BLEEDING DUE TO HORMONAL IMBALANCE

Beginning on the 16th or 21st day of your menstrual cycle, you will take 5 to 10 milligrams daily for 5 to 10 days. Make sure you discuss what effect this will have on your menstrual cycle with your doctor. You should have bleeding 3 to 7 days after you stop taking Provera.

### Overdosage

Although no specific information is available, any medication taken in excess can have serious consequences. If you suspect an overdose of Provera, seek medical attention immediately.

*Brand name:*

# Prozac

*Pronounced: PRO-zak*
*Generic name: Fluoxetine hydrochloride*

### Why is this drug prescribed?

Prozac is prescribed for the treatment of depression—that is, a continuing depression that interferes with daily functioning. The symptoms of major depression often include changes in appetite, sleep habits, and mind/body coordination; decreased sex drive; increased fatigue; feelings of guilt or worthlessness; difficulty concentrating; slowed thinking; and suicidal thoughts.

Prozac is also prescribed to treat obsessive-compulsive disorder. An obsession is a thought that won't go away; a compulsion is an action done over and over to relieve anxiety.

Prozac is thought to work by adjusting the balance of the brain's natural chemical messengers. It has also been used to treat obesity and eating disorders.

### Most important fact about this drug

Serious, sometimes fatal, reactions have been known to occur when Prozac is used in combination with other antidepressant drugs known as MAO inhibitors, including Nardil and Parnate; and when Prozac is discontinued and an MAO inhibitor is started. Never take Prozac with one of these drugs or within 14 days of discontinuing therapy with one

of them; and allow 5 weeks or more between stopping Prozac and starting an MAO inhibitor. Be especially cautious if you have been taking Prozac in high doses or for a long time.

If you are taking any prescription or nonprescription drugs, notify your doctor before taking Prozac.

### How should you take this medication?

Prozac should be taken exactly as prescribed by your doctor.

Prozac usually is taken once or twice a day. To be effective, it should be taken regularly. Make a habit of taking it at the same time you do some other daily activity.

■ *If you miss a dose...*
Take the forgotten dose as soon as you remember. If several hours have passed, skip the dose. Never try to "catch up" by doubling the dose.
■ *Storage instructions...*
Store at room temperature.

### What side effects may occur?

Side effects cannot be anticipated. If any develop or change in intensity, inform your doctor as soon as possible. Only your doctor can determine if it is safe for you to continue taking Prozac.

■ *More common side effects may include:*
Abnormal dreams, abnormal thinking, agitation, allergic reaction, anxiety, bronchitis, chest pain, chills, cough, diarrhea, dizziness, drowsiness and fatigue, dry mouth, flu symptoms, frequent urination, hay fever, headache, inability to fall or stay asleep, increased appetite, indigestion, itching, joint pain, lack or loss of appetite, light-headedness, limb pain, muscle pain, nausea, nervousness, sinus inflammation, sore throat, stomach /intestinal disorder, sweating, tremors, weakness, weight loss, yawning
■ *Less common side effects may include:*
Abnormal ejaculation, abnormal gait, abnormal stoppage of menstrual flow, acne, altered sense of taste, amnesia, apathy, arthritis, asthma, bone pain, breast cysts, breast pain, brief loss of consciousness, bursitis, chills and fever, confusion, conjunctivitis, convulsions, dark, tarry stool, decreased sex drive, difficulty in swallowing, dilation of pupils, dry skin, ear pain, eye pain, exaggerated feeling of well-being, excessive bleeding, facial swelling due to fluid retention,

fever, fluid retention, fluttery heartbeat, gas, hair loss, hallucinations, hangover effect, hiccups, high or low blood pressure, hives, hostility, infection, inflammation of the esophagus, inflammation of the gums, inflammation of the stomach lining, inflammation of the tongue, inflammation of the vagina, intolerance of light, involuntary movement, irrational ideas, irregular heartbeat, jaw or neck pain, lack of muscle coordination, low blood pressure upon standing, low blood sugar, migraine headache, mouth inflammation, muscle spasm, neck pain and rigidity, nosebleed, ovarian disorders, paranoid reaction, pelvic pain, pneumonia, rapid breathing, rapid heartbeat, ringing in the ears, severe chest pain, skin inflammation, skin rash, thirst, tooth problems, twitching, uncoordinated movements, urinary disorders, vague feeling of bodily discomfort, vertigo, vision disturbances, vomiting, weight gain

■ *Rare side effects may include:*

Antisocial behavior, blood in urine, bloody diarrhea, bone disease, breast enlargement, cataracts, colitis, coma, deafness, decreased reflexes, dehydration, double vision, drooping of eyelids, duodenal ulcer, enlarged abdomen, enlargement of liver, enlargement or increased activity of thyroid gland, excess growth of coarse hair on face, chest, etc., excess uterine or vaginal bleeding, extreme muscle tension, eye bleeding, female milk production, fluid accumulation and swelling in the head, fluid buildup in larynx and lungs, gallstones, glaucoma, gout, heart attack, hepatitis, high blood sugar, hysteria, inability to control bowel movements, increased salivation, inflammation of eyes and eyelids, inflammation of fallopian tubes, inflammation of testes, inflammation of the gallbladder, inflammation of the small intestine, inflammation of tissue below skin, kidney disorders, lung inflammation, menstrual disorders, miscarriage, mouth sores, muscle inflammation or bleeding, muscle spasms, painful sexual intercourse for women, psoriasis, rashes, reddish or purplish spots on the skin, reduction of body temperature, rheumatoid arthritis, seborrhea, shingles, skin discoloration, skin inflammation and disorders, slowing of heart rate, slurred speech, spitting blood, stomach ulcer, stupor, suicidal thoughts, taste loss, temporary cessation of breathing, tingling sensation around the mouth, tongue discoloration and swelling, urinary tract disorders, vomiting blood, yellow eyes and skin

## Why should this drug not be prescribed?

If you are sensitive to or have ever had an allergic reaction to Prozac or similar drugs such as Paxil and Zoloft, you should not take this medication. Make sure that your doctor is aware of any drug reactions that you have experienced.

Do not take this drug while using an MAO inhibitor. (See "Most important fact about this drug.")

## Special warnings about this medication

Unless you are directed to do so by your doctor, do not take this medication if you are recovering from a heart attack or if you have kidney or liver disease or diabetes.

Prozac may cause you to become drowsy or less alert and may affect your judgment. Therefore, driving or operating dangerous machinery or participating in any hazardous activity that requires full mental alertness is not recommended.

While taking this medication, you may feel dizzy or light-headed or actually faint when getting up from a lying or sitting position. If getting up slowly doesn't help or if this problem continues, notify your doctor.

If you develop a skin rash or hives while taking Prozac, discontinue use of the medication and notify your doctor immediately.

Prozac should be used with caution if you have a history of seizures. You should discuss all of your medical conditions with your doctor before taking this medication.

The safety and effectiveness of Prozac have not been established in children.

## Possible food and drug interactions when taking this medication

Combining Prozac with MAO inhibitors is dangerous.

Do not drink alcohol while taking this medication.

If Prozac is taken with certain other drugs, the effects of either could be increased, decreased, or altered. It is especially important to check with your doctor before combining Prozac with the following:

Carbamazepine (Tegretol)
Diazepam (Valium)
Digitoxin (Crystodigin)

Drugs that act on the central nervous system (brain and spinal cord) such as Xanax
Flecainide (Tambocor)
Lithium (Eskalith)
Other antidepressants (Elavil)
Phenytoin (Dilantin)
Tryptophan
Vinblastine (Velban)
Warfarin (Coumadin)

### Special information if you are pregnant or breastfeeding

The effects of Prozac during pregnancy have not been adequately studied. If you are pregnant or plan to become pregnant, inform your doctor immediately. This medication appears in breast milk, and breastfeeding is not recommended while you are taking Prozac.

### Recommended dosage

ADULTS

The usual starting dose is 20 milligrams per day, taken in the morning. Your doctor may increase your dose after several weeks if no improvement is observed. People with kidney or liver disease, the elderly, and those taking other drugs may have their dosages adjusted by their doctor.

Dosages above 20 milligrams daily should be taken once a day in the morning or in 2 smaller doses taken in the morning and at noon.

The usual daily dose for depression ranges from 20 to 60 milligrams. For obsessive-compulsive disorder the customary range is 20 to 60 milligrams per day, though a maximum of 80 milligrams is sometimes prescribed.

### Overdosage

Any medication taken in excess or in combination with other drugs can cause symptoms of overdose. If you suspect an overdose, seek medical attention immediately.

■ *Symptoms of Prozac overdose include:*
Agitation, nausea, restlessness, vomiting

*Brand name:*

# Psorcon

*Pronounced: SORE-kon*
*Generic name: Diflorasone diacetate*

### Why is this drug prescribed?

Psorcon is prescribed for the relief of the inflammatory and itching symptoms of skin disorders that respond to the topical application (applied directly to the skin) of steroids (hormones produced by the body that have potent anti-inflammatory effects).

### Most important fact about this drug

When you use Psorcon, you inevitably absorb some of the medication through your skin and into the bloodstream. Too much absorption can lead to unwanted side effects elsewhere in the body. To keep this problem to a minimum, avoid using large amounts of Psorcon over large areas, and do not cover it with airtight dressings such as plastic wrap or adhesive bandages unless specifically told to by your doctor.

### How should you use this medication?

Use this medication exactly as prescribed.

Psorcon is for use only on the skin. Be careful to keep it out of your eyes.

■ *If you miss a dose...*
Apply it as soon as you remember. If it is almost time for the next dose, skip the one you missed and go back to your regular schedule.
■ *Storage instructions...*
Store at room temperature.

### What side effects may occur?

Side effects cannot be anticipated. If any develop or change in intensity, inform your doctor as soon as possible. Only your doctor can determine if it is safe for you to continue taking Psorcon.

■ *Side effects may include:*
Burning, dryness, eruptions resembling acne, excessive discoloring of the skin, excessive growth of hair, inflammation of hair follicles, inflammation around the mouth, irritation, itching, prickly heat, secondary infection, severe inflammation of the skin, softening of the skin, stretch marks, stretching or thinning of the skin

### Why should this drug not be prescribed?

If you are sensitive to or have ever had an allergic reaction to diflorasone diacetate or other drugs of this type (antifungals, steroids), you should not take this medication. Make sure your doctor is aware of any drug reactions you have experienced.

### Special warnings about this medication

Remember that absorption of Psorcon through the skin can affect the whole body. Although it's unusual (most common if Psorcon is spread over large areas of the skin), you could develop symptoms of steroid excess such as weight gain, reddening and rounding of the face and neck, growth of excess body and facial hair, high blood pressure, emotional disturbances, loss of energy due to high blood sugar, and increase in frequency of urination.

Do not use this drug for any disorder other than the one for which it was prescribed.

The treated skin area should not be bandaged, covered, or wrapped unless otherwise directed by your doctor. Avoid covering a treated area with waterproof diapers or plastic pants. They can cause unwanted absorption of Psorcon.

If an irritation or allergic reaction develops while you are using Psorcon, notify your doctor.

## Possible food and drug interactions when taking this medication

No interactions with food or other drugs have been reported.

## Special information if you are pregnant or breastfeeding

If you are pregnant or plan to become pregnant, inform your doctor before using Psorcon. It is not known whether this medication appears in breast milk. If this drug is essential to your health, your doctor may advise you to discontinue breastfeeding until treatment with this medication is finished.

## Recommended dosage

ADULTS

A thin film of Psorcon ointment should be applied to the affected area from 1 to 3 times a day, depending on the severity or resistant nature of the condition.

Your doctor may recommend airtight bandages for the management of psoriasis (chronic skin disorder) or stubborn skin conditions. If an infection develops, you should stop using airtight dressings.

CHILDREN

Your doctor will limit the use of Psorcon for your child to the least amount that is effective. Long-term treatment may interfere with the growth and development of children.

## Overdosage

An acute overdosage is unlikely with the use of Psorcon; however, long-term or prolonged use can produce side effects throughout your body. If you suspect an overdose, seek medical attention immediately.

*Brand name:*

# Pyridium

*Pronounced: pie-RI-di-um*
*Generic name: Phenazopyridine hydrochloride*

## Why is this drug prescribed?

Pyridium is a urinary tract analgesic that helps relieve the pain, burning, urgency, frequency, and irritation caused by infection, trauma, catheters, or various surgical procedures in the lower urinary tract. Pyridium is indicated for short-term use and can only relieve symptoms; it is not a treatment for the underlying cause of the symptoms.

## Most important fact about this drug

Pyridium produces an orange to red color in urine, and may stain fabric. Staining of contact lenses has also been reported.

## How should you take this medication?

Take Pyridium after meals, exactly as prescribed.

■ *If you miss a dose...*
Take it as soon as you remember. If it is almost time for your next dose, skip the one you missed and go back to your regular schedule. Never take 2 doses at the same time.
■ *Storage instructions...*
Store at room temperature.

## What side effects may occur?

Side effects cannot be anticipated. If any occur or change in intensity, inform your doctor as soon as possible. Only your doctor can determine if it is safe for you to continue taking Pyridium.

■ *Side effects may include:*
Headache, itching, rash, severe allergic reaction (rash, difficulty breathing, fever, rapid heartbeat, convulsions), upset stomach

## Why should this drug not be prescribed?

Pyridium should be avoided if you have kidney disease, or if you are sensitive to or have ever had an allergic reaction to it.

## Special warnings about this medication

If your skin or the whites of your eyes develop a yellowish tone, it may indicate that your kidneys are not eliminating the medication as they should. Notify your doctor immediately. If you are older, your doctor will watch you more closely, since the kidneys work less effectively as we age.

## Possible food and drug interactions when taking this medication

No interactions have been reported.

## Special information if you are pregnant or breastfeeding

The effects of Pyridium during pregnancy have not been adequately studied. If you are pregnant or plan to become pregnant, inform your doctor immediately. To date, there is no information on whether Pyridium appears in breast milk. If this medication is essential to your health, your doctor may advise you to stop breastfeeding until your treatment with Pyridium is finished.

## Recommended dosage

ADULTS

The usual dose is two 100-milligram tablets or one 200-milligram tablet 3 times a day after meals.

You should not take Pyridium for more than 2 days if you are also taking an antibiotic for the treatment of a urinary tract infection.

## Overdosage

Any medication taken in excess can have serious consequences. If you suspect an overdose, seek emergency medical treatment immediately.

■ *Symptoms of Pyridium overdose may include:*
Blood disorders, bluish skin color, impaired kidney and liver function

---

*Generic name:*

# Quazepam

*See Doral, page 176.*

---

*Brand name:*

# Questran

*Pronounced: KWEST-ran*
*Generic name: Cholestyramine*
*Other brand name: Questran Light*

## Why is this drug prescribed?

Questran is used to lower cholesterol levels in the blood of people with primary hypercholesterolemia (too much LDL cholesterol). Hypercholesterolemia is a genetic condition characterized by a lack of the LDL receptors that remove cholesterol from the bloodstream.

This drug is also prescribed for people with hypertriglyceridemia, a condition in which an excess of fat is stored in the body.

However, Questran is usually prescribed only when a low-fat, low-sugar, and low-cholesterol diet does not lower cholesterol levels enough.

This drug may also be prescribed to relieve itching associated with gallbladder obstruction.

It is available in two forms: Questran and Questran Light. The same instructions apply to both.

## Most important fact about this drug

Questran is usually prescribed only if diet, exercise, and weight-loss fail to bring your cholesterol levels under control. It's important to remember that Questran is a supplement—not a substitute—for these other measures. To get the full benefit of the medication, you need to stick to the diet and exercise program prescribed by your doctor. All these efforts to keep your cholesterol levels normal are important because together they may lower your risk of heart disease.

## How should you take this medication?

Never take Questran in its dry form. Always mix it with water or other liquids *before* taking it. For Questran, use 2 to 6 ounces of liquid per packet or level scoopful; for Questran Light, use 2 to 3 ounces. Soups or fruits with a high moisture content, such as applesauce or crushed pineapple, can be used in place of beverages.

■ *If you miss a dose...*
Take the forgotten dose as soon as you remember. If it is almost time for the next dose, skip the one you missed and go back to your regular schedule. Never try to "catch up" by doubling the dose.
■ *Storage instructions...*
Store at room temperature. Protect from moisture and high humidity.

## What side effects may occur?

Side effects cannot be anticipated. If any develop or change in intensity, inform your doctor as soon as possible. Only your doctor can determine if it is safe for you to continue taking Questran.

The most common side effect of Questran is constipation.

■ *Less common or rare side effects may include:*
Abdominal discomfort, anemia, anxiety, arthritis, asthma, backache, belching, black stools, bleed-

ing around the teeth, blood in the urine, brittle bones, burnt odor to urine, dental cavities, diarrhea, difficulty swallowing, dizziness, drowsiness, fainting, fatigue, fluid retention, gas, headache, heartburn, hiccups, hives, increased sex drive, increased tendency to bleed due to vitamin K deficiency, indigestion, inflammation of the eye, inflammation of the pancreas, irritation around the anal area, irritation of the skin and tongue, joint pain, lack or loss of appetite, muscle pain, nausea, night blindness due to vitamin A deficiency, painful or difficult urination, rash, rectal bleeding and/or pain, ringing in the ears, shortness of breath, sour taste, swollen glands, tingling sensation, ulcer attack, vertigo, vitamin D deficiency, vomiting, weight gain or loss, wheezing

## Why should this drug not be prescribed?

If you are sensitive to or have ever had an allergic reaction to Questran or similar drugs such as Colestid, you should not take this medication. Make sure that your doctor is aware of any drug reactions that you have experienced.

Unless you are directed to do so by your doctor, do not take this medication if you are being treated for gallbladder obstruction.

## Special warnings about this medication

If you have phenylketonuria, a genetic disorder, check with your doctor before taking Questran because this product contains phenylalanine.

If you are being treated for any disease that contributes to increased blood cholesterol, such as hypothyroidism (reduced thyroid function), diabetes, nephrotic syndrome (kidney and blood vessel disorder), dysproteinemia, or obstructive liver disease, consult with your doctor before taking this medication.

Questran should begin to reduce cholesterol levels during the first month of therapy. If adequate reduction of cholesterol is not obtained, this medication should be discontinued. Therefore, it is important that your doctor check your progress regularly.

The use of this medication may produce or worsen constipation and aggravate hemorrhoids. If this happens, inform your doctor. Only your doctor can determine if your dose needs to be reduced or discontinued.

The prolonged use of Questran may change acidity in the bloodstream, especially in younger and smaller individuals in whom the doses are relatively higher. Again, it is important that you or your child be checked by your doctor on a regular basis.

## Possible food and drug interactions when taking this medication

If Questran is taken with certain other drugs, the effects of either could be increased, decreased, or altered. It is especially important to check with your doctor before taking Questran with the following:

Chlorothiazide (Diuril)
Digitalis (Lanoxin, Crystodigin)
Oral diabetes drugs such as DiaBeta and Diabinese
Penicillin G (Pentids, others)
Phenobarbital
Phenylbutazone (Butazolidin)
Propranolol (Inderal)
Tetracycline (Achromycin V)
Thyroid medication such as Synthroid
Warfarin (Coumadin)

Your doctor may recommend that you take other medications at least 1 hour before or 4 to 6 hours after you take Questran.

If you are taking a drug such as digitalis (Lanoxin), stopping Questran could be hazardous, since you might experience exaggerated effects of the other drug. Consult your doctor before discontinuing Questran.

This drug may interfere with normal digestion and absorption of fats, including fat-soluble vitamins such as A, D, and K. If supplements of vitamins A, D, and K are essential to your health, your doctor may prescribe an alternative form of these vitamins.

There are no special considerations regarding alcohol use with this medication.

## Special information if you are pregnant or breastfeeding

The effects of Questran during pregnancy have not been adequately studied. If you are pregnant or plan to become pregnant, inform your doctor immediately. Because this medication can interfere with vitamin absorption, it may have an effect on nursing infants. If this drug is essential to your health, your doctor may advise you to discontinue breastfeeding until your treatment is finished.

## Recommended dosage

ADULTS

The recommended starting dose is 1 single-dose packet or 1 level scoopful, 1 to 2 times daily. The usual maintenance dosage is a total of 2 to 4 packets or scoopfuls daily divided into 2 doses preferably at mealtime (usually before meals). The maximum daily dose is 6 packets or scoopfuls. Although the recommended dosing schedule is 2 times daily, your doctor may ask you to take Questran in up to 6 smaller doses per day.

CHILDREN

Experience with the use of Questran in infants and children is limited. If this medication is essential to your child's health, follow your doctor's recommended dosing schedule.

## Overdosage

No ill effects from an overdose have been reported. The main potential harm of an overdose would be obstruction of the stomach and intestines. If you suspect an overdose, seek medical attention immediately.

Brand name:

# Quibron-T/SR

See Theo-Dur, page 538.

Generic name:

# Quinapril

See Accupril, page 1.

Brand name:

# Quinidex Extentabs

Pronounced: KWIN-i-deks Eks-TEN-tabs
Generic name: Quinidine sulfate

## Why is this drug prescribed?

Quinidex Extentabs are used to correct certain types of irregular heart rhythms and to slow an abnormally fast heartbeat.

## Most important fact about this drug

It is important to take only the prescribed amount of this medication—no more and no less. Try to keep your doses at regularly spaced intervals, and be sure not to miss any.

## How should you take this medication?

Quinidex Extentabs should be taken whole, not crushed or chewed, with a full glass of water, milk, or other liquid. Take them exactly as prescribed.

You should take this medication while you are sitting up or standing. This will make it easier to swallow the tablets.

■ *If you miss a dose...*
Take it as soon as you remember, if it is within 2 hours of your scheduled time. If you do not remember until later, skip the dose you missed and go back to your regular schedule. Do not take 2 doses at once.

■ *Storage instructions...*
Store at room temperature in a tightly closed container, away from light.

## What side effects may occur?

Side effects cannot be anticipated. If any develop or change in intensity, inform your doctor as soon as possible. Only your doctor can determine if it is safe for you to continue taking Quinidex Extentabs.

■ *More common side effects include:*
Abdominal pain, diarrhea, hepatitis, inflammation of the esophagus (gullet), loss of appetite, nausea, vomiting

■ *Less common or rare side effects may include:*
Allergic reaction (symptoms include: swelling of face, lips, tongue, throat, arms, and legs, sore throat, fever and chills, difficulty swallowing, chest pain), anemia, apprehension, asthma attack, blind spots, blood clots, blurred vision, changes in skin pigmentation, confusion, delirium, depression, dilated pupils, disturbed color perception, double vision, eczema, excitement, fainting, fever, fluid retention, flushing, headache, hearing changes, hepatitis, hives, inability to breathe, intense itching, intolerance to light, irregular heartbeats, joint pain, lack of coordination, low blood pressure, lupus erythematosus (inflammation of connective tissue), mental decline, muscle pain, night blindness, psoriasis, rash, reddish or purplish spots below the skin, skin eruptions and scaling, skin sensitivity to light, vertigo, vision changes

Another possible side effect is a sensitivity reaction called cinchonism. Symptoms include ringing in the ears, loss of hearing, dizziness, light-headedness, headache, nausea, and disturbed vision.

## Why should this drug not be prescribed?

Quinidex Extentabs should not be prescribed for certain heartbeat irregularities, including one known as heart block. This drug should also be avoided if you have myasthenia gravis (abnormal muscle weakness), or if you are sensitive to or have ever had an allergic reaction to quinidine or cinchona derivatives. (Quinidine comes from the bark of the cinchona tree.)

## Special warnings about this medication

If you have poorly controlled heart disease or circulatory problems, Quinidex should be used cautiously. It can cause low blood pressure, slow heartbeat, or heart block.

Your doctor will carefully monitor your use of this medication if you have partial heart block. It can produce complete heart block.

If you have one or more fainting spells, notify your doctor at once.

Use Quinidex Extentabs cautiously if you have kidney or liver disease. Your doctor will check your blood count and liver and kidney function periodically during long-term therapy.

There have been cases of liver damage due to quinidine sensitivity. If you develop an unexplained fever, especially when you begin taking quinidine, your doctor will monitor your liver function for the first 4 to 8 weeks of therapy. Symptoms usually disappear when quinidine is stopped.

There have been rare cases of severe allergic reaction to quinidine, especially during the first few weeks of therapy. Discuss any allergic reactions you have experienced with your doctor.

Do not confuse Quinidex with quinine, which although related, is used to treat nighttime leg cramps and malaria.

## Possible food and drug interactions
## when taking this medication

Concentrations of digoxin (Lanoxin) in your blood may increase or even double when this drug is taken with Quinidex Extentabs. Your doctor may need to reduce the amount of digoxin you take.

If Quinidex Extentabs are taken with certain other drugs, the effects of either could be increased, decreased, or altered. It is especially important to check with your doctor before combining Quinidex Extentabs with the following:

Amiodarone (Cordarone)
Antacids containing magnesium, such as Maalox and Mylanta
Antispasmodic drugs such as Bentyl
Aspirin
Beta-blocking blood pressure medications such as Inderal and Tenormin
Blood thinners such as Coumadin
Certain antidepressants such as Elavil and Tofranil
Certain diuretic drugs such as Diamox and Daranide
Cimetidine (Tagamet)
Decamethonium
Disopyramide (Norpace)
Ketoconazole (Nizoral)
Major tranquilizers such as Stelazine and Thorazine
Nifedipine (Procardia)
Phenobarbital
Phenytoin (Dilantin)
Physostigmine (Antilirium)
Ranitidine (Zantac)
Reserpine (Diupres)
Rifampin (Rifadin)
Sodium bicarbonate
Sucralfate (Carafate)
Thiazide diuretics such as Dyazide and HydroDIURIL
Verapamil (Calan)

## Special information
## if you are pregnant or breastfeeding

The effects of Quinidex Extentabs during pregnancy have not been adequately studied. If you are pregnant or plan to become pregnant, inform your doctor immediately. Quinidex appears in breast milk and can affect a nursing infant. If this medication is essential to your health, your doctor may advise you to discontinue breastfeeding until your treatment is finished.

## Recommended dosage

ADULTS

The usual dosage is 1 or 2 Quinidex Extentabs every 8 to 12 hours.

CHILDREN

The safety and effectiveness of this drug in children have not been established.

## Overdosage

Any medication taken in excess can have serious consequences. If you suspect an overdose, seek medical treatment immediately.

■ *The symptoms of Quinidex Extentabs overdose may include:*
Abnormal heart rhythms, changes in heart function, coma, decreased breathing, decreased production of urine, fluid in the lungs, low blood pressure, seizures

*Generic name:*

# Quinidine sulfate

See Quinidex Extentabs, page 456.

*Generic name:*

# Ramipril

See Altace, page 15.

*Generic name:*

# Ranitidine

See Zantac, page 598.

*Brand name:*

# Reglan

Pronounced: REG-lan
Generic name: Metoclopramide hydrochloride

## Why is this drug prescribed?

Reglan increases the contractions of the stomach and small intestine, helping the passage of food. It is given to treat the symptoms of diabetic gastroparesis, a condition in which the stomach does not contract. These symptoms include vomiting, nausea, heartburn, feeling of indigestion, persistent fullness after meals, and appetite loss. Reglan is also used, for short periods, to treat heartburn in people with gastroesophageal reflux disorder (backflow of stomach contents into the esophagus). In addition, it is given to prevent nausea and vomiting caused by cancer chemotherapy and surgery.

## Most important fact about this drug

Reglan may cause mild to severe depression. If you have suffered from depression in the past, make sure your doctor is aware of it. Reglan may not be the best drug for you.

## How should you take this medication?

Reglan is usually taken 30 minutes before a meal. If you suffer from heartburn that occurs only intermittently or only at certain times of day, your doctor may want you to schedule your Reglan therapy around those times.

You will probably take Reglan for only 4 to 12 weeks. Continuous treatment beyond 12 weeks is not recommended.

If you have diabetic "lazy stomach" (gastric stasis) that tends to recur, your doctor may want you to take Reglan at the first sign of a recurrence.

■ *If you miss a dose...*
Take it as soon as you remember. If it is almost time for your next dose, skip the one you missed and go back to your regular schedule. Do not take 2 doses at once.

■ *Storage instructions...*
Store at room temperature.

## What side effects may occur?

Side effects cannot be anticipated. If any develop or change in intensity, inform your doctor as soon as possible. Only your doctor can determine if it is safe for you to continue taking Reglan.

■ *More common side effects may include:*
Drowsiness, fatigue, restlessness
■ *Less common or rare side effects may include:*
Breast development in males, confusion, continual discharge of milk from the breasts, depression, diarrhea, dizziness, fluid retention, frequent urination, hallucinations, headache, high or low blood pressure, high fever, hives, impotence, inability to hold urine, insomnia, menstrual irregularities, nausea, rapid or slow heartbeat, rash, rigid muscles, slow movement, swollen tongue or throat, tremor, vision problems, wheezing, yellowed eyes and skin

In addition, Reglan may cause symptoms similar to those of Parkinson's disease, such as slow movements, rigidity, tremor, or a mask-like facial appearance.

Reglan may produce tardive dyskinesia, a syndrome of jerky or writhing involuntary movements, particularly of the tongue, face, mouth, or jaw. Reglan may also cause involuntary movements of the arms and legs, and sometimes loud or labored breathing.

Reglan may cause intense restlessness with associated symptoms such as anxiety, agitation, foot-tapping, pacing, inability to sit still, jitteriness, and insomnia. These symptoms may disappear as your body gets used to Reglan, or if your dosage is reduced.

## Why should this drug not be prescribed?

Do not take Reglan if you are sensitive to it or have ever had an allergic reaction to it.

You should not take Reglan if you have a condition such as obstruction, perforation, or hemorrhage of the stomach or small bowel that might be aggravated by increased stomach and small-bowel movement.

If you have pheochromocytoma (a nonmalignant tumor that causes hypertension), do not take Reglan; it could trigger a dangerous jump in blood pressure.

Do not take Reglan if you have epilepsy; it could increase the frequency and severity of seizures.

If you are taking a drug that is likely to cause side effects such as tremors, jerks, grimaces, or writhing movements, do not take Reglan; it could make such symptoms more severe.

Reglan is not recommended for patients under 18 years of age.

## Special warnings about this medication

If you have Parkinson's disease, you should be given Reglan cautiously or not at all, since the drug may make your Parkinson's symptoms worse.

Because Reglan may make you drowsy and impair your coordination, you should not drive, climb, or perform hazardous tasks until you know how the medication affects you.

Use Reglan with caution if you have high blood pressure.

## Possible food and drug interactions
## when taking this medication

If Reglan is taken with certain other drugs, the effects of either could be increased, decreased, or altered. It is especially important to check with your doctor before combining Reglan with the following:

Acetaminophen (Tylenol)
Alcoholic beverages
Antispasmodic drugs such as Bentyl and Pro-
  Banthine

Cimetidine (Tagamet)
Cyclosporine (Sandimmune)
Digoxin (Lanoxin)
Insulin
MAO inhibitor antidepressants such as Nardil and
  Parnate
Levodopa (Dopar, Sinemet)
Narcotic painkillers such as Percocet and Demerol
Sleeping pills such as Dalmane, Halcion, and
  Restoril
Tetracycline (Achromycin, Sumycin, others)
Tranquilizers such as Valium and Xanax

If you take insulin for diabetes, your insulin dosage or dosing schedule may have to be adjusted while you are taking Reglan.

## Special information
## if you are pregnant or breastfeeding

The effects of Reglan during pregnancy have not been adequately studied. If you are pregnant or plan to become pregnant, inform your doctor immediately. Reglan should be used during pregnancy only if it is clearly needed. Reglan appears in breast milk. Your doctor may recommend that you discontinue Reglan while you are breastfeeding your baby.

## Recommended dosage

ADULTS

*Symptoms of Gastroesophageal Reflux*
The usual dose is 10 milligrams to 15 milligrams of Reglan, up to 4 times a day, 30 minutes before each meal and at bedtime, depending upon the symptoms being treated and the effectiveness of the dose. Treatment usually lasts no longer than 12 weeks.

If symptoms occur only intermittently or at specific times of the day, your doctor may give you a single dose of up to 20 milligrams as a preventive measure.

*Symptoms Associated with Diabetic Gastroparesis or Gastric Stasis*
The usual dose is 10 milligrams 30 minutes before each meal and at bedtime for 2 to 8 weeks.

OLDER ADULTS

*Relief of Symptomatic Gastroesophageal Reflux*
Older adults may need only 5 milligrams per dose.

## Overdosage

Any medication taken in excess can have serious consequences. If you suspect an overdose, seek medical attention immediately.

■ *Symptoms of Reglan overdose may include:*
Disorientation, drowsiness, involuntary movements

*Brand name:*

# Relafen

*Pronounced: REL-ah-fen*
*Generic name: Nabumetone*

## Why is this drug prescribed?

Relafen, a nonsteroidal anti-inflammatory drug, is used to relieve the inflammation, swelling, stiffness, and joint pain associated with rheumatoid arthritis and osteoarthritis (the most common form of arthritis).

## Most important fact about this drug

You should have frequent checkups with your doctor if you take Relafen regularly. Ulcers or internal bleeding can occur with or without warning.

## How should you take this medication?

Relafen can be taken with or without food. Take it exactly as prescribed.

■ *If you miss a dose...*
Take the forgotten dose as soon as you remember. If it is almost time for your next dose, skip the one you missed and go back to your regular schedule. Never take a double dose.

■ *Storage instructions...*
Keep this medication in the container it came in, tightly closed, and away from moist places and direct light. It can be stored at room temperature.

## What side effects may occur?

Side effects cannot be anticipated. If any develop or change in intensity, inform your doctor as soon as possible. Only your doctor can determine whether it is safe for you to continue taking Relafen.

■ *More common side effects may include:*
Abdominal pain, constipation, diarrhea, dizziness, fluid retention, gas, headache, indigestion, itching, nausea, rash, ringing in ears

■ *Less common side effects may include:*
Dry mouth, fatigue, inability to fall or stay asleep, increased sweating, inflammation of the mouth, inflammation of the stomach, nervousness, sleepiness, vomiting

■ *Rare side effects may include:*
Agitation, anxiety, confusion, dark, tarry, bloody stools, depression, difficult or labored breathing, difficulty swallowing, fluid retention, general feeling of illness, hives, increase or loss of appetite, large blisters, pins and needles, pneumonia or lung inflammation, sensitivity to light, severe allergic reactions, skin peeling, stomach and intestinal inflammation and/or bleeding, tremor, ulcers, vaginal bleeding, vertigo, vision changes, weakness, weight gain, yellow eyes and skin

## Why should this drug not be prescribed?

Do not take this medication if you are sensitive to or have ever had an allergic reaction to Relafen, or if you have had asthma attacks, hives or other allergic reactions caused by Relafen, aspirin, or other nonsteroidal anti-inflammatory drugs.

## Special warnings about this medication

Stomach and intestinal ulcers can occur without warning. Remember to get regular check-ups.

Make sure the doctor knows if you have kidney or liver disease. Relafen should be used with caution.

This drug can cause fluid retention and swelling. It should be used with caution if you have congestive heart failure or high blood pressure.

Relafen can cause increased sensitivity to sunlight.

## Possible food and drug interactions when taking this medication

If Relafen is taken with certain other drugs, the effects of either could be increased, decreased, or altered. It is especially important to check with your doctor before combining Relafen with blood-thinning drugs such as Coumadin and aspirin.

Other drugs with which Relafen could possibly interact include:

Diuretics (HydroDIURIL, Lasix)
Lithium (Lithonate)
Methotrexate

## Special information
## if you are pregnant or breastfeeding

The effects of Relafen during pregnancy have not been adequately studied. If you are pregnant or plan to become pregnant, inform your doctor immediately. Relafen may appear in breast milk and could affect a nursing infant. If this medication is essential to your health, your doctor may advise you to discontinue breastfeeding until your treatment with Paxil is finished.

## Recommended dosage

ADULTS

The usual starting dose is 1000 milligrams taken as a single dose. Dosage may be increased up to 2000 milligrams per day, taken once or twice a day.

CHILDREN

The safety and effectiveness of this drug in children have not been established.

## Overdosage

Any medication taken in excess can have serious consequences. If you suspect an overdose, seek medical attention immediately.

*Brand name:*

# Renova

*See Retin-A and Renova, page 462.*

*Generic name:*

# Reserpine, Hydralazine, and Hydrochlorothiazide

*See Ser-Ap-Es, page 494.*

*Brand name:*

# Restoril

*Pronounced: RES-tah-rill*
*Generic name: Temazepam*

## Why is this drug prescribed?

Restoril is used for the relief of insomnia (difficulty in falling asleep, waking up frequently at night, or waking up early in the morning). It belongs to a class of drugs known as benzodiazepines.

## Most important fact about this drug

Sleep problems are usually temporary, requiring treatment for only a short time, usually 1 or 2 days and no more than 2 to 3 weeks. Insomnia that lasts longer than this may be a sign of another medical problem. If you find you need this medicine for more than 7 to 10 days, be sure to check with your doctor.

## How should you take this medication?

Take this medication exactly as directed; never take more than the prescribed amount.

■ *If you miss a dose...*
  Take only as needed.
■ *Storage instructions...*
  Keep this medication in the container it came in, tightly closed, and out of the reach of children. Store it at room temperature.

## What side effects may occur?

Side effects cannot be anticipated. If any develop or change in intensity, inform your doctor as soon as possible. Only your doctor can determine if it is safe for you to continue taking Restoril.

■ *More common side effects may include:*
  Dizziness, drowsiness, fatigue, headache, nausea, nervousness, sluggishness
■ *Less common or rare side effects may include:*
  Abdominal discomfort, abnormal sweating, agitation, anxiety, backache, blurred vision, burning eyes, confusion, constant, involuntary movement of the eyeball, depression, diarrhea, difficult or labored breathing, dry mouth, exaggerated feeling of well-being, fluttery or throbbing heartbeat, hallucinations, hangover, increased dreaming, lack of coordination, loss of appetite, loss of equilibrium, loss of memory, nightmares, overstimulation, restlessness, tremors, vertigo, vomiting, weakness
■ *Side effects due to rapid decrease in or abrupt withdrawal from Restoril:*
  Abdominal and muscle cramps, convulsions, feeling of discomfort, inability to fall asleep or stay asleep, sweating, tremors, vomiting

## Why should this drug not be prescribed?

If you are pregnant or plan to become pregnant, you should not take this medication. It poses a potential risk to the developing baby.

### Special warnings about this medication

When you take Restoril every night for more than a few weeks, it loses its effectiveness to help you sleep. This is known as tolerance. You can also develop physical dependence on this drug, especially if you take it regularly for more than a few weeks, or take high doses.

When you first start taking Restoril, until you know whether the medication will have any "carry over" effect the next day, use extreme care while doing anything that requires complete alertness such as driving a car or operating machinery.

If you are severely depressed or have suffered from severe depression, in the past, consult your doctor before taking this medication.

If you have kidney or liver problems or chronic lung disease, make sure your doctor is aware of it.

After you stop taking Restoril, you may have more trouble sleeping than you had before you started taking it. This is called "rebound insomnia" and should clear up after 1 or 2 nights.

### Possible food and drug interactions when taking this medication

Restoril may intensify the effects of alcohol. Do not drink alcohol while taking this medication.

If Restoril is taken with certain other drugs, the effects of either could be increased, decreased, or altered. It is especially important to check with your doctor before combining Restoril with the following:

Antidepressant drugs such as Elavil, Nardil, Parnate, and Tofranil
Antihistamines such as Benadryl
Barbiturates such as phenobarbital and Seconal
Major tranquilizers such as Mellaril and Thorazine
Narcotic pain relievers such as Percocet and Demerol
Oral contraceptives
Tranquilizers such as Valium and Xanax

### Special information if you are pregnant or breastfeeding

Do not take Restoril if you are pregnant or planning to become pregnant. There is an increased risk of birth defects. This drug may appear in breast milk and could affect a nursing infant. If this medication is essential to your health, your doctor may advise you to discontinue breastfeeding until your treatment with this medication is finished.

### Recommended dosage

ADULTS

The usual recommended dose is 15 milligrams at bedtime; however, 7.5 milligrams may be all that is necessary, while some people may need 30 milligrams. Your doctor will tailor your dose to your needs.

CHILDREN

The safety and effectiveness of Restoril have not been established in children under 18 years of age.

OLDER ADULTS

The doctor will prescribe the smallest effective amount in order to avoid side effects such as oversedation, dizziness, confusion, and lack of muscle coordination. The usual starting dose is 7.5 milligrams.

### Overdosage

Any medication taken in excess can cause symptoms of overdose. If you suspect an overdose, seek medical attention immediately.

■ *The symptoms of Restoril overdose may include:* Coma, confusion, diminished reflexes, loss of coordination, low blood pressure, labored or difficult breathing, seizures, sleepiness, slurred speech

*Brand names:*

# Retin-A and Renova

*Pronounced: Ret-in-A, Re-NO-va*
*Generic name: Tretinoin*

### Why is this drug prescribed?

Both Retin-A and Renova contain the skin medication tretinoin. Retin-A is used in the treatment of acne. Renova is prescribed to reduce fine wrinkles, discoloration, and roughness on facial skin (as part of a comprehensive program of skin care and sun avoidance).

### Most important fact about this drug

While using Retin-A or Renova, exposure to sunlight, including sunlamps, should be kept to a minimum. If you have a sunburn, do not use either medication until you have fully recovered. Use of sunscreen products (at least SPF 15) and protective clothing over treated areas is recommended when exposure to the sun cannot be avoided. Weather extremes, such as wind and cold, may be irritating and should also be avoided while using Retin-A or Renova.

### How should you use this medication?

Retin-A gel, cream, or liquid should be applied once a day, at bedtime, to the skin where acne appears, using enough to cover lightly the affected area. The liquid may be applied using a fingertip, gauze pad, or cotton swab. If you use gauze or cotton, avoid oversaturation, which might cause the liquid to run into areas where treatment is not intended.

Apply Renova once a day, before you go to bed. Use only enough to lightly cover the affected area. Before you use Renova, wash your face with a mild soap, pat your skin dry, and wait 20 to 30 minutes. Then apply a dab of Renova cream the size of a pea and spread it lightly over your face, avoiding your eyes, ears, nostrils, and mouth.

You may use cosmetics while being treated with either Retin-A or Renova; however, you should thoroughly cleanse the areas to be treated before applying the medication.

■ *If you miss a dose...*
Resume your regular schedule the next day.
■ *Storage instructions...*
Store at ordinary room temperature. Do not freeze Renova.

### What side effects may occur?

If you have sensitive skin, the use of Retin-A may cause your skin to become excessively red, puffy, blistered, or crusted. If this happens, notify your doctor, who may recommend that you discontinue Retin-A until your skin returns to normal, or adjust the medication to a level that you can tolerate.

An unusual darkening of the skin or lack of color of the skin may occur temporarily with repeated application of Retin-A.

Side effects of Renova are generally not severe and may include burning, dry skin, itching, peeling, redness, and stinging.

### Why should this drug not be prescribed?

If you are sensitive to or have ever had an allergic reaction to either of these products, avoid using them.

The safety and effectiveness of long-term use of Retin-A in the treatment of disorders other than acne have not been established.

The safety and effectiveness of Renova have not been established in children under age 18, adults over age 50, and people with heavily pigmented skin, nor in periods of greater than 48 weeks of daily use.

### Special warnings about this medication

Both products should be kept away from the eyes, mouth, angles of the nose, and mucous membranes.

If use of either product causes an abnormal irritation, redness, or peeling of the skin where it has been applied, notify your doctor. He may suggest that you use the medication less frequently, discontinue use temporarily, or discontinue use altogether.

If you have eczema (skin inflammation consisting of itching and small blisters that ooze and crust over) or other chronic skin conditions, use these products with extreme caution, as either may cause severe irritation.

If a sensitivity reaction or chemical irritation occurs, notify your doctor. He may suggest that you discontinue using the medication.

Both Retin-A and Renova may cause a brief feeling of warmth or slight stinging when applied.

During the early weeks of therapy, a worsening of acne may occur due to the action of Retin-A on deep, previously unseen areas of inflammation. This is not a reason to discontinue therapy, but do notify your doctor if it occurs.

Retin-A gel is flammable and should be kept away from heat and flame.

Renova will not eliminate wrinkles, repair damage done by the sun, or reverse the aging process.

After you stop using Renova, it is best to continue using a sunscreen and avoiding the sun.

### Possible food and drug interactions when taking this medication

If Retin-A is taken with certain other drugs, the effects of either could be increased, decreased, or altered. It is especially important to check with your doctor before combining Retin-A with the following:

Preparations containing sulfur (ointments and other preparations used to treat skin disorders and infections)
Resorcinol (a drug, used in ointments to treat acne, that causes skin to peel)
Salicylic acid (a drug that kills bacteria and fungi and causes skin to peel)

"Resting" your skin is recommended between use of the above preparations and treatment with Retin-A.

Do not use Renova if you are taking other drugs that increase sensitivity to sunlight. These include:

Certain antibiotics, including Cipro, Noroxin, and tetracycline
Major tranquilizers such as Thorazine and Mellaril
Sulfa drugs such as Bactrim and Septra
Thiazide drugs (water pills) such as Diuril and HydroDIURIL

Caution should be exercised when using Retin-A or Renova in combination with other topical medications, medicated or abrasive soaps and cleansers, soaps and cosmetics that have a strong drying effect, products with high concentrations of alcohol, astringents, spices, or lime, permanent wave solutions, electrolysis, hair depilatories or waxes, or other preparations that may dry or irritate the skin.

### Special information
### if you are pregnant or breastfeeding

If you are pregnant or plan to become pregnant, do not use these products. It is not known whether the drug appears in breast milk. Use with caution when breastfeeding.

### Recommended dosage

RETIN-A

Apply once a day at bedtime.

Results should be noticed after 2 to 3 weeks of treatment. More than 6 weeks of treatment may be needed before definite beneficial effects are seen.

Once acne has responded satisfactorily, it may be possible to maintain the improvement with less frequent applications or other dosage forms. However, any change in formulation, drug concentration, or dose frequency should be closely monitored by your doctor to determine your tolerance and response.

RENOVA

Apply just enough to lightly cover the affected area once daily at bedtime. Do not apply more than the recommended amount; it will not improve results and may cause increased discomfort. You will see the most improvement during the first 24 weeks of therapy. After that, Renova will simply maintain

the improvement. When therapy is stopped, the improvement will gradually diminish.

### Overdosage

Applying either Retin-A or Renova excessively will not produce faster or better results, and marked redness, peeling, or discomfort could occur.

*Brand name:*

# Retrovir

*Pronounced: reh-troh-VEER*
*Generic name: Zidovudine*

### Why is this drug prescribed?

Retrovir is prescribed for adults infected with human immunodeficiency virus (HIV). HIV causes the immune system to break down so that it can no longer respond effectively to infection. This virus leads to the fatal disease known as acquired immune deficiency syndrome (AIDS). Retrovir slows down the progress of HIV. Combining Retrovir with other drugs such as Hivid can help slow the progression.

Retrovir is also prescribed for HIV-infected children over 3 months of age who have symptoms of HIV or who have no symptoms but, through testing, have shown evidence of impaired immunity.

Retrovir taken during pregnancy often prevents transmission of HIV from mother to child.

Signs and symptoms of HIV disease are significant weight loss, fever, diarrhea, infections, and problems with the nervous system.

### Most important fact about this drug

The long-term effects of treatment with zidovudine are unknown. However, treatment with this drug may lead to blood diseases, including granulocytopenia (a severe blood disorder characterized by a sharp decrease of certain types of white blood cells called granulocytes) and severe anemia requiring blood transfusions. This is especially true in people with more advanced HIV and those who start treatment later in the course of their infection.

Also, because Retrovir is not a cure for HIV infections or AIDS, those who are infected may continue to develop complications, including opportunistic infections (infections not usually seen in humans that develop when the immune system falters). Therefore, frequent blood counts by your doctor are strongly advised. Notify your doctor immediately of any changes in your general health.

## How should you take this medication?

Take this medication exactly as prescribed by your doctor. Do not share this medication with anyone and do not exceed your recommended dosage. Take it at even intervals every 4 hours around the clock (children every 6 hours).

If you are pregnant, take the drug 5 times a day.

■ *If you miss a dose...*
Take it as soon as you remember. If it is almost time for your next dose, skip the one you missed and go back to your regular schedule. Do not take 2 doses at once.

■ *Storage instructions...*
Capsules should be stored at room temperature, away from light and moisture. Syrup should be stored at room temperature, away from light.

## What side effects may occur?

Side effects cannot be anticipated. If any develop or change in intensity, inform your doctor as soon as possible. Only your doctor can determine if it is safe for you to continue taking Retrovir.

The frequency and severity of side effects associated with the use of Retrovir are greater in people whose infection is more advanced when treatment is started. Sometimes it is difficult to distinguish side effects from the underlying signs of HIV disease or the infections caused by HIV.

■ *More common side effects may include:*
Change in sense of taste, constipation, diarrhea, difficult or labored breathing, dizziness, fever, general feeling of illness, inability to fall or stay asleep, indigestion, loss of appetite, muscle pain, nausea, rash, severe headache, sleepiness, stomach and intestinal pain, sweating, tingling or pins and needles, vomiting, weakness

■ *Less common side effects may include:*
Acne, anxiety, back pain, belching, bleeding from the rectum, bleeding gums, body odor, changeable emotions, chest pain, chills, confusion, cough, decreased mental sharpness, depression, difficulty swallowing, dimness of vision, excess sensitivity to pain, fainting, fatigue, flu-like symptoms, frequent urination, gas, hearing loss, hives, hoarseness, increase in urine volume, inflammation of the sinuses or nose, itching, joint pain, light intolerance, mouth sores, muscle

spasm, nervousness, nosebleed, painful or difficult urination, sore throat, swelling of the lip, swelling of the tongue, tremor, twitching, vertigo

## Why should this drug not be prescribed?

If you have ever had a life-threatening allergic reaction to Retrovir or any of its ingredients, you should not take this drug.

## Special warnings about this medication

This drug has been studied for only a limited period of time. Long-term safety and effectiveness are not known, especially for people who are in a less advanced stage of AIDS or AIDS-related complex (the condition that precedes AIDS), and for those using the drug over a prolonged period of time.

If you develop a blood disease, you may require a blood transfusion, and your doctor may reduce your dose or take you off the drug altogether. Make sure your doctor monitors your blood count on a regular basis.

The use of Retrovir has *not* been shown to reduce the risk of transmission of HIV to others through sexual contact or blood contamination or to nursing infants.

Retrovir should be used with extreme caution by people who have a bone marrow disease.

Some people taking Retrovir develop a sensitization reaction, often signaled by a rash. If you notice a rash developing, notify your doctor.

Because little data are available concerning the use of this drug in people with impaired kidney or liver function, check with your doctor before using Retrovir if you have either problem.

## Possible food and drug interactions when taking this medication

If Retrovir is taken with certain other drugs, the effects of either could be increased, decreased, or altered. It is especially important to check with your doctor before combining Retrovir with the following:

Acetaminophen (Tylenol)
Amphotericin B (Fungizone, a drug used to treat fungal infections)
Aspirin
Atovaquone (Mepron)
Dapsone (a drug used to treat leprosy)
Doxorubicin (Adriamycin, a cancer drug)
Fluconazole (Diflucan)
Flucytosine (Ancobon)

Indomethacin (Indocin)
Interferon (Intron A, Roferon-A)
Pentamidine (NebuPent, Pentam)
Phenytoin (Dilantin, an anticonvulsant)
Probenecid (Benemid, an antigout drug)
Valproic acid (Depakene)
Vinblastine (Velban, a cancer drug)
Vincristine (Oncovin, a cancer drug)

The combined use of phenytoin and Retrovir will be monitored by your doctor because of the possibility of seizures.

## Special information
## if you are pregnant or breastfeeding

The effects of Retrovir during pregnancy are under study. Use during pregnancy has been shown to protect the developing baby from contracting HIV. If you are pregnant or plan to become pregnant, inform your doctor immediately. This drug may appear in breast milk and could affect a nursing infant. If this medication is essential to your health, your doctor may advise you to discontinue breast-feeding until your treatment is finished. Women infected with HIV risk passing the virus on to a nursing infant.

## Recommended dosage

ADULTS

All dosages of Retrovir must be very closely monitored by your physician. The following dosages are general; your physician will tailor the dose to your specific condition.

*Capsules and Syrup*

For adults who have symptoms of HIV infection, including AIDS, the usual starting dose is 200 milligrams (two 100-milligram capsules or 4 teaspoonfuls of syrup) taken every 4 hours. After 1 month, your doctor may reduce your dose to 100 milligrams taken every 4 hours.

For adults who have HIV infection but no symptoms, the usual dose is 100 milligrams taken every 4 hours while awake.

If you are pregnant, the usual dosage is 100 milligrams in capsules or syrup 5 times a day, beginning between 14 and 34 weeks of pregnancy, until you go into labor. You will then be given the drug intravenously until the baby is born. The baby will get Retrovir until it is 6 weeks old.

If you are taking Retrovir and Hivid, the usual doses are 200 milligrams of Retrovir with 0.75 milligrams of Hivid every 8 hours.

CHILDREN

The usual starting dose for children 3 months to 12 years of age is determined by body size. While the dose should not exceed 200 milligrams every 6 hours, it must still be individually determined. Safety and efficacy have not been determined for infants under 3 months of age.

## Overdosage

Any medication taken in excess can have serious consequences. If you suspect an overdose, seek emergency medical treatment immediately.

■ *Symptoms of Retrovir overdose may include:*
   Nausea, vomiting

*Brand name:*

# ReVia

*Pronounced: reh-VEE-uh*
*Generic name: Naltrexone hydrochloride*

## Why is this drug prescribed?

ReVia is prescribed to treat alcohol dependence and narcotic addiction. ReVia is not a cure and must be used as part of a comprehensive treatment program that includes professional counseling, support groups, and close medical supervision.

## Most important fact about this drug

Before taking ReVia for narcotic addiction, you must be drug-free for at least 7 to 10 days. You must also be free of any drug withdrawal symptoms. If you think you are still in withdrawal, be sure to tell your doctor, since taking ReVia while narcotics are still in your system could cause serious physical problems. Your doctor will perform tests to confirm your drug-free condition.

## How should you take this medication?

It is important to take ReVia on schedule as directed by your doctor, and to follow through with your counseling and support group therapy. If you take even small doses of heroin or other narcotic drugs while taking ReVia, the medication will not be effective. Large doses of heroin or other narcotic drugs combined with ReVia can be fatal.

■ *If you miss a dose...*
   Take the missed dose as soon as possible. If you do not remember until the next day, skip the missed dose and go back to your regular dosing schedule. Do not take 2 doses at once.

■ *Storage instructions...*
Protect from light.

## What side effects may occur?

Side effects cannot be anticipated. If any side effects develop or change in intensity, tell your doctor immediately. Only your doctor can determine whether it is safe for you to continue taking ReVia.

■ *More common side effects of treatment for alcoholism may include:*
Dizziness, fatigue, headache, nausea, nervousness, sleeplessness, vomiting
■ *Less common side effects of treatment for alcoholism may include:*
Anxiety, sleepiness
■ *More common side effects of treatment for narcotic addiction may include:*
Abdominal pain/cramps, anxiety, difficulty sleeping, headache, joint and muscle pain, low energy, nausea and/or vomiting, nervousness
■ *Other side effects of treatment for narcotic addiction may include:*
Acne, athlete's foot, blurred vision and aching, burning, or swollen eyes, chills, clogged and aching ears, cold sores, cold feet, confusion, constipation, cough, decreased potency, delayed ejaculation, depression, diarrhea, disorientation, dizziness, dry mouth, fatigue, feeling down, fever, fluid retention, frequent urination, gas, hair loss, hallucinations, head "pounding", heavy breathing, hemorrhoids, hoarseness, "hot spells", increased appetite, increased blood pressure, increased energy, increased mucus, increased or decreased sexual interest, increased thirst, irregular or fast heartbeat, irritability, itching, light sensitivity, loss of appetite, nightmares, nosebleeds, oily skin, pain in shoulders, legs, or knees, pain in groin, painful urination, paranoia, restlessness, ringing in ears, runny nose, shortness of breath, side pains, sinus trouble, skin rash, sleepiness, sneezing, sore throat, stuffy nose, swollen glands, tremor, throbbing heartbeat, twitching, ulcer, weight loss or gain, yawning

## Why should this drug not be prescribed?

If you are sensitive to or have ever had an allergic reaction to ReVia, you should not take it. If you have acute hepatitis (liver disease) or liver failure,

do not start therapy with ReVia. Remember, too, that you must be narcotic-free before beginning ReVia therapy.

## Special warnings about this medication

Since ReVia may cause liver damage when taken at high doses, if you develop symptoms that may signal possible liver problems, such as abdominal pain lasting more than a few days, white bowel movements, dark urine, or yellowing of your eyes, you should stop taking ReVia immediately and see your doctor as soon as possible. Your doctor may periodically test your liver function while you are on ReVia therapy. If you are narcotic-dependent and accidentally take ReVia, you may experience severe withdrawal symptoms lasting up to 48 hours, including confusion, sleepiness, hallucinations, vomiting, and diarrhea. If this occurs, seek help immediately. Ask your doctor to give you a Revia medication card to alert medical personnel that you are taking ReVia in case of an emergency. Carry this card with you at all times. If you do require medical treatment, be sure to tell the doctor that you are taking ReVia. You should also tell your dentist and pharmacist that you are taking ReVia. The safety of ReVia in children under 18 years of age has not been established.

## Possible food and drug interactions when taking this medication

Since studies to evaluate this interaction of ReVia with drugs other than narcotics have not been performed, do not take any medications, either over-the-counter or prescription, without first notifying your doctor. Do not use Antabuse while you are taking ReVia; both drugs can damage your liver. Do not take Mellaril (a drug used to treat depression and anxiety) while on ReVia therapy, as the combination may cause you to feel very sleepy and sluggish. While taking ReVia avoid medicines that contain narcotics, including cough and cold preparations, such as Actifed-C, Ryna-C, and Dimetane-DC; antidiarrheal medications such as Lomotil; and narcotic painkillers such as Percodan, Tylox, and Tylenol No. 3.

## Special information if you are pregnant or breastfeeding

The effects of ReVia during pregnancy have not been adequately studied. If you are pregnant or are planning to become pregnant, tell your doctor immediately. ReVia should be used during pregnancy only if clearly needed. ReVia may appear in breast milk. If this medication is essential to your health, your doctor may tell you to discontinue breastfeeding your baby until your treatment with ReVia is finished.

## Recommended dosage

ALCOHOLISM

The usual starting dose is 50 milligrams once a day.

NARCOTIC DEPENDENCE

The usual starting dose is 25 milligrams once a day. If no withdrawal symptoms occur, the doctor may increase the dosage to 50 milligrams a day.

## Overdosage

Any medication taken in excess can have serious consequences. If you suspect an overdose of ReVia, seek medical attention immediately.

Brand name:

# Rheumatrex

See Methotrexate, page 316.

Brand name:

# Rhinocort

Pronounced: RYE-no-kort
Generic name: Budesonide

## Why is this drug prescribed?

Rhinocort is an anti-inflammatory steroid medication. It is prescribed for relief of the symptoms of hay fever and other nasal inflammations.

## Most important fact about this drug

Because steroids can suppress the immune system, people taking Rhinocort may become more susceptible to infections, and their infections could be more severe. Anyone taking Rhinocort or other corticosteroids who has not had infections such as chickenpox and measles should avoid exposure to them. If you are taking Rhinocort and are exposed, tell your doctor immediately.

## How should you take this medication?

Rhinocort is prescribed as a nasal inhaler. Instructions for use are provided with the product. Do not use doses that are larger than recommended.

Relief of symptoms usually occurs 24 hours to a few days after starting Rhinocort. If symptoms do not improve within 3 weeks, or if nasal irritation worsens, contact your physician.

Shake the Rhinocort container well before using it. Do not use near an open flame.

Rhinocort is to be used within 6 months after opening it.

■ *If you miss a dose...*
  Take the forgotten dose as soon as you remember. If it is almost time for your next dose, skip the one you missed and go back to your regular schedule. Never take two doses at the same time.
■ *Storage instructions...*
  Do not store near an open flame or heat above 120 degrees Fahrenheit. Do not store in areas of high humidity.

## What side effects may occur?

Side effects cannot be anticipated. If any develop or change in intensity, inform your doctor as soon as possible. Only your doctor can determine if it is safe for you to continue taking Rhinocort.

■ *More common side effects may include:*
  Increased coughing, irritation of the nasal passages, nosebleeds, sore throat
■ *Less common side effects may include:*
  Bad taste in mouth, dry mouth, facial swelling, hoarseness, indigestion, inflammation of the skin, itching, nasal sores or pain, nausea, rash, reduced sense of smell, yeast infection of the vagina or mouth, wheezing

## Why should this drug not be prescribed?

If you develop an infection of your nose and throat, stop using Rhinocort and call your doctor. If you already have tuberculosis or any other kind of infection, be sure your doctor knows about it. If you are sensitive to or have ever had an allergic reaction to Rhinocort or any of its ingredients, you should not take this medication.

## Special warnings about this medication

If you have been taking a steroid in tablet form, such as prednisone, and are switched to Rhinocort, you may have symptoms of withdrawal, such as joint or muscle pain, lethargy, and depression. If you have been taking another steroid for a long time for asthma, your asthma may get worse if your medication is cut back too quickly. Using

Rhinocort with another steroid drug can decrease the body's normal ability to make its own steroid chemicals.

### Possible food and drug interactions when taking this medication

Talk to your doctor before using Rhinocort if you already take prednisone or any other steroid medication.

### Special information
### if you are pregnant or breastfeeding

The effects of Rhinocort during pregnancy have not been adequately studied. If you are pregnant or plan to become pregnant, inform your doctor immediately. Rhinocort should be used during pregnancy only if clearly needed. The effects of Rhinocort on the infants of women who breastfeed also are unknown. Your doctor may have you stop breastfeeding while you are taking this drug.

### Recommended dosage

The usual recommended starting dose for adults and children 6 years of age and older is 256 micrograms a day, either as two sprays in each nostril twice a day, morning and evening, or as four sprays in each nostril once a day in the morning. Your doctor may lower the dose once relief of symptoms occurs. Rhinocort is not recommended for use in children with nasal irritation not due to allergies.

### Overdosage

Any medication taken in excess can have serious consequences. If you suspect an overdose, seek medical attention immediately.

Symptoms of Rhinocort overdose stem from a condition called hypercorticism, when the body produces an excess of its own steroid chemicals.

■ *Symptoms of overdose may include:*
Diabetes, excess hair growth, fatigue and weakness, fluid retention, impotence, lack of menstrual periods, skin discoloration

*Brand name:*

# Ridaura

Pronounced: ri-DOOR-ah
Generic name: Auranofin

### Why is this drug prescribed?

Ridaura, a gold preparation, is given to help treat rheumatoid arthritis. Ridaura is taken by mouth, unlike other gold compounds, which are given by injection. It is recommended only for people who have not been helped sufficiently by nonsteroidal anti-inflammatory drugs (Anaprox, Dolobid, Indocin, Motrin, and others). Ridaura should be part of a comprehensive arthritis treatment program that includes non-drug forms of therapy.

You are most likely to benefit from Ridaura if you have active joint inflammation, especially in the early stages.

### Most important fact about this drug

Unlike anti-inflammatory medications, Ridaura does not take effect immediately. In fact, you may have to wait for 3 to 6 months to get any benefit from Ridaura. Ridaura prevents or suppresses joint swelling, but does not cure rheumatoid arthritis.

### How should you take this medication?

Read the patient information sheet provided with Ridaura, and take the medication exactly as prescribed.

You should observe good oral hygiene during therapy with Ridaura.

■ *If you miss a dose...*
If you take 1 dose a day, take the missed dose as soon as you remember. If you do not remember until the next day, skip the dose you missed and go back to your regular schedule.

If you take more than 1 dose a day, take the missed dose as soon as you remember. If it is almost time for your next dose, skip the one you missed and go back to your regular schedule.

Do not take 2 doses at once.

■ *Storage instructions...*
Store at room temperature in a tightly closed, light-resistant container.

### What side effects may occur?

Side effects cannot be anticipated. If any side effects develop or change in intensity, tell your doctor immediately. Only your doctor can determine whether it is safe for you to continue taking Ridaura. Ridaura causes loose stools or diarrhea in about half of all people who take it; there may also be indigestion, abdominal pain and gas, loss of appetite, vomiting, or nausea.

■ *Other commonly reported side effects include:*
Blood-cell abnormalities which may result in bleeding, bronchitis, easy bruising, fever, gold

dermatitis (inflammation of skin), itching, metallic taste, pinkeye, rash, sores in the mouth

■ *Less common or rare side effects may include:*
Altered sense of taste, anemia, black or bloody stools, blood in the urine, constipation, difficulty swallowing, fluid retention and swelling, hair loss, hives, inflammation of the tongue or gums, intestinal inflammation with ulcers, stomach or intestinal bleeding, yellowed eyes and skin

### Why should this drug not be prescribed?

Do not take Ridaura if you have ever had any of the following reactions to a medication containing gold:

Anaphylaxis (life-threatening allergic reaction)
Blood or bone marrow abnormality
Fibrosis (scar tissue formation) in the lungs
Serious bowel inflammation
Skin peeling off in sheets

### Special warnings about this medication

You should be monitored especially closely while taking Ridaura if you have any of the following:

History of a bone marrow abnormality
Inflammatory bowel disease
Kidney disease
Liver disease
Skin rash

Your doctor may order periodic blood and urine tests to check for unwanted effects.

Like other medications containing gold, Ridaura may cause serious blood abnormalities. If you start to bruise easily, or develop small red or purplish skin discolorations, see your doctor. He or she will have you stop taking Ridaura and will do some blood tests, including a platelet count.

Ridaura may cause protein or microscopic amounts of blood to spill into your urine. If a urine test shows that this is happening, your doctor will take you off of Ridaura immediately.

Gold compounds may cause your skin to become more sensitive to sunlight, so you may need to limit your exposure to the sun and wear a sunscreen.

### Possible food and drug interactions when taking this medication

If Ridaura is taken with certain other drugs, the effects of either could be increased, decreased, or altered. It is especially important to check with your doctor before combining Ridaura with the following:

Penicillamine (Cuprimine)
Phenytoin (Dilantin)

### Special information if you are pregnant or breastfeeding

If you are pregnant or plan to become pregnant, inform your doctor immediately. Because Ridaura may cause birth defects, it should not be taken during pregnancy.

Likewise, you should not take Ridaura while breastfeeding; although there are no data on Ridaura, injected gold appears in breast milk. If you are a new mother, you may have to choose between taking Ridaura and breastfeeding your baby.

### Recommended dosage

The usual dosage of Ridaura is 6 milligrams daily in a single dose or divided into 2 smaller doses. After 6 months, your doctor may increase the dose to 9 milligrams, divided into 3 doses. Ridaura is prescribed only for adults.

### Overdosage

Any medication taken in excess can have serious consequences. If you suspect an overdose of Ridaura, seek medical attention immediately.

---

*Generic name:*

# Rifampin, Isoniazid, and Pyrazinamide

See Rifater, page 470.

---

*Brand Name:*

# Rifater

*Pronounced: RIF-a-tur*
*Generic ingredients: Rifampin, Isoniazid, Pyrazinamide*

### Why is this drug prescribed?

Rifater is a combination antibiotic used to treat the initial phase of tuberculosis. After a 2-month period, your doctor may prescribe another combination of antituberculosis drugs (Rifamate), which can be continued for longer periods.

## Most important fact about this drug

Isoniazid, one of the components of Rifater, some-times causes liver damage. Contact your doctor immediately if you develop yellowing of the eyes or skin, fatigue, weakness, loss of appetite, nausea, or vomiting.

## How should you take this medication?

Take Rifater exactly as prescribed. Do not stop without consulting your doctor. It is important to take all of the drug prescribed for you, even if you feel better, and not to miss any doses.

Take Rifater on an empty stomach, either 1 hour before or 2 hours after a meal, with a full glass of water. Wait at least 1 hour before taking an antacid, as antacids may interfere with the drug.

If needed, your doctor may suggest taking vitamin $B_6$ while you are on Rifater therapy.

■ *If you miss a dose...*
Take it as soon as you remember. If it is almost time for the next dose, skip the one you missed and go back to your regular schedule. Never take 2 doses at once.

■ *Storage instructions...*
Store at room temperature. Protect from moisture.

## What side effects may occur?

Side effects cannot be anticipated. If any develop or change in intensity, tell your doctor as soon as pos-sible. Only your doctor can determine if it is safe for you to continue taking Rifater.

■ *More common side effects may include:*
Angina (crushing chest pain), anxiety, bone pain, chest pain, chest tightness, cough, coughing up blood, diabetic coma, diarrhea, difficult breath-ing, digestive pain, fast, fluttery heartbeat, head-ache, hepatitis, hives, itching, joint pain, nausea, numbness or tingling of the legs, rash, reddened skin, skin peeling or flaking, sleeplessness, sweating, swelling of the legs, vomiting, yellow-ing of skin and eyes

■ *Less common side effects may include:*
High or persistent fever, ringing in ears, vertigo

## Why should this drug not be prescribed?

Do not take this medication if you have ever had an allergic reaction to or are sensitive to rifampin, iso-niazid, or pyrazinamide. If you have serious liver disease or have ever had a severe side effect from isoniazid (such as fever, chills, and arthritis), do not take Rifater. Also, if you have a history of liver disease or have had acute and painful joint swelling (gout), avoid this drug.

## Special warnings about this medication

Rifater may cause your urine, sputum, sweat, and tears to turn a red-orange color. This is to be expected and is not harmful. The drug may also permanently discolor contact lenses.

Since Rifater may cause eye problems, you should have a complete eye examination before starting therapy and periodically during Rifater treatment.

Limit the amount of alcohol you drink while on this medicine. Daily users of alcohol may be more prone to liver problems.

Use this medicine with caution if you have dia-betes or kidney disease.

When rifampin, one of the drugs in Rifater, is taken at high doses (more than 600 milligrams) once or twice a week, it is likely that side effects may increase, including "flu-like" symptoms such as fever, chills, fatigue, weakness, upset stomach, and shortness of breath.

## Possible food and drug interactions when taking this medication

If Rifater is taken with certain other drugs, the effects could be increased, decreased, or altered. Consider another form of birth control if you are taking oral contraceptives, since Rifater lowers their effectiveness. Also check with your doctor before combining Rifater with the following:

Antacids such as Maalox or Tums
Anticonvulsants such as Dilantin, Depakene,
    Mysoline, Tegretol
Barbiturates such as phenobarbital and Nembutal
Blood pressure medicines such as Inderal,
    Tenormin, and Vasotec
Blood thinners such as Coumadin
Chloramphenicol (Chloromycetin)
Ciprofloxacin (Cipro)
Clofibrate (Atromid-S)
Cotrimoxazole (Bactrim, Septra)
Cycloserine (Seromycin)
Cyclosporine (Sandimmune)
Dapsone
Diabetes medications such as Diabinese and
    Orinase
Disulfiram (Antabuse)

Fluconazole (Diflucan)

Haloperidol (Haldol)

Heart medications such Calan, Cardizem, Lanoxin, Norpace, Mexitil, Procardia, Quinidex, and Tonocard

Itraconazole (Sporanox)

Ketoconazole (Nizoral)

Levodopa (Sinemet)

Narcotic analgesics such as Darvon, Demerol, Percocet, Percodan

Nortriptyline (Pamelor)

Probenecid (Benemid)

Progestins such as Megace

Steroid drugs such as Deltasone and Prelone

Sulfasalazine (Azulfidine)

Theophylline (Theolair, Slo-Phyllin, Theo-Dur)

Tranquilizers such as Valium and Xanax

Foods such as cheese, fish, and red wine may cause reactions if you are taking a medicine containing isoniazid. Call your doctor immediately if fast or fluttery heartbeat, flushing, sweating, headache, or light-headedness occurs while you are taking this medication.

## Special information
### if you are pregnant or breastfeeding

If you are pregnant or plan to become pregnant, tell your doctor immediately. You may need to discontinue the drug. If needed for preventive treatment, Rifater should be started after delivery. An ingredient in Rifater may cause postnatal hemorrhaging in the mother and baby when given during the last few weeks of pregnancy.

Rifater can pass into breast milk and may affect the nursing infant. Your doctor may recommend that you stop breastfeeding until your treatment with Rifater is finished.

## Recommended dosage

ADULTS

Take once a day, as follows:

If you weigh 97 pounds or less: 4 tablets
If you weigh 98 to 120 pounds: 5 tablets
If you weigh 121 pounds or more: 6 tablets

CHILDREN

Safety and effectiveness in children under the age of 15 have not been established.

## Overdosage

Any medication taken in excess can have serious consequences. An untreated overdose of Rifater can be fatal. If you suspect an overdose, seek medical attention immediately.

■ *Symptoms of Rifater overdose may include:*
Blurred vision, coma, dizziness, hallucinations, increasing tiredness or sluggishness, liver enlargement or tenderness, nausea, seizures, slurring of speech, shallow or difficult breathing, stupor, vomiting, yellow eyes and skin

*Brand name:*

# Risperdal

*Pronounced: RIS-per-dal*
*Generic name: Risperidone*

## Why is this drug prescribed?

Risperdal is prescribed to treat severe mental illnesses such as schizophrenia.

## Most important fact about this drug

Risperdal may cause tardive dyskinesia, a condition that causes involuntary muscle spasms and twitches in the face and body. This condition can become permanent and is most common among older people, especially women. Tell your doctor immediately if you begin to have any involuntary movement. You may need to discontinue Risperdal therapy.

## How should you take this medication?

Do not take more or less of this medication than prescribed or use it for longer than the prescribed term of treatment as this may cause unwanted side effects.

Risperdal may be taken with or without food.

■ *If you miss a dose...*
Take it as soon as you remember. If it is almost time for your next dose, skip the one you missed and go back to your regular schedule. Do not take 2 doses at once.

■ *Storage instructions...*
Store at room temperature. Protect from light and moisture.

## What side effects may occur?

Side effects cannot be anticipated. If any develop or change in intensity, tell your doctor as soon as possible. Only your doctor can determine if it is safe for you to continue taking Risperdal.

■ *More common side effects may include:*
Abdominal pain, abnormal walk, agitation, aggression, anxiety, chest pain, constipation, coughing, decreased activity, diarrhea, difficulty with orgasm, diminished sexual desire, dizziness, dry skin, erection and ejaculation problems, excessive menstrual bleeding, fever, headache, inability to sleep, increased dreaming, increased duration of sleep, indigestion, involuntary movements, joint pain, lack of coordination, nasal inflammation, nausea, overactivity, rapid heartbeat, rash, reduced salivation, respiratory infection, sleepiness, sore throat, tremor, underactive reflexes, urination problems, vomiting, weight gain

■ *Less common side effects may include:*
Abnormal vision, back pain, dandruff, difficult or labored breathing, increased saliva, sinus inflammation, toothache

## Why should this drug not be prescribed?
If you are sensitive to or have ever had an allergic reaction to Risperdal or other major tranquilizers, you should not take this medication.

## Special warnings about this medication
You should use Risperdal cautiously if you have kidney, liver, or heart diseases, seizures, breast cancer, thyroid disorders, or any other diseases that affect the metabolism (conversion of food into energy and tissue), or if you are exposed to extremes of temperature.

Be aware that Risperdal may mask signs and symptoms of drug overdose and of conditions such as intestinal obstruction, brain tumor, and Reye's syndrome (a dangerous neurological condition that may follow viral infections, usually occurring in children).

Risperdal may cause Neuroleptic Malignant Syndrome (NMS), a condition marked by muscle stiffness or rigidity, fast heartbeat or irregular pulse, increased sweating, high fever, and high or low blood pressure. Unchecked, this condition can prove fatal. Call your doctor immediately if you notice any of these symptoms. Risperdal therapy should be discontinued.

This drug may impair your ability to drive a car or operate potentially dangerous machinery. Do not participate in any activities that require full alertness if you are unsure of your ability.

Risperdal can cause orthostatic hypotension (low blood pressure when rising to a standing position), with dizziness, rapid heartbeat, and fainting, especially when you first start to take it.

## Possible food and drug interactions when taking this medication
If Risperdal is taken with certain other drugs, the effects of either can be increased, decreased, or altered. It is especially important to check with your doctor before combining Risperdal with the following:

Blood pressure medicines such as Aldomet,
    Procardia, and
Vasotec
Bromocriptine mesylate (Parlodel)
Carbamazepine (Tegretol)
Clozapine (Clozaril)
Levodopa (Sinemet, Dopar)
Quinidine (Quinidex)

Risperdal tends to increase the effect of blood pressure medicines.

You may experience drowsiness and other potentially serious effects if Risperdal is combined with alcohol and other drugs that slow the central nervous system such as Valium, Percocet, Demerol, or Haldol.

Check with your doctor before taking any new medications.

## Special information if you are pregnant or breastfeeding
The safety and effectiveness of Risperdal during pregnancy have not been adequately studied. If you are pregnant or plan to become pregnant, tell your doctor immediately. It is not known whether Risperdal appears in breast milk. If this medication is essential to your health, your doctor may advise you to discontinue breastfeeding until your treatment with this medication is finished.

## Recommended dosage
ADULTS

The usual starting dose is 1 milligram twice a day, with increases to 2 milligrams by the second day and 3 milligrams by the third day. Your doctor may further adjust the dosage at intervals of 1 week. For the longer term, dosage ranges from 4 to 6 milligrams daily, divided into 2 equal doses.

If you have a liver or kidney disease, your doctor will have you start with one-half of a 1-milligram tablet twice daily and may then increase your dosage by one-half tablet per dose.

### CHILDREN

The safety and effectiveness of Risperdal in children have not been established.

### OLDER ADULTS

Older adults generally take Risperdal at lower doses. The usual starting dose is one-half of a 1-milligram tablet twice daily. Your doctor may increase the dose gradually.

## Overdosage

Any medication taken in excess can have serious consequences. If you suspect an overdose of Risperdal, seek medical attention immediately.

■ *Symptoms of Risperdal overdose may include:*
Drowsiness, low blood pressure, rapid heartbeat, sedation

*Generic name:*
# Risperidone

*See Risperdal, page 472.*

*Brand name:*
# Ritalin

*Pronounced: RIT-ah-lin*
*Generic name: Methylphenidate hydrochloride*

## Why is this drug prescribed?

Ritalin is a mild central nervous system stimulant used in the treatment of attention deficit disorders in children. (This is a general term for several behavior problems previously known as minimal brain dysfunction in children; other names being used are hyperkinetic child syndrome, minimal brain damage, minimal cerebral dysfunction, and minor cerebral dysfunction.) Ritalin is also occasionally used in adults to treat narcolepsy (an uncontrollable desire to sleep).

This drug should be given as an integral part of a total treatment program that includes psychological, educational, and social measures. Symptoms of attention deficit disorder include continual prob-

lems with moderate to severe distractibility, short attention span, hyperactivity, emotional changeability, and impulsiveness.

## Most important fact about this drug

Excessive doses of Ritalin over a long period of time can produce addiction. It is also possible to develop tolerance to the drug, so that larger doses are needed to produce the original effect. Because of these dangers, be sure to check with your doctor before making any change in dosage; and withdraw the drug only under your doctor's supervision.

## How should you take this medication?

Follow your doctor's directions carefully.

Ritalin is available in standard and sustained-release tablets (Ritalin-SR). It is recommended that Ritalin be taken 30 to 45 minutes before meals. If the drug interferes with sleep, give the child the last dose before 6 p.m. Ritalin-SR tablets should be swallowed whole, never crushed or chewed.

■ *If you miss a dose...*
Give it to the child as soon as you remember. Give the remaining doses for the day at regularly spaced intervals. Do not give 2 doses at once.
■ *Storage instructions...*
Keep out of reach of children. Store below 86°F. in a tightly closed, light-resistant container. Protect Ritalin-SR from moisture.

## What side effects may occur?

Side effects cannot be anticipated. If any develop or change in intensity, inform your doctor as soon as possible. Only your doctor can determine if it is safe for you to continue giving Ritalin.

■ *More common side effects may include:*
Inability to fall or stay asleep, nervousness

These side effects can usually be controlled by reducing the dosage and omitting the drug in the afternoon or evening.

In children, loss of appetite, abdominal pain, weight loss during long-term therapy, inability to fall or stay asleep, and abnormally fast heartbeat are more common side effects.

■ *Less common or rare side effects may include:*
Abdominal pain, abnormal heartbeat, abnormal muscular movements, blood pressure changes, chest pain, dizziness, drowsiness, fever, headache, hives, jerking, joint pain, loss of appetite,

nausea, palpitations (fluttery or throbbing heart-beat), pulse changes, rapid heartbeat, reddish or purplish skin spots, skin reddening, skin inflammation with peeling, skin rash, Tourette's syndrome (severe twitching), weight loss during long-term treatment

## Why should this drug not be prescribed?

This drug should not be prescribed for anyone experiencing anxiety, tension, and agitation, since the drug may aggravate these symptoms.

Anyone sensitive or allergic to this drug should not take it.

This medication should not be taken by anyone with the eye condition known as glaucoma, anyone who suffers from tics (repeated, involuntary twitches), or someone with a family history of Tourette's syndrome (severe and multiple tics).

Ritalin is not intended for use in children whose symptoms may be caused by stress or a psychiatric disorder.

Ritalin should not be used for the prevention or treatment of normal fatigue, nor should it be used for the treatment of severe depression

## Special warnings about this medication

Your doctor will do a complete history and evaluation before prescribing Ritalin. He or she will take into account the severity of the symptoms, as well as your child's age.

Ritalin should not be given to children under 6 years of age; safety and effectiveness in this age group have not been established.

There is no information regarding the safety and effectiveness of long-term Ritalin treatment in children. However, suppression of growth has been seen with the long-term use of stimulants, so your doctor will watch your child carefully while he or she is taking this drug.

Blood pressure should be monitored in anyone taking Ritalin, especially those with high blood pressure.

Some people have had visual disturbances such as blurred vision while being treated with Ritalin.

The use of Ritalin by anyone with a seizure disorder is not recommended. Be sure your doctor is aware of any problem in this area.

## Possible food and drug interactions when taking this medication

If Ritalin is taken with certain other drugs, the effects of either can be increased, decreased, or altered. It is especially important to check with your doctor before combining Ritalin with the following:

Antiseizure drugs such as phenobarbital, Dilantin and Mysoline

Antidepressant drugs such as Tofranil, Anafranil, and Norpramin

Blood thinners such as Coumadin

Drugs that restore blood pressure, such as EpiPen

Guanethidine (Ismelin)

MAO inhibitors (antidepressant drugs such as Nardil and Parnate)

Phenylbutazone

## Special information
## if you are pregnant or breastfeeding

The effects of Ritalin during pregnancy have not been adequately studied. If you are pregnant or plan to become pregnant, inform your doctor immediately. It is not known if Ritalin appears in breast milk. If this medication is essential to your health, your doctor may advise you to discontinue nursing your baby until your treatment with this medication is finished.

## Recommended dosage

ADULTS

*Tablets*

The average dosage is 20 to 30 milligrams a day, divided into 2 or 3 doses, preferably taken 30 to 45 minutes before meals. Some people may need 40 to 60 milligrams daily, others only 10 to 15 milligrams. Your doctor will determine the best dose.

*SR Tablets*

Ritalin-SR tablets keep working for 8 hours. They may be used in place of Ritalin tablets if they deliver a comparable dose over an 8-hour period.

CHILDREN

Ritalin should not be given to children under 6 years of age.

Your doctor will start your child on small doses, then increase the dose gradually at weekly intervals. Your child should not take more than 60 milligrams in a day. If you do not see any improvement over a period of 1 month, check with your doctor. He or she may wish to discontinue the drug.

*Tablets*

The usual starting dose is 5 milligrams taken twice a day, before breakfast and lunch; your doctor will increase the dose by 5 to 10 milligrams a week.

*SR Tablets*

Ritalin-SR tablets continue working for 8 hours. Your doctor will decide if SR tablets should be used in place of Ritalin tablets.

Your doctor will periodically discontinue this drug in order to reassess your child's condition. Drug treatment should not, and need not, be indefinite and usually can be discontinued after puberty.

### Overdosage

If you suspect an overdose, seek medical attention immediately.

■ *Symptoms of Ritalin overdose may include:*
Agitation, confusion, convulsions (may be followed by coma), delirium, dryness of mucous membranes, enlarging of the pupil of the eye, exaggerated feeling of elation, extremely elevated body temperature, flushing, hallucinations, headache, high blood pressure, irregular or rapid heartbeat, muscle twitching, sweating, tremors, vomiting

*Generic name:*

# Ritonavir

*See Norvir, page 376.*

*Brand name:*

# Robaxin

*Pronounced: Ro-BAKS-in*
*Generic name: Methocarbamol*

### Why is this drug prescribed?

Robaxin is prescribed, along with rest, physical therapy, and other measures, for the relief of pain due to severe muscular injuries, sprains, and strains.

### Most important fact about this drug

Robaxin is not a substitute for the rest or physical therapy needed for proper healing.

Although the drug may temporarily make an injury feel better, do not let that tempt you into pushing your recovery. Lifting or exercising too soon may further damage the muscle.

### How should you take this medication?

Take Robaxin exactly as prescribed. Do not take a larger dose or use more often than directed.

■ *If you miss a dose...*
If only an hour or so has passed, take it as soon as you remember. If you do not remember until later, skip the dose and go back to your regular schedule. Do not take 2 doses at once.
■ *Storage instructions...*
Store at room temperature in a tightly closed container.

### What side effects may occur?

Side effects cannot be anticipated. If any develop or change in intensity, inform your doctor as soon as possible. Only your doctor can determine if it is safe for you to continue taking Robaxin.

■ *Side effects may include:*
Blurred vision, dizziness, drowsiness, fever, headache, hives, itching, light-headedness, nasal congestion, nausea, "pinkeye", rash

### Why should this drug not be prescribed?

If you are sensitive to or have ever had an allergic reaction to Robaxin or other drugs of this type, you should not take this medication. Make sure your doctor is aware of any drug reactions you have experienced.

### Special warnings about this medication

Robaxin causes drowsiness and blurred vision. Exercise extra caution while driving or performing tasks that require mental alertness.

Avoid or be careful using alcoholic beverages.

Robaxin may darken urine to brown, green, or black.

### Possible food and drug interactions when taking this medication

If Robaxin is taken with certain other drugs, the effects of either can be increased, decreased, or altered. It is especially important to check with your doctor before combining Robaxin with drugs that slow the nervous system, including:

Narcotic pain relievers such as Percocet and
  Tylenol with Codeine
Sleep aids such as Halcion and Seconal
Tranquilizers such as Xanax and Valium

## Special information
## if you are pregnant or breastfeeding

The effects of Robaxin during pregnancy have not been adequately studied. If you are pregnant or plan to become pregnant, inform your doctor immediately. It is not known if this drug appears in breast milk. If this medication is essential to your health, your doctor may advise you to discontinue breastfeeding your baby until your treatment is finished.

## Recommended dosage

### ADULTS

*Robaxin*

The usual starting dose is 3 tablets taken 4 times a day. The usual long-term dose is 2 tablets taken 4 times a day.

*Robaxin-750*

The usual starting dose is 2 tablets taken 4 times a day. The usual long-term dose is 1 tablet taken every 4 hours or 2 tablets taken 3 times a day.

### CHILDREN

The safety and effectiveness of Robaxin have not been established in children under 12 years of age.

## Overdosage

Any drug taken in excess can have dangerous consequences. If you suspect an overdose of Robaxin, seek emergency medical treatment immediately.

---

*Brand name:*

# Rocaltrol

*Pronounced: Ro-CAL-trol*
*Generic name: Calcitriol*

## Why is this drug prescribed?

Rocaltrol is a synthetic form of vitamin D used to treat people on dialysis who have hypocalcemia (abnormally low blood calcium levels) and resulting bone damage. Rocaltrol is also prescribed to treat low blood calcium levels in people who have hypoparathyroidism (decreased functioning of the parathyroid glands). When functioning correctly, these glands help control the level of calcium in the blood.

## Most important fact about this drug

While you are taking Rocaltrol, your doctor may want you to follow a special diet or take calcium supplements. This is an important part of your therapy. On the other hand, too high a calcium level can be harmful. If you are already taking any medications containing calcium or calcium supplements, make sure you doctor knows about it.

## How should you take this medication?

Be sure to get enough fluids and avoid dehydration while taking Rocaltrol.

■ *If you miss a dose...*
If you take 1 dose every other day, and you remember before the next day, take the forgotten dose immediately, then go back to your regular schedule. If you do not remember until the next day, take the dose immediately, skip a day, then go back to your regular schedule.

If you take 1 dose every day, take it as soon as you remember. Then go back to your regular schedule. If you do not remember until the next day, skip the dose you missed and go back to your regular schedule.

If you take Rocaltrol more than once a day, take the forgotten dose as soon as you remember. If it is almost time for your next dose, skip the one you missed and go back to your regular schedule.

Do not take 2 doses at once.

■ *Storage instructions...*
Keep away from heat and light. Keep out of reach of children.

## What side effects may occur?

Side effects cannot be anticipated. If any develop or change in intensity, inform your doctor as soon as possible. Only your doctor can determine if it is safe for you to continue taking Rocaltrol.

■ *More common side effects occurring early may include:*
Bone pain, constipation, dry mouth, extreme sleepiness, headache, metallic taste, muscle pain, nausea, vomiting, weakness

■ *More common side effects occurring later may include:*
Abnormal thirst, decreased sex drive, elevated blood cholesterol levels, excessive urination, extremely high body temperature, high blood pressure, inflamed eyes, intolerance to light, irregular heartbeat, itchy skin, kidney problems, loss of appetite, nighttime urination, runny nose, weight loss, yellowish skin

■ *Rare side effects may include:*
Mental disturbances, red patches (irregular or circular shape) on arms and hands

Excessive amounts of Vitamin D may cause abnormally high calcium levels in the blood.

### Why should this drug not be prescribed?
You should not use Rocaltrol if you have high blood levels of calcium, or if you have vitamin D poisoning.

### Special warnings about this medication
You should not take additional doses of vitamin D while taking Rocaltrol. People who are on dialysis should not take antacids containing magnesium (such as Maalox) while taking Rocaltrol.

Your doctor will monitor your calcium levels while you are taking Rocaltrol.

While taking Rocaltrol, you should have an adequate daily intake of calcium, either from foods (such as milk and dairy products) or from a calcium supplement. Your doctor will estimate your daily calcium intake before you take this drug to see if you will require more calcium.

### Possible food and drug interactions when taking this medication
If Rocaltrol is taken with certain other drugs, the effects of either could be increased, decreased, or altered. It is especially important to check with your doctor before combining Rocaltrol with the following:

Antacids containing magnesium, such as Maalox
Calcium supplements
Cholestyramine (Questran)
Digitalis (Lanoxin)
Vitamin D pills

### Special information if you are pregnant or breastfeeding
The effects of Rocaltrol during pregnancy have not been adequately studied. If you are pregnant or plan to become pregnant, inform your doctor immediately. Pregnant women should use Rocaltrol only if the possible benefit outweighs any possible risk to the unborn baby.

Rocaltrol may appear in breast milk. Because it may affect a nursing infant, you should not use Rocaltrol while you are breastfeeding.

### Recommended dosage
ADULTS

*For People on Dialysis*
The suggested beginning dose is 0.25 microgram daily. Your doctor may increase the dose.

People with normal or only slightly low blood calcium levels may find it helpful to take 0.25 microgram every other day.

*For Low Calcium Levels Due to Hypoparathyroidism*
The suggested beginning dose is 0.25 microgram daily, taken in the morning. Your doctor may increase the dose.

For most adults, regular doses ranging from 0.5 to 2 micrograms daily are effective.

CHILDREN

*For Low Calcium Levels Due to Hypoparathyroidism*
The starting dose is 0.25 microgram, taken in the morning.

For most children 6 years and older, doses ranging from 0.5 to 2 micrograms per day are effective.

Children from 1 to 5 years old are usually given 0.25 to 0.75 microgram a day.

### Overdosage
Any medication taken in excess can have serious consequences. Severe overdosage of Rocaltrol may cause serious effects, such as extremely high blood levels of calcium. If you suspect an overdose, seek medical help immediately.

■ *Symptoms of Rocaltrol overdose may include:*
Coma, confusion, extreme drowsiness

*Brand name:*

# Rogaine

*Pronounced: ROW-gain*
*Generic name: Minoxidil*

### Why is this drug prescribed?
Rogaine is a hair growth stimulant. It is applied directly to the scalp, and is used to treat baldness in men and thinning hair in women. Previously available only by prescription, it can now be purchased over the counter.

## Most important fact about this drug

Rogaine must be used twice a day for at least 4 months before new hair growth can be expected. If you stop using Rogaine you will probably shed the new hair within a few months. Larger or more frequent doses do not speed up or increase hair growth, but do increase the possibility of side effects.

## How should you use this medication?

Use this medication exactly as directed. Do not use more than is recommended. Applying too much increases the chance of side effects.

You may wash your hair before applying Rogaine but your hair and scalp should be dry before applying the medication. Be sure to apply Rogaine directly to the scalp; applying it to the hair will not help the hair grow.

After you apply Rogaine, it must remain on the scalp for at least 4 hours so it can be properly absorbed.

If you use your fingertips to apply Rogaine, be sure to wash your hands thoroughly when you are finished. You may see a slight residue on your hair after the Rogaine dries. This is harmless and does not affect Rogaine's action.

Do not get the medication on other parts of your body.

■ *If you miss a dose...*
Resume your regular schedule with the next application. Do not increase the amount you apply.

■ *Storage instructions...*
The spray attachment or applicator can be left on the bottle when not in use. It will not leak. The spray extender need be removed only when traveling. Store at room temperature out of reach of children.

## What side effects may occur?

Side effects cannot be anticipated. If any develop or change in intensity, inform your doctor as soon as possible. Only your doctor can determine if it is safe for you to continue using Rogaine.

■ *More common side effects may include:*
Itching or irritation of the scalp

■ *Less common side effects may include:*
Aches and pains, arthritis symptoms, anxiety, back pain, blood disorders, bone fractures, bronchitis, changes in blood pressure, changes in pulse rate, chest pain, depression, diarrhea, dizziness, dry skin/scalp flaking, ear infections, eczema, exhaustion, facial swelling, faintness, fluid retention, genital infections and irritation, growth of excess body hair and facial hair in women, headache, hives, increased hair loss, light-headedness, menstrual and breast changes, nausea, pinkeye (conjunctivitis), pounding heartbeat, redness of skin, runny nose, sexual dysfunction, sinus inflammation, vision changes, vomiting, weight gain

## Why should this drug not be prescribed?

Rogaine should not be used if you are under 18 years of age or have ever had an allergic reaction to this medication. If you experience sudden or patchy hair loss and have no family history of gradual hair loss, Rogaine is probably not for you. Instead, check with your doctor. An underlying disease or drug reaction may be at work.

Do not apply Rogaine if your scalp is inflamed, infected, irritated, or painful.

## Special warnings about this medication

Rogaine is for external use only.

You should have a healthy, normal scalp before starting treatment with Rogaine.

Even though Rogaine is applied to your skin, it is absorbed into your bloodstream. If you use more medication than is recommended or suffer from irritations on your scalp, side effects can occur elsewhere in your body. In tablet form, minoxidil, a high blood pressure medication, can cause salt and water retention, generalized and local fluid retention, rapid heartbeat, angina (crushing pain, usually in the chest, accompanied by a choking feeling), and inflammation of the sac that surrounds the heart. Although the likelihood is very small, these symptoms could possibly occur with the use of Rogaine, and people with heart disease would be at particular risk. Rogaine could also have adverse effects when used by people taking medications to lower their blood pressure.

Rogaine contains alcohol. Be careful not to get it in your eyes. If it gets into your eyes or on sensitive parts of your skin, wash the area well with cool tap water. If the irritation does not subside, contact your doctor.

Rogaine should not be used with other topical medications, such as steroids, that increase skin absorption, or with petroleum jelly.

Hair loss may actually continue for 2 weeks after you start treatment with Rogaine. If you continue to shed hair after that, consult your doctor.

Some people using Rogaine, especially women, have experienced growth of hair on the face—including the forehead and temples. Be very careful to apply the medication only to your scalp.

### Possible food and drug interactions when using this medication

No interactions with Rogaine have been reported.

### Special information
### if you are pregnant or breastfeeding

If you are pregnant or plan to become pregnant, check with your doctor before using Rogaine. Also check if you plan to breastfeed your baby.

### Recommended dosage

ADULTS

Apply 1 milliliter of Rogaine to the total affected areas of the scalp 2 times a day. The total daily dosage should not be more than 2 milliliters. Make sure the hair and scalp are dry before applying the medication. It could take up to 4 months of twice-daily use to see results. If hair regrowth occurs, continue to apply Rogaine 2 times a day for additional or continued hair regrowth.

### Overdosage

Any medication taken in excess can have serious consequences. If you suspect an overdose, seek medical attention immediately.

Brand name:

# Rolaids

See Antacids, page 30.

Brand name:

# Rowasa

*Pronounced: ROH-ace-ah*
*Generic name: Mesalamine*
*Other brand names: Pentasa, Asacol*

### Why is this drug prescribed?

Rowasa Suspension Enema, Pentasa, and Asacol are used to treat mild to moderate ulcerative colitis (inflammation of the large intestine and rectum).

Rowasa Suspension Enema is also prescribed for inflammation of the lower colon, and inflammation of the rectum.

Rowasa Suppositories are used to treat inflammation of the rectum.

### Most important fact about this drug

Mesalamine, the active ingredient in these products, has been known to cause side effects such as:

Bloody diarrhea
Cramping
Fever
Rash
Severe headache
Sudden, severe stomach pain

If you develop any of these symptoms, stop taking this medication and consult your doctor.

### How should you use this medication?

*To Use Rowasa Suspension Enema*

1. Rowasa Suspension Enema comes in boxes of 7 bottles each. After the foil on the box has been unwrapped, all Rowasa Suspension Enemas should be used promptly, following your doctor's instructions. The Suspension Enema is normally off-white to tan in color, but may darken over time once its foil cover is unwrapped. You may still use the enema if it is slightly discolored, but do not use Rowasa Suspension Enema if it is dark brown. If you have any questions about using Rowasa Suspension Enema, contact your doctor.
2. Use Rowasa Suspension Enema at bedtime.
3. Shake the bottle thoroughly.
4. Uncover the applicator tip.
5. You may find it easier to use Rowasa Suspension Enema if you lie down on your left side, extending your left leg and bending your right leg forward for a comfortable balance. An alternative position is to squat with your knees to your chest.
6. Pointing the applicator tip up, gently insert the tip into the rectum.
7. Squeeze the bottle steadily to discharge the contents.
8. The enema should be retained all night (8 hours) for best results.

*To Use Rowasa Suppositories*

1. Rowasa Suppositories should be used twice a day.

2. You should handle the suppositories as little as possible, because they are designed to melt at body temperature.

3. Remove one suppository from the strip of suppositories.

4. While holding the suppository upright, carefully remove the foil wrapper.

5. Using gentle pressure, insert the suppository (with the pointed end first) completely into the rectum.

6. The suppository should be retained for 1 to 3 hours or longer for best results.

*To take Pentasa or Asacol*
Swallow the capsule or tablet whole. Do not break, crush, or chew it before swallowing.

You may notice what looks like small beads in your stool. These are just empty shells that are left after the medication has been absorbed into your body. However, if this continues, check with your doctor.

■ *If you miss a dose...*
Take it as soon as you remember. If it is almost time for your next dose, skip the one you missed and go back to your regular schedule. Never take 2 doses at the same time.

■ *Storage instructions...*
Store these products at room temperature.

### What side effects may occur?
Side effects cannot be anticipated. If any side effects develop or change in intensity, tell your doctor immediately. Only your doctor can determine whether it is safe to continue using this medication.

■ *More common side effects of Rowasa Suspension Enema may include:*
Flu-like symptoms, gas, headache, nausea, stomach pain/cramps

■ *Less common side effects of Rowasa Suspension Enema may include:*
Back pain, bloating, diarrhea, dizziness, fever, hemorrhoids, itching, leg/joint pain, pain on insertion of enema tip, rash, rectal pain, sore throat, tiredness, weakness

■ *Rare side effects of Rowasa Suspension Enema may include:*
Constipation, hair loss, insomnia, swelling of the arms or legs, urinary burning

■ *More common side effects of Rowasa Suppositories may include:*
Diarrhea, dizziness, gas, headache, stomach pain

■ *Less common side effects of Rowasa Suppositories may include:*
Acne, cold symptoms, fever, inflammation of the colon, nausea, rash, rectal pain, swelling, weakness

■ *More common side effects of Pentasa and Asacol may include:*
Diarrhea, headache, nausea

■ *Less common or rare side effects of Pentasa and Asacol may include:*
Abdominal pain, abdominal swelling, acne, belching, blood in the urine, bloody diarrhea, breast pain, bruising, conjunctivitis, constipation, depression, difficulty sleeping, difficulty swallowing, dizziness, dry skin, duodenal ulcer, eczema, fever, fluid retention, general feeling of illness, hair loss, hives, inflammation of the pancreas, itching, joint pain, Kawasaki-like syndrome (rash, swollen glands, fever, mouth inflammation, strawberry tongue), lack or loss of appetite, leg cramps, menstrual irregularities, mouth sores and infections, muscle pain, nail problems, palpitations (rapid, fluttery heartbeat), rash, rectal bleeding, sensitivity to light, skin eruptions, sleepiness, stomach and intestinal bleeding, stool changes, sweating, thirst, tingling or pins and needles, ulcer of the esophagus, uncontrollable bowel movements, urinary frequency, weakness, worsening of ulcerative colitis, vomiting

### Why should this drug not be prescribed?
These products should not be used by anyone who is allergic or sensitive to mesalamine or their other ingredients.

Pentasa and Asacol should not be used if you are allergic or sensitive to salicylates (aspirin).

### Special warnings about this medication
Your doctor should check your kidney function while you are taking mesalamine, especially if you have a history of kidney disease or you are using other anti-inflammatory drugs such as Dipentum.

You should use mesalamine cautiously if you are allergic to sulfasalazine (Azulfidine). If you develop a rash or fever, you should stop using the medication and notify your doctor.

Some people using mesalamine have developed flare-ups of their colitis.

Rare cases of pericarditis, in which the membrane surrounding the heart becomes inflamed, have been reported with products containing mesalamine. Symptoms may include chest, neck, and shoulder pain, and shortness of breath.

Rowasa Suspension Enema contains a sulfite that may cause allergic reactions in some people. These reactions may include shock and severe, possibly fatal asthma attacks. Most people aren't sensitive to sulfites. However, some people with asthma might be sensitive and should take any medication containing sulfites cautiously.

Rowasa Suspension Enema may stain clothes and fabrics.

### Possible food and drug interactions when taking this medication

If these products are taken with certain other drugs, the effects of either could be increased, decreased, or altered. It is especially important to check with your doctor before combining Rowasa Suspension Enema or Rowasa Suppositories with sulfasalazine (Azulfidine).

### Special information if you are pregnant or breastfeeding

Pregnant women should use mesalamine only if clearly needed. Mesalamine has been found in breast milk. If this medication is essential to your health your doctor may advise you to discontinue breastfeeding until your treatment is finished.

### Recommended dosage

ADULTS

*Rowasa Suspension Enema*
The usual dose is 1 rectal enema (60 milliliters) per day, preferably used at bedtime and retained for about 8 hours. Treatment time usually lasts from 3 to 6 weeks, although improvement may be seen within 3 to 21 days.

*Rowasa Suppositories*
The usual dose is one rectal suppository (500 milligrams) 2 times a day. To get the most benefit from a Rowasa Suppository, it should be retained for 1 to 3 hours or longer. Treatment time usually lasts from 3 to 6 weeks, although improvement may be seen within 3 to 21 days.

*Pentasa Capsules*
The usual dose is 4 capsules taken 4 times a day for a total of 16 capsules daily.

*Asacol Tablets*
The recommended dose is 2 tablets 3 times a day for 6 weeks.

CHILDREN

Safety and effectiveness in children have not been established.

### Overdosage

There have been no proven reports of serious effects resulting from overdoses of Rowasa. An overdose of Pentasa or Asacol could cause any of the following symptoms:

Confusion, diarrhea, drowsiness, headache, hyperventilation, ringing in the ears, sweating, vomiting

Any medication taken in excess can have serious consequences. If you suspect an overdose, seek medical attention immediately.

Brand name:

# Roxicet

See Percocet, page 407.

Brand name:

# Rufen

See Motrin, page 337.

Brand name:

# Ru-Tuss Tablets

Pronounced: ROO-tus
Generic ingredients: Phenylephrine hydrochloride, Phenylpropanolamine hydrochloride, Chlorpheniramine maleate, Hyoscyamine sulfate, Atropine sulfate, Scopolamine hydrobromide

### Why is this drug prescribed?

Ru-Tuss is an antihistamine/decongestant that relieves the runny, stuffy nose, nasal drip, itching, watery eyes, and scratchy, itchy throat caused by allergies, colds, and other irritations of the sinus, nose, and upper respiratory tract. Chlorpheniramine, the antihistamine, relieves watery eyes, dries up post-nasal drip, and reduces sneezing. Phenylephrine and phenylpropanolamine combine to reduce congestion and make breathing easier. Hyoscyamine, atropine, and scopolamine, commonly called belladonna alkaloids, enhance the drying effects of Ru-Tuss.

### Most important fact about this drug

Ru-Tuss tablets may cause drowsiness. Do not drive, operate machinery or participate in any hazardous activity that requires full mental alertness until you know how you react to this medication.

### How should you take this medication?

Take this medication exactly as prescribed. The tablets act continuously for 10 to 12 hours. Tablets should be swallowed whole, not crushed or chewed.

If this medicine dries out your mouth, sucking on hard candy or chewing gum may help.

■ *If you miss a dose...*
Take it as soon as you remember. If it is almost time for your next dose, skip the one you missed and go back to your regular schedule. Never take 2 doses at the same time.

■ *Storage instructions...*
Store it at room temperature.

### What side effects may occur?

Side effects cannot be anticipated. If any develop or change in intensity, inform your doctor as soon as possible. Only your doctor can determine if it is safe for you to continue taking Ru-Tuss.

■ *Side effects may include:*
Allergic reactions (rash, hives), blood disorders, blurred vision, constipation, diarrhea, difficulty sleeping (insomnia), dilated pupils, dizziness, drowsiness, dry mouth, dry nose and other mucous membranes, exhaustion, faintness, frequent urination, giddiness, headache, hyperirritability, increased chest congestion, itching, lack of coordination, loss of appetite, low blood pressure/high blood pressure, nausea, nervousness, painful or difficult urination, pounding heartbeat, rapid heartbeat, ringing in the ears, stomach upset, tightness in the chest, vision changes, vomiting

### Why should this drug not be prescribed?

Ru-Tuss should be avoided if you are pregnant, if you are sensitive to or have ever had an allergic reaction to antihistamines or any of the ingredients in this medication, if you have glaucoma or bronchial asthma, or if you are taking antidepressant drugs known as MAO inhibitors (Nardil, for example). Ru-Tuss should not be given to children under 12 years of age.

### Special warnings about this medication

This medication can make you feel drowsy. Be careful driving, operating machinery, or using appliances.

Ru-Tuss should be used with care if you have a bladder obstruction, high blood pressure, cardiovascular disease, or an overactive thyroid.

### Possible food and drug interactions when taking this medication

Ru-Tuss may increase the effects of alcohol. Do not drink alcohol while taking this medication.

Do not take Ru-Tuss while taking antidepressant drugs such as Nardil and Parnate.

If Ru-Tuss is taken with certain other drugs, the effects of either could be increased, decreased, or altered. It is especially important to check with your doctor before combining Ru-Tuss with the following:

Sleep medications such as Halcion and Dalmane
Tranquilizers such as Xanax and Valium

### Special information if you are pregnant or breastfeeding

Ru-Tuss is not recommended for use by pregnant women. If you are pregnant or plan to become pregnant, notify your doctor immediately.

### Recommended dosage

ADULTS AND CHILDREN 12 YEARS OR OLDER

The usual dosage is 1 tablet in the morning and 1 tablet in the evening. This drug is not recommended for children under 12.

### Overdosage

Any medication taken in excess can have serious consequences. Convulsions and death may occur from antihistamine overdose in children and infants. If you suspect an overdose, seek medical treatment immediately.

■ *Symptoms of Ru-Tuss overdose may include:*
Coma, delirium, fever, rapid breathing, respiratory failure, stupor

*Brand name:*

# Rynatan

*Pronounced: RYE-nuh-tan*
*Generic ingredients: Phenylephrine tannate,*
*Chlorpheniramine tannate, Pyrilamine tannate*

## Why is this drug prescribed?

Rynatan is an antihistamine/decongestant that relieves runny nose and nasal congestion caused by the common cold, inflamed sinuses, hay fever, and other upper respiratory conditions. Chlorpheniramine and pyrilamine, the antihistamines in the combination, reduce itching and swelling and dry up secretions from the eyes, nose, and throat. Phenylephrine, the decongestant, reduces congestion and makes breathing easier.

## Most important fact about this drug

This medication can make you drowsy. You should not drive or operate dangerous machinery or participate in any hazardous activity that requires full mental alertness until you know how you react to Rynatan.

## How should you take this medication?

Take this medication exactly as prescribed.

■ *If you miss a dose...*
Take it as soon as you remember. If it is almost time for the next dose, skip the one you missed and go back to your regular schedule. Do not take 2 doses at once.
■ *Storage instructions...*
Store at room temperature in a tightly closed container.

## What side effects may occur?

Side effects cannot be anticipated. If any develop or change in intensity, inform your doctor as soon as possible. Only your doctor can determine if it is safe for you to continue taking Rynatan.

■ *Side effects may include:*
Drowsiness, dry nose, mouth, and throat, excessive calm (sedation), stomach and intestinal problems

## Why should this drug not be prescribed?

Rynatan should not be given to newborn babies, or used by nursing mothers or people who are sensitive to or have ever had an allergic reaction to any of its ingredients or to similar antihistamine and decongestant combinations.

## Special warnings about this medication

Use Rynatan with care if you have high blood pressure, heart disease, circulatory problems, an overactive thyroid gland, diabetes, the eye condition known as narrow-angle glaucoma, or an enlarged prostate gland.

If you are taking a drug classified as an MAO inhibitor, such as the antidepressants Nardil and Parnate, or have taken one within the past two weeks, you should avoid taking Rynatan.

The antihistamines in Rynatan are more likely to cause dizziness, sedation, and low blood pressure in elderly people. Antihistamines also can cause excitement, especially in children.

## Possible food and drug interactions when taking this medication

Rynatan may increase the effects of alcohol. Do not drink alcohol while taking this medication.

If Rynatan is taken with certain other drugs, the effects of either could be increased, decreased, or altered. It is especially important to check with your doctor before combining Rynatan with the following:

Drugs classified as MAO inhibitors, including the antidepressants Nardil and Parnate
Sedatives such as Halcion and Dalmane
Tranquilizers such as Xanax and Valium

## Special information if you are pregnant or breastfeeding

The effects of Rynatan during pregnancy have not been adequately studied. If you are pregnant or plan to become pregnant, notify your doctor immediately. Rynatan should not be taken if you are breastfeeding.

## Recommended dosage

RYNATAN TABLETS

*Adults*
The usual dosage is 1 or 2 tablets every 12 hours.

RYNATAN-S PEDIATRIC SUSPENSION

*Children Over Age 6:*
The usual dosage is 1 to 2 teaspoonfuls (5 to 10 milliliters) every 12 hours.

*Children Aged 2 to 6:*
The usual dosage is one-half to 1 teaspoonful (2.5 to 5 milliliters) every 12 hours.

*Children Under Age 2:*
Your doctor will determine the dose.

### Overdosage

Any medication taken in excess can have serious consequences. Antihistamine overdose in young children can lead to convulsions and death. If you suspect an overdose, seek medical treatment immediately.

Symptoms of Rynatan overdose range from sedation to overstimulation (from restlessness to convulsions).

*Brand name:*

# Rythmol

*Pronounced: RITH-mol*
*Generic name: Propafenone*

### Why is this drug prescribed?

Rythmol is used to help correct certain life-threatening heartbeat irregularities (ventricular arrhythmias).

### Most important fact about this drug

There is a possibility that Rythmol may cause new heartbeat irregularities or make the existing ones worse. Rythmol is therefore used only for serious problems, and should be accompanied by periodic electrocardiograms (EKGs) prior to and during treatment. Discuss this with your doctor.

### How should you take this medication?

Rythmol may be taken with food or on an empty stomach.

Take Rythmol exactly as prescribed. It works best when there is a constant amount of the drug in the blood, so you should take it at evenly spaced intervals.

■ *If you miss a dose...*
Unless otherwise instructed by your doctor, take the forgotten dose as soon as possible. However, if it is almost time for your next dose or more than 4 hours have passed, skip the missed dose and go back to your regular schedule. Never take a double dose.

■ *Storage instructions...*
Keep this medication in the container it came in, tightly closed, away from direct light, at room temperature.

### What side effects may occur?

Side effects cannot be anticipated. If any develop or change in intensity, inform your doctor as soon as possible. Only your doctor can determine if it is safe for you to continue taking Rythmol.

The most common side effects affect the digestive, cardiovascular, and nervous systems. The most serious are heartbeat abnormalities.

■ *More common side effects may include:*
Constipation, dizziness, heartbeat abnormalities, nausea, unusual taste in the mouth, vomiting

■ *Other side effects may include:*
Abdominal pain or cramps, anemia, angina (chest pain), anxiety, blood disorders, blurred vision, breathing difficulties, bruising, cardiac arrest, coma, confusion, congestive heart failure, depression, diarrhea, dreaming abnormalities, drowsiness, dry mouth, eye irritation, fainting or near fainting, fatigue, fever, flushing, gas, hair loss, headache, heart palpitations, heartbeat abnormalities (rapid, irregular, slow), hot flashes, impotence, increased blood sugar, indigestion, inflamed esophagus, stomach, or intestines, insomnia, itching, joint pain, kidney disease, kidney failure, lack of coordination, liver dysfunction, loss of appetite, loss of balance, low blood pressure, memory loss, muscle cramps, muscle weakness, numbness, pain, psychosis, rash, red or purple spots on the skin, ringing in the ears, seizures, speech abnormalities, sweating, swelling due to fluid retention, tingling or pins and needles, tremor, unusual smell sensations, vertigo, vision abnormalities, weakness

### Why should this drug not be prescribed?

Do not take Rythmol if you have ever had an allergic reaction to or are sensitive to it. Your doctor will not prescribe Rythmol if you are suffering from any of the following conditions:

Abnormally slow heartbeat
Certain heartbeat irregularities, such as atrioventricular block or "sick sinus" syndrome, that have not been corrected by a pacemaker
Cardiogenic shock (shock due to a weak heart)
Chronic bronchitis or emphysema
Congestive heart failure that is not well controlled
Mineral (electrolyte) imbalance
Severe low blood pressure

## Special warnings about this medication

If you have congestive heart failure, this condition must be brought under full medical control before you start taking Rythmol.

If you have a pacemaker, the pacemaker's settings must be monitored—and possibly reprogrammed—while you are taking Rythmol.

There is some risk that Rythmol may interfere with your body's normal ability to manufacture blood cells. Too few white blood cells may cause signs and symptoms that mimic infection. If you experience fever, chills, or sore throat while taking Rythmol—especially during the first 3 months of treatment—notify your doctor right away.

Rythmol may cause a lupus-like illness characterized by rashes and arthritic symptoms. If you have been taking Rythmol and testing shows that your blood contains ANA (antinuclear antibodies), your doctor may want to discontinue the medication.

## Possible food and drug interactions when taking this medication

If Rythmol is taken with certain other drugs, the effects of either could be increased, decreased, or altered. It is especially important to check with your doctor before combining Rythmol with the following:

Beta blockers such as Inderal and Lopressor
Cimetidine (Tagamet)
Digitalis (Lanoxin)
Local anesthetics (such as Novocain used during dental work)
Quinidine (Cardioquin)
Warfarin (blood thinners such as Coumadin)

## Special information if you are pregnant or breastfeeding

If you are pregnant or plan to become pregnant, inform your doctor immediately. Because of a possible risk of birth defects, Rythmol is not recommended during pregnancy unless the benefit to the mother outweighs the potential risk to the unborn baby.

It is not known whether Rythmol appears in breast milk. You are advised not to take Rythmol if you are nursing a baby. If treatment with Rythmol is essential to your health, your doctor may advise you to stop breastfeeding until your treatment is finished.

## Recommended dosage

### ADULTS

In most cases, treatment with Rythmol begins in the hospital.

Your doctor will tailor your dosage according to your individual condition and the presence of other disorders.

The usual initial dose of Rythmol is 150 milligrams every 8 hours. Your doctor may increase the dosage depending on how you respond to the initial dosage. The maximum recommended daily dosage of Rythmol is 900 milligrams.

### CHILDREN

Safety and effectiveness have not been established in children.

### OLDER ADULTS

The doctor will increase the dosage more slowly at the beginning of treatment.

## Overdosage

Any medication taken in excess can have serious consequences. If you suspect an overdose of Rythmol, seek medical attention immediately.

■ *Symptoms of Rythmol overdose, which are usually most severe within the first 3 hours of taking the medication, may include:*
Convulsions (rarely), heartbeat irregularities, low blood pressure, sleepiness

*Generic name:*

# Salsalate

*See Disalcid, page 168.*

*Brand name:*

# Sandimmune

*Pronounced: SAN-dim-ewn*
*Generic name: Cyclosporine*
*Other brand name: Neoral*

## Why is this drug prescribed?

Sandimmune is given after organ transplant surgery to help prevent rejection of organs (kidney, heart, or liver) by holding down the body's immune system. It is also used to treat long-term rejection in people previously treated with other immunosuppressant drugs, such as Imuran. Neoral is a newer formulation of cyclosporine.

Some doctors also prescribe Sandimmune to treat alopecia areata (localized areas of hair loss), aplastic anemia (shortage of red and white blood cells and platelets), Crohn's disease (chronic inflammation of the digestive tract), and nephropathy (kidney disease). Sandimmune is sometimes used in the treatment of severe skin disorders, including psoriasis and dermatomyositis (inflammation of the skin and muscles causing weakness and rash). The drug is also used in procedures involving bone marrow, the pancreas, and the lungs.

Sandimmune is always given with prednisone or a similar steroid. It is available in capsules and liquid, or as an injection.

### Most important fact about this drug

If you take Sandimmune orally over a period of time, your doctor will monitor your blood levels of cyclosporine to make sure your body is receiving the correct amount of Sandimmune. The reason for this repeated testing is that the absorption of this drug in the body is erratic. Constant monitoring is necessary to prevent toxicity due to overdosing or to prevent possible organ rejection due to underdosing. It is important to note that Sandimmune may need to be taken by mouth for an indefinite period following surgery.

### How should you take this medication?

Take the Sandimmune capsule or oral liquid at the same time every day. You may take the medication either with a meal or between meals, but be consistent.

To make Sandimmune oral liquid more palatable, you may mix it with room-temperature milk, chocolate milk, or orange juice. Neoral oral solution may be mixed with room-temperature orange or pineapple juice. It does not taste good in milk. Use a container made of glass, not plastic. Never let the mixture stand; drink it as soon as you prepare it. To make sure you get your full dose, rinse the glass with a little more liquid and drink that too.

You should maintain good dental hygiene and see your dentist frequently for cleaning to prevent tenderness, bleeding, and gum enlargement.

After you use the dosage syringe to transfer the oral solution to a glass, dry the outside of the syringe with a clean towel and put it away. Do not rinse or wash it. If you do have to clean it, make sure it is thoroughly dry before you use it again.

You may notice an odor when you open the capsule container; this is nothing to worry about and will soon dissipate.

■ *If you miss a dose...*
If fewer than 12 hours have passed, take it as soon as you remember. If it is almost time for the next dose, skip the one you missed and go back to your regular schedule. Do not take 2 doses at once.

■ *Storage instructions...*
Store both the capsules and the oral solution below 86°F; do not store the liquid in the refrigerator. Keep the liquid from freezing. Sandimmune liquid, once opened, must be used within 2 months.

### What side effects may occur?

Side effects cannot be anticipated. If any appear or change in intensity, inform your doctor immediately. Only your doctor can determine if it is safe for you to continue taking Sandimmune. The principal side effects of Sandimmune are high blood pressure, hirsutism (unusual growth of hair), kidney damage, excessive growth of the gums, and tremor.

■ *Other common side effects may include:*
Abdominal discomfort, acne, convulsions, cramps, diarrhea, flushing, headache, liver damage, lymph system tumor, nausea, numbness or tingling, sinus inflammation, vomiting

■ *Less common side effects may include:*
Allergic reactions, anemia, appetite loss, blood disorders, brittle fingernails, confusion, conjunctivitis (pinkeye), fever, fluid retention, hearing loss, hiccups, high blood sugar, muscle pain, peptic ulcer, ringing in the ears, stomach inflammation

■ *Rare side effects may include:*
Anxiety, blood in the urine, breast development in males, chest pain, constipation, depression, hair breaking, heart attack, itching, joint pain, lymph disorders, mouth sores, night sweats, sluggishness, stomach and upper intestinal bleeding, swallowing difficulty, tingling, visual disturbance, weakness, weight loss

### Why should this drug not be prescribed?

Do not take these products if you have ever had an allergic reaction to them. Avoid Sandimmune by injection if you have ever had an allergic reaction to an injection of the drug or you are especially sensitive to castor oil.

### Special warnings about this medication

When your immune system is suppressed by Sandimmune, you are at increased risk of infection and of certain malignancies, including skin cancer and lymph system cancer.

High-dose Sandimmune is toxic to the liver and kidneys and may cause serious kidney damage. Because this toxicity has symptoms similar to those of transplant rejection, you must be monitored closely. If your body is trying hard to reject a transplanted organ, your doctor will probably allow the rejection to occur rather than give you a very high dose of Sandimmune.

Sandimmune and Neoral are not directly interchangeable. Your doctor may need to adjust the dosage if you switch.

If you take large doses of a prednisone-like drug called methylprednisolone (Medrol) along with Sandimmune, you may be at increased risk of convulsions.

Use a barrier method of contraception, such as diaphragms or condoms, during Sandimmune therapy. Do not use oral contraceptive pills without your doctor's approval.

Do not try to change dosage forms without consulting your doctor.

### Possible food and drug interactions when taking this medication

Avoid getting vaccinations and immunizations while you are taking Sandimmune. The drug may make vaccinations less effective or increase your risk of contracting an illness from a live vaccine.

Avoid grapefruit and grapefruit juice while taking this drug.

If Sandimmune is taken with certain other drugs, the effects of either could be increased, decreased, or altered. It is especially important to check with your doctor before combining Sandimmune with the following:

Allopurinol (Zyloprim)
Amphotericin B (Fungizone, Abelcet)
Bromocriptine (Parlodel)
Calcium-blocking heart and blood pressure medications such as Calan, Cardene, Procardia, and Cardizem

Carbamazepine (Tegretol)
Cimetidine (Tagamet)
Clarithromycin (Biaxin)
Danazol (Danocrine)
Diclofenac (Voltaren, Cataflam)
Digoxin (Lanoxin, Lanoxicaps)
Erythromycin (E.E.S., Erythrocin, others)
Fluconazole (Diflucan)
Gentamicin (Garamycin)
Itraconazole (Sporanox)
Ketoconazole (Nizoral)
Lovastatin (Mevacor)
Melphalan (Alkeran)
Methylprednisolone (Depo-Medrol, Medrol, Solu-Medrol)
Metoclopramide (Reglan)
Nafcillin (Unipen)
Octreotide (Sandostatin)
Phenobarbital
Phenytoin (Dilantin)
Potassium-sparing diuretics (Dyrenium, Midamor, Aldactone)
Prednisolone (Delta-Cortef, Prelone)
Ranitidine (Zantac)
Rifampin (Rifadin, Rifamate, Rimactane)
Ticlopidine (Ticlid)
Tobramycin (Nebcin)
Trimethoprim/sulfamethoxazole (Bactrim, Septra)
Vancomycin (Vancocin)

### Special information if you are pregnant or breastfeeding

The effects of Sandimmune in pregnancy have not been adequately studied. If you are pregnant or plan to become pregnant, inform your doctor immediately. Sandimmune should be used during pregnancy only if the benefit justifies the potential risk to the unborn child. Since Sandimmune appears in breast milk, it should not be used during breastfeeding. If you are a new mother, you may need to choose between taking Sandimmune and breastfeeding your baby.

### Recommended dosage

Your doctor will tailor your dosage of Sandimmune in accordance with your body's response. Expect a single dose of 15 milligrams per 2.2 pounds of body weight 4 to 12 hours before a transplant and 1 dose daily for 1 to 2 weeks after the operation. After that, the doctor may keep you on a daily dose of 5 to 10 milligrams per 2.2 pounds of body weight.

The dosage of Neoral depends on the type of transplant and the other drugs you are taking. It is always taken twice a day.

## Overdosage

Although no specific information is available, an overdose of Sandimmune would be expected to cause liver and kidney problems. Any medication taken in excess can have serious consequences. If you suspect an overdose of Sandimmune, seek medical attention immediately.

*Generic name:*

# Saquinavir

See Invirase, page 263.

*Brand name:*

# Sectral

*Pronounced: SEK-tral*
*Generic name: Acebutolol hydrochloride*

## Why is this drug prescribed?

Sectral, a type of medication known as a beta blocker, is used in the treatment of high blood pressure and abnormal heart rhythms. When used to treat high blood pressure, it is effective used alone or in combination with other high blood pressure medications, particularly with a thiazide-type diuretic. Beta blockers decrease the force and rate of heart contractions, thus reducing pressure within the circulatory system.

## Most important fact about this drug

If you have high blood pressure, you must take Sectral regularly for it to be effective. Since blood pressure declines gradually, it may be several weeks before you get the full benefit of Sectral; and you must continue taking it even if you are feeling well. Sectral does not cure high blood pressure; it merely keeps it under control.

## How should you take this medication?

Sectral can be taken with or without food. Take it exactly as prescribed, even if your symptoms have disappeared.

Try not to miss any doses. If this medication is not taken regularly, your condition may worsen.

■ *If you miss a dose...*
Take the forgotten dose as soon as you remember. If it's within 4 hours of your next scheduled dose, skip the one you missed and go back to your regular schedule. Never take 2 doses at the same time.

■ *Storage instructions...*
Store at room temperature. Keep the container tightly closed. Protect from light.

## What side effects may occur?

Side effects cannot be anticipated. If any develop or change in intensity, inform your doctor as soon as possible. Only your doctor can determine if it is safe for you to continue taking Sectral.

■ *More common side effects may include:*
Abnormal vision, chest pain, constipation, cough, decreased sexual ability, depression, diarrhea, dizziness, fatigue, frequent urination, gas, headache, indigestion, joint pain, nasal inflammation, nausea, shortness of breath or difficulty breathing, strange dreams, swelling due to fluid retention, trouble sleeping, weakness

■ *Less common or rare side effects may include:*
Abdominal pain, anxiety, back pain, burning eyes, cold hands and feet, conjunctivitis, dark urine, excessive urination at night, eye pain, fever, heart failure, impotence, itching, loss of appetite, low blood pressure, muscle pain, nervousness, painful or difficult urination, rash, slow heartbeat, throat inflammation, vomiting, wheezing

## Why should this drug not be prescribed?

If you have heart failure; inadequate blood supply to the circulatory system (cardiogenic shock), heart block (a type of irregular heartbeat), or a severely slow heartbeat, you should not take this medication.

## Special warnings about this medication

If you have had severe congestive heart failure in the past, Sectral should be used with caution.

Sectral should not be stopped suddenly. This can cause increased chest pain and heart attack. Dosage should be gradually reduced.

If you suffer from asthma, seasonal allergies, other bronchial conditions, coronary artery disease, or kidney or liver disease, this medication should be used with caution.

Ask your doctor if you should check your pulse while taking Sectral. This medication can cause your heartbeat to become too slow.

This medication may mask the symptoms of low blood sugar or alter blood sugar levels. If you are diabetic, discuss this with your doctor.

Notify your doctor or dentist that you are taking Sectral if you have a medical emergency, or before you have any surgery.

Tell your doctor if you are taking over-the-counter cold medications and nasal drops. They may interact with Sectral.

If you experience difficulty breathing, or develop hives or large areas of swelling, seek medical attention immediately. You may be having a serious allergic reaction to the medicine.

### Possible food and drug interactions when taking this medication

If Sectral is taken with certain other drugs, the effects of either could be increased, decreased, or altered. It is especially important to check with your doctor before combining Sectral with the following:

Albuterol (the airway-opening drug Ventolin)
Certain blood pressure medicines such as reserpine (Diupres)
Certain over-the-counter cold remedies and nasal drops such as Afrin, Neo-Synephrine, and Sudafed
Nonsteroidal anti-inflammatory drugs such as Motrin and Voltaren
Oral diabetes drugs such as Micronase

### Special information if you are pregnant or breastfeeding

The effects of Sectral during pregnancy have not been adequately studied. If you are pregnant or plan to become pregnant, inform your doctor immediately. Sectral appears in breast milk and could affect a nursing infant. If this medication is essential to your health, your doctor may advise you to discontinue breastfeeding until your treatment with Sectral is finished.

### Recommended dosage

ADULTS

*Hypertension*
The usual initial dose for mild to moderate high blood pressure is 400 milligrams per day. It may be taken in a single daily dose or in 2 doses of 200 milligrams each. The usual daily dosage ranges from 200 to 800 milligrams.

People with severe high blood pressure may take up to 1,200 milligrams per day divided into 2 doses. Sectral may be taken alone or in combination with another high blood pressure medication.

*Irregular heartbeat*
The usual starting dosage is 400 milligrams per day divided into 2 doses. Your doctor may gradually increase the dose to 600 to 1,200 milligrams per day. If your doctor wants you to stop taking this medication, he or she will have you taper off over a period of 2 weeks.

CHILDREN

The safety and effectiveness of Sectral have not been established in children.

OLDER ADULTS

Your doctor will determine the dosage based on your particular needs. Do not take more than 800 milligrams per day.

### Overdosage

Any medication taken in excess can have serious consequences. If you suspect an overdose, seek medical attention immediately.

*There is no specific information available on Sectral; however, overdose symptoms seen with other beta blockers include:*
Difficulty breathing, extremely slow heartbeat, irregular heartbeat, low blood pressure, low blood sugar, seizures, severe congestive heart failure

*Brand names:*

# Seldane and Seldane-D

*Pronounced: SELL-dane*
*Generic name: Terfenadine*

### Why is this drug prescribed?

Seldane is an antihistamine that relieves the sneezing, runny nose, stuffiness, itching, and tearing eyes caused by hay fever. Another form of the drug, Seldane-D, also contains pseudoephedrine, which relieves nasal stuffiness.

Antihistamines work by decreasing the effects of histamine, a chemical the body releases in response to certain irritants. Histamine narrows air passages in the lungs and contributes to inflammation. Antihistamines reduce itching and swelling and dry up secretions from the nose, eyes, and throat.

## Most important fact about this drug

Seldane is chemically different from other antihistamines and causes significantly less drowsiness.

## How should you take this medication?

Take Seldane and Seldane-D only as needed. Do not take more than your doctor has prescribed.

■ *If you miss a dose...*
If you are taking Seldane regularly, take the missed dose as soon as you remember. If it is almost time for the next dose, skip the one you missed and go back to your regular schedule. Never take two doses at the same time.

■ *Storage instructions...*
Store at room temperature. Protect from moisture and extreme heat. Keep out of reach of children.

## What side effects may occur?

Side effects cannot be anticipated. If any develop or change in intensity, inform your doctor as soon as possible. Only your doctor can determine if it is safe for you to continue taking Seldane or Seldane-D.

■ *More common side effects of Seldane may include:*
Drowsiness, fatigue, headache, stomach and intestinal problems (nausea, vomiting, change in bowel habits)

■ *Less common or rare side effects of Seldane may include:*
Confusion, cough, depression, dizziness, dry mouth/nose/throat, excessive or spontaneous flow of milk, fainting, frequent urination, hair thinning or loss, hepatitis, hives, increased appetite, irregular heartbeat, insomnia, itching, low blood pressure, menstrual disorders and pain, nightmares, nosebleed, palpitations, rapid heartbeat, seizures, sensitivity to light, severe allergic reaction (anaphylactic shock), sore throat, sweating, tingling or pins and needles, tremor, vision changes, weakness, wheezing

■ *More common side effects of Seldane-D may include:*
Drowsiness, dry mouth, nose, and throat, headache, insomnia, loss of appetite, nausea, nervousness

■ *Less common or rare side effects of Seldane-D may include:*
Blurred vision, change in bowel habits, change in taste, confusion, cough, depression, disorientation, dizziness, excessive or spontaneous flow of milk, fatigue, flare-up of psoriasis, frequent urination, hair loss, hepatitis, hives, increased appetite, increased energy, increased physical activity, irregular heartbeat, irritability, itching, menstrual disorders, muscle twitches, nightmares, nose bleeds, palpitations, rapid heartbeat, rash, restlessness, seizures, sensitivity to light, severe allergic reaction, sore throat, stomach and intestinal upset, sweating, tingling or pins and needles, tremors, upper respiratory infection, vision problems, vomiting, weakness, wheezing

## Why should this drug not be prescribed?

Rare, serious, heart-related side effects have been reported when Seldane or Seldane-D is used with erythromycin (PCE, E-Mycin), itraconazole (Sporanox), ketoconazole (Nizoral), clarithromycin (Biaxin), or troleandomycin (Tao). Do not combine Seldane or Seldane-D with any of these drugs.

Do not take Seldane or Seldane-D if you have liver disease, or if you are sensitive to or have ever had an allergic reaction to the drug.

In addition, Seldane-D should be avoided by nursing mothers, people with severe high blood pressure or heart disease, and people taking the antidepressant drugs known as MAO inhibitors (Nardil, Parnate, others).

## Special warnings about this medication

Seldane and Seldane-D should be used cautiously if you have liver disease or heart disease. An irregular heartbeat can develop. Heartbeat irregularities also can occur when Seldane and Seldane-D are taken with a number of other medications such as bepridil (Vascor), probucol (Lorelco), astemizole (Hismanal), diuretics (water pills), and certain drugs used to treat mental problems. If you develop an irregular heartbeat, stop taking Seldane and notify your doctor. If you have diabetes, glaucoma, or an enlarged prostate, you should take Seldane-D with caution.

## Possible food and drug interactions when taking this medication

If Seldane or Seldane-D is taken with certain other drugs, the effects of either could be increased, decreased, or altered. It is especially important to check with your doctor before combining Seldane or Seldane-D with the following:

Amiodarone (Cordarone)
Astemizole (Hismanal)
Bepridil (Vascor)
Clarithromycin (Biaxin)
Disopyramide (Norpace)
Erythromycin (PCE, E-Mycin)
Itraconazole (Sporanox)
Ketoconazole (Nizoral)
Probucol (Lorelco)
Procainamide (Pronestyl, Procan)
Quinidine (Quinaglute, Quinidex)
Troleandomycin (Tao Capsules)

In addition, Seldane-D may interact with the following:

MAO Inhibitors (antidepressant drugs such as Nardil and Parnate)
Mecamylamine (Inversine)
Methyldopa (an ingredient in some blood pressure medications)
Reserpine (Diupres)

### Special information
### if you are pregnant or breastfeeding

The effects of Seldane and Seldane-D during pregnancy have not been adequately studied. If you are pregnant or plan to become pregnant, inform your doctor immediately.

If you are breastfeeding, Seldane is not recommended and Seldane-D absolutely should not be taken. Animal studies have shown decreased weight gain in developing babies exposed to this drug.

### Recommended dosage

ADULTS AND CHILDREN 12 AND OLDER

*Seldane*
The usual dose is 1 tablet (60 milligrams) 2 times a day.

*Seldane-D*
The usual dose is 1 tablet swallowed whole, morning and night.

CHILDREN

The safety and effectiveness of Seldane and Seldane-D in children below the age of 12 have not been established.

### Overdosage

Any medication taken in excess can have serious consequences. If you suspect an overdose, seek medical attention immediately.

■ *Symptoms of Seldane and Seldane-D overdose may include:*
Changes in heartbeat, confusion, fainting, headache, irregular heartbeat, nausea, seizures

*Generic name:*

# Selegiline

See Eldepryl, page 189.

*Brand name:*

# Semprex-D

Pronounced: SEM-precks-D
Generic ingredients: Acrivastine, Pseudoephedrine hydrochloride

### Why is this drug prescribed?

Semprex-D is an antihistamine and decongestant drug that relieves sneezing, running nose, itching, watery eyes, and stuffy nose caused by seasonal allergies such as hay fever.

### Most important fact about this drug

Semprex-D may cause drowsiness. Do not drive or operate dangerous machinery or participate in any hazardous activity that requires full mental alertness until you know how you react to this medication.

### How should you take this medication?

Take Semprex-D exactly as prescribed by your doctor. Do not take more of this drug or use it more often than your doctor recommends.

■ *If you miss a dose...*
Take it as soon as you remember. If it is almost time for your next dose, skip the one you missed and go back to your regular schedule. Never take 2 doses at the same time.

■ *Storage instructions...*
Store at room temperature in a dry place; protect the drug from light.

### What side effects may occur?

Side effects cannot be anticipated. If any develop or change in intensity, inform your doctor as soon as

possible. Only your doctor can determine if it is safe for you to continue taking Semprex-D.

■ *Side effects may include:*
Cough, dizziness, drowsiness, dry mouth, headache, indigestion, menstrual problems, nausea, nervousness, skin eruptions, sleeplessness, sore throat, weakness, wheezing

Severe allergic reactions are rare. There have been isolated reports of swelling of the throat, lips, neck, face, hands, or feet. Pseudoephedrine, one of the ingredients of this drug, has also been known to cause rapid or fluttery heartbeat.

## Why should this drug not be prescribed?
You should not take Semprex-D if you are sensitive to or have ever had an allergic reaction to acrivastine, pseudoephedrine, or similar drugs such as Actifed, Dimetane, Trinalin, or Seldane-D. Make sure your doctor is aware of any drug reactions you have experienced.

Avoid using Semprex-D if you have extremely high blood pressure or severe heart problems.

Do not take this drug within 14 days of taking any antidepressant drug known as an MAO inhibitor, including Nardil, Parnate, and Marplan.

## Special warnings about this medication
Use this drug with caution if you have high blood pressure, diabetes, heart problems, peptic ulcer or other stomach problems, or an enlarged prostate gland. Use Semprex-D with care, too, if you have increased eye pressure, an overactive thyroid gland, or kidney disease. Make sure the doctor has taken these conditions into account.

Antihistamines are more likely to cause dizziness, extreme calm (sedation), bladder obstruction, and low blood pressure in the elderly (over age 60). The elderly are also more likely to have more side effects from the decongestant (pseudoephedrine) in Semprex-D.

## Possible food and drug interactions when taking this medication
If Semprex-D is taken with certain other drugs, the effects of either could be increased, decreased, or altered. It is especially important to check with your doctor before combining this drug with the following:

Alcoholic beverages
Antidepressants classified as MAO inhibitors, including Nardil, Marplan, and Parnate
Blood pressure medications such as Inderal and Lopressor
Other antihistamines such as Actifed, Seldane-D, and Entex
Other decongestants such as Quibron and Rynatan

## Special information if you are pregnant or breastfeeding
The effects of Semprex-D during pregnancy have not been adequately studied. If you are pregnant or plan to become pregnant, tell your doctor immediately.

It is not known whether acrivastine appears in breast milk, but pseudoephedrine does. If the drug is essential to your health, your doctor may tell you to stop nursing until your treatment is finished.

## Recommended dosage
ADULTS

The usual dose for adults and children 12 years of age and older is 1 capsule, taken by mouth, every 4 to 6 hours, 4 times a day.

CHILDREN

The safety and effectiveness of Semprex-D in children less than 12 years old have not been established.

## Overdosage
Although there have been few reports of overdosage with Semprex-D, overdosage with similar drugs has caused a variety of serious symptoms. If you suspect an overdose of Semprex-D, seek medical attention immediately.

■ *Symptoms of overdose may include:*
Anxiety, convulsions, difficult breathing, drowsiness, fear, hallucinations, heart failure with low blood pressure, irregular heartbeat, loss of consciousness, painful urination, paleness, restlessness, sleeplessness, tenseness, trembling, weakness

*Brand name:*

# Septra

*See Bactrim, page 50.*

*Brand name:*

# Ser-Ap-Es

*Pronounced: Sir-AP-ess*
*Ingredients: Serpasil (reserpine), Apresoline (hydralazine hydrochloride), Esidrix (hydrochlorothiazide)*

## Why is this drug prescribed?

Ser-Ap-Es is a combination drug used in the treatment of high blood pressure. It combines two high blood pressure medications—Serpasil and Apresoline—with a thiazide diuretic, Esidrix. Serpasil and Apresoline improve blood flow throughout your body. Esidrix helps your body produce and eliminate more urine, which also helps lower blood pressure.

## Most important fact about this drug

You must take Ser-Ap-Es regularly for it to be effective. Since blood pressure declines gradually, it may be several weeks before you get the full benefit of Ser-Ap-Es; and you must continue taking it even if you are feeling well. Ser-Ap-Es does not cure high blood pressure; it merely keeps it under control.

## How should you take this medication?

Take Ser-Ap-Es exactly as prescribed by your doctor, even if your symptoms have disappeared.

Try not to miss any doses. If this medication is not taken regularly, your condition may worsen.

■ *If you miss a dose...*
Take the forgotten dose as soon as you remember. If it is almost time for the next dose, skip the one you missed and go back to your regular schedule. Never try to "catch up" by doubling the dose.
■ *Storage instructions...*
Ser-Ap-Es can be stored at room temperature. Use the container it came in.

## What side effects may occur?

Side effects cannot be anticipated. If any develop or change in intensity, inform your doctor as soon as possible. Only your doctor can determine if it is safe for you to continue taking Ser-Ap-Es.

■ *Side effects may include:*
Anemia, anxiety, blockage in the intestines, blood disorders, blurred vision, breast development in males, breast engorgement, change in

potassium levels (dry mouth, excessive thirst, weak or irregular heartbeat, muscle pain or cramps), chills, conjunctivitis, constipation, cramping (stomach and intestinal), crushing chest pain (angina), deafness, decreased sex drive, depression, diarrhea, difficult or labored breathing, difficult or painful urination, disorientation, dizziness, dizziness when standing up, drowsiness, dry mouth, enlarged spleen, eye disorders, fainting, fever, fluid in the lungs, fluid retention, flushing, glaucoma, headache, hepatitis, high blood sugar, hives, impotence, inflammation of the lungs, inflammation of the pancreas, inflammation of the salivary glands, irregular heartbeat, irritation of the stomach, itching, joint pain, loss of appetite, low blood pressure, muscle aches, muscle cramps, muscle spasm, nasal congestion, nausea, nervousness, nightmares, nosebleeds, numbness, parkinsonian syndrome (tremors, muscle weakness, shuffling walk, stooped posture, drooling), pounding heartbeat, rapid heartbeat, rash, red or purple skin discoloration, respiratory distress, restlessness, skin peeling, skin sensitivity to light, slow heartbeat, sugar in the urine, teary eyes, tingling or pins and needles, tremors, vertigo, vision changes, vomiting, weakness, weight gain, yellow eyes and skin

## Why should this drug not be prescribed?

If you are being treated for depression you should avoid this medication.

Ser-Ap-Es should not be prescribed if you have an active peptic ulcer, ulcerative colitis (chronic inflammation of the large intestine and rectum), coronary artery disease, or rheumatic heart disease, or if you are unable to urinate, or are receiving electroshock therapy. Make sure your doctor is aware of all your medical problems.

If you are sensitive to or have ever had an allergic reaction to Ser-Ap-Es, any of its ingredients, or sulfa drugs, do not take this medication. Inform your doctor of any drug reactions you have experienced.

## Special warnings about this medication

Diuretics can cause your body to lose too much potassium. Signs of an excessively low potassium level include muscle weakness and rapid or irregular heartbeat. To boost your potassium level, your doctor may recommend eating potassium-rich foods such as bananas and orange juice, or may prescribe a potassium supplement.

Ser-Ap-Es can cause depression. It can last for several months after you have stopped taking the drug, and it can be severe. If you develop any signs of depression—despondency, waking early in the morning, loss of appetite, impotence, loss of self-esteem—contact your doctor immediately.

If you have a history of peptic ulcer, ulcerative colitis, or gallstones you should use this medication cautiously.

Some people have developed symptoms similar to those of lupus erythematosus, a disease characterized by rash, fever, and sometimes the symptoms of arthritis. These symptoms usually disappear when the Ser-Ap-Es is discontinued.

If you already have lupus erythematosus, Ser-Ap-Es may activate or worsen its symptoms.

If you have coronary artery, kidney, or liver disease, you should be carefully monitored while taking Ser-Ap-Es.

This medication may mask the symptoms of low blood sugar or alter blood sugar levels. If you are diabetic, discuss this with your doctor.

Allergic reactions are more likely to occur if you have a history of allergies or bronchial asthma.

In rare cases, abnormal amounts of uric acid in the blood may develop while taking this medication, leading to an attack of gout.

Notify your doctor or dentist that you are taking Ser-Ap-Es if you have a medical emergency, or before you have surgery or dental treatment.

### Possible food and drug interactions when taking this medication

If Ser-Ap-Es is taken with certain other drugs, the effects of either could be increased, decreased, or altered. It is especially important to check with your doctor before combining Ser-Ap-Es with the following:

ACTH (adrenal hormone)
Amphetamines such as Dexedrine
Antidepressant drugs such as Elavil and Norpramin
Cholestyramine (Questran)
Colestipol (Colestid)
Digitalis (Lanoxin)
Drugs that stimulate the central nervous system
   such as
Cylert and Desoxyn

Drugs that stimulate the sympathetic nervous system such as epinephrine, ephedrine, isoproterenol, metaraminol, tyramine, and phenylephrine
Insulin
Lithium (Eskalith)
MAO inhibitors (antidepressant drugs such as Nardil and Parnate)
Nonsteroidal anti-inflammatory drugs (arthritis drugs and painkillers such as Motrin)
Norepinephrine (Levophed)
Other high blood pressure drugs such as Aldomet and Hyperstat
Quinidine (Quinidex)
Steroids such as Deltasone

### Special information if you are pregnant or breastfeeding

The effects of Ser-Ap-Es during pregnancy have not been adequately studied. If you are pregnant or plan to become pregnant, notify your doctor immediately. Ser-Ap-Es appears in breast milk and could seriously affect a nursing infant. If this medication is essential to your health, your doctor may advise you to discontinue breastfeeding until your treatment is finished.

### Recommended dosage

ADULTS

Your doctor will determine the dosage according to your specific needs. You should not take more than 0.25 milligram of reserpine daily (the amount in 2½ tablets).

CHILDREN

The safety and effectiveness of this drug in children have not been established.

### Overdosage

Any medication taken in excess can have serious consequences. If you suspect an overdose, seek medical attention immediately.

■ *Symptoms of Ser-Ap-Es overdose may include:*
Coma, confusion, constricted pupils, cramps of the calf muscles, decreased amounts of urine, diarrhea, dizziness, drowsiness, fatigue, flushing, headache, heart attack, inability to urinate, increased amounts of urine, increased salivation, irregular heartbeat, low blood pressure, low body

temperature, nausea, rapid heartbeat, severe loss of fluid, shock, slow heartbeat, slowed breathing, thirst, tingling or pins and needles, vomiting, weakness

Brand name:

# Serax

Pronounced: SER-aks
Generic name: Oxazepam

## Why is this drug prescribed?

Serax is used in the treatment of anxiety disorders, including anxiety associated with depression.

This drug seems to be particularly effective for anxiety, tension, agitation, and irritability in older people. It is also prescribed to relieve symptoms of acute alcohol withdrawal.

Serax belongs to a class of drugs known as benzodiazepines.

## Most important fact about this drug

Serax can be habit-forming or addicting and can lose its effectiveness over time, as you develop a tolerance for it. You may experience withdrawal symptoms if you stop using the drug abruptly. When discontinuing the drug, your doctor will reduce the dose gradually.

## How should you take this medication?

Take Serax exactly as prescribed.

■ *If you miss a dose...*
If you remember within an hour or so, take the dose immediately. If you do not remember until later, skip the dose you missed and go back to your regular schedule. Do not take 2 doses at once.
■ *Storage instructions...*
Store at room temperature in a tightly closed container.

## What side effects may occur?

Side effects cannot be anticipated. If any develop or change in intensity, inform your doctor as soon as possible. Only your doctor can determine if it is safe for you to continue taking Serax. Your doctor should periodically reassess the need for this drug.

■ *More common side effects may include:*
Drowsiness
■ *Less common or rare side effects may include:*
Blood disorders, change in sex drive, dizziness, excitement, fainting, headache, hives, liver prob-

lems, loss or lack of muscle control, nausea, skin rashes, sluggishness or unresponsiveness, slurred speech, swelling due to fluid retention, tremors, vertigo, yellowed eyes and skin
■ *Side effects due to rapid decrease or abrupt withdrawal from Serax:*
Abdominal and muscle cramps, convulsions, depressed mood, inability to fall or stay asleep, sweating, tremors, vomiting

## Why should this drug not be prescribed?

If you are sensitive to or have ever had an allergic reaction to Serax or other tranquilizers such as Valium, you should not take this medication. Make sure your doctor is aware of any drug reactions you have experienced.

Anxiety or tension related to everyday stress usually does not require treatment with Serax. Discuss your symptoms thoroughly with your doctor.

Serax should not be prescribed if you are being treated for mental disorders more serious than anxiety.

## Special warnings about this medication

Serax may cause you to become drowsy or less alert; therefore, you should not drive or operate dangerous machinery or participate in any hazardous activity that requires full mental alertness until you know how this drug affects you.

This medication may cause your blood pressure to drop. If you have any heart problems, consult your doctor before taking this medication.

The 15 milligram tablet of this drug contains the coloring agent FD&C Yellow No. 5, which may cause an allergic reaction. If you are sensitive to aspirin or susceptible to allergies, consult your doctor before taking the tablet.

## Possible food and drug interactions when taking this medication

Serax may intensify the effects of alcohol. It may be best to avoid alcohol while taking this medication.

If Serax is taken with certain other drugs, the effects of either could be increased, decreased, or altered. It is especially important to check with your doctor before combining Serax with the following:

Antihistamines such as Benadryl
Narcotic painkillers such as Percocet and Demerol
Sedatives such as Seconal and Halcion
Tranquilizers such as Valium and Xanax

## Special information
## if you are pregnant or breastfeeding

Do not take Serax if you are pregnant or planning to become pregnant. There is an increased risk of birth defects. Serax may appear in breast milk and could affect a nursing infant. If this drug is essential to your health, your doctor may advise you to stop breastfeeding until your treatment with this medication is finished.

## Recommended dosage

### ADULTS

*Mild to Moderate Anxiety with Tension, Irritability, Agitation*
The usual dose is 10 to 15 milligrams 3 or 4 times per day.

*Severe Anxiety, Depression with Anxiety, or Alcohol Withdrawal*
The usual dose is 15 to 30 milligrams, 3 or 4 times per day.

### CHILDREN

This medication is not intended for use in children under 6 years of age. Dosage guidelines for children 6 to 12 years of age have not been established. Your doctor will adjust the dosage to fit the child's needs.

### OLDER ADULTS

The usual starting dose is 10 milligrams, 3 times a day. Your doctor may increase the dose to 15 milligrams 3 or 4 times a day, if needed.

## Overdosage

An overdose of Serax can be fatal. If you suspect an overdose, seek medical attention immediately.

- *Symptoms of mild Serax overdose may include:*
  Confusion, drowsiness, lethargy
- *Symptoms of more serious overdose may include:*
  Coma, hypnotic state, lack of coordination, limp muscles, low blood pressure

*Brand name:*

# Serophene

*See Clomiphene Citrate, page 99.*

*Generic name:*

# Sertraline

*See Zoloft, page 610.*

*Brand name:*

# Serzone

*Pronounced: sur-ZONE*
*Generic name: Nefazodone hydrochloride*

## Why is this drug prescribed?

Serzone is prescribed for the treatment of depression severe enough to interfere with daily functioning. Possible symptoms include changes in appetite, sleep habits, and mind/body coordination, decreased sex drive, increased fatigue, feelings of guilt or worthlessness, difficulty concentrating, slowed thinking, and suicidal thoughts.

## Most important fact about this drug

It may be several weeks before you feel the full antidepressant effect of Serzone. Once you do begin to feel better, it is important to keep taking the drug.

## How should you take this medication?

Take Serzone exactly as prescribed by your doctor. It may take several weeks before you begin to feel better; once you do, it is important to keep taking the drug as prescribed. Your doctor should check your progress periodically.

- *If you miss a dose...*
  Take it as soon as you remember. If it is within 4 hours of your next dose, skip the one you missed and go back to your regular schedule. Do not take 2 doses at once.
- *Storage instructions...*
  Store at room temperature in a tightly closed container.

## What side effects may occur?

Side effects cannot be anticipated. If any develop or change in intensity, tell your doctor as soon as possible. Only your doctor can determine if it is safe for you to continue taking Serzone.

- *More common side effects may include:*
  Blurred or abnormal vision, confusion, constipation, dizziness, dry mouth, light-headedness, nausea, sleepiness, weakness
- *Less common side effects may include:*
  Abnormal dreams, cough, decreased concentration, diarrhea, dizziness on getting up, flu-like symptoms, headache, increased appetite, water retention

■ *Rare side effects may include:*
Breast pain, chills, decreased sex drive, difficulty urinating, fever, frequent urination, lack of coordination, ringing in ears, stiff neck, taste change, thirst, urinary tract infection, vaginal inflammation

## Why should this drug not be prescribed?

If you are sensitive to or have ever had an allergic reaction to Serzone or similar drugs, such as Desyrel, you should not take this medication.

Serious, sometimes fatal reactions have occurred when Serzone is used in combination with other antidepressant drugs known as MAO inhibitors, including Nardil and Parnate. Never take Serzone with one of these drugs; and do not begin therapy with Serzone within 14 days of discontinuing treatment with one of them. Also, allow at least 7 days between the last dose of Serzone and the first dose of an MAO inhibitor.

## Special warnings about this medication

Your doctor will prescribe Serzone with caution if you have a history of seizures or mania (extreme agitation or excitability) or heart or liver disease. Serzone should also be used with caution is you have had a heart attack or stroke, or suffer from dehydration. Be sure to discuss all of your medical problems with your doctor before taking Serzone.

Serzone may cause you to become drowsy or less alert and may affect your judgment. Do not drive or operate dangerous machinery or participate in any hazardous activity that requires full mental alertness until you know how the drug affects you.

Before having surgery, dental treatment, or any diagnostic procedure requiring anesthesia, tell the doctor or dentist you are taking Serzone. If you develop an allergic reaction such as a skin rash or hives while taking Serzone, notify your doctor. If you are male and experience a prolonged or inappropriate erection while taking Serzone, discontinue this drug and call your doctor.

If you have ever been addicted to drugs, tell your doctor before you start Serzone.

## Possible food and drug interactions when taking this medication

If Serzone is taken with certain other drugs, the effects of either could be increased, decreased, or altered. It is especially important to check with your doctor before combining Serzone with the following:

Alcohol
Antidepressants classified as MAO inhibitors, including Nardil and Parnate
Astemizole (Hismanal)
Digoxin (Lanoxin)
Sleep aids such as Halcion and Dalmane
Terfenadine (Seldane)
Tranquilizers such as Adapin and Xanax

## Special information if you are pregnant or breastfeeding

The effects of Serzone during pregnancy have not been adequately studied. If you are pregnant or are planning to become pregnant, tell your doctor immediately. Serzone should be used during pregnancy only if clearly needed. Serzone may appear in breast milk. If this medication is essential to your health, your doctor may tell you to discontinue breastfeeding until your treatment with Serzone is finished.

## Recommended dosage

### ADULTS

The usual starting dose for Serzone is 200 milligrams a day, divided into 2 doses. If needed, your doctor may increase your dose gradually to 300 to 600 milligrams a day.

### CHILDREN

The safety and effectiveness of Serzone have not been established in children under 18 years of age.

### OLDER ADULTS

The usual starting dose for the old or debilitated is 100 milligrams a day, taken in 2 doses. Your doctor will adjust the dose according to your response.

## Overdosage

Any medication taken in excess can have serious consequences. If you suspect an overdose, seek medical attention immediately.

■ *Symptoms of Serzone overdose include:*
Nausea, sleepiness, vomiting

*Brand name:*

# Silvadene Cream 1%

*Pronounced: SIL-vuh-deen*
*Generic name: Silver sulfadiazine*

## Why is this drug prescribed?

Silvadene Cream 1% is applied directly to the skin. The cream is used along with other medications to prevent and treat wound infections in people with second- and third-degree burns. It is effective against a variety of bacteria as well as yeast.

### Most important fact about this drug

Silvadene is a sulfa derivative. If burn wounds cover extensive areas of the body, Silvadene may be absorbed into the bloodstream, and if you have ever had an allergic reaction to sulfa drugs, such as Bactrim or Septra, this could lead to a similar reaction. Make sure your doctor is aware of any drug reactions you have experienced.

### How should you use this medication?

Silvadene cream is for external use only.

Bathe the burned area daily.

You should continue using Silvadene Cream until the area has healed or is ready for skin grafting.

Clean your skin and apply Silvadene with a sterile, gloved hand. Apply a thin layer (about one-sixteenth of an inch) to the affected area.

■ *If you miss a dose...*
Keep the burn areas covered with Silvadene at all times. Reapply the medicine if it is rubbed or washed off.
■ *Storage instructions...*
Silvadene can be stored at room temperature.

### What side effects may occur?

Side effects cannot be anticipated. If any side effects develop or change in intensity, tell your doctor immediately. Only your doctor can determine whether it is safe for you to continue using Silvadene.

■ *Side effects may include:*
Areas of dead skin, burning sensation, red and raised rash on the body, skin discoloration

### Why should this drug not be prescribed?

You should not use Silvadene if you are allergic to sulfa drugs such as Bactrim or Septra.

Do not use Silvadene at the end of pregnancy, on premature infants, or on newborn infants during the first 2 months of life.

### Special warnings about this medication

Make sure your doctor knows about any kidney or liver problems you may have. If either organ becomes impaired, it may be necessary to stop using Silvadene.

There is a small chance of fungal infection when using Silvadene.

### Possible food and drug interactions when using this medication

If Silvadene is used with certain other drugs, the effects of either could be increased, decreased, or altered. It is especially important to check with your doctor before combining Silvadene with the following:

Topical enzyme preparations such as Panafil and Santyl, that contain collagenase, papain, or sutilains

### Special information if you are pregnant or breastfeeding

If you are pregnant or plan to become pregnant, inform your doctor immediately.

The safety of Silvadene during pregnancy has not been fully studied, but you definitely should not take this drug at the end of your pregnancy, as it can lead to complications for the baby.

Although it is not known whether Silvadene appears in breast milk, other sulfa drugs are excreted in breast milk and can cause harm to a nursing infant. If this medication is essential to your health, your doctor may advise you to stop breastfeeding until your treatment is finished.

### Recommended dosage

Apply Silvadene Cream 1% to the affected area once or twice daily to a thickness of one-sixteenth of an inch. Treatment with Silvadene should be continued until your doctor is satisfied that healing has occurred or determines that the burn site is ready for grafting.

### Overdosage

Any medication taken in excess can have serious consequences. If you suspect an overdose, seek medical treatment immediately.

*Generic name:*

# Silver sulfadiazine

*See Silvadene Cream 1%, page 498.*

*Generic name:*

# Simvastatin

*See Zocor, page 608.*

*Brand name:*

# Sinemet CR

*Pronounced: SIN-uh-met see-are*
*Generic ingredients: Carbidopa, Levodopa*

### Why is this drug prescribed?

Sinemet CR is a controlled-release tablet that may be given to help relieve the muscle stiffness, tremor, and weakness caused by Parkinson's disease. It may also be given to relieve Parkinson-like symptoms caused by encephalitis (brain fever), carbon monoxide poisoning, or manganese poisoning.

Sinemet CR contains two drugs, carbidopa and levodopa. The drug that actually produces the anti-Parkinson's effect is levodopa. Carbidopa prevents vitamin $B_6$ from destroying levodopa, thus allowing levodopa to work more efficiently.

Parkinson's drugs such as Sinemet CR relieve the symptoms of the disease, but are not a permanent cure.

### Most important fact about this drug

There is also a regular, non-controlled-release form of this medication, which is called Sinemet. Over a period of hours, Sinemet CR, the controlled-release form, gives a smoother release of the drug than regular Sinemet. If you have been taking regular Sinemet, be aware that you may need a somewhat higher dosage of Sinemet CR to get the same degree of relief. Your first morning dose of Sinemet CR may take as much as an hour longer to start working than your first morning dose of regular Sinemet.

### How should you take this medication?

Take Sinemet CR after meals, rather than before or between meals. Swallow the tablets whole without chewing or crushing them.

Sinemet CR releases its ingredients slowly over a period of 4 to 6 hours. It is important to follow a careful schedule, taking your doses at the same time every day.

You should not change the prescribed dosage or add another product for Parkinson's disease without first consulting your doctor.

Sinemet CR works best when there is a constant amount in the blood. Try not to miss any doses, and take them at evenly spaced intervals day and night.

■ *If you miss a dose...*
If you forget to take a dose, take it as soon as you remember. If it is almost time for your next dose, skip the one you missed and go back to your regular schedule. Do not take 2 doses at once.

■ *Storage instructions...*
Store at room temperature in a tightly closed container.

### What side effects may occur?

Side effects from Sinemet CR cannot be anticipated. If any develop or change in intensity, inform your doctor immediately.

Only your doctor can determine if it is safe for you to continue taking Sinemet CR.

■ *More common side effects may include:*
Confusion, hallucinations, nausea, uncontrollable twitching or jerking

■ *Less common or rare side effects may include:*
Abdominal or stomach pain, abnormal dreams, agitation, anemia, anxiety, back pain, bitter taste, bizarre breathing patterns, bleeding from stomach, blurred vision, burning sensation of tongue, chest pain, clumsiness in walking, common cold, constipation, convulsions, cough, dark sweat, dark urine, delusions, depression, diarrhea, disorientation, dizziness, dizziness upon rising from a sitting or lying position, dream abnormalities, drooling, drowsiness, dry mouth, euphoria, eyelid twitching, faintness, falling, fatigue, fever, flatulence, fluid retention, flushing, hair loss, headache, heart attack, heart palpitations, heartburn, hiccups, high or low blood pressure, hoarseness, hot flashes, increased hand tremor, insomnia or other sleep problems, irregular heartbeat, leg pain, locked jaw, loss of appetite, malignant melanoma, memory problems, mental changes, muscle cramps, muscle twitching, nervousness, numbness, "on-off" phenomena, paralysis of certain muscles and unwanted movement of others, paranoia, persistent erection, phlebitis (swelling of a vein), rash, shortness of breath, shoulder pain, slowed physical movements, sore throat, speech impairment, stomach ulcer, suicidal tendencies, swallowing difficulties, sweating, teeth-grinding, tingling or pins and needles, upper respiratory infection, upset stomach, urinary frequency, urinary incontinence, urinary retention, urinary tract infec-

tions, weakness, weight loss or gain, writhing or flailing movements, vomiting

## Why should this drug not be prescribed?

Do not take Sinemet CR if you are sensitive to or have ever had an allergic reaction to its ingredients.

Sinemet CR should not be prescribed if you have a suspicious, undiagnosed mole or a history of melanoma.

## Special warnings about this medication

Make sure your doctor knows if you have any of the following:

Bronchial asthma
Cardiovascular or lung disease (severe)
Endocrine (glandular) disorder
History of heart attack or heartbeat irregularity
History of active peptic ulcer
Kidney disorder
Liver disorder
Wide-angle glaucoma (pressure in the eye)

Your doctor will monitor your liver, blood, kidney and heart functions during extended therapy with Sinemet CR.

If you have been taking levodopa alone, you should stop taking levodopa for at least 8 hours before starting to take Sinemet CR.

The carbidopa contained in Sinemet CR cannot eliminate side effects caused by levodopa. Since carbidopa helps levodopa reach your brain, Sinemet CR may, in fact, produce some levodopa side effects—particularly twitching, jerking, or writhing—sooner and at a lower dosage than levodopa alone or even regular Sinemet. If such involuntary movements develop while you are taking Sinemet CR, you may need a dosage reduction.

Like levodopa, Sinemet CR may cause depression. Make sure your doctor knows if you have mental or emotional problems.

Muscle rigidity, high temperature, and mental changes may occur when Sinemet CR is reduced suddenly or discontinued. If you stop taking this medication abruptly, your doctor should monitor your condition carefully.

## Possible food and drug interactions when taking this medication

If Sinemet CR is taken with certain other drugs, the effects of either could be increased, decreased, or altered. It is especially important to check with your doctor before combining Sinemet CR with the following:

Antacids such as Di-Gel, Maalox, and Mylanta
Antiseizure drugs such as Dilantin
Antispasmodic drugs such as Artane and Cogentin
Antihypertensives such as Aldomet and Clonidine
Iron products such as Feosol
Isoniazid (Nydrazid)
Major tranquilizers such as Haldol, Mellaril, and Thorazine
MAO inhibitor antidepressants such as Nardil and Parnate
Methionine drugs such as Odor-Scrip and Pedameth
Metoclopramide (Reglan)
Papaverine (Pavabid)
Pyridoxine (Vitamin $B_6$)
Tranquilizers such as Dalmane, Valium and Xanax
Tricyclic antidepressants such as Elavil and Tofranil

If you have been taking an MAO inhibitor antidepressant such as Marplan, Nardil, or Parnate, you must discontinue it at least 2 weeks before starting to take Sinemet CR.

## Special information if you are pregnant or breastfeeding

If you are pregnant or plan to become pregnant, inform your doctor immediately. Sinemet CR should be used during pregnancy only if the benefit outweighs the potential risk to the unborn child. It is not known whether Sinemet CR appears in breast milk. If this medication is essential to your health, your doctor may advise you to stop nursing your baby until your treatment with this drug is finished.

## Recommended dosage

Your doctor will tailor your individual dosage carefully, depending on your response to previous therapy and symptoms.

ADULTS

For patients with mild to moderate symptoms, the initial recommended dose is 1 tablet of Sinemet CR taken 2 times a day.

Starting doses should be spaced out every 4 to 8 hours and then adjusted to each patient's individual response.

The usual long-term dose is 2 to 8 tablets per day, taken in divided doses every 4 to 8 hours during the waking day.

Higher doses (12 or more tablets per day) and shorter intervals (less than 4 hours) have been used, but are not usually recommended.

When doses of Sinemet CR are given at intervals of less than 4 hours, and/or if the divided doses are not equal, it is recommended that the smaller doses be given at the end of the day.

An interval of at least 3 days between dosage adjustments is recommended.

Dosage adjustment of Sinemet CR may be necessary if your doctor prescribes additional medications.

CHILDREN

Use of Sinemet CR in children under 18 is not recommended.

### Overdosage

Too much Sinemet CR may cause muscle twitches, inability to open the eyes, or other symptoms of levodopa overdosage. Like other medications, Sinemet CR taken in excess can have serious consequences. If you suspect symptoms of a Sinemet CR overdose, seek medical attention immediately.

*Brand name:*

# Sinequan

*Pronounced: SIN-uh-kwan*
*Generic name: Doxepin hydrochloride*

### Why is this drug prescribed?

Sinequan is used in the treatment of depression and anxiety. It helps relieve tension, improve sleep, elevate mood, increase energy, and generally ease the feelings of fear, guilt, apprehension, and worry most people experience. It is effective in treating people whose depression and/or anxiety is psychological, associated with alcoholism, or a result of another disease (cancer, for example) or psychotic depressive disorders (severe mental illness). It is in the family of drugs called tricyclic antidepressants.

### Most important fact about this drug

Serious, sometimes fatal, reactions have occurred when Sinequan is used in combination with another type of antidepressant called MAO inhibitors. Any drug of this type should be discontinued at least 2 weeks prior to starting treatment with Sinequan, and you should be carefully monitored by your doctor.

If you are taking any prescription or nonprescription drugs, consult your doctor before taking Sinequan.

### How should you take this medication?

Take this medication exactly as prescribed. It may take several weeks for you to feel better.

■ *If you miss a dose...*
If you are taking several doses a day, take the missed dose as soon as you remember, then take any remaining doses for that day at evenly spaced intervals. If it is almost time for your next dose, skip the one you missed and go back to your regular schedule. Never take 2 doses at the same time.

If you are taking a single dose at bedtime and do not remember until the next morning, skip the dose. Do not take a double dose to make up for a missed one.

■ *Storage instructions...*
Store at room temperature.

### What side effects may occur?

Side effects cannot be anticipated. If any develop or change in intensity, inform your doctor as soon as possible. Only your doctor can determine if it is safe for you to continue taking Sinequan.

The most common side effect is drowsiness.

■ *Less common or rare side effects may include:*
Blurred vision, breast development in males, bruises, buzzing or ringing in the ears, changes in sex drive, chills, confusion, constipation, diarrhea, difficulty urinating, disorientation, dizziness, dry mouth, enlarged breasts, fatigue, fluid retention, flushing, fragmented or incomplete movements, hair loss, hallucinations, headache, high fever, high or low blood sugar, inappropriate breast milk secretion, indigestion, inflammation of the mouth, itching and skin rash, lack of muscle control, loss of appetite, loss of coordination, low blood pressure, nausea, nervousness, numbness, poor bladder control, rapid heartbeat, red or brownish spots on the skin, seizures, sensitivity to light, severe muscle stiffness, sore throat, sweating, swelling of the testicles, taste disturbances, tingling sensation, tremors, vomiting, weakness, weight gain, yellow eyes and skin

### Why should this drug not be prescribed?

If you are sensitive to or have ever had an allergic reaction to Sinequan or similar antidepressants, you should not take this medication. Make sure that your doctor is aware of any drug reactions that you have experienced.

Unless you are directed to do so by your doctor, do not take this medication if you have the eye condition known as glaucoma or difficulty urinating.

### Special warnings about this medication

Sinequan may cause you to become drowsy or less alert; driving or operating dangerous machinery or participating in any hazardous activity that requires full mental alertness is not recommended.

Notify your doctor or dentist that you are taking Sinequan if you have a medical emergency, and before you have surgery or dental treatment.

### Possible food and drug interactions when taking this medication

Alcohol increases the danger in a Sinequan overdose. Do not drink alcohol while taking this medication.

Never combine Sinequan with other antidepressants known as MAO inhibitors. Drugs in this category include Nardil and Parnate.

If you are switching from Prozac, wait at least 5 weeks after your last dose of Prozac before starting Sinequan.

If Sinequan is taken with certain other drugs, the effects of either could be increased, decreased, or altered. It is especially important to check with your doctor before combining Sinequan with the following:

Antidepressants that act on serotonin, such as
    Prozac, Zoloft, and Paxil
Other antidepressants such as Elavil and Serzone
Carbamazepine (Tegretol)
Cimetidine (Tagamet)
Clonidine (Catapres)
Flecainide (Tambocor)
Guanethidine (Ismelin)
Major tranquilizers such as Compazine, Mellaril,
    and Thorazine
Propafenone (Rythmol)
Quinidine (Quinidex)
Tolazamide (Tolinase)

### Special information if you are pregnant or breastfeeding

The effects of Sinequan during pregnancy have not been adequately studied. If you are pregnant or planning to become pregnant, inform your doctor

immediately. Sinequan may appear in breast milk and could affect a nursing infant. If this medication is essential to your health, your doctor may advise you to discontinue breastfeeding your baby until your treatment is finished.

### Recommended dosage

ADULTS

The starting dose for mild to moderate illness is usually 75 milligrams per day. This dose can be increased or decreased by your doctor according to individual need. The usual ideal dose ranges from 75 milligrams per day to 150 milligrams per day, although it can be as low as 25 to 50 milligrams per day. The total daily dose can be given once a day or divided into smaller doses. If you are taking this drug once a day, the recommended dose is 150 milligrams at bedtime.

The 150-milligram capsule strength is intended for long-term therapy only and is not recommended as a starting dose.

For more severe illness, gradually increased doses of up to 300 milligrams may be required as determined by your doctor.

CHILDREN

Safety and effectiveness have not been established for use in children under 12 years of age.

OLDER ADULTS

A once-a-day dosage should be carefully adjusted by your doctor, depending upon the severity of your illness.

### Overdosage

■ *Symptoms of Sinequan overdose may include:*
Blurred vision, coma, convulsions, decreased intestinal movement, dilated pupils, drowsiness, excessive dryness of mouth, high or low body temperature, irregular or rapid heartbeat, low or high blood pressure, overactive reflexes, severe breathing problems, stupor, urinary problems

If you experience any of these symptoms, seek medical attention immediately.

*Brand name:*

# Slo-bid

*See Theo-Dur, page 538.*

*Brand name:*

# Slow-K

*See Micro-K, page 323.*

*Generic name:*

# Sodium fluoride

*See Luride, page 302.*

*Brand name:*

# Sodium Sulamyd

Pronounced: SOH-dee-um SOO-lah-mid
Generic name: Sulfacetamide sodium
Other brand name: Bleph-10

### Why is this drug prescribed?

Sodium Sulamyd is used in the treatment of eye inflammations, corneal ulcer, and other eye infections. It may be used along with an oral sulfa drug to treat a serious eye infection called trachoma.

### Most important fact about this drug

Sodium Sulamyd is similar to oral sulfa drugs such as Bactrim, Gantanol, and Gantrisin. If you are allergic to any of these medications, you may also be allergic to Sodium Sulamyd. In addition, if you have taken one of these medications in the past, you may have developed a "hidden" allergy to sulfa drugs that might show up when you take Sodium Sulamyd. Be alert for a rash, itching, or other signs of allergy. If any of these symptoms develop, stop taking Sodium Sulamyd immediately and consult your doctor.

### How should you use this medication?

Sodium Sulamyd is available in eyedrop and ointment form. Use it exactly as prescribed. Your doctor may tell you to use both the eye drops and the ointment.

To apply Sodium Sulamyd, pull down your lower eyelid to form a pouch, then squeeze in the medication. To avoid contaminating the eye drops or the ointment, do not touch your eye with the dropper bottle or the tip of the tube. Keep the dropper bottle or tube poised slightly above your eye as you instill the drops or squeeze out the ointment.

■ *If you miss a dose...*
Apply it as soon as you remember. If it is almost time for your next dose, skip the one you missed and go back to your regular schedule.

■ *Storage instructions...*
Store at room temperature. Protect the ointment from excessive heat.

### What side effects may occur?

Side effects cannot be anticipated. If any develop or change in intensity, inform your doctor as soon as possible. Only your doctor can determine if it is safe for you to continue taking this medication.

Sodium Sulamyd may irritate your eye, causing stinging and burning. The irritation usually lasts only a short time. If it is very painful or lasts for a long time, you may have to stop using the medication.

In rare cases, people using Sodium Sulamyd have developed a severe blistering skin rash. Be alert for skin reactions. If a rash appears, stop using Sodium Sulamyd and call your doctor.

### Why should this drug not be prescribed?

Do not use Sodium Sulamyd if you have ever had an allergic reaction to or are sensitive to this medication or any other sulfa drug.

### Special warnings about this medication

Stay in close touch with your doctor while using Sodium Sulamyd. In some cases, an eye ointment may actually delay healing of the cornea. If you have a pus-producing eye infection, the pus may inactivate Sodium Sulamyd. Since sulfa drugs do not kill fungi, it is possible to develop a fungus infection in your eye while using Sodium Sulamyd.

### Possible food and drug interactions when taking this medication

Sodium Sulamyd should not be used with medications containing silver. Check with your doctor if you are unsure of any medications you are taking.

### Special information if you are pregnant or breastfeeding

If you are pregnant or plan to become pregnant, inform your doctor immediately. There is no information about the safety of Sodium Sulamyd during pregnancy.

It is not known whether Sodium Sulamyd appears in breast milk. If Sodium Sulamyd is essential to your health, it may be necessary to stop breastfeeding during treatment.

## Recommended dosage

SODIUM SULAMYD OPHTHALMIC SOLUTION 30%

*Inflamed Eyes or Corneal Ulcer*
Place 1 drop inside the lower eyelid every 2 hours or less frequently; your doctor will determine the schedule according to the severity of the infection.
*Trachoma (Contagious Inflammation)*
Use 2 drops every 2 hours.

SODIUM SULAMYD OPHTHALMIC SOLUTION 10%

Place 1 or 2 drops inside the lower eyelid every 2 or 3 hours during the day, less often at night.

SODIUM SULAMYD OPHTHALMIC
OINTMENT 10%

Apply a small amount of the ointment 4 times daily and at bedtime. The ointment may be used at the same time as either of the solutions.

## Overdosage

Although no specific information is available on overdose with Sodium Sulamyd, any medication used in excess can have serious consequences. If you suspect you may have used too much Sodium Sulamyd, seek medical attention immediately.

*Brand name:*

# Sof-Lax

*See Colace, page 107.*

*Brand name:*

# Soma

*Pronounced: SOE-muh*
*Generic name: Carisoprodol*

## Why is this drug prescribed?

Soma is used, along with rest, physical therapy, and other measures, for the relief of acute, painful muscle strains and spasms.

## Most important fact about this drug

Soma alone will not heal your muscles. You need to follow the program of physical therapy, rest, or exercise that your doctor prescribes. Do not attempt any more physical activity than your doctor recommends, even though Soma temporarily makes it seem feasible.

## How should you take this medication?

Take Soma exactly as prescribed by your doctor.

■ *If you miss a dose...*
Take it as soon as you remember if only an hour or so has passed. If you do not remember until later, skip the dose you missed and go back to your regular schedule. Do not take 2 doses at once.
■ *Storage instructions...*
Store at room temperature in a tightly closed container.

## What side effects may occur?

Side effects cannot be anticipated. If any develop or change in intensity, inform your doctor as soon as possible. Only your doctor can determine if it is safe for you to continue taking Soma.

■ *Side effects may include:*
Agitation, depression, dizziness, drowsiness, facial flushing, fainting, headache, hiccups, inability to fall or stay asleep, irritability, light-headedness upon standing up, loss of coordination, nausea, rapid heart rate, stomach upset, tremors, vertigo, vomiting

Allergic reactions usually seen between the first and fourth doses of Soma in patients who have never taken this drug before include: itching, red welts on the skin, and skin rash. A more severe allergic reaction may include symptoms such as asthmatic attacks, dizziness, fever, low blood pressure, shock, stinging of the eyes, swelling due to fluid retention, and weakness.

## Why should this drug not be prescribed?

If you are sensitive to or have ever had an allergic reaction to Soma or drugs of this type, such as meprobamate (Miltown), you should not take this medication. Make sure your doctor is aware of any drug reactions you have experienced.

Unless you are directed to do so by your doctor, do not take this medication if you have porphyria (an inherited blood disorder).

## Special warnings about this medication

In rare cases, the first dose of Soma may cause unusual symptoms that appear within minutes or hours of taking the medication. Symptoms reported include: agitation, confusion, disorientation, dizziness, double vision, enlargement of pupils, extreme weakness, exaggerated feeling of well-being, lack of coordination, speech problems, temporary loss of vision, and temporary paralysis of arms and legs. These symptoms usually subside within a few hours. If you experience any of them, contact your doctor immediately.

Soma may impair the mental or physical abilities you need to drive a car or operate dangerous machinery. Do not participate in hazardous activities until you know how this drug affects you.

If you have a history of drug dependence, make sure your doctor is aware of it before you start taking this medication.

Withdrawal symptoms, including abdominal cramps, chilliness, headache, insomnia, and nausea, have occurred in people who suddenly stop taking Soma.

Take this drug cautiously if you have any kidney or liver problems.

### Possible food and drug interactions when taking this medication

Soma may intensify the effects of alcohol. Be careful drinking alcoholic beverages while you are taking this medication.

If Soma is taken with certain other drugs, the effects of either could be increased, decreased, or altered. It is especially important to check with your doctor before combining Soma with the following:

Antidepressant drugs such as Elavil, Tofranil, and Nardil
Major tranquilizers such as Haldol, Stelazine, and Thorazine
Sedatives such as Nembutal and Halcion
Tranquilizers such as Librium, Valium, and Xanax

### Special information if you are pregnant or breastfeeding

The effects of Soma during pregnancy have not been adequately studied. If you are pregnant or plan to become pregnant, inform your doctor immediately. This drug appears in breast milk and could affect a nursing infant. If this medication is essential to your health, your doctor may advise you to discontinue breastfeeding until your treatment is finished.

### Recommended dosage

ADULTS

The usual dosage of Soma is one 350-milligram tablet, taken 3 times daily and at bedtime.

CHILDREN

The safety and effectiveness of this drug have not been established in children under 12 years of age.

### Overdosage

A severe overdose of Soma can be fatal. If you suspect an overdose, seek medical help immediately.

■ *Symptoms of Soma overdose may include:*
Breathing difficulty, coma, shock, stupor

*Brand name:*

# Sorbitrate

See Isordil, page 264.

*Brand name:*

# Spectazole Cream

*Pronounced: SPEK-tah-zole*
*Generic name: Econazole nitrate*

### Why is this drug prescribed?

Spectazole cream is prescribed for fungal skin diseases commonly called ringworm (tinea). It is used to treat athlete's foot (tinea pedis), "jock itch" (tinea cruris), a fungus infection of the entire body (tinea corporis), and a skin infection that causes yellow- or brown-colored skin eruptions (tinea versicolor). It is also prescribed for yeast infections of the skin caused by candida fungus (cutaneous candidiasis).

### Most important fact about this drug

Do not use Spectazole in or near the eyes.

### How should you use this medication?

Use Spectazole Cream exactly as prescribed by your doctor.

Continue using the medication for the full time prescribed even if your symptoms have been relieved.

When applied, the cream should completely cover the affected area.

■ *If you miss a dose...*
Apply it as soon as you remember. If it is almost time for your next dose, skip the one you missed and go back to your regular schedule.
■ *Storage instructions...*
Store at room temperature.

## What side effects may occur?

Side effects cannot be anticipated. If any develop or change in intensity, inform your doctor as soon as possible. Only your doctor can determine whether it is safe for you to continue using Spectazole.

■ *More common side effects may include:*
Burning, itching, skin redness, stinging
■ *Less common or rare side effects may include:*
Itching rash

## Why should this drug not be prescribed?

Spectazole Cream should not be used if you are sensitive to it or have ever had an allergic reaction to any of its ingredients.

## Special warnings about this medication

If you develop an irritation or an allergic reaction to Spectazole, stop using the cream and inform your doctor.

Spectazole is only for external use.

## Possible food and drug interactions when taking this medication

No interactions have been reported.

## Special information if you are pregnant or breastfeeding

Spectazole should be used during the first trimester (3 months) of pregnancy only if it is essential to your health, and during the remainder of your pregnancy only if your doctor feels it is clearly needed. If you are pregnant or plan to become pregnant, inform your doctor immediately. Spectazole may appear in breast milk and could affect a nursing infant. If this medication is essential to your health, your doctor may advise you to stop breastfeeding until your treatment with Spectazole is finished.

## Recommended dosage

ATHLETE'S FOOT, JOCK ITCH, TINEA CORPORIS, TINEA VERSICOLOR

Apply sufficient Spectazole Cream to completely cover the affected area once a day. Athlete's foot is treated for 1 month; jock itch and tinea corporis are treated for 2 weeks. Tinea versicolor is usually treated for 2 weeks.

CUTANEOUS CANDIDIASIS

Apply sufficient Spectazole Cream to completely cover the affected area 2 times a day, once in the morning and once in the evening. Cutaneous candidiasis is treated for 2 weeks.

## Overdosage

Although no specific information is available on Spectazole Cream overdosage, any medication used in excess can have serious consequences. If you suspect an overdose, seek medical attention immediately.

*Generic name:*

# Spironolactone

*See Aldactone, page 11.*

*Generic name:*

# Spironolactone with Hydrochlorothiazide

*See Aldactazide, page 9.*

*Brand name:*

# Spirozide

*See Aldactazide, page 9.*

*Brand name:*

# Sporanox

*Pronounced: SPORE-ah-nocks*
*Generic name: Itraconazole*

## Why is this drug prescribed?

Sporanox is used to treat three types of serious fungal infection: blastomycosis, histoplasmosis, and aspergillosis. Blastomycosis can affect the lungs, bones, and skin. Histoplasmosis can affect the lungs, heart, and blood. Aspergillosis can affect the lungs, kidneys, and other organs. Sporanox is also used against fungal infections in people with weak immune systems, such as AIDS patients.

## Most important fact about this drug

Be sure to take Sporanox for as long as your doctor prescribes. It will take 3 months or more to cure the infection completely. If you stop taking Sporanox too soon, the infection may return.

## How should you take this medication?

Take Sporanox exactly as prescribed. To make sure the capsules are properly absorbed, you should take them after a full meal. A cola drink can help some people absorb the drug better. Continue taking Sporanox until all the medication is gone. Do not take antacids for at least 2 hours after you take Sporanox.

■ *If you miss a dose...*
Take the forgotten dose as soon as you remember. If it is almost time for the next dose, skip the one you missed and go back to your regular schedule. Never try to "catch up" by doubling the dose.

■ *Storage instructions...*
Store at room temperature. Protect from light and moisture.

### What side effects may occur?
Side effects cannot be anticipated. If any develop or change in intensity, inform your doctor as soon as possible. Only your doctor can determine if it is safe for you to continue taking Sporanox.

■ *More common side effects may include:*
Diarrhea, fatigue, fever, headache, high blood pressure, nausea, rash, swelling due to water retention, vomiting

■ *Less common side effects may include:*
Abdominal pain, decreased sexual drive, dizziness, extreme sleepiness, feeling of general discomfort, hives, itching, loss of appetite, reproductive disorders such as male impotence, sleepiness

■ *Rare side effects may include:*
Depression, gas, hepatitis, male breast development, male breast pain, ringing in the ears, severe allergic reaction, skin peeling, sleeplessness

### Why should this drug not be prescribed?
If you are sensitive to or have ever had an allergic reaction to Sporanox or similar antifungal drugs such as Nizoral, you should not take this medication. Make sure that your doctor is aware of any drug reactions that you have experienced.

Serious heart problems, such as irregular heartbeats and even death, have occurred in people who have taken Sporanox at the same time as Seldane or Hismanal. Never take these drugs with Sporanox, and avoid Propulsid and Halcion as well.

### Special warnings about this medication
If you have liver disease, your doctor should monitor your liver function periodically while you are taking Sporanox. If you develop such symptoms

of liver disease as unusual fatigue, loss of appetite, nausea, vomiting, jaundice, dark urine, or pale stool, report them to your doctor so that the appropriate laboratory testing can be performed.

### Possible food and drug interactions when taking this medication
If Sporanox is taken with certain other drugs, the effects of either could be increased, decreased, or altered. It is especially important to check with your doctor before combining Sporanox with any of the following:

Astemizole (Hismanal)
Blood-thinning drugs such as Coumadin
Calcium channel blockers such as Cardene and
   Norvasc
Cisapride (Propulsid)
Cyclosporine (Sandimmune, Neoral)
Digoxin (Lanoxin)
$H_2$ antagonists such as Tagamet and Zantac
Isoniazid
Lovastatin (Mevacor)
Midazolam (Versed)
Oral diabetes medications such as DiaBeta,
   Diabinese, Glucotrol, Micronase, Orinase, and
   Tolinase
Phenytoin (Dilantin)
Quinidine (Quinidex)
Rifampin (Rifadin, Rimactane)
Simvastatin (Zocor)
Tacrolimus (Prograf)
Terfenadine (Seldane, Seldane-D)
Triazolam (Halcion)

### Special information if you are pregnant or breastfeeding
The effects of Sporanox during pregnancy have not been adequately studied. If you are pregnant or plan to become pregnant, inform your doctor immediately. Sporanox appears in breast milk and could affect a nursing infant. If this medication is essential to your health, your doctor may advise you to discontinue breastfeeding until your treatment with Sporanox is finished.

### Recommended dosage
ADULTS

*Blastomycosis and Histoplasmosis*
The usual dose is two 100-milligram capsules, taken after a full meal once a day. If you feel no

improvement, or if there is evidence that the fungal disease has spread, your doctor will increase the dose 100 milligrams at a time to a maximum of 400 milligrams a day. Daily dosages above 200 milligrams a day should be divided into 2 smaller doses.

### Aspergillosis

The usual dose is 200 to 400 milligrams a day. Treatment usually continues for a minimum of 3 months, until tests indicate that the fungal infection has subsided.

### Overdosage

Any drug taken in excess can have dangerous consequences. If you suspect an overdose, seek emergency medical treatment immediately.

*Generic name:*

# Stavudine

*See Zerit, page 601.*

*Brand name:*

# Stelazine

*Pronounced: STEL-ah-zeen*
*Generic name: Trifluoperazine hydrochloride*

### Why is this drug prescribed?

Stelazine is used to treat severe mental disturbances as well as anxiety that does not respond to ordinary tranquilizers.

### Most important fact about this drug

Stelazine may cause tardive dyskinesia—a condition marked by involuntary muscle spasms and twitches in the face and body. This condition may be permanent and appears to be most common among the elderly, especially women. Ask your doctor for information about this possible risk.

### How should you take this medication?

If taking Stelazine in a liquid concentrate form, you will need to dilute it with a liquid such as a carbonated beverage, coffee, fruit juice, milk, tea, tomato juice, or water. You can also use puddings, soups, and other semisolid foods. Stelazine should be diluted just before you take it.

You should not take Stelazine with alcohol.

■ *If you miss a dose...*
If you take 1 dose a day, take the dose you missed as soon as you remember. Then go back to your regular schedule. If you do not remember until the next day, skip the missed dose and go back to your regular schedule.

If you take more than 1 dose a day, take the dose you missed if it is within an hour or so of the scheduled time. If you do not remember until later, skip the missed dose and go back to your regular schedule. Do not take 2 doses at once.

■ *Storage instructions...*
Store at room temperature. Protect the concentrate from light.

### What side effects may occur?

Side effects cannot be anticipated. If any develop or change in intensity, inform your doctor as soon as possible. Only your doctor can determine if it is safe for you to continue taking Stelazine.

■ *Side effects may include:*
Abnormal secretion of milk, abnormal sugar in urine, abnormalities in movement and posture, agitation, allergic reactions (sometimes severe), anemia, asthma, blood disorders, blurred vision, body rigidly arched backward, breast development in males, chewing movements, constipation, constricted pupils, difficulty swallowing, dilated pupils, dizziness, drooling, drowsiness, dry mouth, ejaculation problems, exaggerated or excessive reflexes, excessive or spontaneous flow of milk, eye problems causing a state of fixed gaze, eye spasms, fatigue, fever or high fever, flu-like symptoms, fluid accumulation and swelling (including the brain), fragmented movements, headache, heart attack, high or low blood sugar, hives, impotence, inability to urinate, increase in appetite and weight, infections, insomnia, intestinal blockage, involuntary movements of tongue, face, mouth, jaw, arms, and legs, irregular blood pressure, pulse, and heartbeat, irregular or no menstrual periods, jitteriness, light-headedness (especially when standing up), liver damage, lockjaw, loss of appetite, low blood pressure, mask-like face, muscle stiffness and rigidity, nasal congestion, nausea, persistent, painful erections, pill-rolling movement, protruding tongue, puckering of mouth, puffing of

cheeks, purple or red spots on the skin, rapid heartbeat, restlessness, rigid arms, feet, head, and muscles, seizures, sensitivity to light, shuffling walk, skin inflammation and peeling, skin itching, pigmentation, reddening, or rash, spasms in jaw, face, tongue, neck, hands, feet, back, and mouth, sweating, swelling of the throat, totally unresponsive state, tremors, twisted neck, weakness, yellowing of skin and whites of eyes

### Why should this drug not be prescribed?

You should not be using Stelazine if you have liver damage, or if you are taking central nervous system depressants such as alcohol, barbiturates, or narcotic pain relievers. Stelazine should not be used if you have an abnormal bone marrow or blood condition.

### Special warnings about this medication

You should use Stelazine cautiously if you have ever had a brain tumor, breast cancer, intestinal blockage, the eye condition called glaucoma, heart or liver disease, or seizures. Be cautious, too, if you are exposed to certain pesticides or extreme heat. Be aware that Stelazine may hide the signs of overdose of other drugs and may make it more difficult for your doctor to diagnose intestinal obstruction, brain tumor, and the dangerous neurological condition called Reye's syndrome.

Tell your doctor if you have ever had an allergic reaction to any major tranquilizer similar to Stelazine.

Dizziness, nausea, vomiting, and tremors can result if you suddenly stop taking Stelazine. Follow your doctor's instructions when discontinuing this drug.

Tell your doctor immediately if you experience symptoms such as a fever or sore throat, mouth, or gums. These signs of infection may signal the need to stop Stelazine treatment. Notify your doctor, too, if you develop flu-like symptoms with fever.

This drug may impair your ability to drive a car or operate potentially dangerous machinery, especially during the first few days of treatment. Do not participate in any activities that require full alertness if you are unsure about your ability.

If you have any trouble with your vision, tell your doctor.

Stelazine concentrate contains a sulfite that may cause allergic reactions in some people, especially in those with asthma.

Stelazine can cause a group of symptoms called Neuroleptic Malignant Syndrome. Signs are high body temperature, rigid muscles, irregular pulse or blood pressure, rapid or abnormal heartbeat, and excessive perspiration.

### Possible food and drug interactions when taking this medication

Extreme drowsiness and other potentially serious effects can result if Stelazine is combined with alcohol, tranquilizers such as Valium, narcotic painkillers such as Percocet, antihistamines such as Benadryl, and barbiturates such as phenobarbital.

If Stelazine is taken with certain other drugs, the effects of either could be increased, decreased, or altered. It is especially important to check with your doctor before combining Stelazine with the following:

Antiseizure drugs such as Dilantin
Atropine (Donnatal)
Blood thinners such as Coumadin
Guanethidine (Ismelin)
Lithium (Lithobid, Eskalith)
Propranolol (Inderal)
Thiazide diuretics such as Dyazide

### Special information if you are pregnant or breastfeeding

Pregnant women should use Stelazine only if clearly needed. The effects of Stelazine during pregnancy have not been adequately studied. If you are pregnant or plan to become pregnant, inform your doctor immediately. Stelazine appears in breast milk and may affect a nursing infant. If this medication is essential to your health, your doctor may have you discontinue breastfeeding while you are taking it.

### Recommended dosage

ADULTS

*Nonpsychotic Anxiety*

Doses usually range from 2 to 4 milligrams daily. This amount should be divided into 2 equal doses and taken twice a day. Do not take more than 6 milligrams a day or take the medication for more than 12 weeks.

*Psychotic Disorders*

The usual starting dose is 4 to 10 milligrams a day, divided into 2 equal doses; doses range from 15 to 40 milligrams daily.

## CHILDREN

Doses are based on the child's weight and the severity of his or her symptoms.

*Psychotic Children 6 to 12 Years Old Who Are Closely Monitored or Hospitalized*
The starting dose is 1 milligram a day, taken all at once or divided into 2 doses. Your doctor will increase the dosage gradually, up to 15 milligrams a day.

## OLDER ADULTS

Older people usually take Stelazine at lower doses. Because you may develop low blood pressure while taking this drug, your doctor will watch you closely. Older people (especially older women) may be more susceptible to tardive dyskinesia—a possibly permanent condition characterized by involuntary muscle spasms and twitches in the face and body. Consult your doctor for information about these potential risks.

### Overdosage

Any medication taken in excess can have serious consequences. If you suspect an overdose of Stelazine, seek medical help immediately.

■ *Symptoms of Stelazine overdose may include:*
Agitation, coma, convulsions, difficulty breathing, difficulty swallowing, dry mouth, extreme sleepiness, fever, intestinal blockage, irregular heart rate, low blood pressure, restlessness

*Brand name:*

# Stimate

*See DDAVP, page 135.*

*Brand name:*

# Stuartnatal Plus

*Pronounced: STU-art NAY-tal plus*
*Generic ingredients: Prenatal vitamins and minerals*
*Other brand names: Materna, Natalins Rx*

### Why is this drug prescribed?

Stuartnatal Plus contains vitamins and minerals including iron, calcium, zinc, and folic acid. The tablets are given during pregnancy and after childbirth to ensure an adequate supply of these critical nutrients. They may also be prescribed to improve a woman's nutritional status before she becomes pregnant.

### Most important fact about this drug

Nutritional supplementation is especially important during pregnancy. Be sure to take Stuartnatal Plus regularly as prescribed.

### How should you take this medication?

Take Stuartnatal Plus exactly as prescribed. The usual dosage is 1 tablet per day with or without food.

■ *If you miss a dose...*
Take it as soon as you remember, then return to your regular schedule.
■ *Storage instructions...*
Store at room temperature, away from excessive heat.

### Why should this drug not be prescribed?

There are no known reasons to avoid this preparation.

### Special information
### if you are pregnant or breastfeeding

Pregnancy and breastfeeding impose special nutritional demands on the mother. A vitamin and mineral supplement can help ensure that there are enough nutrients for both you and your baby.

### Recommended dosage

ADULTS

Before, during, and after pregnancy, take 1 tablet daily, or as directed by your doctor.

### Overdosage

Although no specific overdose information is available, even a nutritional supplement in extremely large amounts can have serious consequences. If you suspect an overdose of Stuartnatal Plus, seek medical attention immediately.

*Generic name:*

# Sucralfate

*See Carafate, page 77.*

*Generic name:*

# Sulfacetamide

*See Sodium Sulamyd, page 504.*

*Generic name:*

# Sulfasalazine

See *Azulfidine, page 48.*

*Generic name:*

# Sulfisoxazole

See *Gantrisin, page 222.*

*Generic name:*

# Sulindac

See *Clinoril, page 98.*

*Generic name:*

# Sumatriptan

See *Imitrex, page 248.*

*Brand name:*

# Sumycin

See *Tetracycline, page 537.*

*Brand name:*

# Suprax

Pronounced: *SUE-praks*
Generic name: *Cefixime*

### Why is this drug prescribed?

Suprax, a cephalosporin antibiotic, is prescribed for bacterial infections of the chest, ears, urinary tract, and throat and for uncomplicated gonorrhea.

### Most important fact about this drug

If you are allergic to either penicillin or cephalosporin antibiotics in any form, consult your doctor *before taking* Suprax. There is a possibility that you are allergic to both types of medication; and if a reaction occurs, it could be extremely severe. If you take the drug and feel signs of a reaction, seek medical attention immediately.

### How should you take this medication?

Suprax can be taken with or without food. If the medication causes stomach upset, take it with meals. Food, however, will slow down the rate at which medication is absorbed into your bloodstream.

If you are taking a liquid form of Suprax, use the specially marked measuring spoon to measure each dose accurately. Shake well before using.

It is important that you finish taking all of this medication even if you are feeling better, in order to obtain the medicine's maximum benefit.

■ *If you miss a dose...*
If you are taking this medication once a day and you forget to take a dose, take it as soon as you remember. Wait at least 10 to 12 hours before taking your next dose. Then return to your regular schedule.

If you are taking this medication 2 times a day and you forget to take a dose, take it as soon as you remember and take your next dose 5 to 6 hours later. Then go back to your regular schedule.

If you are taking this medication 3 times a day and you forget to take a dose, take it as soon as you remember and take your next dose 2 to 4 hours later. Then return to your regular schedule.

■ *Storage instructions...*
Suprax liquid may be kept for 14 days, either at room temperature or in the refrigerator. Keep the bottle tightly closed. Do not store in damp places. Keep out of reach of children and away from direct light and heat. Discard any unused portion after 14 days.

### What side effects may occur?

Side effects cannot be anticipated. If any develop or change in intensity, inform your doctor as soon as possible. Only your doctor can determine if it is safe for you to continue taking Suprax.

■ *More common side effects may include:*
Abdominal pain, gas, indigestion, loose stools, mild diarrhea, nausea, vomiting
■ *Less common side effects may include:*
Colitis, dizziness, fever, headaches, hives, itching, skin rashes, vaginitis
■ *Rare side effects may include:*
Bleeding, decrease in urine output, seizures, severe abdominal or stomach cramps, severe diarrhea (sometimes accompanied by blood), shock, skin redness

## Why should this drug not be prescribed?

If you are sensitive to or have ever had an allergic reaction to Suprax, other cephalosporin antibiotics, or any form of penicillin, you should not take this medication. Make sure that your doctor is aware of any drug reactions that you have experienced.

## Special warnings about this medication

Notify your doctor if you have had allergic reactions to penicillins or other cephalosporin antibiotics.

If you have a history of stomach or intestinal disease such as colitis, check with your doctor before taking Suprax.

If your symptoms of infection do not improve within a few days, or if they get worse, notify your doctor immediately.

If you suffer nausea, vomiting, or severe diarrhea while taking Suprax, check with your doctor before taking a diarrhea medication. Some of these medications, such as Lomotil and Paregoric, may make your diarrhea worse or cause it to last longer.

If you are a diabetic, it is important to note that Suprax may cause false urine-sugar test results. Notify your doctor that you are taking this medication before being tested for sugar in the urine. Do not change diet or dosage of diabetes medication without first consulting with your doctor.

When prescribing Suprax, your doctor may perform laboratory tests to make certain it is effective against the bacteria causing the infection. Some bacteria do not respond to Suprax, so do not give it to other people or use it for other infections.

If you have a kidney disorder, check with your doctor before taking Suprax. You may need a reduced dose of this medication because of your medical condition.

Repeated use of Suprax may result in an overgrowth of bacteria that do not respond to the medication and can cause a secondary infection. Therefore, do not save this medication for use at another time. Take this medication only when directed to do so by your doctor.

## Possible food and drug interactions when taking this medication

No interactions with food or other drugs have been reported.

## Special information
## if you are pregnant or breastfeeding

The effects of Suprax during pregnancy have not been adequately studied. If you are pregnant or plan to become pregnant, inform your doctor immediately. Suprax may appear in breast milk and could affect a nursing infant. If this medication is essential to your health, your doctor may advise you to discontinue breastfeeding your baby until your treatment with this medication is finished.

## Recommended dosage

### ADULTS

*Infections Other Than Gonorrhea*
The usual adult dose is 400 milligrams daily. This may be taken as a single 400 milligram tablet once a day or as a 200-milligram tablet every 12 hours. If you have kidney disease, the dose may be lower.

*Uncomplicated Gonorrhea*
A single 400-milligram oral dose is usually prescribed.

### CHILDREN

The safety and effectiveness of Suprax in children less than 6 months old have not been established. The usual child's dose is 8 milligrams of liquid per 2.2 pounds of body weight per day. This may be given as a single dose or in 2 half doses every 12 hours. Children weighing more than 110 pounds or older than 12 years of age should be treated with an adult dose.

If your child has a middle ear infection (otitis media), your doctor will probably prescribe Suprax suspension. The tablet form is less effective against this type of infection.

### OLDER ADULTS

Your doctor may start you on a low dosage because this drug is eliminated from your body by the kidneys and kidney function tends to decrease with age.

## Overdosage

Any medication taken in excess can cause symptoms of overdose. If you suspect an overdose, seek medical attention immediately.

■ *Symptoms of Suprax overdose may include:*
Blood in the urine, diarrhea, nausea, upper abdominal pain, vomiting

*Brand name:*

# Surmontil

*Pronounced: SIR-mon-til*
*Generic name: Trimipramine maleate*

### Why is this drug prescribed?

Surmontil is used to treat depression. It is a member of the family of drugs known as tricyclic antidepressants.

### Most important fact about this drug

Serious, sometimes fatal, reactions have been known to occur when drugs such as Surmontil are taken with another type of antidepressant called an MAO inhibitor. Drugs in this category include Nardil and Parnate. Do not take Surmontil within 2 weeks of taking one of these drugs. Make sure your doctor and pharmacist know of all the medications you are taking.

### How should you take this medication?

Surmontil may be taken in 1 dose at bedtime. Alternatively, the total daily dosage may be divided into smaller amounts taken during the day. If you are on long-term therapy with Surmontil, the single bedtime dose is preferred.

It is important to take Surmontil exactly as prescribed, even if the drug seems to have no effect. It may take up to 4 weeks for its benefits to appear.

Surmontil can make your mouth dry. Sucking hard candy or chewing gum can help this problem.

■ *If you miss a dose...*

Take it as soon as you remember. If it is almost time for the next dose, skip the one you missed and go back to your regular schedule. Do not take 2 doses at once. If you take Surmontil once a day at bedtime and you miss a dose, do not take it in the morning. It could cause disturbing side effects during the day.

■ *Storage instructions...*

Store at room temperature in a tightly closed container. Capsules in blister strips should be protected from moisture.

### What side effects may occur?

Side effects cannot be anticipated. If any develop or change in intensity, inform your doctor as soon as possible. Only your doctor can determine if it is safe for you to continue taking Surmontil.

■ *Side effects may include:*

Abdominal cramps, agitation, anxiety, black tongue, blocked intestine, blood disorders, blurred vision, breast development in men, confusion (especially in older adults), constipation, delusions, diarrhea, difficulty urinating, dilated pupils, disorientation, dizziness, drowsiness, dry mouth, excessive or spontaneous milk excretion, fatigue, fever, flushing, fluttery or throbbing heartbeat, frequent urination, hair loss, hallucinations, headache, heart attack, high blood pressure, high blood sugar, hives, impotence, increased or decreased sex drive, inflammation of the mouth, insomnia, irregular heart rate, lack of coordination, loss of appetite, low blood pressure, low blood sugar, nausea, nightmares, numbness, peculiar taste in mouth, purple or reddish-brown spots on skin, rapid heartbeat, restlessness, ringing in the ears, seizures, sensitivity to light, skin itching, skin rash, sore throat, stomach upset, stroke, sweating, swelling of breasts, swelling of face and tongue, swelling of testicles, swollen glands, tingling, pins and needles, tremors, visual problems, vomiting, weakness, weight gain or loss, yellowing of the skin and whites of the eyes

### Why should this drug not be prescribed?

Surmontil should not be used if you are recovering from a recent heart attack.

You should not take Surmontil if you are sensitive to it or have ever had an allergic reaction to it or to other similar drugs such as Tofranil.

### Special warnings about this medication

Use Surmontil cautiously if you have a seizure disorder, the eye condition known as glaucoma, heart disease, or a liver disorder. Also use caution if you have thyroid disease or are taking thyroid medication. People who have had problems urinating should also be careful about taking Surmontil.

Nausea, headache, and a general feeling of illness may result if you suddenly stop taking Surmontil. This does not mean you are addicted, but you should follow your doctor's instructions closely when discontinuing the drug.

This drug may impair your ability to drive a car or operate potentially dangerous machinery. Do not participate in any activities that require full alertness if you are unsure of the drug's effect on you.

## Possible food and drug interactions when taking this medication

People who are taking antidepressants known as MAO inhibitors (Parnate and Nardil) should not take Surmontil.

Wait 2 weeks after stopping an MAO inhibitor before you begin taking Surmontil.

If Surmontil is taken with certain other drugs, the effects of either could be increased, decreased, or altered. It is especially important to check with your doctor before combining Surmontil with the following:

Antidepressants such as Desyrel and Wellbutrin
Antidepressants that act on serotonin, such as
 Prozac, Paxil, and Zoloft
Antispasmodic drugs such as Donnatal and
 Cogentin
Cimetidine (Tagamet)
Drugs for heart irregularities, such as Rythmol and
 Tambocor
Guanethidine (Ismelin)
Local anesthetics containing epinephrine
Local decongestants such as Dristan Nasal Spray
Major tranquilizers such as Thorazine and Mellaril
Quinidine (Quinidex, Quinaglute)
Stimulants such as Proventil, Sudafed, and EpiPen
Thyroid medications such as Synthroid

Extreme drowsiness and other potentially serious effects may result if you drink alcoholic beverages while you are taking Surmontil.

## Special information if you are pregnant or breastfeeding

The effects of Surmontil in pregnancy have not been adequately studied. Pregnant women should use Surmontil only when the potential benefits clearly outweigh the potential risks.

## Recommended dosage

### ADULTS

The usual starting dose is 75 milligrams per day, divided into equal smaller doses. Your doctor may gradually increase your dose to 150 milligrams per day, divided into smaller doses. Doses over 200 milligrams a day are not recommended. Doses in long-term therapy may range from 50 to 150 milligrams daily. You can take this total daily dosage at bedtime or spread it throughout the day.

### CHILDREN

Safety and effectiveness of Surmontil in children have not been established.

### OLDER ADULTS AND ADOLESCENTS

Dosages usually start at 50 milligrams per day. Your doctor may increase the dose to 100 milligrams a day, if needed.

## Overdosage

Any medication taken in excess can have serious consequences. An overdose of Surmontil can be fatal. If you suspect an overdose, seek medical help immediately.

■ *Symptoms of Surmontil overdose may include:*
 Agitation, coma, convulsions, difficulty breathing, dilated pupils, discolored bluish skin, drowsiness, heart failure, high fever, involuntary movement, irregular heart rate, lack of coordination, low blood pressure, muscle rigidity, rapid heartbeat, restlessness, shock, stupor, sweating, vomiting

*Brand name:*

# Synalgos-DC

*Pronounced: SIN-al-gose dee-cee*
*Generic ingredients: Dihydrocodeine bitartrate,*
 *Aspirin, Caffeine*

## Why is this drug prescribed?

Synalgos-DC is a narcotic analgesic prescribed for the relief of moderate to moderately severe pain.

## Most important fact about this drug

Narcotics such as Synalgos-DC can be habit-forming or addicting if they are taken over long periods of time.

## How should you take this medication?

Take Synalgos-DC exactly as prescribed. Do not increase the amount you take without your doctor's approval.

Avoid or reduce use of alcohol while taking Synalgos-DC.

■ *If you miss a dose...*
 If you take this drug on a regular schedule, take the forgotten dose as soon as you remember. If it is almost time for your next dose, skip the one you missed and go back to your regular schedule. Do not take 2 doses at once.

■ *Storage instructions...*

Store at room temperature in a tightly closed container.

### What side effects may occur?

Side effects cannot be anticipated. If any develop or change in intensity, inform your doctor as soon as possible. Only your doctor can determine if it is safe for you to continue taking Synalgos-DC.

■ *Side effects may include:*

Constipation, dizziness, drowsiness, itching, light-headedness, nausea, sedation, skin reactions, vomiting

### Why should this drug not be prescribed?

If you are sensitive to or have ever had an allergic reaction to Synalgos-DC, other narcotic pain relievers, or aspirin, you should not take this medication.

Make sure your doctor is aware of any drug reactions you have experienced.

### Special warnings about this medication

Synalgos-DC may cause you to become drowsy or less alert; therefore, you should not drive or operate dangerous machinery or participate in any hazardous activity that requires full mental alertness until you know how this drug affects you.

If you have ever been dependent on or addicted to drugs, consult your doctor before taking Synalgos-DC.

If you are being treated for a stomach ulcer or blood-clotting disorder, consult your doctor before taking this medication.

### Possible food and drug interactions when taking this medication

Synalgos-DC slows brain activity and intensifies the effects of alcohol. Therefore, you should reduce your intake of alcoholic beverages or avoid them altogether.

If Synalgos-DC is taken with certain other drugs, the effects of either could be increased, decreased, or altered. It is especially important to check with your doctor before combining Synalgos-DC with the following:

Narcotic pain relievers such as Percocet and
  Demerol
Sedatives such as Halcion and Seconal
Tranquilizers such as Valium and Xanax

Taking blood thinners such as Coumadin in combination with Synalgos-DC may cause internal bleeding.

The use of Synalgos-DC in combination with antigout medications such as Benemid may alter its effects.

### Special information if you are pregnant or breastfeeding

The effects of Synalgos-DC during pregnancy have not been adequately studied. If you are pregnant or plan to become pregnant, inform your doctor immediately. This drug may appear in breast milk and could affect a nursing infant. If this medication is essential to your health, your doctor may advise you to discontinue breastfeeding until your treatment is finished.

### Recommended dosage

ADULTS

Your doctor will prescribe a dosage based on the severity of your pain and how you respond to this medication. The usual dose of Synalgos-DC is 2 capsules taken every 4 hours as needed.

CHILDREN

The safety and effectiveness of this medication have not been established in children 12 years of age and under.

OLDER ADULTS

Synalgos-DC should be taken with caution by older adults or anyone in a weakened or rundown condition. Therefore, your doctor will adjust the dosage accordingly.

### Overdosage

Although no specific information is available, any medication taken in excess can have serious consequences. If you suspect an overdose of Synalgos-DC, seek medical attention immediately.

*Brand name:*

# Synthroid

*Pronounced: SIN-throid*
*Generic name: Levothyroxine*
*Other brand names: Eltroxin, Levothroid, Levoxyl*

### Why is this drug prescribed?

Synthroid, a synthetic thyroid hormone available in tablet or injectable form, may be given in any of the following cases:

If your own thyroid gland is not making enough hormone;

If you have an enlarged thyroid (a goiter) or are at risk for developing a goiter;

If you need a "suppression test" to determine whether your thyroid gland is making too much hormone;

If you have certain cancers of the thyroid;

If your thyroid production is low due to surgery, radiation, or certain drugs.

### Most important fact about this drug

If you are taking Synthroid to make up for a lack of natural hormone, it is important to take it regularly at the same time every day. You will probably need to take it for the rest of your life.

### How should you take this medication?

Take Synthroid exactly as directed. Take no more or less than the prescribed amount and take it no more or less often than prescribed. Take your dose at the same time every day for consistent effect. Do not use it for any other condition or let anyone else use it for whatever reason.

If a child cannot swallow whole tablets, you may crush a Synthroid tablet and mix it into a spoonful of liquid or sprinkle it over a small amount of food such as cooked cereal or applesauce. Give this mixture while it is very fresh; never store it for future use.

While taking Synthroid, your doctor will perform periodic blood tests to determine whether you are getting the right amount.

■ *If you miss a dose...*
Take it as soon as you remember. If it is almost time for your next dose, skip the one you missed and go back to your regular schedule. Never take 2 doses at the same time. If you miss 2 or more doses in a row, consult your doctor.

■ *Storage instructions...*
Keep this medication in a tightly closed container. Store it at room temperature, away from heat, light, and moisture.

### What side effects may occur?

Side effects from Synthroid, other than overdose symptoms, are rare. People who are treated with Synthroid may initially lose some hair, but this effect is usually temporary. You may have an allergic reaction such as a rash or hives. Children may have an increase in pressure within the skull.

Excessive dosage or a too rapid increase in dosage may lead to overstimulation of the thyroid gland. Notify your doctor immediately if you develop any if the following symptoms.

■ *Symptoms of overstimulation:*
Abdominal cramps, changes in appetite, chest pain, diarrhea, fever, headache, heat intolerance, increased heart rate, irregular heartbeat, irritability, nausea, nervousness, palpitations, sleeplessness, sweating, tremors, weight loss

### Why should this drug not be prescribed?

You should not be treated with Synthroid if you have ever had an allergic reaction to it; your thyroid gland is making too much thyroid hormone; you have had a recent heart attack; or your adrenal glands are not making enough corticosteroid hormone. If you are sensitive to dyes, you can take the Synthroid 50-microgram tablet, which is made without color additives.

Although Synthroid will speed up your metabolism, it is not effective as a weight-loss drug and should not be used as such. An overdose may cause life-threatening side effects, especially if you take Synthroid with an appetite-suppressant medication.

### Special warnings about this medication

Synthroid has profound effects on the body. Make sure your doctor is aware of all your medical problems and allergies.

You should receive low doses of Synthroid, under very close supervision, if you are an older person, or if you suffer from high blood pressure, angina (chest pain caused by a heart condition), or other types of heart disease.

If you have diabetes, or if your body makes insufficient adrenal corticosteroid hormone, Synthroid will tend to make your symptoms worse. If you take medication for any of these disorders, the dosage will probably have to be adjusted once you begin taking Synthroid.

Synthroid may cause seizures at the beginning of treatment, although this is rare.

It may take a few weeks for Synthroid to begin working, and you may not see any change in your symptoms until then.

Tell your doctor or dentist you are taking Synthroid before you have surgery of any kind.

Tell your doctor if you become pregnant while you are taking Synthroid. Your dose may need to be increased.

Do not switch to another brand of levothyroxine without consulting your doctor.

Excessive doses of Synthroid in infants may cause the top of the skull to close too early.

### Possible food and drug interactions when taking this medication

Synthroid can interact with a wide variety of medications. It's advisable to check with your doctor before taking *any* other drug.

### Special information if you are pregnant or breastfeeding

If you need to take Synthroid because of a thyroid hormone deficiency, you can continue to take the medication during pregnancy. Once your baby is born, you may breastfeed while continuing to take carefully regulated doses of Synthroid.

### Recommended dosage

Your doctor will tailor the dosage to meet your individual requirements, taking into consideration the status of your thyroid gland and other medical conditions you may have. He or she will monitor your thyroid hormone level with periodic blood tests.

### Overdosage

If you suspect a Synthroid overdose, seek emergency medical attention immediately. Taken in excess, the drug may have serious consequences.

■ *Symptoms of Synthroid overdose may include:*
Abdominal cramps, chest pain, diarrhea, excessive sweating, fever, headache, heat intolerance, increased appetite, increased pulse and blood pressure, irregular heartbeat, menstrual irregularities, nervousness, palpitations, tremors, weight loss

---

*Generic name:*

# Tacrine

*See Cognex, page 105.*

---

*Brand name:*

# Tagamet

*Pronounced: TAG-ah-met*
*Generic name: Cimetidine*
*Other brand name: Tagamet HB*

### Why is this drug prescribed?

Tagamet is prescribed for the treatment of certain kinds of stomach and intestinal ulcers and related conditions. These include: active duodenal (upper intestinal) ulcers; active benign stomach ulcers; erosive gastroesophageal reflux disease (backflow of acid stomach contents); prevention of upper abdominal bleeding in those who are critically ill; and excess-acid conditions such as Zollinger-Ellison syndrome (a form of peptic ulcer with too much acid). It is also used for maintenance therapy of duodenal ulcer following the healing of active ulcers. Tagamet is known as a histamine blocker.

Some doctors also use Tagamet to treat acne and to prevent stress-induced ulcers. It may also be used to treat chronic hives, herpesvirus infections (including shingles), abnormal hair growth in women, and overactivity of the parathyroid gland.

Tagamet HB is an over-the-counter version of the drug used to relieve heartburn, acid indigestion, and sour stomach.

### Most important fact about this drug

Short-term treatment with Tagamet can result in complete healing of a duodenal ulcer. However, there can be a recurrence of the ulcer after Tagamet has been discontinued. The rate of ulcer recurrence may be slightly higher in people healed with Tagamet rather than other forms of therapy. However, Tagamet is usually prescribed for more severe cases.

### How should you take this medication?

You can take Tagamet with or between meals. Do not take antacids within 1 to 2 hours of a dose of Tagamet. Avoid excessive amounts of caffeine while taking this drug.

It may take several days for Tagamet to begin relieving stomach pain. Be sure to continue taking the drug exactly as prescribed even if it seems to have no effect.

Do not take the maximum daily dose of Tagamet HB for more than 2 weeks continuously without consulting your doctor.

■ *If you miss a dose...*
Take it as soon as you remember. If it is almost time for your next dose, skip the one you missed and go back to your regular schedule. Do not take 2 doses at once.
■ *Storage instructions...*
Store at room temperature in a tightly closed container, away from light.

## What side effects may occur?

Side effects cannot be anticipated. If any develop or change in intensity, inform your doctor as soon as possible. Only your doctor can determine if it is safe for you to continue taking Tagamet.

■ *More common side effects may include:*
Breast development in men, headache

Less common side effects—agitation, anxiety, confusion, depression, disorientation, and hallucinations—may appear in severely ill individuals who have been treated for 1 month or longer. However, these reactions are not permanent and have cleared up within 3 to 4 days of discontinuation of the drug.

■ *Rare side effects may include:*
Allergic reactions, anemia, blood disorders, diarrhea, dizziness, fever, hair loss, impotence, inability to urinate, joint pain, kidney disorders, liver disorders, mild rash, muscle pain, pancreas inflammation, rapid heartbeat, skin inflammation or peeling, sleepiness, slow heart beat

## Why should this drug not be prescribed?

If you have ever had an allergic reaction to Tagamet, do not take this medication.

## Special warnings about this medication

Ulcers may be more difficult to heal if you smoke cigarettes.

If you are being treated for a liver or kidney disorder, make sure the doctor is aware if it.

If you are over 50 years old, have liver or kidney disease, or are severely ill, you may experience temporary mental confusion while taking Tagamet. Notify your doctor.

If you have trouble swallowing or persistent abdominal pain, do not take Tagamet HB; instead, check with your doctor. You may have a serious condition that requires different treatment.

## Possible food and drug interactions when taking this medication

If Tagamet is taken with certain other drugs, the effects of either can be increased, decreased, or altered. It is especially important that you check with your doctor before combining Tagamet with the following:

Antidiabetic drugs such as Micronase and Glucotrol
Antifungal drugs such as Diflucan and Nizoral
Aspirin
Augmentin

Benzodiazepine tranquilizers such as Valium and Librium
Beta-blocking blood pressure drugs such as Inderal and Lopressor
Calcium-blocking blood pressure drugs such as Cardizem, Calan, and Procardia
Chlorpromazine (Thorazine)
Cisapride (Propulsid)
Cyclosporine (Sandimmune)
Digoxin (Lanoxin)
Medications for irregular heartbeat, such as Cordarone, Tonocard, Quinidex, and Procan
Metoclopramide (Reglan)
Metronidazole (Flagyl)
Narcotic pain relievers such as Demerol and Morphine
Nicotine (Nicoderm, Nicorette)
Paroxetine (Paxil)
Pentoxifylline (Trental)
Phenytoin (Dilantin)
Quinine
Sucralfate (Carafate)
Theophylline (Theo-Dur, others)
Warfarin (Coumadin)

Avoid alcoholic beverages while taking Tagamet. This medication increases the effects of alcohol.

Antacids can reduce the effect of Tagamet when taken at the same time. If you take an antacid to relieve the pain of an ulcer, the doses should be separated by 1 to 2 hours.

If you need to take an antifungal drug such as Nizoral, you should take it at least 2 hours before you take Tagamet.

## Special information
## if you are pregnant or breastfeeding

The effects of Tagamet during pregnancy have not been adequately studied. If you are pregnant or plan to become pregnant, notify your doctor immediately. Tagamet appears in breast milk and could affect a nursing infant. If this medication is essential to your health, your doctor may advise you to discontinue breastfeeding until treatment with this drug is finished.

## Recommended dosage

TAGAMET (ADULTS)

*Active Duodenal Ulcer*
The usual dose is 800 milligrams once daily at bedtime. However, other doses shown to be effective are:

300 milligrams 4 times a day with meals and at bedtime

400 milligrams twice a day, in the morning and at bedtime

Most people heal in 4 weeks.

If you require maintenance therapy, the usual dose is 400 milligrams at bedtime.

### Active Benign Gastric Ulcer

The usual dose is 800 milligrams once a day at bedtime or 300 milligrams taken 4 times a day with meals and at bedtime.

### Erosive Gastroesophageal Reflux Disease

The usual dosage is a total of 1,600 milligrams daily divided into doses of 800 milligrams twice a day or 400 milligrams 4 times a day for 12 weeks. The beneficial use of Tagamet beyond 12 weeks has not been firmly established.

### Pathological Hypersecretory Condition

The usual dosage is 300 milligrams 4 times a day with meals and at bedtime. Your doctor may adjust your dosage based on your needs, but you should take no more than 2,400 milligrams per day.

### TAGAMET (CHILDREN)

Safety and effectiveness have not been established in children under 16 years old. However, your doctor may decide that the potential benefits of Tagamet use outweigh the potential risks. Doses of 20 to 40 milligrams per 2.2 pounds of body weight have been used.

### TAGAMET HB

*Heartburn, acid indigestion, sour stomach*
The usual dosage is 2 tablets, taken with water, once or up to twice a day. Do not take more than 4 tablets in 24 hours.

Do not give Tagamet HB to children under 12 years unless your doctor tells you to.

### Overdosage

Information concerning overdosage is limited. However, respiratory failure, an increased heartbeat, exaggerated side effect symptoms or reactions such as unresponsiveness may be signs of Tagamet overdose. If you experience any of these symptoms, notify your doctor immediately.

Brand name:

# Talwin Compound

Pronounced: TAL-win
Generic ingredients: Pentazocine hydrochloride, Aspirin

### Why is this drug prescribed?

Talwin Compound combines the strong analgesic properties of pentazocine and the analgesic, anti-inflammatory, and fever-reducing properties of aspirin. It is used for the relief of moderate pain.

### Most important fact about this drug

Talwin Compound can cause physical and psychological dependence. Do not share Talwin Compound with other people.

### How should you take this medication?

Take Talwin Compound exactly as prescribed by your doctor. Do not increase the amount you take without your doctor's approval.

■ *If you miss a dose...*
And you take this medication on a regular schedule, take the forgotten dose as soon as you remember. If it is almost time for your next dose, skip the one you missed and go back to your regular schedule. Do not take 2 doses at once.
■ *Storage instructions...*
Store away from heat, light, and moisture.

### What side effects may occur?

Side effects cannot be anticipated. If any develop or change in intensity, inform your doctor as soon as possible. Only your doctor can determine if it is safe for you to continue taking Talwin.

■ *More common side effects may include:*
Confusion, disorientation, dizziness, feelings of elation, hallucinations, headache, light-headedness, nausea, sedation, sweating, vomiting

If any of these side effects occur, it may help if you lie down after taking the medication.

■ *Less common side effects may include:*
Blurred vision, constipation, depression, difficulty in focusing, disturbed dreams, fainting, flushing, inability to fall or stay asleep, lowered blood pressure, rapid heart rate, rash, weakness
■ *Rare side effects may include:*
Abdominal distress, chills, diarrhea, excitement, facial swelling, fluid retention, hives, inability to

urinate, irritability, lack or loss of appetite, ringing in the ears, skin peeling, tingling sensation, tremors, troubled or slowed breathing

### Why should this drug not be prescribed?

If you are sensitive to or have ever had an allergic reaction to pentazocine or salicylates (anti-inflammatory drugs such as aspirin), or other drugs of this type, you should not take this medication. Make sure your doctor is aware of any drug reactions you have experienced.

Because there is a possible association between aspirin and the dangerous neurological condition called Reye's syndrome, Talwin should not be given to children and teenagers who have chickenpox or flu, which predispose them to development of the condition.

### Special warnings about this medication

Drug dependence and withdrawal symptoms—if you stop taking the drug abruptly—can occur with the use of pentazocine. If you have a history of drug dependence, Talwin should be used only under the close supervision of your doctor.

Talwin Compound may cause you to become drowsy, dizzy, or less alert; therefore, you should not drive or operate dangerous machinery or participate in any hazardous activity that requires full mental alertness until you know how this drug affects you.

Talwin Compound contains aspirin. If you have a stomach ulcer, consult your doctor before taking this medication. Aspirin may irritate the stomach lining and may cause bleeding.

If you have a kidney or liver disorder, or if you are prone to seizures, consult your doctor before taking Talwin.

Talwin Compound may cause breathing difficulties. If you have severe bronchial asthma or other respiratory problems, check with your doctor before taking this medication.

Talwin should be used with caution if you have had a heart attack or if you are nauseated or are vomiting.

Talwin Compound should be used with extreme caution in patients being treated by a doctor for a head injury. This medication may cause troubled breathing and pressure on the skull from increased brain and spinal fluid—which can be exaggerated by a head injury. This drug may also mask or hide

the pain from head injury, making it difficult for your doctor to treat.

Use Talwin Compound only to relieve pain, not in anticipation of pain.

### Possible food and drug interactions when taking this medication

Talwin Compound slows brain activity and intensifies the effects of alcohol. Limit your intake of alcohol while taking this medication.

If Talwin Compound is taken with certain other drugs, the effects of either could be increased, decreased, or altered. It is especially important to check with your doctor before combining Talwin Compound with the following:

Benzodiazepines such as Valium and Xanax
MAO inhibitors (antidepressants such as Nardil)
Other analgesics (pain relievers such as Demerol)
Sleep aids such as Dalmane and Halcion

The use of these drugs with Talwin Compound increases their sedative or calming effects and may lead to overdose symptoms.

The use of blood thinners such as Coumadin in combination with Talwin Compound may cause bleeding. If you are taking a blood thinner, consult your doctor before taking this drug.

The use of narcotics, including methadone (prescribed for the daily treatment of drug dependence), with Talwin Compound may produce withdrawal symptoms.

### Special information if you are pregnant or breastfeeding

The effects of Talwin Compound during pregnancy have not been adequately studied. Consult your physician before taking Talwin Compound when pregnant. It is not known whether Talwin Compound appears in breast milk. If this medication is essential to your health, your doctor may advise you to discontinue breastfeeding until your treatment is finished.

### Recommended dosage

ADULTS

The usual dose of Talwin Compound is 2 caplets, 3 or 4 times per day.

CHILDREN

The safety and effectiveness of Talwin Compound have not been established in children under 12 years of age.

## Overdosage

Any medication taken in excess can have dangerous consequences. If you suspect an overdose, seek
medical attention immediately.

■ *Symptoms of an overdose of Talwin Compound,*
  *because of its aspirin content, may include:*
  Coma, confusion, convulsions, diarrhea, dizziness, gasping, headache, heavy perspiration,
  nausea, rapid breathing, rapid heart rate, ringing
  in the ears, thirst, vomiting

An inability to breathe may lead to death.

*Brand name:*

# Tambocor

Pronounced: TAM-ba-kore
Generic name: Flecainide acetate

## Why is this drug prescribed?

Tambocor is prescribed to treat certain heart
rhythm disturbances, including paroxysmal atrial
fibrillation (a sudden attack or worsening of irregular heartbeat in which the upper chamber of the
heart beats irregularly and very rapidly) and paroxysmal supraventricular tachycardia (a sudden attack
or worsening of an abnormally fast but regular
heart rate that occurs in intermittent episodes).

## Most important fact about this drug

Tambocor may sometimes cause or worsen heartbeat irregularities and certain heart conditions, such
as heart failure (the inability of the heart to sustain
its workload of pumping blood). Before prescribing
Tambocor, your doctor will explain the risks and
benefits of Tambocor and how he or she will
monitor your condition.

## How should you take this medication?

In almost every case, your doctor will initiate
Tambocor therapy in the hospital.

Take Tambocor exactly as prescribed by your
doctor. Serious heartbeat disturbances may result if
you do not follow your doctor's instructions, if you
miss any regular doses, or if you increase or
decrease the dosage without consulting your doctor.

Your doctor may order regular blood tests to
monitor your therapy.

■ *If you miss a dose...*
  Take it as soon as you remember if it is within 6
  hours of your scheduled time. If you do not

remember until later, skip the dose you missed
and go back to your regular schedule. Do not
take 2 doses at once.

■ *Storage instructions...*
  Store at room temperature in a tightly closed container, away from light.

## What side effects may occur?

Tambocor has a wide variety of possible effects on
the heart, including new or worsened heartbeat
abnormalities, heart attack, congestive heart failure,
and heart block—an interference with the heart's
contraction. If any develop, inform your doctor
immediately. Only your doctor can determine
whether it is safe for you to continue taking
Tambocor.

■ *Other side effects may include:*
  Abdominal pain, angina pectoris (crushing chest
  pain), anxiety, apathy, appetite loss, chest pain,
  confusion, constipation, convulsions, decreased
  sex drive, depression, diarrhea, difficult or
  labored breathing, dizziness (light-headedness,
  faintness, near fainting, unsteadiness), dry
  mouth, edema (accumulation of fluid in the
  tissues), exaggerated feeling of well-being,
  excessive urine, eye pain or irritation, fainting,
  fatigue, fever, flushing, gas, hair loss, headache,
  heart palpitations (fluttery heartbeat), high or low
  blood pressure, hives, impotence, inability to
  urinate, indigestion, insomnia, intolerance of
  light, involuntary eye movements, itching, joint
  pain, lack of coordination, loss of sense of identity, lung inflammation or other conditions,
  malaise (feeling unwell or ill), memory loss,
  morbid dreams, muscle pain, nausea, numbness
  or tingling, paralysis, rash, reduced sensitivity to
  touch, ringing in the ears, skin inflammation and
  peeling, sleepiness, speech problems, stupor,
  sweating, swollen lips, tongue, and mouth, taste
  changes, tremor, twitching, vertigo, vision problems (blurred vision, difficulty in focusing,
  double vision, spots before the eyes), vomiting,
  weakness, wheezing

## Why should this drug not be prescribed?

Your doctor should not prescribe Tambocor if you
have ever had an allergic reaction to it or you are
sensitive to it, if you have heart block (without a
pacemaker), or if your heart cannot supply enough
blood to the body.

## Special warnings about this medication

If you have a pacemaker, you should be monitored very closely while taking Tambocor—your pacemaker may need to be adjusted.

If you have liver disease, Tambocor could build up in your system. Your doctor will prescribe the drug only if the benefits outweigh the risks. In addition, you should have frequent blood tests to make sure your dosage is not too high.

If you have a history of congestive heart failure or a weak heart, you may be at increased risk for dangerous cardiac side effects from Tambocor.

If you have very alkaline urine, perhaps caused by a kidney condition or by a strict vegetarian diet, your body will tend to process and eliminate Tambocor rather slowly and you may need a lower-than-average dosage.

If the potassium levels in your blood are too high or too low, your doctor will want to correct the condition before allowing you to take Tambocor.

If you have kidney failure, your doctor will want to watch you closely.

## Possible food and drug interactions when taking this medication

If Tambocor is taken with certain other drugs, the effects of either could be increased, decreased, or altered. It is especially important to check with your doctor before combining Tambocor with the following:

Amiodarone (Cordarone)
Beta blockers (blood pressure drugs such as
   Inderal, Tenormin, and Sectral)
Carbamazepine (Tegretol)
Cimetidine (Tagamet)
Diltiazem (Cardizem)
Disopyramide (Norpace)
Nifedipine (Procardia)
Phenobarbital
Phenytoin (Dilantin)
Verapamil (Calan, Isoptin)

## Special information if you are pregnant or breastfeeding

The effects of Tambocor during pregnancy have not been adequately studied. If you are pregnant or plan to become pregnant, inform your doctor immediately. Tambocor should be used during pregnancy only if the benefit justifies the potential risk to the unborn child. Tambocor appears in breast milk. Check with your doctor before breastfeeding your baby.

## Recommended dosage

ADULTS

Treatment with Tambocor almost always begins in the hospital.

The usual starting dose is 50 to 100 milligrams every 12 hours, depending on the condition under treatment. Every 4 days, your doctor may increase your dose by 50 milligrams every 12 hours until your condition is under control.

## Overdosage

An overdose of Tambocor is likely to cause slowed or rapid heartbeat, other cardiac problems, fainting, low blood pressure, nausea, vomiting, convulsions, and heart failure. Taken even in moderate excess, Tambocor may have serious consequences and can be fatal. If you suspect an overdose, seek medical attention immediately.

---

*Generic name:*

# Tamoxifen

*See Nolvadex, page 365.*

---

*Brand name:*

# Tavist

*Pronounced: TAV-ist*
*Generic name: Clemastine fumarate*

## Why is this drug prescribed?

Tavist is an antihistamine. Both Tavist and Tavist-1 are used in treatment of the sneezing, runny nose, itching, and watery eyes caused by hay fever. Tavist Tablets also relieve mild allergic skin reactions such as hives and swelling. Antihistamines reduce itching and swelling and dry up secretions from the eyes, nose, and throat.

## Most important fact about this drug

Tavist may cause drowsiness. Be especially careful driving or operating dangerous machinery or participating in any hazardous activity that requires full mental alertness until you know how you react to this medication.

## How should you take this medication?

Tavist should be taken exactly as prescribed.

Tavist may make your mouth dry. Sucking hard candy, chewing gum, or melting bits of ice in your mouth can provide relief.

■ *If you miss a dose...*

If you are taking this medication on a regular schedule, take the forgotten dose as soon as you remember. If it is almost time for your next dose, skip the one you missed and go back to your regular schedule. Do not take 2 doses at once.

■ *Storage instructions...*

Store at room temperature in a tightly closed container, away from light.

## What side effects may occur?

Side effects cannot be anticipated. If any develop or change in intensity, inform your doctor as soon as possible. Only your doctor can determine if it is safe for you to continue taking Tavist.

■ *More common side effects may include:*

Disturbed coordination, dizziness, drowsiness, extreme calm (sedation), sleepiness, upset stomach

■ *Less common or rare side effects may include:*

Acute inflammation of the inner ear, anemia, blurred vision, chills, confusion, constipation, convulsions, diarrhea, difficulty sleeping, difficulty urinating, double vision, dry mouth, nose, and throat, early menstruation, exaggerated sense of well-being, excessive perspiration, excitement, fatigue, frequent urination, headache, hives, hysteria, inability to urinate, increased chest congestion, irregular heartbeat, irritability, loss of appetite, low blood pressure, nausea, nerve inflammation, nervousness, palpitations, rapid heartbeat, rash, restlessness, ringing in the ears, sensitivity to light, severe allergic reaction (anaphylactic shock), stuffy nose, tightness of chest, tingling or pins and needles, tremor, vertigo, vomiting, wheezing

## Why should this drug not be prescribed?

Tavist should be avoided if you are breastfeeding, if you are taking antidepressant drugs known as MAO inhibitors (Nardil, Parnate), or if you have asthma or other breathing problems. If you are sensitive to or have ever had an allergic reaction to clemastine fumarate or other antihistamines with a similar chemical composition, do not take this medication.

## Special warnings about this medication

Use antihistamines very cautiously if you have the eye condition known as narrow-angle glaucoma, a peptic ulcer, intestinal blockage, a bladder obstruction, or an enlarged prostate. Antihistamines can make these problems worse.

Antihistamines are more likely to cause dizziness, sedation, and low blood pressure in the elderly (over age 60).

Use Tavist with care if you have a history of bronchial asthma, heart disease, circulatory problems, an overactive thyroid, or high blood pressure.

## Possible food and drug interactions when taking this medication

Tavist may increase the effects of alcohol. Do not drink alcohol—or at least limit your use—while taking this medication.

If Tavist is taken with certain other drugs, the effects of either could be increased, decreased, or altered. It is especially important to check with your doctor before combining Tavist with the following:

Antidepressant drugs known as MAO inhibitors such as Nardil, Marplan, and Parnate
Sedatives such as Nembutal and Seconal
Tranquilizers such as Xanax and Valium

## Special information if you are pregnant or breastfeeding

The effects of Tavist during pregnancy have not been adequately studied. If you are pregnant or plan to become pregnant, inform your doctor immediately. Tavist should not be used if you are breastfeeding.

## Recommended dosage

TAVIST-1 TABLETS

The recommended starting dose is 1 tablet twice daily. Your doctor may increase the dose to a maximum of 6 tablets daily.

TAVIST TABLETS

The maximum recommended dosage is 1 tablet 3 times daily. Many people do well on a single dose. You should take no more than 3 tablets daily.

TAVIST SYRUP

*Adults and Children 12 Years and Over
For Symptoms of Hay Fever*
The starting dose of Tavist Syrup is 2 teaspoonfuls (1 milligram) 2 times a day. Your doctor may

increase the dosage, but it should not be more than 12 teaspoonfuls (6 milligrams) daily.

### For Hives and Swelling

The starting dose of Tavist Syrup is 4 teaspoonfuls (2 milligrams) twice a day; you should not take more than 12 teaspoonfuls (6 milligrams) daily.

### Children 6 through 11
### For Symptoms of Hay Fever

The starting dose of Tavist Syrup is 1 teaspoonful (0.5 milligram) 2 times per day. Your doctor may increase the dosage to a maximum of 6 teaspoonfuls (3 milligrams) daily.

### For Hives and Swelling

The starting dose of Tavist Syrup is 2 teaspoonfuls (1 milligram) twice a day, not to exceed 6 teaspoonfuls (3 milligrams) daily.

## Overdosage

Any medication taken in excess can have serious consequences. If you suspect an overdose, seek medical treatment immediately.

■ *Symptoms of Tavist overdose may include:*
Coma, convulsions, drowsiness, dry mouth, fever, fixed, dilated pupils, flushing, stimulation, especially in children, stomach and intestinal problems

■ *Symptoms of Tavist overdose in children may include:*
Bluish color to the skin, convulsions, excitement, hallucinations, high body temperature, slow, twisting movements of hand and arms, tremors, twitching, uncoordinated movements

*Brand name:*

# Tegretol

*Pronounced: TEG-re-tawl*
*Generic name: Carbamazepine*
*Other brand names: Epitol, Atretol*

## Why is this drug prescribed?

Tegretol is used in the treatment of seizure disorders, including certain types of epilepsy. It is also prescribed for trigeminal neuralgia (severe pain in the jaws) and pain in the tongue and throat.

In addition, some doctors use Tegretol to treat alcohol withdrawal, cocaine addiction, and emotional disorders such as depression and abnormally aggressive behavior. The drug is also used to treat migraine headache and "restless legs."

## Most important fact about this drug

There are potentially dangerous side effects associated with the use of Tegretol. If you experience symptoms such as fever, sore throat, ulcers in the mouth, easy bruising, or reddish or purplish spots on the skin, you should notify your doctor immediately. These symptoms could be signs of a blood disorder brought on by the drug.

## How should you take this medication?

This medication should only be taken with meals, never on an empty stomach.

Shake the suspension well before using.

■ *If you miss a dose...*
Take it as soon as you remember. If it is almost time for your next dose, skip the one you missed and go back to your regular schedule. Do not take 2 doses at once. If you miss more than 1 dose in a day, check with your doctor.

■ *Storage instructions...*
Store Tegretol at room temperature. Keep the container tightly closed. Protect the tablets from light and moisture. Keep the liquid suspension away from light.

## What side effects may occur?

Side effects cannot be anticipated. If any develop or change in intensity, inform your doctor as soon as possible. Only your doctor can determine if it is safe for you to continue taking Tegretol.

■ *More common side effects, especially at the start of treatment, may include:*
Dizziness, drowsiness, nausea, unsteadiness, vomiting

■ *Other side effects may include:*
Abdominal pain, abnormal heartbeat and rhythm, abnormal involuntary movements, abnormal sensitivity to sound, aching joints and muscles, agitation, anemia, blood clots, blurred vision, chills, confusion, congestive heart failure, constipation, depression, diarrhea, double vision, dry mouth and throat, fainting and collapse, fatigue, fever, fluid retention, frequent urination, hair loss, hallucinations, headache, hepatitis, hives, impotence, inability to urinate, inflammation of the mouth and tongue, inflamed eyes, involuntary movements of the eyeball, itching, kidney

failure, labored breathing, leg cramps, liver disorders, loss of appetite, loss of coordination, low blood pressure, pneumonia, reddened skin, reddish or purplish spots on the skin, reduced urine volume, ringing in the ears, sensitivity to light, skin inflammation and scaling, skin peeling, skin rashes, skin pigmentation changes, speech difficulties, stomach problems, sweating, talkativeness, tingling sensation, worsening of high blood pressure, yellow eyes and skin

## Why should this drug not be prescribed?

You should not use Tegretol if you have a history of bone marrow depression (reduced function), a sensitivity to Tegretol or a sensitivity to tricyclic antidepressant drugs such as amitriptyline (Elavil). You should also not be taking Tegretol if you are on an MAO inhibitor antidepressant such as Nardil or Parnate, or if you have taken such a drug within the past 14 days.

Tegretol is not a simple pain reliever and should not be used for the relief of minor aches and pains.

## Special warnings about this medication

If you have a history of heart, liver, or kidney damage, an adverse blood reaction to any drug, glaucoma, or serious reactions to other drugs, you should discuss this history thoroughly with your doctor before taking this medication.

Anticonvulsant drugs such as Tegretol should not be stopped abruptly if you are taking the medication to prevent major seizures. There exists the strong possibility of continuous epileptic attacks without return to consciousness, leading to possible severe brain damage and death. Only your doctor should determine if and when you should stop taking this medication.

Since dizziness and drowsiness may occur while taking Tegretol, you should refrain from operating machinery or driving an automobile or participating in any high-risk activity that requires full mental alertness until you know how this drug affects you.

The elderly, especially, can become confused or agitated when taking Tegretol.

In very rare cases, some people have had severe, even fatal, skin reactions to Tegretol. Contact your doctor at the first sign of a skin problem.

## Possible food and drug interactions when taking this medication

The use of the antiseizure medications phenobarbital, phenytoin (Dilantin), or primidone (Mysoline) may reduce the effectiveness of Tegretol. Take other anticonvulsants along with Tegretol only if your doctor advises it. The use of Tegretol with other anticonvulsants may change thyroid gland function.

The effectiveness of haloperidol (Haldol) and valproic acid (Depakene) may be reduced when these drugs are taken with Tegretol.

The use of erythromycin, cimetidine (Tagamet), propoxyphene (Darvon), terfenadine (Seldane), isoniazid (Rifamate), fluoxetine (Prozac), or calcium channel blockers such as Calan may raise the amount of Tegretol in the blood to harmful levels.

Lithium (Lithonate) used with Tegretol may cause harmful nervous system side effects.

If you are taking an oral contraceptive and Tegretol, you may experience blood spotting and your contraceptive may not be completely reliable.

The activity of theophylline (Theo-Dur), doxycycline (Vibramycin), phenytoin (Dilantin), and the blood thinner warfarin (Coumadin) may be affected significantly by Tegretol.

## Special information
## if you are pregnant or breastfeeding

There are no adequate safety studies regarding the use of Tegretol in pregnant women. However, there have been reports of birth defects in infants. Therefore, this medication should be used during pregnancy only if the potential benefits justify the potential risk to the fetus. If you are pregnant or plan on becoming pregnant, you should discuss this with your doctor.

Tegretol appears in breast milk. If you are breastfeeding, your doctor may advise you to discontinue doing so if taking Tegretol is essential to your health.

## Recommended dosage

ADULTS

*Seizures*

The usual dose for adults and children over 12 years of age is one 200-milligram tablet taken twice daily or 1 teaspoon 4 times a day. Your doctor may increase the dose at weekly intervals by adding 200-milligram or 2-teaspoon doses to a total of 3 or 4 times per day. Dosage should generally not exceed 1,000 milligrams daily in children 12 to 15 years old and 1,200 milligrams daily for adults and children over 15. The usual daily maintenance dosage range is 800 to 1,200 milligrams.

*Trigeminal Neuralgia*

The usual dose is one 100-milligram tablet twice or one-half teaspoon 4 times on the first day. Your doctor may increase this dose using increments of 100 milligrams every 12 hours or one-half teaspoonful 4 times daily only as needed to achieve freedom from pain. Doses should not exceed 1,200 milligrams daily and are usually in the range of 400 to 800 milligrams a day for maintenance.

## CHILDREN

*Seizures*

The usual dose for children 6 to 12 years old is one 100-milligram tablet twice daily or one-half teaspoon 4 times a day. Your doctor may increase the dose at weekly intervals by adding 100 milligrams or 1 teaspoon 3 or 4 times a day. Total daily dosage should generally not exceed 1,000 milligrams and should be divided into 3 or 4 doses. The usual daily dosage range for maintenance is 400 to 800 milligrams. Safety and effectiveness in children under 6 years of age have not been established.

## OLDER ADULTS

To help determine the ideal dosage, your doctor may decide to periodically check the level of Tegretol in your blood.

### Overdosage

Any medication taken in excess can have serious consequences. If you suspect an overdose, seek medical attention immediately. The first signs and symptoms of an overdose of Tegretol appear after 1 to 3 hours.

■ *The most prominent signs of a Tegretol overdose include:*

Coma, convulsions, dizziness, drowsiness, inability to urinate, involuntary rapid eye movements, irregular or reduced breathing, lack or absence of urine, lack of coordination, low or high blood pressure, muscular twitching, nausea, pupil dilation, rapid heartbeat, restlessness, severe muscle spasm, shock, tremors, unconsciousness, vomiting, writhing movements

*Generic name:*

# Temazepam

*See Restoril, page 461.*

*Brand name:*

# Temovate

*Pronounced: TIM-oh-vate*
*Generic name: Clobetasol propionate*

### Why is this drug prescribed?

Temovate relieves the itching and inflammation of moderate to severe skin conditions. Temovate Scalp Application is used for short-term treatment of scalp conditions; Temovate Cream and Ointment and the super-high potency Emollient Cream and Gel are used for short-term treatment of skin conditions on the body. Temovate is a steroid medication for external use only.

### Most important fact about this drug

When you use Temovate, you inevitably absorb some of the medication through your skin and into the bloodstream. Too much absorption can lead to unwanted side effects elsewhere in the body. To keep this problem to a minimum, avoid using large amounts of Temovate over large areas, and do not cover it with airtight dressings such as plastic wrap or adhesive bandages unless specifically told to by your doctor.

### How should you use this medication?

Use Temovate exactly as directed by your doctor. Remember to avoid covering or bandaging the affected area.

Temovate is for use only on the skin. Be careful to keep it out of your eyes.

A thin layer of cream or ointment should be gently rubbed into the affected area.

■ *If you miss a dose...*

Apply it as soon as you remember. If it is almost time for the next dose, skip the one you missed and go back to your regular schedule.

■ *Storage instructions...*

Store at room temperature. Do not refrigerate the creams or the gel.

### What side effects may occur?

Side effects cannot be anticipated. If any develop or change in intensity, inform your doctor as soon as possible. Only your doctor can determine if it is safe for you to continue using Temovate. This medication is generally well tolerated when used for 2 weeks. However, some side effects have been reported at the affected area.

CREAMS, OINTMENT, GEL

■ *Side effects are infrequent but may include:*
Burning, cracking/fissuring, irritation, itching, numbness of fingers, patches, reddened skin, shrinking of the skin, stinging

SCALP APPLICATION

■ *More frequent side effects may include:*
Burning, stinging
■ *Less frequent side effects may include:*
Eye irritation, hair loss, headache, inflammation, itching, tenderness and/or tightness of the scalp

These additional side effects have been known to result from use of topical steroids and may be particularly apt to occur with the super-high potency Emollient Cream and Gel: Acne, allergic skin inflammation, dryness, excessive hair growth, infection, inflammation around the mouth, loss of skin color, prickly heat, skin softening, streaking.

### Why should this drug not be prescribed?
All forms of Temovate should be avoided if you are sensitive to or have ever had an allergic reaction to clobetasol propionate, other corticosteroids such as Valisone and Topicort, or any of their ingredients. Temovate Scalp Application should not be used if you have a scalp infection.

### Special warnings about this medication
Temovate is a strong corticosteroid that can be absorbed into the bloodstream. It has caused Cushing's syndrome (a disorder characterized by a moon-shaped face, emotional disturbances, high blood pressure, weight gain, and, in women, abnormal growth of facial and body hair) and changes in blood sugar.

This medication should not be used for any condition other than the one for which it was prescribed.

Temovate should not be used by children under 12 years of age.

Treatment should not last for more than 2 weeks.

If you are being scheduled for surgery, let your doctor know you are using Temovate.

### Possible food and drug interactions when using this medication
No interactions have been reported.

### Special information if you are pregnant or breastfeeding
Although Temovate is applied to the skin, there is no way of knowing how much medication is absorbed into the bloodstream. Strong corticosteroids have caused birth defects in animals. Temovate, a strong corticosteroid, should be used only if the potential benefits outweigh the potential risks to the unborn baby; limit use to small amounts, on a limited area, for a short period of time. It is not known whether topical steroids are absorbed in sufficient amounts to appear in breast milk. If Temovate is essential to your health, your doctor may advise you to stop breastfeeding until your treatment with the medication is finished.

### Recommended dosage
ADULTS AND CHILDREN 12 YEARS AND OLDER

Apply the medication to the affected area 2 times a day, once in the morning and once at night. Treatment should not last for more than 2 consecutive weeks, and the affected area should not be covered with a bandage. No more than 50 grams per week (approximately one large tube or bottle) should be used.

### Overdosage
When absorbed into the bloodstream over a prolonged period, Temovate can cause disorders such as Cushing's syndrome. If you suspect an overdose of Temovate, seek medical attention immediately.

*Brand name:*

# Tenex

*Pronounced: TEN-ex*
*Generic name: Guanfacine hydrochloride*

### Why is this drug prescribed?
Tenex is given to help control high blood pressure. This medication reduces nerve impulses to the heart and arteries; this slows the heartbeat, relaxes the blood vessels, and thus reduces blood pressure. Tenex may be given alone or in combination with other high blood pressure medications, especially thiazide diuretics, such as Diuril, Esidrix, or Naturetin.

### Most important fact about this drug
You must take Tenex regularly for it to be effective. Since blood pressure declines gradually, it

may be several weeks before you get the full benefit of Tenex; and you must continue taking it even if you are feeling well. Tenex does not cure high blood pressure; it merely keeps it under control.

## How should you take this medication?

Take Tenex exactly as prescribed by your doctor—usually 1 dose per day. Tenex should be taken at bedtime, since it will probably cause drowsiness.

After 3 or 4 weeks, if your blood pressure is still too high, your doctor may raise the dosage of Tenex. In some cases, you may take 2 evenly spaced doses per day rather than a single dose at bedtime.

■ *If you miss a dose...*
Take the forgotten dose as soon as you remember. This will help to keep the proper amount of medicine in your body. However, if it is almost time for the next dose, skip the one you missed and go back to your regular schedule. Never try to "catch up" by doubling the dose. If you miss taking Tenex for 2 or more days in a row, check with your doctor.

■ *Storage instructions...*
Store Tenex at room temperature. Use the container it came in.

## What side effects may occur?

Side effects cannot be anticipated. If any develop or change in intensity, inform your doctor as soon as possible. Only your doctor can determine whether it is safe for you to continue taking Tenex. This medication will probably make you drowsy, especially when you first begin to take it.

■ *More common side effects may include:*
Constipation, dizziness, dry mouth, fatigue, headache, impotence, sleepiness, weakness

■ *Less common or rare side effects may include:*
Abdominal pain, amnesia, breathing difficulties, chest pain, confusion, conjunctivitis (red, puffy eyes), decreased sex drive, depression, diarrhea, difficulty swallowing, fainting, heart palpitations, indigestion, insomnia, itching, leg cramps, malaise (vague feeling of being sick), nausea, numbness or tingling of the skin, purplish spots on the skin, rash and peeling, ringing in the ears, "runny" nose, skin inflammation, slow heartbeat, stuffy nose, sweating, taste alterations, upset stomach, urinary incontinence, vision disturbance

Some of these side effects may lessen or disappear as your body gets used to Tenex.

## Why should this drug not be prescribed?

Do not take Tenex if you are sensitive to it or have ever had an allergic reaction to it.

Tenex is not recommended for controlling the severe high blood pressure that accompanies toxemia of pregnancy (a disorder of pregnant women characterized by a rise in blood pressure, swelling, and leakage of protein into urine).

## Special warnings about this medication

While taking Tenex, you should be monitored very closely by your doctor if you have any of the following medical conditions:

Chronic kidney or liver failure
Heart disease
History of stroke
Recent heart attack

Since Tenex causes drowsiness and may also make you dizzy, do not drive, climb, or perform hazardous tasks until you find out exactly how the medication affects you.

While taking Tenex, use alcoholic beverages with care; you may feel intoxicated after drinking only a small amount of alcohol.

If you have kidney damage and also take the antiseizure drug phenytoin (Dilantin), your body may process and eliminate Tenex rather quickly; in that case, you may need fairly frequent doses of Tenex to lower your blood pressure adequately.

If you have been taking Tenex for a while, do not stop taking it without consulting your doctor. Discontinuing abruptly may result in nervousness, rapid pulse, anxiety, heartbeat irregularities, and so-called rebound high blood pressure (higher than before you started taking Tenex). If you do have rebound high blood pressure, it will probably develop 2 to 4 days after your last dose of Tenex. Rebound high blood pressure, if it occurs, will usually diminish and then disappear over a period of 2 to 4 days.

## Possible food and drug interactions when taking this medication

If Tenex is taken with certain other drugs, the effects of either could be increased, decreased, or altered. It is especially important to check with your doctor before combining Tenex with the following:

Barbiturates such as Amytal, Seconal, Tuinal, and others

Benzodiazepines such as Tranxene, Valium, Xanax, and others

Phenothiazines such as Mellaril, Stelazine, Thorazine, and others

Phenytoin (Dilantin)

## Special information
## if you are pregnant or breastfeeding

If you are pregnant or plan to become pregnant, notify your doctor immediately. Tenex should be taken during pregnancy only if clearly needed. It is not known whether Tenex appears in breast milk. Check with your doctor if you plan to breastfeed.

## Recommended dosage

ADULTS

The usual recommended dose of Tenex is 1 milligram daily, taken at bedtime. If necessary, after 3 to 4 weeks your doctor may increase the daily dosage to 2 milligrams.

CHILDREN

The safety and effectiveness of Tenex have not been established in children under 12 years of age.

## Overdosage

Any medication taken in excess can have serious consequences. If you suspect an overdose of Tenex, seek medical attention immediately.

■ *Symptoms of Tenex overdose may include:*
Drowsiness, lethargy, slowed heartbeat, very low blood pressure

*Brand name:*

# Tenoretic

*Pronounced: Ten-or-ET-ic*
*Generic ingredients: Atenolol, Chlorthalidone*

## Why is this drug prescribed?

Tenoretic is used in the treatment of high blood pressure. It combines a beta-blocker drug and a diuretic. Tenoretic can be used alone or in combination with other high blood pressure medications. Atenolol, the beta blocker, decreases the force and rate of heart contractions. Chlorthalidone, the diuretic, helps your body produce and eliminate more urine, which helps in lowering blood pressure.

## Most important fact about this drug

You must take Tenoretic regularly for it to be effective. Since blood pressure declines gradually, it may be several weeks before you get the full benefit of Tenoretic; and you must continue taking it even if you are feeling well. Tenoretic does not cure high blood pressure; it merely keeps it under control.

## How should you take this medication?

Tenoretic can be taken with or without food.

Take this medication exactly as prescribed by your doctor, even if your symptoms have disappeared.

Try not to miss any doses. If this medication is not taken regularly, your condition may worsen.

■ *If you miss a dose...*
Take the forgotten dose as soon as you remember. If it's within 8 hours of your next scheduled dose, skip the one you missed and go back to your regular schedule. Never take two doses at the same time.
■ *Storage instructions...*
Store Tenoretic at room temperature in the container it came in.

## What side effects may occur?

Side effects cannot be anticipated. If any develop or change in intensity, inform your doctor as soon as possible. Only your doctor can determine if it is safe for you to continue taking Tenoretic.

■ *More common side effects may include:*
Dizziness, fatigue, nausea, slow heartbeat
■ *Less common or rare side effects may include:*
Blood disorders, constipation, cramping, decreased sexual ability, depression, diarrhea, difficult or labored breathing, dizziness when getting up, drowsiness, excessive thirst, hair loss, headache, high blood sugar, hives, impotence, light-headedness, loss of appetite, low potassium leading to symptoms like dry mouth, muscle pain or cramps, muscle spasm, Peyronie's disease (deformity of the penis), psoriasis-like rash, rash, reddish or purplish spots on skin, restlessness, skin sensitivity to light, sluggishness or unresponsiveness, stomach irritation, sugar in the urine, tingling or pins and needles, tiredness, vertigo, visual disturbances, vomiting, weak or irregular heartbeat, weakness, worsening of psoriasis, yellow eyes and skin

## Why should this drug not be prescribed?

If you have a slow heartbeat; a history of serious heart block (conduction disorder); inadequate blood supply to the circulatory system (cardiogenic shock); heart failure; or inability to urinate; or if you are sensitive to or have ever had an allergic reaction to Tenoretic, its ingredients or similar drugs, or to other sulfonamide-derived drugs, you should not take this medication.

## Special warnings about this medication

If you have a history of congestive heart failure, Tenoretic should be used with caution.

Tenoretic should not be stopped suddenly. It can cause increased chest pain and heart attack. When stopping the drug, your physician will gradually reduce your dosage.

When taking Tenoretic, if you suffer from asthma, seasonal allergies or other bronchial conditions, or liver or kidney disease, your doctor should monitor you more carefully.

Ask your doctor if you should check your pulse while taking Tenoretic. This medication can cause your heartbeat to become too slow.

This medication may mask the symptoms of low blood sugar or alter blood sugar levels. If you are diabetic, discuss this with your doctor.

Tenoretic can cause you to become drowsy or less alert; therefore, activity that requires full mental alertness is not recommended until you know how you respond to the drug.

Make sure the doctor knows that you are taking Tenoretic if you have a medical emergency, or plan to have surgery.

## Possible food and drug interactions when taking this medication

If Tenoretic is taken with certain other drugs, the effects of either could be increased, decreased, or altered. It is especially important to check with your doctor before combining Tenoretic with the following:

Blood pressure medicines containing reserpine
Clonidine (Catapres)
Epinephrine (EpiPen)
Insulin
Lithium( Eskalith)
Nasal decongestants
Other blood pressure drugs

## Special information if you are pregnant or breastfeeding

When taken during pregnancy, Tenoretic may cause harm to the developing baby. If you are pregnant, or plan to become pregnant, inform your doctor immediately. Tenoretic appears in breast milk and could affect a nursing infant. If this medication is essential to your health, your doctor may advise you to discontinue breastfeeding until your treatment with this medication is finished.

## Recommended dosage

ADULTS

Dosage is always individualized.

The usual starting dosage is 1 Tenoretic 50 tablet taken once a day. Your doctor may increase the dosage to 1 Tenoretic 100 tablet taken once a day. Your doctor may gradually add other high blood pressure medications.

Your doctor will adjust your dosage if your kidney function is impaired.

CHILDREN

The safety and effectiveness of Tenoretic have not been established in children.

## Overdosage

Any medication taken in excess can have serious consequences. If you suspect an overdose, seek medical attention immediately.

■ *No specific information on Tenoretic is available, but common symptoms of overdose with the drug's atenolol component are:*
Congestive heart failure, constricted airways, low blood pressure, low blood sugar, slow heartbeat, sluggishness, wheezing
■ *Symptoms of overdose with the chlorthalidone component include:*
Dizziness, nausea, weakness

*Brand name:*

# Tenormin

*Pronounced: Ten-OR-min*
*Generic name: Atenolol*

## Why is this drug prescribed?

Tenormin, a type of medication known as a beta blocker, is used in the treatment of high blood pressure, angina pectoris (chest pain, usually caused by lack of oxygen to the heart due to clogged arteries), and heart attack. When used for high blood pressure it is effective alone or combined with other high blood pressure medications, particularly with a thiazide-type diuretic. Beta blockers decrease the force and rate of heart contractions.

Occasionally doctors prescribe Tenormin for treatment of alcohol withdrawal, prevention of migraine headache, and bouts of anxiety.

### Most important fact about this drug

If you have high blood pressure, you must take Tenormin regularly for it to be effective. Since blood pressure declines gradually, it may be several weeks before you get the full benefit of Tenormin; and you must continue taking it even if you are feeling well. Tenormin does not cure high blood pressure; it merely keeps it under control.

### How should you take this medication?

Tenormin can be taken with or without food. Take it exactly as prescribed, even if your symptoms have disappeared.

Try not to miss any doses, especially if you are taking Tenormin once a day. If this medication is not taken regularly, your condition may worsen.

■ *If you miss a dose...*
Take the forgotten dose as soon as you remember. If it's within 8 hours of your next scheduled dose, skip the one you missed and go back to your regular schedule. Never take 2 doses at the same time.

■ *Storage instructions...*
Store Tenormin at room temperature; protect from light.

### What side effects may occur?

Side effects cannot be anticipated. If any develop or change in intensity, inform your doctor as soon as possible. Only your doctor can determine if it is safe for you to continue taking Tenormin.

■ *More common side effects may include:*
Dizziness, fatigue, nausea, slow heartbeat

■ *Less common or rare side effects may include:*
Depression, diarrhea, difficult or labored breathing, dizziness upon standing up, drowsiness, headache, heart failure, impotence, light-headedness, low blood pressure, penile deformity, psoriasis-like rash, red or purple spots on the skin, rapid heartbeat, slow heartbeat, sluggishness,

temporary hair loss, tiredness, vertigo, wheezing, worsening of psoriasis

### Why should this drug not be prescribed?

If you have heart failure, inadequate blood supply to the circulatory system (cardiogenic shock), heart block (conduction disorder), or a severely slow heartbeat, you should not take this medication.

### Special warnings about this medication

If you have a history of severe congestive heart failure, Tenormin should be used with caution.

Tenormin should not be stopped suddenly. It can cause increased chest pain and heart attack. Dosage should be gradually reduced.

If you suffer from asthma, seasonal allergies, or other bronchial conditions, coronary artery disease or kidney disease, this medication should be used with caution.

Ask your doctor if you should check your pulse while taking Tenormin. This medication can cause your heartbeat to become too slow.

This medication may mask the symptoms of low blood sugar or alter blood sugar levels. If you are diabetic, discuss this with your doctor.

Notify your doctor or dentist that you are taking Tenormin if you have a medical emergency, and before you have surgery or dental surgery.

Tenormin may cause harm to a developing baby when taken during pregnancy. If you are pregnant or become pregnant while taking this medication, inform your doctor immediately.

### Possible food and drug interactions when taking this medication

If Tenormin is taken with certain other drugs, the effects of either could be increased, decreased, or altered. It is especially important to check with your doctor before combining Tenormin with the following:

Ampicillin (Omnipen, others)
Calcium-containing antacids such as Tums
Calcium-blocking blood pressure drugs such as
  Calan and Cardizem
Certain blood pressure drugs such as reserpine
  (Diupres)
Clonidine (Catapres)
Epinephrine (EpiPen)
Insulin
Oral diabetes drugs such as Micronase
Quinidine (Quinidex)

## Special information
## if you are pregnant or breastfeeding

The use of Tenormin during pregnancy may cause harm to a developing baby. If you are pregnant, become pregnant, or plan to become pregnant, inform your doctor immediately. Tenormin appears in breast milk and could affect a nursing infant. If this medication is essential to your health, your doctor may advise you to discontinue breastfeeding until your treatment is finished.

## Recommended dosage

### ADULTS

*Hypertension*

The usual starting dose is 50 milligrams a day in 1 dose, alone or with a diuretic. Full effects should be seen in 1 to 2 weeks. Dosage may be increased to a maximum of 100 milligrams per day in one dose. Your doctor can and may use this medication with other high blood pressure medications.

*Angina Pectoris*

The usual starting dose is 50 milligrams in 1 dose a day. Full effects should be seen in 1 week. Dosage may be increased to a maximum of 100 milligrams per day. In some cases, a single dose of 200 milligrams per day may be given. Dosage will be individualized by your doctor.

*Heart Attack*

This medication may be used in the acute treatment of heart attack in both injectable and tablet form. Your doctor will determine the proper dosage.

### CHILDREN

The safety and effectiveness of Tenormin have not been established in children.

### OLDER ADULTS

The doctor will determine the dosage for an older individual, according to his or her needs, especially in the case of reduced kidney function.

## Overdosage

Any medication taken in excess can have serious consequences. If you suspect an overdose, seek medical attention immediately.

■ *Symptoms of Tenormin overdose may include:*
Congestive heart failure, constricted airways, low blood pressure, low blood sugar, slow heartbeat, sluggishness, wheezing

*Brand name:*

# Tenuate

*Pronounced: TEN-you-ate*
*Generic name: Diethylpropion hydrochloride*

## Why is this drug prescribed?

Tenuate, an appetite suppressant, is prescribed for short-term use (a few weeks) as part of an overall diet plan for weight reduction. It is available in two forms: immediate-release tablets (Tenuate) and controlled-release tablets (Tenuate Dospan). Tenuate should be used with a behavior modification program.

## Most important fact about this drug

Tenuate will lose its effectiveness within a few weeks. When this begins to happen, you should discontinue the medicine rather than increase the dosage.

## How should you take this medication?

Take this medication exactly as prescribed. Tenuate may be habit-forming and can be addicting.

If you are taking Tenuate Dospan (the controlled release formulation), do not crush or chew the tablets. Swallow the medication whole.

■ *If you miss a dose...*
If you are taking the immediate-release form of Tenuate, go back to your regular schedule at the next meal.

If you are taking Tenuate Dospan, take the missed dose as soon as you remember. If you do not remember until the next day, skip the dose. Never take 2 doses at once.

■ *Storage instructions...*
Store at room temperature in a tightly closed container. Protect from excessive heat.

## What side effects may occur?

Side effects cannot be anticipated. If any develop or change in intensity, inform your doctor as soon as possible. Only your doctor can determine if it is safe for you to continue using Tenuate.

■ *Side effects may include:*
Abdominal discomfort, abnormal redness of the skin, anxiety, blood pressure elevation, blurred vision, breast development in males, bruising,

changes in sex drive, chest pain, constipation, depression, diarrhea, difficulty with voluntary movements, dizziness, drowsiness, dryness of the mouth, feelings of discomfort, feelings of elation, feeling of illness, hair loss, headache, hives, impotence, inability to fall or stay asleep, increased heart rate, increased seizures in epileptics, increased sweating, increased volume of diluted urine, irregular heartbeat, jitteriness, menstrual upset, muscle pain, nausea, nervousness, overstimulation, painful urination, palpitations, pupil dilation, rash, restlessness, shortness of breath or labored breathing, stomach and intestinal disturbances, tremors, unpleasant taste, vomiting

## Why should this drug not be prescribed?

If you are sensitive to or have ever had an allergic reaction to Tenuate or other appetite suppressants, you should not take this medication. Make sure your doctor is aware of any drug reactions you have experienced.

Do not take this drug if you have severe hardening of the arteries, an overactive thyroid, glaucoma, or severe high blood pressure, or if you are agitated, have a history of drug abuse or are taking an MAO inhibitor (antidepressant drug such as Nardil) or have taken one within the last 14 days.

## Special warnings about this medication

Tenuate or Tenuate Dospan may impair your ability to engage in potentially hazardous activities. Therefore, make sure you know how you react to this medication before you drive, operate dangerous machinery, or do anything else that requires alertness or concentration.

If you have heart disease or high blood pressure, use caution when taking this medication.

This drug may increase convulsions in some epileptics. Your doctor should monitor you carefully if you have epilepsy.

Psychological dependence has occurred while taking this drug. Talk with your doctor if you find you are relying on this drug to maintain a state of well-being.

The abrupt withdrawal of this medication following prolonged use at high doses may result in extreme fatigue, mental depression, and sleep disturbances.

## Possible food and drug interactions when taking this medication

Tenuate or Tenuate Dospan may interact with alcohol unfavorably. Do not drink alcohol while taking this medication.

If Tenuate or Tenuate Dospan is taken with certain other drugs, the effects of either could be increased, decreased, or altered. It is especially important that you consult your doctor before combining Tenuate with the following:

Blood pressure medications such as Ismelin
Insulin
Phenothiazine drugs such as the major tranquilizer
   Thorazine

## Special information if you are pregnant or breastfeeding

The effects of Tenuate or Tenuate Dospan during pregnancy have not been adequately studied. If you are pregnant or plan to become pregnant, inform your doctor immediately. This drug appears in breast milk. If the medication is essential to your health, your doctor may advise you to discontinue breastfeeding until your treatment is finished.

## Recommended dosage

### ADULTS

*Tenuate Immediate-Release*
The usual dosage is one 25-milligram tablet taken 3 times a day, 1 hour before meals; you may take 1 tablet in the middle of the evening, if you want, to overcome night hunger.

*Tenuate Dospan Controlled-Release*
The usual dosage is one 75-milligram tablet taken once daily, swallowed whole, in midmorning.

### CHILDREN

Safety and effectiveness have not been established in children below 12 years of age.

## Overdosage

Any medication taken in excess can have serious consequences. If you suspect an overdose, seek emergency medical treatment immediately.

■ *Symptoms of Tenuate overdose may include:*
Abdominal cramps, assaultiveness, confusion, depression, diarrhea, elevated blood pressure, fatigue, hallucinations, irregular heartbeat, lowered blood pressure, nausea, overreactive reflexes, panic state, rapid breathing, restlessness, tremors, vomiting

Brand name:

# Terazol

Pronounced: TER-uh-zawl
Generic name: Terconazole

## Why is this drug prescribed?

Terazol is prescribed to treat candidiasis (a yeast-like fungal infection) of the vulva and vagina.

## Most important fact about this drug

Keep using Terazol for the full time of treatment, even if the infection seems to have disappeared. If you stop too soon, the infection could return. You should continue using this medicine during your menstrual period.

## How should you use this medication?

Follow these steps to apply Terazol:

1. Load the applicator to the fill line with cream, or unwrap a suppository, wet it with warm water, and place it in the applicator as shown in the instructions you received with the product.
2. Lie on your back with knees drawn up.
3. Gently insert the applicator high into the vagina and push the plunger.
4. Withdraw the applicator and wash it with soap and water.

To protect your clothing, wear a sanitary napkin. Do not use tampons because they will absorb the medicine. Wear cotton underwear—avoid synthetic fabrics such as rayon or nylon. Do not douche unless your doctor tells you to do so.

Dry the genital area thoroughly after a shower, bath, or swim. Change out of a wet bathing suit or damp workout clothes as soon as possible. Moisture encourages the growth of yeast.

Try not to scratch. It can cause more irritation and can spread the infection.

■ *If you miss a dose...*
Apply it as soon as you remember. If it is almost time for your next dose, skip the one you missed and go back to your regular schedule.
■ *Storage instructions...*
Store at room temperature.

## What side effects may occur?

Side effects cannot be anticipated. If any develop or change in intensity, inform your doctor as soon as possible. Only your doctor can determine if it is safe for you to continue using Terazol.

■ *More common side effects may include:*
Abdominal pain, body pain, burning, genital pain or irritation, headache, menstrual pain
■ *Less common side effects may include:*
Chills, fever, itching

## Why should this drug not be prescribed?

If you have ever had an allergic reaction to or are sensitive to terconazole or any other ingredients of Terazol, you should not use this medication. Make sure your doctor is aware of any drug reactions you have experienced.

## Special warnings about this medication

If irritation, an allergic reaction, fever, chills, or flu-like symptoms develop while using this medication, notify your doctor.

To avoid re-infection while using Terazol, either avoid sexual intercourse or make sure your partner uses a non-latex condom.

Terazol 3 suppositories can interact with latex products such as diaphragms and certain type of condoms. Use some other method of birth control while you are using Terazol.

## Possible food and drug interactions when taking this medication

No interactions have been reported.

## Special information if you are pregnant or breastfeeding

Since Terazol is absorbed from the vagina, it should not be used during the first trimester (first 3 months) of pregnancy unless your doctor considers it essential to your health. It is not known whether this drug appears in breast milk. Your doctor may advise you to discontinue breastfeeding your baby while using this medication.

## Recommended dosage

ADULTS

*Terazol 3 and Terazol 7 Vaginal Cream*
The recommended dose is 1 full applicator (5 grams) of cream inserted into the vagina once daily at bedtime. Apply Terazol 3 for 3 consecutive days; apply Terazol 7 for 7.

*Terazol 3 Vaginal Suppositories*
The recommended dose is 1 suppository inserted into the vagina once daily at bedtime for 3 consecutive days.

CHILDREN

Safety and effectiveness have not been established in children.

## Overdosage

There has been no reported overdose of this ication. Any medication used in excess, however, can have serious consequences. If you suspect an overdose of Terazol, seek medical attention immediately.

*Generic name:*

# Terazosin

*See Hytrin, page 243.*

*Generic name:*

# Terbutaline

*See Brethine, page 63.*

*Generic name:*

# Terconazole

*See Terazol, page 535.*

*Generic name:*

# Terfenadine

*See Seldane and Seldane-D, page 490.*

*Brand name:*

# Tessalon

*Pronounced: TESS-ah-lon*
*Generic name: Benzonatate*

## Why is this drug prescribed?

Tessalon is taken for relief of a cough.

## Most important fact about this drug

Tessalon should be swallowed whole, not chewed.

## How should you take this medication?

Tessalon perles (soft capsule form) should be swallowed whole. If chewed, they can produce a temporary numbness of the mouth and throat that could cause choking or a severe allergic reaction.

■ *If you miss a dose...*
Take the forgotten dose as soon as you remember. If it is almost time for your next dose, skip the one you missed and go back to your regular schedule. Never double the dose.

■ *Storage instructions...*
Store Tessalon at room temperature.

## What side effects may occur?

Side effects cannot be anticipated. If any occur or change in intensity, inform your doctor as soon as possible. Only your doctor can determine if it is safe to continue taking Tessalon.

■ *Side effects may include:*
Allergic reactions, burning sensation in the eyes, constipation, dizziness, extreme calm (sedation), headache, itching, mental confusion, nausea, numbness in chest, skin eruptions, stuffy nose, upset stomach, vague "chilly" feeling, visual hallucinations

## Why should this drug not be prescribed?

Tessalon should not be used if you are sensitive to or have ever had an allergic reaction to benzonatate or similar drugs (such as local anesthetics).

## Special warnings about this medication

Remember to swallow Tessalon perles whole.

## Possible food and drug interactions when taking this medication

There have been rare occurrences of bizarre behavior, including confusion and visual hallucinations, when Tessalon is taken with other prescribed drugs. Check with your doctor before taking Tessalon with other medications.

## Special information if you are pregnant or breastfeeding

The effects of Tessalon during pregnancy have not been studied adequately. Tessalon should be used during pregnancy only if clearly needed. If you are pregnant or plan to become pregnant, notify your doctor immediately. It is unknown if Tessalon appears in breast milk and could affect a nursing infant. If this medication is essential to your health, your doctor may advise you to stop breastfeeding until your treatment with Tessalon ends.

## Recommended dosage

CHILDREN OVER AGE 10 AND ADULTS

The usual dose is a 100-milligram perle 3 times per day, as needed. The maximum dose is 600 milligrams, or 6 perles, a day.

## Overdosage

If capsules are chewed or allowed to dissolve in the mouth, numbness of the mouth and throat will develop rapidly. Symptoms of restlessness and tremors may be followed by convulsions.

If you suspect a Tessalon overdose, seek medical attention immediately.

*Generic name:*

# Tetracycline

*Pronounced: TET-ra-SY-clin*
*Brand name: Sumycin*

## Why is this drug prescribed?

Tetracycline, a "broad-spectrum" antibiotic, is used to treat bacterial infections such as Rocky Mountain spotted fever, typhus fever, and tick fevers; upper respiratory infections; pneumonia; gonorrhea; amoebic infections; and urinary tract infections. It is also used to help treat severe acne and to treat trachoma (a chronic eye infection) and conjunctivitis (pinkeye). Tetracycline is often an alternative drug for people who are allergic to penicillin.

## Most important fact about this drug

Tetracycline should not be used during the last half of pregnancy or in children under the age of 8. It may damage developing teeth and cause permanent discoloration.

## How should you take this medication?

Tetracycline should be taken exactly as prescribed by your doctor. Be sure to use the entire prescription. If you are taking a liquid form of the drug, shake well before using.

Do not use outdated tetracycline. Outdated tetracycline is highly toxic to the kidneys.

Do not take antacids containing aluminum, calcium, or magnesium (e.g., Mylanta, Maalox) while taking this medication. They will affect the absorption of the drug.

Take tetracycline 1 hour before or 2 hours after meals. Foods, milk, and some other dairy products affect absorption of the drug.

Tetracycline should be continued for at least 24 to 48 hours after your symptoms have subsided.

■ *If you miss a dose...*

Take it as soon as you remember. If it is almost time for your next dose and you take tetracycline once a day (e.g., for acne), take the dose you missed, and then take the next one 10 to 12 hours later; if you take it twice a day, take the dose you missed, and then take the next one 5 to 6 hours later; if you take 3 or more doses a day, take the one you missed, and then take the next one 2 to 4 hours later. Then go back to your regular schedule.

■ *Storage instructions...*

Store capsules at room temperature. Keep the liquid form of tetracycline in the refrigerator, but do not allow it to freeze.

## What side effects may occur?

Side effects cannot be anticipated. If any occur or change in intensity, inform your doctor as soon as possible. Only your doctor can determine if it is safe for you to continue taking tetracycline.

■ *More common side effects may include:*

Anemia, blood disorders, blurred vision and headache (in adults), bulging soft spot on the head (in infants), diarrhea, difficult or painful swallowing, dizziness, extreme allergic reactions, genital or anal sores or rash, hives, inflammation of large bowel, inflammation of the tongue, inflammation of the upper digestive tract, increased sensitivity to light, loss of appetite, nausea, rash, ringing in the ears, swelling due to fluid accumulation, vision disturbance, vomiting

■ *Less common or rare side effects may include:*

Inflamed skin, inflammation of the penis, liver poisoning, muscle weakness, peeling, skin eruptions, throat sores and inflammation

## Why should this drug not be prescribed?

Do not take this medication if you are sensitive to or have ever had an allergic reaction to any tetracycline medication.

## Special warnings about this medication

If you have kidney disease, make sure the doctor knows about it. A lower than usual dose of tetracycline may be needed.

Tetracycline drugs can make you more prone to sunburn when you are in sunlight or ultraviolet light. Take appropriate precautions.

Some adults may develop a headache and blurred vision while taking tetracycline, and infants may develop a bulging soft spot on the head.

Contact your doctor if you experience or notice these symptoms. They usually disappear soon after the medication is stopped.

As with other antibiotics, use of this medication may cause other infections to develop. Contact your doctor if this occurs.

If you are taking tetracycline over an extended period of time, your doctor will perform blood, kidney, and liver tests periodically.

### Possible food and drug interactions when taking this medication
If tetracycline is taken with certain other drugs, the effects of either could be increased, decreased, or altered. It is especially important to check with your doctor before combining tetracycline with the following:

Antacids containing aluminum, calcium, or magnesium, such as Mylanta and Maalox
Blood thinners such as Coumadin
Oral contraceptives
Penicillin (Amoxil, Pen-Vee K, others)

### Special information if you are pregnant or breastfeeding
Tetracycline is not recommended for use during pregnancy. It can affect the development of the unborn child's bones and teeth. If you are pregnant or plan to become pregnant, inform your doctor immediately. Tetracycline appears in breast milk and may affect a nursing infant. If this medication is essential to your health, your doctor may recommend that you stop breastfeeding until your treatment is finished.

### Recommended dosage
Your doctor will adjust your dose on the basis of the condition to be treated, your age, and risk factors such as kidney problems.

You should use this drug for at least 24 to 48 hours after symptoms and fever have subsided. For a streptococcal infection, doses should be taken for at least 10 days.

#### ADULTS
For most infections, the usual daily dose is 1 to 2 grams divided into 2 or 4 equal doses, depending on severity.

*For treatment of brucellosis*
The usual dose is 500 milligrams 4 times daily for 3 weeks; the drug should be accompanied by streptomycin.

*For treatment of syphilis*
You should take a total of 30 to 40 grams, divided into equal doses over a period of 10 to 15 days.

Gonorrhea patients sensitive to penicillin can take tetracycline, starting with 1.5 grams, followed by 0.5 gram every 6 hours for 4 days, to a total dosage of 9 grams.

*For urethral, endocervical, or rectal infections in adults caused by* Chlamydia trachomatis
The usual dose is 500 milligrams, 4 times a day, for at least 7 days.

#### CHILDREN 8 YEARS OF AGE AND ABOVE
The usual daily dose is 10 to 20 milligrams per pound of body weight divided into 2 or 4 equal doses.

### Overdosage
Any medication taken in excess can have serious consequences. Seek medical attention immediately if you suspect an overdose of tetracycline.

*Brand name:*
# Thalitone
*See Hygroton, page 242.*

*Brand name:*
# Theochron
*See Theo-Dur, page 538.*

*Brand name:*
# Theo-Dur
Pronounced: THEE-a-door
Generic name: Theophylline
Other brand names: Quibron-T/SR, Slo-bid, T-Phyl, Theochron, Uni-Dur, Uniphyl

### Why is this drug prescribed?
Theo-Dur, an oral bronchodilator medication, is given to prevent or relieve symptoms of asthma, chronic bronchitis, and emphysema. The active ingredient of Theo-Dur, theophylline, is a chemical cousin of caffeine. It opens the airways by relaxing the smooth muscle that lines the tubes and blood vessels in the lungs.

## Most important fact about this drug

Theo-Dur is a controlled-release medication. For an acute attack you should take an immediate-release medication instead of more Theo-Dur. If you develop *status asthmaticus* (a severe breathing difficulty that does not clear up with your usual medications), do not take extra Theo-Dur; instead, seek medical treatment immediately. Since even a little extra Theo-Dur may constitute an overdose, you should be treated in a place where close monitoring is possible.

Individual doses are determined by a person's response (a decrease in symptoms of asthma). In order to avoid overdosing or underdosing, your doctor will perform regular tests to determine the amount of Theo-Dur in your bloodstream.

You should not change from Theo-Dur to another brand without first consulting your doctor or pharmacist. Products manufactured by different companies may not be equally effective.

## How should you take this medication?

Take Theo-Dur exactly as prescribed by your doctor.

This drug is available in two forms. The extended-release tablets should be swallowed whole, not crushed or chewed. The tablets of some brands are scored; if the doctor prescribes a partial dosage, these tablets should be broken only at the score. You may take the tablets with or without food. If you are taking them on a once-a-day basis, do not take the dose at night.

The other form, Theo-Dur Sprinkle sustained-action capsules, must be taken either one hour before or two hours after a meal. You may take the capsule whole or open it and empty the contents onto a spoonful of food that is soft but not hot. Without chewing, immediately swallow the spoonful of food and follow it with a glass of cool water or juice. Always take the complete contents of the capsule.

When taking Theo-Dur, you should avoid large amounts of caffeine-containing beverages, such as tea or coffee.

■ *If you miss a dose...*
   Take it as soon as you remember. If it is almost time for your next dose, skip the one you missed and go back to your regular schedule. Never take two doses at the same time.

■ *Storage instructions...*
   Store at room temperature. Keep the container tightly closed. Protect from excessive heat, light, and moisture. Make sure this medicine is kept out of reach of children.

## What side effects may occur?

Side effects from Theo-Dur cannot be anticipated. Nausea and restlessness may occur when you first start to take Theo-Dur, but will probably disappear as your body becomes used to the drug. If side effects persist, see your doctor; the dosage may be too high.

■ *Other side effects may include:*
   Convulsions, diarrhea, disturbances of heart rhythm, excitability, flushing, frequent urination, hair loss, headache, heart palpitations, high blood sugar, irritability, low blood pressure, muscle twitching, nausea, rapid breathing, rapid heartbeat, rash, restlessness, sleeplessness, stomach pain, vomiting, vomiting blood

Theo-Dur may cause or worsen heartbeat abnormalities. While you are taking this medication, any significant change in your heart rate or rhythm should be investigated promptly and thoroughly.

## Why should this drug not be prescribed?

Do not take Theo-Dur if you have ever had an allergic reaction to it or similar drugs.

Do not take Theo-Dur if you have an active peptic ulcer. If you have epilepsy, you should be taking the correct dosage of antiseizure medication when you start treatment with Theo-Dur.

## Special warnings about this medication

If you are a smoker, your body will tend to process and get rid of Theo-Dur rather quickly; thus, you may need to take more frequent doses than a nonsmoker. Even if you quit smoking, this quick-clearance effect may linger for 6 months to 2 years.

You should take Theo-Dur cautiously and under close medical supervision if you are over 55, especially if you are a male with chronic lung disease.

You should also take Theo-Dur cautiously and under close supervision if you have had a sustained high fever, or if you have heart disease or kidney or liver failure, high blood pressure, low blood oxygen, alcoholism, or a history of stomach ulcers.

## Possible food and drug interactions when taking this medication

If Theo-Dur is taken with certain other drugs, the effects of either could be increased, decreased, or altered. It is especially important to check with your doctor before combining Theo-Dur with the following:

Allopurinol (Lopurin, Zyloprim)
Cimetidine (Tagamet)
Ciprofloxacin (Cipro)
Ephedrine (in medications such as Primatene and Rynatuss)
Erythromycin (E.E.S., ERYC, Erythrocin, and others)
Lithium carbonate (Eskalith, Lithobid, and others)
Norfloxacin (Noroxin)
Oral contraceptives
Phenytoin (Dilantin)
Propranolol (Inderal)
Rifampin (Rifadin, Rifamate, Rimactane)
Sucralfate (Carafate)
Troleandomycin (Tao)

## Special information if you are pregnant or breastfeeding

If you are pregnant or plan to become pregnant, inform your doctor immediately. Theo-Dur should not be taken during pregnancy unless it is clearly needed, and unless the benefits to the mother outweigh the potential risk to the developing child.

Theo-Dur does find its way into breast milk; it may make a nursing baby irritable or harm the baby in other ways. If you are a new mother, you will probably need to choose between breastfeeding and taking Theo-Dur.

## Recommended dosage

### ADULTS

*Theo-Dur Extended Release Tablets*
The usual initial dose is 1 Theo-Dur 200-milligram tablet every 12 hours. If this is not effective, your doctor will gradually increase the dose until you respond, up to a maximum of 900 milligrams per day. Once you have adjusted to the medication, your doctor may be able to put you on a once-a-day dose schedule.

*Theo-Dur Sprinkle*
The usual initial dose is no more than 200 milligrams every 12 hours. If this is not effective, your doctor will gradually increase the dose until you

respond, up to a maximum of 900 milligrams per day. If a dose every 12 hours is inconvenient, your doctor may divide the daily total into 3 small doses taken every 8 hours.

### CHILDREN UNDER 16 YEARS OLD

*Theo-Dur Extended Release Tablets*
For children under 55 pounds, a liquid preparation is recommended to establish proper dosage before switching to Theo-Dur tablets. Maximum regular daily dosages are calculated by body weight as follows:

55 through 76 pounds—500 milligrams
77 through 154 pounds—600 milligrams

*Theo-Dur Sprinkle*
For children under 55 pounds, a liquid preparation is recommended to establish proper dosage before switching to Theo-Dur Sprinkle. Maximum regular daily dosages are calculated by body weight as follows:

Children 6 through 8—24 milligrams per 2.2 pounds
Children 9 through 11—20 milligrams per 2.2 pounds
Children 12 through 15—18 milligrams per 2.2 pounds

## Overdosage

Most of the symptoms listed in the "side effects" section are actually caused by slight overdosage.

Be aware that a flu shot, influenza itself, or another viral infection may make your usual dose of Theo-Dur act like an overdose. Consult your doctor if you anticipate getting a flu shot, or if you think you have the flu; you may need a temporary dosage reduction.

A mild overdose of Theo-Dur may cause nausea and restlessness. A larger overdose may not give any warning before causing serious heartbeat irregularities, convulsions, or even death. If at any time you suspect symptoms of an overdose of Theo-Dur, seek medical attention immediately.

*Generic name:*

# Theophylline

*See Theo-Dur, page 538.*

*Brand name:*

# Theragran

*See Multivitamins, page 341.*

*Brand name:*

# Theroxide

*See Desquam-E, page 150.*

*Generic name:*

# Thioridazine

*See Mellaril, page 313.*

*Generic name:*

# Thiothixene

*See Navane, page 351.*

*Brand name:*

# Thorazine

*Pronounced: THOR-ah-zeen*
*Generic name: Chlorpromazine*

## Why is this drug prescribed?

Thorazine is used for the reduction of symptoms of psychotic disorders such as schizophrenia; for the short-term treatment of severe behavioral disorders in children, including explosive hyperactivity and combativeness; and for the hyperenergetic phase of manic-depressive illness (severely exaggerated moods).

Thorazine is also used to control nausea and vomiting, and to relieve restlessness and apprehension before surgery. It is used as an aid in the treatment of tetanus, and is prescribed for uncontrollable hiccups and acute intermittent porphyria (attacks of severe abdominal pain sometimes accompanied by psychiatric disturbances, cramps in the arms and legs, and muscle weakness).

## Most important fact about this drug

Thorazine may cause tardive dyskinesia—a condition marked by involuntary muscle spasms and twitches in the face and body. This condition may be permanent, and appears to be most common

among the elderly, especially women. Ask your doctor for information about this possible risk.

## How should you take this medication?

If taking Thorazine in a liquid concentrate form, you will need to dilute it with a liquid such as a carbonated beverage, coffee, fruit juice, milk, tea, tomato juice, or water. Puddings, soups, and other semisolid foods may also be used. Thorazine will taste best if it is diluted immediately prior to use. You should not take Thorazine with alcohol.

Do not take antacids such as Gelusil at the same time as Thorazine. Leave at least 1 to 2 hours between doses of the two drugs.

■ *If you miss a dose...*

If you take Thorazine once a day, take the dose you missed as soon as you remember. If you do not remember until the next day, skip the dose, then go back to your regular schedule.

If you take more than 1 dose a day, take the one you missed as soon as you remember if it is within an hour or so of the scheduled time. If you do not remember until later, skip the dose, then go back to your regular schedule.

Never take 2 doses at once.

■ *Storage instructions...*

Store away from heat, light, and moisture. Do not freeze the liquid. Since the liquid concentrate form of Thorazine is light-sensitive, it should be stored in a dark place, but it does not need to be refrigerated.

## What side effects may occur?

Side effects cannot be anticipated. If any develop or change in intensity, inform your doctor as soon as possible. Only your doctor can determine if it is safe for you to continue taking Thorazine.

■ *Side effects may include:*

Abnormal secretion of milk, abnormalities in movement and posture, agitation, anemia, asthma, blood disorders, breast development in males, chewing movements, constipation, difficulty breathing, difficulty swallowing, dizziness, drooling, drowsiness, dry mouth, ejaculation problems, eye problems causing fixed gaze, fainting, fever, flu-like symptoms, fluid accumulation and swelling, headache, heart attack, high or low blood sugar, hives, impotence, inability to urinate, inability to move or talk, increase of appetite, infections, insomnia, intestinal blockage, involuntary movements of arms and legs, tongue, face, mouth, or jaw, irregular blood pressure, pulse, and heartbeat, irregular or no menstrual periods, jitteriness, light-headedness (on standing up), lockjaw, mask-like face, muscle stiffness and rigidity, narrow or dilated pupils, nasal congestion, nausea, pain and stiffness in the neck, persistent, painful erections, pill-rolling motion, protruding tongue, puckering of the mouth, puffing of the cheeks, rapid heartbeat, red or purple spots on the skin, rigid arms, feet, head, and muscles (including the back), seizures, sensitivity to light, severe allergic reactions, shuffling walk, skin inflammation and peeling, sore throat, spasms in jaw, face, tongue, neck, mouth, and feet, sweating, swelling of breasts in women, swelling of the throat, tremors, twitching in the body, neck, shoulders and face, twisted neck, visual problems, weight gain, yellowed skin and whites of eyes

### Why should this drug not be prescribed?

You should not be using Thorazine if you are taking substances that slow down mental function such as alcohol, barbiturates, or narcotics.

You should not take Thorazine if you have ever had an allergic reaction to any major tranquilizer containing phenothiazine.

### Special warnings about this medication

You should use Thorazine cautiously if you have ever had: asthma; a brain tumor; breast cancer; intestinal blockage; emphysema; the eye condition known as glaucoma; heart, kidney, or liver disease; respiratory infections; seizures; or an abnormal bone marrow or blood condition; or if you are exposed to pesticides or extreme heat. Be aware that Thorazine can mask symptoms of brain tumor, intestinal blockage, and the neurological condition called Reye's syndrome.

Stomach inflammation, dizziness, nausea, vomiting, and tremors may result if you suddenly stop taking Thorazine. Follow your doctor's instructions closely when discontinuing Thorazine.

Thorazine can suppress the cough reflex; you may have trouble vomiting.

This drug may impair your ability to drive a car or operate potentially dangerous machinery. Do not participate in any activities that require full alertness if you are unsure about your ability.

This drug can increase your sensitivity to light. Avoid being out in the sun too long.

Thorazine can cause a group of symptoms called Neuroleptic Malignant Syndrome, which can be fatal. Some symptoms are extremely high body temperature, rigid muscles, mental changes, irregular pulse or blood pressure, rapid heartbeat, sweating, and changes in heart rhythm.

If you are on Thorazine for prolonged therapy, you should see your doctor for regular evaluations, since side effects can get worse over time.

### Possible food and drug interactions when taking this medication

If Thorazine is taken with certain other drugs, the effects of either could be increased, decreased, or altered. It is especially important to check with your doctor before combining Thorazine with the following:

Anesthetics
Antacids such as Gelusil
Antiseizure drugs such as Dilantin
Antispasmodic drugs such as Cogentin
Atropine (Donnatal)
Barbiturates such as phenobarbital
Blood-thinning drugs such as Coumadin
Captopril (Capoten)
Cimetidine (Tagamet)
Diuretics such as Dyazide
Epinephrine (EpiPen)
Guanethidine (Ismelin)
Lithium (Lithobid, Eskalith)
MAO inhibitors (antidepressants such as Nardil and
    Parnate)
Narcotics such as Percocet
Propranolol (Inderal)

Extreme drowsiness and other potentially serious effects can result if Thorazine is combined with alcohol and other mental depressants such as narcotic painkillers like Demerol.

Because Thorazine prevents vomiting, it can hide the signs and symptoms of overdose of other drugs.

### Special information if you are pregnant or breastfeeding

The effects of Thorazine during pregnancy have not been adequately studied. If you are pregnant or plan to become pregnant, notify your doctor.

Pregnant women should use Thorazine only if clearly needed. Thorazine appears in breast milk and may affect a nursing infant. If this medication is essential to your health, your doctor may advise you not to breastfeed until your treatment is finished.

## Recommended dosage

### ADULTS

*Psychotic Disorders*

Your doctor will gradually increase the dosage until symptoms are controlled. You may not see full improvement for weeks or even months.

Initial dosages may range from 30 to 75 milligrams daily. The amount is divided into equal doses and taken 3 or 4 times a day. If needed, your doctor may increase the dosage by 20 to 50 milligrams at semiweekly intervals.

*Nausea and Vomiting*

The usual tablet dosage is 10 to 25 milligrams, taken every 4 or 6 hours, as needed.

One 100-milligram suppository can be used every 6 to 8 hours.

*Uncontrollable Hiccups*

Dosages may range from 75 to 200 milligrams daily, divided into 3 or 4 equal doses.

*Acute Intermittent Porphyria*

Dosages may range from 75 to 200 milligrams daily, divided into 3 or 4 equal doses.

### CHILDREN

Thorazine is generally not prescribed for children younger than 6 months.

*Severe Behavior Problems, Nausea, and Vomiting*

Dosages are based on the child's weight.

Oral: The daily dose is one-quarter milligram for each pound of the child's weight, taken every 4 to 6 hours, as needed.

Rectal: the usual dose is one-half milligram per pound of body weight, taken every 6 to 8 hours, as necessary.

### OLDER ADULTS

In general, older people take lower dosages of Thorazine, and any increase in dosage will be gradual. Because of a greater risk of low blood pressure, your doctor will watch you closely while you are taking Thorazine. Older people (especially older women) may be more susceptible to tardive dyskinesia—a possibly permanent condition characterized by involuntary muscle spasms and twitches in the face and body. Consult your doctor for information about these potential risks.

## Overdosage

Any medication taken in excess can have serious consequences. An overdose of Thorazine can be fatal. If you suspect an overdose, seek medical help immediately.

■ *Symptoms of Thorazine overdose may include:*
Agitation, coma, convulsions, difficulty breathing, difficulty swallowing, dry mouth, extreme sleepiness, fever, intestinal blockage, irregular heart rate, low blood pressure, restlessness

*Generic name:*

# Thyroid Hormones

*See Armour Thyroid, page 34.*

*Brand name:*

# Tigan

*Pronounced: TIE-gan*
*Generic name: Trimethobenzamide hydrochloride*

## Why is this drug prescribed?

Tigan is prescribed to control nausea and vomiting.

## Most important fact about this drug

Antiemetics (drugs that prevent or lessen nausea and vomiting) are not recommended for the treatment of simple vomiting in children. Use of Tigan in children should be limited to prolonged vomiting caused by a known disease.

Caution should always be exercised when using this drug in children, since there may be a link between the use of antiemetic drugs to treat symptoms of viral illnesses such as chickenpox and the development of Reye's syndrome, which is a potentially fatal childhood disease of the brain.

## How should you take this medication?

Take this medication exactly as prescribed.

If you are using the suppository form of Tigan and find it is too soft to insert, you can firm it up by chilling it in the refrigerator for about 30 minutes or running cold water over it before removing the wrapper.

To insert a suppository, first remove the wrapper and moisten the suppository with cold water. Then lie down on your side and use a finger to push the suppository well up into the rectum.

■ *If you miss a dose...*
Take it as soon as you remember. If it is almost time for your next dose, skip the one you missed and go back to your regular schedule. Do not take 2 doses at once.

■ *Storage instructions...*
Store away from heat, light, and moisture.

### What side effects may occur?
Side effects cannot be anticipated. If any develop or change in intensity, inform your doctor as soon as possible. Only your doctor can determine if it is safe for you to continue taking Tigan.

■ *Side effects may include:*
Allergic-type skin reactions, blurred vision, coma, convulsions, depression, diarrhea, disorientation, dizziness, drowsiness, headache, muscle cramps, severe muscle spasm, tremors, yellowed eyes and skin

### Why should this drug not be prescribed?
If you are sensitive to or have ever had an allergic reaction to Tigan do not take this medication. Do not use the suppositories if you are allergic to benzocaine or other local anesthetics. Make sure your doctor is aware of any drug reactions you have experienced.

Unless you are directed to do so by your doctor, do not use suppositories in premature or newborn infants.

### Special warnings about this medication
Tigan may cause you to become drowsy or less alert. Do not drive or operate dangerous machinery or participate in any hazardous activity that requires full mental alertness until you know how you respond to this drug.

Reye's syndrome has been associated with the use of Tigan during viral illnesses in children. Reye's syndrome is characterized by severe, persistent vomiting, sluggishness, irrational behavior, and a progressive brain disorder leading to coma, convulsions, and death.

Caution should be exercised when taking Tigan—especially in children, the elderly, or those in a weakened or run-down condition— if you have a severe illness accompanied by high fever, inflammation of the brain (encephalitis), inflammation of the stomach and intestines (gastroenteritis), or dehydration.

Severe vomiting should not be treated with Tigan alone. Your doctor should emphasize restoration of body fluids, the relief of fever, and the relief of the disease causing the vomiting. However, the overconsumption of fluids may result in cerebral edema (excessive accumulation of fluid in the brain).

The antinausea effects of Tigan may make it difficult to diagnose such conditions as appendicitis and may mask signs of drug poisoning due to overdosage of other drugs.

### Possible food and drug interactions when taking this medication
The use of alcohol in combination with this drug may produce an unfavorable reaction.

Caution should be exercised when taking Tigan in combination with central nervous system drugs such as phenothiazines (tranquilizers and antiemetics), barbiturates such as phenobarbital, and drugs derived from belladonna, such as Donnatal, if you are dehydrated or have a severe disease with fever, inflammation of the stomach, intestines, or brain.

### Special information if you are pregnant or breastfeeding
The effects of Tigan during pregnancy or breastfeeding have not been adequately studied. If you are pregnant or plan to become pregnant, inform your doctor immediately. If you are breastfeeding your baby, consult your doctor before taking this medication.

### Recommended dosage
Dosage will be adjusted by your doctor according to your illness, the severity of your symptoms, and how well you do on the drug.

ADULTS

*Capsules*
The usual dosage is one 250-milligram capsule taken 3 or 4 times per day, as determined by your doctor.

*Suppositories*

The recommended dosage is 1 suppository (200 milligrams) inserted into the rectum 3 or 4 times per day, as determined by your doctor.

CHILDREN

*Capsules*

The usual dosage for children weighing 30 to 90 pounds is one or two 100-milligram capsules taken 3 or 4 times per day, as determined by the doctor.

*Suppositories*

The usual dosage for children weighing under 30 pounds is half a suppository (100 milligrams), inserted into the rectum 3 or 4 times a day, as determined by your doctor.

The usual dosage for children weighing 30 to 90 pounds is one-half to one 200-milligram suppository rectally 3 or 4 times a day, as determined by the doctor.

*Pediatric Suppositories*

The usual dosage for children weighing under 30 pounds is 1 suppository (100 milligrams) rectally 3 or 4 times a day, as determined by the doctor.

The usual dosage for children weighing 30 to 90 pounds is 1 to 2 suppositories (100 milligrams to 200 milligrams) rectally 3 or 4 times a day, as determined by the doctor.

### Overdosage

Although no specific information is available, any medication taken in excess can have serious consequences. If you suspect a Tigan overdose, seek medical attention immediately.

*Brand name:*

# Tilade

*Pronounced: TILE-aid*
*Generic name: Nedocromil sodium*

### Why is this drug prescribed?

Tilade is an anti-inflammatory medication prescribed for use on a regular basis to control asthma symptoms in people with mild to moderate bronchial asthma.

### Most important fact about this drug

Tilade must be used regularly to be effective, even if you have no symptoms. It improves your condition, but won't help during an acute attack.

### How should you take this medication?

Proper inhalation of Tilade is essential for it to be effective. Make sure you understand how to use the medication correctly, and take it exactly as prescribed.

Tilade Inhaler should not be used with other mouthpieces.

■ *If you miss a dose...*
To work properly, Tilade must be inhaled every day at regular intervals. If you miss a dose, take it as soon as you remember. If it is almost time for your next dose, skip the one you missed and go back to your regular schedule. Do not take double doses.

■ *Storage instructions...*
Store Tilade Inhaler at room temperature. Because the contents are under pressure, do not puncture, incinerate, or place near heat.

### What side effects may occur?

Side effects cannot be anticipated. If any develop or change in intensity, inform your doctor as soon as possible. Only your doctor can determine if it is safe for you to continue using Tilade.

■ *More common side effects may include:*
Chest pain, coughing, headache, nausea, inflamed nose, sore throat, unpleasant taste, upper respiratory tract infection, wheezing

■ *Less common side effects may include:*
Abdominal pain, bronchitis, diarrhea, difficult or labored breathing, difficulty speaking, dizziness, dry mouth, fatigue, increased sputum, indigestion, viral infection, vomiting

### Why should this drug not be prescribed?

Tilade Inhaler should not be used if you are sensitive to or have ever had an allergic reaction to nedocromil sodium or any of Tilade's other ingredients. Make sure your doctor is aware of any drug reactions you have experienced.

### Special warnings about this medication

This medication will not stop an asthma attack. However, you should continue to take it during an attack, along with a bronchodilator (a medication that increases air flow to your lungs) to relieve the acute symptoms.

Medications that are inhaled can cause coughing and wheezing in some people. If you experience these symptoms, stop taking Tilade and notify your doctor immediately.

## Possible food and drug interactions when taking this medication
No interactions have been reported.

## Special information if you are pregnant or breastfeeding
The effects of Tilade during pregnancy have not been adequately studied. If you are pregnant or plan to become pregnant, notify your doctor immediately. Tilade may appear in breast milk and could affect a nursing infant. If this medication is essential to your health, your doctor may advise you to discontinue breastfeeding until your treatment is finished.

## Recommended dosage
ADULTS AND CHILDREN 12 YEARS OF AGE AND OVER

The recommended dose is 2 inhalations 4 times a day at regular intervals. If you are doing well on that dosage, your doctor may try reducing the dose after a time.

CHILDREN

The safety and effectiveness of Tilade Inhaler have not been established in children under 12 years of age.

## Overdosage
Any medication taken in excess can have serious consequences. If you suspect an overdose, seek medical attention immediately.

*Generic name:*

# Timolol

*See Timoptic, page 546.*

*Brand name:*

# Timoptic

*Pronounced: Tim-OP-tic*
*Generic name: Timolol*
*Other brand name: Betimol*

## Why is this drug prescribed?
Timoptic is a topical medication (applied directly in the eye) that effectively reduces internal pressure in the eye. Timoptic is used in the treatment of glaucoma to lower elevated eye pressure that could damage vision and, with other glaucoma medications, to further reduce pressure in the eye.

## Most important fact about this drug
Although Timoptic eyedrops are applied only to the eye, the medication is absorbed and may have effects in other parts of the body. If you have diabetes, asthma, or other respiratory disease, or decreased heart function, make sure your doctor is aware of the problem.

## How should you use this medication?
Timoptic should be used exactly as prescribed by your doctor.

If you are using Timoptic in Ocudose, use the medication as soon as you open the individual unit and throw out any leftover solution.

If you are using Timoptic-XE, invert the closed container and shake it once—and only once—before each use.

If you need to use other eye medications along with Timoptic-XE, use them at least 10 minutes before you instill Timoptic-XE. Allow 5 minutes with Betimol.

Handle the Timoptic solution carefully to avoid contamination. Do not let the tip of the dispenser actually touch the eye.

*To administer Timoptic, follow these steps:*
1. Wash your hands thoroughly.
2. Gently pull your lower eyelid down to form a pocket.
3. Brace the bottle against the bridge of your nose or your forehead.
4. Tilt your head back and squeeze the medication into your eye.
5. Close your eyes gently.
6. Keep your eyes closed for 1 to 2 minutes.

■ *If you miss a dose...*
  If you use Timoptic once a day, apply it as soon as you remember. If you do not remember until the next day, skip the dose you missed and go back to your regular schedule. Do not take 2 doses at once. If you use it more than once a day, apply it as soon as you remember. If it is almost time for your next dose, skip the one you missed and go back to your regular schedule. Do not take 2 doses at once.

■ *Storage instructions...*
  Store at room temperature, protected from light. Keep from freezing.

## What side effects may occur?

Side effects cannot be anticipated. If any side effects develop or change in intensity, tell your doctor immediately. Only your doctor can determine whether it is safe to continue using this medication. If Timoptic is absorbed into the bloodstream, it can cause additional side effects.

The most common side effects are burning and stinging on instillation of the drug.

■ *Other side effects may include:*

Abnormal overflow of tears, allergic reactions, anxiety, blurred or abnormal vision, cataracts, chest pain, common cold, confusion, conjunctivitis (pinkeye), cough, depression, diarrhea, difficult or labored breathing, disorientation, dizziness, double vision, drooping eyelid, dry mouth, eye discharge, eye dryness or irritation and inflammation, eye pain or itching and tearing, fainting, fatigue, fluid in the lungs, hair loss, hallucinations, headache, heart failure, high blood pressure, hives, impotence, inability to breathe, increase in signs/symptoms of myasthenia gravis (severe muscle weakness), indigestion, inflammation or swelling of the eyelid, intolerance of light, irregular heartbeat, loss of appetite, low blood pressure, nausea, nervousness, pain, pain or swelling in arms and legs, rash, sensation of a foreign body in the eye, sinus inflammation, sleepiness, slow heartbeat, stroke, stuffy nose, throbbing or fluttering heartbeat, tingling or pins and needles, upper respiratory infection, visual disturbances, weakness, wheezing, worsened angina pectoris (crushing chest pain)

## Why should this drug not be prescribed?

Do not use Timoptic if you have bronchial asthma, a history of bronchial asthma, or other serious breathing disorders such as emphysema, slow heartbeat, heart block (conduction disorder), active heart failure, or inadequate blood supply to the circulatory system (cardiogenic shock), or if you have ever had an allergic reaction or are sensitive to Timoptic or any of its ingredients.

## Special warnings about this medication

Use Timoptic cautiously if you have a history of heart failure or poor circulation to the brain.

Tell your doctor if you have any type of allergy. The frequency and severity of allergic reactions may increase while you are using Timoptic.

Timoptic may mask the symptoms of low blood sugar. If you are diabetic, discuss this possibility with your doctor.

Tell your doctor or dentist that you are using Timoptic if you have a medical emergency or before you have surgery or dental treatment.

Timoptic may mask symptoms of an overactive thyroid. If your doctor suspects you have excessive thyroid function, he or she will manage your case carefully to avoid such symptoms as rapid heartbeat, which can occur when the drug is withdrawn too abruptly.

Timoptic's antiglaucoma effects may decrease if you use the medication for a long time.

Some older individuals may be more sensitive to this product than younger people. If you develop an eye infection, check with your doctor. You may need to stop using Timoptic.

## Possible food and drug interactions when using this medication

If Timoptic is used with certain other drugs, the effects of either could be increased, decreased, or altered. It is especially important to check with your doctor before combining Timoptic with the following:

Epinephrine (EpiPen)
Catecholamine-depleting drugs, such as blood pressure drugs that contain reserpine (Serpasil)
Calcium antagonists such as Cardizem and Isoptin
Digitalis (Lanoxin)

Timoptic should not be used with other topical beta blockers and should be used with caution if you are taking oral beta blockers such as Inderal and Tenormin.

## Special information if you are pregnant or breastfeeding

If you are pregnant or plan to become pregnant, inform your doctor immediately. No information is available about the safety of using Timoptic during pregnancy.

Timolol appears in breast milk and may harm a nursing infant. If using Timoptic is essential to your health, your doctor may advise you to stop breastfeeding until your treatment is finished.

### Recommended dosage

ADULTS

Your doctor will tailor an individual Timoptic dosage depending on your medical condition and how you responded to any previous glaucoma treatment.

The usual recommended initial dose is to place 1 drop of 0.25 percent Timoptic in the affected eye(s) twice a day. If you do not respond satisfactorily to this dosage, your doctor may tell you to place 1 drop of 0.5 percent Timoptic in the affected eye(s) twice a day.

The usual dose of Timoptic-XE is 1 drop of either 0.25 percent or 0.5 percent in the affected eye(s) once a day. Invert the closed container and shake it once before you use it.

The usual dose of Betimol is 1 drop of either 0.25 percent or 0.5 percent in the affected eye(s) twice a day.

### Overdosage

Seek medical treatment immediately if you think you might have used too much Timoptic. Call your local poison control center or your doctor for assistance.

■ *Symptoms of Timoptic overdose may include:*
Dizziness, headache, heart failure, shortness of breath, slow heartbeat, wheezing

*Generic name:*

# Tobramycin

*See Tobrex, page 548.*

*Brand name:*

# Tobrex

*Pronounced: TOE-breks*
*Generic name: Tobramycin*
*Other brand name: Aktob*

### Why is this drug prescribed?

Tobrex is an antibiotic applied to the eye to treat bacterial infections.

### Most important fact about this drug

In order to clear up your infection completely, keep using Tobrex for the full time of treatment, even if your symptoms have disappeared.

### How should you use this medication?

To apply Tobrex eye drops:

1. Wash your hands thoroughly.
2. Gently pull your lower eyelid down to form a pocket between your eye and eyelid.
3. Brace the bottle on the bridge of your nose or your forehead.
4. Do not let the applicator tip touch your eye or any other surface.
5. Tilt your head back and squeeze the medication into the eye.
6. Close your eyes gently.
7. Keep your eyes closed for 1 to 2 minutes.
8. Do not rinse the dropper.
9. If you are using another eye drop wait 5 to 10 minutes before applying it.

To apply the ointment form of this medication:

1. Tilt your head back.
2. Place a finger on your cheek just under your eye and gently pull down until a "V" pocket is formed between your eyeball and your lower lid.
3. Place about half an inch of Tobrex in the "V" pocket. Do not let the tip of the tube touch the eye.
4. Look downward before closing your eye.

■ *If you miss a dose...*
Apply it as soon as you remember. If it is almost time for your next dose, skip the one you missed and go back to your regular schedule.
■ *Storage instructions...*
Store Tobrex at room temperature, away from heat, or in the refrigerator. Do not allow to freeze.

### What side effects may occur?

Side effects cannot be anticipated. If any develop or change in intensity, inform your doctor as soon as possible. Only your doctor can determine if it is safe for you to continue to take Tobrex.

■ *Side effects may include:*
Abnormal redness of eye tissue, allergic reactions, lid itching, lid swelling

### Why should this drug not be prescribed?

If you are sensitive to or have ever had an allergic reaction to Tobrex or any of its ingredients, you should not use this medication. Make sure your doctor is aware of any drug reactions you have experienced.

## Special warnings about this medication

If you experience an allergic reaction to this medication, discontinue use and inform your doctor.

Continued or prolonged use of Tobrex may result in a growth of bacteria that do not respond to this medication and can cause a secondary infection.

Ophthalmic ointments may slow healing of wounds of the cornea.

## Possible food and drug interactions when taking this medication

If you are taking any other prescription antibiotics for your eyes, check with your doctor before using Tobrex. Using this medication with certain other antibiotics in your system may cause an overdose.

## Special information if you are pregnant or breastfeeding

The effects of Tobrex during pregnancy have not been adequately studied. If you are pregnant or plan to become pregnant, inform your doctor immediately. Tobrex may appear in breast milk. Your doctor may advise you to discontinue breastfeeding until your treatment with this medication is finished.

## Recommended dosage

ADULTS

*Solution*

If the infection is mild to moderate, place 1 or 2 drops into the affected eye(s) every 4 hours. In severe infections, place 2 drops into the eye(s) every hour until there is improvement. Then you will be instructed to use less medication before you stop using it altogether.

*Ointment*

If the infection is mild to moderate, apply a half-inch ribbon into the affected eye(s) 2 or 3 times per day. In severe infections, apply a half-inch ribbon into the affected eye(s) every 3 or 4 hours until there is improvement. Then use less medication before stopping altogether.

CHILDREN

Your doctor will tailor a dose for the child.

## Overdosage

Any medication used in excess can have serious consequences. If you suspect an overdose, seek medical assistance immediately.

■ *Symptoms of Tobrex overdose may be similar to side effects. They include:*
Corneal redness and inflammation, excessive eye tearing, lid itching and swelling

---

*Generic name:*

# Tocainide

*See Tonocard, page 553.*

*Brand name:*

# Tofranil

*Pronounced: toe-FRAY-nil*
*Generic name: Imipramine hydrochloride*

## Why is this drug prescribed?

Tofranil is used to treat depression. It is a member of the family of drugs called tricyclic antidepressants.

Tofranil is also used on a short term basis, along with behavioral therapies, to treat bed-wetting in children aged 6 and older. Its effectiveness may decrease with longer use.

Some doctors also prescribe Tofranil to treat bulimia, attention deficit disorder in children, obsessive-compulsive disorder, and panic disorder.

## Most important fact about this drug

Serious, sometimes fatal, reactions have been known to occur when drugs such as Tofranil are taken with another type of antidepressant called an MAO inhibitor. Drugs in this category include Nardil and Parnate. Do not take Tofranil within 2 weeks of taking one of these drugs. Make sure your doctor and pharmacist know of all the medications you are taking.

## How should you take this medication?

Tofranil may be taken with or without food.

You should not take Tofranil with alcohol.

Do not stop taking Tofranil if you feel no immediate effect. It can take from 1 to 3 weeks for improvement to begin.

Tofranil can cause dry mouth. Sucking hard candy or chewing gum can help this problem.

■ *If you miss a dose...*
If you take 1 dose a day at bedtime, contact your doctor. Do not take the dose in the morning because of possible side effects.

If you take 2 or more doses a day, take the forgotten dose as soon as you remember. If it is almost time for your next dose, skip the one you missed and go back to your regular schedule. Do not take 2 doses at once.

■ *Storage instructions...*
Store at room temperature in a tightly closed container.

## What side effects may occur?

Side effects cannot be anticipated. If any develop or change in intensity, inform your doctor as soon as possible. Only your doctor can determine if it is safe for you to continue taking Tofranil.

■ *Side effects may include:*

Abdominal cramps, agitation, anxiety, black tongue, bleeding sores, blood disorders, blurred vision, breast development in males, confusion, congestive heart failure, constipation or diarrhea, cough, fever, sore throat, delusions, dilated pupils, disorientation, dizziness, drowsiness, dry mouth, episodes of elation or irritability, excessive or spontaneous flow of milk, fatigue, fever, flushing, frequent urination or difficulty or delay in urinating, hair loss, hallucinations, headache, heart attack, heart failure, high blood pressure, high or low blood sugar, high pressure of fluid in the eyes, hives, impotence, increased or decreased sex drive, inflammation of the mouth, insomnia, intestinal blockage, irregular heartbeat, lack of coordination, light-headedness (especially when rising from lying down), loss of appetite, nausea, nightmares, odd taste in mouth, palpitations, purple or reddish-brown spots on skin, rapid heartbeat, restlessness, ringing in the ears, seizures, sensitivity to light, skin itching and rash, stomach upset, stroke, sweating, swelling due to fluid retention (especially in face or tongue), swelling of breasts, swelling of testicles, swollen glands, tendency to fall, tingling, pins and needles, and numbness in hands and feet, tremors, visual problems, vomiting, weakness, weight gain or loss, yellowed skin and whites of eyes

■ *The most common side effects in children being treated for bed wetting are:*

Nervousness, sleep disorders, stomach and intestinal problems, tiredness

■ *Other side effects in children are:*

Anxiety, collapse, constipation, convulsions, emotional instability, fainting

## Why should this drug not be prescribed?

Tofranil should not be used if you are recovering from a recent heart attack.

People who take antidepressant drugs known as MAO inhibitors, such as Nardil and Parnate, should not take Tofranil. You should not take Tofranil if you are sensitive or allergic to it.

## Special warnings about this medication

You should use Tofranil cautiously if you have or have ever had: narrow-angle glaucoma (increased pressure in the eye); difficulty in urinating; heart, liver, kidney, or thyroid disease; or seizures. Also be cautious if you are taking thyroid medication.

General feelings of illness, headache, and nausea can result if you suddenly stop taking Tofranil. Follow your doctor's instructions closely when discontinuing Tofranil.

Tell your doctor if you develop a sore throat or fever while taking Tofranil.

This drug may impair your ability to drive a car or operate potentially dangerous machinery. Do not participate in any activities that require full alertness if you are unsure about your ability.

This drug can make you sensitive to light. Try to stay out of the sun as much as possible while you are taking it.

If you are going to have elective surgery, your doctor will take you off Tofranil.

## Possible food and drug interactions when taking this medication

If Tofranil is taken with certain other drugs, the effects of either could be increased, decreased, or altered. It is especially important to check with your doctor before combining Tofranil with the following:

Albuterol (Proventil, Ventolin)
Antidepressants that act on serotonin, including
    Prozac, Paxil and Zoloft
Antispasmodic drugs such as Cogentin
Barbiturates such as Nembutal and Seconal
Blood pressure medications such as Ismelin,
    Catapres and Wytensin
Carbamazepine (Tegretol)
Central nervous system depressants such as Xanax
    and Valium
Cimetidine (Tagamet)
Decongestants such as Sudafed
Epinephrine (EpiPen)
Flecainide (Tambocor)
Major tranquilizers such as Mellaril and Thorazine
Methylphenidate (Ritalin)
Norepinephrine
Other antidepressants such as Elavil and Pamelor
Phenytoin (Dilantin)
Propafenone (Rythmol)
Quinidine (Quinaglute)
Thyroid medications such as Synthroid

Extreme drowsiness and other potentially serious effects can result if Tofranil is combined with alcohol or other mental depressants, such as narcotic painkillers (Percocet), sleeping medications (Halcion), or tranquilizers (Valium).

If you are switching from Prozac, wait at least 5 weeks after your last dose of Prozac before starting Tofranil.

## Special information
## if you are pregnant or breastfeeding

The effects of Tofranil during pregnancy have not been adequately studied. Pregnant women should use Tofranil only when the potential benefits clearly outweigh the potential risks. If you are pregnant or plan to become pregnant, inform your doctor immediately. Tofranil may appear in breast milk and could affect a nursing infant. If this medication is essential to your health, your doctor may advise you to stop breastfeeding until your treatment is finished.

## Recommended dosage

### ADULTS

The usual starting dose is 75 milligrams a day. The doctor may increase this to 150 milligrams a day. The maximum daily dose is 200 milligrams.

### CHILDREN

Tofranil is not to be used in children to treat any condition but bedwetting, and its use will be limited to short-term therapy. Safety and effectiveness in children under the age of 6 have not been established.

Total daily dosages for children should not exceed 2.5 milligrams for each 2.2 pounds of the child's weight.

Doses usually begin at 25 milligrams per day. This amount should be taken an hour before bedtime. If needed, this dose may be increased after 1 week to 50 milligrams (ages 6 through 11) or 75 milligrams (ages 12 and up), taken in one dose at bedtime or divided into 2 doses, 1 taken at mid-afternoon and 1 at bedtime.

### OLDER ADULTS AND ADOLESCENTS

People in these two age groups should take lower doses. Dosage starts out at 30 to 40 milligrams per day and can go up to no more than 100 milligrams a day.

## Overdosage

Any medication taken in excess can have serious consequences. An overdose of Tofranil can cause death. It has been reported that children are more sensitive than adults to overdoses of Tofranil. If you suspect an overdose, seek medical help immediately.

■ *Symptoms of Tofranil overdose may include:*
Agitation, bluish skin, coma, convulsions, difficulty breathing, dilated pupils, drowsiness, heart failure, high fever, involuntary writhing or jerky movements, irregular or rapid heartbeat, lack of coordination, low blood pressure, overactive reflexes, restlessness, rigid muscles, shock, stupor, sweating, vomiting

*Generic name:*

# Tolbutamide

*See Orinase, page 385.*

*Brand name:*

# Tolectin

*Pronounced: toe-LEK-tin*
*Generic name: Tolmetin sodium*

## Why is this drug prescribed?

Tolectin is a nonsteroidal anti-inflammatory drug used to relieve the inflammation, swelling, stiffness, and joint pain associated with rheumatoid arthritis and osteoarthritis (the most common form of arthritis). It is used for both acute episodes and long-term treatment. It is also used to treat juvenile rheumatoid arthritis.

## Most important fact about this drug

You should have frequent checkups with your doctor if you take Tolectin regularly. Ulcers or internal bleeding can occur without warning.

## How should you take this medication?

If Tolectin upsets your stomach, it may be taken with food or an antacid, and with a full glass of water. It may also help to prevent upset if you avoid lying down for 20 to 30 minutes after taking the drug.

Take this medication exactly as prescribed by your doctor.

■ *If you miss a dose...*
Take it as soon as you remember. If it is almost time for your next dose, skip the one you missed and go back to your regular schedule. Never take 2 doses at the same time.

■ *Storage instructions...*
Store at room temperature in a tightly closed container, away from light.

## What side effects may occur?

Side effects cannot be anticipated. If any develop or change in intensity, inform your doctor as soon as possible. Only your doctor can determine if it is safe for you to continue taking Tolectin.

■ *More common side effects may include:*
Abdominal pain, change in weight, diarrhea, dizziness, gas, headache, heartburn, high blood pressure, indigestion, nausea, stomach and intestinal upset, swelling due to fluid retention, vomiting, weakness

■ *Less common or rare side effects may include:*
Anemia, blood in urine, chest pain, congestive heart failure, constipation, depression, drowsiness, fever, hepatitis, hives, inflammation of the mouth or tongue, kidney failure, painful urination, peptic ulcer, purple or reddish spots on skin, ringing in the ears, severe allergic reactions, skin irritation, stomach inflammation, stomach or intestinal bleeding, urinary tract infection, visual disturbances, yellow eyes or skin

## Why should this drug not be prescribed?

If you are sensitive to or have ever had an allergic reaction to Tolectin, aspirin, or other nonsteroidal anti-inflammatory drugs, or if you have had asthma, hives, or nasal inflammation caused by aspirin or other nonsteroidal anti-inflammatory drugs, you should not take this medication. Make sure your doctor is aware of any drug reactions you have experienced.

## Special warnings about this medication

Tolectin can cause kidney problems, especially if you are elderly, suffer from heart failure or liver disease, or take diuretics.

This drug can also affect the liver. If you develop symptoms such as yellow skin and eyes, notify your doctor. You should be taken off Tolectin.

Do not take aspirin or any other anti-inflammatory medications while taking Tolectin unless your doctor tells you to do so.

Tolectin can cause visual disturbances. If you experience a change in your vision, inform your doctor.

Tolectin prolongs bleeding time. If you are taking blood-thinning medication, this drug should be taken with caution.

This drug can increase water retention. Use with caution if you have heart disease or high blood pressure.

Tolectin causes some people to become drowsy or less alert. If it has this effect on you, driving or operating dangerous machinery or participating in any hazardous activity that requires full mental alertness is not recommended.

## Possible food and drug interactions when taking this medication

If Tolectin is taken with certain other drugs, the effects of either could be increased, decreased, or altered. It is especially important to check with your doctor before combining Tolectin with the following:

Aspirin
Blood thinners such as Coumadin
Carteolol (Cartrol)
Diuretics such as Lasix
Glyburide (Micronase)
Lithium (Lithonate)
Methotrexate

## Special information if you are pregnant or breastfeeding

The effects of Tolectin during pregnancy have not been adequately studied. If you are pregnant or plan to become pregnant, inform your doctor immediately. Tolectin appears in breast milk and could affect a nursing infant. If this medication is essential to your health, your doctor may advise you to discontinue breastfeeding until your treatment is finished.

## Recommended dosage

ADULTS

*Rheumatoid Arthritis or Osteoarthritis*
The starting dosage is usually 1,200 milligrams a day divided into 3 doses of 400 milligrams each. Take 1 dose when you wake up and 1 at bedtime, and 1 sometime in between. Your doctor may adjust the dosage after 1 to 2 weeks. Most people will take a total daily dosage of 600 to 1,800 milligrams usually divided into 3 doses.

You should see the benefits of Tolectin in a few days to a week.

## CHILDREN

The starting dose for children 2 years and older is usually a total of 20 milligrams per 2.2 pounds of body weight per day, divided into 3 or 4 smaller doses. Your doctor will advise you on use in children. The usual dose ranges from 15 to 30 milligrams per 2.2 pounds per day.

The safety and effectiveness of Tolectin have not been established in children under 2 years of age.

## Overdosage

Although no specific information is available, any medication taken in excess can have serious consequences. If you suspect an overdose of Tolectin, seek medical attention immediately.

*Generic name:*

# Tolmetin

*See Tolectin, page 551.*

*Brand name:*

# Tonocard

*Pronounced: TAH-nuh-card*
*Generic name: Tocainide hydrochloride*

## Why is this drug prescribed?

Tonocard is used to treat severe irregular heartbeat (arrhythmias). Arrhythmias are generally divided into two main types: heartbeats that are faster than normal (tachycardia), or heartbeats that are slower than normal (bradycardia). Irregular heartbeats are often caused by drugs or disease but can occur in otherwise-healthy people with no history of heart disease or other illness. Tonocard works differently from other antiarrhythmic drugs, such as quinidine (Quinidex), procainamide (Procan SR), and disopyramide (Norpace). It is similar to lidocaine (Xylocaine) and is effective in treating ventricular arrhythmias (irregular heartbeats that occur in a particular part of the heart).

## Most important fact about this drug

Tonocard can cause serious blood and lung disorders in some patients, especially in the first 3 months of treatment. Be sure to notify your doctor if any of the following occurs: painful or difficult breathing, wheezing, cough, easy bruising or bleeding, tremors, palpitations, rash, soreness or ulcers in the mouth, sore throat, fever, and chills.

## How should you take this medication?

It is important to take Tonocard on a regular schedule, exactly as prescribed by your doctor. Try not to miss any doses. If this medication is not taken regularly, your condition can worsen.

■ *If you miss a dose...*
   If less than 2 hours have passed, take the forgotten dose as soon as you remember. If you are more than 2 hours late, skip the dose. Never try to "catch up" by taking a double dose.
■ *Storage instructions...*
   Keep the container tightly closed, and store it at room temperature. Protect from extreme heat.

## What side effects may occur?

Side effects cannot be anticipated. If any develop or change in intensity, inform your doctor as soon as possible. Only your doctor can determine if it is safe for you to continue taking Tonocard.

■ *More common side effects may include:*
   Confusion/disorientation, dizziness/vertigo, diarrhea/loose stools, excessive sweating, hallucinations, increased irregular heartbeat, lack of coordination, loss of appetite, nausea, nervousness, rash/skin eruptions, tingling or pins and needles, tremor, vision disturbances, vomiting
■ *Less common side effects may include:*
   Arthritis, anxiety, chest pain, congestive heart failure, drowsiness, exhaustion, fatigue, headache, hearing loss, hot/cold feelings, involuntary eyeball movement, joint pain, low blood pressure, muscle pain, pounding heartbeat, rapid heartbeat, ringing in ears, sleepiness, slow heartbeat, sluggishness, unsteadiness, walking disturbances
■ *Rare side effects may include:*
   Abdominal pain/discomfort, agitation, allergic reactions, anemia, angina, blood clots in lungs, blood disorders, changes in blood counts, changes in heart function, chills, cinchonism (a sensitivity reaction with symptoms including ringing in the ears, loss of hearing, dizziness, light-headedness, headache, nausea, and/or disturbed vision), cold hands and feet, coma, constipation, decreased mental ability, decreased

urination, depression, difficulty breathing, difficulty speaking, difficulty sleeping, difficulty swallowing, disturbed behavior, disturbed dreams, dizziness on standing, double vision, dry mouth, earache, enlarged heart, fainting, fever, fluid in lungs, fluid retention, flushing, general bodily discomfort, hair loss, heart attack, hepatitis, hiccups, high blood pressure, hives, increased stuttering, increased urination, lung disorders, memory loss, muscle cramps, muscle twitching/spasm, myasthenia gravis, neck pain or pain extending from the neck, pallor, pneumonia, seizures, skin peeling, slurred speech, smell disturbance, stomach upset, taste disturbance, thirst, weakness, yawning, yellow eyes and skin

### Why should this drug not be prescribed?

If you have heart block (conduction disorder) and do not have a pacemaker, or if you are sensitive to or have ever had an allergic reaction to Tonocard or certain local anesthetics such as Xylocaine, do not take this medication.

### Special warnings about this medication

Be alert for signs of the blood and lung disorders that can occur early in your treatment. (See "Most important fact about this drug.")

If you have congestive heart failure, make sure the doctor is aware of it. Tonocard could worsen this condition.

Also make certain that the doctor is aware of any kidney or liver problems that you have. You will need to be monitored more carefully.

Before any kind of surgery, including dental surgery and emergency treatment, make sure the surgeon knows that you are taking Tonocard.

### Possible food and drug interactions when taking this medication

If Tonocard is taken with certain other drugs, the effects of either could be increased, decreased, or altered. It is especially important to check with your doctor before combining Tonocard with any of the following:

The anesthetic Lidocaine (Xylocaine)
The blood pressure medicine Metoprolol
    (Lopressor)
Other antiarrhythmics such as Quinidex, Procan,
    Mexitil

### Special information
### if you are pregnant or breastfeeding

The effects of Tonocard during pregnancy have not been adequately studied. However, animal studies have shown an increase in stillbirths and spontaneous abortions. If you are pregnant or plan to become pregnant, inform your doctor immediately. Tonocard may appear in breast milk and could affect a nursing infant. If this medication is essential to your health, your doctor may advise you to discontinue breastfeeding until your treatment is finished.

### Recommended dosage

ADULTS

Dosages of Tonocard must be adjusted according to its effects on each individual. Your doctor should monitor you carefully to determine if the dosage you are taking is working properly. He may divide your doses further or make other changes, such as shortening the time between doses, if side effects occur.

The usual starting dose is 400 milligrams every 8 hours.

The usual dose range is between 1,200 and 1,800 milligrams total per day divided into 3 doses. This medication can be taken in 2 doses a day with careful monitoring by your doctor.

Doses beyond 2,400 milligrams per day are rarely used.

Some people, particularly those with reduced kidney or liver function, may be treated successfully with less than 1,200 milligrams per day.

CHILDREN

The safety and effectiveness of this drug in children have not been established.

### Overdosage

Any medication taken in excess can have serious consequences. If you suspect an overdose, seek medical attention immediately.

There are no specific reports of Tonocard overdose. However, the first and most important signs of overdose would be expected to appear in the central nervous system. Disorders of the stomach and intestines might follow. Convulsions and heart and lung slowing or stopping might occur.

*Brand name:*

# Topicort

*Pronounced: TOP-i-court*
*Generic name: Desoximetasone*

## Why is this drug prescribed?

Topicort is a synthetic steroid medication in cream, gel, or ointment form that relieves the inflammation and itching caused by a variety of skin conditions.

## Most important fact about this drug

When you use Topicort, you may absorb some of the medication through your skin and into the bloodstream. Too much absorption can lead to unwanted side effects elsewhere in the body. To keep this problem to a minimum, avoid using large amounts of Topicort over large areas, do not use it for extended periods of time, and do not cover it with airtight dressings such as plastic wrap or adhesive bandages unless specifically told to by your doctor.

Children may absorb more medication than adults do.

## How should you use this medication?

Topicort is for use only on the skin. Be careful to keep it out of your eyes.

Apply a thin coating of Topicort to the affected area. Rub in gently.

The treated area should not be covered unless your doctor has told you to do so.

If Topicort is being used for an infant or toddler with a genital rash, make sure the diapers or plastic pants are not too tight, so that air can circulate.

■ *If you miss a dose...*
Use Topicort only as needed, in the smallest amount required for relief.

■ *Storage instructions...*
Store Topicort at room temperature.

## What side effects may occur?

Side effects cannot be anticipated. If any develop or change in intensity, inform your doctor as soon as possible. Only your doctor can determine if it is safe for you to continue using Topicort. The side effects listed below occur infrequently, but may occur more often if the treated area is covered with a bandage.

■ *Side effects may include:*
Acne-like pimples, blackheads, blistering, burning of the skin, dryness, excessive growth of hair, infection, inflammation of the hair follicles, irritation, itching, loss of skin pigmentation, prickly heat, skin inflammation around the mouth, rash, redness, stretch marks on the skin, thinning of the skin

## Why should this drug not be prescribed?

Do not use Topicort if you are sensitive to it or have ever had an allergic reaction to any of its ingredients.

## Special warnings about this medication

Remember to avoid getting Topicort in your eyes. Do not use Topicort to treat any condition other than the one for which it was prescribed.

Long-term use of steroids such as Topicort may interfere with the growth and development of children. They may also develop headaches, or bulging at the top of the head.

Avoid covering a treated area with tight waterproof diapers or plastic pants. They can increase unwanted absorption of Topicort.

If your skin becomes irritated or infected, stop using Topicort and call your doctor.

## Possible food and drug interactions when using this medication

No interactions have been reported.

## Special information if you are pregnant or breastfeeding

Topicort should not be used over large areas, in large amounts, or for long periods of time during pregnancy unless the benefit outweighs any potential risk to the unborn child. If you are pregnant or plan to become pregnant, inform your doctor immediately.

It is not known whether topical steroids are absorbed in sufficient amounts to appear in breast milk. If your doctor considers Topicort essential to your health, he or she may advise you to stop breastfeeding until your treatment with the medication is finished.

## Recommended dosage

ADULTS

Apply a thin film of Topicort cream, gel, or ointment to the affected area 2 times a day. Rub in gently.

CHILDREN

Use the least amount of Topicort necessary to relieve symptoms. Ask your doctor for specific instructions.

## Overdosage

Large doses of steroids such as Topicort applied over a large area or for a long time, especially when the treated area is covered, can cause increases in blood sugar and Cushing's syndrome, a condition characterized by a moon-shaped face, emotional disturbances, high blood pressure, weight gain, and, in women, baldness or growth of body and facial hair. Cushing's syndrome may also trigger the development of diabetes. If left uncorrected, Cushing's syndrome may become serious. If you suspect your use of Topicort has led to this problem, seek medical attention immediately.

*Brand name:*

# Toradol

*Pronounced: TOH-rah-dol*
*Generic name: Ketorolac tromethamine*

### Why is this drug prescribed?

Toradol, a nonsteroidal anti-inflammatory drug, is used to relieve moderately severe, acute pain. It is prescribed for a limited amount of time (no more than 5 days), not for long-term therapy.

### Most important fact about this drug

Toradol can cause serious side effects, including ulcers and internal bleeding. Never take it for more than 5 days.

### How should you take this medication?

Toradol works fastest when taken on an empty stomach, but an antacid can be taken if it causes upset. Take this medication exactly as prescribed.

Take Toradol with a full glass of water. Also, do not lie down for about 20 minutes after taking it. This will help to prevent irritation of your upper digestive tract.

■ *If you miss a dose...*
If you take Toradol on a regular schedule, take it as soon as you remember. If it is almost time for your next dose, skip the one you missed and go back to your regular schedule. Never take 2 doses at the same time.

■ *Storage instructions...*
Store at room temperature, away from excessive humidity and light.

### What side effects may occur?

Side effects cannot be anticipated. If any develop or change in intensity, inform your doctor as soon as possible. Only your doctor can determine if it is safe for you to continue using Toradol.

■ *More common side effects may include:*
Diarrhea, dizziness, drowsiness, headache, indigestion, nausea, stomach and intestinal pain, swelling due to fluid retention

■ *Less common side effects may include:*
Abdominal fullness, constipation, gas, high blood pressure, inflammation of the mouth, itching, rash, red or purple spots on the skin, sweating, vomiting

■ *Rare side effects may include:*
Abnormal dreams, allergic reactions, anemia, asthma, belching, black stools, blood in the urine, convulsions, difficult or labored breathing, exaggerated feeling of well-being, fainting, fever, fluid in the lungs, flushing, gastritis (inflammation of the lining of the stomach), hallucinations, hearing problems, hives, increased appetite, kidney failure, kidney inflammation, loss of appetite, low blood pressure, nosebleeds, pallor, peptic ulcer, rapid heartbeat, skin inflammation and flaking, skin peeling, stomach and intestinal bleeding, swelling of the throat or tongue, thirst and dry mouth, tremors, urinary problems, vertigo, vision problems, weight gain, yellow skin and eyes

### Why should this drug not be prescribed?

Do not take Toradol if it has ever given you an allergic reaction. Also avoid this medication if you have ever had an allergic reaction—such as nasal polyps (tumors), swelling of the face, limbs, and throat, hives, wheezing, light-headedness—to aspirin or other nonsteroidal anti-inflammatory drugs (NSAIDs) such as Motrin.

Do not take Toradol if you have ever had a peptic ulcer or stomach or intestinal bleeding. Avoid it if you have severe kidney disease or bleeding problems.

Never combine this drug with aspirin, NSAIDs, or probenecid. Make sure your doctor is aware of any drug reactions you have experienced.

### Special warnings about this medication

Remember that Toradol has been known to cause peptic ulcers and bleeding. Contact your doctor immediately if you suspect a problem.

This drug should be used with caution if you have kidney or liver disease. It may cause liver inflammation or kidney problems in some people.

Toradol is not recommended for long-term use, since side effects increase over time. This medication should be taken for no more than 5 days.

If you are an older adult, use this drug cautiously.

Toradol can increase water retention. If you have heart disease or high blood pressure, use this drug with care.

This medication can prolong bleeding time. If you are taking blood-thinning medication, take Toradol with caution.

## Possible food and drug interactions when using this medication

If Toradol is taken with certain other drugs, the effects of either could be increased, decreased, or altered. It is especially important to check with your doctor before combining Toradol with the following:

ACE inhibitor drugs such as Vasotec and Capoten
Antidepressants such as Prozac
Antiepileptic drugs (Dilantin, Tegretol)
Aspirin and other nonsteroidal anti-inflammatory
    drugs such as Motrin
Blood thinners such as Coumadin
Diuretics such as Lasix and Dyazide
Lithium (Lithonate)
Major tranquilizers such as Navane
Methotrexate (Rheumatrex)
Probenecid (Benemid)
Tranquilizers such as Xanax

## Special information if you are pregnant or breastfeeding

The effects of Toradol during pregnancy have not been adequately studied. If you are pregnant or plan to become pregnant, inform your doctor immediately. Toradol appears in breast milk and could affect a nursing infant. This medication should not be used while you are breastfeeding.

## Recommended dosage

### ADULTS

Your doctor will give you Toradol intravenously or intramuscularly to start, then have you switch to the tablets. You will take 2 tablets for the first dose (20 milligrams) and then 1 tablet (10 milligrams) every 4 to 6 hours. You should not take more than 40 milligrams per day and should not take Toradol for more than 5 days in all.

### CHILDREN

The safety and effectiveness of Toradol in children under age 16 have not been established.

### OLDER ADULTS

Doses are usually lower for people over 65, those with kidney problems, and those who weigh less than 110 pounds. Your doctor will tailor the best dosage for you.

## Overdosage

Although no specific information is available, any medication taken in excess can have serious consequences. If you suspect an overdose, seek medical attention immediately.

■ *Symptoms of Toradol overdose may include:*
    Abdominal pain, peptic ulcer

*Brand name:*

# Totacillin

*See Omnipen, page 381.*

*Brand name:*

# T-Phyl

*See Theo-Dur, page 538.*

*Generic name:*

# Tramadol

*See Ultram, page 574.*

*Brand name:*

# Trandate

*See Normodyne, page 368.*

*Brand name:*

# Transderm-Nitro

*See Nitroglycerin, page 361.*

*Brand name:*

# Tranxene

*Pronounced: TRAN-zeen*
*Generic name: Clorazepate dipotassium*
*Other brand names: Tranxene-SD, Tranxene-SD*
*Half Strength*

## Why is this drug prescribed?

Tranxene belongs to a class of drugs known as benzodiazepines. It is used in the treatment of anxiety disorders and for short-term relief of the symptoms of anxiety.

It is also used to relieve the symptoms of acute alcohol withdrawal and to help in treating certain convulsive disorders such as epilepsy.

## Most important fact about this drug

Tranxene can be habit-forming if taken regularly over a long period. You may experience withdrawal symptoms if you stop using this drug abruptly. Consult your doctor before discontinuing Tranxene or making any change in your dose.

## How should you take this medication?

Tranxene should be taken exactly as prescribed by your doctor.

■ *If you miss a dose...*
Take it as soon as you remember if it is within an hour or so of your scheduled time. If you do not remember until later, skip the dose you missed and go back to your regular schedule. Do not take 2 doses at once.
■ *Storage instructions...*
Store at room temperature. Protect from excessive heat.

## What side effects may occur?

Side effects cannot be anticipated. If any develop or change in intensity, inform your doctor as soon as possible. Only your doctor can determine if it is safe for you to continue taking Tranxene.

■ *More common side effects may include:*
Drowsiness
■ *Less common or rare side effects may include:*
Blurred vision, depression, difficulty in sleeping or falling asleep, dizziness, dry mouth, double vision, fatigue, genital and urinary tract disorders, headache, irritability, lack of muscle coordination, mental confusion, nervousness, tremors, skin rashes, slurred speech, stomach and intestinal disorders, tremor

■ *Side effects due to rapid decrease or abrupt withdrawal from Tranxene may include:*
Abdominal cramps, convulsions, diarrhea, difficulty in sleeping or falling asleep, hallucinations, impaired memory, irritability, muscle aches, nervousness, tremors, vomiting

## Why should this drug not be prescribed?

If you are sensitive to or have ever had an allergic reaction to Tranxene, you should not take this medication. Make sure your doctor is aware of any drug reactions you have experienced.

Do not take this medication if you have the eye condition known as acute narrow-angle glaucoma.

Anxiety or tension related to everyday stress usually does not require treatment with such a strong drug. Discuss your symptoms thoroughly with your doctor.

Tranxene is not recommended for use in more serious conditions such as depression or severe psychological disorders.

## Special warnings about this medication

Tranxene may cause you to become drowsy or less alert; therefore, you should not drive or operate dangerous machinery or participate in any hazardous activity that requires full mental alertness until you know how this drug affects you.

If you are being treated for anxiety associated with depression, your doctor will have you take a low dose of this medication. Do not increase your dose without consulting your doctor.

The elderly and people in a weakened condition are more apt to become unsteady or oversedated when taking Tranxene.

## Possible food and drug interactions when taking this medication

Tranxene slows down the central nervous system and may intensify the effects of alcohol. Do not drink alcohol while taking this medication.

If Tranxene is taken with certain other drugs, the effects of either could be increased, decreased, or altered. It is especially important to check with your doctor before combining Tranxene with the following:

Antidepressant drugs known as MAO inhibitors (Nardil, Parnate) and other antidepressants such as Elavil and Prozac
Barbiturates such as Nembutal and Seconal
Narcotic pain relievers such as Demerol and Percodan
Major tranquilizers such as Mellaril and Thorazine

## Special information
## if you are pregnant or breastfeeding

The effects of Tranxene during pregnancy have not been adequately studied. However, because there is an increased risk of birth defects associated with this class of drug, its use during pregnancy should be avoided. Tranxene may appear in breast milk and could affect a nursing infant. If this medication is essential to your health, your doctor may advise you to discontinue breastfeeding until your treatment with this medication is finished.

## Recommended dosage

ANXIETY

*Adults*

The usual daily dosage is 30 milligrams divided into several smaller doses. A normal daily dose can be as little as 15 milligrams. Your doctor may increase the dosage gradually to as much as 60 milligrams, according to your individual needs.

Tranxene can also be taken in a single bedtime dose. The initial dose is 15 milligrams, but your doctor will adjust the dosage to suit your individual needs.

Tranxene-SD, a 22.5-milligram tablet, and Tranxene-SD Half Strength, an 11.25-milligram tablet, can be taken once every 24 hours. Your doctor may switch you to this form of the drug after you have been taking Tranxene for several weeks.

*Older Adults*

The usual starting dose is 7.5 to 15 milligrams per day.

ACUTE ALCOHOL WITHDRAWAL

Tranxene can be used in a multi-day program for relief of the symptoms of acute alcohol withdrawal.

Dosages are usually increased in the first 2 days from 30 to 90 milligrams and then reduced over the next 2 days to lower levels. After that, your doctor will gradually lower the dose still further, and will take you off the drug when you are ready.

WHEN USED WITH ANTIEPILEPTIC DRUGS

Tranxene can be used in conjunction with antiepileptic drugs. Follow the recommended dosages carefully to avoid drowsiness.

*Adults and Children over 12 Years Old*

The starting dose is 7.5 milligrams 3 times a day. Your doctor may increase the dosage by 7.5 milligrams per week to a maximum of 90 milligrams a day.

*Children 9 to 12 Years Old*

The starting dose is 7.5 milligrams twice a day. Your doctor may increase the dosage by 7.5 milligrams a week to a maximum of 60 milligrams a day.

Safety and effectiveness in children under 9 years of age have not been established.

## Overdosage

Any medication taken in excess can have serious consequences. If you suspect an overdose, seek medical treatment immediately.

■ *Symptoms of Tranxene overdose may include:*
Coma, low blood pressure, sedation

*Generic name:*

# Trazodone

*See Desyrel, page 150.*

*Brand name:*

# Trental

*Pronounced: TREN-tall*
*Generic name: Pentoxifylline*

## Why is this drug prescribed?

Trental is a medication that reduces the viscosity or "stickiness" of your blood, allowing it to flow more freely. It helps relieve the painful leg cramps caused by "intermittent claudication," a condition resulting from poor blood supply to the leg muscles caused by hardening of the arteries.

Some doctors also prescribe Trental for dementia, strokes, circulatory and nerve problems caused by diabetes, and Raynaud's syndrome (a disorder of the blood vessels in which exposure to cold causes the fingers and toes to turn white). The drug is also used to treat impotence and to increase sperm motility in infertile men.

## Most important fact about this drug

Trental can ease the pain in your legs and make walking easier but should not replace other treatments such as physical therapy or surgery.

## How should you take this medication?

Trental comes in controlled-release tablets. Do not break, crush, or chew the tablets; swallow them whole. Take Trental exactly as prescribed.

■ *If you miss a dose...*
Take it as soon as you remember. If it is almost time for your next dose, skip the one you missed and go back to your regular schedule. Never take 2 doses at the same time.

■ *Storage instructions...*
Keep this medication in the container it came in, tightly closed and away from light. Store it at room temperature.

## What side effects may occur?

Side effects cannot be anticipated. If any develop or change in intensity, inform your doctor as soon as possible. Only your doctor can determine if it is safe for you to continue taking Trental.

Trental's side effects are fairly uncommon.

■ *Side effects may include:*
Allergic reaction (symptoms include: swelling of face, lips, tongue, throat, arms, or legs, sore throat, fever and chills, difficulty swallowing, chest pain), anxiety, bad taste in the mouth, blind spot in vision, blurred vision, brittle fingernails, chest pain (sometimes crushing), confusion, conjunctivitis (pinkeye), constipation, depression, difficult or labored breathing, dizziness, dry mouth/thirst, earache, excessive salivation, flu-like symptoms, fluid retention, general body discomfort, headache, hives, indigestion, inflammation of the gallbladder, itching, laryngitis, loss of appetite, low blood pressure, nosebleeds, rash, seizures, sore throat/swollen neck glands, stuffy nose, tremor, vomiting, weight change

## Why should this drug not be prescribed?

Do not take Trental if you have recently had a stroke or bleeding in the retina of your eye.

If you are sensitive to or have ever had an allergic reaction to Trental, caffeine, theophylline (medication for asthma or other breathing disorders), or theobromine, do not take this medication. Make sure that your doctor is aware of any drug reactions that you have experienced.

## Special warnings about this medication

If you are taking a blood thinner, or have recently had surgery, peptic ulcers, or other disorders that involve bleeding, the doctor should test your blood periodically.

Most people tolerate Trental well, but there have been occasional cases of crushing chest pain, low blood pressure, and irregular heartbeat in people with heart disease and brain disorders.

## Possible food and drug interactions when taking this medication

If Trental is taken with certain other drugs, the effects of either could be increased, decreased, or altered. It is especially important to check with your doctor before combining Trental with the following:

Blood pressure medications such as Vasotec and Cardizem SR
Blood-thinning drugs such as Coumadin
Clot inhibitors such as Persantine
Theophylline (Theo-Dur)
Ulcer medicines such as Tagamet

## Special information if you are pregnant or breastfeeding

The effects of Trental during pregnancy have not been adequately studied. If you are pregnant or plan to become pregnant, inform your doctor immediately. Trental appears in breast milk and could affect a nursing infant. If this medication is essential to your health, your doctor may advise you to discontinue breastfeeding until your treatment with this medication is finished.

## Recommended dosage

ADULTS

The usual dosage of Trental in controlled-release tablets is one 400-milligram tablet 3 times a day with meals.

While the effect of Trental may be seen within 2 to 4 weeks, it is recommended that treatment be continued for at least 8 weeks.

Any stomach or central nervous system (affecting the brain and spinal cord) side effects are related to the dose. If any of these side effects occur, the dosage should be lowered to 1 tablet, 2 times a day, for a total of 800 milligrams a day. If side effects persist at this lower dosage, your doctor may consider stopping this drug.

CHILDREN

The safety and effectiveness of this drug in children have not been established.

## Overdosage

Any medication taken in excess can have serious consequences. If you suspect symptoms of a Trental overdose, seek medical attention immediately. Symptoms appear within 4 to 5 hours and may last for 12 hours.

■ *Symptoms of Trental overdose may include:*
Agitation, convulsions, fever, flushing, loss of consciousness, low blood pressure, sleepiness

*Generic name:*

# Tretinoin

*See Retin-A and Renova, page 462.*

*Generic name:*

# Triamcinolone

*See Azmacort, page 46.*

*Generic name:*

# Triamterene with Hydrochlorothiazide

*See Maxzide, page 309.*

*Brand name:*

# Triavil

*Pronounced: TRY-uh-vill*
*Generic ingredients: Amitriptyline hydrochloride, Perphenazine*

## Why is this drug prescribed?

Triavil is used to treat anxiety, agitation, and depression. Triavil is a combination of a tricyclic antidepressant (amitriptyline) and a tranquilizer (perphenazine).

Triavil can also help people with schizophrenia (distorted sense of reality) who are depressed and people with insomnia, fatigue, loss of interest, loss of appetite, or a slowing of physical and mental reactions.

## Most important fact about this drug

Triavil may cause tardive dyskinesia—a condition marked by involuntary muscle spasms and twitches in the face and body. This condition may be permanent and appears to be most common among the elderly, especially women. Ask your doctor for information about this possible risk.

## How should you take this medication?

Triavil may be taken with or without food. You should not take it with alcohol.

■ *If you miss a dose...*
Take it as soon as you remember. If it is within 2 hours of your next dose, skip the one you missed and go back to your regular schedule. Do not take 2 doses at once.

■ *Storage instructions...*
Store at room temperature in a tightly closed container. Protect Triavil 2-10 tablets from light.

## What side effects may occur?

Side effects cannot be anticipated. If any develop or change in intensity, inform your doctor as soon as possible. Only your doctor can determine if it is safe for you to continue taking Triavil.

■ *Side effects may include:*
Abnormal secretion of milk, abnormalities of movements and posture, anxiety, asthma, black tongue, blood disorders, blurred vision, body rigidly arched backward, breast development in males, change in pulse rate, chewing movements, coma, confusion, constipation, convulsions, delusions, diarrhea, difficulty breathing, difficulty concentrating, difficulty swallowing, dilated pupils, disorientation, dizziness, drowsiness, dry mouth, eating abnormal amounts of food, ejaculation failure, episodes of elation or irritability, excessive or spontaneous flow of milk, excitement, exhaustion, eye problems, eye spasms, eyes in a fixed position, fatigue, fever, fluid accumulation and swelling (including throat and brain, face and tongue, arms and legs), frequent urination, hair loss, hallucinations, headache, heart attacks, hepatitis, high blood pressure, high fever, high or low blood sugar, hives, impotence, inability to stop moving, inability to urinate, increased or decreased sex drive, inflammation of the mouth, insomnia, intestinal blockage, intolerance to light, involuntary jerky movements of tongue, face, mouth, lips, jaw, body, or arms and legs, irregular blood pressure, pulse, and heartbeat, irregular menstrual periods, lack of coordination, light-headedness upon standing up, liver problems, lockjaw, loss or increase of appetite, low blood pressure, muscle stiffness, nasal congestion, nausea, nightmares, odd taste in the mouth, overactive reflexes, pain and stiffness around neck, palpitations, protruding tongue, puckering of the mouth, puffing of the cheeks, purple-reddish-brown spots on skin, rapid heartbeat, restlessness, rigid arms, feet,

head, and muscles, ringing in the ears, salivation, sedation, seizures, sensitivity to light, severe allergic reactions, skin rash or inflammation, scaling, spasms in the hands and feet, speech problems, stomach upset, stroke, sweating, swelling of breasts, swelling of testicles, swollen glands, tingling, pins and needles, and numbness in hands and feet, tremors, twisted neck, twitching in the body, neck, shoulders, and face, uncontrollable and involuntary urination, urinary problems, visual problems, vomiting, weakness, weight gain or loss, writhing motions, yellowed skin and whites of eyes

## Why should this drug not be prescribed?

You should not be using Triavil if you are taking drugs that slow down the central nervous system, including alcohol, barbiturates, analgesics, antihistamines, or narcotics.

Triavil should not be used if you are recovering from a recent heart attack, or if you have an abnormal bone marrow condition. Avoid Triavil if you have ever had an allergic reaction to phenothiazines or amitriptyline.

People who are taking antidepressant drugs known as MAO inhibitors (including Nardil and Parnate) should not take Triavil.

## Special warnings about this medication

Before using Triavil, tell your doctor if you have ever had: the eye condition known as glaucoma; difficulty urinating; breast cancer; seizures; heart, liver, or thyroid disease; or if you are exposed to extreme heat or pesticides. Be aware that Triavil may mask signs of brain tumor, intestinal blockage, and overdose of other drugs.

Nausea, headache, and a general ill feeling can result if you suddenly stop taking Triavil. Follow your doctor's instructions closely when discontinuing Triavil. If your dose is gradually reduced, you may experience irritability, restlessness, and dream and sleep disturbances, but these effects will not last.

This drug may impair your ability to drive a car or operate potentially dangerous machinery. Do not participate in any activities that require full alertness if you are unsure about your ability.

If you develop a fever that has no other cause, stop taking Triavil and call your doctor.

## Possible food and drug interactions when taking this medication

If Triavil is taken with certain other drugs, the effects of either could be increased, decreased, or altered. It is especially important to check with your doctor before combining Triavil with the following:

Airway-opening drugs such as Proventil
Antiseizure drugs such as Dilantin
Antidepressant drugs classified as MAO inhibitors, including Nardil and Parnate
Antihistamines such as Benadryl
Antispasmodic drugs such as Bentyl
Atropine (Donnatal)
Barbiturates such as phenobarbital
Blood-thinning drugs such as Coumadin
Cimetidine (Tagamet)
Disulfiram (Antabuse)
Epinephrine (EpiPen)
Ethchlorvynol (Placidyl)
Fluoxetine (Prozac)
Furazolidone (Furoxone)
Guanethidine (Ismelin)
Major tranquilizers such as Haldol
Narcotic analgesics such as Percocet
Thyroid medications such as Synthroid

Extreme drowsiness and other potentially serious effects can result if Triavil is combined with alcohol or other central nervous system depressants such as narcotics, painkillers, and sleep medications.

## Special information if you are pregnant or breastfeeding

Triavil may cause false-positive results on pregnancy tests. Triavil should not be used by pregnant women or mothers who are breastfeeding.

## Recommended dosage

Your doctor will individualize your dose.

You should not take more than 4 tablets of Triavil 4-50 or 8 tablets of any other strength in one day. It may be a few days to a few weeks before you notice any improvement.

ADULTS

*For Non-Psychotic Anxiety and Depression*
The usual dose is 1 tablet of Triavil 2-25 or 4-25 taken 3 or 4 times a day, or 1 tablet of Triavil 4-50 taken twice a day.

*For Anxiety in People with Schizophrenia*
The usual dose is 2 tablets of Triavil 4-25 taken 3 times a day. Your doctor may tell you to take another tablet of Triavil 4-25 at bedtime, if needed.

If you need to keep taking Triavil, your doctor will probably have you take 1 tablet of Triavil 2-25 or 4-25 from 2 to 4 times a day or 1 tablet of Triavil 4-50 twice a day.

CHILDREN

Children should not use Triavil.

OLDER ADULTS AND ADOLESCENTS

*For Anxiety*
The usual dose is 1 tablet of Triavil 4-10, taken 3 or 4 times a day. People in these age groups usually take Triavil at lower doses.

### Overdosage
Any medication taken in excess can have serious consequences. An overdose of Triavil can be fatal. If you suspect an overdose, seek medical help immediately.

■ *Symptoms of Triavil overdose may include:*
Abnormalities of posture and movements, agitation, coma, convulsions, dilated pupils, drowsiness, extreme low body temperature, eye movement problems, high fever, heart failure, overactive reflexes, rapid or irregular heartbeat, rigid muscles, stupor, very low blood pressure, vomiting

*Brand name:*

# Triaz

See Desquam-E, page 150.

*Generic name:*

# Triazolam

See Halcion, page 234.

*Brand name:*

# Tridesilon

Pronounced: tri-DESS-ill-on
Generic name: Desonide
Other brand name: DesOwen

### Why is this drug prescribed?
Tridesilon is a steroid preparation that relieves the itching and inflammation of a variety of skin problems. It is applied directly to the skin.

### Most important fact about this drug
When you use Tridesilon, you inevitably absorb some of the medication through your skin and into the bloodstream. Too much absorption can lead to unwanted side effects elsewhere in the body. To keep this problem to a minimum, avoid using large amounts of Tridesilon over large areas, and do not cover it with airtight dressings such as plastic wrap or adhesive bandages unless specifically told to by your doctor.

### How should you use this medication?
Use Tridesilon exactly as directed by your doctor. Shake lotion well before using.

Tridesilon is for use only on the skin. Be careful to keep it out of your eyes.

Remember to avoid wrapping the treated area with bandages or other coverings unless your doctor has told you to do so.

■ *If you miss a dose...*
Apply it as soon as you remember. If it is almost time for the next dose, skip the one you missed and go back to your regular schedule.
■ *Storage instructions...*
Store at room temperature.

### What side effects may occur?
Side effects cannot be anticipated. If any develop or change in intensity, notify your doctor as soon as possible. Only your doctor can determine if it is safe for you to continue using Tridesilon. Many of the side effects listed below are rare, but may occur more often if the affected area is covered with a bandage or treated for a long time.

■ *Side effects may include:*
Acne, additional infections, allergic reactions of the skin, burning and stinging, dryness, excessive hair growth, irritation, itching, loss of skin color, prickly heat, rash, scaly skin, skin inflammation around the mouth, skin loss, skin peeling or redness, skin softening, stretch marks, worsening of the condition
■ *Side effects that may occur in children include:*
Delayed weight gain, headaches, slowed growth

### Why should this drug not be prescribed?
You should not take this medication if you are sensitive or allergic to any of its ingredients.

Because steroid medications may interfere with their growth and development, children should be given the lowest strength that provides effective therapy. Safety and effectiveness of DesOwen in children have not been established.

### Special warnings about this medication

If an irritation develops, or if your skin condition does not heal within 2 weeks, inform your doctor.

Avoid covering a treated area with waterproof diapers or plastic pants. They can increase unwanted absorption of Tridesilon.

Large doses of steroids applied over a large area, and long-term use of these preparations, especially when the treated areas are covered, can cause increases in blood sugar or sugar in the urine, Cushing's syndrome (a condition characterized by a moon-shaped face, emotional disturbances, high blood pressure, weight gain, and, in women, growth of body hair), and effects on the adrenal gland, pituitary, and hypothalamus.

### Possible food and drug interactions when using this medication

No interactions have been reported.

### Special information
### if you are pregnant or breastfeeding

Although Tridesilon is applied to the skin, there is no way of knowing how much medication is absorbed into the bloodstream. The more powerful steroids have caused birth defects in animals. In general, these preparations should not be used extensively, in large amounts, or for prolonged periods of time by pregnant women. They should be used only if the potential benefits outweigh the potential risks to the unborn baby. If you are pregnant or plan to become pregnant, inform your doctor immediately. It is not known whether steroid creams and ointments are absorbed in sufficient amounts to appear in breast milk. If your doctor considers Tridesilon essential to your health, he or she may advise you to stop breastfeeding until your treatment with the medication is finished.

### Recommended dosage

ADULTS AND CHILDREN

Tridesilon should be applied to the affected area as a thin film, from 2 to 4 times a day, depending on the severity of the condition. Apply DesOwen 2 or 3 times daily.

A bandage or other covering may be prescribed by your doctor to apply over the affected area for psoriasis or conditions that are not responding as well as expected.

### Overdosage

Any medication taken in excess can have serious consequences. With overuse or misuse of Trides-

ilon, too much medicine can enter the body, causing increases in blood sugar and Cushing's syndrome, with symptoms such as a moon-shaped face, emotional disturbances, high blood pressure, weight gain, and, in women, growth of body and facial hair.

*Generic name:*

# Trifluoperazine

*See Stelazine, page 509.*

*Generic name:*

# Trihexyphenidyl

*See Artane, page 35.*

*Brand name:*

# Trilisate

*Pronounced: TRILL-ih-sate*
*Generic name: Choline magnesium trisalicylate*

### Why is this drug prescribed?

Trilisate, a nonsteroidal, anti-inflammatory medication, is prescribed for the relief of the signs and symptoms of rheumatoid arthritis (chronic joint inflammation disease), osteoarthritis (degenerative joint disease), and other forms of arthritis. This drug is used in the long-term management of these diseases and especially for flare-ups of severe rheumatoid arthritis.

Trilisate may also be prescribed for the treatment of acute painful shoulder, for mild to moderate pain in general, and for fever.

In children, this medication is prescribed for severe conditions—such as juvenile rheumatoid arthritis—that require relief of pain and inflammation.

### Most important fact about this drug

Because there is a possible association between the development of the rare but serious neurological disorder known as Reye's syndrome and the use of medicines containing salicylates or aspirin, Trilisate should not be used by children or teenagers who have chickenpox or flu symptoms unless otherwise advised by their doctor.

### How should you take this medication?

Trilisate is available in tablet or liquid form. Take Trilisate exactly as prescribed by your doctor.

■ *If you miss a dose...*
If you take Trilisate on a regular schedule, take the forgotten dose as soon as you remember. If it is almost time for your next dose, skip the one you missed and go back to your regular schedule. Do not take 2 doses at once.

■ *Storage instructions...*
Store at room temperature.

## What side effects may occur?

Side effects cannot be anticipated. If any develop or change in intensity, inform your doctor as soon as possible. Only your doctor can determine if it is safe for you to continue taking Trilisate.

■ *More common side effects may include:*
Constipation, diarrhea, heartburn, indigestion, nausea, ringing in the ears, stomach pain and upset, vomiting

■ *Less common side effects may include:*
Dizziness, drowsiness, headache, hearing impairment, light-headedness, sluggishness

■ *Rare side effects may include:*
Asthma, blood in the stool, bruising, confusion, distorted sense of taste, hallucinations, hearing loss, hepatitis, hives, inflammation of the upper gastric tract, itching, loss of appetite, nosebleed, rash, skin eruptions or discoloration, stomach or intestinal ulcers, swelling due to fluid accumulation, weight gain

## Why should this drug not be prescribed?

If you are sensitive to or have ever had an allergic reaction to Trilisate or drugs of this type, such as aspirin, you should not take this medication. Make sure your doctor is aware of any drug reactions you have experienced.

## Special warnings about this medication

Use Trilisate with caution if you have severe or recurring kidney or liver disorder, gastritis (inflammation of the stomach lining), or a stomach or intestinal ulcer. Consult your doctor regarding any medical problems you may have.

If you are an asthmatic allergic to aspirin, tell your doctor before taking Trilisate.

It may be 2 to 3 weeks before you feel the effect of this medication.

## Possible food and drug interactions when taking this medication

If Trilisate is taken with certain other drugs, the effects of either could be increased, decreased, or altered. It is especially important to check with your doctor before combining Trilisate with the following:

Antacids such as Gaviscon and Maalox
Antigout medications
Blood-thinners such as Coumadin
Carbonic anhydrase inhibitors such as acetazolamide (Diamox) used to treat heart failure, the eye condition called glaucoma, and certain convulsive disorders
Diabetes medications such as insulin, Micronase, and Tolinase
Methotrexate, an anticancer drug
Other salicylates used to reduce fever, inflammation, and pain such as aspirin
Phenytoin (the anticonvulsant Dilantin)
Steroids such as prednisone
Valproic acid (the anticonvulsant Depakene)

## Special information if you are pregnant or breastfeeding

The effects of Trilisate during pregnancy have not been adequately studied. If you are pregnant or plan to become pregnant, inform your doctor immediately. This drug does appear in breast milk and could affect a nursing infant. If this medication is essential to your health, your doctor may advise you not to breastfeed until your treatment is finished.

## Recommended dosage

ADULTS

In rheumatoid arthritis, osteoarthritis, more severe arthritis, and acute painful shoulder, the recommended starting dose is 1,500 milligrams taken 2 times a day or 3,000 milligrams taken once a day. Your doctor will adjust the dosage based on your response to this medication.

If you have a kidney disorder, your doctor will monitor you and adjust your dose accordingly.

For mild to moderate pain or to reduce a high fever, the usual dosage is 2,000 to 3,000 milligrams per day divided into 2 equal doses as recommended by your doctor.

CHILDREN

For reduction of inflammation or pain, the recommended dose for children is determined by weight. The usual dose for children who weigh 81 pounds or less is 50 milligrams per 2.2 pounds of body weight, taken twice a day. For heavier children, the usual dose is 2,250 milligrams per day, divided into 2 doses.

Trilisate liquid can be taken by younger children and by adults who are unable to swallow a tablet.

OLDER ADULTS

The usual dosage is 2,250 milligrams divided into 3 doses of 750 milligrams each.

### Overdosage

Any medication taken in excess can have serious consequences. If you suspect an overdose, seek medical treatment immediately. An overdose of Trilisate can be fatal.

■ *Symptoms of Trilisate overdose may include:*
Confusion, diarrhea, dizziness, drowsiness, headache, hearing impairment, rapid breathing, ringing in the ears, sweating, vomiting

*Generic name:*

# Trimethobenzamide

*See Tigan, page 543.*

*Generic name:*

# Trimethoprim with Sulfamethoxazole

*See Bactrim, page 50.*

*Generic name:*

# Trimipramine

*See Surmontil, page 514.*

*Brand name:*

# Trimox

*See Amoxil, page 22.*

*Brand name:*

# Trinalin Repetabs

*Pronounced: TRIN-uh-lin*
*Generic ingredients: Azatadine maleate,*
    *Pseudoephedrine sulfate*

### Why is this drug prescribed?

Trinalin Repetabs is a long-acting antihistamine/decongestant that relieves nasal stuffiness and middle ear congestion caused by hay fever and ongoing nasal inflammation. It can be used alone or with antibiotics and analgesics such as aspirin or acetaminophen. Azatadine, the antihistamine in the combination, reduces itching and swelling and dries up secretions from the nose, eyes, and throat. Pseudoephedrine, the decongestant, reduces nasal congestion and makes breathing easier.

### Most important fact about this drug

Trinalin Repetabs may cause drowsiness. You should not drive or operate dangerous machinery or participate in any hazardous activity that requires full mental alertness until you know how you react to this medication.

### How should you take this medication?

Take this medication as indicated; do not take more than your doctor has prescribed.

■ *If you miss a dose...*
If you take Trinalin on a regular schedule, take the forgotten dose as soon as you remember. If it is almost time for your next dose, skip the one you missed and go back to your regular schedule. Do not take 2 doses at once.
■ *Storage instructions...*
Store at room temperature in a cool place.

### What side effects may occur?

Side effects cannot be anticipated. If any develop or change in intensity, inform your doctor as soon as possible. Only your doctor can determine if it is safe for you to continue taking Trinalin.

■ *Side effects may include:*
Abdominal cramps, acute inflammation of the inner ear, anemia, anxiety, blood disorders, blurred vision, chest pain, chills, confusion, constipation, convulsions, diarrhea, difficulty breathing, dilated pupils, disturbed coordination, dizziness, dry mouth, nose, and throat, early menstruation, exaggerated feeling of well-being,

excessive perspiration, excitement, extreme calm (sedation), fatigue, fear, fluttery heartbeat, frequent urination, hallucinations, headache, high blood pressure, hives, hysteria, increased chest congestion, increased sensitivity to light, insomnia, irregular heartbeat, irritability, loss of appetite, low blood pressure, nausea, nervousness, painful or difficult urination, pale skin, rapid heartbeat, rash, restlessness, ringing in the ears, severe allergic reaction, sleepiness, stuffy nose, tension, tightness in chest, tingling or pins and needles, tremor, upset stomach, urinary retention, vertigo, vomiting, weakness, wheezing

## Why should this drug not be prescribed?

Trinalin should be avoided if you have narrow-angle glaucoma or difficulty urinating, if you are taking antidepressant drugs known as MAO inhibitors or have stopped taking them within the past 10 days, if you have severe high blood pressure, severe heart disease, or an overactive thyroid, or if you are sensitive to or have ever had an allergic reaction to any of its ingredients.

This drug should not be used to treat asthma and other lower respiratory tract diseases.

## Special warnings about this medication

Trinalin should be used with care if you have a peptic ulcer or other upper intestinal obstruction, bladder obstruction due to an enlarged prostate or other bladder problems, a history of bronchial asthma, heart disease, high blood pressure, increased eye pressure, or diabetes.

Pseudoephedrine can be habit-forming at high doses. Remember that this medication can make you feel drowsy. Be careful driving, operating machinery, or using appliances.

Trinalin may cause dizziness, extreme calm (sedation), and low blood pressure in people aged 60 and over. It is also more likely to cause such side effects as confusion, convulsions, hallucinations, and death in this age group.

## Possible food and drug interactions when taking this medication

Alcohol may increase the effects of Trinalin. Do not drink alcohol while taking this medication.

If Trinalin is taken with certain other drugs, the effects of either could be increased, decreased, or altered. It is especially important to check with your doctor before combining Trinalin with the following:

Antacids such as Maalox
Barbiturates such as phenobarbital
Beta-blocking blood pressure drugs such as Tenormin and Inderal
Blood thinners such as Coumadin
Digitalis (Lanoxin)
Drugs for depression such as Prozac and Elavil
High blood pressure drugs such as Aldomet and Inversine
Kaolin (Kaopectate)
MAO inhibitor drugs (antidepressants such as Nardil and Parnate)
Sedatives such as Nembutal and Seconal
Tranquilizers such as Xanax and Valium

## Special information if you are pregnant or breastfeeding

Although the effects of Trinalin during pregnancy have not been adequately studied, antihistamines have caused severe reactions in premature and newborn babies when used in the last 3 months of pregnancy. If you are pregnant or plan to become pregnant, notify your doctor immediately. Trinalin may appear in breast milk and could affect a nursing infant. If this medication is essential to your health, your doctor may advise you to discontinue breastfeeding until your treatment with Trinalin is finished.

## Recommended dosage

ADULTS AND CHILDREN AGED 12 AND OVER:

The usual dosage is 1 tablet twice a day.
Children under age 12 should not take Trinalin.

## Overdosage

Any medication taken in excess can have serious consequences. An overdose of Trinalin can be fatal. If you suspect an overdose, seek medical attention immediately.

■ *Symptoms of Trinalin overdose may include:*
Anxiety, bluish color caused by lack of oxygen, blurred vision, chest pain, coma, convulsions, decreased mental alertness, delusions, difficulty sleeping, difficulty urinating, dizziness, excitement, extreme calm (sedation), exaggerated sense of well-being, fluttery heartbeat, giddiness, hallucinations, headache, high blood pressure/ low blood pressure, irregular heartbeat, lack of muscle coordination, muscle tenseness, muscle

weakness, nausea, perspiration, rapid heartbeat, restlessness, ringing in the ears, temporary interruption of breathing, thirst, tremors, vomiting

■ *Overdose symptoms more common in children may include:*
Dry mouth, fixed, dilated pupils, flushing, overstimulation, stomach and intestinal problems, very high body temperature

Brand name:
# Triphasil

*See Oral Contraceptives, page 382.*

Brand name:
# T-Stat

*See Erythromycin, Topical, page 198.*

Brand name:
# Tums

*See Antacids, page 30.*

Brand name:
# Tussionex

*Pronounced: TUSS-ee-uh-nex*
*Generic ingredients: Hydrocodone polistirex,*
  *Chlorpheniramine polistirex*

## Why is this drug prescribed?
Tussionex Extended-Release Suspension is a cough-suppressant/antihistamine combination used to relieve coughs and the upper respiratory symptoms of colds and allergies. Hydrocodone, a mild narcotic similar to codeine, is believed to work directly on the cough center. Chlorpheniramine, an antihistamine, reduces itching and swelling and dries up secretions from the eyes, nose, and throat.

## Most important fact about this drug
This medication can cause considerable drowsiness and make you less alert. You should not drive or operate machinery or participate in any activity that requires full mental alertness until you know how you react to Tussionex.

## How should you take this medication?
Tussionex should be taken exactly as prescribed.

It should not be diluted with other liquids or mixed with other drugs. Shake well before using.

■ *If you miss a dose...*
If you take Tussionex on a regular schedule, take the forgotten dose as soon as you remember. If it is almost time for your next dose, skip the one you missed and go back to your regular schedule. Do not take 2 doses at once.
■ *Storage instructions...*
Store at room temperature in a tightly closed container.

## What side effects may occur?
Side effects cannot be anticipated. If any develop or change in intensity, inform your doctor as soon as possible. Only your doctor can determine if it is safe for you to continue taking Tussionex.

■ *Side effects may include:*
Anxiety, constipation, decreased mental and physical performance, difficulty breathing, difficulty urinating, dizziness, drowsiness, dry throat, emotional dependence, exaggerated feeling of depression, extreme calm (sedation), exaggerated sense of well-being, fear, itching, mental clouding, mood changes, nausea, rash, restlessness, sluggishness, tightness in chest, vomiting

## Why should this drug not be prescribed?
Do not take Tussionex if you are sensitive to or have ever had an allergic reaction to hydrocodone or chlorpheniramine. Make sure your doctor is aware of any drug reactions you have experienced.

## Special warnings about this medication
Tussionex contains a mild narcotic that can cause dependence and tolerance when the drug is used for several weeks. However, it is unlikely that dependence will develop when Tussionex is used for the short-term treatment of a cough.

Like all narcotics, Tussionex may produce slowed or irregular breathing. If you have lung disease or a breathing disorder, use this medication cautiously.

Use Tussionex with care if you have the eye condition known as narrow-angle glaucoma, asthma, an enlarged prostate gland, urinary difficulties, an intestinal disorder, liver or kidney disease, an underactive thyroid gland, or Addison's disease (a disorder of the adrenal glands), or if you have recently suffered a head injury.

Extra caution should be used when giving Tussionex to the elderly and those in a weakened condition.

Remember that Tussionex can cause drowsiness.

Narcotics can cause intestinal blockage or mask a severe abdominal condition.

### Possible food and drug interactions when taking this medication

Tussionex may increase the effects of alcohol. Do not drink alcohol while taking this medication.

If Tussionex is taken with certain other drugs, the effects of either could be increased, decreased, or altered. It is especially important to check with your doctor before combining Tussionex with the following:

Antispasmodic medications such as Bentyl and Cogentin
Major tranquilizers such as Thorazine and Compazine
MAO inhibitor drugs (antidepressant drugs such as Nardil and Parnate)
Medications for anxiety such as Xanax and Valium
Medications for depression such as Elavil and Prozac
Other antihistamines such as Benadryl
Other narcotics such as Percocet and Demerol

### Special information if you are pregnant or breastfeeding

The safety of Tussionex during pregnancy has not been adequately studied. However, babies born to mothers who have been taking narcotics regularly before delivery will be born addicted. If you are pregnant or plan to become pregnant, inform your doctor immediately. Tussionex may appear in breast milk and could affect a nursing infant. If this medication is essential to your health, your doctor may recommend that you stop breastfeeding until your treatment with Tussionex is finished.

### Recommended dosage

ADULTS

The usual dose is 1 teaspoonful (5 milliliters) every 12 hours. Do not take more than 2 teaspoonfuls in 24 hours.

CHILDREN AGED 6 TO 12

The usual dose is one-half teaspoonful every 12 hours. Do not take more than 1 teaspoonful in 24 hours.

Tussionex is not recommended for children under 6 years old.

### Overdosage

Any medication taken in excess can have serious consequences. A narcotic overdose can be fatal. If you suspect an overdose, seek medical treatment immediately.

■ *Symptoms of Tussionex overdose may include:*
Blue skin color due to lack of oxygen, cardiac arrest, cold and clammy skin, decreased or difficult breathing, extreme sleepiness leading to stupor or coma, low blood pressure, muscle flabbiness, slow heartbeat, temporary cessation of breathing

*Brand name:*

# Tussi-Organidin NR

*Pronounced: TUSS-ee or-GAN-i-din*
*Generic ingredients: Guaifenesin, Codeine phosphate*
*Other brand name: Brontex*

### Why is this drug prescribed?

Tussi-Organidin NR is used to relieve coughs and chest congestion in adults and children. It contains guaifenesin, which helps thin and loosen mucus in the lungs, making it easier to cough up. It also contains a cough suppressant, the narcotic codeine.

### Most important fact about this drug

Tussi-Organidin NR may cause you to become drowsy or less alert. Alcohol will intensify this effect. Driving, operating dangerous machinery, or participating in any hazardous activity that requires your full mental alertness is not recommended until you know how you react to this medication.

### How should you take this medication?

Take Tussi-Organidin NR exactly as described. When giving the liquid to a child, use a calibrated dropper to measure the dose.

■ *If you miss a dose...*
Take the missed dose as soon as you remember. If it is almost time for your next dose, skip the one you missed and go back to your regular schedule. Never take 2 doses at once.
■ *Storage instructions...*
Store at room temperature in a tightly closed container, away from light.

## What side effects may occur?

Side effects cannot be anticipated. If any side effects develop or change in intensity, tell your doctor as soon as possible. Only your doctor can determine whether it is safe to continue taking Tussi-Organidin NR.

■ *More common side effects may include:*
Constipation, nausea, pinpoint pupils of the eye, vomiting
■ *Less common side effects may include:*
Dizziness, headache, rash

At higher doses, this medication may also cause light-headedness, drowsiness, slowed breathing, and an exaggerated sense of well-being.

## Why should this drug not be prescribed?

Do not take Tussi-Organidin NR if you are allergic to codeine or guaifenesin.

## Special warnings about this medication

Because it contains codeine, Tussi-Organidin NR may cause drug dependence and tolerance with continued use.

Do not use this product in children under 2 years of age. Be cautious if the child has an allergy.

Do not take Tussi-Organidin NR for the constant cough brought on by smoking, asthma, chronic bronchitis, or emphysema unless your doctor recommends it. If your cough lasts for more than 1 week, tends to come back, or is accompanied by fever, rash, or persistent headache, check with your doctor.

Be sure to tell the doctor if you have any breathing problems, a severe abdominal condition, kidney or liver problems, an underactive thyroid gland, or an enlarged prostate. Also alert the doctor if you suffer from seizures, have had a head injury, or have recently had stomach, intestinal, or urinary tract surgery.

## Possible food and drug interactions when taking this medication

If Tussi-Organidin NR is taken with certain other drugs, the effects of either could be increased, decreased, or altered. It is especially important to check with your doctor before combining Tussi-Organidin NR with the following:

Alcohol
Antihistamines such as Actifed or Benadryl
Drugs used to treat anxiety or depression, such as
　Librium and Prozac
Sedatives such as Dalmane

## Special information
## if you are pregnant or breastfeeding

If you are pregnant or plan to become pregnant, inform your doctor immediately. The safety of Tussi-Organidin NR, during pregnancy has not been established. Tussi-Organidin NR should not be taken if you are breastfeeding.

## Recommended dosage

ADULTS AND CHILDREN 12 YEARS AND OLDER

*Tussi-Organidin NR*
The usual dosage is 2 teaspoonfuls every 4 hours, not to exceed 12 teaspoonfuls in 24 hours.

*Brontex*
The usual dosage is 1 tablet or 4 teaspoonfuls every 4 hours.

CHILDREN 6 TO 12 YEARS OF AGE

*Tussi-Organidin NR*
The usual dosage is 1 teaspoonful every 4 hours, not to exceed 6 teaspoonfuls in 24 hours.

*Brontex*
The usual dosage is 2 teaspoonfuls every 4 hours. Do not give tablets.

CHILDREN 2 TO 6 YEARS OF AGE

*Tussi-Organidin NR*
Your doctor will determine the dosage according to weight. The recommended total daily dosage is 1 milligram per 2.2 pounds of body weight, divided into 4 small doses.

## Overdosage

Any medication taken in excess can have serious consequences. If you suspect an overdose, seek medical treatment immediately.

■ *Symptoms of Tussi-Organidin NR overdose may include:*
Alternate periods of not breathing and rapid, deep breathing, bluish skin coloration, cold and clammy skin, constriction of the pupils of the eye, delirium, delusions, double vision, excitement, extreme sleepiness progressing to stupor or coma, flaccid muscles, hallucinations, low blood pressure, restlessness, slow, shallow, or labored breathing, slow heartbeat, speech disturbances, vertigo

*Brand name:*

# Tylenol

*Pronounced: TIE-len-all*
*Generic name: Acetaminophen*
*Other brand names: Panadol, Aspirin Free*
  *Anacin*

## Why is this drug prescribed?

Tylenol is a fever- and pain-reducing medication that is widely used to relieve simple headaches and muscle aches; the minor aches and pains associated with the common cold; backache; toothache; minor pain of arthritis; and menstrual cramps.

Children's Tylenol is used to relieve fever, pain and discomfort due to colds, flu, teething, immunizations, and tonsillectomy.

## Most important fact about this drug

Do not use Tylenol to relieve pain for more than 10 days, or to reduce fever for more than 3 days unless your doctor has specifically told you to do so.

## How should you take this medication?

Follow the dosing instructions on the label. Do not take more Tylenol than is recommended.

■ *If you miss a dose...*
  Take this medication only as needed.
■ *Storage instructions...*
  Store at room temperature. Keep the liquid form from freezing.

## What side effects may occur?

Tylenol is relatively free of side effects. Rarely, an allergic reaction may occur. If you develop any allergic symptoms such as rash, hives, swelling, or difficulty breathing, stop taking Tylenol immediately and notify your doctor.

## Special warnings about this medication

Remember that Tylenol should not be used for more than 10 days for pain, or 3 days for fever. Children's Tylenol should not be used for more than 5 days for pain, or 3 days for fever. If pain or fever persists or gets worse, if new symptoms develop, or if there is any redness or swelling, contact your doctor. These symptoms could indicate a more serious illness.

If you generally drink 3 or more alcoholic beverages per day, check with your doctor about using Tylenol and other acetaminophen-containing products, and never take more than the recommended dosage. There is a possibility of damage to the liver when large amounts of alcohol and acetaminophen are combined.

## Possible food and drug interactions when taking this medication

If Tylenol is taken with certain other drugs the effects of either could be increased, decreased, or altered. It is especially important to check with your doctor before combining Tylenol with the following:

Alcohol
Cholestyramine (Questran)
Isoniazid (Nydrazid)
Nonsteroidal anti-inflammatory drugs such as
  Dolobid and Motrin
Oral Contraceptives
Phenytoin (Dilantin)
Warfarin (Coumadin)
Zidovudine (Retrovir)

Tylenol should not be used with other products containing acetaminophen.

## Special information if you are pregnant or breastfeeding

As with all medications, ask your doctor or health care professional whether it is safe for you to use Tylenol while you are pregnant or breastfeeding.

## Recommended dosage

ADULTS AND CHILDREN 12 YEARS AND OLDER

*Tylenol Regular Strength*
The usual dose is 2 caplets or tablets every 4 to 6 hours. Do not take more than 12 caplets or tablets in 24 hours.

*Tylenol Extended Relief*
The usual dose is 2 caplets every 8 hours, not to exceed 6 caplets in any 24 hour period. Swallow each caplet whole. Do not crush, chew, or dissolve the caplets.

CHILDREN 6 TO 12 YEARS OLD

*Tylenol Regular Strength*
One-half to 1 caplet or tablet every 4 to 6 hours. Children in this age group should not be given more than 5 doses in 24 hours.

*Children's Tylenol*
All doses of Children's Tylenol may be repeated every 4 hours, but not more than 5 times daily.

Chewable tablets: The usual dose for children 6 to 8 years of age is 4 tablets; 9 to 10 years, 5 tablets; 11 to 12 years, 6 tablets. Elixir and suspension liquid: (A special cup for measuring dosage is provided.) The usual dose for children 6 to 8 years of age is 2 teaspoons; 9 to 10 years, 2½ teaspoons; 11 to 12 years, 3 teaspoons.

CHILDREN UNDER 6 YEARS OLD

*Regular Strength Tylenol*
Consult your physician or health care professional.

*Children's Tylenol*
All doses of Children's Tylenol may be repeated every 4 hours, but not more than 5 times daily. Children under 2 years old should be given Children's Tylenol only on the advice of a physician. Chewable tablets: The usual dose for children 2 to 3 years of age is 2 tablets; 4 to 5 years, 3 tablets. Elixir and suspension liquid: (A special cup for measuring dosage is provided.) The usual dose for children 4 to 11 months of age is ½ teaspoon; 12 to 23 months, ¾ teaspoon; 2 to 3 years, 1 teaspoon; 4 to 5 years, 1½ teaspoons.

*Infants' Tylenol Drops and Suspension Drops*
The usual dose for children 0 to 3 months of age is 0.4 milliliter; 4 to 11 months, 0.8 milliliter; 12 to 23 months, 1.2 milliliters; 2 to 3 years, 1.6 milliliters; 4 to 5 years, 2.4 milliliters.

## Overdosage

Any medication taken in excess can have serious consequences. If you suspect an overdose, seek medical attention immediately. Massive doses of Tylenol may cause liver damage.

■ *Symptoms of Tylenol overdose may include:*
Excessive perspiration, exhaustion, general discomfort, nausea, vomiting

*Brand name:*

# Tylenol with Codeine

*Pronounced: TIE-len-awl with CO-deen*
*Generic ingredients: Acetaminophen, Codeine phosphate*
*Other brand name: Phenaphen with Codeine*

## Why is this drug prescribed?

Tylenol with Codeine, a narcotic analgesic, is used to treat mild to moderately severe pain. It contains two drugs—acetaminophen and codeine. Acetaminophen, an antipyretic (fever-reducing) analgesic, is used to reduce pain and fever. Codeine, a narcotic analgesic, is used to treat pain that is moderate to severe.

People who are allergic to aspirin can take Tylenol with Codeine.

## Most important fact about this drug

Tylenol with Codeine contains a narcotic (codeine) and, even if taken in prescribed amounts, can cause physical and psychological addiction if taken for a long enough time.

Addiction may be more of a risk for a person who has been addicted to alcohol or drugs. Be sure to follow your doctor's instructions carefully when taking Tylenol with Codeine (or any other drugs that contain a narcotic).

## How should you take this medication?

Tylenol with Codeine may be taken with meals or with milk (but not with alcohol).

■ *If you miss a dose...*
If you take this medication on a regular schedule, take the forgotten dose as soon as you remember. If it is almost time for your next dose, skip the one you missed and go back to your regular schedule. Do not take 2 doses at once.
■ *Storage instructions...*
Store away from heat, light, and moisture. Keep the liquid from freezing.

## What side effects may occur?

Side effects cannot be anticipated. If any develop or change in intensity, inform your doctor as soon as possible. Only your doctor can determine if it is safe for you to continue taking Tylenol with Codeine.

■ *More common side effects may include:*
Dizziness, light-headedness, nausea, sedation, shortness of breath, vomiting
■ *Less common side effects may include:*
Abdominal pain, allergic reactions, constipation, depressed feeling, exaggerated feeling of well-being, itchy skin
■ *Rare side effects may include:*
Decreased breathing (when Tylenol with Codeine is taken at higher doses)

## Why should this drug not be prescribed?

You should not use Tylenol with Codeine if you are sensitive to either acetaminophen (Tylenol) or codeine.

## Special warnings about this medication

You should take Tylenol with Codeine cautiously and only according to your doctor's instructions, as you would take any medication containing a narcotic. Make sure your doctor is aware of any problems you have had with drug or alcohol addiction.

Tylenol with Codeine tablets contain a sulfite that may cause allergic reactions in some people. These reactions may include shock and severe, possibly life-threatening, asthma attacks. People with asthma are more likely to be sensitive to sulfites.

If you have experienced a head injury, consult your doctor before taking Tylenol with Codeine.

If you have stomach problems, such as an ulcer, check with your doctor before taking Tylenol with Codeine. Tylenol with Codeine may obscure the symptoms of stomach problems, making them difficult to diagnose and treat.

If you have ever had liver, kidney, thyroid, or adrenal disease, difficulty urinating, or an enlarged prostate, consult your doctor before taking Tylenol with Codeine.

If you generally drink 3 or more alcoholic beverages per day, check with your doctor before using Tylenol with Codeine and other acetaminophen-containing products, and never take more than the recommended dosage. There is a possibility of damage to the liver when large amounts of alcohol and acetaminophen are combined.

This drug may cause drowsiness and impair your ability to drive a car or operate potentially dangerous machinery. Do not participate in any activities that require full attention when using this drug until you are sure of its effect on you.

## Possible food and drug interactions when taking this medication

Alcohol may increase the sedative effects of Tylenol with Codeine. Therefore, do not drink alcohol while you are taking this medication.

If Tylenol with Codeine is taken with certain other drugs, the effects of either could be increased, decreased, or altered. It is especially important to check with your doctor before combining Tylenol with Codeine with the following:

Antidepressants such as Elavil, Nardil, Parnate, and Tofranil
Drugs that control spasms, such as Cogentin
Major tranquilizers such as Clozaril and Thorazine
Other narcotic painkillers such as Darvon
Tranquilizers such as Xanax and Valium

## Special information if you are pregnant or breastfeeding

It is not known if Tylenol with Codeine could injure a baby, or if it could affect a woman's reproductive capacity. Using any medication that contains a narcotic during pregnancy may cause babies to be born with a physical addiction to the narcotic. If you are pregnant or plan to become pregnant, you should not take Tylenol with Codeine unless the potential benefits clearly outweigh the possible dangers. As with other narcotic painkillers, taking Tylenol with Codeine shortly before delivery (especially at higher dosages) may cause some degree of breathing difficulty in the mother and newborn.

Some studies (but not all) have reported that codeine appears in breast milk and may affect a nursing infant. Therefore, nursing mothers should use Tylenol with Codeine only if the potential gains are greater than the potential hazards.

## Recommended dosage

ADULTS

Dosage will depend on how severe your pain is and how you respond to the drug.

*To Relieve Pain*
A single dose may contain from 15 milligrams to 60 milligrams of codeine phosphate and from 300 to 1,000 milligrams of acetaminophen. The maximum dose in a 24-hour period should be 360 milligrams of codeine phosphate and 4,000 milligrams of acetaminophen. Your doctor will determine the amounts of codeine phosphate and acetaminophen taken in each dose. Doses may be repeated up to every 4 hours.

Single doses above 60 milligrams of codeine do not give enough pain relief to balance the increased number of side effects.

Adults may also take Tylenol with Codeine elixir (liquid). Tylenol with Codeine elixir contains 120 milligrams of acetaminophen and 12 milligrams of codeine phosphate per teaspoonful.

The usual adult dose is 1 tablespoonful every 4 hours as needed.

CHILDREN

The safety of Tylenol with Codeine elixir has not been established in children under 3 years old.

Children 3 to 6 years old may take 1 teaspoonful 3 or 4 times daily.

Children 7 to 12 years old may take 2 teaspoonsful 3 or 4 times daily.

OLDER ADULTS

Older people and anyone in a weakened or rundown condition should use Tylenol with Codeine cautiously.

### Overdosage

Any medication taken in excess can cause symptoms of overdose. Severe overdosage of Tylenol with Codeine can cause death. If you suspect an overdose, seek medical attention immediately.

■ *Symptoms of Tylenol with Codeine overdose may include:*

Bluish skin, cold and clammy skin, coma due to low blood sugar, decreased, irregular, or stopped breathing, extreme sleepiness progressing to stupor or coma, general bodily discomfort, heart attack, kidney failure, liver failure, low blood pressure, muscle weakness, nausea, slow heartbeat, sweating, vomiting

*Brand name:*

# Tylox

*See Percocet, page 407.*

*Brand name:*

# Ultracef

*See Duricef, page 179.*

*Brand name:*

# Ultram

*Pronounced: UL-tram*
*Generic name: Tramadol hydrochloride*

### Why is this drug prescribed?

Ultram is prescribed to relieve moderate to moderately severe pain.

### Most important fact about this drug

You should not drive a car, operate machinery, or perform any other potentially hazardous activities until you know how this drug affects you.

### How should you take this medication?

It's important to take Ultram exactly as prescribed. Do not increase the dosage or length of time you take this drug without your doctor's approval.

■ *If you miss a dose...*

Take it as soon as you remember. However, if it is almost time for your next dose, skip the one you missed and go back to your regular schedule. Never take 2 doses at once.

■ *Storage instructions...*

Store in a tightly closed container at room temperature.

### What side effects may occur?

Side effects cannot be anticipated. If any develop or change in intensity, tell your doctor as soon as possible. Only your doctor can determine if it is safe for you to continue taking Ultram.

■ *More common side effects may include:*

Agitation, anxiety, bloating and gas, constipation, convulsive movements, diarrhea, dizziness, drowsiness, dry mouth, feeling of elation, hallucinations, headache, indigestion, itching, nausea, nervousness, sweating, tremor, vomiting, weakness

■ *Less common side effects may include:*

Abdominal pain, confusion, coordination problems, feeling of illness, flushing, frequent urination, inability to urinate, loss of appetite, menopausal symptoms, rash, sleeping problems, visual problems

■ *Rare side effects may include:*

Accidental injury, allergic reaction, altered taste, amnesia, difficult or labored breathing, difficulty concentrating, dizziness or light-headedness upon standing, fainting, feeling of "pins and needles", hives, menstrual problems, mental sluggishness or clouding, painful urination, rapid heartbeat, seizures, weight loss

### Why should this drug not be prescribed?

Avoid Ultram if it has ever given you an allergic reaction. Also avoid Ultram after taking large doses of sleeping pills such as Halcion, Dalmane, and Restoril; narcotic pain relievers such as Demerol, morphine, Darvon, and Percocet; or psychotherapeutic drugs such as antidepressants and tranquilizers. And do not take Ultram after drinking excessive amounts of alcohol.

## Special warnings about this medication

If you have stomach problems such as an ulcer, make sure your doctor is aware of them. Ultram may hide the symptoms, making them difficult to diagnose and treat.

If you have become dependent on such drugs as Percocet, Demerol, or morphine, you may experience withdrawal symptoms when you switch to Ultram.

Do not take more than the recommended dose of Ultram, since larger doses may cause seizures, especially if you have epilepsy or are taking medications that increase the risk of seizures. Among the medications with this effect are the type of antidepressants called MAO inhibitors (Nardil, Parnate) and major tranquilizers such as Loxitane and Stelazine.

If you have liver or kidney disease, be sure your doctor knows about it. Your dosage may have to be reduced.

Before you have any kind of surgery, make sure the doctor knows you are taking Ultram.

If you have experienced a head injury, consult your doctor before taking Ultram. The medication's effects may be stronger and could hide warning signs of serious trouble.

## Possible food and drug interactions when taking this medication

Ultram may increase the drowsiness caused by alcohol. Do not drink alcohol while taking this medication.

If Ultram is taken with certain other drugs, the effects of either could be increased, decreased, or altered. It is especially important to check with your doctor before combining Ultram with the following:

Antidepressant drugs known as MAO inhibitors (Nardil, Parnate)
Carbamazepine (Tegretol)
Major tranquilizers such as Thorazine and Stelazine
Narcotic pain relievers (Demerol, morphine, Darvon, Percocet)
Quinidine (Quinidex)
Sleeping pills (Halcion, Dalmane, Restoril)
Tranquilizers (Valium, Xanax)

## Special information if you are pregnant or breastfeeding

The effects of Ultram during pregnancy have not been adequately studied. If you are pregnant or plan to become pregnant, tell your doctor immediately. Ultram appears in breast milk and may affect a nursing infant. If this medication is essential to your health, your doctor may advise you to discontinue breastfeeding until your treatment is finished.

## Recommended dosage

### ADULTS

The usual starting dose of Ultram is 50 to 100 milligrams every 4 to 6 hours, depending on the severity of pain. The most you should take is 400 milligrams a day (300 milligrams for those over age 75).

For people with kidney problems, the usual starting dose is 50 to 100 milligrams every 12 hours; and the maximum per day is 200 milligrams. For those with cirrhosis, the usual dose is 50 milligrams every 12 hours.

### CHILDREN

Safety and effectiveness in children under 16 years of age have not been established.

## Overdosage

An overdose of Ultram can be fatal. If you suspect an overdose, seek emergency medical treatment immediately.

■ *Symptoms of Ultram overdose include:*
   Difficult or slowed breathing, seizures

*Brand name:*

# Ultrase

*See Pancrease, page 392.*

*Brand name:*

# Uni-Dur

*See Theo-Dur, page 538.*

*Brand name:*

# Uniphyl

*See Theo-Dur, page 538.*

*Brand name:*

# Univasc

*Pronounced: YOO-ni-vask*
*Generic name: Moexipril Hydrochloride*

### Why is this drug prescribed?

Univasc is used in the treatment of high blood pressure. It is effective when used alone or with thiazide diuretics that help rid the body of excess water. Univasc belongs to a family of drugs called angiotensin-converting enzyme (ACE) inhibitors. It works by preventing the transformation of a hormone in your blood called angiotensin I into a more potent substance that increases salt and water retention in your body. Univasc also enhances blood flow throughout your blood vessels.

### Most important fact about this drug

You must take Univasc regularly for it to be effective. Since blood pressure declines gradually, it may be several weeks before you get the full benefit of Univasc; and you must continue taking it even if you are feeling well. Univasc does not cure high blood pressure; it merely keeps it under control.

### How should you take this medication?

Univasc should be taken 1 hour before a meal. Try to get in the habit of taking your medication at the same time each day, such as 1 hour before breakfast, so that it is easier to remember. Always take Univasc exactly as prescribed.

■ *If you miss a dose...*
Take the forgotten dose as soon as you remember. If it is almost time for the next dose, skip the one you missed and go back to your regular schedule. Never try to "catch up" by doubling the dose.

■ *Storage instructions...*
Store at room temperature in a tightly closed container, away from moisture.

### What side effects may occur?

Side effects cannot be anticipated. If any develop or change in intensity, tell your doctor as soon as possible. Only your doctor can determine if it is safe for you to continue taking Univasc.

■ *More common side effects may include:*
Cough, diarrhea, dizziness, "flu-like" symptoms

If you develop swelling of your face, around the lips, tongue, or throat; swelling of arms and legs; sore throat, fever, and chills; or difficulty breathing or swallowing, stop taking the drug and contact your doctor immediately. You may need emergency treatment.

■ *Less common side effects may include:*
Fatigue, flushing, muscle pain, rash, sore throat

■ *Rare side effects may include:*
Abdominal pain, anemia, anxiety, changes in appetite and weight, changes in taste, chest pain, constipation, difficult or labored breathing, difficulty sleeping, drowsiness, dry mouth, fainting, feeling of illness, fluid retention, heart attack, hives, irregular heart rhythm, itching, joint pain, kidney problems, light-headedness on standing up, liver disease, low blood pressure, mood changes, nervousness, rash or skin disease, reduced amount of urine, ringing in ears, sensitivity to light, stroke, sweating, swelling of the arms, face, legs, throbbing, fluttery heartbeat, vomiting, wheezing

### Why should this drug not be prescribed?

If you have ever had an allergic reaction to Univasc or other ACE inhibitors such as Capoten, Vasotec, and Zestril, you should not take this medication.

### Special warnings about this medication

Your doctor will check your kidney function when you start taking Univasc and watch it carefully for the first few weeks.

Univasc can cause low blood pressure, especially if you are taking high doses of diuretics. You may feel light-headed or faint, especially during the first few days of therapy. If these symptoms occur, contact your doctor. Your dosage may need to be adjusted or discontinued. If you actually faint, stop taking the drug and contact your doctor immediately.

If you have congestive heart failure or other heart or circulatory disorders, use this drug with caution. Be cautious, too, if you have kidney disease, diabetes, or a collagen-vascular disease such as lupus erythematosus or scleroderma.

Excessive sweating, severe diarrhea, or vomiting could make you lose too much water, causing your blood pressure to become too low. Call your doctor if you have any of those conditions.

If you notice a yellow coloring to your skin or the whites of your eyes, stop taking the drug and notify your doctor immediately. You could be developing liver problems.

If you are using bee or wasp venom to prevent severe reactions to stings, you may have an allergic reaction to Univasc.

Some people on dialysis have had an allergic reaction to this type of drug (ACE inhibitor).

If you develop a persistent, dry cough, tell your doctor. It may be due to the medication and, if so, will disappear if you stop taking Univasc. If you develop a sore throat or fever, you should contact your doctor immediately. It could indicate a more serious illness.

Do not take potassium supplements or salt substitutes containing potassium without talking to your doctor first. In a medical emergency and before you have surgery, notify your doctor or dentist that you are taking Univasc.

## Possible food and drug interactions when taking this medication

If Univasc is taken with certain other drugs, the effects of either could be increased, decreased, or altered. It is especially important to check with your doctor before combining Univasc with the following:

Diuretics (Diuril, Hydrodiuril, Lasix)
Potassium supplements (Slow-K)
Potassium-sparing diuretics (Aldactone, Moduretic, Maxzide)
Lithium (Eskalith, Lithobid)

## Special information if you are pregnant or breastfeeding

Univasc can cause injury or death to developing and newborn babies if taken during the second and third trimesters of pregnancy. If you are pregnant and are taking Univasc, contact your doctor immediately. It is not known whether Univasc appears in human breast milk. Therefore, Univasc should be used with caution if you are breastfeeding.

## Recommended dosage

### ADULTS

For people not taking a diuretic drug, the usual starting dose is 7.5 milligrams taken once a day, an hour before a meal. The dosage after that can range from 7.5 to 30 milligrams per day, taken in either a single dose or divided into 2 equal doses daily. The maximum dose is 60 milligrams per day. Your doctor will closely monitor the effect of this drug and adjust it according to your individual needs.

People already taking a diuretic should stop taking it, if possible, 2 to 3 days before starting Univasc. This reduces the possibility of fainting or light-headedness. If the diuretic cannot be discontinued, the starting dosage of Univasc should be 3.75 milligrams. If Univasc alone does not control your blood pressure, your doctor will have you start taking a diuretic again.

For people with kidney problems, the usual starting dose is 3.75 milligrams a day; your doctor may gradually raise the dose to a maximum of 15 milligrams a day.

### CHILDREN

The safety and effectiveness of Univasc have not been established in children.

## Overdosage

Although there is no specific information available, a sudden drop in blood pressure would be the most likely symptom of Univasc overdose.

If you suspect an overdose, seek medical attention immediately.

*Brand name:*

# Urised

*Pronounced: YOUR-i-said*
*Generic ingredients: Methenamine, Methylene blue, Phenyl salicylate, Benzoic acid, Atropine sulfate, Hyoscyamine*

## Why is this drug prescribed?

Urised relieves lower urinary tract discomfort caused by inflammation or diagnostic procedures. It is used to treat urinary tract infections including cystitis (inflammation of the bladder and ureters), urethritis (inflammation of the urethra), and trigonitis (inflammation of the mucous membrane of the bladder). Methenamine, the major component of this drug, acts as a mild antiseptic by changing into formaldehyde in the urinary tract when it comes in contact with acidic urine.

## Most important fact about this drug

Urised may give a blue to blue-green color to urine and discolor stools as well.

## How should you take this medication?

If dry mouth occurs, hard candy or gum, saliva substitute, or crushed ice may provide temporary relief.

Take this medication exactly as prescribed; do not take more than the recommended dose.

Drinking plenty of fluids will help the medication work better and relieve discomfort.

■ *If you miss a dose...*
Take it as soon as you remember. If it is almost time for your next dose, skip the one you missed and go back to your regular schedule. Never take 2 doses at the same time.

■ *Storage instructions...*
Store Urised at room temperature, in a dry place.

## What side effects may occur?

Side effects cannot be anticipated. If any develop or change in intensity, inform your doctor as soon as possible. Only your doctor can determine if it is safe for you to continue taking Urised.

■ *Side effects with long-term use may include:*
Acute urinary retention (in men with an enlarged prostate), blurry vision, difficulty urinating, dizziness, dry mouth, flushing, rapid pulse, skin rash

## Why should this drug not be prescribed?

Urised should be avoided if you have glaucoma, a bladder blockage, cardiospasm, or a disorder that obstructs the passage of food through the stomach. Also avoid Urised if you are sensitive to or have ever had an allergic reaction to any of its ingredients.

## Special warnings about this medication

Urised should be used cautiously if you have heart disease or have ever had a reaction to medications that are chemically similar to atropine.

Your doctor may ask you to check your urine with phenaphthazine paper to see if it is acidic. Urine acidifiers, such as vitamin C, may be recommended if the urine is not acidic enough.

## Possible food and drug interactions when taking this medication

If Urised is taken with certain other drugs, the effects of either could be increased, decreased, or altered. It is especially important to check with your doctor before combining Urised with the following:

Acetazolamide (Diamox)
Potassium supplements such as Slow-K
Sodium bicarbonate antacids such as Alka-Seltzer
Sulfa drugs such as Gantrisin, Gantanol, Bactrim, and Septra

Drugs and foods that produce alkaline urine (such as sodium bicarbonate, antacids, and orange juice) should be limited.

## Special information if you are pregnant or breastfeeding

The effects of Urised during pregnancy have not been adequately studied. If you are pregnant or plan to become pregnant, inform your doctor immediately. Urised may appear in breast milk and could affect a nursing infant. If this medication is essential to your health, your doctor may advise you to stop breastfeeding until your treatment with Urised ends.

## Recommended dosage

ADULTS

The usual dose is 2 tablets, 4 times a day.

CHILDREN 6 YEARS AND OLDER

The dosage must be determined by your doctor.

CHILDREN UNDER 6 YEARS

Use is not recommended in children under 6 years old.

## Overdosage

Any medication taken in excess can have serious consequences. If you suspect an overdose, seek medical treatment immediately.

■ *Symptoms of Urised overdose may include:*
Abdominal pain, bladder and abdominal irritation, bloody diarrhea, bloody urine, burning pain in throat and mouth, circulatory collapse, coma, dilated pupils (large pupils), dizziness, dry nose, mouth, and throat, elevated blood pressure, extremely high body temperature, headache, hot, dry, flushed skin, painful and frequent urination, pallor (paleness), pounding heartbeat (pounding sensation against the chest), rapid heartbeat (increased pulse rate), respiratory failure, ringing in ears, sweating, vomiting, weakness, white sores in mouth

*Brand name:*

# Urispas

*Pronounced: YOUR-eh-spaz*
*Generic name: Flavoxate hydrochloride*

### Why is this drug prescribed?

Urispas prevents spasms in the urinary tract and relieves the painful or difficult urination, urinary urgency, excessive nighttime urination, pubic area pain, frequency of urination, and inability to hold urine caused by urinary tract infections. Urispas is taken in combination with antibiotics to treat the infection.

### Most important fact about this drug

Urispas can cause blurred vision and drowsiness. Be careful driving, operating machinery, or performing any activity that requires complete mental alertness until you know how you will react to this medication.

### How should you take this medication?

Take this medication exactly as prescribed. Urispas may make your mouth dry. Sucking on a hard candy, chewing gum, or melting bits of ice in your mouth can provide relief.

■ *If you miss a dose...*
Take it as soon as you remember. If it is almost time for your next dose, skip the one you missed and go back to your regular schedule. Do not take 2 doses at once.

■ *Storage instructions...*
Store away from heat, light, and moisture.

### What side effects may occur?

Side effects cannot be anticipated. If any develop or change in intensity, notify your doctor as soon as possible. Only your doctor can determine whether it is safe for you to continue taking Urispas.

■ *Side effects may include:*
Allergic skin reactions, including hives, blurred vision and vision changes, drowsiness, dry mouth, fluttery heartbeat, headache, high body temperature, mental confusion (especially in the elderly), nausea, nervousness, painful or difficult urination, rapid heartbeat, vertigo, vomiting

### Why should this drug not be prescribed?

You should not take Urispas if you have stomach or intestinal blockage, muscle relaxation problems (especially the sphincter muscle), abdominal bleeding, or urinary tract blockage.

### Special warnings about this medication

Use Urispas cautiously if you have the eye condition known as glaucoma.

### Possible food and drug interactions when taking this medication

No interactions involving Urispas have been noted.

### Special information if you are pregnant or breastfeeding

The effects of Urispas during pregnancy have not been adequately studied. If you are pregnant or plan to become pregnant, inform your doctor immediately. Urispas may appear in breast milk and could affect a nursing infant. If this medication is essential to your health, your doctor may advise you to stop breastfeeding until your treatment is finished.

### Recommended dosage

ADULTS AND CHILDREN OVER AGE 12

The usual dose of Urispas is one or two 100-milligram tablets 3 or 4 times a day.

When your symptoms have improved, your doctor may reduce the dosage.

CHILDREN

Safety and effectiveness of Urispas in children under 12 years of age have not been established.

### Overdosage

Any medication taken in excess can have serious consequences. If you suspect an overdose of Urispas, seek medical attention immediately.

■ *Symptoms of Urispas overdose may include:*
Convulsions, decreased ability to sweat, (warm, red skin, dry mouth, and increased body temperature), hallucinations, increased heart rate and blood pressure, mental confusion

*Generic name:*

# Ursodiol

*See Actigall, page 6.*

*Generic name:*

# Valacyclovir

*See Valtrex, page 581.*

*Brand name:*

# Valium

*Pronounced: VAL-ee-um*
*Generic name: Diazepam*

### Why is this drug prescribed?

Valium is used in the treatment of anxiety disorders and for short-term relief of the symptoms of anxiety. It belongs to a class of drugs known as benzodiazepines.

It is also used to relieve the symptoms of acute alcohol withdrawal, to relax muscles, to relieve the uncontrolled muscle movements caused by cerebral palsy and paralysis of the lower body and limbs, to control involuntary movement of the hands (athetosis), to relax tight, aching muscles, and, along with other medications, to treat convulsive disorders such as epilepsy.

### Most important fact about this drug

Valium can be habit-forming or addictive. You may experience withdrawal symptoms if you stop using this drug abruptly. Discontinue or change your dose only on your doctor's advice.

### How should you take this medication?

Take this medication exactly as prescribed. If you are taking Valium for epilepsy, make sure you take it every day at the same time.

■ *If you miss a dose...*
Take it as soon as you remember if it is within an hour or so of the scheduled time. If you do not remember until later, skip the dose you missed and go back to your regular schedule. Never take 2 doses at the same time.

■ *Storage instructions...*
Store away from heat, light, and moisture.

### What side effects may occur?

Side effects cannot be anticipated. If any develop or change in intensity, inform your doctor as soon as possible. Only your doctor can determine if it is safe for you to continue taking Valium.

■ *More common side effects may include:*
Drowsiness, fatigue, light-headedness, loss of muscle coordination

■ *Less common or rare side effects may include:*
Anxiety, blurred vision, changes in salivation, changes in sex drive, confusion, constipation, depression, difficulty urinating, dizziness, double

vision, hallucinations, headache, inability to hold urine, low blood pressure, nausea, over-stimulation, rage, seizures (mild changes in brain wave patterns), skin rash, sleep disturbances, slow heartbeat, slurred speech and other speech problems, stimulation, tremors, vertigo, yellowing of eyes and skin

■ *Side effects due to rapid decrease in dose or abrupt withdrawal from Valium:*
Abdominal and muscle cramps, convulsions, sweating, tremors, vomiting

### Why should this drug not be prescribed?

If you are sensitive to or have ever had an allergic reaction to Valium, you should not take this medication.

Do not take this medication if you have the eye condition known as acute narrow-angle glaucoma.

Anxiety or tension related to everyday stress usually does not require treatment with such a powerful drug as Valium. Discuss your symptoms thoroughly with your doctor.

Valium should not be prescribed if you are being treated for mental disorders more serious than anxiety.

### Special warnings about this medication

Valium may cause you to become drowsy or less alert; therefore, you should not drive or operate dangerous machinery or participate in any hazardous activity that requires full mental alertness until you know how this drug affects you.

If you have liver or kidney problems, use this medication cautiously.

### Possible food and drug interactions when taking this medication

Valium slows down the central nervous system and may intensify the effects of alcohol. Do not drink alcohol while taking this medication.

If Valium is taken with certain other drugs, the effects of either could be increased, decreased, or altered. It is especially important to check with your doctor before combining Valium with any of the following:

Antiseizure drugs such as Dilantin
Antidepressant drugs such as Elavil and Prozac
Barbiturates such as phenobarbital
Cimetidine (Tagamet)
Digoxin (Lanoxin)
Disulfiram (Antabuse)

Fluoxetine (Prozac)
Isoniazid (Rifamate)
Levodopa (Larodopa, Sinemet)
Major tranquilizers such as Mellaril and Thorazine
MAO inhibitors (antidepressant drugs such as Nardil)
Narcotics such as Percocet
Omeprazole (Prilosec)
Oral contraceptives
Propoxyphene (Darvon)
Ranitidine (Zantac)
Rifampin (Rifadin)

### Special information
### if you are pregnant or breastfeeding

Do not take Valium if you are pregnant or planning to become pregnant. There is an increased risk of birth defects.

If this medication is essential to your health, your doctor may advise you to discontinue breast-feeding until your treatment is finished.

### Recommended dosage

#### ADULTS

*Treatment of Anxiety Disorders and Short-Term Relief of the Symptoms of Anxiety*
The usual dose, depending upon severity of symptoms, is 2 milligrams to 10 milligrams 2 to 4 times daily.

*Acute Alcohol Withdrawal*
The usual dose is 10 milligrams 3 or 4 times during the first 24 hours, then 5 milligrams 3 or 4 times daily as needed.

*Relief of Muscle Spasm*
The usual dose is 2 milligrams to 10 milligrams 3 or 4 times daily.

*Convulsive Disorders*
The usual dose is 2 milligrams to 10 milligrams 2 to 4 times daily.

#### CHILDREN

Valium should not be given to children under 6 months of age.

The usual starting dose for children over 6 months is 1 to 2.5 milligrams 3 or 4 times a day. Your doctor may increase the dosage gradually if needed.

#### OLDER ADULTS

The usual dosage is 2 milligrams to 2.5 milligrams once or twice a day, which your doctor will increase as needed. Your doctor will limit the dosage to the smallest effective amount because older people are more apt to become oversedated or uncoordinated.

### Overdosage

Any medication taken in excess can have serious consequences. If you suspect an overdose, seek medical attention immediately.

■ *Symptoms of Valium overdose may include:*
Coma, confusion, diminished reflexes, sleepiness

---

*Generic name:*

# Valproic acid

*See Depakene, page 146.*

---

*Brand name:*

# Valtrex

*Pronounced: VAL-trex*
*Generic name: Valacyclovir hydrochloride*

### Why is this drug prescribed?

Valtrex is used to treat herpes zoster, also known as shingles, in adults. It is also prescribed for repeated attacks of genital herpes.

### Most important fact about this drug

Valtrex should not be used by people whose immune system is not healthy, such as those with HIV infection or those who have undergone a bone marrow or kidney transplant. Valtrex can cause serious side effects, including death, in such people.

### How should you use this medication?

If you are taking Valtrex for shingles, you should start using it as soon as possible after your doctor has made a diagnosis. It's best to see a doctor and start the drug within 48 hours of first noticing the rash. If you wait more than 72 hours after you first get a herpes zoster rash, the medication may not be effective.

If you are using Valtrex for genital herpes, begin taking it at the first sign of an attack. The medication may not be effective if you wait longer than 24 hours. You may take Valtrex with or without food.

■ *If you miss a dose...*
Take it as soon as you remember. If it is almost time for your next dose, skip the one you missed

and go back to your regular schedule. Do not take two doses at the same time.

■ *Storage instructions...*
Store at room temperature.

## What side effects may occur?
Side effects cannot be anticipated. If any develop or change in intensity, inform your doctor as soon as possible. Only your doctor can determine if it is safe for you to continue using Valtrex.

■ *Side effects may include:*
Abdominal pain, appetite loss, constipation, diarrhea, dizziness, headache, nausea, vomiting, weakness

## Why should this drug not be prescribed?
Do not use Valtrex if your immune system is compromised because of HIV infection, bone marrow transplant, or kidney transplant. Also avoid Valtrex if you are sensitive to it or the similar drug acyclovir (Zovirax).

## Special warnings about this medication
If your kidneys are not functioning properly, or you are taking drugs that may damage the kidneys such as Neomycin or Streptomycin, Valtrex can make your condition worse or affect your central nervous system (brain and spinal cord).

Valtrex is not intended for use in children.

## Possible food and drug interactions when taking this medication
If you are taking Valtrex with certain other drugs, the effect of either drug could be increased, decreased, or altered. Check with your doctor before combining Valtrex with cimetidine (Tagamet) and/or probenecid (Benemid).

## Special information
## If you are pregnant or breastfeeding
The effects of Valtrex during pregnancy and breastfeeding have not been adequately studied. If you are pregnant or plan to become pregnant, notify your doctor immediately. If you are nursing and need to use Valtrex, your doctor may advise you to discontinue breastfeeding while using the medication.

## Recommended dosage
SHINGLES

The usual dose is 1 gram (two 500-milligram caplets) 3 times a day for 7 days.

If your kidneys are not functioning well, your doctor will reduce the dosage.

RECURRENT GENITAL HERPES

The usual dose is one 500-milligram tablet twice a day for 5 days.

## Overdosage
There are no reports of overdose with Valtrex. However, any medication taken in excess can have serious consequences.

*Brand name:*

# Vancenase

*See Beclomethasone, page 53.*

*Brand name:*

# Vanceril

*See Beclomethasone, page 53.*

*Brand name:*

# Vaseretic

*Pronounced: Vaz-err-ET-ik*
*Generic ingredients: Enalapril maleate,*
*    Hydrochlorothiazide*

## Why is this drug prescribed?
Vaseretic is used in the treatment of high blood pressure. It combines an ACE inhibitor with a thiazide diuretic. Enalapril, the ACE inhibitor, works by preventing a chemical in your blood called angiotensin I from converting into a more potent form that increases salt and water retention in your body. Enalapril also enhances blood flow throughout your blood vessels. Hydrochlorothiazide, a diuretic, prompts your body to produce and eliminate more urine, which helps in lowering blood pressure.

## Most important fact about this drug
You must take Vaseretic regularly for it to be effective. Since blood pressure declines gradually, it may be several weeks before you get the full benefit of Vaseretic; and you must continue taking it even if you are feeling well. Vaseretic does not cure high blood pressure; it merely keeps it under control.

## How should you take this medication?
Take this medication exactly as prescribed by your doctor.

■ *If you miss a dose...*
Take it as soon as you remember. If it is almost time for your next dose, skip the one you missed and go back to your regular schedule. Never take 2 doses at the same time.

■ *Storage instructions...*
Keep container tightly closed. Store at room temperature and protect from moisture. Keep out of reach of children.

## What side effects may occur?
Side effects cannot be anticipated. If any develop or change in intensity, inform your doctor as soon as possible. Only your doctor can determine if it is safe for you to continue taking Vaseretic.

■ *More common side effects may include:*
Cough, diarrhea, dizziness, drop in blood pressure upon standing up, fatigue, headache, impotence, low potassium levels (leading to symptoms such as dry mouth, excessive thirst, weak or irregular heartbeat, muscle pain or cramps), muscle cramps, nausea, rash, tingling or pins and needles, weakness

■ *Less common or rare side effects may include:*
Abdominal pain, abnormal skin sensations such as numbness, prickling, or burning, allergic reactions, arthritis, back pain, black stools, blisters, blood clots in lungs, blurred vision, bronchitis, chest pain, confusion, conjunctivitis, constipation, decrease in sex drive, depression, disturbances in heart rhythm, dry eyes, dry mouth, excessive sweating, fainting, fluid in lungs, flushing, gas, gout, heart attack, hepatitis, hives, hoarseness, inability to sleep, indigestion, inflammation of mouth and tongue, inflammation of the pancreas, itching, joint pain, kidney failure, liver failure, loss of appetite, loss of coordination, loss of hair, low blood pressure, muscle cramps, nervousness, rapid heartbeat, rash, restlessness, ringing in ears, runny nose, sensitivity to light, shortness of breath, sleepiness, sore throat, stroke, tearing, urinary tract infection, vomiting, yellow eyes and skin

## Why should this drug not be prescribed?
If you are sensitive to or have ever had an allergic reaction to enalapril, hydrochlorothiazide, or similar drugs, or if you are sensitive to other sulfa drugs, you should not take this medication.

If you have a history of angioedema (swelling of face, extremities, and throat) or inability to urinate, you should not take this medication. Tell your doctor of all allergic reactions you have experienced.

## Special warnings about this medication
If you develop swelling of your face, eyes, lips, tongue, or throat; swelling of your arms and legs; or difficulty swallowing, you should contact your doctor immediately. You may need emergency treatment.

If you are taking bee or wasp venom to prevent an allergic reaction to stings, you may have a severe allergic reaction to Vaseretic.

If you develop chest pain, a sore throat, or fever you should contact your doctor immediately. It could indicate a more serious illness.

If you are taking Vaseretic, a complete assessment of your kidney function should be done. Kidney function should continue to be monitored. Some people on dialysis have had a severe allergic reaction to Vaseretic.

If you have liver disease or lupus erythematosus (a form of rheumatism), Vaseretic should be used with caution.

If your skin or the whites of your eyes turn yellow, stop taking Vaseretic and notify your doctor at once.

If you have severe congestive heart failure, you should be carefully watched for low blood pressure.

Excessive sweating, dehydration, severe diarrhea, or vomiting could cause you to lose too much water and cause your blood pressure to become too low. Be careful when exercising and in hot weather.

Vaseretic can cause some people to become drowsy or less alert. If it has this effect on you, driving or operating dangerous machinery or participating in any hazardous activity that requires full mental alertness is not recommended.

If you are diabetic, blood sugar levels should be monitored.

Vaseretic may increase your sensitivity to sunlight. Be careful to avoid overexposure.

## Possible food and drug interactions when taking this medication
Vaseretic may intensify the effects of alcohol. Do not drink alcohol while taking this medication.

If Vaseretic is taken with certain other drugs, the effects of either could be increased, decreased, or altered. It is especially important to check with your doctor before combining Vaseretic with the following:

Alcohol
Barbiturates such as phenobarbital
Certain other antihypertensives
Corticosteroids such as prednisone
Digitalis (Lanoxin)
Insulin
Lithium (Eskalith, Lithonate)
Narcotics (Percocet)
Nonsteroidal anti-inflammatory drugs such as
    Naprosyn, Advil, and Motrin
Norepinephrine
Oral antidiabetic drugs such as Micronase
Potassium supplements (K-Lyte, K-Tab, others)
Potassium-containing salt substitutes
Potassium-sparing diuretics such as Midamor

## Special information
## if you are pregnant or breastfeeding
Vaseretic can cause birth defects, prematurity, and death to the newborn baby. If you are pregnant or plan to become pregnant and are taking Vaseretic, contact your doctor immediately to discuss the potential hazard to your unborn child. Vaseretic appears in breast milk and could affect a nursing infant. If this medication is essential to your health, your doctor may advise you to discontinue breastfeeding until your treatment is finished.

## Recommended dosage
### ADULTS

Dosages of this drug are always individualized. Your doctor will determine what works best for you. This medication can and may be used in combination with other high blood pressure medications, and dosages will be adjusted accordingly. Dosages will also be modified and carefully monitored in people with reduced kidney function.

Once your doctor has determined that your blood pressure is stable, the usual starting dose is 1 or 2 tablets once a day. Maximum daily dosage is 2 tablets.

Diuretic use should, if possible, be stopped before using Vaseretic. If not, your doctor may give an initial dose under his or her supervision before any further medication is prescribed.

### CHILDREN

The safety and effectiveness of Vaseretic in children have not been established.

## Overdosage
Any medication taken in excess can cause symptoms of overdose. If you suspect an overdose, seek medical attention immediately.

No specific information on treatment of Vaseretic overdose is available.

■ *Symptoms of a Vaseretic overdose may include:*
    Dehydration, low blood pressure

*Brand name:*

# Vasotec

*Pronounced: VAZ-oh-tek*
*Generic name: Enalapril maleate*

## Why is this drug prescribed?
Vasotec is a high blood pressure medication known as an ACE inhibitor. It works by preventing a chemical in your blood called angiotensin I from converting into a more potent form that increases salt and water retention in your body. It is effective when used alone or in combination with other medications, especially thiazide-type diuretics. It is also used in the treatment of congestive heart failure, usually in combination with diuretics and digitalis, and is prescribed as a preventive measure in certain conditions that could lead to heart failure.

## Most important fact about this drug
If you have high blood pressure, you must take Vasotec regularly for it to be effective. Since blood pressure declines gradually, it may be several weeks before you get the full benefit of Vasotec; and you must continue taking it even if you are feeling well. Vasotec does not cure high blood pressure; it merely keeps it under control.

## How should you take this medication?
Vasotec can be taken with or without food.

Do not use salt substitutes containing potassium without first consulting your doctor.

Take this medication exactly as prescribed by your doctor.

■ *If you miss a dose...*
    Take it as soon as you remember. If it is almost time for your next dose, skip the one you missed

and go back to your regular schedule. Never take two doses at the same time.

■ *Storage instructions...*

Keep container tightly closed. Store at room temperature and protect from moisture.

## What side effects may occur?

Side effects cannot be anticipated. If any develop or change in intensity, inform your doctor as soon as possible. Only your doctor can determine if it is safe for you to continue taking Vasotec.

■ *Side effects may include:*

Abdominal pain, abnormal skin sensations such as numbness or prickling, anaphylactoid reactions (severe allergic reactions), angina pectoris (chest pain, often accompanied by a feeling of choking or impending death), angioedema (swelling of face, lips, tongue, throat, arms and legs, difficulty swallowing), asthma, blisters, blood abnormalities, blood clots or foreign material in the lungs, blurred vision, breast enlargement in males, bronchitis, confusion, constipation, cough, dark, tarry stool containing blood, decreased urination, depression, diarrhea, difficulty breathing, difficulty sleeping, digestive difficulty and stomach discomfort, dizziness, dizziness upon standing, dry eyes, dry mouth, excessive perspiration, fainting, fatigue, flank pain, fluid in lungs, flushing, hair loss, headache, heart palpitations, heart rhythm disturbances, hepatitis, herpes zoster, hives, impotence, inflammation of the mouth, inflammation of the tongue, itching, lack of muscle coordination, liver failure, loss of appetite, loss of sense of smell, low blood pressure, low blood pressure upon standing, muscle cramps, nausea, nervousness, pinkeye (conjunctivitis), pneumonia, pounding heartbeat, rapid or slow heartbeat, rash, red skin (like sunburn), ringing in ears, runny nose, sensitivity to light, sleepiness, sore throat and hoarseness, stroke, taste alteration, tearing, tingling or pins and needles or burning sensation, upper respiratory infection, upset stomach, urinary tract infection, vertigo, vomiting, weakness, wheezing

## Why should this drug not be prescribed?

If you are sensitive or have ever had an allergic reaction to Vasotec or similar drugs, or if you have a history of angioedema (swollen throat and difficulty swallowing) related to previous treatment with ACE inhibitors, you should not take this medication. Make sure that your doctor is aware of any drug reactions that you have experienced.

## Special warnings about this medication

Vasotec has been known to cause a serious allergic reaction called angioedema. The symptoms are swelling of the face, lips, tongue, or throat; swelling of arms and legs; and difficulty swallowing or breathing. If you notice any of these symptoms, call your doctor immediately.

If you are taking bee or wasp venom to prevent an allergic reaction to stings, you may have a severe allergic reaction to Vasotec.

If you are taking high doses of diuretics and Vasotec, you may develop excessively low blood pressure. You are at special risk if you have heart disease, kidney disease, or a potassium or salt imbalance. Some people on kidney dialysis have had a severe allergic reaction to Vasotec.

There have been cases of serious blood disorders reported with the use of Captopril, another ACE inhibitor drug. Your doctor should check your blood regularly while you are taking Vasotec.

ACE inhibitors can cause fetal abnormalities and fetal and newborn deaths when used in pregnancy during the second and third trimesters.

When pregnancy is detected, Vasotec should be discontinued as soon as possible.

If you develop a sore throat or fever, you should contact your doctor immediately. It could indicate a more serious illness. Also, if your skin and the whites of your eyes turn yellow, contact your doctor at once.

Excessive sweating, dehydration, severe diarrhea, or vomiting could cause you to lose too much water, causing your blood pressure to drop dangerously. Be careful when exercising or when exposed to excessive heat.

## Possible food and drug interactions when taking this medication

If Vasotec is taken with certain other drugs, the effects of either could be increased, decreased, or altered. It is especially important to check with your doctor before combining Vasotec with the following:

Diuretics such as Lasix and HydroDIURIL
Lithium (Eskalith, Lithobid)
Potassium-containing salt substitutes

Potassium-sparing diuretics such as Aldactazide
and Moduretic
Potassium supplements such as K-Lyte and K-Tab

### Special information
### if you are pregnant or breastfeeding

Vasotec can cause birth defects, prematurity, and
death to the developing or newborn baby. If you are
pregnant or plan to become pregnant, inform your
doctor immediately. Vasotec may appear in breast
milk and could affect a nursing infant. If this medication is essential to your health, your doctor may
advise you to stop breastfeeding until your treatment with Vasotec is finished.

### Recommended dosage

ADULTS

*Hypertension*

The usual starting dose for people not using diuretics is 5 milligrams, taken once a day. The usual
dose is 10 to 40 milligrams per day, taken as a
single dose or divided into 2 smaller doses.

If you are taking a diuretic, your physician
may ask you to stop for 2 to 3 days before using
Vasotec. Otherwise, he or she may give an initial
dose of 2.5 milligrams of Vasotec under medical
supervision before any further medication is
prescribed.

If you have a kidney disorder, your dosage will
be adjusted according to its severity.

*To Treat Heart Failure*

This medication can be used in conjunction with
digitalis and diuretics in people with heart disease.
The usual starting dose is 2.5 milligrams twice
a day.

The usual regular dose is 2.5 to 20 milligrams
each day, taken in 2 separate doses. The maximum
daily dose is 40 milligrams, in 2 separate doses.

*To Prevent Heart Failure*

The usual starting dose is 2.5 milligrams twice a
day, to be gradually increased to 20 milligrams a
day divided into smaller doses.

CHILDREN

The safety and effectiveness of Vasotec in children
have not been established.

### Overdosage

Any medication taken in excess can have serious
consequences. If you suspect symptoms of a
Vasotec overdose, seek medical attention immediately.

A sudden drop in blood pressure is the primary
effect of a Vasotec overdose.

*Brand name:*

# V-Cillin K

*See Penicillin V Potassium, page 403.*

*Brand name:*

# Veetids

*See Penicillin V Potassium, page 403.*

*Brand name:*

# Velosulin

*See Insulin, page 258.*

*Generic name:*

# Venlafaxine

*See Effexor, page 184.*

*Brand name:*

# Ventolin

*See Proventil, page 446.*

*Generic name:*

# Verapamil

*See Calan, page 70.*

*Brand name:*

# Verelan

*See Calan, page 70.*

*Brand name:*

# Vibramycin

*See Doryx, page 177.*

*Brand name:*

# Vibra-Tabs

See Doryx, page 177.

*Brand name:*

# Vicodin

*Pronounced: VY-koe-din*
*Generic ingredients: Hydrocodone bitartrate,*
*Acetaminophen*
*Other brand names: Anexsia, Co-Gesic, Hydrocet,*
*Lorcet, Lortab, Zydone*

### Why is this drug prescribed?

Vicodin combines a narcotic analgesic (painkiller) and cough reliever with a non-narcotic analgesic for the relief of moderate to moderately severe pain.

### Most important fact about this drug

Vicodin can be habit-forming. If you take this drug over a long period of time, you can become mentally and physically dependent on it, and you may find the drug no longer works for you at the prescribed dosage.

### How should you take this medication?

Take Vicodin exactly as prescribed. Do not increase the amount you take or the frequency without your doctor's approval. Do not take this drug for any reason other than the one prescribed.

Do not give this drug to others who may have similar symptoms.

■ *If you miss a dose...*
If you take Vicodin regularly, take the forgotten dose as soon as you remember. If it is almost time for your next dose, skip the one you missed and go back to your regular schedule. Do not take 2 doses at once.

■ *Storage instructions...*
Store at room temperature in a tightly closed container, away from light.

### What side effects may occur?

Side effects cannot be anticipated. If any develop or change in intensity, inform your doctor as soon as possible. Only your doctor can determine if it is safe for you to continue taking Vicodin.

■ *More common side effects may include:*
Dizziness, light-headedness, nausea, sedation, vomiting

If these side effects occur, it may help if you lie down after taking the medication.

■ *Less common or rare side effects may include:*
Allergic reactions, anxiety, blood disorders, constipation, decreased mental and physical capability, difficulty urinating, drowsiness, fear, mental clouding, mood changes, restlessness, skin rash, sluggishness, troubled, irregular, or slowed breathing

### Why should this drug not be prescribed?

If you are sensitive to or have ever had an allergic reaction to hydrocodone or acetaminophen (Tylenol), you should not take this medication. Make sure your doctor is aware of any drug reactions you have experienced.

### Special warnings about this medication

Vicodin may make you drowsy, less alert, or unable to function well physically. Do not drive a car, operate machinery, or perform any other potentially dangerous activities until you know how this drug affects you.

Use caution in taking Vicodin if you have a head injury. Narcotics tend to increase the pressure of the fluid within the skull, and this effect may be exaggerated by head injuries. Side effects of narcotics can interfere in the treatment of people with head injuries.

Use Vicodin with caution if you have a severe liver or kidney disorder, an underactive thyroid gland, Addison's disease (a disease of the adrenal glands), an enlarged prostate, or urethral stricture (narrowing of the tube carrying urine from the bladder).

The elderly or those in a weakened condition should be careful using this drug, since it contains a narcotic.

Narcotics such as Vicodin may interfere with the diagnosis and treatment of people with abdominal conditions.

Hydrocodone suppresses the cough reflex; therefore, be careful using Vicodin after an operation or if you have a lung disease.

High doses of hydrocodone may produce troubled, irregular, or slowed breathing; if you are sensitive to this drug, you are more likely to experience this effect.

### Possible food and drug interactions when taking this medication

Hydrocodone slows the nervous system. Alcohol can intensify this effect.

If hydrocodone is taken with certain other drugs, the effects of either may be increased, decreased, or altered. It is especially important to check with your doctor before combining Vicodin with the following:

Antianxiety drugs such as Valium and Librium
Antidepressants such as Elavil, Nardil, and Tofranil
Antihistamines such as Tavist
Drugs that control muscle spasms, such as Cogentin
Major tranquilizers such as Thorazine and Haldol
Other narcotic analgesics such as Demerol
Other nervous system depressants such as Halcion
   and Restoril

### Special information if you are pregnant or breastfeeding

The effects of Vicodin in pregnancy have not been adequately studied. Do not take this drug if you are pregnant or plan to become pregnant unless you are directed to do so by your doctor. Drug dependence occurs in newborns when the mother has taken this drug regularly prior to delivery. If you take it shortly before delivery, the baby's breathing may be slowed. Acetaminophen does, and hydrocodone may, appear in breast milk and could affect a nursing infant. If this medication is essential to your health, your doctor may advise you to discontinue breastfeeding your baby until your treatment is finished.

### Recommended dosage

ADULTS

Your doctor will adjust the dosage according to the severity of the pain and the way the medication affects you.

The dosages given below are for Vicodin and Vicodin ES only. If your doctor prescribes other brands, your daily dose may vary.

The usual dose of Vicodin is 1 or 2 tablets taken every 4 to 6 hours for pain as needed. The total dose should not exceed 8 tablets a day.

The usual dose of Vicodin ES is 1 tablet every 4 to 6 hours for pain as needed. The total dose should not exceed 5 tablets a day.

CHILDREN

The safety and effectiveness of Vicodin have not been established in children.

### Overdosage

Any medication taken in excess can have serious consequences. A severe overdose of Vicodin can be fatal. If you suspect an overdose, seek emergency medical treatment immediately.

■ *Symptoms of a Vicodin overdose include:*
Blood disorders, bluish tinge to skin, cold and clammy skin, extreme sleepiness progressing to a state of unresponsiveness or coma, general feeling of bodily discomfort, heart problems, heavy perspiration, kidney problems, limp muscles, liver failure, low blood pressure, nausea, slow heartbeat, troubled or slowed breathing, vomiting

Brand name:

# Vi-Daylin

See Multivitamins, page 341.

Brand name:

# Viokase

See Pancrease, page 392.

Brand name:

# Visken

Pronounced: VIS-kin
Generic name: Pindolol

### Why is this drug prescribed?

Visken, a type of medication known as a beta blocker, is used in the treatment of high blood pressure. It is effective alone or combined with other high blood pressure medications, particularly with a thiazide-type diuretic. Beta blockers decrease the force and rate of heart contractions.

### Most important fact about this drug

You must take Visken regularly for it to be effective. Since blood pressure declines gradually, it may be several weeks before you get the full benefit of Visken; and you must continue taking it even if you are feeling well. Visken does not cure high blood pressure; it merely keeps it under control.

### How should you take this medication?

Visken can be taken with or without food.

Take this medication exactly as prescribed, even if your symptoms have disappeared. Try not to miss any doses. If this medication is not taken regularly, your condition may worsen.

■ *If you miss a dose...*
Take it as soon as you remember. If it's within 4 hours of your next scheduled dose, skip the one you missed and go back to your regular schedule. Never take 2 doses at the same time.

■ *Storage instructions...*
Store Visken at room temperature in a tightly closed, light-resistant container.

### What side effects may occur?
Side effects cannot be anticipated. If any develop or change in intensity, inform your doctor as soon as possible. Only your doctor can determine if it is safe for you to continue taking Visken.

■ *More common side effects may include:*
Abdominal discomfort, chest pain, difficult or labored breathing, dizziness, fatigue, joint pain, muscle pain or cramps, nausea, nervousness, strange dreams, swelling due to fluid retention, tingling or pins and needles, trouble sleeping, weakness

■ *Less common or rare side effects may include:*
Hallucinations, heart failure, itching, palpitations, rapid heartbeat, rash

### Why should this drug not be prescribed?
If you have bronchial asthma; severe congestive heart failure; inadequate blood supply to the circulatory system (cardiogenic shock); heart block (a heart irregularity); or a severely slow heartbeat, you should not take this medication.

### Special warnings about this medication
If you have had severe congestive heart failure in the past, Visken should be used with caution.

Visken should not be stopped suddenly. It can cause increased chest pain and heart attack. Dosage should be gradually reduced.

If you suffer from asthma, chronic bronchitis, emphysema, seasonal allergies or other bronchial conditions, coronary artery disease, or kidney or liver disease, this medication should be used with caution.

Ask your doctor if you should check your pulse while taking Visken. This medication can cause your heartbeat to become too slow.

This medication may mask the symptoms of low blood sugar in diabetics or alter blood sugar levels. If you are diabetic, discuss this with your doctor.

Visken may cause you to become disoriented. If it has this effect on you, driving or operating dangerous machinery or participating in any hazardous activity that requires full mental alertness is not recommended.

If you have a history of severe allergic reactions, inform your doctor before taking Visken.

Notify your doctor or dentist that you are taking Visken if you have a medical emergency and before you have surgery or dental treatment.

### Possible food and drug interactions when taking this medication
If Visken is taken with certain other drugs, the effects of either could be increased, decreased, or altered. It is especially important to check with your doctor before combining Visken with the following:

Airway-opening drugs such as Proventil and Ventolin
Blood pressure drugs such as reserpine
Digoxin (Lanoxin)
Epinephrine (EpiPen)
Hydrochlorothiazide (HydroDIURIL)
Insulin or oral antidiabetic agents such as Micronase
Nonsteroidal anti-inflammatory drugs such as Motrin
Ritodrine (Yutopar)
Theophylline (Theo-Dur, others)
Thioridazine (Mellaril)
Verapamil (Calan, Verelan)

### Special information if you are pregnant or breastfeeding
The effects of Visken during pregnancy have not been adequately studied. If you are pregnant or plan to become pregnant, inform your doctor immediately. Visken appears in breast milk and could affect a nursing infant. If this medication is essential to your health, your doctor may advise you to discontinue breastfeeding until your treatment with this medication is finished.

### Recommended dosage
ADULTS

Your doctor will determine the dosage according to your specific needs.

The usual starting dose is 5 milligrams, 2 times per day, alone or with other high blood pressure medication. Your blood pressure should be lower in

1 to 2 weeks. If blood pressure is not reduced sufficiently within 3 to 4 weeks, your doctor may increase your total daily dosage by 10 milligrams at a time, at 3 to 4 week intervals, up to a maximum of 60 milligrams a day.

CHILDREN

The safety and effectiveness of Visken have not been established in children.

ELDERLY

The doctor will determine dosage for an elderly individual based on his or her particular needs.

### Overdosage

Any medication taken in excess can have serious consequences. If you suspect an overdose, seek medical attention immediately.

■ *Symptoms of Visken overdose may include:*
Bronchospasm (spasm of the air passages), excessively slow heartbeat, heart failure, low blood pressure

---

*Brand name:*

# Vistaril

*See Atarax, page 38.*

---

*Generic name:*

# Vitamins with Fluoride

*See Poly-Vi-Flor, page 424.*

---

*Brand name:*

# Volmax Extended-Release Tablets

*See Proventil, page 446.*

---

*Brand name:*

# Voltaren

*Pronounced: vol-TAR-en*
*Generic name: Diclofenac sodium*
*Other brand name: Cataflam (Diclofenac Potassium)*

### Why is this drug prescribed?

Voltaren and Cataflam, nonsteroidal anti-inflammatory drugs, are used to relieve the inflammation, swelling, stiffness, and joint pain associated with rheumatoid arthritis, osteoarthritis (the most common form of arthritis), and ankylosing spondylitis (arthritis and stiffness of the spine). Cataflam is also used in the treatment of menstrual pain.

### Most important fact about this drug

You should have frequent checkups with your doctor if you take Voltaren regularly. Ulcers or internal bleeding can occur without warning.

### How should you take this medication?

To minimize stomach upset and related side effects, your doctor may recommend taking this medicine with food, milk, or an antacid. However, this may delay onset of relief.

Take this drug with a full glass of water. Also, do not lie down for about 20 minutes after taking it. This will help to prevent irritation in your upper digestive tract.

Take this medication exactly as prescribed.

■ *If you miss a dose...*
If you take this medicine on a regular schedule, take it as soon as you remember. If it is almost time for your next dose, skip the one you missed and go back to your regular schedule. Do not take 2 doses at once.
■ *Storage instructions...*
Store at room temperature. Keep the container tightly closed and protect from moisture.

### What side effects may occur?

Side effects cannot be anticipated. If any develop or change in intensity, inform your doctor as soon as possible. Only your doctor can determine if it is safe for you to continue taking Voltaren.

■ *More common side effects may include:*
Abdominal pain or cramps, constipation, diarrhea, dizziness, headache, indigestion, nausea
■ *Less common side effects may include:*
Abdominal bleeding, abdominal swelling, fluid retention, gas, itching, peptic ulcers, rash, ringing in the ears
■ *Rare side effects may include:*
Anaphylaxis (severe allergic reaction), anemia, anxiety, appetite change, asthma, black stools, blood disorders, bloody diarrhea, blurred vision, changes in taste, colitis, congestive heart failure, decrease in white blood cells, decreased urine production, depression, double vision, drowsi-

ness, dry mouth, hair loss, hearing loss (temporary), hepatitis, high blood pressure, hives, inability to sleep, inflammation of mouth, irritability, kidney failure, low blood pressure, nosebleed, red or purple skin discoloration and itching, sensitivity to light, skin eruptions and inflammation, scaling, or peeling, Stevens-Johnson syndrome (a severe form of skin eruption), swelling of eyelids, lips, and tongue, swelling of the throat due to fluid retention, vague feeling of illness, vision changes, vomiting, yellow eyes and skin

## Why should this drug not be prescribed?

If you are sensitive to or have ever had an allergic reaction to Voltaren or Cataflam, or if you have had asthma attacks, hives, or other allergic reactions caused by aspirin or other nonsteroidal anti-inflammatory drugs, you should not take this medication. Make sure your doctor is aware of any drug reactions you have experienced.

## Special warnings about this medication

Remember this medication has been known to cause peptic ulcers and bleeding. Contact your doctor immediately if you suspect a problem.

This drug should be used with caution if you have heart failure, kidney problems, or liver disease, and it can cause liver inflammation in some people.

If you are taking blood-thinning medication or diuretics, use this drug with caution.

Use with caution if you have heart disease or high blood pressure. This drug can increase water retention.

If you experience nausea, fatigue, lethargy, itching, yellowed eyes and skin, tenderness in the upper right area of your abdomen, or flu-like symptoms, notify your doctor at once.

## Possible food and drug interactions when taking this medication

If Voltaren or Cataflam are taken with certain other drugs, the effects of either could be increased, decreased, or altered. It is especially important to check with your doctor before combining Voltaren with the following:

Aspirin
Blood thinners such as Coumadin
Carteolol (Cartrol)
Cyclosporine (Sandimmune)

Digitalis drugs such as Lanoxin
Diuretics such as Dyazide, Midamor, and Lasix
Insulin or oral antidiabetes medications such as
 Micronase
Lithium (Lithonate)
Methotrexate

## Special information
## if you are pregnant or breastfeeding

The effects of Voltaren during pregnancy have not been adequately studied. If you are pregnant or plan to become pregnant, inform your doctor immediately. Voltaren appears in breast milk and could affect a nursing infant. If this medication is essential to your health, your doctor may advise you to discontinue breastfeeding until your treatment with Voltaren is finished.

## Recommended dosage

ADULTS

*Osteoarthritis*

The usual dose is 100 to 150 milligrams a day, divided into smaller doses of 50 milligrams 2 or 3 times a day (for Voltaren or Cataflam) or 75 milligrams twice a day (for Voltaren).

*Rheumatoid Arthritis*

The usual dose is 150 to 200 milligrams a day, divided into smaller doses of 50 milligrams 3 or 4 times a day (for Voltaren or Cataflam) or 75 milligrams twice a day (for Voltaren).

People with rheumatoid arthritis should not take more than 225 milligrams a day.

*Ankylosing Spondylitis*

The usual dose is 100 to 125 milligrams a day, divided into smaller doses of 25 milligrams 4 times a day, with another 25 milligrams at bedtime if necessary.

*Menstrual pain and discomfort*

The usual starting dose of Cataflam is 50 milligrams 3 times a day, although some women will take 100 milligrams for the first dose, followed by 50-milligram doses. After the first day, you should not take more than 150 milligrams in a day.

CHILDREN

The safety and effectiveness of Voltaren have not been established in children.

## Overdosage

Any medication taken in excess can have serious consequences. If you suspect an overdose, seek medical attention immediately.

■ *The symptoms of Voltaren overdose may include:*
Acute kidney failure, drowsiness, loss of consciousness, lung inflammation, vomiting

*Generic name:*

# Warfarin

*See Coumadin, page 118.*

*Brand name:*

# Wellbutrin

*Pronounced: Well-BEW-trin*
*Generic name: Bupropion hydrochloride*

## Why is this drug prescribed?

Wellbutrin, a relatively new antidepressant medication, is given to help relieve certain kinds of major depression.

Major depression involves a severely depressed mood (for 2 weeks or more) accompanied by sleep and appetite disturbances, agitation or lack of energy, feelings of guilt or worthlessness, decreased sex drive, inability to concentrate, and perhaps thoughts of suicide.

Unlike the more familiar tricyclic antidepressants, such as Elavil, Tofranil, and others, Wellbutrin tends to have a somewhat stimulating effect.

## Most important fact about this drug

Although Wellbutrin occasionally causes weight gain, a more common effect is weight loss: Some 28 percent of people who take this medication lose 5 pounds or more. If depression has already caused you to lose weight, and if further weight loss would be detrimental to your health, Wellbutrin may not be the best antidepressant for you.

## How should you take this medication?

Take Wellbutrin exactly as prescribed by your doctor. The usual dosing regimen is 3 equal doses spaced evenly throughout the day. Allow at least 6 hours between doses. Your doctor will probably start you at a low dosage and gradually increase it; this helps minimize side effects.

Since Wellbutrin may impair your coordination or judgment, do not drive or operate dangerous machinery until you find out how the medication affects you.

If Wellbutrin works for you, your doctor will probably have you continue taking it for at least several months.

Avoid alcoholic beverages.

■ *If you miss a dose...*
Take it as soon as you remember. If it is within 4 hours of your next dose, skip the one you missed and go back to your regular schedule. Never take 2 doses at the same time.

■ *Storage instructions...*
Store at room temperature. Protect from light and moisture.

## What side effects may occur?

Side effects cannot be anticipated. If any develop or change in intensity, inform your doctor as soon as possible. Only your doctor can determine if it is safe for you to continue taking Wellbutrin.

Seizures are perhaps the most worrisome side effect.

■ *More common side effects may include:*
Agitation, constipation, dizziness, dry mouth, excessive sweating, headache, nausea, vomiting, skin rash, sleep disturbances, tremor

■ *Other side effects may include:*
Acne, bed-wetting, blisters in the mouth and eyes (Stevens-Johnson syndrome), blurred vision, breathing difficulty, chest pain, chills, complete or almost complete loss of movement, confusion, dry skin, episodes of over-activity, elation, or irritability, extreme calmness, fatigue, fever, fluid retention, flu-like symptoms, gum irritation and inflammation, hair color changes, hair loss, hives, impotence, incoordination and clumsiness, indigestion, itching, increased libido, menstrual complaints, mood instability, muscle rigidity, painful ejaculation, painful erection, retarded ejaculation, ringing in the ears, sexual dysfunction, suicidal ideation, thirst disturbances, toothache, urinary disturbances, weight gain or loss

## Why should this drug not be prescribed?

Do not take Wellbutrin if you are sensitive to or have ever had an allergic reaction to it.

Since Wellbutrin causes seizures in some people, do not take it if you have any type of seizure disorder.

You should not take Wellbutrin if you currently have, or formerly had, an eating disorder. For some reason, people with a history of anorexia nervosa or bulimia seem to be more likely to experience Wellbutrin-related seizures.

Do not take Wellbutrin if, within the past 14 days, you have taken a monoamine oxidase inhibitor (MAO inhibitor) type of antidepressant, such as Nardil or Parnate. This particular drug combination could cause you to experience a sudden, dangerous rise in blood pressure.

### Special warnings about this medication

If you take Wellbutrin, you may be vulnerable to seizures if your dosage is too high or if you ever suffered brain damage or experienced seizures in the past.

Do not take other medications that might help trigger seizures (e.g., antipsychotics, other antidepressants).

If you have been taking Valium or a similar tranquilizer but are ready to stop, taper off gradually rather than quitting abruptly.

### Possible food and drug interactions when taking this medication

Do not drink alcohol while you are taking Wellbutrin; an interaction between alcohol and Wellbutrin could increase the possibility of a seizure.

If Wellbutrin is taken with certain other drugs, the effects of either could be increased, decreased, or altered. It is especially important to check with your doctor before combining Wellbutrin with the following:

Dilantin
Levodopa (Larodopa)
Major Tranquilizers such as Thorazine and Mellaril
MAO inhibitors (antidepressants such as Parnate and Nardil)
Other antidepressants such as Elavil and Tofranil
Phenobarbital (Luminal)
Tagamet
Tegretol

### Special information if you are pregnant or breastfeeding

If you are pregnant or plan to become pregnant, notify your doctor immediately. Wellbutrin should be taken during pregnancy only if clearly needed.

Wellbutrin may pass into breast milk and cause serious reactions in a nursing baby; therefore, if you are a new mother, you may need to discontinue breastfeeding while you are taking this medication.

### Recommended dosage

No single dose of Wellbutrin should exceed 150 milligrams.

ADULTS

At the beginning, your dose will probably be 200 milligrams per day, taken as 100 milligrams 2 times a day. After at least 3 days at this dose, your doctor may increase the dosage to 300 milligrams per day, taken as 100 milligrams 3 times a day, with at least 6 hours between doses. This is the usual adult dose. The maximum recommended dosage is 450 milligrams per day taken in doses of no more than 150 milligrams each.

CHILDREN

The safety and effectiveness in children under 18 years old have not been established.

OLDER ADULTS

Because they are more sensitive to antidepressant drugs, older people may find smaller doses satisfactory.

### Overdosage

Any medication taken in excess can have serious consequences. If you suspect an overdose of Wellbutrin, seek medical attention immediately.

■ *Symptoms of Wellbutrin overdose may include:*
 Hallucinations, heart failure, loss of consciousness, rapid heartbeat, seizures
■ *An overdose that involves other drugs in combination with Wellbutrin may also cause these symptoms:*
 Breathing difficulties, coma, fever, rigid muscles, stupor

*Brand name:*

# Wymox

*See Amoxil, page 22.*

*Brand name:*

# Wytensin

*Pronounced: why-TEN-sin*
*Generic name: Guanabenz acetate*

### Why is this drug prescribed?

Wytensin is used in the treatment of high blood pressure. It is effective used alone or in combination with a thiazide type of diuretic. Wytensin begins to lower blood pressure within 60 minutes after taking a single dose and may slow your pulse rate slightly.

### Most important fact about this drug

You must take Wytensin regularly for it to be effective. Since blood pressure declines gradually, it may be several weeks before you get the full benefit of Wytensin; and you must continue taking it even if you are feeling well. Wytensin does not cure high blood pressure; it merely keeps it under control.

### How should you take this medication?

Wytensin may be taken with or without food. Take it exactly as prescribed.

■ *If you miss a dose...*
Take it as soon as you remember. If it is almost time for the next dose, skip the one you missed and go back to your regular schedule. Do not take 2 doses at the same time. If you forget the medication 2 or more times in a row, contact your doctor.

■ *Storage instructions...*
Store at room temperature, in a tightly closed container, away from light.

### What side effects may occur?

Side effects cannot be anticipated. If any develop or change in intensity, inform your doctor as soon as possible. Only your doctor can determine if it is safe for you to continue taking Wytensin.

■ *More common side effects may include:*
Dizziness, drowsiness, dry mouth, headache, weakness

■ *Less common side effects may include:*
Abdominal discomfort, aches in arms and legs, anxiety, blurred vision, breast development in males, changes in taste, chest pain, constipation, decreased sex drive, depression, diarrhea, fluid retention, frequent urination, impotence, irregular heartbeat, itching, lack of muscle coordination, muscle aches, nausea, pounding heartbeat, rash, shortness of breath, sleep disturbances, stomach pain, stuffy nose, vomiting

■ *Rare side effects may include:*
Heartbeat irregularities

### Why should this drug not be prescribed?

Do not take Wytensin if you are sensitive to it or have ever had an allergic reaction to it.

### Special warnings about this medication

Wytensin can make you drowsy or less alert. Driving or operating dangerous machinery or participating in any hazardous activity that requires full mental alertness is not recommended until you know how this drug affects you.

If you have severe heart disease, stroke or related disorders, or severe liver or kidney failure, or if you have recently had a heart attack, this drug should be used with caution.

Your doctor will monitor your blood pressure if you have disorders of the kidney or liver.

### Possible food and drug interactions when taking this medication

Wytensin may intensify the effects of alcohol. Use of alcohol should be avoided.

If Wytensin is taken with certain other drugs, the effects of either could be increased, decreased, or altered. It is especially important to check with your doctor before combining Wytensin with the following:

Antihistamines such as Benadryl, Clor-Trimeton, and Tavist
Drugs that depress the central nervous system such as Halcion, Valium, and phenobarbital

### Special information if you are pregnant or breastfeeding

The effects of Wytensin during pregnancy have not been adequately studied, but it may affect the fetus. If you are pregnant or plan to become pregnant, inform your doctor immediately. Wytensin may appear in breast milk and could affect a nursing infant. If this medication is essential to your health, your doctor may advise you to discontinue breastfeeding until your treatment is finished.

### Recommended dosage

ADULTS

Your doctor will adjust the dosage of this medication to meet your individual needs.

The usual starting dose is 4 milligrams 2 times per day, whether Wytensin is used alone or with a thiazide type of diuretic.

Your doctor may increase the dosage in increments of 4 to 8 milligrams per day every 1 to 2 weeks, depending on your response.

The maximum reported dose has been 32 milligrams twice daily, but doses as high as this are rarely needed.

CHILDREN

The safety and effectiveness of this drug have not been established in children under 12 years of age.

OLDER ADULTS

Older adults should use this drug with caution.

## Overdosage

Any medication taken in excess can have serious consequences. If you suspect an overdose, seek medical attention immediately.

■ *Symptoms of Wytensin overdose may include:*
Excessive contraction of the pupils, irritability, low blood pressure, sleepiness, slow heartbeat, sluggishness

*Brand name:*

# Xanax

*Pronounced: ZAN-ax*
*Generic name: Alprazolam*

## Why is this drug prescribed?

Xanax is a tranquilizer used in the short-term relief of symptoms of anxiety or the treatment of anxiety disorders. Anxiety disorder is marked by unrealistic worry or excessive fears and concerns.

Xanax is also used in the treatment of panic disorder, which appears as unexpected panic attacks and may be accompanied by a fear of open spaces called agoraphobia. Only your doctor can diagnose panic disorder and best advise you about treatment. Anxiety associated with depression is also responsive to Xanax.

Some doctors prescribe Xanax to treat alcohol withdrawal, fear of open spaces and strangers, depression, irritable bowel syndrome, and premenstrual syndrome.

## Most important fact about this drug

Tolerance and dependence can occur with the use of Xanax. You may experience withdrawal symptoms if you stop using the drug abruptly. Only your doctor should advise you to discontinue or change your dose.

## How should you take this medication?

Xanax may be taken with or without food. Take it exactly as prescribed.

■ *If you miss a dose...*
If you are less than 1 hour late, take it as soon as you remember. Otherwise skip the dose and go back to your regular schedule. Never take 2 doses at the same time.
■ *Storage instructions...*
Store Xanax at room temperature.

## What side effects may occur?

Side effects cannot be anticipated. If any develop or change in intensity, inform your doctor as soon as possible. Only your doctor can determine if it is safe for you to continue taking Xanax. Your doctor should periodically reassess the need for this drug.

Side effects to Xanax are usually seen at the beginning of treatment and disappear with continued medication. However, if dosage is increased, side effects will be more likely.

■ *More common side effects may include:*
Abdominal discomfort, abnormal involuntary movement, agitation, allergies, anxiety, blurred vision, chest pain, confusion, constipation, decreased or increased sex drive, depression, diarrhea, difficult urination, dream abnormalities, drowsiness, dry mouth, fainting, fatigue, fluid retention, headache, hyperventilation (too frequent or too deep breathing), inability to fall asleep, increase or decrease in appetite, increased or decreased salivation, impaired memory, irritability, lack of coordination, light-headedness, low blood pressure, menstrual problems, muscular twitching, nausea and vomiting, nervousness, palpitations, rapid heartbeat, rash, restlessness, ringing in the ears, sexual dysfunction, skin inflammation, speech difficulties, stiffness, stuffy nose, sweating, tiredness/sleepiness, tremors, upper respiratory infections, weakness, weight gain or loss
■ *Less common or rare side effects may include:*
Abnormal muscle tone, concentration difficulties, decreased coordination, dizziness, double vision,

fear, hallucinations, inability to control urination or bowel movements, infection, itching, loss of appetite, muscle cramps, muscle spasticity, rage, sedation, seizures, sleep disturbances, slurred speech, stimulation, talkativeness, taste alterations, temporary memory loss, tingling or pins and needles, uninhibited behavior, urine retention, warm feeling, weakness in muscle and bone, weight gain or loss, yellow eyes and skin

■ *Side effects due to decrease or withdrawal from Xanax:*
Blurred vision, decreased concentration, decreased mental clarity, diarrhea, heightened awareness of noise or bright lights, impaired sense of smell, loss of appetite, loss of weight, muscle cramps, seizures, tingling sensation, twitching

### Why should this drug not be prescribed?

If you are sensitive to or have ever had an allergic reaction to Xanax or other tranquilizers, you should not take this medication. Make sure that your doctor is aware of any drug reactions that you have experienced.

Do not take this medication if you have been diagnosed with the eye condition called narrow-angle glaucoma.

Anxiety or tension related to everyday stress usually does not require treatment with Xanax. Discuss your symptoms thoroughly with your doctor.

### Special warnings about this medication

Xanax may cause you to become drowsy or less alert; therefore, driving or operating dangerous machinery or participating in any hazardous activity that requires full mental alertness is not recommended.

If you are being treated for panic disorder, you may need to take a higher dose of Xanax than for anxiety alone. High doses of this medication taken for long intervals may cause emotional and physical dependence. It is important that your doctor supervise you carefully when you are using this medication.

Remember that withdrawal symptoms can occur when Xanax is stopped suddenly.

### Possible food and drug interactions when taking this medication

Xanax may intensify the effect of alcohol. Do not drink alcohol while taking this medication.

If Xanax is taken with certain other drugs, the effects of either could be increased, decreased, or altered. It is important to check with your doctor before combining Xanax with the following:

Antihistamines such as Benadryl and Tavist
Carbamazepine (Tegretol)
Certain antidepressant drugs, including Elavil, Norpramin, and Tofranil
Cimetidine (Tagamet)
Digoxin (Lanoxin)
Disulfiram (Antabuse)
Major tranquilizers such as Mellaril and Thorazine
Oral contraceptives
Other central nervous system depressants such as Valium and Demerol

### Special information if you are pregnant or breastfeeding

Do not take this medication if you are pregnant or planning to become pregnant. There is an increased risk of respiratory problems and muscular weakness in your baby. Infants may also experience withdrawal symptoms. Xanax may appear in breast milk and could affect a nursing infant. If this medication is essential to your health, your doctor may advise you to stop breastfeeding until your treatment with this medication is finished.

### Recommended dosage

ADULTS

*Anxiety disorder*
The usual starting dose of Xanax is 0.25 to 0.5 milligram taken 3 times a day. The dose may be increased every 3 to 4 days to a maximum daily dose of 4 milligrams, divided into smaller doses.

*Panic disorder*
You may be given a dose from 1 up to a total of 10 milligrams, according to your needs. The typical dose is 5 to 6 milligrams a day.

The usual starting dose is 0.5 milligram 3 times a day. This dose can be increased by 1 milligram a day every 3 or 4 days.

CHILDREN

Safety and effectiveness have not been established in children under 18 years of age.

OLDER ADULTS

The usual starting dose for an anxiety disorder is 0.25 milligram, 2 or 3 times daily. This dose may be gradually increased if needed and tolerated.

## Overdosage

Any medication taken in excess can have serious consequences. If you suspect an overdose, seek medical attention immediately.

■ *Symptoms of Xanax overdose may include:*
Confusion, coma, impaired coordination, sleepiness, slowed reaction time

An overdose of Xanax, alone or after combining it with alcohol, can be fatal.

*Brand name:*

# Yocon

*Pronounced: YOE-kon*
*Generic name: Yohimbine hydrochloride*
*Other brand name: Yohimex*

## Why is this drug prescribed?

Yocon is used in the treatment of male impotence. The drug is thought to work by stimulating the release of norepinephrine, one of the body's natural chemical regulators. This results in increased blood flow to the penis.

## Most important fact about this drug

Yocon does not work for all men. Your doctor will determine if Yocon can be prescribed for you.

## How should you take this medication?

Take this medication exactly as prescribed.

■ *If you miss a dose...*
Take it as soon as you remember. If it is almost time for your next dose, skip the one you missed and go back to your regular schedule. Never take 2 doses at the same time.

■ *Storage instructions...*
Keep this medication in the container it came in, tightly closed, and out of the reach of children. Store it at room temperature, away from moist places and direct light.

## What side effects may occur?

Side effects cannot be anticipated. If any develop or change in intensity, inform your doctor as soon as possible. Only your doctor can determine if it is safe for you to continue taking Yocon.

■ *Side effects may include:*
Decreased urination, dizziness, flushing, headache, increase in blood pressure, increased heart rate, increased motor activity, irritability, nausea, nervousness, tremor

## Why should this drug not be prescribed?

Yocon should not be used if you have kidney disease, or if you are sensitive to or have ever had an allergic reaction to yohimbine. Make sure your doctor is aware of any drug reactions you have experienced.

## Special warnings about this medication

Yocon is generally not recommended for use by children, the elderly, or men with heart and kidney disease who also have a history of stomach or duodenal ulcer. The drug is also not recommended for men being treated for a psychiatric disorder.

## Possible food and drug interactions when taking this medication

It is important that you consult with your doctor before taking Yocon with drugs for depression such as Elavil or other drugs that change mood.

## Special information if you are pregnant or breastfeeding

Yocon is not recommended for use in women generally and certainly must not be used during pregnancy.

## Recommended dosage

ADULTS

Dosages of this drug are based on experimental research in the treatment of male impotence.

This dosage is one 5.4-milligram tablet, 3 times a day.

If you experience nausea, dizziness, or nervousness, your doctor will reduce the dose to one-half tablet 3 times a day, and then increase it gradually back up to 1 tablet 3 times a day.

CHILDREN

This drug is not for use in children.

OLDER ADULTS

This drug should not be used by older men.

## Overdosage

Any medication taken in excess can cause symptoms of overdose. If you suspect an overdose, seek medical attention immediately. No specific symptoms of Yocon overdose have been reported.

Generic name:

# Yohimbine

*See Yocon, page 597.*

Brand name:

# Yohimex

*See Yocon, page 597.*

Brand name:

# Zantac

Pronounced: ZAN-tac
Generic name: Ranitidine hydrochloride

## Why is this drug prescribed?

Zantac is prescribed for the short-term treatment (4 to 8 weeks) of active duodenal ulcer and active benign gastric ulcer, and as maintenance therapy for gastric or duodenal ulcer, at a reduced dosage, after the ulcer has healed. It is also used for the treatment of conditions in which the stomach produces too much acid, such as Zollinger-Ellison syndrome and systemic mastocytosis, for gastro-esophageal reflux disease (backflow of acid stomach contents) and for healing—and maintaining healing of—erosive esophagitis (severe inflammation of the esophagus).

Some doctors prescribe Zantac to prevent damage to the stomach and duodenum from long-term use of nonsteroidal anti-inflammatory drugs such as Indocin and Motrin, and to treat bleeding of the stomach and intestine. Zantac is also sometimes prescribed for stress-induced ulcers.

## Most important fact about this drug

Zantac helps to prevent the recurrence of gastric or duodenal ulcers and aids the healing of ulcers that do occur.

## How should you take this medication?

Take this medication exactly as prescribed by your doctor. Make sure you follow the diet your doctor recommends.

Dissolve "Efferdose" tablets and granules in 6 to 8 ounces of water before taking them.

You can take an antacid for pain while you are taking Zantac.

■ *If you miss a dose...*
Take it as soon as you remember. If it is almost time for your next dose, skip the one you missed and go back to your regular schedule. Never take 2 doses at the same time.

■ *Storage instructions...*
Store this medication at room temperature in the container it came in, tightly closed and away from moist places and direct light. Keep Zantac Syrup from freezing.

## What side effects may occur?

Side effects cannot be anticipated. If any develop or change in intensity, inform your doctor as soon as possible. Only your doctor can determine if it is safe for you to continue taking Zantac.

■ *More common side effects may include:*
Headache, sometimes severe

■ *Less common or rare side effects may include:*
Abdominal discomfort and pain, agitation, changes in blood count (anemia), changes in liver function, constipation, depression, diarrhea, difficulty sleeping, dizziness, hair loss, hallucinations, heart block, hepatitis, hypersensitivity reactions, inflammation of the pancreas, involuntary movements, irregular heartbeat, joint pain, muscle pain, nausea and vomiting, rapid heartbeat, rash, reduced white blood cells, reversible mental confusion, sleepiness, slow heartbeat, vague feeling of bodily discomfort, vertigo, yellow eyes and skin

## Why should this drug not be prescribed?

If you are sensitive to or have ever had an allergic reaction to Zantac or similar drugs such as Tagamet, you should not take this medication. Make sure that your doctor is aware of any drug reactions that you have experienced.

## Special warnings about this medication

A stomach malignancy could be present, even if your symptoms have been relieved by Zantac.

If you have kidney or liver disease, this drug should be used with caution.

If you have phenylketonuria, you should be aware that the "Efferdose" tablets and granules contain phenylalanine.

## Possible food and drug interactions when taking this medication

If Zantac is taken with certain other drugs, the effects of either could be increased, decreased, or altered. It is especially important to check with your doctor before combining Zantac with the following:

Alcohol
Blood-thinning drugs such as Coumadin
Glipizide (Glucotrol)
Glyburide (DiaBeta, Micronase)
Itraconazole (Sporanox)
Ketoconazole (Nizoral)
Metoprolol (Lopressor)
Midazolam (Versed)
Nifedipine (Procardia)
Phenytoin (Dilantin)
Procainamide (Procan SR)
Sucralfate (Carafate)
Theophylline (Theo-Dur)

## Special information
## if you are pregnant or breastfeeding

The effects of Zantac in pregnancy have not been adequately studied. If you are pregnant or plan to become pregnant, inform your doctor immediately. Zantac appears in breast milk and could affect a nursing infant. If this medication is essential to your health, your doctor may advise you to discontinue breastfeeding until your treatment with this medication is finished.

## Recommended dosage

### ADULTS

*Active Duodenal Ulcer*
The usual starting dose is 150 milligrams 2 times a day or 10 milliliters (2 teaspoonfuls) 2 times a day. Your doctor also might prescribe 300 milligrams or 20 milliliters (4 teaspoonfuls) once a day, after the evening meal or at bedtime, if necessary for your convenience. The dose should be the lowest effective dose. Long-term use should be reduced to a daily total of 150 milligrams or 10 milliliters (2 teaspoonfuls), taken at bedtime.

*Other Excess Acid Conditions (such as Zollinger-Ellison Syndrome)*
The usual dose is 150 milligrams or 10 milliliters (2 teaspoonfuls) 2 times a day. This dose can be adjusted upwards by your doctor.

*Benign Gastric Ulcer and Gastroesophageal Reflux Disease (GERD)*
The usual dose is 150 milligrams or 10 milliliters (2 teaspoonfuls) 2 times a day. To maintain healing of gastric ulcer, this dose is taken once a day at bedtime.

*Erosive Esophagitis*
The usual dose is 150 milligrams or 10 milliliters (2 teaspoonfuls) 4 times a day. Maintenance dosage is 150 milligrams or 10 milliliters (2 teaspoonfuls) twice a day.

### CHILDREN

The safety and effectiveness of Zantac have not been established in children.

## Overdosage

Any medication taken in excess can have serious consequences. If you suspect an overdose, seek medical attention immediately.

Information concerning Zantac overdosage is limited. However, an abnormal manner of walking, low blood pressure, and exaggerated side effect symptoms may be signs of an overdose.

If you experience any of these symptoms, notify your doctor immediately.

*Brand name:*

# Zaroxolyn

*Pronounced: Zar-OX-uh-lin*
*Generic name: Metolazone*
*Other brand name: Mykrox*

## Why is this drug prescribed?

Zaroxolyn is a diuretic used in the treatment of high blood pressure and other conditions that require the elimination of excess fluid from the body. These conditions include congestive heart failure and kidney disease. When used for high blood pressure, Zaroxolyn can be used alone or with other high blood pressure medications. Diuretics prompt your body to produce and eliminate more urine, which helps lower blood pressure.

Zaroxolyn is also occasionally prescribed for kidney stones.

## Most important fact about this drug

If you have high blood pressure, you must take Zaroxolyn regularly for it to be effective. Since blood pressure declines gradually, it may be several weeks before you get the full benefit of Zaroxolyn; and you must continue taking it even if you are feeling well. Zaroxolyn does not cure high blood pressure; it merely keeps it under control.

## How should you take this medication?

Take Zaroxolyn exactly as prescribed. Stopping Zaroxolyn suddenly could cause your condition to worsen.

■ *If you miss a dose...*

Take it as soon as you remember. If it is almost time for the next dose, skip the one you missed and go back to your regular schedule. Do not take 2 doses at the same time.

■ *Storage instructions...*

Store at room temperature in a tightly closed, light-resistant container.

## What side effects may occur?

Side effects cannot be anticipated. If any develop or change in intensity, inform your doctor as soon as possible. Only your doctor can determine if it is safe for you to continue taking Zaroxolyn.

■ *Side effects may include:*

Anemia, bloating of the abdomen, blood clots, blurred vision, chest pain, chills, constipation, depression, diarrhea, dizziness on standing up, dizziness or light-headedness, drowsiness, fainting, fatigue, gout, headache, hepatitis, high blood sugar, hives, impotence, inflammation of the skin, inflammation of the pancreas, joint pain, loss of appetite, low potassium levels (leading to dry mouth, excessive thirst, weak or irregular heartbeat, or muscle pain or cramps), muscle spasms or cramps, nausea, rapid, pounding heartbeat, rash, reddish or purplish spots on the skin, restlessness, sensitivity to light, sugar in the urine, tingling or pins and needles, upset stomach, vertigo, vomiting, weakness, yellow eyes and skin

## Why should this drug not be prescribed?

If you are unable to urinate or have severe liver disease, you should not take this medication.

If you are sensitive to or have ever had an allergic reaction to Zaroxolyn or other diuretics such as HydroDIURIL, you should not take this medication.

## Special warnings about this medication

Diuretics can cause your body to lose too much potassium. Signs of an excessively low potassium level include muscle weakness and rapid or irregular heartbeat. To boost your potassium level, your doctor may recommend eating potassium-rich foods or taking a potassium supplement.

If you are taking Zaroxolyn, your doctor will do a complete assessment of your kidney function and continue to monitor it.

Do not interchange Zaroxolyn and other formulations of metolazone such as Mykrox. The brands vary in potency of action.

If you have liver disease, diabetes, gout, or lupus erythematosus (a disease of the immune system), Zaroxolyn should be used with caution.

If you have had an allergic reaction to sulfa drugs, thiazides, or quinethazone, you may be at greater risk for an allergic reaction to this medication. You can have an allergic reaction to Zaroxolyn even if you have never had allergies or asthma.

Dehydration, excessive sweating, severe diarrhea, or vomiting could deplete your fluids and cause your blood pressure to become too low. Be careful when exercising and in hot weather.

Notify your doctor or dentist that you are taking Zaroxolyn if you have a medical emergency and before you have surgery or dental treatment.

## Possible food and drug interactions when taking this medication

Zaroxolyn may intensify the effects of alcohol. Avoid drinking alcohol while taking this medication.

If Zaroxolyn is taken with certain other drugs, the effects of either could be increased, decreased, or altered. It is especially important to check with your doctor before combining Zaroxolyn with the following:

ACTH
Antidiabetic drugs such as Micronase
Barbiturates such as phenobarbital
Corticosteroids such as prednisone (Deltasone)
Digitalis glycosides such as Lanoxin
Insulin
Lithium (Lithonate)
Loop diuretics such as furosemide (Lasix)
Methenamine (Mandelamine)
Narcotics such as Percocet
Nonsteroidal anti-inflammatory agents such as
    Advil, Motrin, and Naprosyn
Norepinephrine (Levophed)
Other high blood pressure medications such as
    Aldomet
Tubocurarine

## Special information
## if you are pregnant or breastfeeding

The effects of Zaroxolyn during pregnancy have not been adequately studied. If you are pregnant or plan to become pregnant, inform your doctor immediately. Zaroxolyn appears in breast milk and could affect a nursing infant. If this medication is essential to your health, your doctor may advise you to discontinue breastfeeding until your treatment is finished.

## Recommended dosage

### ADULTS

Your doctor will adjust the dosage of this medication to your individual needs and will use the lowest possible dose with the maximum effect. The time it takes for this medication to become effective varies from person to person, depending on the diagnosis.

Most starting doses of this medication will be given once a day.

*Edema Due to Heart or Kidney Disorders*
The usual dosage is 5 milligrams to 20 milligrams once a day.

*Mild to Moderate High Blood Pressure*
The usual dosage is 2.5 milligrams to 5 milligrams once a day.

### CHILDREN

The safety and effectiveness of Zaroxolyn in children have not been established.

## Overdosage

Any medication taken in excess can have serious consequences. If you suspect an overdose, seek medical attention immediately.

■ *Symptoms of Zaroxolyn overdose may include:*
Difficulty breathing, dizziness, dizziness on standing up, drowsiness, fainting, irritation of the stomach and intestines, lethargy leading to coma

*Brand name:*

# Zerit

*Pronounced: ZAIR-it*
*Generic name: Stavudine*

## Why is this drug prescribed?

Zerit is an antiviral drug in capsule form used to treat adults with human immunodeficiency virus (HIV) infection. HIV is the virus that causes the fatal disease AIDS, a breakdown of the immune system. Zerit is prescribed for adults with advanced HIV infection who have already taken other antiviral drugs such as Retrovir (zidovudine, AZT), and who either have not improved on them or have experienced serious side effects or allergic reactions.

## Most important fact about this drug

Zerit is not a cure for HIV infection or AIDS. At present, there is no evidence from studies that Zerit has increased the lifespan of people with HIV or lowered their risk of getting an opportunistic infection. (An opportunistic infection, such as a serious type of pneumonia called *Pneumocystis carinii* pneumonia, occurs only in people with a weak immune system.) People taking Zerit or any other antiviral drug may still develop infections or other complications of HIV infection. Consequently, if you are on Zerit, you should be closely monitored by your doctor and should see a doctor who is experienced in treating people with HIV infection.

## How should you take this medication?

Take this medication at regular 12-hour intervals, exactly as prescribed. You may take it with meals or in between.

■ *If you miss a dose...*
Take the forgotten dose as soon as you remember. If it is almost time for your next dose, skip the one you missed and go back to your regular schedule. Never take two doses at the same time.
■ *Storage instructions...*
Store at room temperature in a tightly closed container.

## What side effects may occur?

Side effects cannot be anticipated. If any develop or change in intensity, inform your doctor as soon as possible. Only your doctor can determine if it is safe for you to continue taking Zerit.

The major side effect associated with the use of Zerit is peripheral neuropathy, a usually temporary condition that causes numbness, tingling, burning, or pain in the feet or hands. If you develop peripheral neuropathy while taking Zerit, your doctor may take you off the drug, especially if your symptoms are severe. Sometimes, symptoms are temporarily worse when people stop taking Zerit.

■ *More common side effects may include:*
Abdominal pain, allergic reaction, anxiety, back pain, chest pain, chills and fever, confusion, conjunctivitis (pinkeye), constipation, depression, diarrhea, difficult or labored breathing, dizziness, flu-like symptoms, general feeling of illness, headache, hives, indigestion, inflammation and sores of the mouth, insomnia, itching, joint pain, loss of appetite, migraine, muscle pain, nausea, nervousness, pain, painful urination, pneumonia, rash, skin tumor, sweating, vision problems, vomiting, weakness, weight gain

■ *Less common or rare side effects may include:*
Asthma, blood in the urine, development of tumors, fainting, frequent urination, genital pain, high blood pressure, impotence, noncancerous skin tumors, painful menstruation, skin inflammation, sleepiness, tremors, vaginal inflammation

### Why should this drug not be prescribed?
If you are sensitive to or have ever had an allergic reaction to Zerit, you should not take this drug.

### Special warnings about this medication
Although Zerit attacks HIV in the bloodstream, people taking the drug can still transmit the virus to others. Zerit has not been shown to reduce the risk of transmitting HIV through sexual contact or exposure to blood.

### Possible food and drug interactions when taking this medication
No interactions have been reported.

### Special information if you are pregnant or breastfeeding
The effects of Zerit during pregnancy have not been adequately studied. Zerit should be used during pregnancy only if it is clearly needed. It is not known if Zerit appears in breast milk. Because it may affect a nursing infant, your doctor may instruct you not to breastfeed if you are taking Zerit.

### Recommended dosage
ADULTS

The recommended starting dose is based on body weight. If you weigh 132 pounds or more, it is 40 milligrams twice a day. If you weigh less than 132 pounds, it is 30 milligrams twice a day.

If your doctor has taken you off Zerit because you have developed peripheral neuropathy, he may start giving you the drug again when your symptoms go away. The recommended dose when resuming Zerit therapy is 20 milligrams twice a day for people weighing 132 pounds or more, and 15 milligrams twice a day for those weighing less.

Your doctor may also give you a lower dose of Zerit if you develop liver or kidney problems.

### Overdosage
Any medication taken in excess can have serious consequences. If you suspect an overdose, seek medical attention immediately.

■ *Symptoms of Zerit overdose may include:*
Peripheral neuropathy, problems with liver functions

*Brand name:*

# Zestoretic

*Pronounced: zest-or-ET-ik*
*Generic ingredients: Lisinopril,*
    *Hydrochlorothiazide*
*Other brand name: Prinzide*

### Why is this drug prescribed?
Zestoretic is used in the treatment of high blood pressure. It combines an ACE inhibitor drug with a diuretic. Lisinopril, the ACE inhibitor, works by limiting production of a substance that promotes salt and water retention in your body. Hydrochlorothiazide, a diuretic, prompts your body to produce and eliminate more urine, which helps in lowering blood pressure. Combination products such as Zestoretic are usually not prescribed until therapy is already under way.

### Most important fact about this drug
You must take Zestoretic regularly for it to be effective. Since blood pressure declines gradually, it may be several weeks before you get the full benefit of Zestoretic; and you must continue taking it even if you are feeling well. Zestoretic does not cure high blood pressure; it merely keeps it under control.

### How should you take this medication?
Zestoretic can be taken with or without food. Take it exactly as prescribed.

■ *If you miss a dose...*
Take the forgotten dose as soon as you remember. If it is almost time for your next dose, skip

the one you missed and go back to your regular schedule. Never take a double dose.

■ *Storage instructions...*
Zestoretic should be stored at room temperature. Keep the container tightly closed.

### What side effects may occur?
Side effects cannot be anticipated. If any develop or change in intensity, inform your doctor as soon as possible. Only your doctor can determine if it is safe for you to continue taking Zestoretic.

■ *More common side effects may include:*
Cough, dizziness, dizziness when standing up, fatigue, headache

■ *Less common side effects may include:*
Asthma, diarrhea, hair loss, impotence, indigestion, low blood pressure, muscle cramps, nausea, rash, tingling or pins and needles, upper respiratory infection, vomiting, weakness

■ *Rare side effects may include:*
Abdominal pain, anemia, arthritis, back pain, back strain, blurred vision, bronchitis, bruising, chest discomfort or pain, common cold, confusion, constipation, decreased sex drive, depression, difficulty breathing, difficulty falling or staying asleep, dry mouth, earache, excessive perspiration, fainting, fever, flu, flushing, foot pain, gas, general feeling of illness, gout, hay fever, heart attack, heartburn, heart rhythm disturbances, hepatitis, hives, itching, joint pain, knee pain, loss of appetite, lung congestion, muscle pain, muscle spasm, nervousness, palpitations, rapid heartbeat, red or purple areas on the skin, reduced urine output, restlessness, ringing in ears, sensitivity to light, shortness of breath, severe allergic reaction, shoulder pain, sinus inflammation, skin inflammation, sleepiness, sore throat, stomach and intestinal cramps, stroke, stuffy nose, swelling of the face, lips, tongue, throat, or arms and legs, trauma, urinary tract infection, vertigo, virus infection, vision abnormality in which objects have a yellowish hue, yellow eyes and skin

### Why should this drug not be prescribed?
If you are sensitive to or have ever had an allergic reaction to lisinopril or hydrochlorothiazide or if you are sensitive to other ACE inhibitor drugs such as Capoten or sulfa drugs such as Gantrisin, you should not take this medication. If you suffered angioedema (swelling of face, lips, tongue, throat, arms, or legs) during previous treatment with an ACE inhibitor, you should not take this medication; if you have ever developed angioedema for any reason, you run a higher risk of developing it while you are taking this kind of drug. You should also avoid Zestoretic if you are unable to urinate. Tell your doctor of all allergic reactions you have experienced.

### Special warnings about this medication
If you develop swelling of your face, lips, tongue, or throat, or of your arms and legs, or have difficulty swallowing or breathing, you should stop taking the drug and contact your doctor immediately. You may need emergency treatment.

Zestoretic may cause your blood pressure to become too low. If you feel light-headed, especially during the first few days of treatment, inform your doctor. If you actually faint, stop taking Zestoretic until you have consulted your doctor.

Do not use salt substitutes containing potassium without first consulting your doctor.

Excessive sweating, dehydration, severe diarrhea, or vomiting could cause you to lose too much water and cause your blood pressure to drop dangerously.

If you develop chest pain, a sore throat, or fever and chills, contact your doctor immediately. It could indicate a more serious illness.

Make sure the doctor knows if you have congestive heart failure, diabetes, liver disease, a history of allergy or bronchial asthma, or lupus erythematosus (an arthritis-like disease sometimes accompanied by rashes). Zestoretic should be used cautiously. If you have kidney disease, your doctor should monitor your kidney function regularly.

If you are undergoing desensitization to bee or wasp venom, Zestoretic may cause a severe allergic reaction.

This medication is not recommended for people on dialysis; severe allergic reactions have occurred.

If you notice a yellowish cast to your skin or eyes, stop taking Zestoretic and contact your doctor immediately.

If you are diabetic, your doctor will want to keep an eye on your blood sugar levels.

Make sure your doctor or dentist knows you are taking Zestoretic before undergoing surgery.

## Possible food and drug interactions when taking this medication

Zestoretic may intensify the effects of alcohol. Do not drink alcohol while taking this medication.

If Zestoretic is taken with certain other drugs, the effects of either could be increased, decreased, or altered. It is especially important to check with your doctor before combining Zestoretic with the following:

Barbiturates such as Nembutal and Seconal
Cholestyramine (Questran)
Colestipol (Colestid)
Corticosteroids such as prednisone
High blood pressure drugs such as Procardia XL and Aldomet
Indomethacin (Indocin)
Insulin
Lithium (Lithonate)
Narcotics such as Darvon and Dilaudid
Nonsteroidal anti-inflammatory drugs such as Naprosyn
Oral antidiabetic drugs such as Micronase
Potassium supplements such as K-Dur and Slow-K
Potassium-containing salt substitutes
Potassium-sparing diuretics such as Midamor

## Special information if you are pregnant or breastfeeding

During the second and third trimester, lisinopril can cause birth defects, prematurity, and death in the fetus and newborn. If you are pregnant or plan to become pregnant, contact your doctor immediately to discuss the potential hazard to your unborn child. Zestoretic may appear in breast milk and could affect a nursing infant. If this medication is essential to your health, your doctor may advise you to discontinue breastfeeding until your treatment with this medication is finished.

## Recommended dosage

### ADULTS

Dosages of this drug are always individualized. Your doctor will determine what works best for you. Dosages will also be modified and carefully monitored if you have reduced kidney function.

### CHILDREN

Safety and effectiveness in children have not been established.

## Overdosage

Any medication taken in excess can have serious consequences. If you suspect an overdose, seek medical treatment immediately.

■ *Symptoms of Zestoretic overdose may include:*
Dehydration, low blood pressure

*Brand name:*

# Zestril

*Pronounced: ZEST-rill*
*Generic name: Lisinopril*
*Other brand name: Prinivil*

## Why is this drug prescribed?

Lisinopril is used in the treatment of high blood pressure. It is effective when used alone or when combined with other high blood pressure medications. It may also be used with other medications in the treatment of heart failure.

Lisinopril is a type of drug called an ACE inhibitor. It works by reducing production of a substance that increases salt and water retention in your body.

## Most important fact about this drug

If you have high blood pressure, you must take lisinopril regularly for it to be effective. Since blood pressure declines gradually, it may be several weeks before you get the full benefit of lisinopril; and you must continue taking it even if you are feeling well. Lisinopril does not cure high blood pressure; it merely keeps it under control.

## How should you take this medication?

Lisinopril can be taken with or without food. Take it exactly as prescribed. Stopping lisinopril suddenly could cause your blood pressure to rise.

■ *If you miss a dose...*
Take the forgotten dose as soon as you remember. If it is almost time for your next dose, skip the one you missed and go back to your regular schedule. Never take 2 doses at the same time.

■ *Storage instructions...*
Store at room temperature, with the container sealed and dry. Avoid excessive heat or freezing cold.

## What side effects may occur?

Side effects cannot be anticipated. If any develop or change in intensity, inform your doctor as soon as

possible. Only your doctor can determine if it is safe for you to continue taking lisinopril.

■ *More common side effects may include:*
Abdominal pain, chest pain, common cold, cough, diarrhea, difficulty in breathing, dizziness, fatigue, headache, itching, low blood pressure, nausea, rash, respiratory infection, vomiting, weakness

■ *Less common or rare side effects may include:*
Anemia, arm pain, arthritis, asthma, back pain, blurred vision, breast pain, bronchitis, burning sensation, changes in heart rhythm, chills, confusion, constipation, coughing up blood, cramps in stomach/intestines, decreased sex drive, dehydration, depression, diabetes, difficult breathing at night, dizziness on standing, double vision, dry mouth, excessive sweating, fainting, feeling of illness, fever, flu, fluid retention, flushing, gas, gout, hair loss, heart attack, heartburn, hepatitis, hip pain, hives, impotence, inability to sleep or sleeping too much, incoordination, indigestion, inflamed stomach, intolerance of light, irregular heartbeat, irritability, joint pain, kidney failure, knee pain, leg pain, little or no urine, "little strokes", liver failure, loss of appetite, lung cancer, memory impairment, muscle pain or cramps, nasal congestion or inflammation, neck pain, nervousness, nosebleed, numbness or tingling, painful breathing, painful urination, pelvic pain, pneumonia, prickling or burning sensation, rapid or fluttery heartbeat, rash, reddening of skin, ringing in ears, runny nose, sensitivity to light, severe allergic reactions, skin eruptions, shoulder pain, sinus inflammation, sleepiness, sore throat, spasm, stroke, sweating, swelling of face or arms and legs, thigh pain, tremor, upset stomach, urinary tract infection, vertigo, virus infection, vision changes, weight loss or gain, wheezing, yellow eyes and skin

### Why should this drug not be prescribed?

If you are sensitive to or have ever had an allergic reaction to lisinopril or other ACE inhibitors, you should not take this medication. Make sure your doctor is aware of any drug reactions you have experienced.

### Special warnings about this medication

If you develop swelling of your face, lips, tongue, or throat, or of your arms and legs, or have difficulty swallowing or breathing, you should contact your doctor immediately. You may need emergency treatment.

If you are being given bee or wasp venom to guard against future reactions, you may have a severe reaction to lisinopril.

If you have kidney disorder or connective tissue disease such as lupus, your doctor may perform periodic blood tests while you are taking this medication.

If you are taking lisinopril, a complete assessment of your kidney function should be done and kidney function should continue to be monitored.

This drug should be used with caution if you are on dialysis. There have been reports of extreme allergic reactions during dialysis in people taking ACE inhibitor medications such as lisinopril.

If you are taking high doses of a diuretic (water pill) and lisinopril, you may develop excessively low blood pressure.

Lisinopril may cause some people to become dizzy, light-headed, or faint, especially if they are taking a water pill at the same time. Do not drive, operate dangerous machinery, or participate in any hazardous activity that requires full mental alertness until you are certain lisinopril does not have this effect on you.

If you develop chest pain, sore throat, fever, and chills, contact your doctor for medical attention.

If your skin and the whites of your eyes turn yellow, stop taking the medication and contact your doctor.

Avoid salt substitutes that contain potassium. Limit your consumption of potassium-rich foods such as bananas, prunes, raisins, orange juice, and whole and skim milk. Ask your doctor for advice on how much of these foods to consume.

Excessive sweating, dehydration, severe diarrhea, or vomiting could cause you to lose too much water and cause your blood pressure to drop dangerously.

### Possible food and drug interactions when taking this medication

If lisinopril is taken with certain other drugs, the effects of either could be increased, decreased, or altered. It is especially important to check with your doctor before combining lisinopril with any of the following:

Diuretics such as HydroDIURIL and Lasix
Indomethacin (Indocin)

Lithium (Lithonate, Eskalith)
Potassium preparations such as K-Phos and Micro-K
Potassium-sparing diuretics such as Aldactone and Midamor

## Special information
## if you are pregnant or breastfeeding

If it is taken during the second and third trimesters, lisinopril can cause birth defects, prematurity, and death in the fetus and newborn. If you are pregnant or plan to become pregnant and are taking lisinopril, contact your doctor immediately to discuss the potential hazard to your unborn child. Lisinopril may appear in breast milk and could affect a nursing infant. If this medication is essential to your health, your doctor may advise you to discontinue breastfeeding until your treatment with this medication is finished.

## Recommended dosage

ADULTS

### Hypertension

For people not on diuretics, the initial starting dose is usually 10 milligrams, taken 1 time a day. After blood pressure is adjusted, dosage is usually 20 to 40 milligrams a day, taken in a single dose.

Diuretic use should, if possible, be stopped before using lisinopril. If not, your physician may give an initial dose of 5 milligrams under supervision before any further medication is prescribed.

People with kidney disorders must be carefully monitored, and dosages will be adjusted to the individual's needs, depending on kidney function.

### Heart failure

The recommended dose is 5 milligrams, once a day, along with diuretics and digitalis. This starting dose should be taken under your doctor's supervision. The usual dosage range is 5 to 20 milligrams taken once a day.

CHILDREN

The safety and effectiveness of lisinopril in children have not been established.

OLDER ADULTS

The physician will adjust the dosage carefully, according to the individual's needs.

## Overdosage

Any medication taken in excess can cause symptoms of overdose. If you suspect an overdose, seek medical attention immediately.

A severe drop in blood pressure is the primary sign of a lisinopril overdose.

*Generic name:*

# Zidovudine

*See Retrovir, page 464.*

*Brand name:*

# Zithromax

*Pronounced: ZITH-roh-macks*
*Generic name: Azithromycin*

## Why is this drug prescribed?

Zithromax is an antibiotic related to erythromycin. It is prescribed to treat certain mild to moderate skin infections; upper and lower respiratory tract infections, including pharyngitis (strep throat), tonsillitis, and pneumonia; and sexually transmitted infections of the cervix or urinary tract.

## Most important fact about this drug

There is a possibility of rare but very serious reactions to Zithromax, including angioedema (swelling of the face, lips, and neck that impedes speaking, swallowing, and breathing) and anaphylaxis (a violent, even fatal allergic reaction). If you develop these symptoms, stop taking Zithromax and call your doctor immediately.

## How should you take this medication?

Take Zithromax at least 1 hour before or 2 hours after a meal. Do not take this medication with food, or with an antacid that contains aluminum or magnesium, such as Di-Gel, Gelusil, Maalox, and others.

Zithromax oral suspension can be taken with or without food. Mix the contents of the packet with 2 ounces of water. Drink it all; then add 2 more ounces of water to the glass, stir again, and drink. This ensures that you are getting all the medication.

Be sure to take all the drug prescribed. If you stop taking Zithromax too soon, some germs may survive and the illness may return.

■ *If you miss a dose...*
Take the forgotten dose as soon as you remember. If you don't remember until the next day, skip the dose and go back to your regular schedule. Never try to "catch up" by doubling the dose.

■ *Storage instructions...*
Zithromax should be stored at room temperature. The packets for oral suspension can also be refrigerated.

## What side effects may occur?
Side effects cannot be anticipated. If any develop or change in intensity, inform your doctor as soon as possible. Only your doctor can determine if it is safe for you to continue taking Zithromax.

■ *More common side effects may include:*
Abdominal pain, diarrhea or loose stools, nausea
■ *Less common side effects may include:*
Blood in the stools, chest pain, dizziness, drowsiness, fatigue, gas, headache, heart palpitations, indigestion, jaundice (yellowing of the skin and the whites of the eyes), kidney infection, light sensitivity, rash, severe allergic reaction including swelling (as in hives), sleepiness, vaginal inflammation, vertigo, vomiting, yeast infection

The single large dose (4 capsules) of Zithromax that is prescribed to treat sexually transmitted infection of the cervix or urinary tract is more likely to cause stomach and bowel side effects than the smaller doses prescribed for a skin or respiratory tract infection.

## Why should this drug not be prescribed?
Do not take Zithromax if you have ever had an allergic reaction to it or to similar antibiotics such as erythromycin (E.E.S., PCE, and others).

## Special warnings about this medication
Like certain other antibiotics, Zithromax may cause a potentially life-threatening form of diarrhea called pseudomembranous colitis. Pseudomembranous colitis may clear up spontaneously when the drug is stopped; if it does not, hospital treatment may be required. If you develop diarrhea, check with your doctor immediately.

If you have a liver problem, your doctor should monitor you very carefully while you are taking Zithromax.

## Possible food and drug interactions when taking this medication
If Zithromax is taken with certain other drugs, the effects of either could be increased, decreased, or altered. It is especially important to check with your doctor before combining Zithromax with antacids containing aluminum or magnesium, such as Maalox and Mylanta.

The following interactions can occur with erythromycin, a similar drug.

Carbamazepine (Tegretol)
Certain antihistamines such as Hismanal and Seldane
Cyclosporine (Neoral and Sandimmune)
Digoxin (Lanoxin, Lanoxicaps)
Ergot-containing drugs such as Cafergot and D.H.E.
Hexobarbital
Lovastatin (Mevacor)
Phenytoin (Dilantin)
Theophylline drugs such as Bronkodyl, Slo-Phyllin, Theo-Dur, and others
Triazolam (Halcion)
Warfarin (Coumadin)

## Special information if you are pregnant or breastfeeding
If you are pregnant or plan to become pregnant, inform your doctor immediately. You should take Zithromax during pregnancy only if it is clearly needed. It is not known whether Zithromax can make its way into breast milk. If the drug is essential to your health, your doctor may advise you to stop breastfeeding until your treatment is finished.

## Recommended dosage
### ADULTS

The usual dose of Zithromax for people aged 16 years and older is 500 milligrams in a single dose the first day. This is followed by 250 milligrams one time each day for the next 4 days. The total amount taken should be 1.5 grams.

For treatment of non-gonococcal urethritis and cervicitis (sexually transmitted disease) due to the organism *Chlamydia trachomatis*, the usual dose is a single gram (1,000 milligrams) one time only. You can take it as four 250-milligram capsules or one 1-gram packet.

### CHILDREN

This medication is not recommended for children under age 16.

## Overdosage
Although no specific information on Zithromax overdose is available, any medication taken in excess can have serious consequences. If you suspect an overdose, seek medical attention immediately.

*Brand name:*

# Zocor

*Pronounced: ZOH-core*
*Generic name: Simvastatin*

## Why is this drug prescribed?

Zocor is a cholesterol-lowering drug. Your doctor may prescribe Zocor in addition to a cholesterol-lowering diet if your blood cholesterol level is too high, and if you have been unable to lower it by diet alone.

In people with high cholesterol and heart disease, Zocor reduces the risk of heart attack and can stave off the need for bypass surgery or angioplasty to clear clogged arteries.

## Most important fact about this drug

Zocor is usually prescribed only if diet, exercise, and weight-loss fail to bring your cholesterol level under control. It's important to remember that Zocor is a supplement to—not a substitute for—those other measures. To get the full benefit of the medication, you need to stick to the diet and exercise program prescribed by your doctor. All these efforts to keep your cholesterol levels normal are important because together they may lower your risk of heart disease.

## How should you take this medication?

Take Zocor exactly as prescribed.

■ *If you miss a dose...*
Take it as soon as you remember. If it is almost time for your next dose, skip the one you missed and go back to your regular schedule. Do not take 2 doses at once.
■ *Storage instructions...*
Store at room temperature.

## What side effects may occur?

Side effects cannot be anticipated. If any develop or change in intensity, inform your doctor as soon as possible. Only your doctor can determine whether it is safe for you to continue taking Zocor.

■ *More common side effects may include:*
Abdominal pain, headache
■ *Less common side effects may include:*
Constipation, diarrhea, gas, nausea, upper respiratory infection, upset stomach, weakness

## Why should this drug not be prescribed?

Do not take Zocor if you have ever had an allergic reaction to it or are sensitive to it.

Do not take Zocor if you have active liver disease.

Do not take Zocor if you are pregnant or plan to become pregnant.

## Special warnings about this medication

Because Zocor may damage the liver, your doctor may order a blood test to check your liver enzyme levels before you start taking the drug. Blood tests will probably be done before your treatment is started, at 6 weeks and 12 weeks after you start taking the drug or your dosage is increased, and at periodic intervals after that. If your liver enzyme levels rise too high, your doctor may tell you to stop taking Zocor.

Since Zocor may cause damage to muscle tissue, be sure to tell your doctor of any unexplained muscle tenderness, weakness, or pain right away, especially if you also have a fever or feel sick. Your doctor may want to do a blood test to check for signs of muscle damage.

## Possible food and drug interactions when taking this medication

If you take Zocor with certain other drugs, the effects of either could be increased, decreased, or altered. It is especially important to check with your doctor before combining Zocor with any of the following:

Blood-thinning drugs such as Coumadin and
    Dicumarol
Cimetidine (Tagamet)
Clofibrate (Atromid-S)
Cyclosporine (Sandimmune, Neoral)
Digoxin (Lanoxin, Lanoxicaps)
Erythromycin (PCE and others)
Gemfibrozil (Lopid)
Itraconazole (Sporanox)
Ketoconazole (Nizoral)
Nicotinic acid
Spironolactone (Aldactone, Aldactazide)

## Special information if you are pregnant or breastfeeding

You must not become pregnant while taking Zocor. This drug lowers cholesterol, and cholesterol is needed for a baby to develop properly. If you do become pregnant while taking Zocor, notify your doctor right away. Based on studies of other cholesterol-lowering drugs, it is assumed that Zocor could appear in breast milk and could cause severe adverse effects in a nursing baby. Do not take Zocor while breastfeeding your baby.

### Recommended dosage

You will have to follow a standard cholesterol-lowering diet before starting treatment with Zocor and continue this diet while using Zocor.

All doses should be adjusted to your individual needs.

ADULTS

The usual starting dose is 5 to 10 milligrams per day, taken as a single dose in the evening. The maximum recommended dose is 40 milligrams per day. Dosage adjustments may be made every 4 weeks, and dose levels should be reduced as cholesterol levels come down.

People with high cholesterol and heart disease may start with 20 milligrams daily taken as a single dose in the evening.

Those who have severe kidney disease should use Zocor with caution. The recommended dose is 5 milligrams per day.

Zocor may be used with other drugs. Your doctor will determine the proper dose based on your individual needs.

OLDER ADULTS

Doses of 20 milligrams per day or less may be sufficient.

### Overdosage

Although no specific information about Zocor overdose is available, any medication taken in excess can have serious consequences. If you suspect an overdose of Zocor, seek medical attention immediately.

*Brand name:*

# Zofran

*Pronounced: ZOH-fran*
*Generic name: Ondansetron hydrochloride*

### Why is this drug prescribed?

Zofran is used for the prevention of nausea and vomiting caused by radiation therapy and chemotherapy for cancer, and, in some cases, to prevent these problems following surgery.

### Most important fact about this drug

To ensure the maximum effect, it is important to take all doses of Zofran exactly as prescribed by your doctor.

### How should you take this medication?

Your doctor will tell you how much drug to take and how often, depending on the type of therapy you will be having.

■ *If you miss a dose...*
 Take the forgotten dose as soon as you remember.
■ *Storage instructions...*
 Store Zofran at room temperature. Protect from light. Keep the drug in the carton it came in.

### What side effects may occur?

Side effects cannot be anticipated. If any develop or change in intensity, inform your doctor as soon as possible. Only your doctor can determine if it is safe for you to continue taking Zofran.

■ *More common side effects may include:*
 Abdominal pain, constipation, diarrhea, dizziness, fatigue, headache
■ *Less common or rare side effects may include:*
 Anaphylaxis (severe allergic reaction), dry mouth, rash, weakness, wheezing

*When Zofran is used to prevent nausea and vomiting after surgery, the following side effects may occur:*
Anxiety, difficulty breathing, difficulty urinating, dizziness, drowsiness, female reproductive disorders, fever, headache, itching, low blood pressure, shivers, slow heartbeat

### Why should this drug not be prescribed?

If you are sensitive to or have ever had an allergic reaction to ondansetron hydrochloride, you should not take this medication. Make sure that your doctor is aware of any drug reactions that you have experienced.

### Special warnings about this medication

There are no special warnings about Zofran.

### Possible food and drug interactions when taking this medication

No interactions with Zofran have been reported.

## Special information
## if you are pregnant or breastfeeding

The effects of Zofran during pregnancy have not been adequately studied. If you are pregnant or plan to become pregnant, inform your doctor immediately. Zofran may appear in breast milk and could affect a nursing infant. If this medication is essential to your health, your doctor may advise you to discontinue breastfeeding until your treatment with this medication is finished.

## Recommended dosage

PREVENTION OF NAUSEA AND VOMITING DUE TO CHEMOTHERAPY

### Adults and Children 12 Years of Age and Older

The recommended dose of Zofran is one 8-milligram tablet taken twice a day. The first dose should be taken 30 minutes before the start of treatment. The other dose should be taken 8 hours after the first dose. One 8-milligram tablet should be taken twice a day (every 12 hours) for 1 to 2 days after completing chemotherapy.

### Children 4 through 11 Years of Age

The recommended dose of Zofran is one 4-milligram tablet taken 3 times a day. The first dose should be taken 30 minutes before the start of chemotherapy. The other 2 doses should be taken 4 and 8 hours after the first dose. One 4-milligram tablet should be taken 3 times a day (every 8 hours) for 1 to 2 days after completing chemotherapy.

PREVENTION OF NAUSEA AND VOMITING DUE TO RADIATION THERAPY

### Adults

The usual dosage is one 8-milligram tablet taken 3 times a day. You will take the first dose 1 to 2 hours before therapy; the other intervals will depend on the type of radiation therapy you are receiving.

### Children

Zofran has not been used for this purpose in children.

PREVENTION OF NAUSEA AND VOMITING AFTER SURGERY

### Adults

The usual dose is two 8-milligram tablets taken 1 hour before undergoing anesthesia.

### Children

Zofran has not been used for this purpose in children.

## Overdosage

There are no specific symptoms of Zofran overdose to report. However, any medication taken in excess can have serious consequences. If you suspect an overdose, seek medical attention immediately.

*Brand name:*

# Zoloft

*Pronounced: ZOE-loft*
*Generic name: Sertraline*

## Why is this drug prescribed?

Zoloft is prescribed for major depression—a persistently low mood that interferes with everyday living. Symptoms may include loss of interest in your usual activities, disturbed sleep, change in appetite, constant fidgeting or lethargic movement, fatigue, feelings of worthlessness or guilt, difficulty thinking or concentrating, and recurrent thoughts of suicide.

Some doctors also prescribe Zoloft for obsessive-compulsive disorders.

Zoloft is thought to work by boosting the amount of serotonin in the brain. Serotonin is one of the brain's natural chemical messengers.

## Most important fact about this drug

Do not take Zoloft within two weeks of taking another type of antidepressant medication known as an MAO inhibitor. Drugs in this category include Nardil and Parnate. When serotonin boosters such as Zoloft are combined with MAO inhibitors, serious and sometimes fatal reactions can occur.

## How should you take this medication?

Take Zoloft exactly as prescribed: once a day, in either the morning or the evening.

Improvement with Zoloft may not be seen for several days to a few weeks.

Zoloft may make your mouth dry. For temporary relief suck a hard candy, chew gum, or melt bits of ice in your mouth.

■ *If you miss a dose...*
Take the forgotten dose as soon as you remember. If several hours have passed, skip the dose. Never try to "catch up" by doubling the dose.

■ *Storage instructions...*
Store at room temperature.

## What side effects may occur?

Side effects cannot be anticipated. If any develop or change in intensity, inform your doctor as soon as possible. Only your doctor can determine if it is safe for you to continue taking Zoloft.

■ *More common side effects may include:*
Agitation, confusion, constipation, diarrhea or loose stools, difficulty with ejaculation, dizziness, dry mouth, fatigue, fluttery or throbbing heartbeat, gas, headache, increased sweating, indigestion, insomnia, nausea, nervousness, sleepiness, tremor, vomiting

■ *Less common or rare side effects may include:*
Abdominal pain, abnormal hair growth, abnormal skin odor, acne, altered taste, anxiety, back pain, bad breath, breast development in males, breast pain or enlargement, bruise-like marks on the skin, changeable emotions, chest pain, cold, clammy skin, conjunctivitis (pinkeye), coughing, difficulty breathing, difficulty concentrating, difficulty swallowing, double vision, dry eyes, enlarged abdomen, excessive menstrual bleeding, eye pain, fainting, feeling faint upon arising from a sitting or lying position, female sexual problems, fever, fluid retention, flushing, frequent urination, hair loss, heart attack, hemorrhoids, hiccups, high blood pressure, hot flushes, increased appetite, increased salivation, inflammation of nose or throat, inflammation of the penis, intolerance to light, itching, joint pains, lack of coordination, lack of menstruation, lack of sensation, loss of appetite, low blood pressure, menstrual problems, middle ear infection, migraine, movement problems, muscle cramps or weakness, muscle pain, need to urinate during the night, nosebleed, pain upon urination, painful menstruation, purple or red spots on the skin, racing heartbeat, rash, ringing in the ears, sensitivity to light, sinus inflammation, skin eruptions or inflammation, sleepwalking, sores on tongue, speech problems, stomach and intestinal inflammation, swelling of the face, swollen wrists and ankles, thirst, tingling or pins and needles, twitching, urinary trouble, vaginal inflammation or discharge, varicose veins, vision problems, weight loss or gain, yawning

■ *Zoloft may also cause mental or emotional symptoms such as:*
Abnormal dreams or thoughts, aggressiveness, exaggerated feeling of well-being, depersonalization ("unreal" feeling), hallucinations, memory loss, paranoia, rapid mood shifts, suicidal thoughts, tooth-grinding, worsened depression

Many people lose a pound or two of body weight while taking Zoloft. This usually poses no problem but may be a concern if your depression has already caused you to lose a great deal of weight.

In a few people, Zoloft may trigger the grandiose, inappropriate, out-of-control behavior called mania or the similar, but less dramatic, "hyper" state called hypomania.

## Why should this drug not be prescribed?

Do not use this drug while taking an MAO inhibitor (see "Most important fact about this drug").

## Special warnings about this medication

If you have a kidney or liver disorder, take Zoloft cautiously and under close medical supervision.

## Possible food and drug interactions when taking this medication

You should not drink alcoholic beverages while taking Zoloft.

If Zoloft is taken with certain other drugs, the effects of either could be increased, decreased, or altered. It is especially important to check with your doctor before combining Zoloft with the following:

Cimetidine (Tagamet)
Diazepam (Valium, Valrelease)
Digitoxin (Crystodigin)
Flecainide (Tambocor)
Lithium (Lithonate)
MAO inhibitors (antidepressant drugs such as Nardil and Parnate)
Other serotonin-boosting drugs such as Paxil and Prozac
Other antidepressants such as Elavil and Serzone
Over-the-counter drugs such as cold remedies
Propafenone (Rythmol)
Tolbutamide (Orinase)
Warfarin (Coumadin)

## Special information if you are pregnant or breastfeeding

The effects of Zoloft during pregnancy have not been adequately studied. If you are pregnant or plan to become pregnant, inform your doctor immediately. Zoloft should be taken during pregnancy only if it is clearly needed. It is not known whether Zoloft appears in breast milk. Caution is advised when using Zoloft during breastfeeding.

### Recommended dosage

ADULTS

The usual starting dose is 50 milligrams once a day, taken either in the morning or in the evening.

Your doctor may increase your dose depending upon your response. You should not take more than 200 milligrams in a day.

### Overdosage

Any medication taken in excess can have serious consequences. If you suspect an overdose, seek medical attention immediately.

■ *Symptoms of Zoloft overdose may include:*
Anxiety, dilated pupils, nausea, rapid heartbeat, sleepiness, vomiting

*Generic name:*

# Zolpidem

See Ambien, page 20.

*Brand name:*

# Zovirax

*Pronounced: zoh-VIGH-racks*
*Generic name: Acyclovir*

### Why is this drug prescribed?

Zovirax liquid, capsules, and tablets, are used in the treatment of certain infections with herpes viruses. These include genital herpes, shingles, and chickenpox. This drug may not be appropriate for everyone, and its use should be thoroughly discussed with your doctor. Zovirax ointment is used to treat initial episodes of genital herpes and certain herpes simplex infections of the skin and mucous membranes.

Some doctors use Zovirax, along with other drugs, in the treatment of AIDS, and for unusual herpes infections such as those following kidney and bone marrow transplants.

### Most important fact about this drug

Zovirax does not cure herpes. However, it does reduce pain and may help the sores caused by

herpes to heal faster. Genital herpes is a sexually transmitted disease. To avoid infecting your partner, forgo intercourse and other sexual contact when visible lesions are present.

### How should you take this medication?

Your medication should not be shared with others, and the prescribed dose should not be exceeded. Zovirax ointment should not be used in or near the eyes.

To reduce the risk of spreading the infection, use a rubber glove to apply the ointment.

■ *If you miss a dose...*
Take it as soon as you remember. If it is almost time for your next dose, skip the one you missed and go back to your regular schedule. Never take 2 doses at the same time.

If you are using the ointment, apply it as soon as you remember and continue your regular schedule.

■ *Storage instructions...*
Store Zovirax at room temperature in a dry place.

### What side effects may occur?

Side effects cannot be anticipated. If any develop or change in intensity, inform your doctor as soon as possible. Only your doctor can determine if it is safe for you to continue taking Zovirax.

■ *More common side effects may include:*
Confusion, constipation, diarrhea, dizziness, fever, fluid retention, general feeling of bodily discomfort, gland enlargement in the groin, hair loss, hallucinations, headache, hives, itching, muscle pain, nausea, pain, skin rash, sleepiness, stomach and intestinal problems, visual abnormalities, vomiting

■ *Less common or rare side effects may include:*
Abdominal pain, anaphylaxis (severe allergic reaction), diarrhea, dizziness, fatigue, gas, headache, inability to sleep, leg pain, loss of appetite, medicinal taste, rash, retention of fluid, sore throat, tingling or pins and needles, vomiting, weakness

■ *Common side effects of Zovirax ointment may include:*
Burning, itching, mild pain, skin rash, stinging, vaginal inflammation

### Why should this drug not be prescribed?

If you are sensitive to or have ever had an allergic reaction to Zovirax or similar drugs, you should not take this medication. Make sure that your doctor is aware of any drug reactions that you have experienced.

### Special warnings about this medication

If you are being treated for a kidney disorder, consult your doctor before taking Zovirax.

Although decreased sperm count has been reported in animals given high doses of Zovirax, this effect has not been documented to occur in humans.

### Possible food and drug interactions when taking this medication

If Zovirax is taken with certain other drugs, the effects of either could be increased, decreased, or altered. It is especially important to check with your doctor before combining Zovirax with the following:

Cyclosporine (Sandimmune, Neoral)
Interferon (Roferon-A)
Probenecid (Benemid)
Zidovudine (Retrovir)

### Special information if you are pregnant or breastfeeding

The effects of Zovirax during pregnancy have not been adequately studied. If you are pregnant or plan to become pregnant, inform your doctor immediately. Zovirax appears in breast milk and could affect a nursing infant. If this medication is essential to your health, your doctor may advise you to discontinue breastfeeding your baby until your treatment with Zovirax is finished.

### Recommended dosage

ADULTS

*For Genital Herpes*
The usual dose is one 200-milligram capsule or 1 teaspoonful of liquid every 4 hours, 5 times daily for 10 days. If the herpes is recurrent, the usual adult dose is 400 milligrams (two 200-milligram capsules, one 400-milligram tablet or 2 teaspoonfuls) 2 times daily for up to 12 months.

If genital herpes is intermittent, the usual adult dose is one 200-milligram capsule or 1 teaspoon of liquid every 4 hours, 5 times a day for 5 days. Therapy should be started at the earliest sign or symptom.

Ointment: Apply ointment to affected area every 3 hours, 6 times per day, for 7 days. Use enough ointment (approximately one-half inch ribbon of ointment per 4 square inches of surface area) to cover the affected area.

*For Herpes Zoster (Shingles)*
The usual adult dose is 800 milligrams (four 200-milligram capsules, two 400-milligram tablets, or 4 teaspoonfuls of liquid) every 4 hours, 5 times daily for 7 to 10 days.

*For Chickenpox:*
The usual adult dose is 800 milligrams 4 times a day for 5 days.

If you have a kidney disorder, the dose will need to be adjusted by your doctor.

CHILDREN

The usual dose for chickenpox is 20 milligrams per 2.2 pounds of body weight taken orally 4 times daily, for a total of 80 milligrams per 2.2 pounds, for 5 days. A child weighing more than 88 pounds should take the adult dose.

The safety and effectiveness of Zovirax have not been established in children under 2 years of age. However, your doctor may decide that the benefits of this medication outweigh the potential risks.

### Overdosage

Zovirax is generally safe; however, there have been cases of kidney disorder in people taking Zovirax orally. Any medication taken in excess can have serious consequences. If you suspect an overdose, seek medical attention immediately.

*Brand name:*

# Zydone

See Vicodin, page 587.

*Brand name:*

# Zyloprim

*Pronounced: ZYE-loe-prim*
*Generic name: Allopurinol*
*Other brand name: Lopurin*

### Why is this drug prescribed?

Zyloprim is used in the treatment of many symptoms of gout, including acute attacks, tophi (collection of uric acid crystals in the tissues, especially around joints), joint destruction, and uric acid stones. Gout is a form of arthritis characterized by increased blood levels of uric acid. Zyloprim works by reducing uric acid production in the body, thus preventing crystals from forming.

Zyloprim is also used to manage the increased uric acid levels in the blood of people with certain cancers, such as leukemia. It is also prescribed to manage some types of kidney stones.

### Most important fact about this drug

Zyloprim will not stop a gout attack that is already underway. However, when taken over a period of several months, this drug will begin to reduce your symptoms. It's important to keep taking it regularly, even if it seems to have no immediate effect.

### How should you take this medication?

Take Zyloprim exactly as prescribed. Your doctor will probably start you on a low dosage, increasing it gradually each week until you reach the dosage that is best for you.

A typical starting dose is one 100-milligram tablet per day. You may want to take Zyloprim immediately after a meal to minimize the risk of stomach irritation.

You should avoid taking large doses of vitamin C because of the increased possibility of kidney stone formation.

While taking Zyloprim you should drink plenty of liquids—10 to 12 glasses (8 ounces each) per day—unless otherwise prescribed by your doctor.

To help prevent attacks of gout, you should also avoid beer, wine, and purine-rich foods such as anchovies, sardines, liver, kidneys, lentils, and sweetbreads.

If you have been taking colchicine and/or an anti-inflammatory drug, such as Anaprox, Indocin, and others, to relieve your gout, your doctor will probably want you to continue taking this medication while your Zyloprim dosage is being adjusted. Later, when you have had no attacks of gout for several months, you may be able to stop taking these other medications.

If you have been taking a drug that promotes the excretion of uric acid in the urine, such as probenecid (Benemid) or sulfinpyrazone (Anturane), to try to prevent attacks of gout, your doctor will probably want to reduce or stop your dosage of this drug while increasing your dosage of Zyloprim.

■ *If you miss a dose...*
Take it as soon as you remember. If it is almost time for your next dose, skip the one you missed and go back to your regular schedule. Do not take 2 doses at once.

■ *Storage instructions...*
Store at room temperature in a cool, dry place, away from light.

### What side effects may occur?

Side effects cannot be anticipated. If any develop or change in intensity, inform your doctor as soon as possible. Only your doctor can determine if it is safe for you to continue taking Zyloprim.

Because a skin reaction, the most common side effect of Zyloprim, may occasionally become severe or even fatal, you should stop taking Zyloprim if you notice even the beginnings of a rash. Such a rash may be itchy or scaly or may make your skin peel off in sheets; it may be accompanied by chills and fever, aching joints, or jaundice.

■ *More common side effects may include:*
Acute attack of gout, diarrhea, nausea, rash

■ *Less common or rare side effects may include:*
Abdominal pain, bruising, chills, fever, hair loss, headache, hepatitis, hives, indigestion, itching, joint pain, kidney failure, loosening of nails, muscle disease, nosebleed, rare skin condition characterized by severe blisters and bleeding on the lips, eyes, or nose, reddish-brown or purplish spots on skin, skin inflammation or peeling, sleepiness, stomach inflammation, taste loss or change, tingling or pins and needles, unusual bleeding, vomiting, yellowing of skin and eyes

### Why should this drug not be prescribed?

Do not take Zyloprim if you have ever had a severe reaction to it in the past.

### Special warnings about this medication

If you notice a rash or other signs of an allergic reaction, stop taking Zyloprim immediately and consult your doctor. In some people, a Zyloprim-induced rash may lead to a serious skin disease, generalized inflammation of a blood or lymph vessel, irreversible liver damage, or even death.

You may experience acute attacks of gout more often in the early stages of Zyloprim therapy, even when normal uric acid levels have been attained. These attacks will become shorter and less severe after several months of therapy.

A kidney problem may turn a normal dose of Zyloprim into an overdose. If you have a kidney disease, or a condition such as diabetes or high blood pressure that may affect your kidneys, your doctor should prescribe Zyloprim cautiously and order periodic blood and urine tests to assess your kidney function.

Because Zyloprim may make you drowsy, do not drive or perform hazardous tasks until you know how the medication affects you.

It may be 2 to 6 weeks before you see any results from this medication.

## Possible food and drug interactions when taking this medication

If Zyloprim is taken with certain other drugs, the effects of either could be increased, decreased, or altered. It is especially important to check with your doctor before combining Zyloprim with the following:

Amoxicillin (Amoxil, Trimox, Wymox)
Ampicillin (Omnipen, Principen)
Azathioprine (Imuran)
Blood thinners such as Coumadin
Cyclosporine (Sandimmune, Neoral)
Drugs for diabetes, such as Diabinese and Orinase
Mercaptopurine (Purinethol)
Probenecid (Benemid, ColBENEMID)
Sulfinpyrazone (Anturane)
Theophylline (Theo-Dur, Slo-Phyllin, and others)
Thiazide diuretics such as HydroDIURIL, Diuril, and others
Vitamin C

## Special information if you are pregnant or breastfeeding

The effects of Zyloprim during pregnancy have not been adequately studied. If you are pregnant or plan to become pregnant, notify your doctor immediately. Zyloprim should be taken during pregnancy only if it is clearly needed.

Zyloprim appears in breast milk; what effect it may have on a nursing baby is unknown. Caution is advised when Zyloprim is taken during breastfeeding.

## Recommended dosage

ADULTS

Your doctor will tailor the dosage of Zyloprim individually to control the severity of symptoms and to bring the uric acid levels to normal or near normal.

*Gout*

The usual starting dose is 100 milligrams once daily. Your doctor may increase your dose by 100 milligrams per day at 1-week intervals until desired results are attained. The average dose is 200 to 300 milligrams per day for mild gout and 400 to 600 milligrams daily for moderate to severe gout. The most you should take in a day is 800 milligrams.

*Recurrent Kidney Stones*

The usual dose is 200 to 300 milligrams daily, divided into smaller doses or taken as one dose.

*Management of Uric Acid Levels in Certain Cancers*

The usual dose is 600 to 800 milligrams daily for 2 to 3 days, together with a high fluid intake.

CHILDREN

The usual recommended dose for children 6 to 10 years of age is 300 milligrams daily for the management of uric acid levels in certain types of cancer. Children under 6 years of age are generally given 150 milligrams daily.

## Overdosage

Although no specific information is available regarding Zyloprim overdosage, any medication taken in excess can have serious consequences. If you suspect an overdose of Zyloprim, seek medical attention immediately.

## CHAPTER 1

# New Hope
# for Heart Patients

Each year heart disease kills twice as many people as cancer and eight times as many people as car accidents or infections. According to the annual National Health and National Nutrition Examination Survey, 43 percent of all deaths recorded each year are caused by heart and other "vascular diseases" such as stroke and kidney failure.

■ Heart disease alone kills more than 940,000 Americans a year.

■ Over 69 million Americans have high blood pressure, coronary heart disease, stroke, or rheumatic heart disease.

■ Total U.S. medical costs for heart disease exceed $100 billion annually.

But the byword among cardiologists and researchers today is hope, tempered by the knowledge that we can and must do much more. The rate of heart disease in the U.S. is still among the highest in the world, due in part to lack of proper diet and exercise, and other unhealthy personal habits like cigarette smoking. So, the battle to defeat heart disease must be fought on two fronts: the research lab and our homes.

Our attention to changing the way we live—reducing personal stress and seeking early detection and treatment—has helped. From 1979 to 1989 the death rate from heart attacks actually declined 23.4 percent. Much of this progress is also due to a fast-paced revolution in the medicines used to treat and prevent heart attacks, strokes, high blood pressure, and related circulatory diseases that combine to produce high risks of death and disability in many individuals.

Exciting new therapies promise to stop heart attacks even before the patient reaches the hospital, reducing the need for expensive and hazardous coronary artery bypass surgery. Other new treatments promise to dissolve dangerous blood clots and reverse the crippling effects of strokes.

What actually happens when someone suffers a heart attack? What causes high blood pressure or angina (suffocating chest pains)? And why are these particular medicines effective against these and similar conditions?

This chapter and chapter two on high blood pressure will help you understand more about your heart medicines and why they can help you if you have heart disease.

## What Is a Heart Attack?

The heart is a remarkably effective muscle. Consider that if your heart beats 80 times a minute, in a single year it will pump blood through your body approximately 42 million times. It also pumps blood through itself. Like any muscle, your heart must also receive a supply of blood in order to work properly.

To get an idea of how hard your heart works, try clenching and unclenching your fist and see how long you can keep it up. You'll quickly find that your hand and arm soon begin to ache. That ache signals that the muscles are overworked. Yet your heart keeps up that pace 24 hours a day, every day, year after year. So it's vitally important to keep a supply of fresh oxygenated blood coming to the heart through open, unclogged blood vessels. The blood vessels that supply your heart with blood are called coronary arteries.

A heart attack occurs when a portion of the heart muscle dies from lack of oxygen. Usually a problem in the coronary arteries is the cause. These arteries are narrow, and their pathway in the heart follows many twists and turns. For a variety of reasons, they tend to become blocked. When the supply of oxygenated blood they deliver is cut off or reduced, you feel pain, just as you did in your hand and arm. When the pain comes from your heart, it's called angina. You can have angina without having a full-blown heart attack, but

## WHAT IS A HEART?

The subject of song and verse, the heart was believed by the ancients to be the seat of the soul and the emotions. Even today we send "heart-shaped" cards (which aren't really shaped anything like hearts) on Valentine's Day and refer to broken-hearted lovers, but modern science tells us that hearts are about as romantic as your car's oil pump. In fact, the heart is a pump—a lumpy mass of muscle about the size of your fist that forces blood first through the lungs to pick up oxygen and then through the body to deliver that oxygen to the body's cells. That's a more mundane job than housing the soul, but vital nonetheless.

The rest of your circulatory system isn't much more difficult

VENA CAVA
(Returns oxygen-depleted blood from the body)

AORTA
(Delivers oxygenated blood to the body)

PULMONARY ARTERY
(Conducts spent blood to the lungs)

RIGHT ATRIUM
(Upper pumping chamber)

PULMONARY VEINS (Return oxygen-rich blood to the heart)

RIGHT VENTRICLE
(Lower pumping chamber)

to understand than the heart. The arteries and veins are essentially tubing carrying the blood where it's needed around the body. But on closer inspection they turn out to be more than simple hoses.

Veins, for instance, have a series of valves that prevent blood from flowing backward as it returns to the heart. Arteries are really a combination of tubing and pump. The walls of the arteries are made up of layers of muscle that expand with every heartbeat and then rebound between heartbeats, giving the circulation an added boost.

The coronary arteries supply blood directly to the muscle tissue that makes up the heart. Like every other part of the body, the heart needs oxygen, and the coronary arteries' sole purpose is to supply it with oxygen-rich blood. They branch off from the aorta (the main artery that emerges from the heart) and snake along the surface of the heart itself.

angina is a danger signal that can mean serious heart disease.

When your arm got sore from squeezing your fist, you probably stopped and gave it a rest. Unfortunately, your heart can't stop for very long without death as the result. So to try to rest, it starts beating with less force, which results in less blood being circulated throughout the body. This causes some of the symptoms of what is commonly called a heart attack: clammy skin, pallor, and profuse perspiration. Along with the pain from the heart attack, there is general weakness as blood flow to the brain decreases. The person suffering the heart attack may feel dizzy or even lose consciousness. If coronary artery blockage is severe enough, the heart stops beating altogether, and, within a few minutes, death occurs.

Heart attacks can vary greatly in severity. The first attack may be mild, or severe enough to be disabling, or even fatal. Some people never experience a subsequent attack, while others experience several before succumbing to a fatal attack. Having a heart attack does not necessarily mean that you may die any minute of heart disease, but it is a strong signal that help is needed to reduce this possibility. So one of the major areas of cardiac research has been the reduction and prevention of coronary artery disease. As a result, we now have dozens of drugs to prevent and reduce the devastating effects of cardiovascular illnesses.

## Your Arteries and Your Heart

What causes the blockages that prevent the heart from working efficiently? How can they be prevented or treated?

Like a system of supply highways running from the suburbs to the central city, the body's arteries are key to the survival of the heart muscle. Each person has miles of veins and arteries that circulate blood to the organs and muscles. Arteries are those blood vessels that carry oxygen-rich blood to the organs and tissues, while veins return blood to the heart. If the highways surrounding the city aren't well maintained, and debris is left along the sides or strewn along the road, traffic is slowed, and the supply system becomes inefficient.

The same problems develop in the body's blood supply system when fatty materials called **cholesterol** start to build up on the walls of the arteries. This narrows the vessels and stiffens their walls,

leading to a condition called atherosclerosis. Like any highway with a closed lane, traffic slows to a crawl. But in this case, what is slowed is the life-sustaining flow of oxygen-rich blood, which creeps to a near standstill.

Together, the narrowing and the hardening of the arteries create a risk of high blood pressure, kidney failure, irregular heart rhythms, and stroke. If the blockage isn't treated, the blood flow slows and eventually stops, causing a heart attack. What makes matters worse is that the arteries clog gradually and produce few symptoms, if any, until it's too late. Often the presence of atherosclerosis may not be noticed, or diagnosed, until a stroke or a heart attack has occurred.

## How We Treat Heart Disease

Beginning in the late 1950s, doctors began to make great strides in the fight against heart disease. In 1959, Swedish doctors implanted the first pacemaker in a 43-year-old man. In 1961, researchers at Johns Hopkins University found that a combination of simple and easily learned resuscitative techniques such as CPR could keep heart-attack victims alive long enough to get them to a hospital and more sophisticated care.

We have learned more about the causes of heart disease and the roles life-style and diet play. In addition, we have now refined surgical techniques like valve replacements and transplants to treat damaged hearts.

Researchers developing medications for heart disease have had a wide range of problems to deal with. We've needed drugs first to forestall heart and vascular disease, then to correct the resulting conditions. Many new drugs have been developed and tested. The first real breakthrough came with the discovery of a surprisingly versatile group of drugs called beta blockers, but we still find extremely useful some drugs discovered more than two centuries ago.

### From Garden to Pharmacy:
### The Discovery of Digitalis

**Digitalis** (Digitoxin and Digoxin) is a drug class that was first discovered 200 years ago by Dr. William Withering in an ingredient in foxglove, a common flower in English gardens. It was used to treat a condition called **dropsy**, which we know today as **congestive heart failure.** It occurs when an overworked heart can't pump enough blood to meet the body's circulatory needs.

A common symptom of congestive heart failure (and several other problems) is swelling, or edema, as doctors call it. This occurs because the kidneys can't eliminate salt from the body as efficiently as they once could. As salt concentrations build up, the body responds by increasing the amount of water in the blood and other body tissues, which causes swelling and puffiness, particularly in the ankles and feet.

Researchers in the 1930s, working with animals and with heart tissue, learned that digitalis affected the heart muscle by invigorating it and causing it to pump with more force. By beating more powerfully and pumping more blood with each beat, the heart doesn't have to beat as quickly. This also explains the drug's other effects. By strengthening

## CLOGGED HIGHWAY TO THE HEART

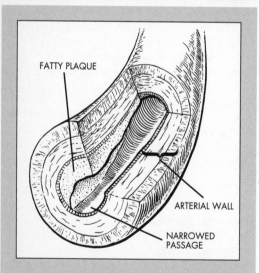

FATTY PLAQUE

ARTERIAL WALL

NARROWED PASSAGE

When fatty deposits of cholesterol and degenerate muscle cells build up on the inside walls of the coronary arteries, heart disease lies ahead. The build-up, known as atherosclerosis, reduces blood flow to the muscles of the heart, ultimately leading to angina. Worse yet, if a blood clot blocks the already narrowed passage, a heart attack may be the result.

the heartbeat, it almost magically reverses the symptoms of congestive heart failure. Blood passes through the kidneys more quickly, enabling them to eliminate the excess fluid and salt; a heart that has enlarged may shrink back toward its normal size. The overall result is an improvement of circulation throughout the body.

Digitalis continues to be an extremely useful drug. Nonetheless, there are limits to what it can do. Today this drug and others may be combined in a comprehensive cardiac care program.

### Quinidine: Remedy from the Past

Quinidine, another important cardiac drug, was discovered quite by chance. The setting was Vienna, just before the First World War. In 1912, a patient appeared at the office of Viennese physician Karl Wenkebach, complaining of an abnormal heartbeat.

Dr. Wenkebach could offer no cure. But, the man insisted a cure was possible, and he himself could provide it. Wenkebach protested; the man insisted. He would, he said, return the next morning with a regular heart rhythm. True to his word, he was back the next morning, and his heartbeat was normal, thanks to quinine, a drug already in wide use for the treatment of malaria.

That was how the *first* of the "antiarrhythmic" drugs that help restore a normal heartbeat was discovered. Today, doctors prefer to use quinidine—a close relative of quinine—rather than quinine itself, because smaller doses are effective and have fewer side effects.

### Nitroglycerin: Help from the Test Tube

**Nitroglycerin** and related drugs trace their ancestry to the chemist's test tube. Amyl nitrite, first synthesized in 1844, was quickly found to cause flushing of the face due to the relaxation of the tiny blood vessels known as capillaries that connect arteries and veins. Twenty-three years later, a young Scottish medical student by the name of Thomas Lauder Brunton suspected that amyl nitrite might also relieve angina by increasing blood flow to the heart. He was right, as he found when he tried the drug on some of his patients. It wasn't long before nitroglycerin, which is chemically similar to amyl nitrite, was discovered to have a similar effect, relaxing the smooth muscles that make up your veins and arteries and allowing

## HEART FACTS

Is it possible to die of a broken heart? Yes, the stress that accompanies the loss of a loved one has, on more than one occasion, triggered a fatal heart attack. Researchers have found that other emotions also can affect the heart. Reducing stress, not only from heart and cardiovascular disease, but also from emotional sources, can be an important factor in improving overall health.

them to dilate. Both drugs are still used for treatment of angina, but nitroglycerin is by far the more common, because it is more easily administered and has fewer side effects.

One new way of delivering nitroglycerin (as well as some other drugs) is by means of a **transdermal patch.** For years doctors have known that nitroglycerin is easily absorbed into the bloodstream through the skin. There are nitroglycerin ointments that can be spread on the skin, tablets that are held under the tongue or in the cheek until they dissolve, and capsules that can be swallowed. The advantage of transdermal patches, which look like big adhesive bandages, is that they regulate the delivery of the drug, providing a constant amount of it for as long as 24 hours at a time.

Other **vasodilators** employed to relax the muscles in the arterial walls are more fully discussed in Chapter Two, "Defusing High Blood Pressure."

There are also drugs used specifically for treating the complications of atherosclerosis elsewhere in the body. One, pentoxifylline (Trental), is known as a hemorheologic agent and helps reduce the cramping that blocked arteries can cause when blood supply to the legs and feet are cut off.

### Beta Blockers: The First Family of Heart Medicines

Various nerve systems in the body stimulate the activity of the heart. The beta-adrenergic system was discovered to be involved in irregular heartbeats. Scientists began looking for a drug that would block the activity of this system and ended up with a drug that became one of the most valuable medications we have.

Propranolol (Inderal) is the granddaddy of the beta-blocker family, and the first of its class to be approved by the Food and Drug Administration (FDA) for use in the United States. At the time of approval, no one knew that propranolol would someday come to play a starring role in the treatment of heart disease. Few suspected that within 15 years it would become one of the most prescribed drugs in America.

In 1967, its sole approved use was for treatment of irregular heartbeats (arrhythmias). Since then the FDA has expanded the approved uses of the drug to include treatment of angina, high blood pressure, and migraine headaches. Doctors have also researched its value for unapproved uses including anxiety and serious thyroid disease.

These multiple uses would have qualified propranolol as one of the most versatile drugs ever discovered, but its most important use was yet to come.

Despite the technology in modern coronary care units, and advances in treatment, doctors knew that people who'd had one heart attack were at increased risk for a second, which could strike at any time, anywhere, far from the help that had been only seconds away while they were in the hospital. And yet doctors couldn't keep their patients in the hospital, waiting for a subsequent heart attack that might never come.

In 1981, cardiologists conducting a study of propranolol found that it helped prevent second heart attacks, and that it reduced mortality rates among heart patients by 26 percent. They were so excited by this discovery that they ended the study nine months early, believing it would be unethical to withhold the drug from the control group of patients. The study's sponsor, the National Heart, Blood, and Lung Institute, estimated that appropriate use of the drug could save hundreds of thousands of lives a year in the United States alone. Thus, propranolol and other drugs in the beta-blocker class have become extremely useful in reducing the pain and suffering of heart disease.

### The Calcium Channel Blockers

When verapamil (Isoptin, Calan), the first calcium channel blocker, was approved by the FDA in 1982, its sole use was for the treatment of arrhythmias (irregular heartbeats), and often it wasn't even the drug of first choice for that condition. If your doctor wanted to give you verapamil, you'd have to be in the hospital to get it, since it was only available in an injectable form. In fact, verapamil was thought to be so unpromising that nobody thought much about how it worked or what beneficial effects it might have other than controlling irregular heartbeats.

This situation changed when cardiologists began to study propranolol and the other beta blockers. Their success with these drugs prompted increased research into other drugs that act upon the heart. When researchers began looking around, they found that verapamil had a lot more potential benefits to offer heart disease victims than anyone had ever guessed.

Your heartbeat is controlled by tiny electrical impulses; that's why doctors sometimes use electronic pacemakers to regulate hearts that don't beat the way they should. Calcium plays a key role in regulating the heart's response to these electrical signals. It flows between the heart cells and surrounding fluid through a sort of chemical revolving door—the calcium channel. The more calcium that gets through the door before the electrical signal comes, the more strongly the heart contracts and the harder it works. Calcium channel blockers, like verapamil and its cousins, don't quite "lock" the revolving door, but they significantly slow it down. This eases the load on a damaged heart and, for many patients, improves heart functioning.

If you suffer from angina, you'll be interested to know that calcium channel blockers have turned out to be among the most effective antianginal medications ever discovered. They help your heart work with less effort; and at the same time, they relax the coronary arteries, improving the supply of oxygen-enriched blood to the heart itself. The result is almost as if the drug told your heart to sit back, relax, and take a few deep breaths.

### Calcium Blockers and the Future

What about the future of this new class of drugs? Researchers are still exploring their potential, and some promising possibilities include the prevention of heart attacks and slowing of atherosclerosis. Other possible uses include treatment of migraine headaches, Raynaud's phenomenon (a condition in which arteries in the extremities spasm, causing pallor), menstrual cramps, and premature labor. Researchers also speculate that calcium channel blockers may someday help in the treatment of strokes, spinal-cord injuries, certain types of kidney failure, and even cancer.

### Cholesterol-Reducing Drugs

One in four Americans is at higher risk for heart disease because of elevated cholesterol levels which are either inherited or acquired due to diet or another disease. Over the past 20 years, physicians and researchers have recognized that high cholesterol levels in both men and women are an important risk factor in cardiovascular diseases. (See your physician to evaluate your own risk levels.) While cholesterol levels can be controlled somewhat by diet alone, adding a medication is the most effective way of lowering them.

Cholesterol-lowering drugs act by preventing the body from manufacturing cholesterol, reducing absorption of dietary cholesterol, or combining with cholesterol to remove it from the bloodstream. Common cholesterol-lowering drugs are Lescol, Lopid, Mevacor, Pravachol, Questran, Zocor, and niacin.

## Hope for the Future:
## Unblocking Clogged Arteries

Heart attacks usually occur because the coronary arteries become clogged by a blood clot, and some of the most promising new drugs work to unclog them directly. These drugs offer an alternative to coronary artery bypass surgery, in which surgeons take lengths of veins from a patient's leg or chest wall and attach them

### CPR SAVES THE DAY

Cardiopulmonary resuscitation, or CPR as it's usually called today, has saved countless lives and is taught in high schools, community centers, and company cafeterias. It's also taught to hospital employees and has become a mainstay of "code blue" techniques that bring hospitalized patients back from the threshold of death.

## THE ROLE OF ADRENALINE

The so-called fight-or-flight response is governed by a complex series of interactions between your mind and body. When your brain perceives a threat, it automatically tells your adrenal glands—small organs that sit atop your kidneys—to start pumping out adrenaline.

The adrenaline, in turn, quickly travels through your bloodstream to all parts of your body, acting as a sort of chemical Paul Revere to warn them that they may soon be called upon to do their best. Your digestive system shuts down, and blood is diverted to the brain, helping you think more quickly. Your muscles are primed to work at peak efficiency—hence the muscular tension that results in shaky knees and twitching muscles—and your breathing becomes faster, bringing more oxygen to the blood. All of this activity is geared to help you either fight or run away. If you decide to fight, the response helps you move and think quickly—to literally stay on your toes. If you decide to run, adrenaline gives you added speed and endurance.

Now let's look specifically at what happens to your heart and cardiovascular system when all that adrenaline hits it.

When you're under stress, your heart starts pounding much harder and faster than usual. That tells you it's working a lot harder, which in turn means it's going to need more oxygen. At the same time, the adrenaline is causing your arteries to squeeze tighter. There are two results. First, your heart has to work that much harder to pump blood through the narrowed arteries, and second, the coronary arteries can't deliver as much oxygen-enriched blood to the heart as usual.

In the normal, healthy person, these effects aren't dangerous, but if the heart is diseased or damaged, they can be disastrous. If the coronary arteries of a diseased heart tighten up, you'll feel pain (angina) which tells you that your heart is starved for oxygen. If they tighten more, or if the heart has to work harder, the oxygen shortage becomes even more severe. The heart falters—parts of it may even die from lack of oxygen—and you experience a heart attack.

---

to the coronary arteries to provide a "detour" around blockages.

While bypass surgery can prevent a heart attack, it's no help for patients who come to the hospital in the midst of an acute heart attack. However, three drugs, t-PA (Activase), streptokinase (Streptase), and anistreplase (Eminase), are now being used to open clogged arteries during and after an attack.

These medications work by dissolving blood clots. Blood passing through arteries filled with arterial plaque tends to clot, cutting off the blood supply to tissues downstream.

Depending upon where they create a blockage, blood clots can cause strokes, heart attacks, or life-threatening pulmonary emboli (blockages in the lung). If these clot-dissolving drugs can be given quickly enough, they can reverse these conditions before heart muscle or lung tissue dies from lack of oxygen.

Streptokinase was the first of these drugs to be used. Sometimes it is used in combination with a technique known as percutaneous transluminal coronary angioplasty (PTCA) that reduces blockages.

Tissue-Plasminogen Activator, or t-PA, was the first "genetically engineered" drug to show promise as a post-heart attack treatment. Scientists created this medication by "splicing" genes together. The drug dissolves clots in as little as 10 minutes—a mere fraction of the time streptokinase needs to work. And since t-PA is derived from human cells, not bacteria, it doesn't stimulate the body's immune system.

Studies of these drugs show that the sooner they are administered, the more effective they will be. In the future, these drugs may be used by Emergency Medical Teams when heart attack victims are being transported to the hospital, thus preventing even more deaths. □

## CHAPTER 2

# Defusing High Blood Pressure

High Blood Pressure or Hypertension is the most common chronic illness in America. The American Heart Association estimates that more than 62 million Americans over the age of six suffer from high blood pressure, and that only a minority of these people have their blood pressure under control. Many don't know they have hypertension, and go untreated, since you can have the disease for years before any symptoms develop. And, because you can be symptom-free, many people think high blood pressure is harmless.

Nothing, in fact, could be further from the truth! Left untreated, hypertension can lead to stroke, heart attack, kidney damage, congestive heart failure, and death.

Uncontrolled mild-to-moderate hypertension will reduce the life expectancy of a typical 35-year-old person by 16 years. Even the mildest form of high blood pressure, "borderline hypertension," can cut your life span by two to four years.

The good news is that more Americans each year are being diagnosed earlier—in routine physicals, workplace screening programs, and health education classes.

Because of extensive research, high blood pressure is actually one of the easiest diseases to diagnose. Breakthroughs in drug treatment described below have saved millions of lives.

## What Is Blood Pressure?

Blood pressure is the measure of the force of your blood moving through your body's "circulatory system." This complex network of veins and arteries contains blood vessels that can be as large as a banana or so narrow that blood cells can barely squeeze through them. Ideally, your blood flows through almost 100,000 miles of arteries and veins in a smooth stream—much like water flowing through your home's faucets into the sink or tub.

Within your body, the beats of your heart create a pressure-driven force that sends your blood moving through the body's arterial pathways in a steady, pulsating rhythm. This "force" is measured to determine your blood pressure level.

With each beat, your heart contracts, sending out a "surge" of pressure into the bloodstream. This surge period is called **"systolic"** from a Greek word meaning "to contract." After the pressure surge, your heart rests for a brief time and "expands" to get ready for another beat. The arteries that have received the surge of blood now rebound, forcing it further through the system. This is called the **"diastolic"** or "expansion" period.

Doctors measure your blood pressure during each of these periods. They often say "your pressure is 120 over 80," or some other combination of numbers. This first number is a measure of the "systolic push" of the heartbeat on the blood. The second number is the "diastolic" measurement of the pressure in your arteries as blood continues to flow through the system while the heart is at rest.

Finding this measurement is easy. Anyone can do it with a simple home monitoring device called a *sphygmomanometer* or blood pressure cuff. Your doctor's device may be a little more sophisticated—with a cuff, a stethoscope, and a pressure gauge—but they all work pretty much the same way. When your pressure is measured, this cuff is tightened to cut off the circulation momentarily. The cuff is loosened, and as the blood begins to flow again, the device measures the systolic and diastolic forces. The measurement is expressed in numbers as though they were a fraction (e.g., 140/90).

## What Do We Mean by "You Have High Blood Pressure"?

After years of study and research around the world, medical experts have reached certain agreements on "average levels" of blood pressure. If your doctor says you have hypertension, or "high blood pressure," he or she is actually comparing your blood pressure levels with the "normal" or average blood pressure of people of your age and sex.

Most physicians agree that in adults, a systolic reading of 100 to 140 and a diastolic reading of 70 to 90 is normal. A reading slightly above those limits—140 to 159 over 90 to 94—is considered mild hypertension. Readings from 160 to 179 over 94 to 114 indicate moderate hypertension. Anything above those limits represents serious high blood pressure. (Blood pressure readings in children vary greatly, and only a physician can determine a "normal" reading for an infant or child.) In general, at least two blood pressure readings should be taken on each of three separate days before a diagnosis of high blood pressure is given.

It's important to remember that high blood pressure is a disease not of the heart but of the arteries. And arterial pressure changes constantly. Normally, blood pressure drops when you sleep and rises when you are subjected to stress, startled by a loud noise, or threatened.

This temporary rise in pressure is the natural result of a complex chemical reaction in the body; and when the events that triggered it subside, your pressure should return to normal. If it doesn't—if it remains high all of the time—it means there is

## LIVING WITH HIGH BLOOD PRESSURE

- Have your pressure monitored frequently—learn to do it yourself.
- Never skip a dose of medication without talking to your doctor. Don't let your prescription run out.
- Report any side effects to your doctor.
- Make your lifestyle changes gradually—but make them.
- Reduce your stress, follow a sensible diet, and get plenty of exercise.

something wrong with your arterial pathways; and you have "hypertension."

## What Causes High Blood Pressure?

There are two types of high blood pressure: **primary (or "essential") hypertension** and **secondary hypertension.** Although the exact cause of primary hypertension isn't known, contributing factors include heredity, obesity, lack of exercise, diet—including salt intake— cigarette smoking, sex, race, age, and even personality. Over 90 percent of all hypertensives fall into the primary category. Secondary hypertension may be linked to kidney disease, endocrine disorders, the use of oral contraceptives, and excessive use of alcohol.

There is some evidence that continual stress can trigger biochemical changes within the body that raise blood pressure and keep it high. However, the common myth that "nerves" or "a case of the jitters" can bring on hypertension simply isn't true. High blood pressure is a disease; and even though it is often "silent," it must be treated promptly, exactly as directed by your physician.

Changes in the arteries can complicate the problem. Normally the arteries are rather springy; in addition to expanding and contracting in rhythm with the heart, they adjust themselves to the volume of the blood and to other conditions within the body, stretching or tightening up as necessary to raise, lower, or maintain blood pressure. Various factors—stress, for instance—as well as diet, heredity, lifestyle, and aging, have a detrimental effect on the arteries. They become less elastic and thus less able to adjust to changes in the body; and they tend to become coated with arterial cholesterol plaque, a fatty deposit that clogs them, just as deposits in your house's pipes can cause your sink to back up.

This condition, called atherosclerosis, can obstruct coronary arteries, and can lead to a stroke if arteries that supply blood to the brain become blocked.

## Drugs That Bring Down Pressure

If high blood pressure is identified early enough, when it is still in its very mildest stages, the first line of defense is an attempt to modify the risk factors associated with it. Of course, we can't do anything about our heredity, age, race, or sex; but we can lose weight, exercise more, stop smoking, and improve our eating habits. We may even be able to alter our personality; your doctor can recommend programs intended to teach Type-A personalities (the hard-driven, success-oriented types who start blowing their horns before the traffic light has changed) how to become easy-going, Type-B personalities.

In most cases, the mainstay of treatment for hypertension is medication. It brings blood pressure down quickly and keeps it down. And although it doesn't cure the disease (if you haven't improved your diet and lifestyle, blood pressure almost always shoots back up when medication is discontinued), it does prevent the serious and even life-threatening complications that can result if high blood pressure is left untreated.

The first step is usually a prescription for one of five types of medication: a diuretic, a beta blocker, an ACE (angiotensin converting enzyme) inhibitor, an angiotensin II receptor antagonist, or a calcium channel blocker. If these drugs, either alone or in combination, fail to bring blood pressure under control, other classes of drugs may be prescribed.

These drugs usually make no difference in the way you feel, so it's easy to forget about them. Nevertheless, it's important to take them faithfully according to the prescribed schedule. If they are not taken on a regular basis, they won't do their hidden, but lifesaving job. Here's a closer look at the various categories that are generally prescribed.

**Diuretics,** such as furosemide (Lasix), chlorothiazide (Diuril), hydrochlorothiazide (Esidrix, HydroDIURIL), and spironolactone (Aldactone), make it difficult for the kidneys to retain water and salt, which are then filtered out into the urine. Increasing the amount of urine reduces the amount of fluid in the bloodstream, and hence the pressure on artery walls. It's like turning on a second faucet in your house and watching the water pressure drop in the first—not a subtle mechanism, to be sure, but it works. Because some important chemicals may be washed out along with the water and salt, a doctor may prescribe supplements—most commonly a potassium supplement—to go with the diuretic.

**Beta blockers** reduce high blood pressure by throttling back the force and speed of the heart. They may also reduce blood pressure by a direct effect on the body's master controls, the central nervous system. Propranolol (Inderal) is the granddaddy of the beta-blocker family, and the first of its class to be approved by the Food and Drug Administration (FDA) for use in the United States. Among the other beta blockers on the market today are: metoprolol (Lopressor), atenolol (Tenormin), and bisoprolol (Zebeta).

**ACE inhibitors**, which include captopril (Capoten), lisinopril (Prinivil, Zestril), quinapril (Accupril), and enalapril (Vasotec), block the production of angiotensin II, a chemical the body produces to raise blood pressure. Angiotensin's normal role is to maintain equilibrium when blood pressure drops. It acts directly on the arteries, tightening them up to raise the pressure. The ACE inhibitors can bring blood pressure down quickly but in very rare cases can cause kidney damage or a reduction in the number of white blood cells (leading to an increased susceptibility to infection).

**Angiotensin II receptor antagonists**, a new class of drugs, work to lower blood pressure by blocking angiotensin from binding to "receptor sites" in the smooth muscles of the blood vessels. This blocking action stops the angiotensin from tightening the arteries and raising the blood pressure. Currently, there are two medications containing an angiotensin II receptor antagonist: Losartan Potassium tablets (Cozaar) and Losartan Potassium with Hydrochlorothiazide (Hyzaar), which combines the medication with a diuretic.

**Calcium channel blockers** are the most widely prescribed drugs in the United States today. Like so many of the other drugs used for hypertension, they act by dilating the arteries and reducing resistance to the flow of blood. They have proved to be beneficial not only for high blood pressure, but also for angina and other problems of a weakened heart. Included in this group are drugs such as diltiazem (Cardizem), isradipine (DynaCirc), and verapamil (Calan).

Recently, the National Heart, Lung and Blood Institute and the National Institute on Aging in Bethesda, Maryland, warned that high doses of the fast-acting form of nifedipine (Procardia, Adalat), which is taken three or four times a day, could possibly increase the risk for potentially fatal heart attack. These findings were based on two studies. The first followed hypertensive patients who had previous heart attacks; the second concentrated on people over the age of 71 who suffered from high blood pressure. All the subjects (except those in the control groups) were taking short-acting nifedipine. Both studies concluded that the risk of heart attack was higher with this drug than with other blood pressure medication. Older people were especially vulnerable: Nearly twice as many were likely to die within five years as those treated with other drugs. Because controversy still surrounds these findings, you should not stop taking this type of nifedipine without consulting your doctor.

In addition to these leading types of blood pressure medication, there are a number of other potent drugs that relax the muscles in the arterial walls, thus lowering blood pressure. Some act directly on the muscles, others work by inhibiting the production or effect of adrenaline, a powerful stimulant released by the body in response to stress. Among the drugs you might encounter are doxazosin (Cardura), clonidine (Catapres), guanfacine (Tenex), hydralazine (Apresoline), methyldopa (Aldomet), minoxidil (Loniten), and prazosin (Minipress).

Though many of the blood pressure drugs are the result of major scientific breakthroughs, it's all too easy to underestimate their value. There's nothing very magical about the way they work, and they don't, on a day-to-day level, make patients feel demonstrably better. In fact, because hypertension is so often a disease without symptoms, we're usually more aware of the drugs' side effects and inconvenience than of their lifesaving properties. But in terms of the number of patients helped, and the number of years added to these patients' lives, these drugs rank among the most important of any in use today. If hypertension is the "silent killer," then these drugs deserve the title "silent saviors." □

**CHAPTER 3**

# Coping with Arthritis

Arthritis has plagued mankind for millennia. Historians have found references to forms of arthritis in Greek and Roman literature, and some even suspect cavemen suffered from it. Today it's so widespread that one in seven people and one in three families are affected by it. More than 37 million Americans of all ages are victims. Frequently we ignore arthritis, calling it simply the "aches and pains" of old age. Or we self-medicate with painkillers, not bothering to seek professional treatment. But make no mistake: Arthritis is a serious, potentially crippling, and even fatal disease. The early warning signs should never be ignored.

## Some Arthritis Facts

■ Women are more likely than men to suffer from arthritis. The disease becomes more prevalent after age 45. Yet it is not a disease exclusively of the elderly, for more than 200,000 children are also affected.

■ Arthritis is a costly disease: It's the leading cause of absenteeism; 45 million work days are lost each year.

■ The estimated yearly cost in lost wages and medical bills is $35 billion (equivalent to one percent of the gross national product).

■ Arthritis patients average eight visits to their doctor each year—twice as many as those suffering from other chronic illnesses like high blood pressure.

■ Approximately six million people are "self-diagnosed" and improperly "self-treated."

## What Is Arthritis?

"Arthritis" literally means *"inflamed joints."* It is an umbrella term for more than 100 different forms of joint disease. However, while arthritis primarily affects the joints, it also attacks muscles and connective tissues surrounding organs. Arthritic disease stems from injuries, defects in the immune system, wear and tear on the joints, infections, or genetic predisposition. Whatever the cause, the effect is much the same in all individuals: Where bones meet in the joints, they are actually disintegrating.

Imagine a machine with well-oiled parts working smoothly, all valves pumping, all parts meshing together. Then, for some reason, one part bends, or the lubricating fluid dries up. Over a period of time, the parts begin to wear down or grind together until something gives way. For a variety of reasons, this is what happens in the joints of your arms, legs, hips, and even your back when they become arthritic. Some forms of arthritis do affect other parts of the body—skin, eyes, and various organ systems—and doctors watch for these symptoms in all patients with arthritic disease.

Many people believe that medicine's only answer for arthritis is use of strong prescription painkillers. And so they "self-medicate," follow "alternative diets," or try unproven "miracle" treatments such as copper bracelets or bee stings. Because arthritis is a disease that frequently comes and goes, these non-medical cures often seem to work. In fact, their success is merely a coincidence.

Fortunately, legitimate therapy is *not* limited to a few potent painkillers. There are many safe and effective medications for arthritis that, when combined with physical therapy, some dietary changes, and regular exercise, can enable most patients to lead normal lives.

## How Do We Treat Arthritis?

Arthritis treatment is determined by the type you have. In general, however, the front line therapy is an analgesic like *aspirin or acetaminophen* or a member of a group of medications called *nonsteroidal anti-inflammatory drugs, or NSAIDs*. Most arthritis sufferers rely on NSAIDs for daily pain relief. While aspirin is still widely used, NSAIDs have fewer gastric side effects and are longer-acting than aspirin, so you have to take fewer pills each day. Strong anti-inflammatory medications such as corticosteroids or immunosuppressive drugs may also be used.

Here's a rundown of treatments for each form of arthritis:

### Osteoarthritis (OA)

Most people will suffer from some form of OA as they grow older, and the joints naturally age through wear and tear. The most notable symptom, a dull aching feeling in the joints, usually appears toward the end of the day. The joints most commonly affected are in the hands, knees, fingers, spine, hips, neck, and feet. OA is a progressive disease and is not usually reversible. However, medication can relieve the symptoms.

Treatment for OA usually starts with a mild drug such as acetaminophen (Tylenol) or aspirin taken every four to six hours as needed. As the disease progresses, symptoms become more severe, and an NSAID such as ibuprofen (Motrin), indomethacin (Indocin), or naproxen (Naprosyn) may be substituted.

If OA pain becomes especially severe, a doctor will sometimes prescribe a short course of narcotic pain relievers such as Tylenol with Codeine. When joints become inflamed, injections of corticosteroids such as cortisone or prednisone can be effective.

Finally, a real exercise program—swimming, golf, walking, tennis, range-of-motion exercises (such as stretching)—is as valuable as medication in keeping joints flexible and mobile. Weight loss to relieve extra stress on joints is also vital to OA care.

### Rheumatoid Arthritis (RA)

Between the ages of 30 and 50, eight times as many women as men develop this crippling form of arthritis. Although we don't know why it develops, researchers suspect that victims have a genetic predisposition.

Unlike OA, RA symptoms are more pronounced in the morning—the joints and muscles tend to stiffen up overnight as you sleep. RA patients may develop swelling in the joints; and this may lead to deformities and, ultimately, total immobility. RA patients may also develop such related symptoms as fever, fatigue, and loss of appetite.

Drug treatment of RA begins with the same types of medications used for OA: aspirin, NSAIDs, and, occasionally, steroids. If these drugs fail to

## THE FIVE BASIC TYPES OF ARTHRITIS

1. Osteoarthritis: The most common form, this disease affects 15.8 million Americans (usually over age 45).
2. Rheumatoid Arthritis: Affects more than 2.1 million people, mostly women.
3. Gout: More frequent among men, with an estimated one million victims.
4. Ankylosing Spondylitis (Spinal Arthritis): More than 300,000 patients, also mostly males.
5. Systemic Lupus Erythematosus: Affecting 131,000 people, usually women.
Other, less common forms include Juvenile Rheumatoid Arthritis, Scleroderma and Arthritis Due to Infection.

control joint inflammation, other, more potent medications are prescribed. Although we don't know why, an antimalarial drug called hydroxychloroquine (Plaquenil) is known to reduce RA inflammation. While the drug seems to work well, it has potentially serious side effects that can cause vision problems, so careful monitoring by your physician and eye doctor is important. Gold salts, injected on a weekly or biweekly basis, can reduce joint inflammation, but, again, serious side effects make them impractical for many patients. Another drug—penicillamine (Depen)—works much like gold salts in reducing symptoms and retarding disease in severe cases of RA, and may cause fewer side effects.

Researchers today are exploring the role that immunosuppressive drugs can play in the treatment of RA. One, azathioprine (Imuran), is approved for use in RA cases. A second, methotrexate (Rheumatrex), is now frequently prescribed as well. Immunosuppressants are very powerful drugs and are used only in extremely serious cases where all else has failed. However, the drugs do relieve joint inflammation very effectively, and may even be lifesavers for patients with severe complications.

Like other forms of arthritis, RA should be treated by both medication and physical therapy, which can help restore some of the lost joint function. Surgical procedures such as hip and knee replacements have enabled many patients to return to a more fully functional lifestyle.

### Gout

Gout, one of the most painful forms of arthritis, is found primarily in men. While we can't cure it, we do have several highly effective treatments to control it. The symptoms of gout are often centered in the big toe, causing it be become swollen and extremely painful; but any joint may be affected. Pain usually occurs when the body is unable to eliminate uric acid, a waste product normally in the blood. If your body produces too much uric acid, or your kidneys aren't working properly to excrete it, an acute gout attack can follow.

Through the ages gout was known as the "disease of kings" because it was believed that a rich (man's) diet caused the disease. This myth is partially true. Diets high in purines (organ meats, fish eggs, sardines, anchovies, beer, and wine) can aggravate gout—but only in people who have trouble dealing with uric acid. Likewise, eliminating these foods may help reduce chances of an attack, but won't cure the underlying cause. Alcohol, too, can cause an attack or make one worse. Your diet and drinking habits should be fully discussed with your doctor when you begin treatment.

In general, gout is controlled or prevented by a number of specific medications that reduce the inflammation caused by the crystal-like deposits of uric acid that form in the toe, or other areas, and precipitate an attack.

Colchicine, a drug developed from the crocus plant, is among the best known anti-gout drugs. It provides quick relief during a gout attack and is also used preventively. In addition, there are two types of second-line treatment: Drugs that lower uric acid levels by increasing output, such as probenecid (Benemid) and sulfinpyrazone (Anturane), and drugs like allopurinol (Zyloprim) that prevent uric acid production. These medications are often supplemented with NSAIDs during acute attacks.

### Ankylosing Spondylitis (AS)

Ankylosing spondylitis (AS), or spinal arthritis, literally means "fused spine," since its basic symptom is an inability to bend the spinal column. Primarily afflicting men, this form of arthritis usually causes severe pain where the base of the spine connects to the pelvis. During the course of the disease, inflammation actually destroys the flexible joints in the lower spine. A certain genetic marker called HLA B-27 signals an increased risk of AS. Patients first experience pain in the lower back and buttocks, fever, and fatigue. Later, they may develop a stooped-over posture. Inflammation of the eyes and valvular heart disease may also occur.

The good news is that most cases of AS are relatively mild and can be treated with NSAIDs and a regular physical therapy program.

### Systemic Lupus Erythematosus (SLE or Lupus)

Though not itself a form of arthritis, lupus is linked to arthritis in more than half the cases. Its victims are teenage girls and young women more often than men. While it is treatable, no cure has been found

## HOW ARTHRITIS DISABLES THE JOINTS

CARTILAGE

HIP JOINT

LIGAMENT

LUBRICATING FLUID

SYNOVIUM

CAPSULE

BONE

THICKENING OF BONE

DEGENERATION OF CARTILAGE

FINGER JOINT

JOINT SPACE NARROWING

EROSION OF BONE HEAD

SWELLING AND INFLAMMATION OF SYNOVIUM AND CAPSULE

**Normal joint:** Where two bones meet, our bodies normally provide a simple and effective lubricating system. Ligaments binding the bones together form a capsule within which a thin membrane called the synovium exudes a fluid lubricant. For good measure, the ends of both bones are cushioned by a smooth layer of cartilage.

**Osteoarthritis:** In this form of arthritis, trouble begins when the protective cushion of cartilage between the bones slowly degenerates. As it disappears, the synovium and the ends of the bones thicken within the joint, leading to the aching stiffness that characterizes the disease.

**Rheumatoid arthritis:** The culprit here is the synovium, which for unknown reasons becomes swollen and inflamed, leading to irreversible damage to the joint's capsule and protective cartilage. Eventually the unprotected ends of the bones themselves begin to erode.

for this largely hereditary and possibly fatal disease. A less serious form of lupus is discoid lupus erythematosus (DLE).

The main symptom of SLE is inflammation of internal connective tissue. DLE, on the other hand, causes a circular rash on the face or skin. Although we don't know why either form occurs, lupus is classified as an immune system disorder. It can cause the body to attack its own organs, including the kidneys, causing high blood pressure and kidney failure; the lungs, causing pleurisy; or even the central nervous system, causing problems ranging from headache to psychosis. The symptoms wax and wane, reappearing with differing degrees of severity.

Once diagnosed, usually through blood tests or a skin biopsy, lupus is treated mainly by reducing its symptoms. NSAIDs, antimalarial drugs, and steroids are frequently used. Immunosuppressive drugs are prescribed for difficult cases. Because sunlight can make lupus symptoms worse in many cases, sunblock or sunscreen should always be worn.

While lupus is a serious, life-threatening disease, patient survival rates have steadily improved over the last decade, due to more effective treatment of related kidney disease and other problems.

### Other Arthritic Disease

**Progressive Systemic Sclerosis**, better known as Scleroderma, is a relatively rare disease that causes thickening of the skin and, like lupus, can affect connective tissue in internal organs. While there is no cure, its symptoms are often relieved by high blood pressure medications like vasodilators (see Chapter 2), steroids, and immunosuppressive drugs.

**Juvenile Rheumatoid Arthritis** is also known as Still's Disease, monarticular juvenile arthritis, or polyarticular juvenile arthritis. This disease, which afflicts children and adolescents, usually has symptoms—aching and swollen joints—similar to other forms of arthritis. Treatment includes pain relief with NSAIDs and analgesics. Steroids and other drugs used to treat adult RA may be needed in some juvenile cases.

**Infectious arthritis** is the name given to arthritis-like symptoms that often occur after severe infections such as Lyme disease or gonorrhea, and viral illnesses such as measles, chickenpox, and mumps. Symptoms usually disappear with treatment of the primary infection by antibiotics or other appropriate drugs.

## Living with Arthritis

Many arthritis victims will suffer for prolonged periods, even the rest of their lives. Often simple skills like dressing, eating, and bathing must be relearned. To make life easier, there are many assistive devices that can be installed in the home, such as "grab bars" to help a person get in and out of the bathtub, and other aids such as large-button phones. Any physical therapist or rehabilitation specialist can make a visit to your home to help determine your needs. Often simply removing dangerous electrical cords or other impediments can prevent the falls and other accidents that damage fragile joints. In general, proper use of medications, exercise, rest, and a good diet will do the most to relieve arthritis symptoms.

Over the past three decades, research breakthroughs have helped reduce the suffering of many afflicted with arthritis. We have learned that certain gene patterns mean a susceptibility to arthritis, making early detection possible. There is now evidence that a genetic marker for osteoarthritis may exist. Researchers are closer to understanding which cells trigger the autoimmune forms of arthritis such as lupus, and what these forms may have in common with other diseases such as diabetes and multiple sclerosis. Even the drugs we take for granted today were the result of years of research. And now on the horizon is a new class of medicines called *leumedins* which block inflamed cells from reaching the joints. □

## CHAPTER 4

# Osteoporosis, Low Back Pain, and Other Bone Disorders

The human skeleton is an intricate framework of 206 bones that give the body its structure and shape. These bones serve as armor for vital organs and soft tissue, a storehouse for minerals, and a birthplace for blood cells. Together, the bones act in concert with the muscles, ligaments, tendons, and other connective tissue to give humans an amazing range of movement.

Most bone diseases are rare, but a few pose serious health problems. Osteoporosis, for example, is a progressive loss of bone substance that affects about 25 million Americans, mostly postmenopausal caucasian women. Osteoarthritis, the most common form of arthritis, is widespread among people over 40. (See Chapter 3, "Coping with Arthritis.") Low back pain, which often results from slipped vertebrae or disks, is the second most frequent cause of lost work for adults under 45 years of age.

## How Bones Are Structured

Bones are made of inorganic salts—including calcium and phosphate—imbedded in collagen fibers. Though solid and seemingly completely formed, bones undergo constant renewal and change. The marrow, or soft center, of certain bones serves as a spawning ground for the many different cells that make up the blood.

There are three types of bones—long, short, and flat or irregular. Long bones include the humerus,

radius, and ulna of the arm; the femur, tibia, and fibula of the leg; and the phalanges, metacarpals, and metatarsals of the hand and foot. The tarsal in the foot and the carpal in the wrist are short bones. Flat bones can be found in the head and also include the ribs, breastbone, and collarbone. Irregular bones are located mostly in the spine; certain others are situated in the head.

## Osteoporosis

In osteoporosis a loss of calcium and phosphate salts causes the bones to become porous, brittle, and easily broken. The vertebrae in the spine may compress, causing the back to become bent and resulting in such conditions as kyphosis (round back) or scoliosis (spinal curvature). A deformed spine usually affects other body parts, particularly nearby organs.

Inadequate dietary intake of calcium, hormonal changes associated with aging, and an inactive lifestyle have all been implicated in the development of osteoporosis. Drug use, alcoholism, lactose intolerance, an overactive thyroid, and faulty calcium absorption may also put people at risk. Other risk factors include premature menopause and the absence or abnormal halt of menstrual periods; a petite, thin build; smoking; a caucasian or oriental background; scoliosis; and a fair complexion.

Menopause, which is accompanied by a sudden, rapid loss of bone minerals, is a particularly critical point in the development of osteoporosis. It's

## OUR 206 BONES

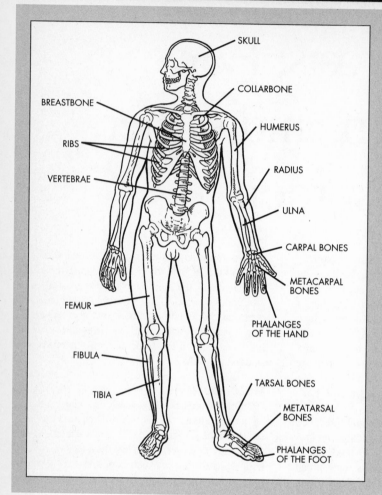

SKULL

COLLARBONE

BREASTBONE

HUMERUS

RIBS

VERTEBRAE

RADIUS

ULNA

CARPAL BONES

METACARPAL BONES

FEMUR

PHALANGES OF THE HAND

FIBULA

TIBIA

TARSAL BONES

METATARSAL BONES

PHALANGES OF THE FOOT

We're conscious of our complex skeletal infrastructure only when something goes awry. The joints are particularly problem-prone; and the spine, with its many joints, gives us the most trouble of all. The effects of osteoporosis may first be seen in the spine. Low back pain arises in the spine. Even neck pain may have its source in the spine. Indeed, where our bones are concerned, back problems are exceeded only by arthritis as a source of pain and suffering.

wise to consult a doctor for guidance at this important juncture. Unfortunately, most people learn they have osteoporosis only after the disease has progressed. Indeed, the first signal is often a sharp pain in the lower back while lifting or bending, which usually indicates the collapse of a vertebra. Some people may show signs of increasing deformity, such as a humped back and a loss of height.

Treatment for osteoporosis is aimed at preventing bone mineral loss. It usually includes physical therapy; an exercise regimen; and estrogen, calcium, vitamin D, and in some cases calcitonin.

## Low Back Pain

The back is a complex structure comprised of vertebrae (irregular bones), disks (cushions between the vertebrae), the spinal cord, nerves, muscles, and ligaments. Back problems may involve any of these components and are usually very distressing and debilitating. Low back pain is one of the most common complaints, affecting four out of five people at some point in their lives.

Osteoporosis or arthritis may be the cause of low back pain. Scoliosis or slippage of one vertebra onto another vertebra (spondylolisthesis) can also cause severe discomfort in the lower back.

Another common cause of low back pain is ruptured, slipped, or herniated disks. Disks have a soft, gelatinous center (nucleus) surrounded by an outer ring (anulus). Trauma, strain, or degeneration may weaken the outer ring so that the center bulges through and impinges on nerve roots in the spine, or on the spinal cord itself.

Herniated disks usually cause severe lower back pain that radiates to the buttocks, legs, and feet. There may also be a loss of feeling and mobility in the affected areas and ultimately weakness and atrophy of leg muscles.

Treatment of herniated disks usually includes a week or more of bed rest, heat treatments, and exercise. Aspirin or another analgesic is usually recommended; cortisone is prescribed in rare instances. Muscle relaxants, such as methocarbamol (Robaxin) or diazepam (Valium), can also be very helpful. If the pain persists, disk surgery may be necessary.

## Neck Pain

Neck pain is another common source of severe discomfort. The neck is less protected than the rest of the spine and thus is more prone to painful and disabling injuries and disorders. As with the lower back, neck pain may result from abnormalities in the muscles, ligaments, and nerves, as well as the joints and bones. Osteoarthritis, rheumatoid arthritis, and cervical degeneration are common causes of pain in this area.

Whiplash injuries, falls, and contact sports can also do real damage to the neck. Careful diagnosis is essential to determine the correct treatment and rehabilitation program. Treatment usually consists of rest, medication, immobilization, exercise, neck braces, and physical therapy. Medications usually include aspirin, nonsteroidal anti-inflammatory drugs (NSAIDs) such as Motrin, other analgesics, and muscle relaxants.

## Scoliosis

The spine's normal curves produce the rounding of the shoulders and the inward curve of the lower back. Scoliosis is an abnormal "s" curving of the spine that gives a person the appearance of slumping to one side. Usually first noticed in the teen years, and more prevalent among girls,

scoliosis often causes one shoulder blade to protrude and one shoulder to be higher than the other. Hips and ribs can also become misaligned.

The treatment of scoliosis is determined by the severity of the deformity and may include exercise, a brace, surgery, or any combination of these measures.

## Carpal Tunnel Syndrome

Carpal tunnel syndrome occurs when the main nerve in the wrist becomes compressed. The compression causes pain and motor difficulties in the hand. The carpal tunnel is a hollow area in the wrist. The median nerve, blood vessels, and flexor tendons of the fingers and thumb all pass through the carpal tunnel. The tunnel is formed by the carpal (wrist) bones and ligaments. Problems arise when the content or structure of the tunnel swells and presses the median nerve against the ligament.

People who use poorly designed tools, assembly-line workers, and typists are prone to carpal tunnel syndrome. This problem can also be brought on by rheumatoid arthritis, pregnancy, kidney failure, acromegaly (a hormonal disorder), menopause, diabetes mellitus, amyloidosis, tuberculosis, myxedema (thyroid hormone disorder), and benign tumors.

Symptoms of carpal tunnel syndrome usually include pain, burning, weakness, tingling, or numbness in one or both hands. Treatment usually consists of wearing braces or splints at night to keep the wrist from bending. NSAIDs and cortisone are often given to reduce swelling. If these methods are not successful, surgery may be required.

## Fractures

Broken bones aren't always serious, but a break almost always is debilitating in some way. A fracture usually affects surrounding tissue, so there is often swelling and additional pain as a result of the extra damage. Since most broken bones are caused by trauma of some kind, shock and emotional distress often occur as well.

Broken bones can cause pain, swelling, deformity, discoloration, tenderness, and loss of function in the affected area. Whether the broken bone is in the skull, nose, jaw, rib, hip, or a limb, all fractures and breaks require immediate treatment by a physician. Proper medical care includes treat-

## THE CARPAL TUNNEL

METACARPAL
BONES 1 - 5

CARPAL BONES

CARPAL BONES

ULNA

RADIUS

Within the complex cluster of bones that form the wrist, a collection of ligaments, tendons, blood vessels, and nerves crowd a narrow passage between the arm and the hand. If repeated stress causes swelling within this tunnel, the main nerve will be squeezed against nearby ligaments and tendons. The well-known carpal tunnel syndrome —pain in the wrist, hand, or forearm — then may follow.

ment of shock and the prevention of blood loss and other serious complications. Realignment of the displaced bones and immobilization with a cast or traction are standard measures.

A local anesthetic such as lidocaine is usually all that's needed to set a broken limb. Analgesics such as meperidine (Demerol) are given to relieve pain; muscle relaxants such as diazepam (Valium) help stretch muscles to make it easier to set the bone. □

**CHAPTER 5**

# Digestive Disorders, Minor and Major

I f we are what we eat, then what we are is only as good as our digestion. When it goes awry, it generally affects our total well-being. Whether it's mild nausea, a nasty virus, or a chronic disorder such as irritable bowel syndrome, a disorder of the digestive tract is usually impossible to ignore. If the condition persists, it can undermine our total health, eventually threatening our very lives.

## How the Digestive System Works

T he gastrointestinal (GI) tract is a long hollow tube stretching from the head to the end of the body, including the mouth, pharynx, esophagus, stomach, small intestine, and large intestine. The salivary glands, liver, gallbladder, and pancreas are also important parts of this far-reaching system.

The main purpose of the GI tract is to break down carbohydrates, fats, and proteins into molecules small enough to be absorbed through cell membranes. In that way, it provides the cells with the necessary energy for life and health.

Digestion begins in the mouth when food is chewed and starch is broken down by ptyalin, an enzyme secreted in saliva. Food then enters the stomach, where it is reduced to tiny particles and further transformed by gastric juices. The solid portion remains in the stomach for one to six hours until it liquefies completely; liquid passes into the duodenum (small intestine), where numerous

enzymes produced by the pancreas, along with bile from the liver, break it down further for absorption. When it finally arrives in the large intestine, all nutritional value has been spent, and the only remaining process is the removal of water before final elimination.

Every section of the GI tract is prone to its own unique disorders—some merely annoying, others potentially fatal. Fortunately, for all but a few we now have simple treatments that will, at the very least, relieve the symptoms.

## Diseases of the Upper GI Tract

R eflux esophagitis is characterized by heartburn, upper abdominal or chest pain, difficulty swallowing, nausea, or belching that leaves an acid taste. It is caused by a backflow of acid stomach contents into the esophagus. Symptoms usually occur within an hour after eating, and are most likely to strike when you lie down, bend, or stoop. It is alleviated by taking antacids or sitting up. It may be aggravated by vigorous exercise, and is often associated with hiatal hernia (protrusion of the stomach above the diaphragm). Severe cases can lead to a narrowing of the esophagus requiring medical therapy.

Liquid antacids are effective for immediate relief of heartburn. Histamine blockers such as Pepcid and Tagamet are now becoming available for heartburn in low, over-the-counter dosage strengths. Medications such as omeprazole

## MAPPING THE GI TRACT

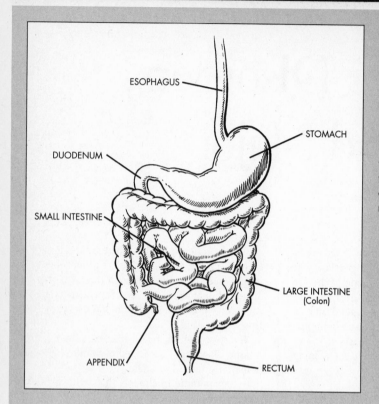

ESOPHAGUS

STOMACH

DUODENUM

SMALL INTESTINE

LARGE INTESTINE
(Colon)

APPENDIX

RECTUM

The digestive tract's convoluted course begins at the mouth, ending yards later at the rectum. In between lie the esophagus, stomach, and small and large intestines. Each segment is vulnerable to a characteristic set of afflictions, ranging from gastritis, gastroenteritis, and ulcers in the upper tract to colitis, diverticulosis, and colon cancer in the lower segments.

(Prilosec) and cisapride (Propulsid) are frequently prescribed to reduce backflow. Since almost anything that increases pressure in the abdomen can cause heartburn, long-term therapy involves ways of reducing that pressure. These include losing weight (for those who are overweight); avoiding tight clothing; remembering not to bend or stoop; and elevating the head of the bed by 30 degrees. Eating smaller meals more often can decrease symptoms. It is also wise to avoid lying down for two to three hours after eating and to forgo foods that increase heartburn—such as chocolate, coffee, tea, citrus fruits, alcohol, and those high in fat—as well as smoking.

**Gastroenteritis** is diarrhea, nausea, vomiting, and abdominal cramping brought on by bacteria, amoebas, parasites, toxins, certain drugs, enzymes, or allergens in foods. Treatment usually includes bed rest, fluids, bismuth-containing products such as Pepto-Bismol, and anti-nausea drugs like trimethobenzamide (Tigan) and prochlorperazine (Compazine). When an infection is the cause, the doctor may also prescribe an antibiotic.

**Chronic gastritis** is inflammation of the stomach lining. It is sometimes caused by eating irritating substances. In elderly people, it is associated with pernicious anemia. Some people with this disorder have no symptoms, but many experience vague pain, a feeling of fullness, loss of appetite, belching, nausea and vomiting. Treatment consists of eliminating the irritating foods, avoiding aspirin, and taking antacids if the condition persists. If pernicious anemia is the underlying cause, the doctor may administer vitamin B$_{12}$. Severe cases may call for other medication.

**Ulcers** can occur in the lower esophagus, stomach, or any part of the small intestine, and are designated by their location. About 80 percent are **duodenal ulcers**, found in the first segment of the small intestine, mostly in men between 20 and 50. Less common are **gastric ulcers**, located in the stomach and found most often in middle-aged and elderly men and chronic users of aspirin, alcohol, and cigarettes. Both types of ulcer can produce heartburn, pain, nausea, indigestion, and, in gastric ulcer, pain after eating a meal. Weight loss is common with gastric ulcers, while the opposite often happens with duodenal ulcers because patients may eat to relieve discomfort. Ulcers are caused by a bacterial infection, and usually can be cured with antibiotics. Over-secretion of gastric acids and stress have long been regarded as contributing factors.

In addition to antibiotics, therapy includes rest and is generally directed toward buffering stomach acid with antacids, as well as reducing acid production with drugs known as histamine H$_2$ blockers, including cimetidine (Tagamet), ranitidine (Zantac), nizatidine (Axid), and famotidine (Pepcid). The doctor may also prescribe drugs such as sucralfate (Carafate) that coat the ulcer without reducing acid. In the future, so-called protective drugs will be available that can heal ulcers and prevent their recurrence.

Whatever form of therapy is employed, close follow-up by either upper endoscopy or X-rays is required. If an ulcer has not healed after two to three months, surgery may be needed.

**Gastric cancer** is more common in males than females, especially those over 40. It has a higher incidence in northern industrial areas and a higher mortality in Japan, Iceland, Chile, and Austria. In the U.S., the incidence has decreased 50 percent in the last 25 years. Dietary patterns—such as heavy consumption of pickled, smoked, or salt-preserved foods and those containing nitrates and nitrous compounds—may be implicated in its development. This disease is also more likely in those with Type A blood and those with a history of gastric cancer in their families. The risk may be reduced by a diet including whole milk, fresh vegetables, and vitamin C. Early signs include indigestion and discomfort, followed by weight and appetite loss, a sensation of fullness after eating, fatigue, and anemia. Surgery, sometimes followed by chemotherapy, is currently the only effective treatment.

## WHERE ULCERS STRIKE

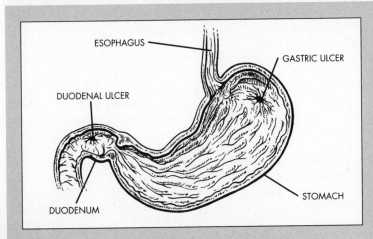

ESOPHAGUS
GASTRIC ULCER
DUODENAL ULCER
STOMACH
DUODENUM

Though we think of ulcers as a stomach problem, the most common variety actually occurs just outside the stomach in the duodenum, or beginning of the small intestine. Others (gastric ulcers) do appear in the stomach; and no part of the intestines is immune to the problem. An ulcer is, essentially, an open sore. We feel pain when stomach acids come in contact with the ulcer's raw, exposed surface.

# Diseases of the Large Intestine

Irritable bowel syndrome occurs more frequently in women under age 35, and often begins in late adolescence. It may be related to psychological stress and is commonly marked by an abnormally active—even spastic—lower bowel. Its symptoms are similar to a number of other illnesses, including diverticulosis and lactose intolerance. These symptoms include uncomfortable abdominal sensations and periodic diarrhea or constipation, sometimes occurring alternately. Some patients come to depend on laxatives and even enemas to alleviate the constipation. For others, the only symptom is painless diarrhea. Treatment includes a diet high in fiber and low in fat. Certain gas-producing foods, such as those in the cabbage family, should be avoided, as should any other suspected irritants. For constipation, a bulk-producing product may be recommended; for diarrhea, diphenoxylate with atropine (Lomotil) or loperamide (Imodium) are possibilities. As a last resort, antispasmodics such as propantheline (Pro-Banthine) may be prescribed.

**Inflammatory bowel disease** is a blanket term covering three serious disorders: ulcerative colitis, proctitis, and Crohn's disease.

Ulcerative colitis is an inflammation of the colon that produces ulceration of the inside wall. Its primary symptom is bloody, chronic diarrhea, often containing pus and mucus, and associated with abdominal pain and weight and appetite loss. When confined to the rectum, it's referred to as ulcerative proctitis. Though there is no known cause of ulcerative colitis, it does tend to run in families and is more common in Jews and caucasians than other ethnic or racial groups.

Sometimes known as ileitis, Crohn's disease is an inflammation of the small and/or large intestine, with accompanying pain, cramping, tenderness, gas, fever, nausea, and diarrhea. Though usually mild, bleeding may occur and may sometimes be massive.

Proctitis, an inflammation of the rectum, is characterized by bloody stools, a frequent urge to defecate but inability to do so, and sometimes diarrhea. Possible causes are ulcerative colitis, Crohn's disease, trauma, infection, or radiation.

Ulcerative colitis and Crohn's disease are generally chronic and have no known cures. Treatment usually consists of symptom relief and reduction of inflammation. When there are acute flare-ups, the patient should avoid stimulants such as caffeine, citrus fruits, and foods high in fiber. Medical therapy includes steroids such as prednisone (Deltasone) and drugs such as olsalazine (Dipentum) that have both anti-inflammatory and antibacterial properties. These medications can control symptoms and often produce long-term remissions. Steroids should be used only when necessary, and under a physician's guidance, to avoid serious side effects. If attacks of ulcerative colitis become severe enough to be life-threatening, surgical removal of the colon can save the patient's life. Surgery also is sometimes performed for very severe complications of Crohn's disease, but will not cure the disease itself.

**Diverticulosis**, a condition most common in men over 40, is present in up to 50 percent of people aged 60. Though generally silent until bleeding and inflammation occur, it can be marked by alternating constipation and diarrhea. The disease occurs when bulging pouches (diverticula) form at weak points in the wall of the colon. If they become inflamed, they can cause severe pain, fever, nausea, and vomiting; if small vessels at the base of the pouch become disrupted, there may be significant intestinal bleeding. When symptoms occur, they can be alleviated by a liquid or bland diet and stool softeners. After symptoms subside, a high-fiber diet is usually effective in preventing recurrence and progression of the disease. When infection is present, treatment includes a broad-spectrum antibiotic and bowel rest.

**Intestinal polyps**, abnormal growths that may occur anywhere in the GI tract, are most often found in the large intestine. Though they generally cause no symptoms, a major sign is rectal bleeding. Polyps are rare in underdeveloped countries, suggesting that our high-fat, low-fiber diets may be partially responsible. They are more frequent in individuals with a family history of polyps or cancer of the colon. No current treatment is known to prevent recurrence. Reducing the fat content of your diet by 25 percent and consuming fiber-containing foods on a daily basis are both recommended. Because polyps are thought to be precursors of colon cancer, it's important to have them removed. This can be done with colonoscopy on an outpatient basis. An annual examination for polyps is advisable from age 50 onward.

**Colon cancer**, silent in its earliest stages, becomes evident as it progresses. Symptoms include bleeding, at times invisible to the naked eye, with resultant anemia, as well as a change in bowel habits, often accompanied by pain, weight and appetite loss, weakness, and a general decline in health. The risk for colon cancer increases with age, doubling with each decade after 40. Its exact causes are unknown, but it appears to be related to diets high in fat and low in fiber, and is known to occur more frequently in those with a family history of colon cancer. Surgery, sometimes followed by chemotherapy and radiation, are the current treatments for this type of cancer.

## Other GI Problems

**H**emorrhoids are dilated veins in the lower rectum and anus. They affect 50 percent of people over age 50. Diets low in fiber are thought to be a major cause. Straining at defecation to evacuate hard stools also seems to promote their development. A high-fiber diet and prompt, strain-free defecation help relieve mildly symptomatic hemorrhoids. Local swelling and pain can be decreased with local anesthetic creams, lotions, or suppositories; astringents; or cold compresses. For those with severe symptoms, rubber band ligation, cryosurgery, injection therapy, or surgical removal may be needed.

**Constipation** is the term given for infrequent or difficult evacuation of small, hard stools, accompanied by mild abdominal discomfort. When the condition is chronic, it may include nausea, stomach rumbling, appetite loss, and malaise. Constipation is a common condition that affects mostly the very young and the aged. While the number of bowel movements is variable in the general population, a normal individual should have at least three per week, or, ideally, one daily.

Treatment for constipation includes laxatives and enemas, a diet high in fiber, and adequate exercise. If these efforts fail, a doctor should be consulted to rule out causes such as drugs, diabetes, hypothyroidism, or colon problems.

**Pancreatitis** is an inflammation of the pancreas. It can occur periodically or chronically. The first sign may be a sudden, severe abdominal pain above the navel, which travels through to the back. Accompanying symptoms may include a low-grade fever, nausea, and vomiting. Pancreatitis in men is commonly associated with alcohol use, trauma, and peptic ulcer; in women, with gallstones and disease of the bile duct. In rare instances, a medication may be the cause.

Patients with an acute attack are hospitalized, given intravenous fluids, and administered painkillers. If the symptoms are caused by gallstones, the gallbladder should be removed. If alcohol is the cause, it should be stopped immediately and completely avoided thereafter. Any drugs that might be responsible should be discontinued.

For patients with chronic pancreatitis, analgesics are often used to treat the severe pain. A low-fat diet, along with pancreatic enzymes, is also sometimes part of the treatment regimen.

It's a little-known fact that sexually transmitted diseases may involve not only the genitalia but also the digestive tract. **Shigellosis, giardiasis,** and **amebiasis** are the most common of the sexually transmitted digestive diseases. They can also be passed along in food and water contaminated by infected individuals who fail to wash their hands properly. Symptoms generally include watery or even bloody diarrhea associated with severe abdominal pain. Without treatment, an attack may last from days to weeks. Therapy depends on the type of infection. These diseases should always be treated by a physician. □

**CHAPTER 6**

# Defeating the Dangers of Respiratory Disease

We can go without water for days and do without food even longer, but without air we will die in a matter of minutes. Breathing, along with the beating of our hearts, is one of the body's most essential functions, and any disruption can be deadly. Even a minor cold, by affecting our normal intake and outflow of air, can make us feel miserable.

Respiratory problems are common—indeed the most common of all physical complaints. Almost everyone experiences infections of the head, throat, and chest. These infections range from colds to influenza and pneumonia, which can be mildly debilitating or seriously life-threatening.

## How The Respiratory System Works

The nose, lungs, and diaphragm are the major respiratory organs. As the diaphragm contracts, the rib cage expands. This action creates negative pressure in the lung cavity, and air is then pulled in through the nose. When the diaphragm stops contracting, the lungs recoil and push the air out. Oxygen is exchanged for carbon dioxide ($CO_2$) in the blood that flows through the capillaries in any one of the lung's 300 million alveoli. Circulating blood then delivers the oxygen to the body's cells in exchange for $CO_2$ and metabolic waste. This trade is known as internal respiration. The lungs subsequently exhale $CO_2$-containing air.

## Colds and Flu

The common cold is aptly named: It ranks as the most prevalent infectious disease in humans. Indeed, the common cold accounts for just about as many trips to the drugstore as any other ailment. And although the common cold tends to be benign and brief, this nuisance illness can lead to more serious bacterial infections.

Colds are almost always caused by viral infections of the upper respiratory tract. Many different families of viruses can cause a common cold, and each family has numerous members. The sheer diversity of causative agents is why it has been impossible to develop a vaccine for the common cold.

Different viruses affect different areas of the respiratory tract and may result in fever, chills, malaise, and lethargy. When a virus causes nasal inflammation, you develop stuffiness or runniness, and sometimes postnasal drip. If the virus travels to the pharynx, you get a sore throat or pharyngitis. If inflammation reaches the vocal cords, you may become hoarse or even lose your voice (laryngitis). If the trachea and main bronchi are involved, you will most likely complain of congestion and coughing, and will also produce sputum. This particular medical condition is called tracheobronchitis or acute bronchitis.

Since there is no cure for colds, treatment focuses on the symptoms. Remedies include aspirin, acetaminophen or ibuprofen, increased fluids, and rest. (Avoid giving aspirin to children.

It may be linked with a dangerous condition called Reye's syndrome.) Decongestants, throat lozenges, nasal sprays, cough medicines, and expectorants are all used and may or may not ease the symptoms of a cold. In some instances, antibiotics are needed to wipe out any accompanying bacterial infection. This is often the case with bronchitis.

**The influenza virus** attacks the respiratory tract with particularly debilitating results. Influenza, often called "flu," commonly causes severe aching in the muscles and joints, chills, headache, fever, discomfort, a dry cough, and exhaustion. The virus typically spreads throughout an entire community, often causing serious complications such as pneumonia, and even death. The good news is that influenza can be prevented if you get an annual vaccination.

The treatment of influenza consists of bed rest, increased fluids, aspirin—or for children, acetaminophen—and an expectorant, such as guaifenesin, to treat the cough. Amantadine, an antiviral agent, has proved helpful in reducing the symptoms and the duration of influenza A, and is also used to help prevent it.

## Pneumonia

Pneumonia, an inflammation of the lungs, is usually caused by viruses, bacteria, fungi, protozoa, mycobacteria, mycoplasma, or rickettsia. Pneumonia is a serious matter because the infection may interfere with the lung's very important function of exchanging oxygen and carbon dioxide in the blood.

Common symptoms of pneumonia are fever, shaking chills, pleuritic (lung) pain, cough, and sputum production. In some cases, the resulting sputum may be minimal and off-white in color. Sometimes the patient produces abundant amounts of yellow, green, or brown sputum.

Viral pneumonia is treated symptomatically with adequate liquids and bed rest. Severe cases may require humidified oxygen therapy and mechanical ventilation. The treatment of bacterial pneumonia must also include appropriate antibiotics. There is a vaccine available to prevent the most common bacterial form of this disease.

## A CLOSE-UP VIEW OF OUR AMAZING LUNGS

ALVEOLI

BRONCHIOLES

BRONCHI

DIAPHRAGM

TRACHEA

LUNG

Though they fill most of the chest, the lungs perform their crucial task at an almost microscopic level. Starting at the trachea, or windpipe, the air passages within the lungs divide and redivide into ever smaller branches, or bronchioles, finally terminating in 300 million minute air sacs called alveoli. It's within these capillary-laced sacs that the air we inhale meets our circulatory system, passing fresh oxygen to the blood and removing waste $CO_2$.

## Chronic Lung Disorders

Chronic obstructive pulmonary disease (COPD), the most common chronic lung disorder, currently afflicts some 17 million Americans. And the incidence of COPD is on the rise. Emphysema, chronic bronchitis, asthma (see chapter on allergies), or any combination of these conditions may result in COPD. Smoking is the most common cause of COPD; recurrent infections and allergies may also predispose an individual to this disorder.

**Emphysema** actually destroys the lung, causing it to lose its elastic properties. As a result, the lungs have trouble expelling air and thus are unable to move air in and out at a normal rate.

**Chronic bronchitis** involves an inflammation of the bronchial tubes and is characterized by excessive mucus production. The symptoms of chronic bronchitis are cough and sputum production. The disease begins with a typical smoker's cough. Each morning, coughing helps to clear the excess mucus from the lungs. As the bronchitis progresses, shortness of breath develops and eventually becomes chronic.

People with COPD can live relatively normal lives for years. Sooner or later, though, they will notice a growing inability to exercise or do strenuous work, along with the onset of a productive cough. The symptoms tend to get worse as time goes by, and the individual becomes more and more prone to respiratory infections, shortness of breath, and reduced pulmonary function.

Treatment consists of relieving the symptoms of COPD, preventing complications, educating smokers to stop, and encouraging all patients to eliminate any airborne irritants. Patients are also taught deep breathing exercises to strengthen muscles used in respiration and are trained to cough effectively. Oxygen therapy is sometimes necessary as well. The medications prescribed for COPD are bronchodilators such as theophylline (Theo-Dur), antibiotics for infections, diuretics (water pills) to eliminate the fluid retention, and corticosteroids (for chronic bronchitis and asthma).

## The Resurgence of TB

Tuberculosis was declining for many years in America; but, unfortunately, this infection is back and on the rise. Some people who contract tuberculosis fail to take their medication properly. It is this lack of compliance that is often cited as the reason for the increasing spread of this dread disease.

Tuberculosis is a serious, chronic infection. In about five percent of those exposed, tuberculosis develops within one year. However, the infection may also lie dormant for years, emerging as tuberculosis when the person is weakened by another serious illness, such as diabetes, leukemia, or Hodgkin's disease, or when immunity is compromised by immunosuppressive drugs or AIDS. Tuberculosis is transmitted through the air, particularly after an infected person coughs.

The initial infection with TB generally does not produce any symptoms. When symptoms do appear, infected individuals are likely to complain of fever, night sweats, loss of appetite, weight loss, and fatigue. In its reactivated phase, TB may be signaled by a cough with discolored sputum production and sometimes pain in the chest. Patients may also cough up blood. Tuberculosis is caused by *Mycobacterium tuberculosis* and as such is treated with daily oral doses of antibiotics for at least nine months. The drugs used most often are isoniazid and rifampin (Rifadin, Rimactane).

The diagnostic test for tuberculosis is called a Tine test or PPD skin test. A positive reading indicates that a person has been exposed to tuberculosis but does not necessarily predict who will ultimately develop active infection. People with positive skin test results can often prevent subsequent illness by faithfully taking a one-year course of antituberculosis antibiotics.

## Childhood Respiratory Diseases

Croup, a childhood disease more common in boys than girls, typically occurs between the ages of three months and three years. This disease usually follows a viral infection and is associated with a harsh, grating, creaking sound upon breathing; hoarse or muffled vocal sounds; labored breathing; and the characteristic sharp, barking cough. Depending on the type of infection, croup may also be accompanied by a sore throat, hoarseness, runny nose, rapid pulse, clammy skin, and breathing marked by sharp inward and outward movement of the spot above the sternum and muscles of the rib cage—like a balloon quickly filling and then losing air.

Treatment for croup usually consists of rest, cool humidification while sleeping, and acetaminophen. If the child has severe respiratory distress, hospitalization and oxygen therapy may be necessary. If a bacterial infection is a factor, the child must also take antibiotics.

**Epiglottitis** is a disorder in which the epiglottis becomes inflamed—often to the point of blocking breathing. Epiglottitis typically strikes children between the ages of two and eight years. It is a critical condition, one that can prove fatal if appropriate emergency treatment is not implemented.

Epiglottitis may begin as a respiratory infection, progressing to complete upper airway obstruction within two to five hours. Symptoms include difficulty in breathing and swallowing, a harsh, grating or creaking sound when breathing, high fever, sore throat, restlessness, irritability, and drooling. Emergency treatment is necessary and includes endotracheal intubation or a tracheotomy, oxygen therapy, and the administration of fluids to prevent dehydration. Patients always receive antibiotics.

For more on childhood diseases, including whooping cough, turn to Chapter 12.

## Other Serious Respiratory Illnesses

Legionnaires' disease got its name from the highly publicized outbreak that occurred in 1976 during an American Legion convention in Philadelphia. Legionnaires' disease is usually an acute bronchopneumonia accompanied by diarrhea, malaise, body aches and headaches, loss of appetite, recurrent chills, and a fever that occurs within 12 to 48 hours and rises as high as 105 degrees. Patients subsequently develop a dry cough that may later produce grayish and sometimes blood-streaked sputum. Other possible symptoms of legionnaires' disease include disorientation, vomiting, nausea, mental sluggishness, and mild, temporary amnesia.

As soon as legionnaires' disease is suspected, antibiotics should be administered immediately.

Erythromycin (E-Mycin), alone or in combination with rifampin (Rifadin), is the preferred treatment for legionnaires' disease. If the patient cannot tolerate erythromycin, the doctor may prescribe doxycycline (Vibramycin)—alone or with rifampin—instead. Treatment may also consist of aspirin or acetaminophen; drugs that increase blood pressure if necessary; fluid replacement; and oxygen therapy.

**Pleurisy** is an inflammation of the tissue that lines the lungs and the inner surface of the chest wall. Pleurisy is usually a complication of pneumonia, but may also result from viruses, tuberculosis, chest trauma, rheumatoid arthritis, systemic lupus erythematosus (a collagen vascular disease), cancer, pulmonary infarction (a blood clot in the lungs), and Dressler's syndrome (a complication of heart attack). Pleurisy is characterized by a sharp, stabbing pain that intensifies with breathing. The pain may at times inhibit movement on the affected side. Breathing is labored. Treatment involves anti-inflammatory drugs, painkillers, bed rest, and, in severe cases, a nerve block.

**Asthma**, a grave respiratory disorder affecting millions, is discussed in the chapter on allergies. To learn about lung cancer, turn to Chapter 7. □

**CHAPTER 7**

# Cancer: Improving the Odds of a Cure

Cancer is the scourge of the late 20th century. Few things raise more fear in our hearts than the diagnosis—or even the mere thought—of this dreaded disease. And though cancer has been claiming more lives each year over the past five decades, the news is not entirely grim.

At the turn of the century, almost no one with cancer could expect to live very long. By the 1930s, not even one in five cancer patients was still alive five years after treatment. In the 1940s, the five-year survival rate was one in four; in the 1960s, one in three Americans survived. Today, about four out of 10 cancer patients live for at least five years after the initial diagnosis.

The survival rate increases substantially with early detection. Cancers of the breast, tongue, mouth, colon, rectum, cervix, prostate, testes, and skin account for half of all new cases. Two-thirds of the people diagnosed with these cancers will pass the five-year survival mark. However, the survival rate could climb as high as 89 percent *if* these cancers were diagnosed early through screening and self-examinations *and* were treated promptly. In other words, of the 1,130,000 Americans who will be diagnosed with cancer this year, an additional 100,000 people would survive.

In addition, many cancers are preventable. Researchers say that up to 90 percent of the estimated 600,000 skin cancers diagnosed annually could be prevented by proper precautions against the sun's rays. All cancers caused by smoking and excessive alcohol use could be prevented entirely. This translates into an estimated 146,000 lung cancer deaths per year and 16,500 cancer deaths related to the heavy consumption of alcohol, often in combination with cigarette use.

## What Is Cancer?

The millions of cells that make up the body normally reproduce in an orderly manner, replacing worn-out tissues and repairing injuries to maintain health. However, certain cells may begin to reproduce abnormally, massing together to form tumors.

If a tumor is benign, it will remain self-contained. A malignant—or cancerous—tumor, on the other hand, will invade neighboring tissues, and can spread through the blood and lymphatic systems to distant parts of the body in a process called metastasis.

Cancer is not one disease, but rather many related diseases. Cancer is typed according to the part of the body where it is located and the kind of cells that comprise it. The most common types of cancer cells and their locations are:

- **Carcinomas** originate in skin tissue or tissues that line the body cavities and such internal organs as the lungs, breast, colon, and intestines.

## SOME CANCER FACTS

- Cancer can occur at any age, but mostly appears in people middle-aged and older.
- Cancer causes more deaths in American children aged one to 14 years than any other disease.
- In the 1980s more than 4.5 million Americans died from cancer.
- About 83 million people alive today—or one in three Americans—will eventually get cancer.
- Cancer cost the United States roughly $104 billion in 1990—including medical expenses and loss of work productivity.
- Approximately 520,000 Americans die of cancer each year.

- **Sarcomas** grow in bones and connective tissues between organs and skin, and sometimes spread into the blood or lymphatic system.
- **Lymphomas** are cancers of the lymphatic system, usually occurring in the lymph nodes.
- **Leukemias** form in the blood or circulatory system, particularly in the bone marrow, which is the site of blood cell production.
- **Myelomas** are tumors of bone marrow cells and frequently form simultaneously in many sites, including the ribs, vertebrae, and pelvic bones.

## The Latest Advances in Diagnosis and Treatment

Cancer is treated by surgery, chemotherapy, radiation, or a combination of these methods. Diagnoses and treatment have become increasingly individualized in recent years. Early detection and the precise staging of therapies have contributed to higher success rates in the battle against cancer.

Many cancers that only recently had poor prognoses are now considered curable. Potentially curable cancers now include acute lymphocytic leukemia in children, Burkitt's lymphoma, Ewing's sarcoma (a form of bone cancer), Wilm's tumor (a kidney cancer in children), Hodgkin's disease, rhabdomyosarcoma (a cancer of certain muscle tissues), testicular cancer, choriocarcinoma (placental cancer), osteogenic sarcoma, and breast cancer.

Current developments also show the promise of improved treatment for many other forms of cancer. For example, the recently discovered importance of oncogenes—the genes in a tumor cell that are associated with the transformation of normal cells into cancerous ones—promises to help predict which tumors are likely to return after surgery. This knowledge can also help identify family members who are at risk.

It has also been found that cancer cells fused genetically with normal cells produce special antibodies that seek out cancer cells. These monoclonal antibodies are being studied for their potential use in diagnosis and treatment.

There are many other advances, including:

- Adjuvant treatment in which drugs are administered postoperatively in early breast and colon cancers to eradicate remaining cancer cells and thus increase cure rates

- Neoadjuvant chemotherapy in which drugs are given to shrink the cancer before surgery

- Synthetic retinoids (cousins of vitamin A) to prevent cancer in high-risk groups or the recurrence of cancer after surgery

- Removal and replacement of sections of bone in bone cancer instead of amputation of entire limbs

- New high-tech diagnostic imaging techniques (magnetic resonance imaging [MRI] and computerized tomography [CT] scans) instead of exploratory surgery in some cases

- Immunotherapy to enhance the body's disease-fighting capabilities (naturally occurring bodily substances, such as interferon, interleukin-2, and biologic response modifiers, are all in trials for this purpose)

- Bone marrow transplants for the treatment of leukemia

## Lung Cancer

The increase in lung cancer largely explains the steady rise in the number of cancer deaths in the United States. Most of the estimated 146,000 deaths caused by lung cancer each year result from cigarette smoking. The incidence in men declined from a high of 86.6 per 100,000 in 1984 to 81.5 in 1988. Unfortunately, the rate in women has been rising steadily, reaching a high of 39.8 per 100,000 in 1988. More women are smoking and, as a result, more women now die of lung cancer than breast cancer, which forty years ago was the leading cause of cancer death in women.

The symptoms of lung cancer include a persistent cough, sputum streaked with blood, chest pain, and recurring pneumonia or bronchitis. Additional risk factors include exposure to industrial chemicals (including arsenic, certain organic chemicals, and asbestos); radiation exposure, including possible residential radon exposure (especially for smokers); and for non-smokers, passive exposure to sidestream cigarette smoke.

Unfortunately, early detection of lung cancer is very difficult. Symptoms often don't appear until the disease is in an advanced stage. If smokers quit when early precancerous cellular changes have already damaged bronchial lining tissue, there is a chance that the disease will not progress. Those who continue to smoke often end up with lung cancer.

The treatment of lung cancer depends on the type and stage of the disease and includes surgery, radiation therapy, and chemotherapy. If the cancer is localized, surgery is the best option. However, because only 18 percent of lung cancers are discovered early enough for surgery, radiation and chemotherapy are often necessary.

In small-cell carcinoma, a large percentage of patients achieve remission with chemotherapy—alone or in combination with radiation—instead of surgery. Small-cell carcinomas have responded to the following combinations: cyclophosphamide, doxorubicin, and vincristine; cyclophosphamide, doxorubicin, vincristine, and etoposide; and etoposide and cisplatin.

Experimental immunotherapy for lung cancer uses BCG vaccine, or *Corynebacterium parvum*. In experimental laser therapy, laser energy is beamed through a bronchoscope to destroy local tumors, which are often the cause of bronchial obstruction and resulting infection.

## Colon Cancer

Colon and rectal cancers are the second leading cause of cancer deaths in the United States, claiming the lives of an estimated 58,300 Americans annually. People at greatest risk are those with a personal or family history of colon or rectal cancer, or of inflammatory bowel disease. High-fat and/or low-fiber diets are also believed to be risk factors.

Symptoms of colon and rectal cancers include rectal bleeding, blood in the stool, and a change in bowel habits that lasts more than two weeks, such as diarrhea alternating with constipation. Early detection methods include a digital rectal exam, a stool test for occult blood—recommended annually for people over 50—and a proctosigmoidoscopy—an examination of the rectum and colon via a hollow lighted tube, which is recommended every three to five years after age 50.

Colon and rectal cancers are treated by surgery, sometimes in combination with radiation. Patients with metastasis, residual disease, recurrent inoperable tumors, or a high risk of recurrence are candidates for chemotherapy. Drugs used in chemotherapy include 5-fluorouracil, levamisole, mitomycin, lomustine, vincristine, and methotrexate. Colostomies are needed only rarely.

## Breast Cancer

This type of cancer attacks one out of every nine American women. Among women aged 40 to 55, it is the leading cause of death.

Every woman is at risk of developing breast cancer. However, women over age 50 and those with a personal or family history are at higher risk. Other risk factors include never having had children and giving birth for the first time after age 30.

Warning signs include persistent breast changes such as a lump, swelling, dimpling, thickening, skin irritations, distortion, retraction, scaliness, pain, discharge, or tenderness of the nipple.

As part of a comprehensive early detection program, every woman should do her own monthly breast examination. Regular clinical examinations are recommended every three years for women

## BREAST CANCER: A CLOSER LOOK

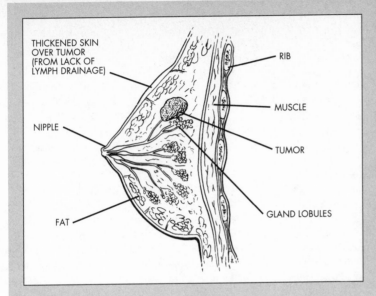

THICKENED SKIN
OVER TUMOR
(FROM LACK OF
LYMPH DRAINAGE)

RIB

MUSCLE

NIPPLE

TUMOR

FAT

GLAND LOBULES

Until fairly sizable, a cancerous breast tumor can easily go unnoticed. That's why monthly self-examinations and regular medical visits are so important: Early treatment can make the difference between a cure and death.

aged 20 to 40 and every year for those over 40. Mammograms can detect cancers too small to feel, and should be done every one or two years for women aged 40 to 49 and every year for women aged 50 and older. Suspicious lumps found on a mammogram should be biopsied for a definitive diagnosis.

Treatment for breast cancer depends on the individual case, and may consist of lumpectomy (local removal of the tumor); mastectomy (surgical removal of the breast); or radiation therapy followed by chemotherapy or hormone manipulation therapy for patients at high risk of metastatic disease.

The most common drugs used in the treatment of breast cancer include methotrexate, 5-fluorouracil, cyclophosphamide, and doxorubicin. The drugs are usually given in combination. Hormone manipulation therapy may consist of administering progesterone or an androgen such as testosterone; anti-estrogen therapy with tamoxifen (Nolvadex); or inhibition of adrenal corticosteroid production with aminoglutethimide (Cytadren).

## Prostate Cancer

Prostate cancer claims an estimated 34,000 lives annually, making it the second leading cause of cancer deaths in men. Prostate cancer is also the next-to-most common form of cancer in men (after skin cancer), with well over 100,000 new cases reported each year.

The incidence of prostate cancer rises with age. More than 80 percent of the cases are diagnosed after the age of 65. Prostate cancer is more prevalent in northwestern Europe and the United States. For some reason, African-Americans currently have the highest incidence of prostate cancer in the world. Dietary fat may be a contributing cause of prostate cancer.

Warning signs appear only after prostate cancer has progressed to an advanced stage. Symptoms include urinary dribbling; inability to urinate; difficulty starting or stopping the urinary stream; frequent urination, especially at night; blood in the urine; pain or burning while urinating; and persistent pain in the lower back, pelvis, or upper thighs. Most of these signs could also be a warning of such benign conditions as infection or prostate enlargement.

As with all cancers, early detection of prostate

cancer is essential. Men over 40 are urged to have rectal examinations annually. Through transrectal ultrasound, a new technique, it is now possible to detect cancers too small to show up on physical examination. A blood test for prostate specific antigen (PSA) can also detect the disease at an early stage.

Surgery or radiation is the primary treatment for localized prostate cancer. Hormonal therapy is used for metastatic disease. Chemotherapy is tried when other types of therapy cannot be used or have failed. It involves various combinations of anti-cancer agents.

## Pancreatic Cancer

Each year some 28,000 cases of pancreatic cancer are discovered; and each year 25,000 Americans die from it. It is the fifth leading cause of cancer deaths.

The incidence of pancreatic cancer rises after age 50, with most cases occurring between the ages of 65 and 79. The risk of pancreatic cancer is twice as high in people who smoke. Other possible predisposing factors include high fat diets, exposure to industrial chemicals, diabetes mellitus, chronic inflammation of the pancreas (pancreatitis), and chronic alcohol abuse.

Pancreatic cancer is a silent disease, producing no symptoms until the advanced stages. The most common warning signs include weight loss, jaundice, abdominal or low back pain, and diarrhea. Others include fever and lesions on the legs. Patients may also experience emotional disturbances such as anxiety and depression, as well as premonitions of life-threatening illness.

Treatment for pancreatic cancer consists of surgery, radiation therapy, and drugs. However, the diagnosis usually comes so late that these therapies are rarely feasible. Drugs used for treating pancreatic cancer are antibiotics, anticholinergics (especially propantheline), antacids, diuretics, insulin, analgesics, and pancreatic enzymes.

## Cancer of the Uterus and Cervix

Each year nearly 40,000 women learn that they have uterine cancer. An additional 13,500 are diagnosed with cancer of the cervix. Of the two, cervical cancer is the more dangerous, causing as many as 4,500 deaths annually. Thanks to regular Pap testing for early detection, the death rate for uterine cancer has shrunk by more than 70 percent in the past 40 years. The incidence of invasive cervical cancer has also decreased steadily, being replaced in frequency by carcinoma

## ANATOMY OF PROSTATE CANCER

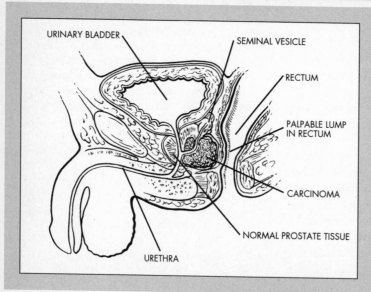

URINARY BLADDER

SEMINAL VESICLE

RECTUM

PALPABLE LUMP IN RECTUM

CARCINOMA

NORMAL PROSTATE TISSUE

URETHRA

Nestled near the bladder and urethra, the prostate gland is frequently the culprit when urinary problems arise. These difficulties are often due to nothing more than prostate enlargement or infection; but cancer is a possibility. Take any urinary irregularity as a signal to visit your doctor or urologist.

in situ, a precancerous condition found mostly in women over the age of 50.

Although all women are at risk for cervical cancer, this type of cancer tends to strike more frequently among women in lower socioeconomic groups. Other risk factors include multiple sex partners, having intercourse at an early age, cigarette smoking, and certain sexually transmitted diseases. Women over 50 are most at risk of getting endometrial cancer, which affects the lining of the uterus.

Warning signs include abnormal vaginal bleeding or an unusual discharge, postcoital pain and bleeding, and for uterine cancer, uterine enlargement.

Treatment consists of surgery and radiation, alone or in combination. Precancerous stages may be treated by cryotherapy, in which cells are destroyed by extreme cold; electrocoagulation, in which tissue is destroyed by intense heat; or by local surgery. Precancerous conditions in the endometrium may be treated with progesterone. Uterine cancer may be treated with doxorubicin, vincristine, cyclophosphamide, and dactinomycin.

## Leukemia

Leukemia is a cancer of the blood-forming tissues in which millions of abnormal white blood cells crowd out normal ones. Though usually considered a childhood disease, leukemia strikes over 25,000 adults annually, compared to 2,500 young people. Leukemia causes some 18,000 deaths in a typical year.

People of all ages and both genders are at risk for leukemia, although those with Down's syndrome and certain other genetic abnormalities tend to experience a higher incidence of this disease. While we don't know what causes leukemia in most cases, excessive exposure to ionizing radiation and certain chemicals are suspected to be contributing factors.

The early warning signs of leukemia include paleness, fatigue, weight loss, a tendency to bruise easily, repeated infections, and hemorrhages such as nosebleeds. Any of these symptoms can appear suddenly in acute leukemia. The progress of chronic leukemia can be slow and produce no symptoms for years.

The treatment of leukemia usually consists of chemotherapy to kill the attacking abnormal blood cells. Treatment varies according to the specific type of leukemia.

Drugs used to treat leukemias include methotrexate, cytarabine, vincristine, prednisone, L-asparaginase, daunorubicin, doxorubicin, thioguanine, cyclophosphamide, amsacrine, and mitoxantrone—alone or in combination.

Treatment of infections associated with the disease may include antifungal, antibacterial, and antiviral drugs. Bone marrow transplants are effective in some cases.

## Skin Cancer

Skin cancer is by far the most common of all cancers, with more than 600,000 cases occurring each year. Fortunately, the vast majority of these cancers are highly curable basal cell or squamous cell cancers. A small minority, however, are the extremely dangerous form called melanoma.

Melanoma is diagnosed in more than 30,000 people in the United States each year. The incidence of melanoma has increased by about four percent a year since 1973.

Excessive exposure to the sun is the greatest risk factor, especially for people with fair complexions. On-the-job exposure to coal tar, pitch, creosote, arsenic compounds, or radium also increases the risk of melanoma.

Early detection is crucial. People should examine their skin regularly for any unusual changes. Any changes in the size or color of a mole or other darkly pigmented spot or growth should be reported to a doctor immediately. Bleeding, scaliness, oozing, or a change in the appearance of a bump or nodule; the spread of pigmentation beyond its border; and any changes in sensation—itchiness, tenderness, or pain—are other warning signals of skin cancer.

Melanoma often begins as a small, mole-like growth that enlarges, changes color, becomes ulcerated, and bleeds easily. A melanoma is usually asymmetrical, has irregular borders and uneven pigmentation, and is larger than six millimeters in diameter.

Skin cancer treatments include surgery; radiation; electrodesiccation, in which the tissue is destroyed by heat; and cryosurgery, in which extreme cold is used to destroy the tissue.

## CANCER IN CHILDREN

About 8,000 cases of pediatric cancer are diagnosed each year; and some 1,500 children die from it annually. The cancer mortality rate for this age-group has declined from 8.3 cases per 100,000 in 1950 to 3.3 per 100,000 in 1988.

Unfortunately, pediatric cancers are often difficult to detect. Consequently, regular medical checkups are advised, and parents should be alert to any unusual, persistent symptoms. Warning signs include localized pain or persistent limping; any unusual mass or swelling; unexplained fever, illness, paleness, or loss of energy; frequent headaches, often with vomiting; a sudden tendency to bruise; sudden eye or vision changes; and excessive, rapid weight loss.

The most common childhood cancers include:
- Leukemia
- Osteogenic Sarcoma and Ewing's Sarcoma (bone cancers)
- Neuroblastoma (usually appears in the abdomen with accompanying swelling)
- Rhabdomyosarcoma (cancer of soft tissue in the head and neck area, genitourinary area, trunk, and extremities)
- Brain cancer
- Lymphomas and Hodgkin's Disease (involving the lymph nodes)
- Retinoblastoma (of the eye)
- Wilm's Tumor (kidney cancer)

## Ovarian Cancer

Ovarian cancer causes more deaths than any other type of cancer affecting the reproductive system. In a typical year, over 20,000 women contract this disease, and more than 12,000 die from it.

The risk of ovarian cancer increases with age. Women over the age of 60 have the highest incidence. Women who have never given birth are twice as likely to develop ovarian cancer as those who have. Early pregnancy and menopause and the use of oral contraceptives seem to offer protection against ovarian cancer.

Ovarian cancer often shows no symptoms until the later stages. Most commonly, women notice an enlarged abdomen. Other symptoms may include vague, unexplained digestive disturbances.

Treatment is altered according to the stage of the disease and consists of varying combinations of surgery, chemotherapy, and radiation. Drugs useful in treating ovarian cancer include chlorambucil, melphalan, cyclophosphamide, cisplatin, and paclitaxel (Taxol).

## Bladder Cancer

Bladder cancer attacks more than 50,000 Americans each year, leading to nearly 10,000 deaths annually. Bladder cancer strikes many more men than women. It is the fourth most common type of cancer in men and the ninth most common in women.

Smoking is the most serious risk factor for bladder cancer, although people who live in urban areas and those exposed to dye, rubber, or leather products at work are also at higher risk.

The most common symptoms of bladder cancer are blood in the urine and increased frequency of urination.

Treatment consists of surgery—alone or in combination with other therapies. Chemotherapy for bladder cancer often consists of 5-fluorouracil, cisplatin, cyclophosphamide, doxorubicin, methotrexate, and vinblastine.

## Other Cancers

Oral cancers kill approximately 8,000 Americans in a typical year. Some 30,000 new cases are diagnosed annually. Cigarette, cigar, or pipe smoking, along with the use of smokeless tobacco and excessive alcohol consumption, are the greatest risk factors for this disease.

The warning signs of oral cancer include a sore that bleeds easily and doesn't heal, a persistent red or white patch, and a lump or thickening. As the disease progresses, the individual might also experience difficulty swallowing, chewing, or moving the tongue.

Oral cancers are principally treated by radiation and surgery.

Cancer can develop in any part of any organ in the body. For example, there are malignant brain tumors, pituitary tumors, laryngeal tumors, thyroid cancer, and spinal neoplasms. Cancer can also occur in the stomach, esophagus, kidney, liver, and gallbladder. Cancers of the genitalia include testicular cancer, penile cancer, vaginal cancer, cancer of the vulva, and fallopian tube cancer. People also develop primary malignant bone tumors, multiple myeloma, Hodgkin's disease (cancer of the lymph nodes), malignant lymphomas, and mycosis fungoides.

Therapy is always determined by the type of cancer, and the extent of its spread at the time of diagnosis. The chance of recovery is largely dependent on the same factors, which is why early detection is so crucially important. Always remember: Finding a cancer before it becomes widespread is the best way of improving your odds of a successful cure. □

## CHAPTER 8

# New Answers for Pain

Pain is the chief reason that people seek medical care. And whether it is a tooth, ear, stomach, head, or back that aches, people all want the same thing—relief. Since ancient times, humanity has been preoccupied with finding ways to relieve pain. For thousands of years, our ancestors had only a few substances (mainly alcohol, opium, and the coca and hemp plants) to help make the pain go away.

But modern pharmacology changed all that. Today, dozens of drugs mercifully eliminate, or at least greatly reduce, the pain that comes with all types of ailments. However, their effectiveness for chronic pain is a different matter. Treating chronic pain is tricky; great care and caution must be exercised because of the potential for side effects and addiction associated with pain-relieving drugs.

## What Is Pain?

Pain is the body's way of telling us that something is wrong. If we place our hand too close to a fire, we feel pain. When a bone is broken or the skin is cut, if we have inflammation from arthritis, or tense muscles from stress, a signal flashes from nerves in the distressed area to a part of the spinal cord where cells called pain receptors are located. These pain receptors send the signal along different tracks in the spinal cord to the brain, where the message of pain is registered.

Pain evokes emotion. Sudden, short-lived pain can cause anxiety; constant, unrelenting pain can leave us seriously depressed. Because of the emotional aspect of pain, treatment may involve much more than common painkillers, particularly for those in constant distress.

## Common Types of Pain

For purposes of treatment, doctors divide pain into the following three basic types:

- Acute pain, which is usually temporary and often the result of injury. Causes of acute pain range from surgery, fractures, infections, and burns to natural events such as childbirth.

- Chronic pain, which is arbitrarily defined as a pain that persists for more than three to six months and threatens to disrupt the patient's normal activities. Chronic pain is associated with a wide range of long-lasting and permanent disorders (see box).

- Cancer pain syndromes, which can result from either the tumor itself or the surgery, radiation, and chemotherapy used during treatment.

In addition to these three major types of general pain, headaches come in so many forms—and have so many causes—that they are considered a category unto themselves (see box).

## Treating Acute Pain

Because this type of pain is often the result of a specific trauma or infection, your doctor's first goal is to eliminate the underlying cause, if at all possible. To relieve the pain while other measures take effect, he or she will draw on a wide array of analgesics, including the following:

- Aspirin, buffered or plain
- Acetaminophen
- Narcotics
- Nonsteroidal anti-inflammatory drugs (NSAIDs), such as Motrin
- Tranquilizers
- Muscle relaxants
- Local anesthetics, applied to the surface or injected

The choice of analgesic varies according to the severity of the pain and the stage of the healing process. Consider, for example, a fracture.

The pain of a fracture results from muscle, nerve, and soft-tissue damage. When the bone is first being set, pain-killing measures vary with the severity of the injury. They can range all the way from general anesthesia to use of a local anesthetic and a narcotic analgesic such as meperidine (Demerol). (A muscle relaxant may be used to help stretch muscles and make it easier to set the bone.)

As the fracture heals, painkillers containing codeine are gradually replaced by milder pain relievers such as aspirin or NSAIDs. Aspirin usually provides sufficient pain relief for strains and sprains. However, if the strain is chronic and

## THE MYRIAD CAUSES OF CHRONIC PAIN

A list of disorders that can lead to chronic pain would be almost endless; but here is a sample of some common culprits:

- Lower back problems, slipped disks, and sciatica
- Arthritis, tendinitis, and bursitis
- Sickle-cell anemia and hemophilia
- Nerve damage caused by diabetes, kidney failure, and many other problems

doesn't respond to local heat application, muscle relaxants may be necessary.

Likewise, the intense pain typically following surgery and childbirth is treated initially with morphine-based analgesics administered intravenously, intramuscularly, or epidurally (in the spine). These measures may be followed with PCA (patient-controlled intravenous agents), then oral painkillers, and finally milder aspirin and acetaminophen compounds.

Treatment for other forms of acute pain varies with the cause. Depending on the severity, pain from burns is treated with anything from aspirin to narcotic-based painkillers. Though pain occurs with most bacterial infections, the first line of treatment is to cure the infection with antibiotics. Analgesics are given only for specific conditions—in the treatment of certain skin infections, for example. The treatment of viral infections ranges from acetaminophen for the head and muscle aches of the flu to codeine compounds for the uncomfortable itching and pain of shingles.

## Treating Chronic Pain

An estimated 80 million Americans suffer from chronic pain. Though narcotic analgesics are extremely effective in easing acute pain, their addictive properties and side effects make these drugs a less desirable choice for long-term use and often undermine the relief they bring. That's why they must be used carefully, if at all, for chronic pain. It is also the reason that other methods have been developed to treat and manage the problem.

Indeed, a new medical specialty known as pain management has emerged in recent years. Pain management employs a wide range of therapies to help people learn to live with pain, using only a minimum of drugs. These alternative treatments include exercise, deep-muscle relaxation training, massage, biofeedback, cognitive therapy for pain control, TENS (Transcutaneous Electrical Nerve Stimulation), neural blockade, steroid therapy, and diet counseling. Because chronic pain usually affects a person's psychological well-being and his or her relationships, individual, group, and family therapy are also advised in most cases.

The full spectrum of analgesics and muscle relaxants are prescribed for chronic pain, although morphine-based drugs are generally replaced with

# HEADACHES

Headaches are the most common pain complaint. Ninety percent of all headaches are caused by tension—muscular, vascular, or a combination of both types. The remaining 10 percent result from underlying intracranial, biological, or psychological disorders. Migraines are severe, throbbing headaches that result from the contraction and expansion of cranial arteries. We don't know what causes migraines, but we do know that they afflict about 10 percent of the population, tend to run in families, and are more prevalent in women.

Most people rely on over-the-counter medications, such as aspirin or acetaminophen, to treat simple headaches. Typically caused by fleeting conditions such as fatigue, emotional strain, menstruation, or environmental stimuli (bright lights, crowds, or noise), these headaches usually subside when the stress ends.

But if a headache persists for more than a few days or recurs over an extended period of time, it should be reported to a physician in order to determine any possible underlying causes. These causes may include glaucoma; diseases of the teeth, scalp, extracranial arteries, external or middle ear; spasms of the shoulder, neck, or face; systemic disease; hypertension; intracranial bleeding; head trauma or tumor; aneurysms; and abscesses. Vasodilators, such as alcohol, histamines, and nitrates, can also cause headaches.

Migraine headaches are characterized by intense localized throbbing that usually spreads. Migraines are often preceded by changes in vision (a flashing blind-spot or the absence of half of the normal field of vision), pins and needles on one side of the body, or impaired speech. The headaches are frequently accompanied by nausea, vomiting, loss of appetite, and sensitivity to light. Sometimes migraines are a symptom of the onset of menopause.

The best treatment for migraines is a shot of the new drug Imitrex taken under the skin or, if Imitrex can't be taken, the older drug ergotamine (Cafergot, Bellergal-S), taken alone or with caffeine. Drug treatment is most effective when the medication is used in the early stages of an attack. If nausea and vomiting are present, ergotamine may be given as a rectal suppository. Propranolol (Inderal) and calcium channel blockers, such as verapamil (Calan, Isoptin) and diltiazem (Cardizem), can help prevent migraines.

The treatment of chronic headaches depends on the type of headache and may include anything from aspirin to codeine or meperidine (Demerol). Acute attacks often respond well to tranquilizers; chronic tension headaches are sometimes alleviated by muscle relaxants. An accurate diagnosis and elimination of underlying causes of the problem are essential. Psychotherapy may be necessary if the headaches are caused by emotional distress.

NSAIDs to minimize the possibility of addiction. Antidepressants have also been found to be effective for some individuals suffering from long-term pain.

To meet the needs of those with chronic cancer pain, doctors are now using a variety of advanced techniques. Painkillers can be delivered through home intravenous infusion systems or implanted epidural catheters. TENS systems may come into play, and neurolytic (nerve-destroying) neural blockade has proved effective for certain patients.

Despite all these advances, there's still no perfect solution for pain. Many of our current medications present one drawback or another, ranging from gastric side effects to the potential of addiction. Nevertheless, there's no denying we now have more ways of providing effective control of pain than could be imagined just a few decades ago. □

**CHAPTER 9**

# Overcoming Emotional and Psychological Problems

Anyone, at any time, can develop an emotional problem. You begin to feel sad, angry, alone, or just frustrated by the problems of everyday life. You lose sleep, become irritable, or simply want to "pull the covers over your head." Ordinarily, simply "venting"—talking with your spouse or a clergyman, friend, or co-worker—is enough to put you in a better frame of mind.

But if things don't turn around, and your ability to function diminishes each day, you may be suffering from something more than a temporary emotional upset. You may have a condition that needs professional treatment.

If so, you will not be alone. According to the National Institute of Mental Health, more than 41 million Americans—nearly 1 in 5—experience a mental disorder at some point in their lives.

■ More than 7 million children and adolescents suffer from psychological problems such as hyperactivity, autism, and conduct disorders.

■ Severe clinical depression, needing professional treatment, strikes more than 10 million people during the course of their lives.

■ Each year, more than 18 million Americans are affected by the most common of all mental problems: anxiety disorder.

■ Nearly 14 million Americans abuse alcohol or illicit drugs to the point of dependence each year.

■ More than 1.5 million people have schizophrenia and need hospitalization or long-term treatment.

■ Perhaps as many as 14 percent of our elderly suffer from some degree of dementia, or loss of mental function.

Studies conducted by the Institute of Medicine show that direct expenditures on health care for mental illness total more than $23 billion a year; substance abuse adds another $17 billion.

But that's only a fraction of the true cost. If mental illness goes undiagnosed, the personal and social consequences can be severe. Suicide is the eighth leading cause of death in the United States and the third leading cause among adolescents and young adults. And the lost workdays, accidents, crime, and reduced productivity that can be traced to untreated mental illness have been estimated to cost us upwards of $250 billion a year.

Much of this suffering and expense could be reduced by early detection and prompt treatment. But unfortunately, as few as one in four who need help seek it. Less than a third of those suffering from depression look for treatment; and less than 10 percent of the children who need help receive it.

Ironically, 80 percent of those suffering from mental illness can be treated effectively with medication and therapy on an outpatient basis.

# What Do We Mean by Mental Illness?

Mental illness is a broad, umbrella-term for a wide range of disorders that can strike anyone. Even today, the term "mentally ill" carries with it a heavy burden of social stigma, embarrassment, and fear. The idea of "losing your mind" remains a terrifying thought.

Yet, given today's improved diagnostic and therapeutic techniques, such fears are usually misplaced. With earlier detection, better diagnosis, and faster, more effective treatment, millions of the "mentally ill" are now able to lead satisfying, productive lives.

Amazingly, only 40 years ago more than a half million profoundly ill people were beyond help, languishing in huge mental hospitals where they were managed with restraints, confinement, and sedation. The stigma attached to "mental illness" was enormous—few people would admit that they or any member of their family suffered from any kind of psychiatric disease.

As a result, most of those who were "neurotic" or "phobic" went untreated, leading lives of hidden desperation. For those who did seek help, psychiatric treatment consisted almost entirely of "talk therapy," or psychoanalysis. The most seriously ill psychotic patients were simply warehoused in the hospitals.

In those days, health-care experts predicted that the number of people confined to mental institutions would more than double in the next few decades. Yet by the mid-1970s the number of psychiatric inpatients had actually dropped by half!

What had happened? Why were they wrong?

The answer is simple. For decades, researchers had concentrated on development of medications to cure infections, heart disease, cancer, and other illnesses, while mental disorders were ignored. But in 1952, chlorpromazine (Thorazine) was tried in schizophrenic patients at low doses. People who suffered from delusions, hallucinations, paranoia, and other symptoms improved almost immediately. For the first time, psychiatrists realized that medication could be a partner with other forms of therapy for mental illness. Once the pharmaceutical floodgates opened, psychiatry changed overnight. A new age of "biopsychiatry" was born that led to tremendous strides in the diagnosis and treatment of mental illness.

# Major Types of Mental Illness

Today, psychiatrists use everything from blood tests and brain scans to complete physical exams and family histories to aid in the diagnosis of mental disorders. Targeting an emotional disorder for accurate treatment is a complicated task, so mental health professionals have created a unique system to help pin down ambiguous psychiatric problems. Hundreds of types of mental illness are cataloged in a book known as *The Diagnostic and Statistical Manual of Mental Disorders* (DSM-IV). Published by the American Psychiatric Association and currently in its fourth edition, DSM-IV, like *Physicians' Desk Reference*, is the "bible" of its discipline. Understanding that the mind is, in effect, an organ system like the heart or kidneys and, like these organs, can develop a disease, was an important breakthrough in diagnosis and treatment.

The DSM-IV breaks psychiatric illness into more than two dozen categories and over 100 sub-categories, each with its own unique set of symptoms. When a patient's symptoms fit within the DSM-IV criteria, a psychiatrist can pinpoint a specific diagnosis. Among the major categories of mental illness listed in the DSM-IV are the following:

- Anxiety Disorders (phobias, panic disorder, post-traumatic stress disorder, obsessive-compulsive disorder)
- Mood Disorders (depression, manic-depressive disorder)
- Schizophrenia
- Developmental Disorders (learning disorders, retardation, autism)
- Disruptive Behavior Disorders (attention deficit hyperactivity disorder, conduct disorder)
- Substance Abuse Disorders (alcoholism, drug dependence)
- Delusional Disorders (delusional paranoia)
- Sexual Disorders
- Sleep Disorders
- Impulse Control Disorders (kleptomania, pyromania)
- Dissociative Disorders (multiple-personality disorder)
- Eating Disorders (anorexia, bulimia)
- Organic Mental Disorders (Alzheimer's disease and other psychiatric diseases that result from

## TEN WARNING SIGNS OF MENTAL ILLNESS

According to the American Psychiatric Association, anyone displaying one or more of these warning signs should be evaluated by a doctor as soon as possible:

1. Marked personality change
2. Inability to cope with problems and daily activities
3. Strange or grandiose ideas
4. Obsessive ideas
5. Prolonged depression and apathy
6. Marked changes in eating or sleeping patterns
7. Thinking or talking about suicide
8. Extreme highs and lows
9. Abuse of alcohol or drugs
10. Excessive anger, hostility, or violent behavior

metabolic problems in the brain or from substance abuse)

Perhaps the most important step in diagnosing any mental illness is for the patient and the family to actually seek help. As with a physical illness, the earlier an emotional or psychiatric problem is detected, the more likely and the easier is the cure. Unfortunately, psychiatric symptoms are far easier to ignore or misinterpret than physiological symptoms. While the criteria for disorders like cancer, arthritis, and high blood pressure are precisely defined, psychological symptoms (e.g., "the blues") are often ambiguous. Coupled with the stigma or "denial" that is common in questions of mental health, this may make an accurate diagnosis harder to achieve.

Still, the meaning of certain specific sets of symptoms is relatively clear. Here's a closer look at the most prevalent types of mental illness.

### Anxiety Disorders

Almost everybody gets anxious. Most of us feel nervous before a test or an important business meeting. The "butterflies" that we all experience from time to time are so common that we tend to ignore them. Yet, for more than 18 million Americans, "anxiety" is so severe that it interferes with their daily functioning.

Actually, a genuine anxiety disorder is marked not by anxiety, but by outright fear. While anxiety is a form of mental tension that we can't really put our finger on, fear is easily recognized. Its symptoms are well known: shakiness, trembling, aching muscles, sweating, chills, dizziness, pounding heart, dry mouth, a lump in the throat.

If you are diagnosed with an anxiety disorder, you suffer from one or more of a group of problems including generalized anxiety disorder, phobias, panic disorders, obsessive-compulsive disorder, and post-traumatic stress disorder.

**Phobias** are the most common of the anxiety disorders. An estimated 5 to 12 percent of the population suffer a psychological and physiological reaction to a place, a situation, or an object that interferes with daily life. The "phobic reaction" is almost a reflex. The victim is filled with dread, horror, and terror. He begins to gasp for breath, shake, and often flees. Some people will go miles out of their way to avoid a phobic situation.

There are hundreds of phobias. For instance, there is "agoraphobia," a phobia that is widely misunderstood. Most think that an "agoraphobic" is simply afraid to leave home. In fact, his real fear is of being alone in public places from which he thinks escape would be difficult or help unavailable if he were hurt or trapped. As a result, agoraphobics stay home rather than risk the terror they've come to expect.

Likewise, people with social phobias aren't antisocial. Rather, they fear that they will do something in a public place that will cause them humiliation. They fear "being watched" while doing almost anything—eating a meal, standing in line at the bank, making small talk at the beach. To some extent, almost everyone has social phobias—nervousness in front of an audience is the most common. However, most of us can cope and get on with it. Someone with a social phobia will, like an agoraphobic, go to any length to avoid placing himself in an "unsafe" situation.

"The Simple Phobias": Make a list of just about anything—dogs, cats, snakes, mice, bats, spiders, insects, dark rooms, heights, closed spaces—and you will find someone with a phobic reaction to it.

**Panic Disorder:** A panic attack is one of the most frightening of all psychological events.

Imagine that you are walking down the street one day, feeling fine, when, out of the blue, you are overcome by an intense fear and foreboding unlike anything you've ever felt before. You are literally frozen to the sidewalk, unable to move. And then it gets worse. You start to shake, sweat, gasp for air. You are sure you are having a heart attack and that you will die the next instant. People stop and stare; some even offer to help. But you can't move or respond. The weight on your chest is growing heavier, and you are now just waiting to die.

And then, as suddenly as it started, it stops. Gone. Since you feel so good, you carry on, ignoring the event—except that you now avoid the street where it happened.

A week goes by and nothing happens, and then another week. You've almost forgotten about the attack completely when, without warning, it hits you again, this time far more intensely. Your body is tingling. You're overcome with nausea. You are so out of control you think you're going insane. If you don't continue to ignore what's happened and instead call a psychiatrist, chances are you'll be told that you are one of nearly 3 million Americans who suffer from the relatively common form of anxiety called "panic disorder," and that the attacks are every bit as real as they seem.

Panic disorder, many researchers think, may be partly a result of genetics—it does run in families—or may be caused by disturbances of the neurotransmitters that form the brain's chemical messenger system. Panic attacks may also be signs of underlying physiologic illness. Researchers often refer to panic attacks as "impostors," because their symptoms may actually be caused by heart disease, thyroid imbalances, or respiratory problems. In fact, more than 40 medical problems can cause panic-like symptoms.

**Obsessive-Compulsive Disorder:** This illness is very much what it sounds like. People who have continual, unwanted thoughts that prevent them from functioning properly are considered "obsessed;" to rid themselves of these nagging ideas, they usually develop "compulsions"—rituals

they must go through before they can move on to another activity. Compulsive rituals include repetitious washing, repeating certain phrases, completing steps in a process over and over, counting and recounting, checking and re-checking to make sure something hasn't been forgotten, excessive neatness, and hoarding of useless items.

The cause of OCD, as it's called, has remained a mystery, despite theories that link it to other disorders, such as depression. Research on a physical cause of the disorder is on the rise; and several effective medications are available, including Anafranil, Luvox, and Prozac.

**Post-Traumatic Stress Disorder:** PTSD was known for years as shell shock or battle fatigue, but we now know that it's not limited to soldiers who've seen too much of war. PTSD is a disorder that can affect anyone who has survived a severe and unusual trauma, such as a hurricane, tornado, flood, or airplane crash. One psychiatrist calls it "aftershock," which is an apt description, because the symptoms of PTSD may surface months after the actual event.

Veterans do remain the main victims of PTSD. The Department of Veterans Affairs estimates that 700,000 to 800,000 of the 3.5 million Vietnam veterans have experienced PTSD. For these vets and other victims, the symptoms are often a "re-experience of the traumatic event . . . also known as flashbacks." In effect, the person replays the emotions he felt during the traumatic event itself. Some of the afflicted develop insomnia, extreme anger, fear and grief, and even an inability to feel any emotions, which leads to withdrawal from society. Some PTSD patients have "survivor's guilt." Others begin to avoid situations that remind them of the traumatic event (flying, for example).

**Treating Anxiety Disorders:** Anxiety disorders are often treated with a combination of psychotherapy and drugs. Once medication has reduced the symptoms of the various anxiety disorders, psychiatrists use behavioral therapy, psychotherapy, and other forms of therapy that are tailored to the patient's personal needs.

The most commonly prescribed medications for anxiety are the benzodiazepine class of drugs, such as Valium and Xanax, and other tranquilizers such as BuSpar. Recently some psychiatrists have been using beta blockers such as propranolol (Inderal) to curb certain forms of anxiety and phobias. (For more on beta blockers, see the chapter on heart disease.)

### Depression

Depression is not just "the blues." Depression is one of the most serious and common of all mental disorders. It is also one of the most treatable—provided the victim seeks treatment. At any time, more than nine million Americans may be suffering from depression. More than 15 percent of Americans are attacked by depression at some time in their lives.

While we've all felt sad at times, we usually get up, go to work, and try to overcome our general discouragement with life. But when these overwhelming feelings of sadness persist—even if for only a few weeks—you may be suffering from a clinical depression, which means you need some professional treatment. Besides a depressed mood or loss of pleasure, symptoms of clinical depression may include appetite and sleep changes, apathy, fatigue, hopelessness, guilt, loss of concentration, and thoughts of suicide.

There are two major kinds of depression: bipolar and unipolar. In bipolar depression, the patient rides a roller coaster of emotions from high to low, leading to the term "manic depression." Unipolar depression, also known as clinical or major depression, lacks bipolar's "highs."

**Treating Depression:** The American Psychiatric Association estimates that 80 to 90 percent of all depression can be treated. The first step is an accurate diagnosis. Along with a physical and lab tests to rule out causes such as reduced thyroid activity, a complete psychiatric history should be taken. And because depression and other major psychiatric problems are side effects of many medications, a good work-up will also include a review of the patient's medications and any illicit drug use.

Once a diagnosis is made, the basic medications used for depression today are:

- **Tricyclic antidepressants** such as Elavil, Tofranil, and Pamelor are prescribed for patients who are in despair, feeling helpless, and unable to feel pleasure.
- **Serotonin uptake inhibitors** such as Prozac, Paxil, and Effexor, all prescribed for uncomplicated depression.
- **Monoamine Oxidase (MAO) Inhibitors** like Nardil and Parnate: These medications are usually used when depressive symptoms are accompanied by symptoms of an anxiety disorder.

## TEN QUESTIONS TO ASK ABOUT ANY INPATIENT TREATMENT PROGRAM

Sometimes mental health problems require hospitalization. This is a serious decision that should not be made without considering the following questions carefully:

1. Is an experienced medical doctor in charge?
2. Does the program provide a total treatment environment, including individual, group, and family therapy?
3. Is a fully qualified staff available, including psychiatrists, psychologists, nurses, and social workers?
4. Does the program use effective diagnostic and laboratory tests to help make correct diagnoses and to evaluate treatment?
5. Does the program provide for family sessions and counseling when necessary? If so, how many family sessions are there?
6. For child and adolescent hospital programs: Does the program offer an accredited school and/or vocational training to prevent children and teens from falling behind in their schoolwork?
7. Are family members encouraged to visit?
8. Are support groups such as Alcoholics Anonymous encouraged?
9. Does the program provide well-defined aftercare through individual or group therapy?
10. How much does the program cost? Will your insurance cover all or part of the treatment, and for how long will your insurance continue?

■**Lithium**: This is the most effective drug for manic depression. However, it can also be used to prevent recurring episodes of depression.

When one of these medications is prescribed, follow-up and continued medical supervision are critical. Blood tests and other metabolic studies are often performed on a regular basis to determine the effect of the drug on the patient. This can be a drawn-out process, because most drugs for depression don't relieve symptoms instantly. Often it takes four to six weeks for a medication to become effective.

Other forms of therapy for depression include interpersonal psychotherapy to help broken relationships, cognitive behavioral therapy to help reverse the patient's negative view of himself and the world, and traditional psychoanalysis. Electroconvulsive therapy—known as ECT or shock therapy—has been used effectively in patients who cannot tolerate the side effects of today's medications, who cannot wait for the medications to work, or who are unable to take drugs for other reasons. While controversial, ECT has proved to be a good treatment option.

### Schizophrenia

One of the most debilitating mental illnesses, schizophrenia often appears first in adolescence. Like alcoholism, diabetes, or high blood pressure, this disease, once it strikes, is usually with the patient for life.

The first signs of schizophrenia may be mild—work performance tails off or the victim stops seeing friends and loved ones. Soon, however, psychotic symptoms surface: hallucinations, paranoia, delusions, disordered thinking. At times, the more severe symptoms abate and the patient is left in a sort of withdrawn state. Some people just lose touch and drift off into another reality.

Some experts believe that the causes of schizophrenia are genetic, but lie dormant until adolescence, when the body undergoes changes that produce the combination of chemicals needed to trip off the disease. Other theories suggest that schizophrenia may be an autoimmune disorder in which the immune system turns on the body itself, or that it's the result of a prenatal viral infection. Whatever the cause proves to be, we still know very little about the disease. But we do know how to treat it on some levels.

**Treating Schizophrenia:** Medications called "antipsychotics," which include Thorazine, Haldol, and Risperdal, seem to be effective in reducing symptoms in up to 80 percent of all patients. Despite severe side effects such as tardive dyskinesia, which afflicts 20 to 30 percent of patients with involuntary movements of the mouth and tongue, these medications combat the hallucinations and delusions that are the hallmarks of schizophrenia. As these symptoms subside, psychotherapy and group therapy for the family and patient can create an environment in which the patient can function once again.

### Childhood Disorders

Mental illness in children and adolescents is particularly painful. Childhood is supposed to be a time of joy, learning, and growth. But a child hampered by learning disabilities, antisocial behavior or severe depression is robbed of one of the most precious periods of life. The greater tragedy is that of the 7.5 million children suffering from some sort of mental disorder, 70 percent do not receive the kind of treatment they need.

■In the past three decades, mental illness, and particularly clinical depression, has led to a doubling of the suicide rate among adolescents and young adults.

■Between 200,000 and 300,000 children suffer from autism—a developmental disorder that prevents learning and other cognitive growth.

■Three to five percent of all children have Attention Deficit Hyperactivity Disorder (ADHD), also known as minimal brain dysfunction, among other names. Basically, these kids can't concentrate, learn, or behave normally. They can't finish a project, don't seem to listen, and require very close supervision. They can be very bright, yet unable to focus their intelligence. Tragically, many are labeled "troublemakers" and shunted aside in schools and homes that don't understand the problem.

■Conduct Disorders (CD) afflict more adolescent boys and girls than any other emotional illness.

As many as nine percent of males and two percent of females are in the grip of violent, socially unacceptable behavior patterns that lead them to destroy property, steal, and make physical or sexual attacks on others. CD may arise from a combination of biological predisposition and environmental influence that is not fully understood. Whatever the cause, CD refers to a specific set of behaviors, not merely to a difficult teenager who's moody and hard to control.

Children also suffer from several forms of anxiety similar to those seen in adults. For example, separation anxiety can lead a child to persistently refuse to leave a parent's side. It may be more apparent when the school years begin, but can strike at any time. Phobias, too are common among children. They include fear of the dark, animals, and certain colors. In fact, according to some estimates, as many as 43 percent of children under age 12 have some sort of exaggerated fear.

**Treating Childhood Disorders:** Curbing mental illness in children is often controversial, since children are harder to treat effectively on an outpatient basis than are adults. Often their problems stem from sexual or physical abuse, drug addiction, genetic conditions, or dysfunctional family environments. If a child is left in the same destructive environment that caused the problem, medication or therapy may not be effective.

Treatment for children almost always includes the entire family. For some problems, such as depression, anxiety, and phobias, the same medications used in adults can, with close supervision by a doctor, be effective in conjunction with family therapy.

Treatment for ADHD involves medications such as Ritalin and Dexedrine, a special educational track that enables the student to remain in school with his peers, and family therapy. Medications enable the child to control his impulsive behavior and perform without loss of attention. The American Psychiatric Association reports that between 70 and 80 percent of ADHD patients "respond to medications when they are properly used." Children with conduct disorders must have treatment that includes behavioral therapy and, when appropriate, medications for underlying depression or ADHD, if present.

There are other mental health problems that affect specific groups such as the elderly (see chapter 23, "Drugs and the Elderly") or teenage girls (anorexia and bulimia), or that result from organic brain damage, such as mental retardation. If you or a loved one suffers from one of these conditions, you should contact a psychiatrist who specializes in its treatment.

Many people define mental illness as "the absence of mental health." After all, we all know when we do or don't "feel good," both mentally and physically. However, as you can see by the variety of disorders, this definition is too simplistic. A mental illness is a specific problem that causes a sustained disruption of your general well-being, behavior, or mood, and interferes with your normal functioning. It can result in *either* psychological or physiological symptoms. The most important things to remember about mental illness are that it can usually be treated effectively, that it is not a sign of weakness or failure, that it is nobody's fault, and that getting help as soon as possible is a vital part of treatment. □

## CHAPTER 10

# OB/GYN Disorders: Causes and Treatments

The term OB/GYN stands for **obstetrics and gynecology**. This is the branch of medicine that deals with pregnancy, childbirth, and women's health problems. "Obstetrics" comes from *obstetrix*, the Latin word for midwife; "gynecology" comes from *gune*, the Greek word for woman.

Some OB/GYN specialists limit their practices to obstetrics. They provide health care to women before, during, and after childbirth. Others concentrate on gynecology, diagnosing and treating disorders of the female reproductive and urinary systems. Some OB/GYNs do both.

Good OB/GYN care is important, both to prevent problems and to treat any existing disease or disorder. For example:

- Pregnant women who do not have regular prenatal checkups run almost double the risk of losing their babies through miscarriage or neonatal (newborn) death.

- Pelvic inflammatory disease (PID) is diagnosed in more than one million women each year. A high percentage of these women require costly hospitalization; many end up permanently infertile.

Regular OB/GYN checkups could save a great deal of expense and avert much personal tragedy.

## Common OB/GYN Disorders and Their Causes

OB/GYN specialists diagnose and treat a wide variety of problems related to menstruation, the urinary tract, the vulva and vagina, the uterus, the ovaries and fallopian tubes, the breasts, and the bone brittleness that sometimes develops after menopause. These physicians also diagnose and treat infertility.

### Menstrual Disorders

**Dysmenorrhea**, or extremely painful menstruation, is a widespread problem, affecting some 10 percent of all women of childbearing age. During menstruation, natural chemicals called prostaglandins make the uterus and its blood vessels contract. Very strong contractions can be painful.

Primary dysmenorrhea occurs when the prostaglandins provoke an overly vigorous uterine response. Secondary dysmenorrhea is caused by such abnormalities as infection, a tumor, or a disorder called endometriosis.

**Premenstrual syndrome (PMS)** occurs just before a woman's monthly period and consists of physical and mental distress. About one in 10 women has PMS severe enough to create problems at work, at home, and in social relationships.

It was once assumed that PMS was simply the

result of an hormonal imbalance. We now know that most women who suffer from PMS have normal hormone levels. A newer theory suggests that PMS may result from an interaction between female hormones and neurotransmitters—chemical messengers manufactured in the brain and nerve cells.

**Endometriosis** (derived from "endometrium," the lining of the uterus) develops when uterine cells migrate and grow elsewhere in the abdominal cavity. The cells may be found on the outside of the uterus, in the ovaries or fallopian tubes, or on the bowels. During menstruation, the endometrial tissue bleeds into the abdomen and causes inflammation, pain, and scarring.

Although we don't know what causes endometriosis, there is some evidence that the condition is inherited.

### Urinary Tract Disorders

**Urinary tract infection (UTI)** is an extremely common condition that occurs in the urethra, bladder, or kidneys. UTIs are usually caused by bacteria originating in the bowels. Friction during intercourse sometimes transfers the bacteria from the vulva (external female genitals) into the urethra (passage to the bladder). The urethra is shorter in women than in men, which makes women more susceptible to UTIs.

**Urinary incontinence** is the chronic leaking of urine. This condition may also involve painful or frequent urination, bedwetting, or the need to urinate frequently throughout the night. Incontinence may be caused by infection, a urinary tract abnormality, estrogen loss after menopause, sagging pelvic muscles, or a neuromuscular disorder.

## THE FEMALE URINARY TRACT: COMMON SITE OF INFECTION

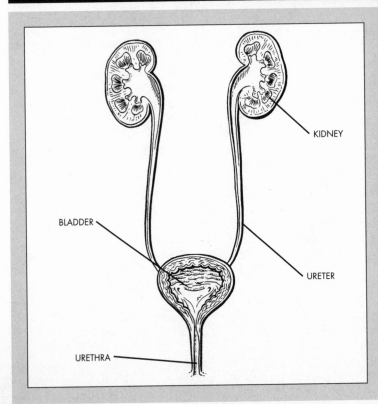

KIDNEY

BLADDER

URETER

URETHRA

A relatively short urethra conspires to increase the risk of urinary tract infections (UTIs) in women. In fact, between the ages of 20 and 50, women suffer 50 times as many UTIs as men. Bacteria traveling up the urethra may attack the bladder or even the kidneys themselves. Infections confined to the bladder are known as cystitis. If bacteria reach the kidneys, a condition called acute bacterial pyelonephritis can result.

## KEY ELEMENTS OF THE FEMALE REPRODUCTIVE SYSTEM

OVARY

FALLOPIAN TUBE

ENDOMETRIUM

UTERUS

CERVIX

VAGINA

VULVA

The female reproductive tract, host to the majority of gynecological disorders, includes the ovaries, uterus, cervix, vagina, and vulva. All are prey to infections; all can fall victim to cancer. Among the most dangerous infections is pelvic inflammatory disease. This condition can lead to a life-threatening tubal pregnancy, in which an egg released from the ovary lodges and develops within the fallopian tube, instead of completing its normal course to the uterus.

### Disorders of the Vulva and Vagina

**Contact dermatitis** of the vulva is a chemical irritation of the skin. The dermatitis may be caused by perfumes or dyes in toilet paper, soap, menstrual pads, or feminine hygiene sprays.

**Genital warts** are caused by the human papillomavirus and are spread through sexual contact. The warts may be flat or raised, painless or painful.

**Genital herpes**, an infection caused by the herpes simplex virus, is also transmitted sexually and causes blisterlike sores in the genital area or other parts of the body.

**Vulvar intraepithelial neoplasia (VIN)**, is an abnormality of cell growth on the vulva. Some women have raised, itchy sores; others notice no symptoms at all. Left untreated, the neoplasia may gradually become cancerous. VIN may be caused by infection with the human papillomavirus—the same virus that causes genital warts.

**Vaginitis**, an inflammation of the vagina, causes redness, itching, discharge, and odor. Some cases of vaginitis stem from infection by bacteria, yeast, or protozoa. Other cases can be traced to antibiotics, birth control pills, frequent douching, tampons, tight or non-breathing pants, obesity, or diabetes.

### Disorders of the Uterus

**Cervicitis** is an inflammation of the cervix, which is the low, narrow end of the uterus. Common in women of childbearing age, it may or may not cause vaginal discharge, pain, tenderness, or slight bleeding between periods.

Some cases of cervicitis are caused by infection with bacteria, protozoa, or a virus; others result from irritation from an IUD or a forgotten tampon. Sometimes the cause is unknown.

**Cervical dysplasia** is an abnormal growth of the cells of the cervix. Like VIN, this condition may eventually turn cancerous if left untreated.

Women who smoke, have multiple sexual partners, have genital warts, or first had sex before the age of 20 are at special risk of developing cervical dysplasia.

**Abnormal uterine bleeding** occurs when menstrual periods are irregular, last longer, or are heavier than usual. Bleeding that occurs between periods may also be deemed "abnormal."

Menopause (the "change of life") and hormonal imbalance are the most common causes of irregular periods. Other possible reasons for abnormal or heavy uterine bleeding include miscarriage; infection of the cervix or uterus; tubal pregnancy; abnormal blood clotting; fibroids; polyps in the uterus; abnormal thickening of the uterine lining; thyroid disease; cancer; an intrauterine contraceptive device (IUD); or birth control pills.

**Pelvic inflammatory disease (PID)** is an infection of the cervix that may spread to the uterus, fallopian tubes, and ovaries. PID affects one woman in seven at some point in life, causing chronic pain and abdominal abscesses. PID is also a leading cause of **tubal pregnancy,** in which the fertilized egg implants in one of the fallopian tubes instead of the uterus. Tubal pregnancy can be a medical emergency. If untreated, a tubal pregnancy may rupture the fallopian tube, causing the embryo to die and possibly endangering the mother's life.

PID usually develops as the result of a sexually transmitted (venereal) disease such as gonorrhea or chlamydial infection. PID may also develop as a result of infection following an abortion, childbirth, or the insertion of an intrauterine contraceptive device (IUD) into the uterus, but such cases are very rare.

**Fibroids** (myomas) are noncancerous growths in or on the uterus. It is estimated that one out of every four or five women over the age of 35 has fibroids. These women may experience longer or heavier periods, irregular vaginal bleeding, abdominal or back pain, or frequent urination.

Although we don't know exactly what causes fibroids, we do know that abnormal growths tend to grow larger under the influence of the female hormone estrogen. For instance, fibroids often

## FIBROIDS: OFTEN UNNOTICED, SURPRISINGLY COMMON

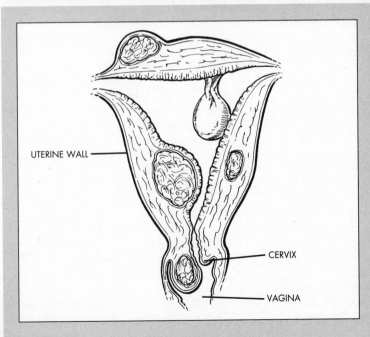

UTERINE WALL

CERVIX

VAGINA

It's estimated that as many as 40 percent of women develop these benign uterine growths by age 40. Few, however, experience any symptoms. If problems such as abnormal bleeding do occur, treatment options include removal of the growths (myomectomy) or the entire uterus (hysterectomy). Fibroids can develop anywhere within the walls of the uterus, or as protrusions attached by a stalk of tissue.

enlarge during pregnancy, when estrogen levels are high. Fibroids may also get bigger in women who use birth control pills with a relatively high estrogen content.

**Uterine cancer** most often affects the endometrium, or lining of the uterus. With early detection, the cure rate is more than 90 percent.

A woman is considered to be at increased risk for uterine cancer if her mother or sister has had the disease, or if she has previously had breast, ovarian, or colon cancer. Other risk factors include endometrial hyperplasia (abnormal thickening of the lining of the uterus); cyst-filled ovaries; irregular ovulation; unusually late menopause; and obesity.

### Disorders of the Ovaries

**Ovarian cysts** are blister-like sacs filled with liquid. They may cause pain during intercourse or at other times. Women may also notice feelings of abdominal pressure and fullness. Most ovarian cysts are noncancerous.

Some ovarian cysts form at the time of ovulation, when the ovary releases an egg cell. Other types of ovarian cysts may result from (or cause) an imbalance of the female hormones estrogen and progesterone, which are produced in the ovaries.

**Ovarian cancer** may affect one or both ovaries. Although two-thirds of the women diagnosed with an early stage of the disease are cured, early ovarian cancer is "silent" and thus very hard to detect. More than three-quarters of all ovarian cancers go undetected until the advanced stages of the disease, when the cure rate is only 5 to 15 percent.

The exact cause of ovarian cancer is unknown. A woman is considered to be at increased risk if her grandmother, mother, or sister has had the disease. Women who have never had children, are infertile, or have previously had cancer of the breast, endometrium, or colon are also at greater risk.

### Disorders of the Breasts

**Fibrocystic breast changes** are noncancerous cysts that develop within the breasts, usually in women aged 25 to 50. The cysts may be small or large, painful or painless.

**Breast cancer** is extremely common and affects one woman out of 9. Early-stage breast cancer is usually curable. That's why OB/GYN specialists urge women to examine their own breasts every month for any lumps, thickenings, or other unusual developments. Many OB/GYNs also advise regular mammograms (breast x-rays) once a woman reaches the age of 40. Others start taking the x-rays at age 50.

### Osteoporosis

**Osteoporosis**, in which bones become fragile and brittle, affects many women who have gone through menopause (the "change of life"). For women with osteoporosis, even a minor fall, a light blow, or a trivial lifting action may be enough to break a bone. Bones in the spine, wrist, hip, and upper thigh are the most likely to break.

The female hormone estrogen helps prevent bone loss. After menopause—or following the surgical removal of the ovaries—the body produces much less estrogen. This sharp drop places women at risk for osteoporosis. For more information, turn to Chapter Four, "Osteoporosis, Low Back Pain, and Other Bone Disorders."

### Infertility

**Infertility** is the inability of a couple to have children. A couple is considered infertile if they fail to conceive after 12 months of trying. About 14 percent of couples in the United States meet this definition. Infertility may be caused by a problem with the man, the woman, or both partners. This is why couples with fertility problems should be diagnosed together.

The common causes of male infertility are sexually transmitted diseases such as gonorrhea or chlamydia; hormonal disorders; damage to the reproductive tract from surgery or disease; certain medications; overheating of the testes from tight clothing, a hot tub, or workplace conditions; and varicose veins in the scrotum.

In women, common causes of infertility are pelvic inflammatory disease (PID); endometriosis; defects or tumors of the uterus; adhesions from past surgery; hormonal imbalance that prevents ovulation; obesity; the use of alcohol, tobacco, or drugs; and the production of antibodies that neutralize the man's sperm.

Thyroid disease, diabetes, or the use of alcohol, tobacco, or marijuana can lead to infertility in both men and women.

## Treatments Focus on Comfort and Function

Treatment for an OB/GYN disorder depends on what's wrong. Some conditions require medication, surgery, or both. In any case, the treatment objective is to ease the woman's discomfort and help her body function more normally.

### When Surgery Is Needed

Common OB/GYN surgical procedures include:

**Dilatation and curettage (D&C)** is performed to help control heavy, prolonged, or irregular bleeding from the uterus. In a D&C, the cervix is stretched open and the lining of the uterus is gently suctioned or scraped. A sample of the lining may later be examined for possible tumors.

**Laparoscopy** is a procedure in which a fiberoptic instrument is inserted through a small incision in the abdomen. The doctor uses an eyepiece to look directly at the uterus, fallopian tubes, and ovaries. During laparoscopy, it is sometimes possible for the doctor to perform a procedure such as draining fluid from an ovarian cyst.

**Laser treatment** uses a laser (high-intensity beam of light) to destroy abnormal tissue—on the cervix, for example.

**Electrosurgical excision** involves using an electrified loop made of fine wire to remove growths on the cervix, vagina, or vulva.

**Electrosurgery** uses heat to destroy abnormal growths.

**Cryotherapy** uses a probe coated with a freezing agent to destroy abnormal growths.

**Myomectomy** is an operation to remove fibroids (benign growths) within the uterus.

**Hysterectomy** is an operation to remove the entire uterus because of abnormal growths.

**Oophorectomy** is the surgical removal of the ovaries.

### When Medication Is Needed

In many cases, **medication** is sufficient to alleviate an OB/GYN problem. For example:

**Antibiotics** are used to treat reproductive organ or urinary tract infections caused by bacteria or protozoa.

**Hormonal therapy** typically includes synthetic estrogen and progesterone, the hormones contained in birth control pills. Hormones may also be used to treat dysmenorrhea (painful menstruation), certain types of vaginitis, and endometriosis. Hormonal treatment can also help prevent or halt osteoporosis. Hormones are given to some patients following breast cancer surgery.

**Diuretics**, or "water pills," help reduce bloating in women who have premenstrual syndrome.

**Antiprostaglandins** prevent menstrual cramps and menstrual-related nausea, diarrhea, and general achiness.

**Antifungal medication** is used to treat vaginal infections caused by yeast.

**Acyclovir (Zovirax)** alleviates the sores and blisters of a genital herpes infection.

**Flavoxate (Urispas)** and similar drugs control abnormal bladder contractions and are useful in treating certain types of urinary incontinence (inability to hold urine).

**Fertility drugs** to bring on ovulation are used to treat certain types of infertility in women.

**Anticancer drugs** are used to treat tumors of the breast, uterus, or ovary, as well as other cancers. □

**CHAPTER 11**

# Birth Control: More Options than Ever

Over the course of a single year, from 60 to 80 percent of the sexually active women who use no form of birth control will get pregnant. To avoid an unwanted pregnancy, some knowledge of birth control is therefore a virtual necessity.

A wide variety of birth control methods is available. Some are extremely effective. Others are less reliable, but may be more appealing to people with particular beliefs or lifestyles. Several reduce the risk of spreading AIDS and other sexually transmitted diseases; others do not. In this chapter, you'll find the strong points and drawbacks of each.

## Birth Control Methods
## That Work Poorly

Among the least effective techniques for preventing pregnancy is withdrawal, in which the man withdraws before he ejaculates. According to the American College of Obstetrics and Gynecology, of all couples who rely on the withdrawal method, one in five will face pregnancy within a year.

Another form of birth control with a poor track record is fertility awareness. Here the woman avoids having intercourse during the days of the month when she is most likely to get pregnant. To determine which days are "unsafe," she keeps track of her past menstrual periods, or notes changes in her basal body temperature or vaginal secretions. The record for this procedure is no better than withdrawal: Chances of pregnancy are one in five within a year.

Both withdrawal and fertility awareness cost nothing or almost nothing, and are accepted by almost all religions. For most women, however, these benefits are outweighed by several disadvantages: the need for continuous self-monitoring, the potential for sexual frustration, and the relatively low reliability these methods provide.

## An Effective—but
## Irrevocable—Alternative

At the opposite end of the spectrum is surgical sterilization, which, short of total abstinence, is unquestionably the most effective form of birth control (though even surgery is not 100 percent reliable).

In female sterilization, or tubal ligation, a doctor seals the fallopian tubes, which carry egg cells from the ovaries to the uterus. In male sterilization, or vasectomy, a doctor seals the vasa deferentia, the tubes that carry sperm from the testicles to the penis.

Although extremely effective, sterilization is meant to be permanent. If the person later changes his or her mind, the operation may be difficult or even impossible to reverse. Sterilization is therefore not a good choice for anyone who might possibly want to have children someday.

## PREGNANCY: THE BEGINNINGS

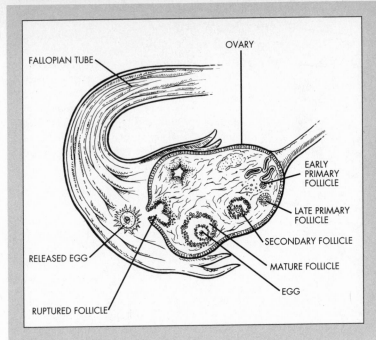

FALLOPIAN TUBE

OVARY

EARLY PRIMARY FOLLICLE

LATE PRIMARY FOLLICLE

SECONDARY FOLLICLE

MATURE FOLLICLE

EGG

RELEASED EGG

RUPTURED FOLLICLE

Human reproduction gets its start in the ovary. Once a month, within one of the two ovaries, a single egg ripens toward maturity. Together with the cells that cluster around it and nourish it, this egg forms a "follicle" moving towards the outer edge. About halfway through the menstrual cycle, the liquid-filled follicle bursts, expelling the mature egg into the fallopian tube. There, if the egg encounters a sperm, conception will take place.

## Contraception: The Other Option

Between withdrawal and sterilization lies contraception, a reversible form of birth control that relies on some kind of equipment, device, or medication. There are three basic kinds of contraception:

**(1) Barrier methods** such as the condom, diaphragm, and cervical cap; or contraceptive foam, jelly, suppositories, and sponges. All of these prevent pregnancy by putting a physical or chemical barrier between the woman's egg and the man's sperm.

**(2) Intrauterine device (IUD),** a small device left in the woman's uterus. By causing changes in the lining of the uterus, the IUD either prevents the man's sperm from fertilizing the woman's egg, or else prevents a fertilized egg from settling into the wall of the uterus.

**(3) Hormonal methods** such as birth control pills and contraceptive implants and shots. These deliver female hormones that prevent monthly ovulation—the release of a mature egg cell from the woman's ovary. The pills are generally taken daily at home. Shots are administered every three months at the doctor's office. Implants, which last up to five years, are also administered at the office.

### How Does Pregnancy Happen?

To understand how the various contraceptives work, it may be useful to recall some facts about pregnancy.

Every month or so, inside a woman's body, one of the ovaries releases a ripe (mature) egg cell. This is called ovulation. The egg cell travels slowly through the fallopian tube to the uterus—a trip that takes several days. It is only during this time that a woman can become pregnant.

When sexual intercourse occurs, some of the millions of sperm cells in the man's semen travel from the vagina to the woman's uterus, or womb,

## THE DIAPHRAGM: A BARRIER METHOD FOR WOMEN

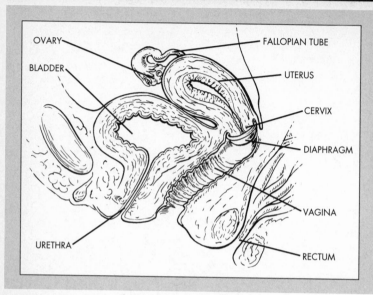

OVARY

FALLOPIAN TUBE

BLADDER

UTERUS

CERVIX

DIAPHRAGM

VAGINA

URETHRA

RECTUM

Stretched across a flexible wire hoop, this shallow rubber cup fits over the cervix, blocking access to the fallopian tubes and the mature egg they may harbor. The device can be inserted prior to love-making, and should be left in place for eight hours afterward. It is usually fitted individually to the woman's vaginal cavity.

and on into her fallopian tubes. There, if the sperm meet a ripe egg cell descending from the ovaries, one of the sperm may unite with the egg cell and fertilize it.

When this happens, the fertilized egg cell continues to advance through the fallopian tube and into the uterus, where it settles into the lining and begins to develop, becoming first an embryo and then a fetus. After nine months of pregnancy, the woman gives birth.

Each of the three basic types of contraception—barrier, IUD, and hormonal—disrupts this process at a different point; and each has unique advantages and disadvantages. Let's consider them in turn.

## Choosing a Contraceptive:
## Barrier Methods

**C**ondom: The condom, a latex or natural-membrane sheath that fits over the erect penis, is a physical barrier to conception. The newly introduced female condom, which combines a diaphragm with a latex liner extending the length of the vagina, serves the same purpose. During ejaculation, both condoms prevent semen from entering the vagina.

One great advantage of latex condoms is that they offer a measure of protection not just against

pregnancy, but also against sexually transmitted diseases such as AIDS, hepatitis B, gonorrhea, syphilis, chlamydia, herpes, and genital warts.

What about disadvantages? Occasionally a condom will break, tear, or slip during sex, allowing sperm-laden semen to spill into the vagina (backup protection with a spermicide can be of value here). Also, some men are reluctant to use a condom, claiming it forces an interruption of intercourse or dulls sexual sensation. Couples who rely on condoms alone are at a two to 12 percent risk of accidental pregnancy.

**Diaphragm or Cervical Cap:** Barrier devices worn by women include the diaphragm, a soft, shallow, rubber cup, and the cervical cap, a small, deep, latex cup shaped like a thimble. After smearing the inside of the diaphragm or cap with contraceptive jelly or cream, the woman inserts the device into her vagina and positions it over her cervix, the opening to her uterus. For the device to be effective she must keep it in place during intercourse and for eight hours afterward.

A diaphragm or cap offers women the advantage of having personal control over contraception. In addition, it can be positioned in advance and need not interrupt love-making. The diaphragm also reduces the risk of pelvic inflammatory disease and certain venereal diseases. And both diaphragm and cap are reusable.

However, as with the condom, these devices do require some preparedness and advance planning. Hence, for women relying on this approach, the risk of accidental pregnancy is six percent to 18 percent.

**Spermicides:** Chemical barriers to conception include spermicidal (sperm-killing) cream, jelly, and foam. These products are measured into an applicator and inserted into the vagina shortly before intercourse. The contraceptive suppository, which is inserted into the vagina and allowed to dissolve, works on the same principle, and provides protection against pregnancy for roughly an hour. The disposable contraceptive sponge contains a spermicide that becomes active when moistened. Placed against the woman's cervix, it protects against pregnancy for up to 24 hours.

An important advantage of spermicidal chemicals is that they kill not just sperm but also certain microbes, possibly including the AIDS virus. However, they do have drawbacks. Certain brands,

in certain people, can cause skin or mucous membrane irritation. And because they taste bad, they can interfere with oral sex. Women who use a spermicide as their sole means of contraception have a three to 21 percent risk of accidental pregnancy.

**Combinations:** It's worth noting that the combination of a condom for the man **plus** a spermicide for the woman offers excellent protection against both pregnancy and many sexually transmitted diseases. The condom-plus-spermicide combination is the logical form of contraception for anyone who has several sexual partners, or whose sexual partner(s) might be infected with the AIDS virus or some other sexually transmitted microbe.

## Choosing a Contraceptive: The Intrauterine Device

The intrauterine device (IUD), a small device that a doctor inserts into a woman's uterus, requires less attention than any other type of contraceptive. Once in place, it provides effortless round-the-clock protection against pregnancy. It

## EFFORTLESS OPTION: THE INTRAUTERINE DEVICE

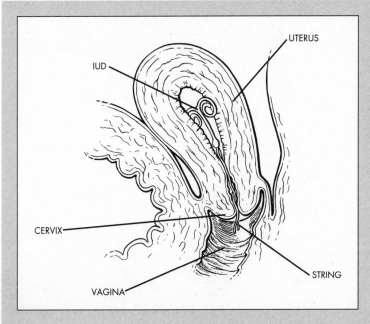

UTERUS

IUD

CERVIX

VAGINA

STRING

The exact reason is unknown, but this small object, when installed in the uterus, prevents conception with better than 95 percent reliability. The device must be inserted by a doctor, but can be left in position for at least a year. The string protruding through the cervix serves to confirm that the IUD has remained properly placed.

deserves consideration by any woman who cannot take birth control pills and is unable or unwilling to use barrier methods consistently.

With the IUD, maintenance is minimal. All the woman need do is check at least once a month to make sure the device is correctly in place. A string attached to the IUD hangs down through the cervix and into the vagina. If this string can be felt with a fingertip, the IUD is still in position.

Of course, even if the IUD seems to be working fine, it periodically must be replaced: every year for the type containing a slow-release female hormone; every eight years for the type wrapped with copper wire.

Although the IUD sounds beautifully simple, it has a number of distinct disadvantages:

1. Insertion of the IUD may briefly be painful, especially for a woman who has never borne a child.

2. After insertion of the IUD, mild uterine cramps and bleeding may continue for days or even weeks.

3. An IUD may make menstrual periods both heavier and more painful.

4. An IUD increases the risk of a pelvic infection, particularly in women with multiple partners; some such infections can cause permanent sterility.

5. There is some risk that the IUD will damage the wall of the uterus.

6. If a woman gets pregnant despite the IUD, she is at increased risk of an ectopic (tubal) pregnancy, which is a life-threatening emergency.

For all these reasons, a woman should **not** use an IUD if she has multiple sex partners or if she has ever had a pelvic infection, a tubal pregnancy, or unexplained bleeding from the uterus.

Surprisingly, it is still uncertain *how* the IUD prevents pregnancy. It may work by irritating the woman's uterus, changing the uterine lining and secretions in ways that disrupt fertilization.

Women who use an IUD have a two to four percent risk of accidental pregnancy.

## Choosing a Contraceptive:

## Hormonal Methods

**P**ills: Birth control pills, used by 32 percent of women of reproductive age, contain synthetic versions of two female hormones: estrogen and progesterone. (The so-called minipill contains synthetic progesterone only.) These hormones prevent a woman's ovaries from releasing a ripe egg cell every month.

A woman who uses this method of contraception should take her pill each day at about the same time. With some brands, there is a pill to take every day of the month. With others, a woman takes a pill for 21 days, stops for seven days, then starts over.

**Shots:** Administered in the doctor's office, the contraceptive shot (Depo-Provera) works in much the same way as the Pill, but need be taken only once every three months. Though Depo-Provera has been in use abroad since 1969, it was not available in the U.S. until 1993.

**Implants:** The contraceptive implant Norplant, also relatively new in the U.S., works on the same hormonal principle. The implant consists of a slow-release female hormone contained in six thin, rubbery capsules. A doctor inserts the capsules beneath the skin on the inside of the woman's upper arm. The gradually released hormone prevents pregnancy round-the-clock for five years. If she wants to get pregnant before the five years are up, she can have the implant removed.

### Pros and Cons of Hormonal Contraception

High reliability is a major advantage of hormonal contraception: The risk of accidental pregnancy is less than 3 percent. The hormones make for lighter and more regular menstrual periods, and reduce the cramps associated with periods. They also lower the statistical risk of tubal pregnancy, pelvic infections, and certain types of cancer (particularly ovarian cancer).

However, not all women are candidates for hormone-based contraception. A woman should use none of the hormonal methods if she has, or has ever had:

■ Breast, uterine, or cervical cancer
■ Blood clots in a leg, lung, or eye
■ Unusual, unexplained vaginal bleeding
■ Angina pectoris (chest pain from a heart condition)
■ A liver tumor of any kind
■ Jaundice while pregnant or taking the pill

One disadvantage of hormonal contraception is the possibility of nausea and vomiting, the most common side effects. Other possible side effects include breast tenderness, bleeding between periods, missed periods, weight gain or loss, depression, headaches, and blurred vision. In most women, the side effects disappear after a month or two. In others, switching to a different brand may diminish the problems.

Rarely, hormonal contraceptives precipitate a serious medical problem: an internal blood clot, stroke, heart attack (in women aged 40 and over), or liver tumor. Cigarette smoking increases the risk that such a problem will develop. So does the presence of high blood pressure, high cholesterol, or diabetes. For these reasons, it is important for any woman who uses a hormonal contraceptive to have regular medical checkups. □

## CHAPTER 12

# Handling Familiar Childhood Infections

With all the sore throats, runny noses, intestinal disorders, and allergies that plague our kids, childhood must sometimes seem like a constant blur of illnesses—especially to the parent doing the nursing. But even though these ailments are debilitating and take an enormous toll on the young patient, most of the problems clear up pretty quickly, are not life-threatening, and carry few long-term effects. (See the appropriate chapters for information on these disorders.)

Even so, parents still need to be particularly vigilant about safeguarding their children's health. The recent rise in the incidence of serious diseases—including whooping cough, rubella, measles, mumps, and hepatitis B—makes a compelling case for keeping vaccinations up-to-date. One of the latest vaccines, now recommended for all newborns, is for hepatitis B, a viral infection that causes an inflamed liver, and may lead to chronic infection and even cancer of the liver.

Routine medical checkups, proper diet, and plenty of rest are also essential to give children the protection they need. When a child falls ill or shows any unexplained or persistent symptoms, prompt medical advice and attention are crucial. This strategy helps keep minor illnesses from getting out of control and ensures early treatment for more serious disorders.

## Treating the Diseases of Childhood

Despite great strides in preventive medicine, many familiar diseases of childhood continue to haunt us. Here's a closer look at the most common, and the ways they are treated today.

### Chickenpox

Chickenpox remains one of the most prevalent childhood diseases, occurring most frequently in those between two and eight years of age. This highly contagious disease begins with a slight fever, loss of appetite, and malaise. Next, the distinctive itchy, blister-like rash appears, usually on the trunk or scalp at first, later spreading over the body. Scratching the blisters may result in scarring, impetigo, boils, and other infections. Children mustn't scratch.

Children must be isolated until the blisters are crusted, usually five to seven days from the time of onset. The contagious period starts one or two days before the rash appears, so keep an eye on your child if he or she has been around someone who later broke out in a rash. The time between exposure and onset of the illness is usually 14 to 16 days. Cases have been known to occur as early as 11 or as late as 20 days after exposure.

Treatment of chickenpox consists of acetaminophen (Tylenol) and daily baths with lukewarm water. The doctor may prescribe an antihistamine such as Benadryl to help reduce itching. Trimming the child's fingernails minimizes the possibility of scarring. Medical care generally isn't necessary unless the child's temperature exceeds 102 degrees, or if the fever lasts for more than four days. In severe cases, acyclovir (Zovirax) may be prescribed. If the rash becomes very warm, red, or tender, the child may have a bacterial infection that requires antibiotics, and a physician should be called. Prompt medical treatment is also necessary if a child shows confusion, nervousness, vomiting, convulsions, lack of responsiveness, poor balance, or increasing sleepiness.

A vaccine for chickenpox (Varivax) is now available. Check with your pediatrician about getting this new type of shot.

## Measles

There is a vaccine for measles, yet the number of cases in the United States rose from fewer than 1,500 in 1983 to 27,672 cases in 1990. Measles may well be *the* most serious communicable disease of childhood, and it is also becoming more prevalent in adolescents and young adults who did not respond to vaccination. Authorities now recommend a second measles, mumps, rubella vaccination after age five.

The incubation period for measles lasts from seven to 14 days. The disease is most communicable during the three to five days before the rash appears. Pre-rash symptoms last four to five days and include malaise, loss of appetite, inflamed eyelids, fever, sensitivity to light, hoarseness, runny nose, and a severe cough. Toward the end of this period, tiny, bluish-gray specks encircled by red appear in the mouth. A day or two after their appearance, the temperature shoots up, the oral spots slough off, and an itchy rash appears behind the ears and on the neck and cheeks.

The final stage of measles is marked by a high fever, puffy, red eyes, extensive rash, and a severe cough. Symptoms usually disappear—and communicability ends—five days after the rash begins.

Treatment of measles consists of bed rest and isolation. Vaporizers and a warm room help relieve respiratory symptoms; taking acetaminophen reduces the fever.

## VACCINES ESSENTIAL FOR YOUR CHILD'S HEALTH

- Polio
- DPT to protect against diphtheria, pertussis (whooping cough), and tetanus
- MMR to protect against measles, mumps, and rubella (German measles)
- Hemophilus Type B to protect against such serious illnesses as meningitis, epiglottitis (inflammation of the epiglottis), and pneumonia
- Hepatitis B
- Chickenpox

## Mumps

Mumps, an acute viral disease, is most common in children between the ages of five and nine years. The disease is transmitted in the saliva of an infected person and has an incubation period of 14 to 24 days.

Mumps begins with a headache, muscle pain, low-grade fever, loss of appetite, and malaise. The next wave of symptoms includes an earache, along with swelling and tenderness in the parotid, and, possibly, other salivary glands. Possible complications include swelling and inflammation of the testicles in males past puberty, abdominal pain, nausea, fever, vomiting, and chills. Meningitis develops in about 10 percent of the cases, but does not usually lead to long-term problems.

Treatment for mumps includes acetaminophen to ease the pain and fever and adequate fluid intake. If swallowing is difficult, it may be necessary to replace the fluids intravenously.

## Whooping Cough

In the past few years, approximately 4,200 cases of whooping cough (Pertussis) have been reported annually in the United States. Whooping cough may produce shock, seizures, pneumonia, and other serious side effects, especially in children younger than 12 months of age.

Whooping cough is highly contagious, and is marked by sudden fits of coughing followed by a high-pitched whooping sound when the child inhales.

The incubation period for whooping cough is seven to 10 days. The first symptoms include thick mucus, a hacking cough, loss of appetite, sneezing, conjunctivitis, listlessness, and, sometimes, a low-grade fever. The next stage is marked by an increasingly spasmodic cough and possible choking on mucus. The characteristic cough may be triggered by respiratory infections that occur months after this illness subsides. Infants often must be hospitalized for supportive care. Antibiotics such as erythromycin are sometimes administered.

### Mononucleosis

Mononucleosis is a viral disease frequently contracted by teenagers. Preschoolers also get mononucleosis, although symptoms may be so mild that the disease is often overlooked. Mononucleosis is caused by the Epstein-Barr virus, which appears intermittently in the mouth of anyone ever infected by it. The disease is usually contracted from someone who is not ill at the time of contact. Symptoms of mononucleosis include fever, sore throat, headache, extreme fatigue, swollen lymph nodes, and possibly a rash. The symptoms tend to subside after six to 10 days, but sometimes may continue for weeks.

Treatment consists of bed rest and acetaminophen. In rare cases, steroids such as prednisone are given if swelling of the tonsils obstructs the airway and makes it hard for the person to breathe.

### Other Childhood Diseases

**Rubella** (German measles) appears most frequently in children between the ages of five and nine years, adolescents, and young adults. The rash is the first sign of disease in children. In adults, the rash, if it develops at all, follows a low-grade fever, loss of appetite, malaise, headache, and swollen glands. In either case, the rash spreads, then disappears rapidly, and usually is completely gone after four to five days. In both children and adults, symptoms may be minimal, or may not appear at all. Treatment includes isolation until the rash disappears plus acetaminophen for pain and fever. Thanks to widespread use of rubella vaccine, the disease is now very rarely seen.

**Reye's syndrome** is a very rare, but acute and extremely serious childhood disease that usually appears one to three days following a viral illness such as an upper respiratory infection or chickenpox. The child typically recovers from the initial infection only to relapse a few days later with intractable vomiting, mild to severe confusion, agitation, and irritability. The syndrome often progresses to coma and is fatal in 20 percent of the cases. Needless to say, you should contact a doctor immediately if any of these symptoms appear. And, since aspirin increases the risk of Reye's syndrome, give your child acetaminophen instead.

**Pinworms** are the most common type of worms found in children. Rectal itching at night is the first—and sometimes the only—symptom. The itching can disturb the child's sleep and result in irritability, skin irritation, and scratching. Treatment usually consists of anti-worm medication such as mebendazole (Vermox).

Other childhood diseases include ringworm, lice, and appendicitis. Children also commonly suffer from allergy, dermatitis, middle-ear infections, anemia, asthma, croup, diarrhea, warts, nosebleeds, and impetigo. □

## CHAPTER 13

# Ear, Nose, and Throat Disorders

Although ear, nose and throat disorders aren't usually fatal, they still can be quite debilitating. Even a minor stuffed nose can make breathing and talking difficult. Ear disorders can disturb our equilibrium or compromise our hearing, impairing our ability to get along in life. Throat ailments can make it hard to eat, breathe and talk.

### How the Ear Works

The organ we loosely refer to as the ear consists of a whole array of parts, including the outer ear, the ear canal, the eardrum (tympanic membrane), the middle ear and inner ear (cochlea), the hearing nerve, and the eustachian tube. Hearing occurs when sound waves strike the eardrum, sending vibrations through a set of tiny bones leading to the inner ear. There the sound is transformed into nerve impulses that then travel to the brain.

To maintain health, air in the middle ear must be at the same atmospheric pressure as that outside the ear. Air reaches the middle ear via the eustachian tube, which is connected to the back of the nose. Air passes through this tube to equalize pressure 1,000 times a day.

### What the Nose Does

The nose is the main entry point of air for the lungs. Inhaled air is cleansed, moisturized, and warmed by the cilia and mucus that line the nasal passages. In addition, when cilia are touched by air, they send nerve impulses to the olfactory areas of the brain, which register our sense of smell. Mucus is produced in the nose, lungs, and sinuses (air pouches that extend from the inside of the nose to the bones of the face and skull).

### A Close Look at the Throat

The throat consists of the pharynx, epiglottis, and larynx. Food travels through the pharynx on the way to the esophagus and stomach. Air passes through the pharynx en route to the trachea and lungs.

When we swallow, food and liquid chewed or manipulated in the mouth is propelled backward by the tongue. It then moves through the pharynx and on to the esophagus and stomach. During this automatic swallowing response, the epiglottis covers the larynx—or voice box—to prevent food from entering the lungs.

With this basic anatomy in mind, let's take a look at the afflictions to which all three of these crucial organs are most prone.

## INSIDE THE EAR

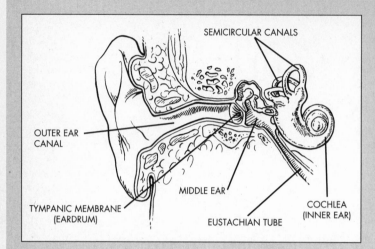

SEMICIRCULAR CANALS

OUTER EAR
CANAL

TYMPANIC MEMBRANE
(EARDRUM)

MIDDLE EAR

EUSTACHIAN TUBE

COCHLEA
(INNER EAR)

The ear boasts two main passageways, one visible, the other hidden. The visible outer ear canal connects the middle and inner ear with the outside world; the hidden eustachian tube travels from the middle ear to the back of the nasal cavity, providing a way to equalize air pressure. Riding atop the inner ear are the semicircular canals, which help us maintain our balance.

## Treating Ear Disorders

Swimmer's ear, or infection of the outer ear canal, is caused by bacteria or fungus that grow when water becomes trapped in that passageway. Symptoms include a feeling of blockage or itching, swelling, pain, foul-smelling discharge, and a temporary partial loss of hearing. Treatment includes acetaminophen (or aspirin for adults) and eardrops containing antibacterial, antifungal, and steroid drugs, such as Cortisporin Otic.

The outer ear canal can also be infected through incorrect use of cotton swabs to clean the ear. Avoid pushing swabs into the canal.

**Otitis media,** or middle ear infection, is a common reason for childhood visits to the doctor; and adults, too, can be at risk. The condition occurs when the eustachian tube becomes inflamed from a cold, a sinus or throat infection, or an allergic reaction, causing fluid to accumulate in the middle ear. If bacteria or viruses take hold, the resulting infection causes pain, an inflamed eardrum, and a buildup of pus and mucus behind the eardrum.

Common symptoms of otitis media are severe ear pain, fever, a feeling of blockage or pressure, and muffled hearing. (Young babies may tug at their ears.) There may also be signs of an upper respiratory tract infection, nausea, vomiting, and dizziness. On the other hand, there may be no symptoms at all.

Prompt treatment of this condition is vital to prevent it from becoming chronic and causing complications. Therapy consists of antibiotics such as ampicillin, amoxicillin, cefaclor, clarithromycin, or the combination drug trimethoprim/sulfamethoxazole (Bactrim). Acetaminophen is used for pain. The doctor may also prescribe antihistamines or pain-relieving eardrops. If these measures are not sufficient, a myringotomy (an incision in the ear drum to allow drainage) may be necessary.

If the eardrum ruptures on its own, the pus drains out of the ear, but may be trapped in the middle ear by the swollen eustachian tube. This condition is known as middle ear fluid or effusion, or serous otitis media. It may become chronic, lasting weeks or months past the original infection, and making the individual vulnerable to frequent recurrences of the acute infection.

**Mastoiditis** is a rare complication of otitis media, usually resulting from the chronic form. It is an infection of the airspace that connects the mastoid sinus to the middle ear. Symptoms include tenderness and a dull ache in the involved area, along with a discharge. This condition requires antibiotics and myringotomy for drainage. If the surrounding bone is diseased, removal of the bones, or mastoidectomy, may be necessary.

**A cholesteatoma** is an abnormal skin growth in the middle ear behind the eardrum. Often the result of repeated infection, cholesteatomas frequently take the form of a cyst or pouch that sheds layers of old skin, causing a buildup inside the ear. If a cholesteatoma grows too large, it can destroy the bones of the middle ear. Symptoms include a feeling of pressure, a foul-smelling discharge, earache, and hearing loss. Dizziness and/or muscle weakness on one side of the face are particularly ominous symptoms, signaling the possibility of serious complications. If they occur, seek medical attention immediately. Treatment consists of antibiotics, ear drops, and careful cleansing of the ear. Large cholesteatomas usually necessitate surgery.

**A perforated eardrum**, often the result of infection or trauma, usually heals spontaneously in a few weeks. If it doesn't, surgery is required. In either circumstance, the eardrum should be observed by a physician and protected from water and trauma.

**Ménière's disease** is a disorder of the inner ear thought to result from an overproduction or malabsorption of the fluids contained therein. Its symptoms are ringing or roaring in the ears, vertigo, and hearing loss. The vertigo is sometimes accompanied by disequilibrium, nausea, and vomiting. Treatment includes meclizine (Antivert) or diazepam (Valium). A low-salt diet and a diuretic may be recommended to reduce frequency of attacks over time.

## Treating Nose Disorders

Nosebleeds are usually not serious, especially in children. Often caused by trauma, they can originate either in the front (anterior) or back (posterior) of the nose. In the former instance, the blood flows out of the nostrils. In the latter, it will flow down the back of the nose and throat even while the patient is standing or sitting. Nosebleeds can also result from acute or chronic infections, polyps, nose-picking, or the inhalation of irritating substances.

Home treatment for an anterior nosebleed includes pinching the nose, pressing firmly toward the face, and holding for five minutes while sitting or lying with head elevated. Ice may also be applied to the nose and cheeks. To prevent rebleeding, the nose should not be picked or blown,

## BEHIND THE NOSE

SINUSES

OLFACTORY NERVES

OPENING OF EUSTACHIAN TUBE

This cut-away view of the nasal cavity reveals a major source of pain and aggravation — the air-filled cavities we call the sinuses. Between the sinuses, hair-like cilia hang from the roof of the nasal cavity, bringing the olfactory nerves in contact with the odors we inhale. Near the juncture of the nasal cavity and the throat below, the entrance of the eustachian tube leads to the middle ear.

the head should be kept at a level higher than the heart, and the person should not strain or bend down.

If re-bleeding occurs, the nose should be cleared of all clots by gently blowing out through the nose. The involved nostril should be sprayed four times with decongestant spray, and the nose should be pinched and held as described above. In addition, a doctor should be contacted.

Since posterior nosebleeds tend to be more serious, they always require a physician's care. If bleeding continues for 10 minutes after pressure is applied, it is considered severe.

Medical care for nosebleeds may include application of epinephrine to the bleeding site, gauze packing, or a nasal balloon catheter. If packing is needed for longer than 24 hours, antibiotics may be necessary.

**A stuffy nose** may be a symptom of allergies, upper respiratory infections, or structural abnormalities. Other less common causes of nasal congestion are a chronic condition called vasomotor rhinitis, thyroid disease, emotional stress, and pregnancy. Used correctly, over-the-counter medications can provide relief for most stuffy noses. Products to consider should include antihistamines, decongestants, or a combination of these agents. Surgery is sometimes necessary to correct structural abnormalities such as a deviated septum.

**Sinusitis** is an infection of the sinuses that may be either acute or chronic. It usually begins with a cold or allergy episode that causes swelling of the mucous membranes and increased production of watery mucus. Because the sinuses are swollen, the mucus tends to build up and become blocked, resulting in the pressure and pain of a sinus headache. The trapped mucus also becomes a breeding ground for bacteria.

Symptoms of sinusitis include characteristic pain in the face, cheeks, forehead and upper teeth; a green or yellow colored and foul-smelling nasal discharge; malaise; fever; and sore throat.

Treatment for sinusitis includes an antibiotic such as Amoxil, Bactrim, or a cephalosporin; decongestants; and occasionally application of a drug such as phenylephrine to constrict the nasal blood vessels. Steam inhalation or heat applications help relieve pain. If sinusitis recurs frequently, it should prompt your doctor to search for an underlying cause, such as structural abnormalities, allergic rhinitis, or immune deficiency.

**Postnasal drip**, the sensation that mucus is dripping downward from the back of the nose into the throat, results from excessive mucus production due to infection, allergies, irritation, swallowing disorders, or structural abnormalities.

Antibiotics may be required to clear up an underlying infection, while antihistamines, decongestants, inhaled corticosteroids, or immunotherapy might be recommended if allergy is the cause. Structural abnormalities such as a deviated septum or septal spur (sharp projection) may require surgery.

**Nasal polyps** are associated with chronic allergies, chronic sinusitis, chronic rhinitis, and nasal infections. The primary symptoms are nasal obstruction and loss of the sense of smell. Medical treatment usually includes inhaled corticosteroids, antihistamines and decongestants (for allergy), and antibiotics (for infection). If this fails to provide complete relief, surgery may be considered.

## Treating Throat Disorders

Pharyngitis or sore throat, one of the most common medical complaints, is caused by viruses 90 percent of the time. The streptococcus bacteria, responsible for strep throat in one in 10 Americans every year, is a common non-viral cause.

Symptoms include soreness, difficulty swallowing, the feeling of having a lump in the throat, and the constant urge to swallow. The infection may also be accompanied by headache, muscle and joint pain, and fever.

Treatment consists of warm salt-water gargles, mildly anesthetic throat lozenges, fluids, painkillers, and rest. If the infection is bacterial, penicillin or a broad-spectrum antibiotic will be required. (See Chapter 17, "Counterattacking Major Infections," for more information about strep.)

**Acute tonsillitis** typically starts out as a mild-to-severe sore throat. Symptoms may then progress to fever, difficulty swallowing, tenderness and swelling of the lymph glands, joint and muscle pain, headache, chills, malaise, and ear pain. In

## WITHIN THE THROAT

TONSILS

PHARYNX

ESOPHAGUS

TONQUE

EPIGLOTTIS

TRACHEA

The site of numerous trouble-some infections, the throat extends from the back of the nasal cavity downward to the trachea (windpipe) and the esophagus (alimentary canal). Called the pharynx in medical terminology, the throat conducts both food and air to the body below. As food passes down the throat to the esophagus, the epiglottis shuts off access to the nearby windpipe.

chronic tonsillitis, the sore throat recurs and is usually accompanied by discolored discharge in the area of the tonsils.

Treatment for acute tonsillitis consists of aspirin (for adults) or acetaminophen, rest, and adequate fluid intake. If the infection is bacterial, antibiotics such as penicillin or erythromycin are necessary. Chronic tonsillitis may require surgical removal of the tonsils.

**Acute or chronic laryngitis** is an inflammation of the vocal cords. It may be caused by a local infection, or can be part of a bacterial or viral upper-respiratory infection. Symptoms include mild to severe hoarseness and even complete loss of the voice. Laryngitis may be accompanied by pain, a dry cough, malaise, swelling in the throat, and fever.

Treatment consists of resting the voice and taking analgesics and anesthetic throat lozenges. If the infection is bacterial, antibiotics are necessary. Hospitalization may be required if acute laryngitis is so severe that the airways become obstructed. □

## CHAPTER 14

# Relief for Common Allergies

Allergies pose a significant and serious health problem in this country. According to conservative estimates, nearly 15 million Americans are plagued by hay fever and 10 million have asthma. Twelve million more Americans suffer from such allergies as eczema and hives, not to mention allergic reactions to food, drugs, and insect stings. Most of these disorders have a hereditary component and tend to run in families.

## What Is An Allergic Reaction?

Basically, an allergic reaction occurs whenever the immune system overreacts to a seemingly harmless substance. Known as allergens, these substances include pollen, mold, house dust, mites, animal saliva and dander (skin shed by cats, dogs, or rabbits), feathers (such as those used in feather pillows), certain foods and drugs, and insect stings.

Allergens are usually absorbed into the body by way of the skin, nasal passages, lungs, or digestive tract. Once inside the body, allergens stimulate the lymphocytes (small white blood cells) to produce what are known as allergic antibodies. The reaction between the allergen and these antibodies, which are attached to certain special cells (mast cells), leads to inflammation of the nose, eyes, lungs, and the digestive tract. A stuffy nose, sneezing, wheezing, skin rash, watery eyes, abdominal cramps, and nausea are some of the most common results.

## Asthma

Although asthma is a common condition that affects all age groups, one-third of all cases occur in children under 10 years old. This means that approximately three million children in the fifth grade and below suffer from this disorder. Not surprisingly, asthma accounts for more school absences than any other chronic childhood illness.

The chief symptoms of asthma include coughing, wheezing, and shortness of breath. An asthma attack may be brought on by any of the previously mentioned allergens or by infections in the sinuses or bronchial tubes. Emotional stress, hormonal changes, irritants such as cigarette smoke, changes in temperature and humidity, and exercise also may trigger an asthmatic episode.

Asthma attacks may begin suddenly with the onset of severe symptoms, or start slowly with a gradually increasing difficulty in breathing. A typical acute asthmatic attack is marked by wheezing, labored breathing, tightness in the chest, and a dry cough. Asthma attacks may produce a feeling of suffocation and an inability to speak without frequent pauses to catch the breath. The victim may also have a rapid pulse, sweat profusely, and turn blue.

Treatment for asthma usually consists of removing the offending allergen or irritant and administering medications that reduce inflammation and open the air passages. For patients with daily symptoms, inhaled steroid drugs such as Azmacort,

Beclovent, Vanceril, and AeroBid are frequently prescribed, as are cromolyn sodium (Intal), nedocromil sodium (Tilade), theophylline (Theo-Dur, Uniphyl), and albuterol (Proventil, Ventolin). For patients hospitalized with a serious attack, airway-opening drugs may be given intravenously.

## Hay Fever

Allergic rhinitis (hay fever) can be brought on at certain seasons by the airborne pollens of trees, grass, and weeds. Other allergens cause hay fever all year. These year-round troublemakers include molds, dust mites, and animal dander.

Hay fever symptoms include sneezing, watery eyes, runny nose, nasal congestion, and an itchy palate and throat. Hay fever can also be accompanied by conjunctivitis (itchy, swollen eyes), malaise, headache, and sinus pain.

The treatment of hay fever consists of removing the environmental antigen, if possible, and implementing drug therapy and immunotherapy (allergy shots). The newer antihistamines, such as terfenadine (Seldane) and loratadine (Claritin), cause less drowsiness and dryness. Topical intranasal steroids, such as flunisolide (Nasalide), beclomethasone (Beconase, Vancenase), and triamcinolone (Nasacort), reduce inflammation and may eliminate the need for oral antihistamines and decongestants.

## Hives and Angioedema

Hives (urticaria) are itchy, red, swollen patches of skin that appear suddenly. Although they may vanish within one to two hours, they can last as long as two days. They frequently occur in clusters, with new clusters forming as others fade. They do not leave scars.

Hives may have an allergic or non-allergic cause; and the exact culprit usually cannot be determined. They are often triggered by a food or a drug. Common foods that cause hives include nuts, shellfish, peanuts, and eggs. Drugs that typically produce hives include penicillin, sulfa, anticonvulsants, aspirin, and nonsteroidal anti-inflammatory drugs (NSAIDs). Tight-fitting clothing that scratches or rubs the skin, activities that increase the body's temperature (warm baths, hot tubs, exercise, or fever), and exposure to cold or sunlight may all cause hives in susceptible individuals.

Angioedema is a condition like hives that occurs in the deeper layers of the skin, most often in the hands, feet, and face. Certain types of hereditary angioedema may cause fatal swelling of the larynx.

Hives and angioedema are treated by avoiding whatever substance has provoked the outbreak, if it can be identified. Antihistamines such as hydroxyzine (Atarax), diphenhydramine (Benadryl), loratadine (Claritin), astemizole (Hismanal), terfenadine (Seldane) and clemastine (Tavist) are used to treat daily occurrences. Oral corticosteroids are considered a last resort.

## Dermatitis

Atopic dermatitis is a form of eczema that often begins in early childhood. It is frequently associated with allergic rhinitis or asthma. Half the cases disappear by adulthood.

We don't know what causes atopic dermatitis. The symptoms in infants include itchy red patches on the face, torso, and lower parts of the limbs. These patchy areas crust, scale, and ooze. A child between the ages of two and four may develop clusters of red or flesh-colored scaly patches or bumps on the elbows, knee creases, ankles, neck, wrists, and feet. The rash becomes more concentrated during adolescence, appearing on the sides of the neck, hands, and face, and the skin becomes more thickened.

People with atopic dermatitis are prone to bacterial skin infections that produce itching and redness. Oozing, crusting ulcers may also occur in some cases.

The goal of treatment is to eliminate the itching. Therapeutic measures typically include application of lubricants and moisturizers while the skin is damp after bathing, plus use of topical corticosteroids, such as fluocinolone acetonide (Synalar). Oral antihistamines such as hydroxyzine (Atarax) and diphenhydramine (Benadryl) help ease the itching.

Allergic contact dermatitis may be caused by poison ivy, oak, or sumac, as well as by exposure to nickel, chrome, mercury, certain cosmetics, and drugs applied to the skin.

Poison ivy produces redness, bumps, and blisters, as well as swelling after the initial contact.

The blisters burst after a few days, releasing a watery liquid, and healing begins. Treatment includes trying to prevent a rash by promptly washing the affected area with soap and water—within five minutes of contact, if possible. If a rash develops, wet, cold compresses and steroid ointments may be advised. Oral steroids may be necessary for severe cases.

## Stings and Anaphylaxis

Stinging insect allergies result when a sensitive individual is stung by a bee, wasp, hornet, yellow jacket, or fire ant. The reaction usually occurs soon after the initial sting and may include wheezing, generalized hives, angioedema, and a sharp drop in blood pressure. The victim may also go into shock and lose consciousness. If not treated immediately, severe reactions may be fatal.

Avoidance is the best strategy for someone with this type of sensitivity. Anyone who has an adverse reaction should consult an allergist for skin testing. Venom immunotherapy could be a lifesaver in the event of a future sting. Sensitive individuals should have injectable epinephrine (EpiPen, Ana-Kit) available in case of an attack.

Anaphylaxis is a severe and potentially life-threatening allergic reaction distinguished by the sudden onset of hives or angioedema, respiratory distress, and a drop in blood pressure. The reaction is caused in susceptible individuals by a variety of allergens, including vaccines; penicillin and other antibiotics; diagnostic chemicals; insect venom; polysaccharides; food (including berries, nuts, seafood, and egg whites); aspirin; and nonsteroidal anti-inflammatory agents. Penicillin is by far the most common culprit. Exercise may also induce anaphylaxis in some people.

Symptoms of anaphylaxis include feelings of impending doom or fright, itching of the skin, nasal congestion and coughing, hives and swelling of tissues in the lips or larynx, wheezing, shortness of breath, low blood pressure, and loss of consciousness. The person's eyes may also itch, swell, and tear. Other symptoms include change of voice, hoarseness, itching of the mouth and throat, sneezing, chest pain and tightness, redness of the skin, cramping of the uterus, a feeling of warmth and flushing, a need to urinate, abdominal cramps, nausea, vomiting, and diarrhea.

Anaphylaxis is an emergency condition that requires an immediate injection of epinephrine. Emergency injection devices such as EpiPen or Ana-Kit could be lifesaving if available for use in an unexpected attack. In any event, if you experience any of these symptoms, seek medical help right away. □

**CHAPTER 15**

# Dealing with Skin Problems

The skin is the body's largest and most visible organ. It reflects a person's general health and performs many important bodily functions. An average-sized person has 20 square feet of skin that serves as the body's front-line defense against injury and bacteria. The skin also regulates body temperature, acts as a sensory and excretory organ, and synthesizes vitamin D when exposed to ultraviolet light. A vast network of blood vessels in the skin provides oxygen and nutrients to sensory and motor nerves and also to skin appendages, including glands, nails, and hair.

Not surprisingly, this complex, exposed organ is vulnerable to many diseases. Each year, as many as seven million people seek medical treatment for newly diagnosed skin diseases. And almost everyone will experience some type of skin problem sooner or later. Skin disorders are usually noticeable and often disfiguring, causing both physical and psychological distress.

## Some Other Skin Facts

- The American Academy of Dermatology reports that one out of four people seeking medical advice about new skin problems is bedridden.

- Teenagers and young adults account for a significant number of dermatology (skin) patients. In highly urban areas, however, a surprisingly large proportion of patients are adults.

- Acne is the leading skin disease, occurring in 20 percent of all patients seeking treatment for skin disorders. Contact skin disorders, such as poison ivy and burns or rashes caused by industrial or household chemicals, are the second most common problem.

- Other common skin disorders include skin cancer, warts, fungal infections, and psoriasis.

- More than three million workdays are lost each year because of skin diseases.

- Chronic skin disease accounts for up to 50 percent of workers compensation claims in some states.

- Skin disease is the fourth largest cause of disability in the Armed Forces, affecting almost seven percent of military personnel.

## The Skin's Architecture

The skin has three major layers—the epidermis, the dermis, and the subcutaneous tissue. The epidermis is the outermost layer of skin. Its main function is to produce the keratin that protects the body against harmful environmental substances and controls water loss. Cells in the epidermis also produce melanin, which gives the skin its color.

The next layer of the skin is the dermis. This layer contains a number of important substances such as collagen and reticulin, which prevent the skin from tearing; elastin, which makes the skin resilient; and jellylike substances that make the skin soft and compressible.

The third layer, subcutaneous tissue, is primarily made up of fat, which provides insulation, shock absorption, and calorie reserves. Both the dermis and the subcutaneous tissue contain sensory and motor nerves.

Among the most common causes of skin disorders are infections, overexposure to sunlight, follicle dysfunction, and hormonal imbalance. Parasites, external substances, cell dysfunction, genetic factors, stress, and aging also cause skin problems. Here are the most common skin disorders and their treatments:

## Acne: The Leading Complaint

Acne typically affects teenagers, occurring during a time of dramatic hormonal shifts and rapid growth. The blackheads, whiteheads, pimples, and boil-like lesions that appear on the face, back, chest, and shoulders are a source of embarrassment and may lead to permanent scarring.

Rising hormone levels during puberty cause the sebaceous glands to enlarge and produce more oil. No one knows why this process causes acne in some people but not in others. However, certain factors are known to contribute to the development of acne. They include oral contraceptives; certain medications, such as steroids, some hormones, iodides, bromides, and lithium; exposure to heavy oils, greases, or tars; trauma or irritation from tight clothing; cosmetics; and emotional stress.

Acne results when small kernels of sebum (oil), skin cells, and bacteria fill up hair follicles, causing blackheads and whiteheads to appear. The sebum ruptures the walls of the follicles, forming pimples and boil-like eruptions in nearby tissue. If the sebum is further altered by bacteria, it may cause even more irritation to the surrounding skin.

Acne is usually treated with an antibacterial agent such as benzoyl peroxide—either alone or in

## A CLOSER LOOK AT THE LARGEST ORGAN

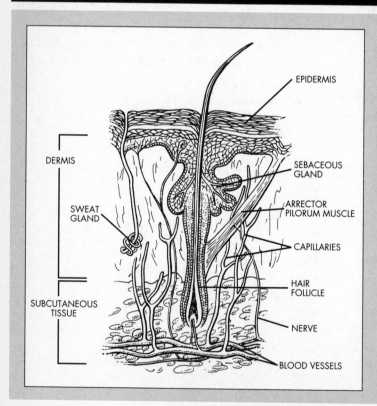

DERMIS

EPIDERMIS

SEBACEOUS GLAND

SWEAT GLAND

ARRECTOR PILORUM MUSCLE

CAPILLARIES

HAIR FOLLICLE

SUBCUTANEOUS TISSUE

NERVE

BLOOD VESSELS

Below the skin's deceptively smooth surface lies a veritable forest of support structures and glands, including nerves, muscles, capillaries, and the sebaceous glands implicated in acne. The epidermis, or top layer, acts as a protective barrier. As its cells are rubbed off and shed, cells in the dermis below are constantly dividing to provide replacements. When this renewal cycle gets out of control, the result is psoriasis.

combination with tretinoin (Retin-A). Oral and topical antibiotics such as tetracycline, erythromycin, and topical clindamycin also help alleviate acne. Accutane (oral isotretinoin), inhibits the secretion of sebum, but has severe side effects and must be used cautiously.

Other acne remedies include injecting cortisone directly into the lesions, estrogen therapy for women, and exposure to ultraviolet light. Proper cleansing techniques also are often part of the therapeutic plan.

## Rosacea and Rhinophyma

Rosacea is a chronic skin disorder that produces flushing and dilation of the small blood vessels in the face. Tiny pimples also appear. As the disease progresses, small, thin, red lines (telangiectasia) may appear on the skin's surface. In advanced cases—and usually only in men—the nose becomes bulbous and red, the cheeks become puffy, and thick bumps develop on the lower half of the nose and adjacent cheek areas. We don't know what causes this condition, which is called rhinophyma, but the problem may be aggravated by stress, infection, vitamin deficiencies, and glandular upset.

Topical steroids as well as topical and oral antibacterial agents are helpful in the treatment of rosacea. Beta blockers can be used to reduce redness and swelling. The dilated blood vessels of telangiectasias can be closed off with a small needle, a laser, or surgery.

Rhinophyma is usually treated with surgery or dermabrasion. Most people with this disorder are advised to avoid alcohol, spicy foods, hot drinks, and smoking, and to stop using facial products that contain alcohol or other irritants.

## Psoriasis: An Array of Treatment Options

Psoriasis affects as many as eight million Americans. Though the cause is unknown, psoriasis results in an overproduction of skin cells. The surplus skin leads to thickening and scaling. The resulting silvery plaques generally appear on the scalp, elbows, knees, and lower back. The severity of psoriasis ranges from mild, undetected forms to rare cases in which the scales cover the entire body. Psoriasis may cause pitting of the fingernail surface, thickening and crumbling of the nail plate, and separation of the nail from the nail bed.

Genetic factors apparently cause a biochemical malfunction that triggers the psoriasis. Skin cells mature in three to four days— much faster than the usual 28 to 30 days—resulting in a flaky buildup. Itching, occasional pain, and embarrassment are the chief complaints of psoriasis sufferers.

Treatment of psoriasis consists of removing the scales by softening them with certain preparations, then gently scrubbing the skin with a soft brush in an oatmeal or salt bath. Other treatments include exposure to ultraviolet type B light (UVB), coal tar preparations, steroid creams, methotrexate (an anticancer drug), anthralin, and PUVA (psoralen in conjunction with UVA exposure). Tegison, a synthetic vitamin A derivative, is sometimes used in conjunction with PUVA, UVB, and topical medications. Low-dosage antihistamines may also be prescribed.

Arthritic symptoms often accompany psoriasis. Aspirin and local heat usually relieve these symptoms. Severe cases may require nonsteroidal antiinflammatory drugs. Psoriasis of the scalp often responds to the use of tar shampoo and steroid lotion. Psoriasis of the fingernail cannot be treated, but usually clears up when the skin lesions subside.

## Dermatitis: Many Forms, Many Remedies

Dermatitis is the general term for any inflammation of the skin. There are many types of dermatitis and many different causes.

**Atopic eczema** affects about three percent of the United States population and often occurs as an allergic reaction to wool, silk, fur, ointment, detergent, perfume, wheat, milk, or eggs. It produces an intensely itchy rash that blisters, oozes, and crusts. In infants, it appears primarily on the face and scalp. When it occurs in adolescents and young adults, it is usually found in the large folds of the hands and feet; elbow bends and backs of knees; and the face, neck, and upper chest.

Doctors usually treat atopic eczema with topical corticosteroids and petrolatum, sedatives, and antihistamines. Oral antibiotics may be prescribed for a secondary infection; ultraviolet light therapy has been helpful in treating severe cases. Patients are instructed to eliminate or avoid allergens, irritants, extreme temperatures, stress, and other possible aggravating factors.

**Seborrheic dermatitis** is another common skin disorder. This chronic condition causes red skin covered by yellowish, greasy-appearing scales and usually occurs on the scalp (where it's known as dandruff), sides of the nose, eyebrows, eyelids, skin behind the ears, and the middle of the chest. Treatment with low-strength topical cortisone preparations usually provides relief. Scalp treatments include frequent shampoos with preparations containing such chemicals as tar, zinc pyrithione, selenium sulfide, sulfur, and/or salicylic acid. Seborrheic dermatitis may be caused or perpetuated by a yeast organism, and antiyeast creams have been used with good results by some people.

Other forms of dermatitis include contact dermatitis, localized neurodermatitis, stasis dermatitis, exfoliative dermatitis, and allergic contact dermatitis (poison ivy, oak, and sumac).

## Infections: Common and Surprisingly Stubborn

Athlete's foot may affect as many as 90 percent of Americans. This fungal infection shows up as sores between the toes, or as a blistering rash on the foot. Another type of athlete's foot manifests itself as a very mild inflammation and dry scaling of the entire sole of the foot, along with infection of the toenails. Treatment consists of dressings of tap water or a weak salt solution. Oral antibiotics and topical and oral antifungal medicines are also used. Other fungal infections of the skin include tinea versicolor and dermatophytosis (ringworm).

Other infection-related skin diseases include herpes and warts—both of which are viral infections; impetigo; folliculitis, furunculosis, carbunculosis, and staphylococcal scalded skin syndrome—all bacterial infections; scabies—caused by the itch mite; cutaneous larva migrans—a reaction to infestation by hookworms and roundworms; and pediculosis—caused by parasitic forms of lice.

Also common are such skin conditions as hives, which are treated with antihistamines and the removal of the offending agent; and vitiligo, a condition in which pigment cells are destroyed, which is treated with repigmentation drugs activated by ultraviolet light.

## Skin Cancer: The Three Major Types

Basal cell carcinoma is the most common form of skin cancer and affects some 400,000 people each year. The tumors appear as small, fleshy, translucent bumps or nodules on the head, neck, hands, or occasionally, on the trunk of the body. These tumors don't grow quickly and don't metastasize (spread to other organs). If left untreated, however, the tumors begin to bleed, crust over, and then repeat the cycle. If treatment is further delayed, basal cell carcinoma can invade the skin and spread, causing significant damage as it extends.

**Squamous cell carcinoma tumors** appear as nodules that ulcerate in the center, or as red, scaly patches on the rim of the ear, face, lips, and mouth. The tumors eventually enlarge into sizable masses and can spread via the blood and lymph systems.

**A malignant melanoma** is the most virulent of all skin cancers. If untreated, it can be fatal; and in the U.S., the increase in new cases tops all other forms of skin cancer.

Malignant melanoma results from the uncontrolled growth of pigment-producing tanning cells. It resembles an oversized, asymmetrical mole and

## WHAT YOU SHOULD KNOW ABOUT SKIN CANCER

Skin cancer is mainly caused by overexposure to ultraviolet light. The rate of skin cancer—the most common of all cancers—is growing at an alarming rate. Recognizing the early signs of the various forms of skin cancer is essential for early detection and successful treatment. All forms of skin cancer are highly curable if caught in time.

is characterized by an irregular border and unusual pigmentation. Any mole larger than a pencil eraser that has these characteristics is cause for concern and should be checked.

As with all skin cancers, malignant melanoma is thought to be linked with excessive exposure to the sun. It also tends to run in families. If a relative has had it, extra caution is advisable.

Malignant melanoma may appear suddenly without warning or may begin near a mole or another dark spot on the skin. Additional warning signs include changes in the surface of a mole, oozing, scaliness, bleeding or the appearance of a bump or nodule; spread of pigment from the border of a mole into the surrounding skin; and changes in sensation, such as pain, tenderness, or itching. If detected early enough, melanoma can usually be cured by surgical removal.

Several options are available for treating basal cell and squamous cell carcinomas. Treatment may involve surgical removal; electrodesiccation (destroying cancerous tissue with a high-frequency current transmitted through a needle electrode); cryosurgery (using cold liquid nitrogen to destroy the cancerous tissue); radiation therapy; and topical chemotherapy. ☐

## CHAPTER 16

# Correcting Glandular Disorders

The endocrine system is a complex network of glands that acts in concert with the nervous system to control and coordinate the myriad chemical reactions associated with storage and release of energy, growth, maturation, reproduction, and behavior. The sheer complexity of this system makes it vulnerable to breakdown, a fact that is reflected in numerous and varied endocrine disorders. The endocrine system's influence on bodily functions is so profound that many body systems may be affected when any of these glands fails to operate properly.

## How Does the Endocrine System Work?

The endocrine system includes the pituitary, thyroid, parathyroid, adrenals, testes, ovaries, pineal, and thymus glands and the islet cells of the pancreas. The endocrine glands function by releasing hormones (or chemical messengers) into the bloodstream. These hormones trigger reactions in specific tissues.

This network of glands is regulated by the hypothalamus—the area at the base of the brain where the endocrine system meets the nervous system—and by the pituitary gland. Together, they generate chemical messages that stimulate the other glands to further activity. When endocrine disorders develop, they usually consist of either hypofunction (underactivity) or hyperfunction (overactivity) of one or more glands. Occasionally, inflammation or development of tumors in a gland leads to trouble as well.

Endocrine hyperfunction and hypofunction may have their source in the hypothalamus, the pituitary, or the target gland itself. Chronic disorders are more common, and generally lead to hypofunction; however, inflammation can cause acute episodic malfunctions. Tumors more commonly occur in the glands themselves, but can appear in other areas of the body, such as the lungs or stomach, where they produce hormones that cause endocrine dysfunction.

## Pituitary Disorders

Hypopituitarism is characterized by growth retardation in children, sexual immaturity, and metabolic dysfunction. Hypopituitarism results from a deficiency of the hormones secreted by the anterior pituitary gland. Panhypopituitarism involves a partial or total failure of all this gland's hormones. These two conditions can be caused by tumors; but they may also result from certain chemicals, congenital defects, irradiation, and changes in blood flow.

Symptoms usually develop gradually and may include impotence, the absence of menstrual periods, infertility, decreased sexual drive, and diabetes insipidus (a state of high urinary output unrelated to the more common diabetes mellitus). Other symptoms are

## THE MAJOR ENDOCRINE GLANDS AND THEIR FUNCTIONS

■ The pituitary gland, located at the base of the brain, produces several hormones, including antidiuretic hormone (ADH), adrenocorticotrophic hormone (ACTH), thyroid-stimulating hormone (TSH), growth-hormone (GH), follicle-stimulating hormones (FSH), luteinizing hormone (LH), and prolactin. The pituitary has been called the master gland because so many of the hormones it produces control the functions of other glands.

■ The thyroid gland, situated at the front of the throat, secretes thyroxine (T4) and tri-iodothyronine (T3), which are essential for growth and development. These two hormones stimulate metabolism and protein synthesis in most of the body's tissues.

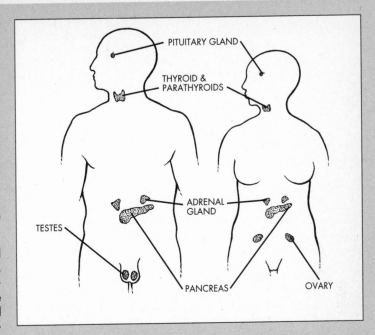

■ The four parathyroid glands are located next to the thyroid glands. The parathyroid glands secrete parathyroid hormone (PTH), which controls phosphorous and calcium metabolism and plays a central role in bone development.

■ The pancreas lies transversely in the abdomen, just behind the stomach. The pancreas secretes digestive juices into the stomach, and two hormones—insulin and glucagon—into the bloodstream. The hormones regulate glucose metabolism. Insulin promotes use of glucose by the body's cells. Glucagon regulates release of stored glucose into the bloodstream.

■ The adrenal glands sit atop the kidneys and are composed of two separate parts—the outer cortex and the inner medulla. The adrenal cortex, which accounts for 90 percent of the adrenals, secretes aldosterone, which causes the kidneys to excrete potassium and retain sodium; and cortisol, corticosterone, and cortisone, which together help the body resist stress; inhibit the immune response; promote normal metabolism of proteins, fats, and carbohydrates; and inhibit inflammation. The adrenal cortex also secretes sex hormones. The adrenal medulla secretes epinephrine and norepinephrine, which produce the body's fight-or-flight response to stress.

■ Men have two testes, which are located in the scrotum outside the abdominal cavity. The testes produce sperm and male hormones—most notably testosterone, which controls the development of the male sex organs.

■ Women have two ovaries, which are situated on either side of the uterus. The ovaries release eggs and secrete female sex hormones. Ovarian hormones include estrogen, which mediates the development of female sex organs and characteristics; and progesterone, which prepares the uterus for pregnancy and readies the breasts for lactation.

hypothyroidism and adrenal insufficiency (Addison's disease). Treatment consists of replacement hormones.

**Hyperpituitarism** results in the extreme overgrowth of the skeleton and is often caused by a tumor. When hyperpituitarism occurs before puberty, the entire body becomes abnormally large. This condition is called gigantism. Postpubertal hyperpituitarism is called acromegaly and produces bone thickening; this rare condition usually strikes between the ages of 30 and 50.

Other symptoms of hyperpituitarism include oily skin, severe headaches, blurred vision, profuse sweating, a loss of peripheral vision, nervous system impairment, and a rapid metabolism. The head and facial features become enlarged and distorted in hyperpituitarism, and the individual may show symptoms of irritability, hostility, and other psychological disturbances.Treatment consists of removing the tumor, followed by hormone replacement if necessary.

## Thyroid Disorders

Hypothyroidism occurs more frequently in women than in men and is diagnosed most often between the ages of 40 and 50. Hypothyroidism, essentially an underproduction of thyroid hormone, can be caused by an insufficiency of the hypothalamus, the pituitary, or the thyroid gland itself.

An underactive thyroid gland may be the result of surgery, inflammation, autoimmune conditions, or insufficient iodine in the diet. Congenital defects may also cause hypothyroidism, and the condition can be a side effect of certain drugs.

The early symptoms of hypothyroidism tend to be vague. They include short-term memory loss, fatigue, lethargy, unexplained weight gain, intolerance to cold, poor wound healing, and constipation. Later signs of hypothyroidism include increased mental instability; puffiness in the face and extremities; thin, dry hair; loss of libido; loss of appetite; hand tremors; and abdominal bloating. If left untreated, hypothyroidism may eventually lead to onset of a life-threatening coma.

Hypothyroidism is treated by replacing the thyroid hormones.

**Hyperthyroidism** is caused by overproduction of thyroid hormone. In Graves' disease, the most common form of hyperthyroidism, patients are likely to have an enlarged thyroid, heat sensitivity,

nervousness, difficulty in concentrating, prematurely gray hair, weight loss, increased appetite, diarrhea, palpitations, tremors, sweating, and, in some cases, bulging eyes. Graves' disease is thought to result from an immune-system malfunction that overstimulates the thyroid. The disease may not become apparent until it is triggered by trauma or by a benign tumor of the thyroid gland.

Hyperthyroidism is treated with antithyroid drugs, surgery, and radioactive iodine. The drugs used to treat hyperthyroidism include methimazole (Tapazole) and propylthiouracil (PTU), which reduce thyroid activity. Surgery and radioactive iodine are both aimed at destroying enough thyroid tissue to reduce hormone secretion to more normal levels.

Other thyroid disorders include thyroiditis, an inflammation of the thyroid gland, and goiter, an enlargement of the thyroid glands.

**Hypoparathyroidism** results from diseased, injured, or congenitally defective parathyroid glands. Injury to the glands most often occurs during surgery involving nearby tissue. Hypoparathyroidism may also be caused by the prolonged, severe magnesium deficiency associated with alcoholism.

Hypoparathyroidism leads to low blood concentrations of calcium, which may cause neuromuscular excitability, including spasms and twitching of the face, hands, and feet; abdominal pain; hair loss; dry skin; and cataracts.

Treatment with vitamin D will usually reverse hypoparathyroidism, although calcium supplementation is sometimes required.

**Hyperparathyroidism**, usually caused by a benign tumor, can lead to kidney problems, bone abnormalities, brittle bones, and chronic low-back pain. People with hyperparathyroidism also show such signs of gastrointestinal discomfort as pain and ulcers, as well as muscle weakness, constipation, depression, psychosis, stupor, and, sometimes, coma. Treatment consists of surgery to remove the tumor or drugs to correct any abnormalities the condition has caused. In some cases, no specific therapy is required.

## Disorders of the Adrenal Glands

Addison's disease (or adrenal insufficiency) usually results from an autoimmune response that destroys the adrenal glands. The symptoms of Addison's disease are loss of appetite, weight loss, fatigue, weakness, vomiting, nausea, and diarrhea. Other signs include a sun-tanned appearance, intolerance for stress, and a craving for salty food. The treatment of Addison's disease entails lifelong replacement of the steroid hormones produced by the adrenals, usually with hydrocortisone or cortisone. Because serious illness or injury may dramatically increase the body's need for adrenal hormones, patients with Addison's disease should wear an identification bracelet in case of emergency.

Cushing's syndrome results from the over-secretion of adrenal hormones, especially cortisol, or from taking synthetic ACTH or steroids. Excessive cortisol production is, in turn, usually brought on by an oversupply of ACTH, possibly due to a tumor that produces ACTH in another organ.

Common symptoms of Cushing's syndrome include fatty deposits on the face, neck, and trunk, and purple streaking on the skin. This syndrome also produces muscle and bone weakness, poor wound healing, peptic ulcer, irritability, mood swings, difficulty sleeping, high blood pressure, suppressed immune response, diabetes, and changes in the reproductive system.

Treatment for Cushing's syndrome may include radiation, drugs, or surgery. Metyrapone (Metopirone) and aminoglutethimide (Cytadren) are among the medications used to reduce cortisol production. □

**CHAPTER 17**

# Counterattacking Major Infections

Our struggle for survival has always entailed a battle against the countless microbes with which we share the earth. Hostile bacteria, viruses, fungi, and parasites invade our bodies and go to war with our immune systems. To fight back, we must call forth all our strength and defenses. Plagues and epidemics are as much a part of our history as any struggle between nations.

Though it may seem hard to believe, prior to the use of penicillin during World War II, physicians had no effective medicines to treat serious infections. Fifty years later, we have more than 100 different antibiotics—including sulfa drugs, synthetic penicillin, and many, many more—to ward off the full spectrum of bacterial diseases. The development of numerous vaccines has virtually wiped out many former killers, both bacterial and viral, in the U.S. and many other developed countries.

Yet infection still plagues us, despite these gains. Many strains of bacteria are now resistant to the drugs that once killed them. Most viruses are impervious to antiviral drugs. Some microorganisms come in so many different forms that a single vaccine just can't cope with them all. Other microorganisms elude treatment by hiding in hard to reach areas such as the central nervous system and bones. Then too, some people today are simply exposed to a wider range of diseases because of our increased mobility, the use of immunosuppres-

sive drugs, and such invasive procedures as surgery and catheterization.

Consequently, infection is still a serious threat, even in our highly advanced society. In Third World countries, infectious diseases continue to cause widespread mortality.

## How Infections Cause Illness

When organisms invade the body, they reproduce and multiply rapidly. In the process, the microorganisms compete with the body's metabolic processes. Some also produce toxins that injure cells. What's more, our own immune response may actually cause even further tissue damage. How sick someone actually gets as a result of the infectious process depends on the type and number of invading organisms and the person's overall health and strength.

## Staph Infections

Staphylococcal bacteria produce a wide range of diseases, causing anything from skin eruptions to blood poisoning (bacteremia) and death. Staphylococcal infections include the following conditions:

**Bacteremia**, the presence of bacteria in the blood, is characterized by a high fever, shaking chills, racing heart, pallor, agitation, and joint pain. It may progress to confusion and stupor, and can be fatal in just 12 hours. Treatment must begin immediately with semi-synthetic penicillin (nafcillin or methicillin) or cephalosporins (cefazolin) given intravenously. People who are allergic to penicillin or are infected by penicillin-resistant organisms must be treated with vancomycin.

The symptoms of **staphylococcal pneumonia** are similar to those of other pneumonias—sudden onset of high fever, cough with yellow or bloody sputum, difficulty in breathing, and chest pain. Treatment consists of the same medication used for bacteremia.

The use of some of these drugs, particularly broad-spectrum antibiotics like cephalosporins, sometimes brings on enterocolitis (inflammation of the intestines). This condition is marked by profuse, watery diarrhea; abdominal pain; nausea; vomiting; and dehydration. If a patient develops enterocolitis, the antibiotics must be stopped at once and replaced with a different drug, such as vancomycin.

**Osteomyelitis** is a bone infection that occurs as a complication of a blood-borne infection, or as a sequel of surgery or trauma. Osteomyelitis may come on rapidly, exhibiting fever, sudden pain, swelling, tenderness, heat, and restricted movement in the affected bone. Its onset can also be insidious, however, with fever as the first warning. Treatment consists of surgery to open and cleanse the wound and large doses of antibiotics for four to eight weeks.

Staphylococcal bacteria are among the most common causes of **food poisoning**. Symptoms of food poisoning include nausea, loss of appetite, diarrhea, vomiting, and abdominal cramps. Since the symptoms typically subside within 18 hours, there's usually no need for treatment unless the person shows signs of dehydration. Full recovery takes one to three days.

Some **skin infections** owe their source to staphylococcal bacteria as well. These infections are manifested by widespread inflammation of soft tissue (cellulitis), and pus-producing or boil-like lesions, sometimes accompanied by fever and discomfort. Treatment includes applying mupirocin ointment (Bactroban), as well as administering oral antibi-

otics (erythromycin, dicloxacillin, or cloxacillin). Severe infections are treated with intravenous oxacillin, methicillin, or nafcillin. Ointments such as bacitracin-neomycin-polymyxin are used to prevent further infection of broken skin.

**Toxic shock syndrome (TSS)** is an acute infection that is sometimes associated with tampon use during menstruation. The symptoms of toxic shock syndrome include a high fever, an abrupt episode of shivering and chills, intense muscle pain, profuse watery diarrhea, headache, and vomiting. A dark red rash appears on the palms and soles within a few hours. Shock may develop within 48 hours.

TSS is treated with antibiotics, such as oxacillin, methicillin, and nafcillin, given intravenously.

## Strep Infections

A total of 21 species of **streptococcal bacteria** have been identified, but three classes—**Groups A, B, and D**—are responsible for most infections.

**Group A** bacteria cause the following infections:

**Streptococcal pharyngitis** accounts for the majority of sore throats caused by bacteria. Children between the ages of five and 10 years get most of these strep throats—mainly from October through April. The symptoms of strep throat may include a fever, severe pain and difficulty swallowing, inflamed tonsils, a sore and red throat, a "strawberry" appearance of the tongue, enlarged lymph nodes, loss of appetite, weakness, malaise, and abdominal discomfort.

Sometimes, however, the symptoms of strep throat are mild, and the infection escapes detection. Left untreated, a strep infection can lead to rheumatic fever.

It is essential that anyone with a strep throat take the full prescription of antibiotics—usually either penicillin or erythromycin. Isolation from others for 24 hours after starting antibiotic therapy is recommended to prevent the disease from spreading.

**Scarlet fever** may occur along with a strep throat, certain wound infections, and blood poisoning.

Children between the ages of two and 10 years are most likely to get scarlet fever. Symptoms include those of strep throat plus a sunburn-like rash that feels like sandpaper to the touch. The rash usually begins on the upper chest and then spreads to the rest of the body. Prompt treatment with an antibiotic is essential.

**Erysipelas** is another type of strep infection. It usually occurs in infants and in adults over 30 years of age. When erysipelas develops, swollen, red, raised lesions with a raised, firm border suddenly appear and spread. Other symptoms include headache, vomiting, fever, and irritability. An antibiotic should be administered promptly. Cold packs and analgesics, such as aspirin and codeine, can alleviate local pain.

Other infections caused by streptococcal A bacteria include **impetigo** (skin lesions with itching and encrustment) and **lymphadenitis** (red-streaked, painful skin lesions with fever, racing heart, and lethargy.) Both infections require treatment with antibiotics.

**Group B streptococcal infections** include newborn and adult forms. The adult form usually occurs after women give birth. Both newborn and adult infections are usually treated by penicillin or ampicillin. **Group D streptococcal** bacteria are frequently implicated in endocarditis, an inflammation of the interior of the heart.

Various strains of strep are among the causes of other diseases, including **pneumonia** (see Chapter 6 on respiratory disorders); **otitis media** (fluid in the middle ear); and **meningitis**. All of these infections are treated with penicillin, amoxicillin, or ampicillin.

## Meningitis

Meningitis occurs most often in children under five years of age and in people living in crowded conditions such as those found in the military or in institutions. In older patients, meningococcal bacteria are a more likely cause than strep. The symptoms are varied and may include sore throat; stiff neck; a sudden, spiking fever; intense headache; chills; muscle pain in the back and legs; racing heart; and a rash. As many as 20 percent of all cases evolve into a severe form of meningitis marked by extreme prostration, intravascular coagulation, skin lesions, and shock. Left untreated, this particular infection may cause respiratory or heart failure and be fatal in just six to 24 hours.

Meningitis must be treated immediately with large doses of penicillin G, ampicillin, or a cephalosporin, such as ceftriaxone or cefotaxime.

## Tetanus

People get tetanus (lockjaw) when a puncture wound becomes contaminated by soil, dust, or animal feces. The incubation period ranges from less than two days in severe cases to three or four weeks in milder cases.

Symptoms include spasms and increased muscle tone near the wound, profuse sweating, and a low-grade fever. Patients also experience an extreme tightening of neck and facial muscles, which produces a grotesque grinning expression; rigidity of abdominal and back muscles; and convulsions.

Treatment must begin within 72 hours after a puncture wound occurs. Patients who have no previous immunization need tetanus immune globulin or tetanus antitoxin for temporary protection, followed by immunization with tetanus toxoid. Those who have not been immunized in the past five years need a booster shot of tetanus toxoid. If tetanus develops, treatment consists of airway maintenance and the use of muscle relaxants, such as diazepam (Valium), or a neuromuscular blocker. High doses of antibiotics (preferably penicillin) are also necessary.

## Intestinal Infections

Salmonella is an extremely common infection—more than two million new cases are reported in the United States each year. Salmonella bacteria are the cause of typhoid fever, and are often the culprits in gastroenteritis (inflammation of the stomach and intestines). Occasionally, they cause blood poisoning and localized infection.

**Gastroenteritis** caused by salmonella is usually contracted by eating contaminated or inadequately processed foods—especially eggs, turkey, duck, and chicken. Other sources include contaminated dry milk, chocolate bars, and contact with infected animals or people. Symptoms typically include diarrhea, nausea, abdominal pain, and fever. Though the infection usually clears up on its own, at times it may progress to intervals of high fever, abscesses, dehydration, and blood poisoning. Treatment for uncomplicated cases includes bed rest and fluid and electrolyte replacement.

**Typhoid fever** is usually contracted by drinking contaminated water, takes three weeks to run its course, and is marked by persistent fever and flu-like symptoms. For this infection, a wide variety of antibiotics may be prescribed.

**Infections by** *Escherichia coli* and other bacteria living in human intestines cause a great deal of diarrheal illness in American children. These infections are also prevalent among travelers to other countries—particularly those visiting Mexico, South America, and Southeast Asia. People with mild infections recover easily. Those with severe infections, however, require prompt fluid and electrolyte replacement to prevent fatal dehydration. This cautious course is especially important for children, who are highly susceptible to dehydration.

Symptoms include the sudden onset of watery diarrhea, abdominal pain, and cramping. Some forms may produce chills, along with blood and pus in the stools. In small children, the stools may be yellow or green, and the child may experience vomiting, irritability, loss of appetite, and listlessness, possibly progressing to severe dehydration, fever, and shock.

Treatment includes rest and correction of fluid and electrolyte imbalances. Intravenous antibiotics are occasionally needed to treat infections in infants.

## Lyme disease

Lyme disease is contracted from the bite of an infected deer tick. A red, enlarging ring is the first sign of infection. This mark may be itchy, but usually causes no irritation. Several days later, a few more lesions may turn up. The blotches last several weeks, and within a few days of their appearance may be joined by a variety of other symptoms including stiff neck, malaise, fatigue, chills, fever, headache, achiness, and muscle pain. Stage two occurs weeks or months later and may include cardiac and neurologic symptoms such as facial palsy. These symptoms may last for months or become chronic. Stage three can begin weeks or years later and is marked by chronic arthritis-like symptoms.

Early treatment may prevent later complications. The usual treatment for adults is a 10- to 20-day course of oral doxycycline or tetracycline, although penicillin, amoxicillin, or cephalosporins may be used instead. Children under eight years of age usually receive oral penicillin or amoxicillin. In advanced stages of the disease, intravenous penicillin or ceftriaxone may be given for two to four weeks.

The list of infectious diseases goes on—diphtheria, listeriosis, botulism, gas gangrene, actinomycosis, dysentery, cholera, poliomyelitis, Colorado tick fever, Rocky Mountain spotted fever, malaria, giardiasis, trichinosis, hookworm—but, happily, most are either rare in this country or easily preventable. If we take full advantage of the immunization measures and advanced antibiotics available today, we now have less to fear than ever before in history. □

**CHAPTER 18**

# Overcoming Kidney Disease

Kidney disease is a major health problem in this country, afflicting some eight million Americans. Kidney and urinary tract diseases together affect an estimated 20 million people, causing more than 95,000 deaths a year and contributing to an additional quarter of a million.

Kidney disorders run the gamut from minor infections to total kidney failure. Kidney disease can cause high blood pressure, anemia, and elevated cholesterol. When chronic, it can lead to depression and sexual dysfunction. Kidney stones, diagnosed in more than one million Americans annually, can be extremely painful and are a significant cause of hospital stays and lost work days. But the picture is not entirely bleak.

Thanks to major medical advances, diagnosis and treatment of kidney problems have improved significantly in the past 30 years. Even people with complete kidney failure can now lead reasonably normal lives because of modern dialysis techniques and new successes in transplantation. Today dialysis keeps alive more than 120,000 Americans who would otherwise perish because of kidney failure. Kidney transplants, first performed in the U.S. some 30 years ago, have saved the lives of thousands more.

## Why Are Your Kidneys So Vital?

Called the "master chemists" of the body, the kidneys keep a variety of elements in balance. When the kidneys become damaged, other organs suffer as well.

It's commonly known that the kidneys remove waste products and excess fluids from the body via the urine, and that they maintain a critical balance of salt, potassium and acid. But most people are unaware that kidneys perform other vital functions as well. For example, the kidneys produce a hormone—erythropoietin or EPO—that stimulates the production of red blood cells. Other kidney hormones help regulate blood pressure and calcium metabolism. The kidneys even synthesize the hormones that control tissue growth.

Anytime the kidneys' ability to remove and regulate water and chemicals is impaired by disease or blockage, fluids and waste products accumulate, ultimately resulting in extreme swelling and symptoms of uremia (an overload of toxic byproducts) or kidney failure. The kidneys' various functions can each be affected separately, so urine output may be normal despite significant kidney disease.

Kidney diseases, which usually involve both kidneys, are categorized as **hereditary, congenital** or **acquired**.

**Inherited kidney disorders** usually begin producing symptoms during the teen to adult years, and are often serious.

**Congenital kidney diseases** typically involve a malformation of the genitourinary tract that can lead to blockages, which, in turn, can cause infection and/or destruction of kidney tissue. Tissue destruction may then lead to chronic kidney failure.

**Acquired kidney disorders** have numerous causes, including blockages, drugs, and toxins. However, diabetes and high blood pressure are by far the most common culprits.

## Inherited Kidney Diseases

The most common inherited disorder is polycystic kidney disease; others include Alport's syndrome, hereditary nephritis, primary hyperoxaluria, and cystinuria.

**Polycystic kidney disease (or PKD)** is marked by the formation of fluid-filled cysts in the kidney tubules. These cysts compress functioning kidney tissue, eventually replacing it. In the most common type of the disease (autosomal dominant PKD), almost half of the patients develop chronic kidney failure between the ages of 40 and 60. The rarer form (autosomal recessive PKD) causes kidney failure in early childhood.

In PKD, both kidneys become enlarged. Patients experience back pain, blood in the urine, kidney stones, recurring bladder or kidney infections, and high blood pressure.

Though there is no cure, careful management of high blood pressure and prompt antibiotic treatment of kidney or bladder infections can prolong life. Exercise to help maintain good physical condition is frequently recommended as part of the

## HOW YOUR AMAZING KIDNEYS WORK

GLOMERULUS

RENAL ARTERY

TUBULE

RENAL VEIN

URETER

The two fist-sized kidneys sit on either side of the spine at the lower end of the rib cage. Each consists of approximately one million nephrons; each nephron contains a filtering apparatus called a glomerulus, which is laced with tiny blood vessels; each glomerulus is attached to a tubule. After blood is filtered in the glomerulus, the remaining fluid passes along the tubule, where chemicals and water are either added or extracted according to the body's needs. The final product of this process is the urine we eliminate.

The kidneys filter and return to the bloodstream about 200 quarts of fluid every 24 hours. Approximately two quarts are eliminated as urine, which flows from the kidneys through the ureter to the bladder, where it is stored for up to eight hours.

treatment program. Since PKD is progressive and often leads to kidney failure, patients are counseled, given emotional support, and prepared for the eventuality of dialysis or transplantation.

## Congenital Kidney Diseases

There are two types of congenital kidney disease. In one, malformations present at birth usually lead to some type of blockage. This disrupts the normal flow of urine, causing it to back up and exert increasing pressure on the kidneys, ultimately leading to permanent damage. In the other form, the muscles of the bladder fail to contract as they should, due to some abnormality in the muscles or their nerve supply.

Though kidney malformations are common, affecting up to 15 percent of the population, they generally don't cause problems. Blockages that can lead to serious kidney difficulties include the narrowing of the upper urinary tract (**ureteropelvic junction obstruction** or **ureteral stenosis**), congenital contracture of the bladder outlet (**vesical neck contracture**), or narrowing of the channel from the bladder to the outside of the body (**urethral stricture**).

Urinary tract blockages require early diagnosis, ordinarily accomplished by injecting dye into the bloodstream or the bladder so that an X-ray can be taken. Specific diagnostic procedures include intravenous urography and retrograde pyelography. (The latter procedure sometimes actually relieves the blockage, eliminating the need for surgery.) Non-invasive diagnostic techniques include renal scans, ultrasound, and CT scans. Some urinary tract blockages can be treated by abdominal surgery; others can be relieved by surgery through the urethra.

## Acquired Kidney Diseases

Inflammation of the kidneys, or nephritis, is the primary characteristic of acquired kidney diseases. In the most common of these, glomerulonephritis (also known as Bright's disease), the glomerulus or filtering part of the kidney becomes inflamed. The disease can be brief and severe, mild and protracted, or rapidly progressive.

**Acute post-streptococcal glomerulonephritis** typically starts about 10 days after the onset of a strep throat or a skin infection such as impetigo. Though more common in children, it can occur at any age.

Most people recover fully, but the few who don't may develop chronic kidney failure within months.

Symptoms include a fall in urine output, "smoke"- or "rust"-colored urine, and a burning sensation when urinating. Swelling of the face, eyelids, and hands due to fluid retention is also common, as are shortness of breath, a cough, and high blood pressure.

Acute post-streptococcal glomerulonephritis usually heals completely within three to 12 months after onset. The only treatment is the relief of symptoms and complications. Accompanying high blood pressure must be treated with an antihypertensive. Fluid retention is controlled with diuretics (water pills), including metolazone (Diulo, Zaroxolyn) or furosemide (Lasix).

**Chronic glomerulonephritis** is a term used for a wide variety of diseases that cause progressive scarring of the kidneys over a long period of time, often without any initial symptoms. Frequently, the only findings in the early stages of the illness are an abnormal urinalysis and high blood pressure. Edema (fluid retention) and persistent high blood pressure appear as the disease progresses. As with the acute form, the accompanying high blood pressure must be treated with medication. A diet restricting protein, sodium, and potassium is also often part of the treatment plan. Steroids and other drugs have been used to treat this disease; their success depends on the underlying cause.

**Rapidly progressive glomerulonephritis (RPGN)** is characterized by a decrease in urine output and progressive decline in kidney function over a three to six month period or less. RPGN has no known cause, appears suddenly, and can quickly lead to kidney failure. RPGN is irreversible once kidney function is severely affected, but the kidneys may recover significantly if treatment is begun early enough.

**Nephrotic Syndrome:** Though not a disease in itself, this condition is often the result of other kidney disorders or more generalized diseases (such as diabetes' mellitus and lupus erythematosus). It is marked by heavy loss of protein in the urine, a low protein level in the blood, an increase in blood cholesterol level, and edema (fluid retention). Prognosis is variable and depends on the underlying cause; in some cases, the condition may progress to end-stage kidney failure.

Some forms of nephrotic syndrome respond to corticosteroids, which significantly reduce the amount of protein lost in the urine. In those cases in which steroids do not help, treatment consists of diuretics to control high blood pressure and swelling due to fluid retention.

**Acquired Kidney Obstructions**: These are generally mechanical in nature. Common causes include an enlarged prostate gland in older men, sagging pelvic muscles in older women, and tumors in the genitourinary organs of both males and females. Kidney stones and scar tissue that develops as a result of infections, x-ray treatment, and surgery may also cause blockage of the urinary tract. Some of these obstructions can be alleviated by surgery and follow-up medical treatment. Tumors are treated with surgery, radiation, and appropriate medications.

**Kidney Stones**: These hard masses appear when certain chemicals in the urine form crystals that stick together. The crystals can grow into a stone as small as a grain of sand or as large as a golf ball. Small stones are passed out of the body with the urine. The larger ones can block urine flow or irritate the lining of the urinary tract. Some individuals with kidney stones have no symptoms, but most usually experience some of the following: severe pain, nausea, and vomiting; burning and a frequent urge to urinate; fever, chills, and weakness; cloudy or foul-smelling urine; blood in the urine; and a blocked flow of urine. Serious infections can result from a blockage.

Specialized x-rays or sound waves (ultrasound) can be used to diagnose and identify the location and size of kidney stones. Since 90 percent of stones are small enough to pass naturally, treatment usually consists of methods to promote this, such as drinking a lot of liquid. Medications that may be prescribed include antibiotics (if an infection develops) and analgesics such as meperidine (Demerol) for pain. Larger stones are often treated by passing a telescopic device into the ureter or bladder and either removing the stones or breaking them into small fragments with lasers or sound waves. Alternatively, larger stones may be broken

down by high-energy shock waves. Only rarely is surgery necessary.

Drinking large amounts of fluids, taking certain medications, and changing the diet may help prevent the formation of new stones.

## Treatment of Kidney Failure

As much as 90 to 95 percent of kidney function can be lost before kidney failure becomes apparent. Symptoms include loss of appetite, nausea and vomiting, extreme fatigue, difficulty sleeping, itching and dry skin, muscle cramps, and twitching. Left untreated, the build-up of waste products in the body can lead to coma, seizure, and death.

Many years ago, kidney failure was inevitably fatal. But modern medicine now offers three life-saving treatments.

In **hemodialysis** an artificial kidney machine carries out the vital functions the kidneys can no longer perform. In this procedure, a person is connected to the machine by plastic tubing that attaches to special blood vessels in the arm or leg. The treatment can be done at home or at a dialysis unit.

In **peritoneal dialysis**, waste products from the blood are flushed from the body with fluid instilled and drained through a catheter that has been surgically placed in the abdomen. Once the catheter is in place, this technique is usually done at home.

Since patients with kidney failure are often anemic, many have to take a substance known as EPO (erythropoietin), the synthetic form of a hormone that helps make red blood cells. Iron supplements are also sometimes required.

**Kidney transplantation**, the third option for people with kidney failure, has shown increasing success in recent years. Depending on the quality of the match between donor and recipient, there is an 80 to 90 percent chance that a transplanted organ will still be functioning one year after the operation. The major complication of a transplant, rejection of the organ, is treated with such medications as steroids, azathioprine, and cyclosporine. Many transplant patients also need blood pressure medication, as well as drugs to prevent ulcers and infections. □

**CHAPTER 19**

# Bringing Urinary Disorders under Control

When functioning properly, the urinary tract is a marvel of efficiency. Throughout every 24-hour period, it thoroughly cleanses approximately 200 quarts of fluid, returning most of it to the circulatory system and eliminating the remaining two quarts as urine through the bladder.

As with most parts of the body, however, when this system breaks down, it causes pain and discomfort. And unfortunately, it breaks down quite frequently. Urinary tract infections (UTIs), second only to respiratory infections in frequency, account for 10 million visits to the doctor each year. One in five women will suffer from cystitis, an inflammation of the bladder, at some time in her life. Twenty percent of women who have a UTI will have a second infection, and 30 percent of those will have yet another. In addition, at least 10 million adults suffer from urinary incontinence (an inability to hold urine) to some degree.

## Some Facts About

## Urinary Tract Disorders
- Women are more prone to UTIs than are men or children.
- Urinary tract problems increase with menopause.
- One to two percent of children develop urinary tract infections.
- Young children have the greatest risk of kidney damage caused by urinary tract infections.

- Certain people who contract one or more urinary tract infections may need further testing to ensure they do not suffer from other health problems.

The kidneys, ureters, bladder, and urethra are the key components of the urinary tract. The kidneys filter waste from the blood (see Chapter 18, "Overcoming Kidney Disease") and eliminate it in the form of urine. The urine travels from the kidneys to the bladder through narrow tubes called ureters. The bladder, a ball-shaped receptacle in the lower abdomen, stores the urine for anywhere from one to eight hours before it is emptied from the body through the urethra.

## Urinary Tract Infections

Urine contains fluids, salts, and waste products. Normally it is sterile. Trouble starts when microorganisms, usually *Escherichia coli* from the digestive tract, cling to the opening of the urethra and multiply. The type of infection that follows depends on whether the bacteria stay in the urethra or travel to the bladder or even the kidneys themselves. Microorganisms called *chlamydia* and *mycoplasma* may also cause UTIs. These infections usually remain limited to the urethra.

The chief causes of UTIs are blockages, changes in hormone levels, prostate enlargement, lowered immunity, catheters, structural abnormalities, and,

## TRACING THE COURSE OF THE URINARY TRACT

Originating at the kidneys, the urinary tract conducts waste fluid down the ureters and into the bladder, where it accumulates until expelled through the urethra. Note the striking difference in the lengths of the male and female urethras. This, more than any other factor, accounts for a woman's greater vulnerability to bladder infections.

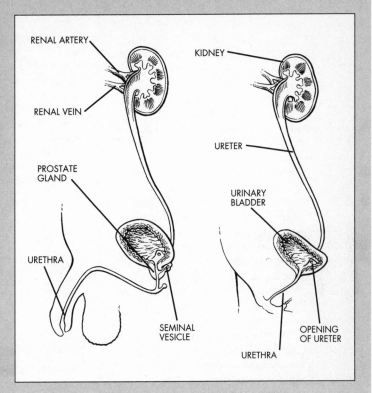

RENAL ARTERY

RENAL VEIN

PROSTATE GLAND

URETHRA

SEMINAL VESICLE

KIDNEY

URETER

URINARY BLADDER

OPENING OF URETER

URETHRA

for some women, sexual intercourse. Women who use a diaphragm are also prone to UTIs.

Symptoms of possible urinary tract infection include:

- A frequent urge to urinate
- A painful, burning sensation in the area of the bladder or urethra during urination
- A feeling of tiredness
- Bladder pain, even when not urinating (caused by pressure above the pubic bone in women and fullness in the rectum in men)
- The passing of only a small amount of urine at a time
- In a few cases, lower back pain, fever, or chills
- Milky or cloudy urine
- Blood in the urine, back pain, or a fever (signs that the infection may have reached the kidneys)

- In children or infants, irritability; loss of appetite; unexplained, persistent fever; incontinence or loose bowels; a change in urinary patterns; or a generally unhealthy appearance

UTIs are treated with antibiotics, usually for seven to 10 days. The regimen may be shorter or longer, however, depending on whether the bladder or kidneys are infected. The drugs most commonly used for bladder infections are trimethoprim (Trimpex), trimethoprim/sulfamethoxazole (Bactrim, Septra), amoxicillin (Amoxil, Trimox, Wymox), nitrofurantoin (Macrodantin), ampicillin and the quinolone antibiotics (Cipro, Floxin, Noroxin, Penetrex, Maxaquin). Longer treatments with tetracycline, trimethoprim/sulfamethoxazole or doxycycline are necessary for infections caused by *Chlamydia* or *Mycoplasma*. Lengthier courses of treatment are also usually recommended for men, in part to treat infection of the prostate gland. Women may receive extended treatment to prevent a recurrence. Pregnant women with UTIs should be treated promptly to avoid premature delivery and the risk of high blood pressure (though only certain drugs are safe to use). Severe kidney infections usually require hospitalization and several weeks of antibiotic treatment.

Women who experience recurrent UTIs often respond to one of the following regimens:

- Low doses of an anti-infective drug such as trimethoprim/sulfamethoxazole or nitrofurantoin daily for six months or longer
- A single dose of an antibiotic after sexual intercourse
- A short course (one or two days) of antibiotics when symptoms first appear

## Urinary Incontinence

Though not a natural consequence of the aging process, urinary incontinence is nevertheless a widespread problem among the elderly. It can be caused by age-related changes in the lower urinary tract or by certain illnesses. The good news is that most cases can be cured or improved with proper diagnosis and treatment.

The specific causes of incontinence are numerous. Though many cases do not fit a clear-cut classification, they generally fall into one of three main categories:

**Stress incontinence** is the most common type among women. Its hallmark is the involuntary loss of urine during physical activity, sneezing, or coughing. The disorder may have its roots in the unique stress that pregnancy places on the urinary tract. However, symptoms may not be noticed until menopause, when the bladder tissues start to sag due to a drop in estrogen levels. Estrogen supplements often improve the condition. Other remedies include Kegel exercises (rhythmic flexing of the muscles surrounding the vagina, anus, and urethra), and surgery to reposition the bladder.

**Urge incontinence** is marked by an urgent, and quickly irresistible desire to urinate. In most cases, uninhibited bladder contractions are at fault. They may be a result of damage to the central nervous system from stroke or diseases such as multiple sclerosis, or may be caused by urinary infections or bladder tumors. A variant of this disorder is **reflex incontinence**, in which unintended urination occurs without feelings of urgency.

**Overflow incontinence** happens when the bladder cannot empty normally and becomes overdistended. This condition usually involves frequent, sometimes nearly constant, urine loss. Causes include neurologic abnormalities such as spinal cord injury and conditions that block outflow such as an enlarged or cancerous prostate or a stricture of the urethra.

Treatment depends on the cause of the problem. Medications prescribed for incontinence include bladder relaxants such as propantheline (Pro-Banthine), flavoxate (Urispas), dicyclomine (Bentyl), oxybutynin (Ditropan), and the antidepressant imipramine (Tofranil). Estrogen replacement therapy is another possibility. Surgery and behavioral techniques such as pelvic muscle exercises, biofeedback, and bladder training may also be employed.

## PREVENTING UTIs

During treatment of UTIs, and to prevent their recurrence, the following measures are usually recommended:

- Drink plenty of fluids, especially water.
- Drink cranberry juice or take supplements of vitamin C daily to keep urine acidic.
- Do not resist the urge to urinate.
- Wipe from front to back and wash the genital area thoroughly with soap and water after defecating to prevent bacteria from the anal area from entering the vagina
- Cleanse the genital area before having sex, and empty the bladder immediately afterward.
- Take showers instead of baths.
- Avoid using feminine hygiene sprays and scented douches; they may cause irritation of the urethra.

## Other Major Urinary Disorders

Interstitial cystitis occurs when the lining of the bladder becomes scarred or even ulcerated, causing pain when the bladder fills and relief when it empties. This condition is treated by stretching the bladder under anesthesia. It can also be treated by instillations of DMSO (dimethyl sulfoxide) into the bladder through a catheter. Researchers are working on many new treatments for this important and disabling condition.

Bladder cancer accounts for two to four percent of all cancers. It is most prevalent in people over age 50 and more common in men than in women. Approximately one-quarter of the people with this disease have no early symptoms. Most, however, experience blood in the urine. Other symptoms include pain after urination; frequent urination, especially at night; and dribbling.

The causes of bladder cancer are thought to include tobacco, nitrates, and aniline dyes.

Superficial bladder tumors can be removed surgically through the urethra by use of a cystoscope. If a tumor has penetrated the bladder wall, however, partial or even total removal of the bladder may be necessary, depending on the tumor's location. □

**CHAPTER 20**

# Dealing with Liver Disease

The largest internal organ, the liver literally keeps you alive. It performs over 100 separate bodily functions; and its sheer complexity makes it susceptible to almost as many different diseases. Fortunately, most are rare. But there are a few that are all too common, including hepatitis, cirrhosis, liver disorders in children, alcohol-related disorders, and liver cancer.

The American Liver Foundation reports that more than 25 million people are afflicted with liver and gallbladder disease each year. Over 27,000 Americans die from cirrhosis annually, making it the country's third leading cause of death for people between the ages of 25 and 59, and the seventh leading cause of death overall. Viruses, hereditary defects, and reactions to drugs and chemicals are among the known causes of liver breakdown. Though few treatments are effective for life-threatening liver disease, avoiding alcohol and other substances known to cause damage can do a lot to safeguard this important organ. A recently developed vaccine against the hepatitis B virus is now being recommended for children and for adults such as health-care workers who are in danger of exposure. (See section below on viral hepatitis.)

The liver is located behind the lower ribs, right below the diaphragm on the right side of the abdomen. In an average-sized man, it is about the size of a football, weighing a little over three pounds.

A miniature refinery, the liver processes many chemicals necessary for the body's overall functioning. For example, it converts carbohydrates, fats, and proteins into chemicals essential for life and growth. It manufactures and exports to other organs some of the substances they need to function properly, such as the bile used by the intestines during digestion. It modifies drugs taken to treat disease so that they can be used more easily by the body. And it cleanses the blood of toxic substances either ingested or produced by the body itself.

But that's only part of the picture. Below are some of the liver's many other important functions:

- Regulates the blood's ability to clot—governs the transport of fat stores

- Stores extra vitamins, minerals, and sugars to prevent shortages

- Produces quick energy as needed

- Controls the production and excretion of cholesterol

- Breaks down alcohol

- Monitors and maintains the right level of numerous chemicals and drugs in the blood

- Maintains and controls hormone balance

- Helps the body resist infection by producing immune factors and cleansing bacteria from the blood
- Stores iron

## The Threat of Viral Hepatitis

Viral hepatitis, a contagious infection of the liver, afflicts more than 70,000 Americans each year. It is usually caused by one of three different organisms.

**Hepatitis A**, formerly known as infectious hepatitis, can be contracted by consuming contaminated water or food, most notably shellfish. Since the virus is eliminated in the stool, it also spreads through improper hand washing, especially by restaurant workers or anyone else who handles food. Although hepatitis A is seldom serious, in one percent of the cases it can cause severe liver failure and death. It does not cause chronic hepatitis and will not lead to cirrhosis or other long-term liver problems.

**Hepatitis B**, formerly known as serum hepatitis, is found in blood and other body fluids such as urine, tears, semen, breast milk, and vaginal secretions. It is usually transmitted in blood, via transfusions, or through illicit injectable-drug use. But it also can be contracted through a minor cut or abrasion, or during such everyday acts as toothbrushing, kissing, or having sex. Infants can contract the disease from the mother at birth, or from the mother's breast milk. Dental work, ear piercing, and tattooing are other ways people can get hepatitis B.

**Type C hepatitis virus** is the cause of a disease known as "non-A, non-B hepatitis," which is also contracted through contact with contaminated blood, or through household or sexual contact with an infected person. It affects approximately 170,000 Americans each year.

Viral hepatitis may produce no symptoms at all. When they occur in type A, they usually begin suddenly and last for several weeks. This period is followed by a convalescent phase of anywhere from two to 12 weeks. Symptoms of viral hepatitis mimic the flu and include mild fever, fatigue, nausea, muscle and joint aches, loss of appetite, vomiting, occasional diarrhea, and vague abdominal pain. Some people also develop a yellow cast to the skin and whites of the eyes known as jaundice, along with dark-colored urine, clay-colored stools, and itching of the skin. The liver may be enlarged and tender.

Patients usually recover completely from hepatitis A and develop a lifelong immunity to it. Immune globulin (IG) should be administered to anyone exposed to type A hepatitis as soon as possible or within two weeks after jaundice appears. This medication is 80 to 90 percent effective in preventing the disease. A vaccine for hepatitis A is now available.

Hepatitis B also frequently has no symptoms; but if they do occur, they are similar to those of hepatitis A. The disease follows an unpredictable course, sometimes incapacitating a person for weeks or months and leading to complications, but usually ending in full recovery. Hepatitis C is similar to hepatitis B, but milder. However, like hepatitis B, it may develop into a chronic form in approximately 30 to 50 percent of those who contract it.

The problem with hepatitis B is that five to 10 percent of those who become infected with this disease become chronic carriers who can spread it to others for an indefinite period of time. At present there are more than a million of these silent carriers in this country, and their number is growing by two to three percent annually. Consequently, authorities recommend that all children and anyone with a high risk of exposure be vaccinated against this dangerous virus.

Chronic carriers usually do not develop chronic hepatitis. If it does develop, however, cirrhosis and primary cancer of the liver can be long-term consequences. An estimated 4,000 people in the United States die from hepatitis B-related cirrhosis annually. Carriers are many times more likely to get liver cancer than are non-carriers.

Treatment for acute hepatitis consists of rest and small, nourishing meals; fluids; and sometimes anti-nausea drugs such as trimethobenzamide (Tigan). Chronic cases of hepatitis B and C are now being treated with interferon, a biotech medicine derived from the human immune system.

# THE GALLBLADDER

The gallbladder stores bile, a substance the liver produces to aid digestion. The most common disorder of the gallbladder is the formation of gallstones. These stones often get stuck in the bile ducts that lead from the gallbladder to the first part of the small intestine, causing the gallbladder to become inflamed. Gallbladder surgery, in which the entire organ is removed, is one of the most common operations in this country. Laparoscopic cholecystectomy, a new procedure that requires only a small incision, has cut down stress and recovery time dramatically. Chenodiol, a recently available drug that dissolves gallstones, is an alternative to surgery. However, due to limited success and troublesome side effects, it is not widely used.

## Other Diseases of the Liver

In cirrhosis, liver cells are damaged and replaced by scar tissue which, as it accumulates, hardens the liver, diminishes blood flow, and causes even more cells to die. The loss of liver function that accompanies this degenerative condition results in gastrointestinal disturbances, jaundice, enlargement of the liver and spleen, emaciation, and accumulation of fluid in the abdomen and other tissues. Over half of the deaths related to cirrhosis are due to alcohol abuse, hepatitis, and other viruses. Chemicals, poisons, too much iron or copper, and blockages of the bile duct also may cause the disease.

Treatment of cirrhosis usually consists of eliminating the underlying cause, if possible, to avoid further damage, and preventing or treating complications. Care is mostly supportive, often including a specialized diet, diuretics (water pills), vitamins, and abstinence from alcohol. For some patients, a liver transplant is now a feasible option.

**Liver abscesses** are caused by bacteria, such as *Escherichia coli* (*E. coli*) or staphylococcus (staph), or by *Entamoeba histolytica*, the parasite that causes amebic dysentery. In either case, the offending organisms destroy liver tissue, leaving a cavity that fills with other infectious organisms, white blood cells, and liquefied liver cells. Common symptoms include shoulder and abdominal pain, fever, weight loss, chills, nausea, vomiting, anemia, and, if there is severe liver damage, jaundice. If the offending organism can't be determined, liver abscesses are treated with long-term antibiotics such as aminoglycosides, cephalosporins, clindamycin, or chloramphenicol. If *E. coli* is causing the infection, treatment includes ampicillin; for *Entamoeba histolytica*, chloroquine (Aralen), or metronidazole (Flagyl) are included.

**Pediatric liver diseases** afflict tens of thousands of children in this country annually, and kill hundreds each year. More than 100 different liver diseases are found in infants and children. Most of these disorders are genetic. Among the more common are:

- **Biliary atresia**, an inadequate bile duct, often fatal but sometimes relieved by surgery;

- **Chronic active hepatitis**, in which scar tissue forms and destroys the liver;

- **Wilson's disease**, in which an abnormally large buildup of copper in the liver is treated with vitamin $B_6$ and d-penicillamine, or, in some cases, corticosteroids such as prednisone;

- **Reye's syndrome**, an acute, often fatal disease secondary to flu or other infections in which fat accumulates in the liver and the patient lapses into coma.

Other serious diseases of the liver, fortunately seen less frequently than these discussed above, include fatty liver, hepatic coma, and liver cancer. □

## CHAPTER 21

# Facing Up to Sexually Transmitted Disease

**S**exually transmitted disease (STD) constitutes a staggering public health problem in the U.S. According to the government's Centers for Disease Control, nearly 12 million new cases are diagnosed annually. Young people aged 15 to 29 have the highest rates of infection. By the age of 21, almost one American in five requires treatment for a disease acquired through sexual contact. Among teenagers who are sexually active, the infection rate is a whopping one in four.

Sexually transmitted diseases are more than just a nuisance. Some of these diseases may be fatal, particularly to women and their unborn babies. Other STDs cause pelvic inflammatory disease, tubal pregnancy, sterility, certain types of cancer, or blindness. Babies whose mothers are infected with STDs may suffer from birth defects or mental retardation.

Although the rates of disease and disability from sexually acquired illnesses are highest among the poor, the impact of STDs on health care spending touches all income levels. Indeed, STDs cost Americans more than $3.5 billion a year. Almost 75 percent of this amount goes to treat pelvic inflammatory disease and its consequences, which include tubal pregnancy and female infertility.

During the 1970s, the government monitored just five sexually transmitted diseases—syphilis, gonorrhea, chlamydial infection/nongonococcal urethritis, pelvic inflammatory disease, and genital herpes/warts.

In the 1980s, however, the mounting AIDS epidemic triggered an explosion of research into and monitoring of diseases that were transmitted sexually. The painstaking study of AIDS taught scientists a great deal about other STDs; and today the federal government recognizes some 50 types of sexually transmitted infection.

Thanks to public awareness campaigns, many people now know how to protect themselves from the AIDS virus by avoiding injection drug use and by faithfully using "safer sex" techniques. Fortunately, this same approach also protects them from the many other disease agents transmitted through sexual contact or some other transfer of bodily fluids.

## Basic Facts About Sexually Transmitted Diseases

**H**ere are a few basic facts everyone should know for his or her own protection:

■ STDs are easily spread through any person-to-person transfer of bodily fluids such as semen, vaginal secretions, or blood.

■ When someone has a sexually transmitted disease, anyone who has sex with that person stands a good chance of becoming infected. Thus, having sex with multiple partners carries a greater risk of disease than staying faithful to a spouse or long-term partner. Even a monogamous relationship isn't necessarily risk-free, however, since one partner could be carrying an infection picked up during a prior sexual encounter.

■ Many sexually transmitted diseases are highly contagious. For example, if a man has gonorrhea, a woman who has sex with him **just once** stands an 80 to 90 percent chance of getting infected. If the man has gonorrhea plus chlamydia, as frequently happens, the woman could be infected with both diseases at the same time.

■ Vaginal intercourse is the classic route of STD infection. However, other important routes include anal sex (among men or man-to-woman), oral sex, sexual abuse of children, and mother-to-baby infection during childbirth.

■ Sexually transmitted diseases weaken the immune system, so a person infected with one STD has a greater risk of acquiring other infections. Unfortunately, recovering from an STD does not make a person immune. Anyone who has had a particular STD is still at risk of getting it again.

■ Men are more likely to show clear symptoms of STDs. Symptoms in women may not be as obvious, and the problem could be misdiagnosed.

■ Many women infected with certain types of STDs have no early symptoms at all and may unknowingly infect sexual partner(s).

■ In the past, gay men have tended to have an above-average rate of infection with STDs. This is largely attributed to promiscuity and may have declined in response to the AIDS epidemic. Additionally, some men are secretly bisexual. If a man picks up an STD from a homosexual encounter, he may then pass the infection on to unsuspecting heterosexual partners.

■ Lesbians have a lower-than-average risk for STDs, since most sexually acquired diseases are not easily spread from woman to woman.

## AIDS: IN A CLASS OF ITS OWN

AIDS, although definitely an STD, has become such an overriding public health concern that it is discussed separately in this book. Turn to Chapter 22.

### Preventive Measures
It is important to distinguish between birth control and prevention of STDs. While birth control pills and IUDs help prevent pregnancy, neither measure offers any worthwhile protection against disease.

Practicing "safer sex" is the most reliable way for sexually active people to protect themselves against STDs. Using a latex condom with a contraceptive foam or jelly is an excellent option. The chemical in the foam or jelly kills some infectious microorganisms along with the sperm. (Warning: People who reach for a tube of contraceptive jelly during sex should make sure they do not accidentally grab a tube of simple lubricating jelly, which has no sperm- or germ-killing ingredients.) It's also wise to think about a partner's sexual history, and avoid intimate contact with people at high risk of infection, such as those with multiple sexual partners.

People who even suspect they might have acquired a sexually transmitted disease should stop having sex until they consult a doctor and find out for sure. If test results show an infection, it is essential to notify *all* sexual partners so they can be tested, too. It is vitally important to follow the treatment exactly as prescribed and to abstain from sexual contact until receiving a clean bill of health.

### How Sexually Transmitted Disease Is NOT Spread
In most cases, people do NOT pick up sexually transmitted diseases from doorknobs, toilet seats, or towels. That's because the microorganisms that cause STDs thrive in a warm, moist environment such as the mucous membranes of the genitals or the mouth. Many of these organisms die soon after being exposed to dry air. (The virulent hepatitis B virus is a notable exception.)

# Common Sexually Transmitted Diseases

As we've seen, the government currently monitors about 50 sexually transmitted diseases. Here is a brief overview of some common STDs (excluding AIDS).

## Gonorrhea

Gonorrhea is an infection caused by the *Gonococcus* bacterium. In men, it is marked by a thick, white discharge from the penis and a burning pain when urinating.

In women, gonorrhea may infect the cervix. There may be mild pain and a discharge. If the urethra is infected, there may be a burning sensation during urination. However, women's symptoms are most often mild or simply unnoticeable. Even so, it is important to treat the infection because gonorrhea can lead to pelvic inflammatory disease (see below).

When gonorrhea is transmitted during anal or oral sex, painful infection of the rectum or throat may occur in both men and women.

## Chlamydia

Infection by the *Chlamydia trachomatis* bacterium is the leading cause of nongonococcal urethritis in men. This condition consists of pain or burning during urination, a thin discharge from the penis, and staining on underwear. Chlamydial infection may also inflame the sperm-collecting tubules in the scrotum and eventually cause sterility. A man infected with Chlamydia may be infected simultaneously with *Ureaplasma urealyticum*, which also causes urethritis.

In women, a chlamydial infection may cause a thin vaginal discharge, pain during urination, or pain in the lower abdomen about 10 to 20 days after exposure. However, women often do not notice any early symptoms. Chlamydia may also lead to pelvic inflammatory disease.

## Pelvic Inflammatory Disease

Pelvic inflammatory disease (PID) is an infection of the uterus, fallopian tubes, or ovaries and usually results from either gonorrhea or chlamydial infection.

The disease typically develops in two stages. First the infection attacks the cervix (the lower part of the uterus). It then spreads to the uterus, fallopian tubes, and ovaries. Sometimes PID starts directly within the uterus when germs gain entry following childbirth, abortion, or the insertion of an intrauterine contraceptive device (IUD). This, however, is rare.

Since PID causes scar tissue to form, there is up to a 25 percent risk of infertility. PID is also the single most common cause of tubal pregnancy, in which a fertilized egg begins to grow while still in the fallopian tube, instead of the uterus. If the tube bursts, the woman could die.

## Genital Warts

Genital warts (condyloma) are caused by the human papillomavirus (HPV) and look much like other warts. They usually occur near the tip of the penis in men. In women, the warts appear on the vulva, in the vagina, on the cervix of the uterus, or near the anus.

Genital warts are flat, hard, and painless when they first appear. If allowed to grow, however, they develop a "cauliflower" appearance and hurt when pressed. Genital warts tend to get bigger during pregnancy. In rare instances, very large warts may interfere with childbirth, making a Caesarean section necessary.

There are several types of HPV. Some types can cause precancerous cell changes in the tissues of a woman's vulva, anus, cervix, or vagina. An invasive cervical cancer can be fatal, which is why women with genital warts should have a Pap test at least once a year.

## Vaginitis

Vaginitis, or inflammation of the vagina, is an extremely common gynecological problem. Some types of vaginitis occur because of irritation from tampons, tight clothing, or frequent douching. Other types develop as a side effect of birth control pills or treatment with antibiotics, which may encourage fungal infections.

Two types of vaginitis, however, can be transmitted sexually: Bacterial vaginosis is caused by an overgrowth of several bacteria; trichomoniasis is caused by a one-celled organism called a protozoon. Although these infections do not carry dire consequences, they do cause burning, itching, discharge, and odor, and should certainly be treated.

In either case, it is important for both sexual partners to be treated at the same time. Men may harbor these organisms without showing any symptoms. Unless both partners are cured, the couple could keep passing the problem back and forth.

### Genital Herpes

Infection by the *Herpes simplex* virus causes red bumps. These bumps change to watery blisters and then rupture, leaving little hollow spots that may ooze or bleed. The first attack is often accompanied by high fever and swollen lymph nodes in the groin.

In men, genital herpes sores may develop on the penis, scrotum, buttocks, anus, or thighs. The sores can also develop inside the urethra (urinary passage),

remaining invisible but possibly causing a thin discharge and painful urination.

Women develop herpes sores on the outer genital area, buttocks, or thighs, or in the vagina or cervix. The sores may cause vaginal discharge, pain during urination, inflammation of the vulva, and aching or pain in the entire genital region.

Herpes sores usually scab over and heal within a week to 10 days, even without treatment. However, because the virus continues to live inside the body, a man or woman can pass on the infection even when the sores have disappeared. Outbreaks of sores may recur periodically. A tingling sensation in the genitals often announces the development of a new outbreak.

Pregnant women infected with herpes are at risk for miscarriage or premature delivery. A woman

## CERVICAL CANCER: A DEADLY STD

NORMAL SURFACE CELLS

BASAL CELLS

CONNECTIVE TISSUE

ATYPICAL CELLS

BASAL CELL HYPERACTIVITY

ATYPICAL CELLS AT THE SURFACE

MALIGNANT CELLS INVADING TISSUES

**Normal cervix:** Like skin, the surface of the cervix is constantly being replaced with new cells from below. Generated by division of the basal cells, these new cells rise as older ones are shed from the surface.

**Cervical dysplasia:** Triggered by an HPV infection, the cervical basal cells may go into overdrive, producing an excessive number of new — but malformed — replacement cells. These cells are not cancerous, but signal the danger of cancer to come.

**Invasive cancer of the cervix:** As the condition progresses, truly malignant cells develop and migrate downward into underlying tissues. Unchecked, the disease can be fatal.

may pass herpes on to her baby during childbirth. This happens rarely, but can cause blindness, brain damage, and infant death.

## Syphilis

The spirochete bacterium *Treponema pallidum* causes syphilis. The infection develops in distinct stages:

The first symptom is often a painless but highly infectious sore called a chancre. The sore develops from nine to 90 days after exposure and is sometimes accompanied by swollen lymph glands in the groin. Chancres may occur on the genitals or on the mouth, lips, breast, anus, or even the fingertips. The chancre often goes unnoticed in women because it develops inside the vagina. Some infected people never do get a chancre sore. Although a chancre disappears within one to five weeks, the syphilis bacteria remain in the body.

Stage two starts a week to six months later and involves a rash, mouth sores, and/or flu symptoms (headache, mild fever, aching joints). By this time, the bacteria have multiplied and spread, and the disease can be transmitted just by kissing.

Stage three, the latent stage, begins approximately a year after initial infection and lasts 10 to 20 years. There are no noticeable signs of the disease during this period, and after several years the disease is no longer contagious. However, the syphilis bacteria may be silently invading the heart, brain, or other organs.

Stage four is the late stage. Depending on which organs have been attacked, the accumulated damage may cause heart disease, blindness, mental illness, or crippling.

If syphilis is not treated during pregnancy, the mother-to-be may pass the disease on to her baby, and the infant could be born dead, deformed, or diseased.

Before syphilis was curable, it was the most dreaded of the sexually transmitted diseases. The advent of penicillin in the 1940s brought a large and gratifying drop in the syphilis rate. The case load plummeted from 575,600 in 1943 to fewer than 68,000 cases in 1985. Unfortunately, rampant prostitution among crack cocaine users has now driven the syphilis rate back up to its highest level since the early 1950s.

## Hepatitis B

Like AIDS, hepatitis B is caused by a virus and can be transmitted via sexual contact, bodily secretions, or blood. But unlike the virus that causes AIDS, hepatitis B is a hardy virus and can remain infectious for quite a while, even in dried blood, saliva, or other secretions.

Hepatitis B begins with flu-like symptoms that disappear as jaundice, the second stage, sets in. The person infected with hepatitis B is thin, weak, lethargic, and irritable and has an enlarged, painful liver. The resulting liver damage is often permanent, and one-fourth of those with hepatitis B eventually die of liver failure.

People who know about hepatitis B fear the virus because it is so easy to catch—especially when compared to AIDS. A hepatitis B vaccine is available, and medical personnel must be inoculated. Unfortunately, the very people most likely to get hepatitis B—intravenous drug users, prostitutes, and sexual partners of infected individuals—generally don't bother to get vaccinated or simply don't know the vaccine exists. That's why the incidence of this serious disease has been rising since 1982.

## Treating Sexually Transmitted Diseases

Once again, the best way to handle sexually transmitted disease is to prevent its spread by faithfully following safety precautions, including "safer sex" techniques.

If an STD does develop, it may be treated with medications, surgical procedures, or possibly both.

For a given STD, it is important to take the right medication exactly as prescribed. For example, even though gonorrhea and chlamydial infections often occur together, they require different medications. Never try to treat a sexually transmitted disease without a doctor's supervision. Using the wrong medication could do more harm than good.

By far the most common group of medications used to treat sexually transmitted diseases are the antibiotics that are available in ever-increasing variety. Sometimes a disease-causing organism "learns" to outwit a given antibiotic, at which point a different one is required. To cope with this ongoing problem, pharmaceutical companies are constantly striving to develop new antibiotics.

Metronidazole, a different type of antimicrobial

medication, is used to combat STDs caused by anaerobic (non-oxygen-dependent) bacteria or protozoa.

Various caustic creams, ointments, and solutions are used to shrink genital warts. Dry ice can be used to freeze and remove them. Laser surgery is also employed.

Although not a cure, acyclovir helps prevent or reduce the severity of genital herpes sores. To remove growths on or in the vagina, cervix, or uterus, electrosurgical excision is an option. □

**CHAPTER 22**

# The Facts about AIDS

No disease is so widely misunderstood or so controversial as Acquired Immunodeficiency Syndrome, better known as AIDS. Myth and controversy swirl around AIDS because it is primarily a sexually transmitted disease, has only recently been identified, and has caused a seemingly sudden surge of fatalities among certain high-risk groups in this country. While it affects far fewer people than high blood pressure, cancer, or heart disease, it has captured our attention because of its abrupt apocalyptic appearance and its almost certain fatal outcome.

AIDS is simple in neither cause nor effect. Basically, it is a life-threatening disruption of the immune system by the Human Immunodeficiency Virus (HIV). This virus progressively weakens the body's ability to fight off disease, opening it to severe infections with both common and exotic organisms, as well as various forms of cancer. In the United States, most cases of AIDS have been traced to the virus called HIV-1.

HIV is particularly dangerous because it can lie hidden for years. Someone infected by HIV may not yet have AIDS, and, in fact, may have no symptoms at all. As symptoms related to the viral infection do begin to appear, the term AIDS-Related Complex (ARC) is often used to describe the situation. Only when the immune system nears total collapse, or specific infections or cancers develop, is a patient said to have AIDS.

HIV has sparked tremendous fear and controversy, not only because of whom it attacks and the way it is transmitted, but because of its hidden nature and lethal results. No virus since polio has garnered so much scientific attention. Researchers have yet to find a cure; but their efforts have paid off with a growing number of medicines that can slow the progress of the infection and prolong the patient's life.

## Our Status Today

AIDS was not recognized until the early 1980s, when frequent reports of unusual lung infections with *Pneumocystis carinii* and a rapidly spreading form of cancer called Kaposi's sarcoma, found primarily in homosexual men, reached the Centers for Disease Control and Prevention in Atlanta, Georgia. The fact that these previously rare diseases were clustered in a single group of people led scientists to suspect that some sort of underlying infection was involved. As more and more people developed the exotic diseases now known to be symptoms of AIDS, it became clear that a "new" illness had surfaced in the U.S. HIV, the virus responsible for AIDS, was first identified by French and American research groups in 1984, and since that time, both public and private organizations have committed considerable resources to combat this disease.

By the end of 1989, there were 115,000 reported cases of AIDS in the United States.

Before the end of 1993, the number had surpassed 340,000, and over 200,000 had died from the disease.

All told, there are an estimated million to a million and a half people infected with HIV in the United States. While only 10 to 20 percent per year will develop the AIDS group of symptoms, all are believed to be capable of transmitting and spreading the virus.

When the AIDS epidemic struck, it first spread within the homosexual community, whose sexual practices put them at especially high risk. Today, AIDS among heterosexuals is also on the rise, accounting for about a third of all cases.

We now know that women who have had sexual relations with bisexuals, as well as injection drug users and certain other populations, are also at high risk for infection. In 1985, only seven percent of AIDS cases were women; now the proportion is over 12 percent. AIDS is the leading cause of death in women between ages 25 and 44 in New York City. Urban teenagers, according to the American Foundation for AIDS Research, are the next group that will develop widespread HIV infection. HIV infections among urban teens admitted to hospitals rose by 250 percent from 1987 to 1991. Between 1991 and 1993 the number of reported cases among teenagers doubled again.

Total annual costs of AIDS were projected at between $5 and $13 billion by the end of 1992. AIDS is now the seventh leading cause of death in the U.S. and is the leading cause of death among injection drug users and hemophiliacs.

According to the Department of Health and Human Services, "Despite the uncertainty about the incidence of HIV infection and the ultimate magnitude of the problem, HIV and AIDS are a growing threat to the health of the nation and will continue to make major demands on health and social systems for many decades."

## The Virus and What It Does

In order to understand AIDS, it's important to know a few basic facts about the "germs" we call viruses. These tiny invaders are especially difficult to repel. While infections by bacteria can be treated with common antibiotics, a viral infection cannot.

Viruses are minute microorganisms that com-

mandeer the machinery of the body's own cells to survive and reproduce. They can take hold in many parts of the body, but under ordinary circumstances are eventually eradicated—or at least held in check—by the immune system. HIV is scientifically termed a *retrovirus*. What makes it so deadly is the fact that it attacks certain key cells of the immune system itself.

These cells, known as "helper" or CD4 lymphocytes, play a central role in the body's defense against infections. But as they are themselves infected and destroyed by HIV, their number declines, and the chance of successful attack by other germs steadily rises. Treatment with an anti-retroviral drug such as zidovudine (AZT, Retrovir) can, at least temporarily, halt this decline. In fact, physicians often monitor a patient's helper lymphocyte count to gauge the success of therapy.

Other cells of the immune system are also liable to HIV attack. Called monocytes and macrophages, these cells may serve to transport the virus to the brain. They may also act as a long-term reservoir of infection.

## How Do You Get AIDS?

Most researchers now agree that HIV is the main cause of AIDS. They also agree that, unlike airborne or animal-transmitted viruses, HIV's primary method of transmission is via a substance that contains the virus or infected cells. In most cases, the vehicle seems to have been male seminal fluid, which enters the body through mucous membranes that become torn during anal or vaginal intercourse. AIDS may also be transmitted in infected transfused blood or menstrual blood, on used needles shared among drug users, through deep puncture wounds in healthcare workers, from mother to baby, and possibly by some other unknown routes.

Fortunately, HIV is not spread through routine social interaction. AIDS is not passed on through casual non-sexual contact—shaking hands, attending school with an HIV-positive person, hugging, or even sharing the same plates and utensils. In general, HIV is passed from men to men or men to women during intercourse, but less readily from women to men.

It is this fact that has misled many people to believe that AIDS is simply a "gay" or "drug addict's" disease. But as we have seen, this is increasingly untrue. And because the infection can go undetected for years, an unsuspecting carrier can pass on the virus to sexual partners unknowingly, until symptoms finally appear.

## What Are the Symptoms of AIDS?

HIV infection poses a difficult diagnostic problem because the blood tests most commonly used don't identify the virus itself, but rather, the presence of antibodies that the body gradually develops to fight the infection. The first test, often referred to as an ELISA (enzyme-linked immunosorbent assay), will, when positive, usually lead to a second test called the Western blot. However, if conducted too soon after exposure, both tests may fail to detect any antibodies—even though the person is already infected and capable of transmitting the virus. For this reason, experts recommend repeat testing for six months (or up to one year) after known or suspected exposure.

When first infected with HIV, a person may experience the same symptoms seen in many other viral infections—fever, sore throat, headache, rash, or a mononucleosis-type illness. For the majority of those infected, however, there may be no symptoms at all.

After this first flare-up, if it occurs, there are usually no symptoms for an extended period—typically five to six years. There is some evidence, however, that for those infected through blood transfusions, the time is much shorter.

While this period wears on, some patients develop shingles, itchy skin lesions, tuberculosis, fungal infections of the mouth (thrush), night sweats, fatigue, or swollen lymph nodes. Then, as damage to the immune system increases, additional problems may appear, including bacterial infections of the blood and lungs, a severe form of pneumonia caused by *Pneumocystis carinii*, various cancers such as lymphoma, severe herpes infections of the genitals or mouth, a fungal form of meningitis, toxoplasmosis involving the brain, and severe diarrhea. Also possible in the more advanced stages of the disease are sight-threatening cytomegalovirus infections of the eyes; generalized infection with *Mycobacterium avium-intracellulare*, or "MAI" (an organism resembling the cause of tuberculosis); and numerous neurological disorders, including progressive dementia.

Finally, in addition to the many bizarre infections that strike only those with failing immune systems, HIV patients are subject to all the more common infections as well, often in their severest forms.

## PREVENTION OF AIDS IS THE BEST CURE

The spread of AIDS can be stopped only by eliminating the behaviors that spread the disease, including high-risk sexual practices and injection drug use. Health-care institutions, such as blood banks and hospitals, have taken steps to protect the blood supply and to reduce risk among health-care workers. However, the most important line of defense against AIDS must come from the people most at risk. Since we are relatively sure of the way AIDS is spread, it is comparatively easy to identify what needs to be done. For your personal safety, always remember the three key precautions:

- Avoid high-risk behavior such as injection drug abuse, sexual promiscuity, and sexual contact with anyone you believe has indulged in such activities. Make certain you know a partner's sexual history. Remember that someone can appear perfectly healthy, yet still be harboring HIV.

- All people who are at risk (i.e. have multiple sexual contacts or a partner with multiple contacts) must practice "safer sex." This means no sexual contact should be unprotected. Latex condoms and spermicidal jellies that can kill the virus should always be used. Sexual practices such as unprotected anal intercourse should be avoided. If you suspect you're at risk, get tested for HIV periodically. Remember that it may take up to six months—or even a year—for the virus to show up. Do not donate blood if unsure of your status.

- Although the blood supply is generally safe in the U.S., you may want to consider banking your own blood prior to elective surgery.

# How Is HIV Infection Treated?

There is still no cure for HIV; but we do have ways of delaying its progress and fighting the "opportunistic" infections that can seize hold in its wake. To control the virus itself, we now have several anti-retroviral drugs. To fend off opportunistic infections, there are potent antibiotics. And, for the future, work continues on a vaccine to fight the virus in those already infected.

Treatment with anti-retroviral drugs is difficult for several reasons. First, the virus usually has time to become well established before any symptoms appear. Second, a drug must be able to attack the virus *within* infected cells, while preventing infection of additional cells. Third, many of the drugs currently in use tend to produce significant side effects. These unwanted side effects impose unavoidable limits on the way the drugs can be used.

In developing anti-retroviral drugs, scientists have taken advantage of critical steps in HIV's life cycle. For example, the first four drugs approved for treating HIV infection—zidovudine (AZT, Retrovir), didanosine (ddI, Videx), zalcitabine (ddC, Hivid) and stavudine (d4t, Zerit)—all act by inhibiting an enzyme (reverse transcriptase) that the virus uses to reproduce. Newer drugs—including indinavir (Crixivan), ritonavir (Norvir), and saquinavir (Invirase)—interfere at a different point in the reproductive cycle, inhibiting the action of an enzyme called HIV protease.

Both types of drug increase the body's supply of vital CD4 white blood cells while reducing the amount of viral RNA circulating in the bloodstream. Because the two types attack the virus in different ways, they are more effective when taken together than when taken individually. In addition, if the virus develops resistance to one type of drug, drugs in the other category will continue to work.

Older drugs such as Retrovir have a proven ability to inhibit the development of dangerous infections and thereby prolong patients' lives. The latest protease inhibitors are too new to have a similar track record; but their effect on CD4 counts and circulating viral RNA is even more encouraging than the older drugs'. Still, the effectiveness of all these drugs is likely to decrease with prolonged use; and although they can hold the virus at bay, none of them is a cure.

To prevent the life-threatening infections that can break through the HIV-weakened immune system, doctors use a variety of antibiotics. For example, the development of the serious pneumonia caused by *Pneumocystis carinii* can be prevented or delayed by medications such as trimethoprim/sulfamethoxazole (Bactrim, Septra), atovaquone (Mepron), or pentamidine (Pentam, NebuPent). Many of the same drugs, usually administered intravenously, are used to treat the infections once they take hold. For some infections, medication may be continued for life because of the high risk of recurrence. Unfortunately, the use of these drugs too may be limited by significant side effects.

Because all of these drugs can, in fact, improve the lives of those with HIV infections, anyone at risk of AIDS owes it to him-or herself to get an HIV test. □

## CHAPTER 23

# Drugs and the Elderly

When it comes to medications, the elderly are just like everyone else—only more so. They have more health problems, take more medicines, get more side effects, and sustain more deaths from improper use. In fact, some two-thirds of all people over age 65 take medication regularly. The elderly spend upwards of $10 billion per year on drugs, about 25 percent of the national pill bill, though they comprise only about 12 to 15 percent of the population. Today more elderly live longer, better lives than ever because of the many new medicines that keep jumpy hearts in line, arteries unclogged, aging bones from breaking, and eyesight from diminishing.

In fact, those over age 65 are among the main beneficiaries of the revolutionary advances in medicine during the twentieth century. Three key developments have especially helped the aging population have healthier and more productive lives: heart and high blood pressure medications, medicines that treat pain and injuries, and medications that overcome the mental health problems encountered in the aged. Medications that fight diabetes and kidney problems have also benefited the elderly.

Along with better nutrition and low cholesterol, low salt diets, the development of drugs that help us as we age has reduced death rates from heart attacks, strokes, and suicides significantly in the past few decades. But medications used by any aging person are truly the proverbial double-edged sword, since as many as 80 percent of the elderly are on confusing multiple-drug regimens. Indeed, some studies show that less than 30 percent of the aged use their drugs properly.

## What Do We Mean By Aging?

Aging isn't just "getting old." It's a process that involves biological, emotional, social, and even financial changes that affect a person's overall health. Disease and mental attitude are the wild cards that affect the speed of the aging process. Certainly, we all know people over age 65 who differ widely in their ability to get around. Some run marathons in their eighties and beyond, and others are so debilitated by illness that just getting up in the morning is a major effort. How do we explain this disparity among older people? Age is less a chronological marker than a combination of factors that determine the overall functioning of people in their mid-sixties and beyond.

First, genetics plays an important part in the aging process. Aging is associated with the development of chronic diseases such as high blood pressure that contribute to wear and tear on the body. Most of us who develop a chronic condition do so because we have a genetic predisposition to the disorder. High cholesterol, heart disease, cancer, diabetes, and other problems "run in families," just as eye color and hair color do. Some experts feel that our body's immune system is also affected by aging, gradually losing its ability to recognize outside threats—a virus, for example—and hence putting us at greater risk of disease.

Emotional and psychological issues have a major impact on overall health and the aging process. Even though an older person is well physically, he may still be at risk for mental illnesses such as Alzheimer's disease, depression, and anxiety. According to the American Psychiatric Association, 15 to 25 percent of the elderly in the U.S. suffer from "significant symptoms of mental illness." The aged—especially elderly men—are more likely to commit suicide than the rest of the population (some 6,000 do each year), but most do not seek professional help. Despite the fact that over one million elderly have some sort of abnormal memory loss (senility or dementia), they are often too embarrassed or too ill to seek help.

Social and financial changes are commonly overlooked as part of the aging process, but they can contribute to both physical and mental illness in the elderly. First of all, many elderly live on fixed budgets. If their income is modest, then every fluctuation in the economy, change in interest rates and cutback in government care has an impact on their lives. This can affect their nutrition (the elderly often skip meals to save money), which can lead to reduced body weight and, in turn, a change in the effects of medications they are taking. If their budget problems are too severe, they may even skip doses or stop their medications entirely.

Many older people also suffer severe stress from radical changes in life-style. Frequently this happens to aging widows who outlive their spouses. Retirement itself can be a source of stress for the elderly, whether financially secure or not. Some who have worked all their lives have no idea how to "slow-down" or may find it hard to adjust to full-time life with their spouses. These massive changes, when added to a heart condition, for example, increase stress on already inefficient organ systems.

## How Does Aging Affect Medication Use?

Despite the eternal search for the "fountain of youth," there are no medications that prevent or "cure" aging. The drugs used by the elderly are the same as those that a younger person might take—yet they can have a far different effect. It doesn't matter whether a person has heart disease or arthritis, osteoporosis, or high blood pressure, the story is the same: Because our organ systems tend to function less efficiently as we age, medications are handled differently by our bodies. Here are some of the most common changes affecting our health and our response to medicines:

- Our stomachs may not absorb food and medication as well as they did before.

- Our kidneys and livers don't eliminate fluids and toxins in the same efficient manner.

- Skin "dries up," making us more vulnerable to bruises.

- Our lung capacity diminishes, which increases risk of pneumonia and diseases caused by smoking or air pollution (emphysema).

- Muscles and joints weaken and wear out, making injury to hips, legs, and wrists more likely from even a simple fall.

- The heart and circulatory system loose peak efficiency.

- The senses we depend on—hearing, sight, taste—change subtly and affect mobility (driving a car) or pleasure (sexuality).

- The body's weight and composition changes, so that "usual" doses of medication require adjustments.

- Our immune systems decline, making us more prone to both infection and cancer.

- Our memories may deteriorate as chemical changes or clogged arteries cause brain cell damage.

All of the above contribute to the potential harm that medications can cause in the aging body. If a kidney can't eliminate a drug after it has done its work, it remains in the body longer, perhaps causing an overdose or an adverse effect. If someone forgets to take a medication that regulates the heart or blood pressure, a stroke or heart attack could be the result.

Any person over the age of 65 who is taking medications in the following categories should be aware of the potential for increased side effects, overdose, and diminished efficacy:

- Antibiotics
- Antihistamines
- Antihypertensives
- Antiulcer medicines
- Blood thinners
- Bronchodilators
- Calcium or potassium supplements
- Cardiac medications
- Corticosteroids
- Estrogens
- Over-the-counter drugs containing alcohol (cough and cold medications) or caffeine
- Pain relievers
- Psychiatric medications
- Skin medications and creams

## Aging, Mental Health and Medications—a Special Note

Among the first signs that a drug may not be working properly in an older person is a change in mood, energy, attitude, or memory. Too often, these alterations are overlooked, ignored, or chalked off to "old age" or senility. Older people may themselves feel that their blue mood is caused by something external such as the death of a friend or simply by boredom. Nothing could be farther from the truth. Virtually every heart medication, blood pressure drug, sleeping pill, and tranquilizer has been known to trigger depressive symptoms.

When a psychological symptom appears in an older person, examine his or her medication or drug use first. Consider, too, factors like alcohol intake, poor nutrition, and hormone imbalance. And never dismiss the possibility that a real psychological problem has developed and may itself require medication. Any older person with feelings of hopelessness, worthlessness, unexplained crying, thoughts of suicide and similar symptoms could be among the five percent of the elderly who have a treatable, reversible depression.

Likewise, up to 15 percent of the aging population suffer from the symptoms of dementia: memory loss, disorientation, and confusion. Dementia can be a side effect of medicines. It may also be related to high blood pressure or conditions like Huntington's disease (a genetic disorder), Parkinson's disease (involuntary tremors), or Creutzfeldt-Jakob disease (a viral infection). Treatment of these can, to a small extent, reverse the dementia. However, some 60 percent of those with symptoms of dementia have Alzheimer's disease, a slow, progressive mental deterioration that, so far, can't be cured.

Alzheimer's disease is a particularly tragic disorder. It can affect people in their forties, but is more common among the elderly. Among the first signs of Alzheimer's are loss of short-term or recent memory—forgetting to shut off a light or the stove, or pick up the kids on time. As the disease gets worse, the person tends to become lost more easily and begins to forget how to do simple tasks like adding up numbers or reading the newspaper. Later on, all mental functions deteriorate, although the body is usually spared.

Treatment today consists largely of keeping the patient nourished, reducing agitation through tranquilizers, and helping the family cope through support groups. There is one medication — Cognex — that can alleviate the symptoms of Alzheimer's in some victims. It's not a cure and doesn't work for many people; but it's definitely worth trying if someone in your family suffers from this devastating disorder.

## Safe Medication Use for the Aged

Safe medication use for the elderly requires vigilance on the part of the older person and those assisting him. It is especially important to keep track of maintenance drugs and make sure they are taken regularly. For a chronic condition such as high blood pressure, these medications are a key to maintaining good health.

Remember, too, that perfectly ordinary medications really can lead to unexpected results—especially in the elderly. Be alert for gradual changes that may signal an unwanted side effect. And guard against harmful drug interactions by making sure the doctor knows about all the medicines the older person is taking, including those prescribed by other doctors and any over-the-counter drugs. □

## APPENDIX 1

# Safe Medication Use

Using medications safely is largely a matter of common sense and caution. The following are general guidelines to keep in mind:

### You and your doctor
■ Tell your doctor everything about your medical history, including reactions to medications you've used in the past.
■ Tell the doctor about any medications you are using now, even if they are over-the-counter drugs.
■ Keep track of your reactions to a medication and report them to your doctor.
■ Ask your doctor what you can do when given a new drug. For example, are there any foods to avoid when taking the drug? Should you avoid alcohol?
■ Never change your dose schedule unless your doctor tells you to do so.
■ Ask about the addiction or dependence potential of any new drug.

### You and your pharmacist
■ See if there are any written instructions that you can take with you.
■ Ask the pharmacist to explain clearly when and how to take the drug.
■ Check the ingredients of over-the-counter drugs you may be taking to ensure that your prescription doesn't interact with them.
■ If you are starting a new medication, ask your pharmacist to fill only half the prescription in case you have an adverse reaction and the drug is stopped.
■ Ask how long the medication remains effective. Don't take it after its expiration date.
■ If you are going on a vacation, make sure your drug can be used in different climates.

### You and your medications
■ Never take someone else's medication; and don't share your own medicines.
■ Check the label each time you take a drug. Don't take a drug in the dark.
■ Keep your medications in a dry, safe spot.
■ Keep each medicine in the bottle from the drug store. Don't mix medicines together in a single bottle.
■ If you think you are pregnant, consult with your doctor before using any medication.
■ Destroy any unused portions of a drug and throw out the bottle.
■ If you need a certain medicine (for instance, insulin) in case of emergency, carry the information with you.

### Your medicines and your children
■ Keep all medications in a locked cabinet or in a spot well out of the reach of children.
■ Ask for child-proof safety bottles.
■ Be alert and awake when giving a child medication.
■ Make sure that children know medications can be dangerous if misused.
■ Keep antidotes such as Syrup of Ipecac on hand.
■ Keep the numbers of your EMS and poison control centers handy. □

## APPENDIX 2

# Poison Control Centers

If there is one phone number that no home should be without, it is the nearest poison control center. The following is a list of regional centers that are certified members of the American Association of Poison Control Centers. To be certified, they must be supervised by a medical director; have pharmacists and nurses available to answer questions; be open 24-hours a day; and be accessible by direct dialing or a toll-free number.

The Centers in each state are listed alphabetically by name. "TTY" numbers are reserved for the hearing impared. "TTD" numbers reach a telecommunications device for the deaf.

## Alabama

**Alabama Poison Center, Tuscaloosa**
408-A Paul Bryant Drive
Tuscaloosa, AL 35401
Emergency Phone:
(800) 462-0800 (AL only) or
(205) 345-0600

**Regional Poison Control Center**
The Children's Hospital of Alabama
1600 Seventh Ave. South
Birmingham, AL 35233-1711
Emergency Phone: (205) 939-9201,
(800) 292-6678 (AL only) or
(205) 933-4050

## Arizona

**Arizona Poison and Drug Information Center**
Arizona Health Sciences Center
1501 N. Campbell Ave., #1156
Tucson, AZ 85724
Emergency Phone:
(800) 362-0101 (AZ only),
(520) 626-6016

**Samaritan Regional Poison Center**
Good Samaritan Regional Medical Center, Ancillary-1
1111 E. McDowell Road
Phoenix, AZ 85006
Emergency Phone: (602) 253-3334

## California

**Central California Regional Poison Control Center**
Valley Children's Hospital
3151 N. Millbrook
Fresno, CA 93703
Emergency Phone:
(800) 346-5922 (Central CA only) or
(209) 445-1222

**Los Angeles County Regional Drug and Poison Information Center**
LAC & USC Medical Center
1200 N. State St.
Los Angeles, CA 90033
Emergency Phone: (213) 222-3212
(800) 777-6476

**San Diego Regional Poison Center**
UCSD Medical Center
200 West Arbor Drive
San Diego, CA 92103-8925
Emergency Phone: (619) 543-6000,
(800) 876-4766
(in 619 area code only)

**San Francisco Bay Area Regional Poison Control Center**
San Francisco General Hospital
1001 Potrero Ave.,
Building 80, Room 230
San Francisco, CA 94110
Emergency Phone: (800) 523-2222

**University of California, Davis, Medical Center Regional Poison Control Center**
2315 Stockton Blvd.
Sacramento, CA 95817
Emergency Phone: (916) 734-3692,
(800) 342-9293 (Northern CA only)

## Colorado

**Rocky Mountain Poison and Drug Center**
8802 E. 9th Ave., Bldg. 752
Denver, CO 80220
Emergency Phone: (303) 629-1123
(303) 739-1127 (TTY)

## Connecticut

**Connecticut Poison Control Center**
University of Connecticut Health Center
263 Farmington Ave.
Farmington, CT 06032
Emergency Phone: (800) 343-2722 (CT)
(203) 679-4346 (TTY)

## District of Columbia

**National Capital Poison Center**
3201 New Mexico Ave, NW
Suite 310
Washington, DC 20016
Emergency Phone:
(202) 625-3333,
(202) 362-8563 (TTY)

## Florida

**Florida Poison Information Center—Jacksonville**
655 West 8th Street
Jacksonville, FL 32209
Emergency Phone: (904) 549-4480
(800) 282-3171 (FL only)

**The Florida Poison Information and Toxicology Resource Center Tampa General Hospital**
Post Office Box 1289
Tampa, FL 33601
Emergency Phone:
(813) 253-4444 (Tampa),
(800) 282-3171 (Florida)

# Georgia

**Georgia Poison Center**
Grady Health System
80 Butler Street S.E.
P.O. Box 26066
Atlanta, GA 30335-3801
Emergency Phone:
(800) 282-5846 (GA only),
(404) 616-9000

# Indiana

**Indiana Poison Center**
Methodist Hospital of Indiana
1701 N. Senate Boulevard
P.O. Box 1367
Indianapolis, IN 46206-1367
Emergency Phone:
(800) 382-9097 (IN only),
(317) 929-2323

# Iowa

**Poison Control Center**
University of Iowa Hospitals and Clinics
200 Hawkins Dr.
Iowa City, IA 52242
Emergency Phone: (800) 272-6477
(IA only)

# Kentucky

**Kentucky Regional Poison Center
of Kosair's Children's Hospital**
P.O. Box 35070
Louisville, KY 40232-5070
Emergency Phone: (502) 629-7275,
(800) 722-5725 (KY only)

# Louisiana

**Louisiana Drug and Poison
Information Center**
Northeast Louisiana University
School of Pharmacy
Monroe, LA 71209-6403
Emergency Phone: (800) 256-9822 (LA)

# Maine

**Maine Poison Center**
Maine Medical Center
22 Bramhall St.
Portland, ME 04102
Emergency Phone: (800) 442-6305 (ME)

# Maryland

**Maryland Poison Center**
20 N. Pine St.
Baltimore, MD 21201
Emergency Phone: (410) 706-7701,
(800) 492-2414 (MD only)

**National Capital Poison Center
(D.C. suburbs only)**
3201 New Mexico Ave, NW
Suite 310
Washington, DC 20016
Emergency Phone: (202) 625-3333,
(202) 362-8563 (TTY)

# Massachusetts

**Massachusetts Poison Control
System**
300 Longwood Ave.
Boston, MA 02115
Emergency Phone: (617) 232-2120,
(800) 682-9211

# Michigan

**Poison Control Center**
Children's Hospital of Michigan
3901 Beaubien Blvd.
Detroit, MI 48201
Emergency Phone: (313) 745-5711

# Minnesota

**Hennepin Regional Poison Center**
Hennepin County Medical Center
701 Park Ave.
Minneapolis, MN 55415
Emergency Phone: (612) 347-3141

**Minnesota Regional
Poison Center**
8100 34th Ave. South, Box 1309
Minneapolis, MN 55440
Emergency Phone: (612) 221-2113

# Mississippi

**Mississippi Regional Poison Control**
University of Mississippi Medical Center
2500 North State St.
Jackson, MS 39216
Emergency Phone: (601) 354-7660

# Missouri

**Cardinal Glennon Children's
Hospital Regional Poison Center**
1465 S. Grand Blvd.
St. Louis, MO 63104
Emergency Phone: (314) 772-5200,
(800) 366-8888

# Montana

**Rocky Mountain Poison
and Drug Center**
8802 E. 9th Ave., Bldg. 752
Denver, CO 80220
Emergency Phone: (303) 629-1123
(303) 739-1127 (TTY)

# Nebraska

**The Poison Center**
8301 Dodge St.
Omaha, NE 68114
Emergency Phone:
(402) 390-5555 (Omaha),
(800) 955-9119 (NE & WY)

# New Hampshire

**New Hampshire Poison
Information Center**
Dartmouth-Hitchcock Medical Center
1 Medical Center Dr.
Lebanon, NH 03756
Emergency Phone: (603) 650-5000,
(800) 562-8236 (NH only)

# New Jersey

**New Jersey Poison Information and
Education System**
201 Lyons Ave.
Newark, NJ 07112
Emergency Phone: (800) 764-7661

# New Mexico

**New Mexico Poison and Drug
Information Center**
University of New Mexico
Albuquerque, NM 87131-1076
Emergency Phone: (505) 843-2551,
(800) 432-6866 (NM only)

# New York

**Hudson Valley Regional Poison
Center**
Phelps Memorial Hospital Center
701 North Broadway
North Tarrytown, NY 10591
Emergency Phone: (800) 336-6997,
(914) 353-1000

**Long Island Regional Poison
Control Center**
Winthrop University Hospital
259 First Street
Mineola, NY 11501
Emergency Phone: (516) 542-2323,
542-2324, 542-2325, 542-3813

**New York City Poison
Control Center**
N.Y.C. Department of Health
455 First Ave., Room 123
New York, NY 10016
Emergency Phone: (212) 340-4494,
(212) P-O-I-S-O-N-S,
TDD: (212) 689-9014

# North Carolina

**Carolinas Poison Center**
1000 Blythe Blvd.
P.O. Box 32861
Charlotte, NC 28232-2861
Emergency Phone: (704) 355-4000,
(800) 84-TOXIN (1-800-848-6946)

# North Dakota

**North Dakota Poison
Information Center**
Meritcare Medical Center
720 North 4th St.
Fargo, ND 58122
Emergency Phone: (701) 234-5575,
(800) 732-2200 (ND)

# Ohio

**Central Ohio Poison Center**
700 Children's Drive
Columbus, OH 43205-2696
Emergency Phone: (614) 228-1323,
(800) 682-7625,
(614) 228-2272 (TTY)

**Cincinnati Drug & Poison
Information Center and Regional
Poison Control System**
231 Bethesda Avenue,
M.L. 144
Cincinnati, OH 45267-0144
Emergency Phone: (513) 558-5111,
800-872-5111 (OH only)

# Oklahoma

**Oklahoma Poison Control Center**
University of Oklahoma and Children's
Hospital of Oklahoma
940 Northeast 13th St.
Oklahoma City, OK 73104
Emergency Phone: (405) 271-5454,
(800) 522-4611 (OK),
(405) 271-1122(TTD)

# Oregon

**Oregon Poison Center**
Oregon Health Sciences University
3181 S.W. Sam Jackson Park Road
Portland, OR 97201
Emergency Phone: (503) 494-8968,
(800) 452-7165 (OR only)

# Pennsylvania

**Central Pennsylvania
Poison Center**
University Hospital
Milton S. Hershey
Medical Center
Hershey, PA 17033
Emergency Phone: (800) 521-6110

**The Poison Control Center**
3600 Market St., Rm. 220
Philadelphia, PA 19104-2641
Emergency Phone: (215) 386-2100

**Pittsburgh Poison Center**
3705 Fifth Avenue
Pittsburgh, PA 15213
Emergency Phone: (412) 681-6669

# Rhode Island

**Rhode Island Poison Center**
593 Eddy St.
Providence, RI 02903
Emergency Phone: (401) 444-5727

# South Carolina

**Palmetto Poison Center**
College of Pharmacy
University of South Carolina
Columbia, SC 29208
Emergency Phone: (803) 777-1117
(800) 922-1117 (SC)

# Tennessee

**Southern Poison Center**
847 Monroe Ave., Suite 230
Memphis, TN 38163
Emergency Phone: (901) 528-6048
(800) 288-9999 (TN only)

# Texas

**North Texas Poison Center**
5201 Harry Hines Blvd.
P.O. Box 35926
Dallas, TX 75235
Emergency Phone: (800) 764-7661

**Southeast Texas Poison Center**
The University of Texas
Medical Branch
Galveston, TX 77550-1175
Emergency Phone:
(409) 765-1420 (Galveston),
(800) 764-7661 (TX only)

# Utah

**Utah Poison Control Center**
410 Chipeta Way, Suite 230
Salt Lake City, UT 84108
Emergency Phone: (801) 581-2151,
(800) 456-7707 (UT only)

# Vermont

**Vermont Poison Center**
Fletcher Allen Health Care
111 Colchester Ave.
Burlington, VT 05401
Emergency Phone: (802) 658-3456

# Virginia

**Blue Ridge Poison Center**
Box 67
Blue Ridge Hospital
Charlottesville, VA 22901
Emergency Phone: (804) 924-5543,
(800) 451-1428

**National Capital Poison Center
(Northern VA only)**
3201 New Mexico Ave, NW
Suite 310
Washington, DC 20016
Emergency Phone:
(202) 625-3333,
(202) 362-8563 (TTY)

# West Virginia

**West Virginia Poison Center**
3110 MacCorkle Ave., S.E.
Charleston, WV 25304
Emergency Phone:
(800) 642-3625 (WV only),
(304) 348-4211

# Wisconsin

**Poison Control Center**
University of Wisconsin
Hospital and Clinics
600 Highland Ave., E5/238
Madison, WI 53792
Emergency Phone: (608) 262-3702
(800) 815-8855 (WI)

# Wyoming

**The Poison Center**
8301 Dodge St.
Omaha, NE 68114
Emergency Phone:
(402) 390-5555 (Omaha),
(800) 955-9119 (NE & WY)

# Disease and Disorder Index

**U**se this index to find out which drugs are available for a specific medical problem. Both brand and generic names are listed; the generic names are shown in italics. Only brands covered in the drug profiles are included.

# General Index

Listed in this index are the diseases, treatments, and other key subjects discussed in the Disease Overview Chapters. Also shown are the names of the entries in the Drug Profile Section. Drugs and diseases mentioned within the text of the profiles are not included in the index.